CONTEMPORARY
PERIODONTICS

CONTEMPORARY PERIODONTICS

Edited by

Robert J. Genco, D.D.S., Ph.D.
Professor and Chairman,
Department of Oral Biology,
State University of New York at Buffalo,
School of Dental Medicine,
Buffalo, New York

Henry M. Goldman, D.M.D., D.Sc. (Hon.), F.A.C.D.
Dean Emeritus,
Boston University, Goldman School of Graduate Dentistry,
Boston, Massachusetts

D. Walter Cohen, D.D.S., F.A.C.D.
President,
The Medical College of Pennsylvania;
Dean Emeritus
and Professor Emeritus of Periodontics,
University of Pennsylvania,
School of Dental Medicine,
Philadelphia, Pennsylvania

with 1232 illustrations, including 2 color plates

THE C. V. MOSBY COMPANY

ST. LOUIS • BALTIMORE • PHILADELPHIA • TORONTO 1990

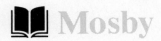

Editor: Robert Reinhardt
Developmental editor: Elaine Steinborn
Project manager: Kathleen L. Teal
Manuscript editor: Judith Bange
Designer: Liz Fett
Production: Ginny Douglas, Judith Bange

Printed in the United States of America

The C.V. Mosby Company
11830 Westline Industrial Drive, St. Louis, Missouri 63146

Library of Congress Cataloging in Publication Data
Contemporary periodontics / edited by Robert J. Genco, Henry M.
  Goldman, D. Walter Cohen.
    p.   cm.
  Rev. ed. of: Periodontal therapy / Henry M. Goldman, D. Walter
Cohen. 6th ed. 1980.
  Includes bibliographical references.
  ISBN 0-8016-1935-1
  1. Periodontics.   I. Genco, Robert J. II. Goldman, Henry M.
(Henry Maurice). III. Cohen, D. Walter (David Walter).
IV. Goldman, Henry M. (Henry Maurice).
Periodontal therapy.
  [DNLM: 1. Periodontal Diseases. 2. Periodontal Diseases — therapy.
WU 240 C761]
RK361.C59   1990
617.6'32 — dc20
DNLM/DLC
  for Library of Congress   89-12194
                                                        CIP

CL/MV 9 8 7 6 5 4

CONTRIBUTORS

Leonard Abrams, D.D.S., F.A.C.D.
Clinical Professor of Periodontology,
University of Pennsylvania,
School of Dental Medicine,
Philadelphia, Pennsylvania

Gary C. Armitage, D.D.S., M.S.
Professor and Chairman, Division of Periodontology,
University of California, San Francisco,
School of Dentistry,
San Francisco, California

Harold S. Baumgarten, D.M.D.
Clinical Assistant Professor of Restorative Dentistry,
University of Pennsylvania, School of Dental Medicine,
Philadelphia, Pennsylvania

Sally A. Buchanan, M.S., D.D.S.
Assistant Clinical Professor, Department of Stomatology,
University of California, San Francisco,
School of Dentistry,
San Francisco, California

Brian A. Burt, B.D.S., M.P.H., Ph.D.
Director, Program in Dental Public Health,
and Chairman, Department of Community Health Programs,
The University of Michigan, School of Public Health;
Professor of Dentistry, The University of Michigan,
School of Dentistry,
Ann Arbor, Michigan

Raul G. Caffesse, D.D.S., M.S.
Dr. Odont., Professor and Chairman, Periodontics;
Director, Advanced Education Program in Periodontics,
The University of Texas Health Science Center at
Houston, Dental Branch,
Houston, Texas

Daniel P. Casullo, D.M.D., P.C.
Associate Professor, Department of Oral Rehabilitation;
Director of General Practice Fellowship Program,
University of Pennsylvania, School of Dental Medicine,
Philadelphia, Pennsylvania

Lars A. Christersson, D.D.S.
Associate Professor, Department of Oral Biology,
State University of New York at Buffalo,
School of Dental Medicine,
Buffalo, New York

Sebastian G. Ciancio, D.D.S.
Professor and Chairman, Department of Periodontology,
State University of New York at Buffalo,
School of Dental Medicine; Clinical Professor of
Pharmacology, State University of New York at Buffalo,
School of Medicine and Biomedical Sciences,
Buffalo, New York

Ronald B. Cogen, D.D.S., Ph.D.
Professor of Periodontics, University of Alabama,
School of Dentistry,
Birmingham, Alabama

D. Walter Cohen, D.D.S., F.A.C.D.
President, The Medical College of Pennsylvania;
Dean Emeritus and Professor Emeritus of Periodontics,
University of Pennsylvania,
School of Dental Medicine,
Philadelphia, Pennsylvania

Ernesto De Nardin, Ph.D.
Research Assistant Professor, Department of Oral
Biology, State University of New York at Buffalo,
School of Dental Medicine,
Buffalo, New York

Cyril Evian, B.D.S., D.M.D.
Assistant Professor of Periodontics,
University of Pennsylvania,
School of Dental Medicine,
Philadelphia, Pennsylvania

Steven Garrett, D.D.S., M.S.
Associate Professor of Periodontics,
Loma Linda University, School of Dentistry,
Loma Linda, California

Robert J. Genco, D.D.S., Ph.D.
Professor and Chairman, Department of Oral Biology,
State University of New York at Buffalo,
School of Dental Medicine,
Buffalo, New York

Henry M. Goldman, D.M.D., D.Sc. (Hon.), F.A.C.D.
Dean Emeritus, Boston University,
Goldman School of Graduate Dentistry,
Boston, Massachusetts

Charles H. Goodman, D.D.S., M.S.
Assistant Professor and
Coordinator of Graduate Periodontics,
Northwestern University, School of Dentistry,
Chicago, Illinois

John C. Greene, D.M.D., M.P.H.
Professor and Dean, University of California,
San Francisco, School of Dentistry,
San Francisco, California

Deborah Greenspan, B.D.S.
Associate Clinical Professor, Division of Oral Medicine,
Department of Stomatology, University of California,
San Francisco, School of Dentistry,
San Francisco, California

John S. Greenspan, B.D.S., Ph.D., F.R.C.Path.
Professor and Chairman,
Department of Stomatology; Director,
Oral AIDS Center and AIDS Specimen Bank,
University of California, San Francisco,
School of Dentistry,
San Francisco, California

Benjamin F. Hammond, D.D.S., Ph.D.
Professor of Microbiology,
Associate Dean for Academic Affairs,
University of Pennsylvania, School of Dental Medicine,
Philadelphia, Pennsylvania

Thomas M. Hassell, D.D.S., Dr. Med. Dent., Ph.D.
Professor and Chairman of Periodontology,
University of Florida, College of Dentistry,
Gainesville, Florida

Ernest Hausmann, D.M.D., Ph.D.
Professor of Oral Biology, Department of Oral Biology
and Periodontal Disease Clinical Research Center,
State University of New York at Buffalo,
School of Dental Medicine,
Buffalo, New York

William H. Hiatt, D.D.S.
Clinical Professor of Periodontics,
University of Colorado, School of Dentistry;
Associate Clinical Professor, Department of Surgery,
University of Colorado, School of Medicine;
Private Practice,
Denver, Colorado

Murray W. Hill, B.D.Sc., M.Sc., Ph.D.
Dows Institute for Dental Research,
The University of Iowa, College of Dentistry,
Iowa City, Iowa

Vincent J. Iacono, D.M.D.
Professor, Department of Periodontics,
State University of New York at Stony Brook,
School of Dental Medicine,
Stony Brook, New York

Marjorie Jeffcoat, D.M.D.
Professor and Chair, Department of Periodontics,
University of Alabama at Birmingham,
School of Dentistry,
Birmingham, Alabama

William J. Killoy, D.D.S., M.S.
Professor and Chairman, Department of Periodontics,
University of Missouri–Kansas City, School of Dentistry,
Kansas City, Missouri

Niklaus P. Lang, D.D.S., Dr. Odont. H.C., M.S.,
Ph.D.
Professor and Chairman,
Department of Comprehensive Dental Care,
University of Berne, School of Dental Medicine,
Berne, Switzerland

Michael J. Levine, D.D.S., Ph.D.
Professor, Department of Oral Biology and
Dental Research Institute, State University of New York
at Buffalo, School of Dental Medicine,
Buffalo, New York

Max A. Listgarten, D.D.S.
Professor and Chairman, Department of Periodontics,
University of Pennsylvania, School of Dental Medicine,
Philadelphia, Pennsylvania

Harald Löe, D.D.S., Dr. Odont.
Director, National Institute of Dental Research,
Bethesda, Maryland

Walter J. Loesche, D.M.D., Ph.D.
Professor of Dentistry and Professor of Microbiology,
University of Michigan, School of Dentistry,
Ann Arbor, Michigan

Ian C. Mackenzie, B.D.S., Ph.D.
Professor of Periodontology;
Director, Dental Science Institute, The University of Texas
Health Science Center at Houston, Dental Branch,
Houston, Texas

Irwin D. Mandel, D.D.S.
Professor of Dentistry; Director,
Center for Clinical Research in Dentistry,
Columbia University, School of Dental and Oral Surgery,
New York, New York

Lucinda B. McKechnie, R.D.H.
Continuing Education Faculty,
University of Pennsylvania, School of Dental Medicine,
Philadelphia, Pennsylvania; Faculty,
The Institute for Advanced Dental Studies,
Swampscott, Massachusetts

Edith Morrison, M.P.H., D.P.H.
Associate Professor, Department of Periodontics,
The University of Texas Health Science Center at Houston,
Dental Branch,
Houston, Texas

Joseph M. Mylotte, M.D.
Associate Professor of Medicine and Microbiology,
State University of New York at Buffalo,
School of Medicine and Biomedical Sciences;
Chief of Infectious Diseases,
Veterans Administration Medical Center,
Buffalo, New York

Patricia A. Murray, D.M.D., Ph.D.
Assistant Professor, Division of Periodontology,
Department of Stomatology, University of California,
San Francisco, School of Dentistry,
San Francisco, California

Mirdza Neiders, D.D.S., M.S.
Professor, Department of Stomatology,
Interdisciplinary Sciences, and Oral Biology,
State University of New York at Buffalo,
School of Dental Medicine,
Buffalo, New York

Russell Nisengard, D.D.S., Ph.D.
Professor, Departments of Periodontology and
Microbiology, State University of New York at Buffalo,
Schools of Dental Medicine and Medicine,
Buffalo, New York

Steven R. Potashnick, D.D.S.
Assistant Professor, Department of Periodontics,
Northwestern University, School of Dentistry;
Section Chief, Restorative Dentistry,
Michael Reese Hospital and Medical Center; Private Practice,
Chicago, Illinois

Paul B. Robertson, D.D.S., M.S., F.A.C.D.
Dean, Faculty of Dentistry,
University of British Columbia, Vancouver,
British Columbia, Canada

Peter J. Robinson, D.D.S., Ph.D.
Professor and Chairman of Periodontics,
Northwestern University, School of Dentistry,
Chicago, Illinois

Louis F. Rose, D.D.S., M.D.
Professor of Medicine and Surgery; Chief,
Division of Dental Medicine,
The Medical College of Pennsylvania;
Professor of Periodontics, University of Pennsylvania,
School of Dental Medicine,
Philadelphia, Pennsylvania

Edwin S. Rosenberg, B.D.S., H.D.D., D.M.D.
Professor of Periodontics, University of Pennsylvania,
School of Dental Medicine; Professor of Medicine,
The Medical College of Pennsylvania,
Philadelphia, Pennsylvania

Louis E. Rossman, D.M.D.
Chairman and Program Director, Division of
Endodontics, Albert Einstein Medical Center, Northern
Division; Clinical Assistant Professor of Endodontics,
University of Pennsylvania, School of Dental
Medicine; Clinical Assistant Professor of Medicine
(Dental Medicine), The Medical College of
Pennsylvania, Philadelphia, Pennsylvania; Director,
American Board of Endodontics

Frank A. Scannapieco, D.M.D., M.S.
Postdoctoral Fellow, Department of Oral Biology and
Dental Research Institute,
State University of New York at Buffalo,
School of Dental Medicine,
Buffalo, New York

Jay S. Seibert, D.D.S., M.Sc.D.
Professor of Periodontics, University of Pennsylvania,
School of Dental Medicine,
Philadelphia, Pennsylvania

Knut A. Selvig, D.D.S., M.S., Ph.D.
Professor, Department of Dental Research,
University of Bergen, School of Dentistry,
Bergen, Norway

Aubrey Sheiham, B.D.S., Ph.D.
Professor of Community Dental Health and Dental
Practice, University College, The Dental School, and
London Hospital Medical College,
London, England

Lindsey A. Sherwood, R.D.H., B.A.
Instructor, Department of Periodontics,
University of Pennsylvania, School of Dental Medicine,
Philadelphia, Pennsylvania

Beatrice E. Siegrist, M.S., D.D.S.
Assistant Professor, University of Berne,
School of Dental Medicine,
Berne, Switzerland

Barbara J. Steinberg, D.D.S.
Clinical Assistant Professor of Oral Medicine,
University of Pennsylvania, School of Dental Medicine,
Philadelphia, Pennsylvania

Victor P. Terranova, D.M.D., Ph.D.
Director, Laboratory of Tumor Biology and
Connective Tissue Research; Associate Professor
of Dentistry, Columbia University, School of
Dental and Oral Surgery, New York, New York

Robert L. Vanarsdall, Jr., D.D.S.
Associate Professor of Orthodontics and Periodontics;
Chairman, Department of Orthodontics,
University of Pennsylvania, School of Dental Medicine,
Philadelphia, Pennsylvania

Steven D. Vincent, D.D.S., M.S.
Assistant Professor, Department of Oral Pathology and
Diagnosis, The University of Iowa, College of Dentistry,
Iowa City, Iowa

Arnold S. Weisgold, D.D.S., F.A.C.D.
Clinical Professor of Restorative Dentistry; Director of
Postdoctoral Periodontal Prosthesis, University of
Pennsylvania, School of Dental Medicine,
Philadelphia, Pennsylvania

Ray C. Williams, D.M.D.
Associate Professor and Head, Department of
Periodontology, Harvard School of Dental Medicine,
Boston, Massachusetts

Mark E. Wilson, Ph.D.
Associate Professor, Department of Oral Biology,
State University of New York at Buffalo,
School of Dental Medicine,
Buffalo, New York

James R. Winkler, D.D.S., Ph.D.
Assistant Professor, Division of Periodontology,
Department of Stomatology, University of California,
San Francisco, School of Dentistry,
San Francisco, California

Irene R. Woodall, R.D.H., M.A., Ph.D.
Director of Clinical Studies, Vipont Pharmaceutical, Inc.,
Fort Collins, Colorado; Clinical Associate Professor,
Department of Applied Dentistry,
University of Colorado, School of Dentistry,
Denver, Colorado

Joseph J. Zambon, D.D.S., Ph.D.
Associate Professor of Periodontology and Oral Biology;
Director of Postgraduate Periodontology,
State University of New York at Buffalo,
School of Dental Medicine,
Buffalo, New York

To my wife, Sandra; my children, Deborah, Michael, Robert, Caroline, and Julie; my parents and grandchildren.

R.J.G.

To my wife, Dorothy; my children, Richard and Jerry; my parents and grandchildren.

H.M.G.

To my wife, Betty Ann; my children, Jane, Martin, Amy, and Joanne; my parents and grandchildren.

D.W.C.

PREFACE

Drs. Henry Goldman and Walter Cohen have been pioneers in periodontology and wrote the first edition of *Periodontal Therapy,* the precursor of this text, in 1959. They advocated that periodontology be an integral part of general practice, long before it became fashionable to do so.

The six editions of *Periodontal Therapy* were edited by Drs. Goldman and Cohen. During the past 55 years, Dr. Goldman's numerous contributions to dental medicine have earned the respect of colleagues around the world. Since his first volume in 1940 entitled *Periodontia,* he has been considered by many as the "father of modern periodontics." His major efforts toward dental education, such as establishing the only private dental school in the United States since World War II and constantly teaching at all levels, have made him a legend in his own time. It is fitting that two generations of former graduate students join him in this endeavor. Recently Dr. Goldman retired from academics and practice, and the task of editing *Contemporary Periodontics* was taken up by Dr. Robert Genco along with Drs. Goldman and Cohen.

This text has been completely rewritten, as reflected by the new title. With the substantial decline in dental caries and the aging of the population, more emphasis has been given to periodontal therapy. This text is directed to the needs of dentists and dental students and residents who are addressing this emphasis in periodontology.

This book has been reorganized to cover those major advances in periodontology that most affect clinical dentistry. These advances include:

1. The recognition of specific bacteria associated with periodontal disease, which has led to major advances in antiinfective therapy, chemical prophylaxis with antiplaque agents, and bacteriologic diagnosis and monitoring
2. The recognition that the neutrophil is a key protective cell, and that diseases or conditions that decrease neutrophil protective function (e.g., diabetes, stress, AIDS) place patients at risk for periodontal disease
3. Regeneration of the periodontal attachment apparatus, which is more predictable with demineralized bone graft materials and barrier membranes
4. Clarification of the importance of integrating therapies such as occlusal therapy and endosseous root-form implants with periodontal therapy

At the same time, an effort has been made to emphasize the tried-and-true concepts and methodologies that Drs. Goldman and Cohen introduced to periodontology several decades ago. The theme that periodontics is a phase of clinical practice that must be an integral part of general dentistry has been maintained, and this was facilitated in part by the fact that Dr. Genco was a student of Drs. Goldman and Cohen at the University of Pennsylvania in the mid 1960s. This book has been prepared with the same overall intention of the earlier text; that is, to present periodontics in a comprehensive manner to dental students and graduate students, as well as to the practitioner.

In the present text chapters have been grouped into four parts:

Part I The Nature of Periodontal Tissues in Health and Disease

Part II Antiinfective and Adjunctive Management of Periodontal Diseases

Part III Management of Advanced Periodontal Diseases

Part IV Future Directions and Controversial Questions in Periodontal Therapy

The first three parts deal with state-of-the-art concepts and technologies in periodontics—the tried and proven procedures. Specific procedures are discussed, and those recommended described in detail to provide the student and practitioner with practical information leading to their use in clinical practice. In Part IV on future therapy, current cutting-edge technologies are presented, some of which may become state-of-the-art in the future. References have been carefully selected to represent those key studies that are either historic or of current scientific or clinical relevance.

Part I has been greatly expanded to give extensive information about the anatomy, structure, and biochemistry of the periodontal tissues, as well as changes seen with development and aging. Emphasis here is on new information on the biochemistry of the connective tissue matrix, bone, and cell biology in an effort to help us understand wound healing and regeneration of the periodontal tissues. Periodontal diseases are presented in a chapter that gives a useful classification that builds on older classifications and adds new concepts. There is also a chapter on epidemiology that aids greatly in our understanding of disease patterns as they affect the practice of periodontology. Extensive chapters cover the etiology of periodontal disease, wherein detailed discussions of plaques, calculus, and periodontopathic organisms are presented. Since antimicrobial therapy has become a useful adjunct in treatment of periodontal disease, a chapter on the antimicrobial sensitivity of periodontal pathogens is also provided. The discussion of the pathogenesis of periodontal disease has been expanded to include chapters on host response to periodontal infections, as well as a discussion of trauma from occlusion. A series of chapters then follow on the effects of systemic conditions on periodontal disease, both gingivitis and periodontitis. In these chapters concise descriptions are given of systemic diseases in which neutrophils are abnormal and periodontal disease is more severe; of skin and mucous membrane diseases that affect the oral tissues; and of periodontal changes associated with infectious diseases such as viral infections and AIDS.

Part II deals with antiinfective and adjunctive therapy. Here treatment of periodontal infections by eliminating the causative organisms is stressed, a departure from older resective concepts where elimination of the anatomic defects left by periodontal disease was the primary rationale for therapy. A detailed description of antiinfective therapy, its role in the treatment plan, and the role of other therapies used to complement or supplement antiinfective therapy is presented. Prevention and surgical procedures directed to suppressing infectious periodontal diseases are also given. Specific considerations in the treatment of ANUG, juvenile periodontitis, and periodontal abscesses are presented for those unique conditions. Occlusal therapy as an adjunct to periodontal therapy is described.

Part III on management of advanced periodontal diseases goes into detail on periodontal surgical procedures and their current rationale. There is also a chapter on regenerative therapy in which new procedures, including use of barrier membranes for guided tissue regeneration and the newer bone graft materials, are described in detail. Prosthetic considerations in periodontics are also discussed, with pontic design and preprosthetic surgery described. A chapter on osseointegrated endosseous root-form implants has been added, since we believe that implants are a state-of-the-art technology and represent viable options for many patients who suffer from severe periodontal disease that jeopardizes their oral health. Throughout the book the incorporation of treatment-planning principles based on the option of implants is included.

In Part IV on future directions, chapters on antiinfective therapy, regenerative therapy, antiinflammatory therapy, measurements, and predicted trends in disease patterns are presented. A chapter on controversies in periodontics is also provided so that students of periodontology come away with the realization that although we have a large body of state-of-the-art proven methodologies, there are still many areas in which paradigms are evolving and information is incomplete.

In conclusion, the remarkable developments over the last two decades in the understanding of periodontal disease and periodontal therapy are incorporated in this text. A major shift in paradigm from resective therapy directed to eliminating periodontal pockets or providing physiologic contours only, to the new concept of treating periodontal diseases by suppressing the causative bacteria (i.e., antiinfective therapy) is found throughout the book. At the same time, periodontal surgical procedures and their contemporary rationale are extensively described. The rationale for periodontal surgery is not simply resective but may be to achieve regeneration of lost tissue support, to provide contours that can be maintained infection-free, for cosmetics or in preparation for prosthetics. Regenerative therapy and the role of implants are two fairly new important areas in the management of periodontal patients and are also included. Extensive discussion of the role of occlusion and occlusal therapy in periodontal disease, as well as the role of systemic conditions, is also presented.

ACKNOWLEDGMENTS

This text results from the collaboration and inspiration of many individuals whom we wish now to acknowledge. We would like to thank our wives, Sandra Genco, Dorothy Goldman, and Betty Ann Cohen, and our children for their inspiration, support, and patience with the many hours we have spent away from our families during the preparation of the book.

The success of the book is highly dependent on the integrity, inspiration, and extra efforts of our contributors, and we thank them. We also express our sincere appreciation to many of these individuals with whom we have collaborated in our research who have made major contributions of clinical relevance summarized in this textbook. We are proud and pleased to have been asked by the C.V. Mosby Company to prepare this edition. We would like to thank the Mosby staff, including Robert Reinhardt, Elaine Steinborn, Kathleen Teal, Judi Bange, Liz Fett, and Ginny Douglas for their able assistance in the editing and publication of this text.

We would also like to thank our office staff. A special thanks to Rose Parkhill for her very careful attention to all the details of manuscript tracking, proofreading, and communications that were critical to the success of this textbook. We would also like to thank Denise Nicosia for transcribing the chapters to computer disks and Paul Dressel, artist/illustrator, who was responsible for providing many of the illustrations.

Robert J. Genco

Henry M. Goldman

D. Walter Cohen

CONTENTS

Part I

The Nature of Periodontal Tissues in Health and Disease

Chapter 1

THE GINGIVA
Structure and function

Harald Löe
Max A. Listgarten
Victor P. Terranova

ANATOMY

The gingiva is that part of the oral mucous membrane that covers the alveolar processes and the cervical portions of the teeth. It has been divided traditionally into the *free* and the *attached gingiva*. The line of division between the two is an imaginary line between the bottom of the *gingival sulcus* and the visible gingival surface opposite it. The attached gingiva then extends apically from this point to the *mucogingival junction*. Apical to this line the alveolar mucosa is continuous without any demarcation into the mucous membrane of the cheek, lip, and floor of the oral cavity (Figs. 1-1 to 1-3). It should be noted here that the gingival sulcus as observed in histologic sections of well-preserved tissue blocks is not necessarily the same entity as the gingival sulcus determined by sounding with a clinical probe.

In fully erupted teeth the gingival margin is located on the enamel approximately 0.5 to 2 mm coronal to the cervix (Fig. 1-4). In human teeth the gingival margin seldom forms a knife-edged termination against the tooth, but is rounded. A shallow furrow is usually found between the gingival margin and the tooth surface. This is the entrance to, or orifice of, the gingival sulcus. The clinically healthy gingival sulcus rarely exceeds 2 to 3 mm. However, the depth of the gingival sulcus that is obtained by measurement with a periodontal probe may differ significantly from that of a gingival sulcus as observed in well-preserved histologic specimens. Since the depth of the *histologic gingival sulcus* at strictly normal sites is a negligible fraction of the total width of the attached gingiva, it has been suggested that the use of the qualifying terms *free* and *attached* in reference to the gingiva be discontinued. Furthermore, since periodontal probing does not accurately reflect the depth of the histologic sulcus, the readings provided by the periodontal probe would be more accurately described by a term such as *probing depth* or *probeable depth* of the gingival sulcus, rather than by the current terminology, *sulcus depth*. The term *pocket* should be reserved for pathologically altered sulci, the probing depth of which may exceed 3 mm.

In fully developed and erupted teeth the gingival sulcus is lined coronally with *sulcular epithelium*, the nonkeratinized extension of the *oral epithelium* into the sulcus. The bottom of the sulcus is formed by the coronal surface of the *junctional epithelium*. The junctional epithelium unites the gingival connective tissue with the enamel surface

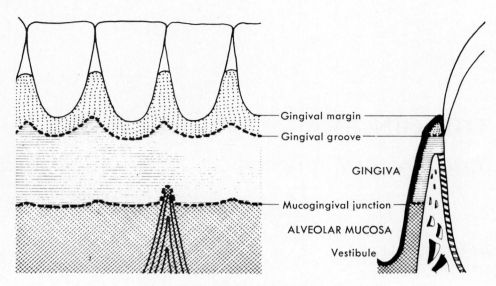

Fig. 1-1.   Anatomic relationships of normal gingiva.

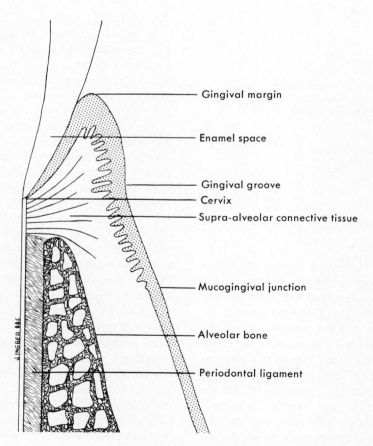

Fig. 1-2.   Anatomic relationships of marginal periodontium.

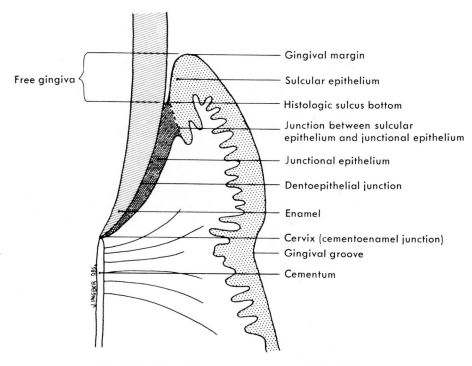

Gingival margin

Sulcular epithelium

Histologic sulcus bottom

Junction between sulcular
epithelium and junctional epithelium

Junctional epithelium

Dentoepithelial junction

Enamel

Cervix (cementoenamel junction)

Gingival groove

Cementum

Free gingiva

Fig. 1-3. Histologic relationships of marginal gingiva.

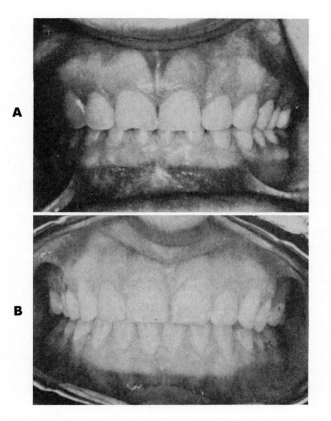

Fig. 1-4. Dentitions of a 38-year-old individual, **A,** and a 40-year-old individual, **B,** showing physiologic form of gingival tissue.

from the cervix, or neck, of the tooth and with the bottom of the gingival sulcus (see Fig. 1-3). The length of the junctional epithelium rarely exceeds 2 to 3 mm.

The margin of the gingiva describes a wavy course around the four surfaces of the tooth, with the gingival margin on the interdental surfaces constituting the most occlusally located part of the gingiva. The steepness of the arcuate form varies in accordance with the course of the cementoenamel junction (CEJ) in different teeth. In anterior teeth the gingival papilla is the interdental extension of the gingiva; the form and size are determined by the contact relationships of the adjacent teeth, the course of the CEJ, and the width of the interdental surfaces. The interdental papillae of anterior teeth have the shape of a pyramid, the base of which is an imaginary horizontal plane through the region of the CEJ. From this base the facial and oral parts of the marginal gingiva and the mesial and distal surfaces attached to the tooth form the steep sides of the pyramid. The four surfaces join at the tip of the papilla. In the premolar and molar regions the papilla is more rounded in the facio-oral direction.

In some instances the interdental gingiva may consist of two papillae: one facial to and one oral to the contact point or contact area. This configuration of the interdental gingiva has been described as a saddle, or *col,* in the facio-oral dimension. Such a smooth saddlelike depression of the interdental gingiva is frequently found in children. In the normal periodontium the tip of the interdental papilla is

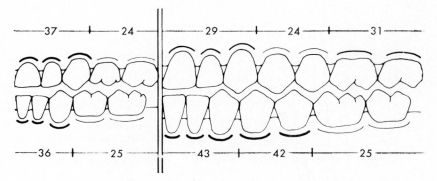

Fig. 1-5. Frequency of occurrence (%) of gingival groove on different teeth in deciduous *(left)* and permanent *(right)* dentitions. (From Ainamo J and Löe H: J Periodontol 37:5, 1966.)

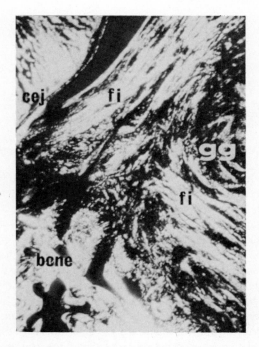

Fig. 1-6. Histologic section of marginal epithelium of a monkey. Well-defined fan-shaped fiber bundles emerge from cementum between cementoenamel junction *(cej)* and alveolar crest *(bone)*. Epithelial ridge corresponding to gingival groove *(gg)* is situated in angle produced by fiber arrangements *(fi)*. (From Ainamo J and Löe H: J Periodontol 37:5, 1966.)

always that part of the gingiva located nearest the incisal or occlusal surface of the tooth.

The *gingival groove* is a shallow groove that runs parallel to and at a distance of 0.5 to 2 mm from the margin of the gingiva. It may be found both on the facial and on the oral aspects of the gingiva. Less than half of all normal gingivae show a gingival groove (Fig. 1-5). Its presence or absence does not seem to depend on whether the gingival margin is located on the enamel, since the gingival groove frequently occurs in teeth where the gingival margin is confined to various levels below the CEJ. Measurements indicate that the distance from the gingival margin to the gingival groove roughly corresponds to the distance from the apical extension of the junctional epithelium.

The presence or absence, as well as the location, of the groove is dependent on the distinctness of the fan-shaped arrangement of the supraalveolar collagenous fibers running from the cementum into the gingiva. There seems to be no correlation between the occurrence of a gingival groove and the mechanical effects of mastication. It is believed that the special configuration of the fiber system arises when a certain number of dimensional relationships exist between the different anatomic features of the marginal periodontium (Fig. 1-6). The facts that the gingival groove persists during mild and moderate inflammation and that less than half of all normal gingivae exhibit a gingival groove indicate that a groove is not directly related to the health of the marginal gingiva. Consequently, the presence of a gingival groove cannot be used as a criterion for normal gingiva (Ainamo and Löe, 1966).

The oral and vestibular surfaces of the healthy marginal gingiva, including the tip of the interdental papilla, are covered with keratinized or parakeratinized epithelium. They are firm, frequently stippled, and pink. The gingiva extends from the gingival margin to the level of the mucogingival junction. It comprises an epithelial lining and the supraalveolar connective tissue. The *gingival epithelium* has three components: *oral, sulcular,* and *junctional.* The connective tissue core attaches the gingiva to the cementum and the alveolar bone (see Figs. 1-2 and 1-6).

Except for the hard palate, which is entirely covered with masticatory mucosa, the width of the gingiva varies from 1 to 9 mm. The gingiva is widest around the maxillary and mandibular incisors and decreases toward the canine region and the lateral segments (Fig. 1-7). The narrowest zone of gingiva is found in the region of the maxillary and mandibular first premolars and usually in con-

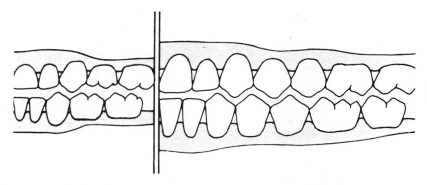

Fig. 1-7. Variation in width of attached gingiva in primary *(left)* and permanent *(right)* teeth. (From Ainamo J and Löe H: J Periodontol 37:5, 1966.)

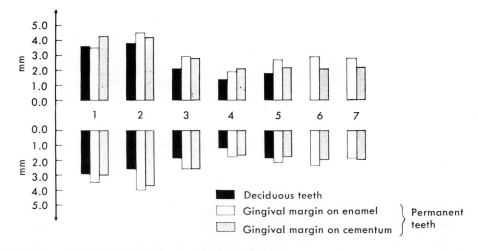

Fig. 1-8. Mean width (in millimeters) of attached gingiva in primary and permanent dentitions. (From Ainamo J and Löe H: J Periodontol 37:5, 1966.)

nection with frenum and muscle attachments. The pattern of variation is approximately the same in deciduous and permanent teeth (Fig. 1-8).

The gingiva is firm and resilient because of the tight attachment of the fibers of the supraalveolar connective tissue to the cementum and bone (Fig. 1-9). The gingiva is covered by a keratinized or parakeratinized epithelium, the surface of which presents minute depressions and elevations, giving the surface an orange-peel appearance. This stippling of the gingiva may vary considerably within the normal range. It varies with age, being less conspicuous in childhood than in adult life. It is more common on the facial than on the lingual surfaces.

The alveolar mucosa is relatively sharply delineated from the attached gingiva at the mucogingival junction. It covers the basal part of the alveolar process and continues without demarcation into the vestibular fornix or the floor of the mouth. In contrast to the attached gingiva, the alve-

olar mucosa is but loosely attached to the periosteum and is therefore highly movable. The surface of the alveolar mucosa is smooth. It is covered by nonkeratinized epithelium and is markedly redder than the attached gingiva.

GINGIVAL EPITHELIUM

The gingival surface is covered with a stratified squamous epithelium. In humans this epithelium (oral epithelium of the gingiva) is normally of the keratinizing type. The epithelium of the dentogingival junction is not keratinized.

The oral epithelium of the gingiva is fairly uniform in thickness and character. The border between the epithelium and the underlying lamina propria of the connective tissue is uneven and characterized by deep epithelial ridges that surround fingerlike connective tissue papillae (Fig. 1-10, *A*). These ridges and papillae, as they appear in histologic preparations, represent interdigitating pegs or folds

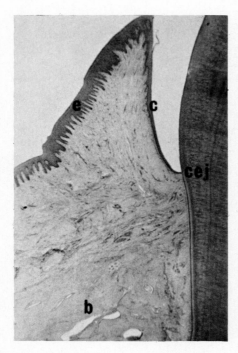

Fig. 1-9. Histologic section of marginal periodontium. *e,* Surface epithelium; *c,* junctional epithelium; *cej,* cementoenamel junction; *b,* alveolar bone.

that tend to run horizontally and parallel to the surface of the gingiva (Löe and Karring, 1971) (Fig. 1-10, *B).*

The oral epithelium of the gingiva is, like epidermis, subdivided into several layers of cells (Fig. 1-11). In the *basal layer (stratum basale, stratum germinativum)* all cells are adjacent to the connective tissue, from which they are separated by a basement membrane *(basal lamina)* (Fig. 1-12). The cells are relatively small and more or less cuboidal. The next several layers of cells constitute the *prickle cell layer (stratum spinosum),* so named because the relatively large, polyhedral cells in this layer have short cytoplasmic processes resembling spines, which connect with the processes of adjacent cells. The cellular processes are merely connected to one another by specialized cell-cell junctions. Superficial to the stratum spinosum are several layers of flattened cells that form the *granular layer (stratum granulosum).* The cytoplasm of these cells characteristically displays *keratohyaline granules* that have been associated with keratin formation. The most superficial layer is the *cornified layer (stratum corneum),* which consists of closely packed, flattened cells that have lost their nuclei and most other organelles as they became keratinized. These cells contain primarily densely packed tonofilaments (Schroeder and Theilade, 1966).

Electron microscopic studies have shown that the basal cells reside on a basement membrane consisting of an

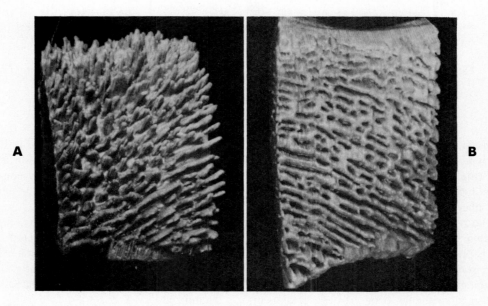

Fig. 1-10. Three-dimensional models of epithelium-connective tissue boundary of gingiva. Connective tissue papillae, **A,** are arranged in rows running predominantly parallel to gingival margin *(top).* In some areas papillae tend to fuse and form horizontal ridges *(lower right corner).* Epithelium, **B,** shows a pattern corresponding to that of connective tissue. Smooth parallel ridges running horizontally are connected by vertical cross ridges. Ridges are pitted at intervals corresponding to distribution of connective tissue papillae. (×200.) (From Löe H and Karring T: Scand J Dent Res 79:315, 1971. © 1971 Munksgaard International Publishers, Ltd., Copenhagen, Denmark.)

amorphous, moderately dense layer, the *lamina densa,* approximately 40 to 60 nm thick, which is rich in type IV collagens. The lamina densa is separated from the epithelial cell membrane by the *lamina lucida,* a space 25 to 45 nm wide, which is rich in laminin. The basement membrane is a structural entity of epithelial origin. The cytoplasmic membrane of the basal cells covers the numerous fingerlike extensions of the cell that protrude into the underlying connective tissue (Figs. 1-12 and 1-13). The cytoplasm of the basal cells generally contains a relatively high concentration of organelles and other cytoplasmic constituents. *Tonofibrils* are regularly seen in the basal cells. They are composed of finer elements, the *tonofilaments,* which measure approximately 5 nm in diameter.

Specialized connective tissue fibrils have been described in close association with a variety of basement membranes, including those of the gingival epithelium. These so-called *anchoring fibrils* are composed of types V and VII collagen and connect the lamina densa to the underlying connective tissue (Fig. 1-13).

The cells of the spinous layer (stratum spinosum) are

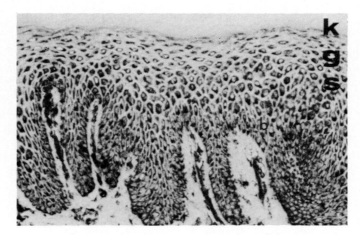

Fig. 1-11. Frozen sections of human attached gingiva (5μm thick) incubated to show glutamic dehydrogenase activity. *b,* Basal layer; *s,* spinous layer; *g,* granular layer; *k,* keratinized surface layer. (From Löe H and Nuki K: J Periodont Res 1:43, 1967. © 1967 Munksgaard International Publishers, Ltd., Copenhagen, Denmark.)

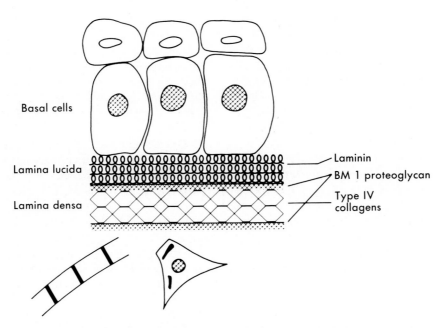

Fig. 1-12. Schematic representation of basement membrane.

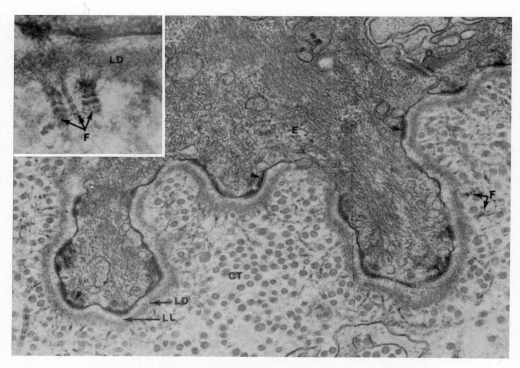

Fig. 1-13.   Gingiva. Basement lamina joining epithelial cell *(E)* to underlying connective tissue *(CT)* consists of finely granular lamina densa *(LD)* separated from cell membrane by clear lamina lucida *(LL)*. Hemidesmosomes *(arrows)* connect epithelial cell to basement lamina. Anchoring fibrils *(F)* may participate in joining basement lamina to underlying connective tissue. *D,* Desmosome joining adjacent epithelial cells. (× 33,000.) *Inset:* Higher magnification of anchoring fibrils *(F)* and their relationship to lamina densa *(LD).* (× 110,000.) (From Listgarten M: Unpublished data, 1967.)

generally larger than the basal cells. They contain fewer cytoplasmic organelles and relatively more tonofibrils than the basal cells (Fig. 1-14). In the superficial layers the tonofibrils become concentrated on the periphery of the cell and increase in number. In the stratum corneum the cells are densely packed with tonofilaments. The peripheral cytoplasm tends to become condensed against the inner leaflet of the cell membrane, thereby giving the latter a thickened appearance. Lipid droplets may be present within the cell, but other cytoplasmic organelles are infrequently recognized.

Both basal and spinous cells have an irregular contour. Numerous cytoplasmic processes protrude from the entire cell periphery, giving the cell surface a jagged appearance (Fig. 1-15). The cell membranes of adjacent cells are generally found in close apposition to each other. This results in narrow and irregular intercellular spaces between the cells.

Adjacent cells are attached to each other by specialized portions of the cell membrane. The most common type of junction is the *desmosome* (Fig. 1-16). It consists of two adjacent attachment plaques—one from each cell—that are separated by an interval approximately 30 nm wide

that contains three dense lamellae. Intracellular tonofilaments converge toward the internal surface of the attachment plaques (Fig. 1-17). The desmosome and a portion of the cytoplasm from each of the adjacent cells constitute the "intercellular bridge" of classic histology (Fig. 1-18). *Tight junctions (maculae occludentes),* which are also found in the gingival epithelium, are formed by fusion of the external leaflets of adjacent cell membranes. The area of fusion appears to be of a size and shape similar to that of a desmosome (Fig. 1-19). The connection of one cell to another depends on the chemical and physical forces that determine the properties of various cell junctions. It is possible that the intercellular substance, which contains polysaccharides, proteins, and some lipid, may also play a part in the adhesion of adjacent cells (Fig. 1-20).

In the granular layer (stratum granulosum) the cells become flattened in a plane parallel to the gingival surface. The tonofibrils become more prominent than in the stratum spinosum. Keratohyaline granules, up to 1 μm in diameter, round in shape, and electron dense, appear in the cytoplasm (Fig. 1-21). There is a further decrease in the number of mitochondria. Smaller *membrane-coating granules,* approximately 0.1 μm in diameter, can be observed

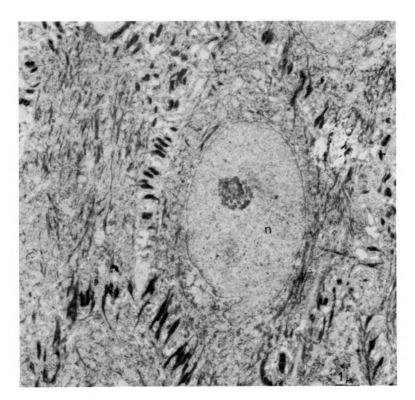

Fig. 1-14. Spinous epithelial cells, Tonofilaments *(t)* are seen in cytoplasm around nucleus *(n)* and extending toward periphery of cytoplasm. (From Schroeder H and Theilade J: J Periodont Res 1:95, 1966. © 1966, Munksgaard International Publishers, Ltd., Copenhagen, Denmark.)

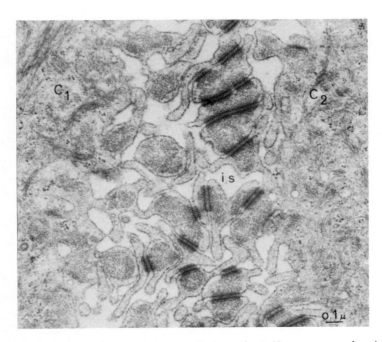

Fig. 1-15. Relationship between two adjacent cells *(c₁ and c₂). Numerous cytoplasmic processes protrude from cell periphery into intercellular space (is),* giving cell surface a jagged appearance. (From Schroeder H and Theilade J: J Periodont Res 1:95, 1966. © 1966, Munksgaard International Publishers, Ltd., Copenhagen, Denmark.)

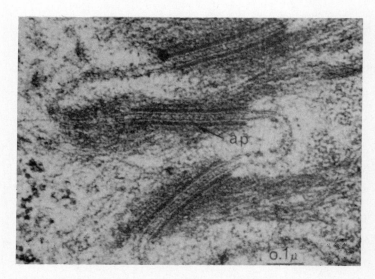

Fig. 1-16. Typical desmosomes consisting of attachment plaque areas of two adjacent cells separated by a 20 to 30 nm wide laminated space. Attachment plaques *(ap)* from two adjacent cells and laminated intercellular space constitute desmosome. (From Schroeder H and Theilade J: J Periodont Res 1:95, 1966. © 1966 Munksgaard International Publishers, Ltd., Copenhagen, Denmark.)

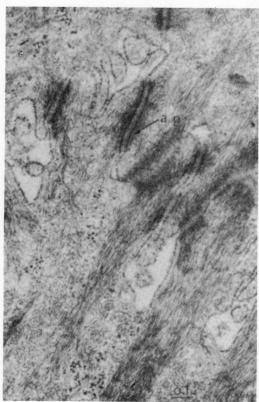

Fig. 1-17. At intervals cell membrane is thickened, and adjacent intracellular cytoplasm is condensed. Such areas are designated attachment plaques *(ap)*. Intracellular tonofibrils *(t)* terminate at internal aspect of attachment plaque. (From Schroeder H and Theilade J: J Periodont Res 1:95, 1966. © 1966 Munksgaard International Publishers, Ltd., Copenhagen, Denmark.)

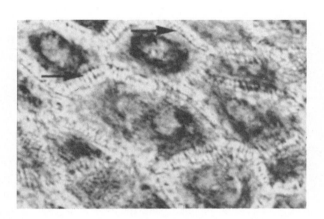

Fig. 1-18. Intercellular bridges *(arrows)* crossing between prickle cells.

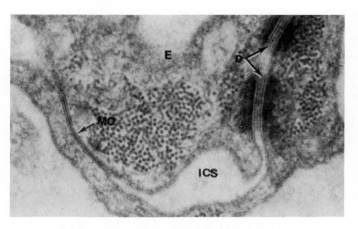

Fig. 1-19. Desmosomes *(D)* and tight junction (macula occludens, *MO*) connecting adjacent portions of gingival epithelial cells *(E)*. Note relationship of inner and outer leaflet of cell membranes to each type of junction. *ICS,* Intercellular space. (×67,000.) (From Listgarten M: Unpublished data, 1967.)

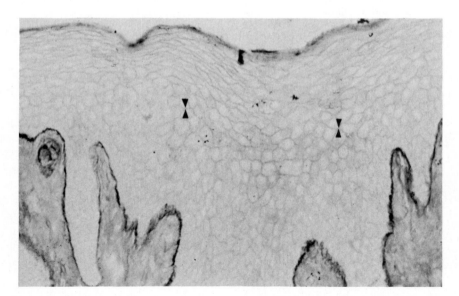

Fig. 1-20. Keratinized epithelium of attached gingiva (5μm thick) stained in periodic acid-Schiff (PAS). Note heavy PAS-positive material of basement membrane and PAS-positive material of intercellular substance of epithelium *(arrows)*. (From Löe H: Unpublished data, 1962.)

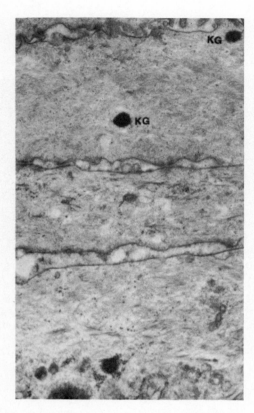

Fig. 1-21. Stratum granulosum. Note diminution of cytoplasmic organelles from bottom of illustration to top and appearance of keratohyaline granules *(KG)*. Membrane-coating granules are not apparent in this section. Note thickening of cell membranes. (×10,000.) (From Listgarten M: Unpublished data, 1964.)

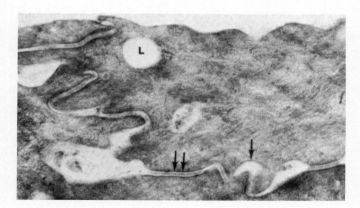

Fig. 1-22. Superficial cell of stratum corneum. Densely packed tonofilaments and lipid droplets *(L)* are prime constituents of cell interior. Thickened inner leaflet of plasmalemma *(single arrow)* is nearly as broad as attachment plaque of desmosomes *(double arrow)*. (×30,000.) (From Listgarten M: Unpublished data, 1966.)

in close proximity to the most superficial cell membrane. The content of these granules appears to contribute to the material within the narrow intercellular spaces characteristically noted at this level. The desmosomes become oriented more or less parallel to the cell surface.

At the inferior border of the cornified layer (stratum corneum) the cells undergo a sudden transition into keratinized cells. This is characterized by an increased prominence of the tonofilaments, which are closely packed together and form the predominant morphologic constituent of the cell. Clear, rounded bodies probably representing lipid droplets appear within the cytoplasm. The remaining organelles and the nucleus disappear. Concomitant with these alterations, the cell membrane appears to undergo a marked thickening of the inner leaflet of the membrane, which becomes about as thick as the attachment plaque of the desmosomes, with which it is continuous (Fig. 1-22). The outer leaflet is frequently interrupted and difficult to identify. The superficial cells desquamate as a result of intradesmosomal disruption (Schroeder and Theilade, 1966).

GINGIVAL SULCUS AND DENTOGINGIVAL JUNCTION

The soft tissue wall of the gingival sulcus is lined coronally with sulcular epithelium. The apical part of the soft tissue wall and the bottom of the sulcus are formed by the coronal surface of the junctional epithelium (see Fig. 1-3).

The junctional epithelium consists of a thin layer of epithelium that joins the gingival connective tissue to the tooth surface. In recently erupted teeth this epithelium extends from the bottom of the gingival sulcus to the apical border of the enamel. It consists of a band varying in thickness from 15 to 30 cells in the vicinity of the gingival sulcus to as few as 1 cell at its apical extension in the cervical area. The cells immediately adjacent to the gingival connective tissue and the cells located in the most apical portion of the junctional epithelium have characteristics in common with basal epithelial cells, including the ability to divide. The remaining cells that are oriented in a plane parallel to the long axis of the tooth are morphologically similar to cells of the lower stratum spinosum.

The histologic appearance of junctional epithelium is different from that of the keratinized oral epithelium. It is thinner and lacks well-developed epithelial ridges. Consequently, the basement membrane bordering on the subepithelial connective tissue follows a relatively straight course. However, in the normal gingiva of adult individuals, epithelial ridges and connective tissue papillae are frequently encountered beneath the sulcular epithelium lining the coronal portion of the sulcus. Provided that no signs of inflammation or other pathologic conditions are present, this should be regarded as normal. Junctional epithelium does not contain a stratum granulosum or stratum corneum. Histochemical stains also have shown that cells of the normal junctional epithelium do not show any tendency toward keratinization. The cells of the junctional epithelium are oriented with their long axis parallel to the tooth surface. The coronal surface of the junctional epithelium represents its free surface, since it is the surface from which desquamation takes place. This surface forms the floor and part of the apical portion of the lateral wall of the gingival sulcus (Fig. 1-23).

Whereas the orifice of the gingival sulcus is bound by the tooth surface on one side and sulcular epithelium on the other, the bottom of the sulcus is frequently surrounded by epithelium on all sides. This is due to the per-

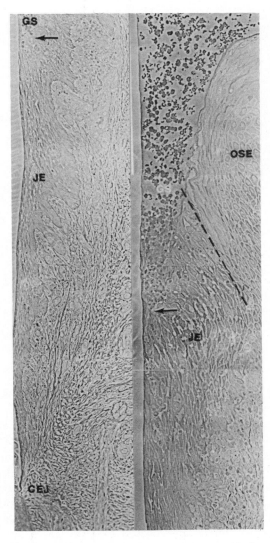

Fig. 1-23. Gingival sulcus *(GS)* and junctional epithelium *(JE)*. Epithelial attachment extends from bottom of gingival sulcus *(arrow)* to apical border of enamel *(CEJ)*. Dotted line indicates junction of oral sulcular epithelium *(OSE)* and junctional epithelium *(JE)*. Phase-contrast micrograph. (From Schroeder HE and Listgarten MA: In Wolsky A, editor: Monographs in developmental biology, vol 2, Fine structure of the developing epithelial attachment of human teeth, Basel, Switzerland, 1971, S Karger.)

sistence of junctional epithelial cells on the tooth surface for a distance of approximately 100 μm coronal to the sulcus bottom (Fig. 1-24).

The epithelial lining of the coronal portion of the lateral wall of the gingival sulcus resembles the gingival epithelium covering the external surface of the gingiva in all respects with the exception that it does not become fully keratinized. Unlike junctional epithelium, which is composed almost entirely of stratum spinosum–type cells, this epithelium is stratified in the pattern generally observed in other oral epithelia. The surface cells are flattened and exhibit a tendency toward partial keratinization (Figs. 1-24 and 1-25).

Electron microscopically, the junctional epithelial cells are moderately rich in rough-surfaced endoplasmic reticulum and mitochondria. They have well-developed Golgi regions and relatively few tonofibrils. The intercellular spaces are relatively larger and the number of desmosomes fewer than in the stratum spinosum of the gingival epithelium.

The sulcular epithelium is ultrastructurally similar to the oral epithelium of the gingiva described previously, except that the superficial cells may retain some organelles and exhibit focal accumulations of glycogen in addition to the lipid droplets typically found in the superficial cells of oral epithelium (Fig. 1-25). The compacted tonofilaments characteristically noted in keratinized epithelial cells are also present, but more loosely arranged, in the superficial cell layers of the sulcular epithelium (Schroeder and Listgarten, 1971).

SUPRAALVEOLAR CONNECTIVE TISSUE

The supraalveolar connective tissue comprises the mesodermal structures of the gingiva coronal to the crest of the alveolar bone. It consists primarily of cells, fibers, nerve processes, and blood vessels embedded in a dense connective tissue. The main cell is the fibroblast, which synthesizes the basic elements of the connective tissue. Other cells normally found include undifferentiated mesenchymal cells, mast cells, and macrophages. The predominant connective tissue fibers are of two distinct types: *collagen* and *elastin fibers*. *Reticular fibers* are numerous beneath the basement membrane in a narrow area adjacent to the epithelium. Reticular fibers are also found in tissue investing blood vessels. They appear to be composed of a special variety of collagen. *Oxytalan fibers,* so named because of their resistance to acid digestion, are found throughout the periodontal connective tissue but do not seem to contribute significantly to the attachment of the teeth. Their origin, chemical composition, and function are as yet unknown. They probably represent a form of immature elastic fiber, consisting of the microfibrillar component of the mature elastin fiber without the amorphous elastin. *Anchoring fibrils,* which have been described in close association with the connective tissue side

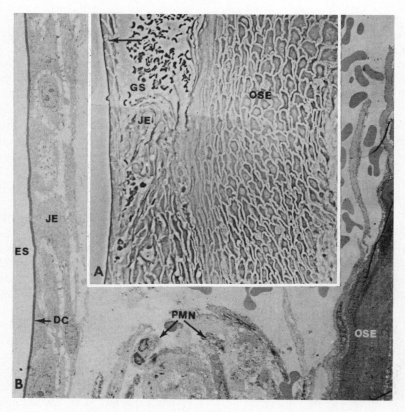

Fig. 1-24. Gingival sulcus. **A,** Phase-contrast micrograph illustrating bottom of gingival sulcus *(GS)* bound by oral sulcular epithelium *(OSE)* laterally, free surface of junctional epithelium *(JE)* beneath, and junctional epithelial cells still clinging to enamel surface *(arrow)*. **B,** Electron micrograph of serial section showing tendency of oral sulcular epithelium *(OSE)* to keratinize and presence of a dental cuticle *(DC)* between junctional epithelial cells *(JE)* still clinging to tooth and enamel space *(ES)*. Bottom of sulcus consists of desquamating junctional epithelial cells and polymorphonuclear leukocytes *(PMN)* in various stages of disintegration. (**A** ×360; **B** ×2400.) (From Schroeder HE and Listgarten MA: In Wolsky A, editor: Monographs in developmental biology, vol 2, Fine structure of the developing epithelial attachment of human teeth, Basel, Switzerland, 1971, S Karger.)

of epithelial basement laminae, consist of types V and VII collagen (see Fig. 1-13).

The most conspicuous parts of the gingival connective tissue are the collagen fibers. Some of these fibers are distributed in a haphazard arrangement throughout the connective tissue ground substance. Others are arranged in coarse bundles that exhibit a distinct orientation. The fiber bundles have been given names according to their general direction and coarseness (Fig. 1-26). Each of the fiber arrangements consists of collagenous fiber bundles built up from numerous fibers. According to current nomenclature, these fiber systems should not be termed *fibers*. The terms *circular fibers, transseptal fibers,* and so on, however, have been adapted into the professional language and are also used in the following description with the understanding that they are systems of collagen fiber bundles (Fig. 1-26).

The *circular fibers* belong to the free gingiva and encircle the tooth in a ringlike fashion.

The *dentogingival fibers* are part of a fan-shaped fiber system that emerges from the supraalveolar part of the cementum of the entire circumference of the tooth. The dentogingival branch of this system sweeps outward and upward and terminates in the marginal gingiva. Another group emerges from the same area, but it passes outward beyond the alveolar crest in an apical direction into the mucoperiosteum of the attached gingiva. These are the *dentoperiosteal fibers.*

An *interpapillary* group of fibers has also been described that runs in an orovestibular direction from the vestibular to the oral interdental papillae of posterior teeth.

The architecture of the gingival and interdental ligaments of clinically healthy young adult marmosets was studied by Page et al. (1974). The gingivae were free of

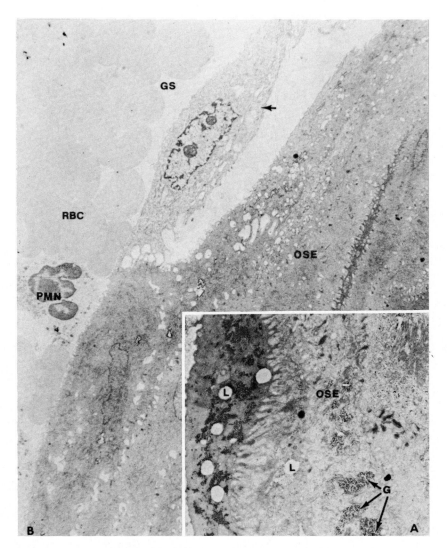

Fig. 1-25. Oral sulcular epithelium *(OSE)* that lines lateral wall of gingival sulcus *(GS)* shows partially keratinized surface cells, one of which *(arrow)* is desquamating into sulcus. *Inset:* Glycogen particles *(G)* are present in surface cells, as well as in deeper layers. *RBC,* Red blood cells from surgical hemorrhage; *PMN,* polymorphonuclear leukocyte; *L,* lipid droplets. (**A** ×4300; **B** ×6000.) (From Schroeder HE and Listgarten MA: In Wolsky A, editor: Monographs in developmental biology, vol 2, Fine structure of the developing epithelial attachment of human teeth, Basel, Switzerland, 1971, S Karger.)

histologic manifestations of inflammatory gingival disease. In addition to the fiber groups previously described (Fig. 1-26), *semicircular fibers* were found to arise from the cementum near the CEJ, traverse the free marginal, facial, and lingual gingivae, and insert into a comparable position on the opposite side of the tooth at a level just apical to the circular fibers. *Intergingival fibers* course in the free marginal gingiva on both the facial and lingual surfaces of the teeth; also, *transgingival fibers* arise from the cementum of one tooth and extend into the marginal gingiva of an adjacent tooth.

The *transseptal fibers* (Fig. 1-26) extend from the supraalveolar cementum of one tooth mesiodistally through the interdental gingiva above the septum of the alveolar bone to the cementum of the adjacent tooth.

The *lamina propria* of the attached gingiva is a layer of dense connective tissue into which most of the above-mentioned fiber systems enter, but that, in addition, contains numerous other bundles of fibers of more or less well-defined orientation. Some of the latter fibers provide for the firm attachment of the lamina propria to the periosteum of the alveolar process.

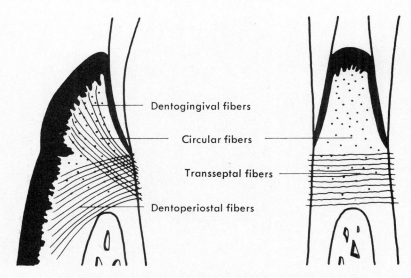

Dentogingival fibers

Circular fibers

Transseptal fibers

Dentoperiostal fibers

Fig. 1-26. Fiber arrangements of gingival connective tissue.

The gingival fibers, as well as the principal fibers of the periodontal ligament, consist mainly of bundles of collagen fibrils embedded in a ground substance. The fibrils are composed of aggregated collagen molecules.

The basic structure of the type I collagen molecule is a rodlike molecule approximately 300 nm long and 1.5 nm in diameter. It is composed of three polypeptide chains, the alpha chains, each approximately 100,000 molecular weight, wrapped together in a right-handed helix.

There are at least four types of collagen, which are differentiated according to their alpha-chain composition. The alpha chains are currently classified as alpha-1 or alpha-2 chains, depending on their elution position from chromatography columns. In addition, the alpha-1 chains are subdivided further, according to the sequence of the amino acids along their length, into "types" I to IV.

The most common form of collagen in the body is the collagen of skin, mucous membranes, bone, dentin, and cementum. Under the electron microscope it appears as well-defined fibrils with a characteristic axial periodicity of approximately 70 nm. This form of collagen is referred to as type I collagen. Type I collagen molecules are composed of two alpha-1 type I chains and one alpha-2 chain. The structural formula for type I collagen is $[\alpha 1(I)]_2 \alpha 2$.

Other types of collagen that have been recognized include collagen from cartilage, which is designated as type II, with the structural formula $[\alpha 1(II)]_3$; collagen from fetal skin and reticular fibers, which contains type III $[\alpha 1(III)]_3$ collagen; and type IV collagen, which is found in basement membranes, with the structural formula $[\alpha 1(IV)]_3$.

Type I collagen is the only form that has been shown to contain both alpha-1 and alpha-2 chains. It is able to form, by lateral aggregation of the collagen molecules, striated collagen fibrils with a distinct periodicity.

Two unusual amino acids characterize the collagen protein: hydroxyproline and hydroxylysine. The hydroxyproline content of tissues in general is taken as a measure of their collagen content.

Between the collagenous elements is found an interfibrillar, amorphous ground substance. Histochemical and chemical analyses have disclosed that the ground substance is characterized by the presence of certain polysaccharide-protein complexes, or proteoglycans. Proteoglycans that contain a relatively high proportion of protein are also called *glycoproteins.* When carbohydrates predominate, the proteoglycans are called *mucopolysaccharides* or *glycosaminoglycans,* the latter term having largely replaced the former. Glycosaminoglycans consist of linear carbohydrate chains linked by covalent bonds to a protein core. Some of these molecules are sulfated (e.g., chondroitin sulfates); others do not contain sulfate (e.g., hyaluronic acid).

It is difficult to precisely specify the function of the ground substance. But its important role in the maintenance of normal tissue physiology is probably best demonstrated by the fact that the ground substance constitutes the immediate environment of the cells. Any substance vital to cells must pass from the blood vessels through this substance to reach the cells.

Deviations from normal as to chemical composition and physical state of the ground substance will consequently reflect on both the cellular physiology and the rheology.

BLOOD SUPPLY OF THE GINGIVA

The blood supply of the gingival tissues is derived mainly from supraperiosteal vessels originating from the lingual, mental, buccinator, and palatine arteries. These vessels give off branches along the facial and oral surfaces of the alveolar bone (Karring and Löe, 1967) (Fig. 1-27).

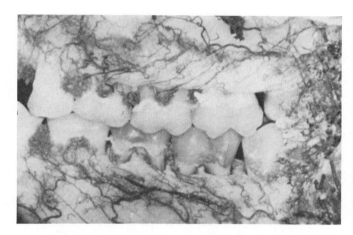

Fig. 1-27. Corrosion preparation of left buccal maxillary and mandibular segments of a monkey injected with cold-setting colored acrylic through carotid artery. Gingival branches of buccal and facial arteries are shown. (From Karring T and Löe H: J Periodont Res 2:74, 1967. © 1967 Munksgaard International Publishers, Ltd., Copenhagen, Denmark.)

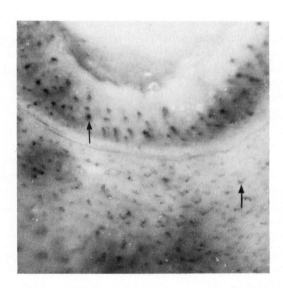

Fig. 1-28. Small blood vessels *(arrows)* terminating in loops at connective tissue–epithelium interface of buccal gingiva. (From Glavind L and Löe H: J Periodont Res 2:74, 1967. © 1967 Munksgaard International Publishers, Ltd., Copenhagen, Denmark.)

The superficial portions of these vessels are readily seen through the vestibular and oral mucosa (Glavind and Löe, 1967) (Fig. 1-28). Also, branches of the alveolar arteries penetrating the interdental septa or emerging from the periodontal ligament contribute to the gingival blood supply. These branches anastomose with the periosteal ones and form the vascular bed of the gingiva. Because of the keratinized surface layer of the gingiva, blood vessels are not commonly seen with the naked eye.

The nutritional supply to the gingival epithelium is via capillaries terminating in groups immediately below the basement membrane (Fig. 1-29). Microscopic studies of the gingival surface in vivo have shown that there are approximately 50 capillaries per square millimeter, each of which terminates in a loop in the peripheral part of the connective tissue papillae adjacent to the epithelial border. Wide variations in number exist, however, between teeth as well as between different individuals. However, longitudinal studies show that within a particular gingival region the same vascular pattern persists over a long period of time. This indicates that under normal conditions the blood supply is quite consistent with respect to the number, distribution, and size of the blood vessels (Karring and Löe, 1967).

Next to the sulcular and junctional epithelia, the terminal blood vessels form a plexus that extends under the epithelial surface from the gingival margin to the apical extension of the junctional epithelium (Fig. 1-30) (Egelberg, 1966).

Most of the vessels in the gingival connective tissue are arterioles, capillaries, and small veins. Occasionally, small arteries are seen in the connective tissue of oral mucosa. The overall diameter of an arteriole is of the order of 100 μm. The walls of the arterioles consist of three more or less well-defined layers. The *intima* is a simple layer of endothelial cells. Sometimes a small amount of connective tissue may be interposed between this and the media, which is made up of circularly arranged smooth muscle fibers. Occasionally in the larger arterioles the *adventitia* may consist of collagenous and elastic fibers forming an external elastic lamina.

The change from arteriole to capillary is a gradual one, during which both the diameter and the thickness of the wall of the arteriole decrease. The capillary wall is made up of a single layer of endothelial cells arranged end to end and held together by specialized junctions and an intercellular cementing substance. The diameter of the capil-

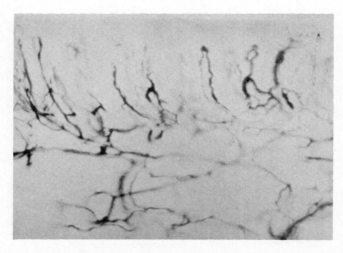

Fig. 1-29. Terminating vessels immediately below basement membrane in attached gingiva. Animal was injected with carbon serum. (From Karring T and Löe H: J Periodont Res 2:74, 1967. © 1967 Munksgaard International Publishers, Ltd., Copenhagen, Denmark.)

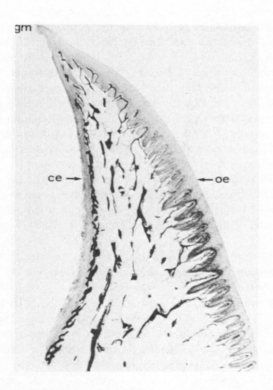

Fig. 1-30. Clinically healthy gingiva of a dog (buccolingual section) showing a layer of blood vessels in close apposition to junctional epithelium *(ce)*. Animal was injected with carbon gelatin. *gm,* Gingival margin; *oe,* oral epithelium. (From Egelberg J: J Periodont Res 1:63, 1966. © 1966 Munksgaard International Publishers, Ltd., Copenhagen, Denmark.)

lary is approximately 10 μm. The endothelial cells as observed in electron micrographs are surrounded by an amorphous basement lamina. The basement lamina is too thin to be observed by the light microscope. However, a layer containing thin connective tissue filaments surrounds the basement lamina and separates the blood vessel from the surrounding collagenous matrix. It is probable that the basement lamina, together with this adjacent region, constitutes what at the level of the light microscope is termed the *basement membrane.*

Normally the transport of substances between the circulatory system and the tissues take place across the capillary wall at a rate that meets the requirements of the particular part of the tissue at any given moment. Under normal conditions water and electrolytes diffuse through the capillary wall. This diffusion is made possible by the slightly high hydrostatic pressure within the vessel as compared with that outside. Normally, high molecular weight substances from plasma do not leak out into the tissue fluid. Nevertheless, it is evident that plasma proteins under physiologic conditions are found in the extravascular compartment.

The necessary adjustment of capillary circulation and the alteration of the capillary wall to allow for this transfer are controlled by indirect and direct mechanisms. Although the capillaries are indirectly controlled by nervous mechanisms to some degree, the major regulation of permeability is dependent on general and local chemical mechanisms. The accumulation of locally formed metabolites (e.g., histamine), as well as a lack of oxygen, increased carbon dioxide tension, and corresponding change in pH, causes dilation and increased permeability. For shorter periods of oxygen deprivation, the rate of filtration through the capillary wall may be increased several times, and the endothelium may be so permeable that protein molecules may also pass through with ease. As the capil-

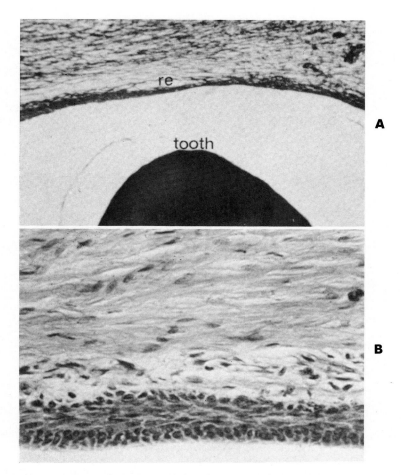

Fig. 1-31. Unerupted tooth during formation. **A,** Note reduced enamel epithelium *(re)* encircling crown. **B,** Reduced enamel epithelium consists of shortened ameloblasts and cellular derivatives from other cell layers of enamel organ.

laries dilate, fresh blood flows through the area, removing the waste material and bringing a new supply of oxygen. The attraction of metabolites into the venous blood is made possible through the fact that the osmotic pressure of blood is somewhat greater than the osmotic pressure of tissue fluid.

HISTOGENESIS OF THE DENTOGINGIVAL JUNCTION

Recent evidence indicates that after the enamel matrix is deposited, the ameloblasts become shortened but continue to function for a period of time in a resorptive capacity during maturation of the enamel. The epithelial cells derived from the enamel organ, including the reduced ameloblasts and cells adjacent to their proximal (external) surface, form the *reduced enamel epithelium* (Fig. 1-31). In normal human teeth prior to eruption, the reduced enamel epithelium forms an almost complete covering over the external surface of the enamel. In the cervical region of the crown, minor interruptions in the lining may

occur that allow the formation of relatively thin, irregularly shaped layers of cementum over the exposed enamel surface. These afibrillar cementum patches are frequently devoid of typical collagen fibrils. In sections they may appear as cementum "spurs" that overlap the apical border of the enamel (Fig. 1-32) or as "islands" of afibrillar cementum on the cervical enamel surface.

The reduced enamel epithelium is normally composed of several layers of cells that are arranged with their long axes parallel to the enamel surface. As the tooth erupts and approaches the oral epithelium covering the alveolar ridge, the outer cell layers of the reduced enamel epithelium covering the tip of the crown begin to divide. The reduced ameloblasts cannot divide, since they have lost the ability to do so shortly after their differentiation from preameloblasts. As the crown is about to break into the oral cavity, the reduced enamel epithelium appears to fuse with the oral epithelium.

At this stage the enamel surface is partly covered with epithelium, the coronal part of which may be morphologi-

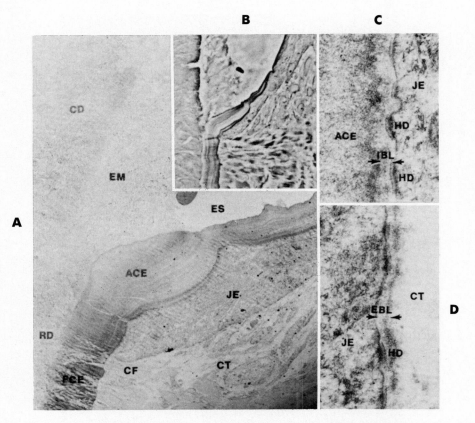

Fig. 1-32. Cervical region of tooth, **A,** Electron micrograph illustrating fibrillar root cementum *(FCE)* covering root dentin *(RD)*. Cervical enamel surface is covered by a layer of afibrillar cementum that does not contain collagen fibrils *(ACE)*. Junctional epithelium *(JE)* is attached to outer surface of collagen fibrillar "spur" and extends apically up to fibrillar cementum of root. A collagen fiber *(CF)* immediately below it extends from gingival connective tissue *(CT)* into fibrillar root cementum. *CD,* Crown dentin; *EM,* enamel matrix; *ES,* enamel space. **B,** Phase-contrast micrograph of serial section of **A** for orientation. **C,** Junction of junctional epithelium *(JE)* with collagen fibrils *(ACE)*. Note presence of hemidesmosomes *(HD* and an internal basement lamina *(IBL)*. **D,** Junction of junctional epithelium *(JE)* with gingival connective tissue *(CT)*. This region is similar to **C** and contains hemidesmosomes and an external basement lamina *(EBL)*. (**A** × 1800; **B** ×420; **C** ×45,000.) (From Schroeder HE and Listgarten MA: In Wolsky A, editor: Monographs in developmental biology, vol 2, Fine structure of the developing epithelial attachment of human teeth, Basel, Switzerland, 1971, S Karger.)

cally similar to junctional epithelium, and the apical portion to reduced enamel epithelium (Fig. 1-33). Shortly after the crown enters the oral cavity, the epithelium over the enamel becomes entirely composed of junctional epithelium, which may form a band several millimeters wide around the crown. With further eruption the crown is gradually uncovered until the tooth has reached the plane of occlusion.

As the crown surface is uncovered, the width of the junctional epithelial band diminishes, since in the normal state the apical extension remains more or less stabilized at the level of the cervical region.

Some investigators have claimed that the reduced enamel epithelium is displaced by cells derived primarily from oral epithelial cells that proliferate in an apical direction and replace the reduced enamel epithelium. Electron microscopic and autoradiographic data suggest that the junctional epithelium is produced primarily by proliferation of the outer cells of the reduced enamel epithelium. The reduced ameloblasts become flattened and assume the morphologic characteristics of squamous epithelial cells. Because they have lost the ability to divide, they are eventually displaced by the outer cells of the reduced enamel epithelium that give rise to most of the junctional epithelium. This occurs as part of the normal physiologic turnover of the cells in junctional epithelium. Oral epithelium may initially contribute to the formation of only the most coronal portion of the junctional epithelium. In some

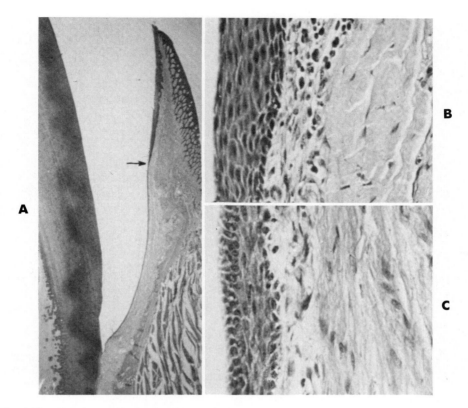

Fig. 1-33. Erupting tooth, **A,** showing gradual replacement of reduced enamel epithelium, **C,** by junctional epithelium, **B.**

erupted teeth a *dental cuticle* may be noted between the junctional epithelium and the adjacent tooth surface (Fig. 1-34). The origin and nature of this structure are not clear. As the junctional epithelium assumes a more apical position in relation to the tooth surface during the years that follow tooth emergence into the oral cavity, the dental cuticle may become exposed to the oral environment while remaining attached to the tooth surface in the vicinity of the gingival sulcus. In this location it may subsequently become colonized by bacteria or worn off.

Although the oral epithelium may play a limited role in the initial formation of the junctional epithelium, it is capable, when called on, of regenerating a completely new junctional epithelium (e.g., after gingivectomy).

CONNECTION BETWEEN EPITHELIUM AND ENAMEL

The nature of the relationship between epithelium and enamel has been the subject of controversy for many years. Until 1921 the epithelium was not believed to be connected to the enamel surface. The gingival sulcus was thought of as a space lined by an extension of the oral epithelium into the sulcus, the epithelium tapering toward the cervix of the tooth where it ended in the form of a linear

junction. In 1921 Gottlieb reported that the epithelium was attached to the enamel surface. Gottlieb stated that during completion of enamel formation the ameloblasts produced a specialized layer of material that he named the "primary enamel cuticle." Subsequently, the ameloblasts were thought to degenerate, followed by the cells of the stratum intermedium and stellate reticulum. The outer enamel epithelium was believed to change from a simple epithelium into a stratified squamous keratinizing epithelial layer; the keratin layer formed an "organic union" between the epithelium and the primary enamel cuticle covering the enamel surface. Gottlieb referred to the keratinized layer as the "secondary enamel cuticle." Subsequently, this name was changed to the current term, *dental cuticle*. Although Gottlieb originally postulated the presence of a keratinized cuticle between the epithelium and the enamel surface, subsequent histochemical and electron microscopic studies have indicated that this material is not composed of keratin.

Another view, proposed by Becks (1929), postulated that the odontogenic epithelium did not persist but degenerated and was replaced by epithelial cells proliferating from the oral epithelium. The degenerating odontogenic epithelium was thought to keratinize and form the second-

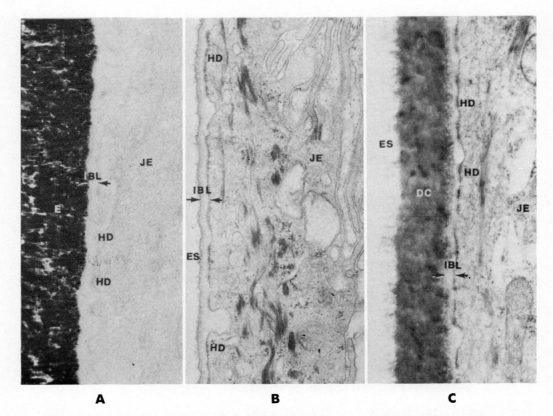

Fig. 1-34. Ultrastructure of epithelial attachment. **A,** Junctional epithelium *(JE)* is attached to undemineralized enamel *(E)* by internal basement lamina *(IBL)* and hemidesmosomes *(HD)*. **B,** Similar section to that shown in **A** except that tissue was first demineralized. *ES,* Enamel space; *IBL,* internal basement lamina; *HD,* hemidesmosomes; *JE,* junctional epithelium. **C,** Dental cuticle *(DC)* is interposed between enamel space *(ES)* and internal basement lamina *(IBL)* of junctional epithelium *(JE)*. *HE,* Hemidesmosomes. (× 14,000.) (From Schroeder HE and Listgarten MA: In Wolsky A, editor: Monographs in developmental biology, vol 2, Fine structure of the developing epithelial attachment of human teeth, Basel, Switzerland, 1971, S Karger.)

ary cuticle, which established a firm union with the primary cuticle. A later theory rejected the concept of a secondary cuticle as a medium of structural continuity between the two tissues and suggested that the new epithelial cells arising from the oral epithelium attached themselves to the enamel by means of tonofibrils inserted into the primary cuticle. This was not corroborated by subsequent electron microscopic data (Schroeder and Listgarten, 1971).

Based on the consideration that Gottlieb's histologic concept of the epithelial attachment did not coincide with clinical observations, Waerhaug (1960) set out to investigate the discrepancy. Waerhaug noted that thin steel blades could be inserted through the gingival sulcus to the region of the CEJ with relative ease. On the basis of these and related experiments, Waerhaug restated the view held to be valid prior to Gottlieb, that no structural continuity existed between gingiva and enamel and that the bottom of the gingival sulcus was located at the CEJ. Waerhaug be-

lieved that the epithelium was only weakly adherent to the enamel surface and described the epithelium surrounding the neck of the tooth as an "epithelial cuff."

Electron microscopic and autoradiographic studies have provided a clearer understanding of the nature of the dentoepithelial interface. Toward the end of enamel maturization, the plasmalemma of the ameloblasts in contact with the enamel surface develops *hemidesmosomes*. The space between the cell membrane and the enamel surface is occupied by a *basement lamina* joining the cells to the enamel surface. The hemidesmosomes and the basement lamina are believed to form the attachment apparatus joining the epithelium to the tooth. A similar attachment apparatus is also found between the external surface of the reduced enamel epithelium and the surrounding connective tissue. The basement lamina facing the tooth surface is referred to as the *internal basement lamina,* whereas the basement lamina facing the connective tissue is called the *external basement lamina.* The biologic mechanism that unites epithelial cells to the tooth surface may be properly described as the *epithelial attachment*. This term should not be used to describe an epithelium such as the junctional epithelium or reduced enamel epithelium. Its morphologically recognizable components consist of hemidesmosomes and the internal basement lamina.

Electron microscopic studies have revealed the presence of hemidesmosomes and a basement lamina at the interface of a large variety of epithelial membranes and the underlying connective tissue. It has been shown that epithelial cells grown in tissue culture are also capable of synthesizing such an apparatus against the surface on which they are cultured. It has also been demonstrated that junctional epithelial cells are able to attach to artificial endosseous tooth implants by means of hemidesmosomes and basement lamina. The basement lamina consists of carbohydrate-protein complex, the exact composition of which may vary in different sites of the body. The main protein component of basement laminae has been identified as a form of collagen peculiar to basement laminae. It is one of at least four different types of collagen, which have been defined previously. It is known as type IV collagen, whereas the collagen fibrils commonly observed in the connective tissue of the periodontium and in the organic matrix of bone, dentin, and cementum are composed of type I collagen. The basement lamina material serves as a glue that attaches the epithelial cell to the underlying surface. The strength of this attachment may be greater in the immediate vicinity of hemidesmosomes. Despite the presence of an epithelial attachment, the cells appear to be capable of moving in relation to the underlying stratum. An analogous situation exists when two glass plates are held together by a film of water. They cannot be readily pulled apart, although they slide easily over each other.

As the tooth erupts into the oral cavity, the enamel surface is covered with a layer of reduced enamel epithelium characterized by the presence of recognizable ameloblasts in contact with the enamel surface. Ultrastructurally, these cells may be identified by the presence of large numbers of mitochondria, invaginated nuclei frequently surrounded by pigmentlike granules in the perinuclear cytoplasm, and their attachment to the enamel surface via hemidesmosomes and the internal basement lamina. After eruption most of the reduced ameloblasts undergo a morphologic change, so that they begin to resemble squamous epithelial cells. Most of the mitochondria are lost, and the nucleus assumes a more ovoid shape. The cytoplasm, with its tonofibrils, Golgi region, and other cytoplasmic components, becomes indistinguishable from that of typical squamous epithelial cells. In addition to their cytoplasmic reorganization, these cells become flattened and indistinguishable from the epithelial cells found in the mature junctional epithelium. At the same time, the cells external to the transformed ameloblasts proliferate, thereby causing an increased thickening of the epithelium. These cells eventually displace the transformed ameloblasts and become in turn attached to the enamel surface through hemidesmosomes and internal basement lamina.

When reduced ameloblasts can no longer be recognized as such within the epithelium lining the enamel surface, the epithelium becomes known as the *junctional epithelium*. The morphology of the attachment apparatus of the junctional epithelium to the enamel surface is identical to that connecting the reduced enamel epithelium to the enamel. In erupted teeth an electron-dense dental cuticle may be found in close association with the junctional epithelium. When present, it is generally found between the enamel surface and the junctional epithelium (see Fig. 1-34). It may also appear as an intervening layer between the surface of afibrillar cementum patches and the junctional epithelium. Its origin and nature are not known at the present time. It is clear, however, that this material is not a keratinized layer, as originally suggested by Gottlieb.

The nature of the connection between the junctional epithelium and the tooth surface is such that mechanical stresses to this region result in tears within the epithelium rather than in a clean separation of the epithelium from the tooth surface. Because the cell turnover rate in this region is relatively high (the junctional epithelium replaces itself approximately every 7 days), minor tears can be readily repaired within that period of time. Cells in the junctional epithelium pass from the basal layer through the epithelial lining to become desquamated in the gingival sulcus.

In ideal situations the junctional epithelium may be attached to the tooth all the way from the most apical border of the enamel to a level approaching the gingival margin. In such cases the depth of the histologic sulcus may approach 0 mm. The clinical sulcus depth as determined with periodontal probing may considerably disagree with the histologic sulcus depth. This is apparently due to tearing of the epithelium by the periodontal probe. The depth of such tears may vary with such factors as width of the junctional epithelium, local inflammation, contour of the dentoepithelial junction, size of the probe, and direction and force applied to it. It should be clear at this point that the probeable depth of a sulcus and the histologic sulcus depth are two distinct entities that should not be equated with each other, particularly in the presence of an inflammatory infiltrate.

SULCULAR FLUID

The flow of tissue fluid through the sulcular epithelium and the possible biologic function of this fluid have been subjects of considerable research during the last 25 years. After intravenous injection or oral administration of fluorescein, which labels plasma proteins, Brill and Björn (1959) and Brill and Brönnestam (1960) recovered the dye at the orifice of the gingival sulci. The fluid was collected on filter paper strips that were either inserted into the sulci or adapted to bridge the orifice of the facial aspect of the gingival sulci (Figs. 1-35, 1-36, and 1-37). The results indicated that a fluid containing small molecules might pass from the subepithelial tissues into the gingival crevice and out into the oral cavity. Other epithelial surfaces of the mouth did not allow the passage of tissue fluid.

Immunoelectrophoretic analyses have disclosed that at least seven different plasma proteins are present in this fluid. Both alpha-1 and alpha-2 globulins, as well as beta and gamma globulins and fibronectin, have been identified.

A series of similar experiments have tended to show that the flow of fluid has an intimate relationship with capillary permeability and that it passes from the subepithelial connective tissues between or through the cells of the junctional epithelium (Brill and Brönnestam, 1960).

The amount of fluid from normal gingivae is minimal. It increases after mechanical stimulation of the gingivae or after intravenous injection of histamine. If bacteria or other particulate materials are introduced into the sulcus, they are expelled with the fluid within minutes, provided that they are not mechanically retained. Also, in these instances the flow of fluid is increased. The suggestion has been made that the flushing effect that is produced in this way may form an important part of the local defense mechanism, since the outward flow can normally prevent the penetration of foreign particulate matter into the gingival sulcus.

In gingival inflammation the rate of outward flow is markedly increased. Obviously this fluid must be considered not simply as a filtrate from tissues with normal metabolism, but as an inflammatory exudate. Because of the almost invariable presence of an inflammatory reaction at the gingival margin and the regular finding of neutrophilic leukocytes in the sulcular fluid, it has been difficult to accept the presence of sulcular fluid as part of the normal, noninflamed gingiva. In fact, studies have shown that strictly normal human gingiva does not exhibit a flow of fluid. Nor does mechanical stimulation of the periodontium produce a flow of fluid from normal sulci. Inflamed gingiva, on the other hand, regularly shows the presence of fluid, the amount of which varies with the severity of the inflammation. These results tend to show that the fluid that oozes out between the gingiva and the tooth is closely related to tissue changes in the area.

This relationship has been confirmed in a longitudinal study of the development of gingivitis (Fig. 1-38). During this experiment, gingivae that at the start did not exhibit any flow of fluid began to do so as soon as increased bac-

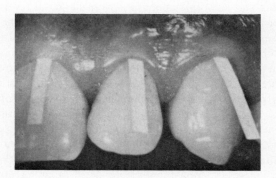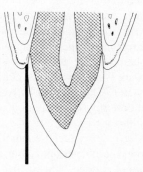

Fig. 1-35. Intrasulcular sampling of exudate. Note that strip is placed at entrance of sulcus. (From Löe H and Holm-Pedersen P: Periodontics 3:171, 1965.)

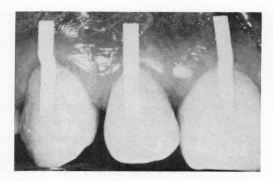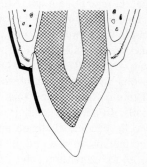

Fig. 1-36. Extrasulcular sampling method. (From Löe H and Holm-Pedersen P: Periodontics 3:171, 1965.)

terial activity developed in the region. The amount of fluid increased steadily throughout the experimental period, and maximal flow occurred shortly before clinically observable gingivitis developed. As soon as gingival inflammation lessened as a result of local treatment, a corresponding decrease in the flow of fluid occurred. Finally, a few days after gingival inflammation had resolved, the flow of fluid ceased (Löe and Holm-Pedersen, 1965).

Based on the observations that (1) inflammatory cells are regularly present in sulcular fluid, (2) the chemical composition is different from tissue fluid, and (3) the passage of fluid is closely related to the area of inflammation, the sulcular fluid should be considered an inflammatory exudate rather than a physiologic secretion. The relatively narrow intercellular spaces of the sulcular epithelium,

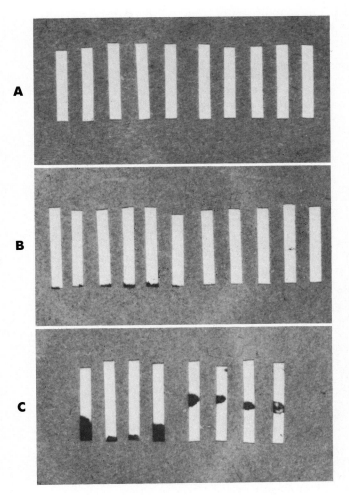

Fig. 1-37. Strips of filter paper used for collecting gingival exudate. Strips on left half of illustrations were used to collect intrasulcular samples. Treating strips with ninhydrine shows absence of fluid in teeth with clinically normal gingiva, **A,** traces or small amounts of exudate in teeth with slightly inflamed gingiva, **B,** and increased amount of exudate in teeth with moderate gingival inflammation, **C.** (From Löe H and Holm-Pedersen P: Periodontics 3:171, 1965.)

which are generally free of leukocytes, and the tendency demonstrated by the surface cells toward keratinization suggest that the coronal portion of the sulcus lined by sulcular epithelium is relatively more impermeable to the passage of sulcular fluid or leukocytes than the apical portion lined by junctional epithelium.

The finding that the flow of fluid regularly starts before structural changes can be ascertained at the clinical level and persists some time after clinical inflammation has subsided indicates that exudation is discernible before gingival inflammation can be clinically assessed. It is possible, therefore, that the absence or presence of fluid may represent the best available clinical means of establishing the distinction between normal and subclinically inflamed gingivae.

DEFENSE MECHANISMS OF GINGIVA

Recent periodontal research has furnished substantial evidence that bacterial irritation is essential for the development and maintenance of marginal periodontal inflammation. As in any other infection, the clinical manifestations of the disease are dependent on the aggressive properties of the microorganisms and the capability of the host to withstand the aggression.

Although particulate material may not find ready ingress into the sulcular and junctional epithelia, it is likely that soluble products originating in the gingival sulcus can diffuse into the connective tissue via the junctional epithelium. The role played by the epithelium in protecting the underlying connective tissue from damaging substances originating in the oral cavity appears to be less dependent on the so-called seal at the dentoepithelial junction (epithelial attachment) than on the permeability of the junctional epithelium (Fig. 1-39). Although bacterial plaque may extend to the very bottom of the gingival sulcus, individual microorganisms may not necessarily be able to penetrate the epithelial barrier. However, their soluble products may enter the connective tissue via the large intercellular spaces of the junctional epithelium and give rise to an inflammatory response in the region immediately subjacent to the permeable portion of the junctional epithelium. This would explain the localization of the earliest inflammatory lesion in close proximity to the junctional epithelium (Schroeder and Listgarten, 1971).

Besides structural protection, the local defense against exogenous attack generally rests on mechanical, chemical, and cellular mechanisms. The efficacy of the mechanical factor is probably best illustrated by the lubricating action of saliva and the continuous desquamation of superficial epithelial cells, which prevent bacteria from settling en masse on the oral mucosa. The cleansing effect of the saliva on the gingival area seems rather insignificant. Recent experiments actually indicate that an effective self-cleansing of the marginal parts of human teeth does not occur, not even during prolonged mastication of a diet

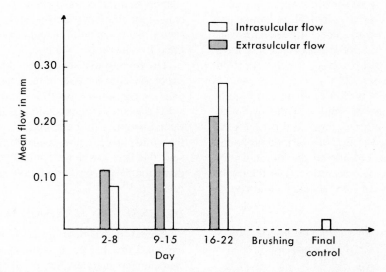

Fig. 1-38. Mean flow of gingival exudate of 15 teeth after withdrawal of all oral hygiene measures in eight individuals. Teeth showed no flow at start of experiment. During period of no cleansing, all teeth developed flow of exudate, amount of which increased throughout experimental period. As soon as tooth cleansing was reintroduced, flow of fluid decreased and finally disappeared. (From Löe H and Holm-Pedersen P: Periodontics 3:171, 1965.)

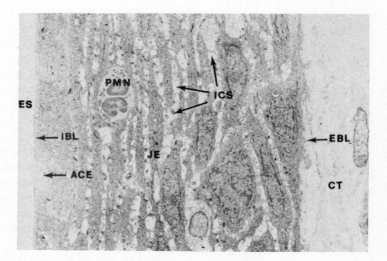

Fig. 1-39. Junctional epithelium *(JE)*. Intercellular spaces *(ICS)* are wider than in normal gingival epithelium and may contain polymorphonuclear leukocytes *(PMN)*, particularly in close proximity to sulcus. Cells are attached to each other by relatively few desmosomes. Sulcular exudate probably percolates through intercellular spaces rather than through internal basement lamina *(IBL)*, joining epithelium to tooth surface. *ACE,* Afibrillar cementum island; *ES,* enamel space; *EBL,* external basement lamina; *CT,* gingival connective tissue. (× 2000.) (From Schroeder HE and Listgarten MA: In Wolsky A, editor: Monographs in developmental biology, vol 2, Fine structure of the developing epithelial attachment of human teeth, Basel, Switzerland, 1971, S Karger.)

consisting of hard food. Some cleansing effect has been ascribed to the sulcular fluid inasmuch as it has been shown that the fluid is able to expel bacteria and particles that have gained entrance into the sulcus. From this it has been inferred that the fluid to some extent may also resist the introduction of foreign material into the gingival sulcus (Löe et al., 1965).

The presence of immunoglobulins in the sulcular fluid may indicate that it possesses antibacterial properties. It has also been demonstrated that polymorphonuclear leukocytes (PMNs) are consistently found in this fluid. There can be little doubt about the phagocytic properties of these cells as long as they are lodged in the epithelium or the connective tissue. However, since microorganisms are frequently deposited in comparatively large numbers outside the gingival tissues on the tooth or gingival surface, phagocytosis at this site may not be clinically significant.

It is likely that the most important defense mechanism of the dentoepithelial junction resides in the inflammatory reaction that manifests itself initially as gingivitis. It remains to be shown whether the resulting sulcular exudate and the leukocytes it contains possess any immunologic or phagocytic properties that may be of significance in this process. Variations in the protective efficacy of the inflammatory process and the composition of the microbial flora may be the chief causes of differences in susceptibility to periodontal disease.

APICAL SHIFT OF THE DENTOGINGIVAL JUNCTION

When the tooth has reached the occlusal plane, the gingival sulcus is located approximately over the gingival third of the crown. The junctional epithelium extends from this point apically to the region of the cervix. Apical to this point and along the entire circumference of the root, the Sharpey fibers anchored into the cementum attach the tooth to the bone. This is the ideal arrangement of the periodontium.

Many investigators, starting with Gottlieb (1921, 1943), hold that this state of affairs is merely a transitional stage and that the epithelium, as age progresses, is apt to proliferate in an apical direction. In so doing, it establishes a new firm union (epithelial attachment) with the cementum surface. This apical shift of the dentogingival junction has been termed *passive eruption*. Passive eruption is thought to continue at a varying rate throughout life.

The apical shift of the bottom of the gingival sulcus may be accompanied by an increase in sulcus depth. In other instances a shallow sulcus may remain, in which case a recession of the marginal gingiva has taken place concomitantly with the downgrowth of the epithelium. Why marginal atrophy occurs in some instances, whereas in others deepening of the sulcus takes place, has not been explained. In any event, downgrowth of the sulcular epithelium below the CEJ, with or without gingival recession,

represents a significant change in the periodontium that, from a functional point of view, results in a loss of fibrous attachment and functional support of the teeth.

Gottlieb (1943) and others have considered passive eruption as a physiologic process that is continuous throughout life at a rate corresponding to the occlusal movement of the teeth in compensation for attrition. The latter process is known as *active eruption*. Active and passive eruptions have been thought to occur simultaneously; the purpose of passive eruption is to keep the clinical crown at an adequate length.

Basically, any apical proliferation of cells of the junctional epithelium along the cementum surface presupposes a breakdown of the uppermost Sharpey's fibers. According to Gottlieb, loss of fiber attachment occurs as a result of devitalization of the cementum. His belief was that attached fibers lived and functioned for a certain length of time and then died, leaving behind a devitalized cementum. The vitality of the cementum was considered to be a matter of age of the tissue. The evidence to support this view has never been substantiated.

The fate of the fiber attachment seems to be entirely dependent on the state of the supraalveolar connective tissue. A simple degeneration of its fibers as part of a physiologic process has not been demonstrated and seems very unlikely. On the other hand, collagen from any location in the body has a certain turnover (i.e., collagen fibrils and fibers are dissolved and replaced by new ones at corresponding rates). The turnover of periodontal collagen does not differ in any respect from similar collagen elsewhere in the body. These processes are physiologic processes that aim at the maintenance of tissue, and they cannot be held responsible for the permanent destruction of periodontal fibers.

It has been suggested that a permanent dissolution of the collagen fibers may be brought about by an enzymatic action of the epithelial cells.

The cells have been shown to synthesize both a type IV collagenase (or gelatinase) and a type I collagenase. Fibroblasts also may contribute specific proteases. However, the major contribution of neutral protease are the PMNs.

Variations of specific dietary components do not seem to cause downgrowth of sulcular epithelium. Not even in vitamin C deficiency, where connective tissue metabolism is seriously altered, are these fibers destroyed to the extent that a downgrowth of epithelium can take place.

The concept of passive eruption as a physiologic process seems to derive mainly from microscopic examination of human teeth of different ages, in which it is regularly seen that the bottoms of sulci in the teeth of adults are situated at varying levels below the CEJ. In view of the fact that nearly all civilized adult patients have or have had a history of periodontal tissue inflammation, the use of specimens without a known history may be of doubtful value as a basis for investigating this problem.

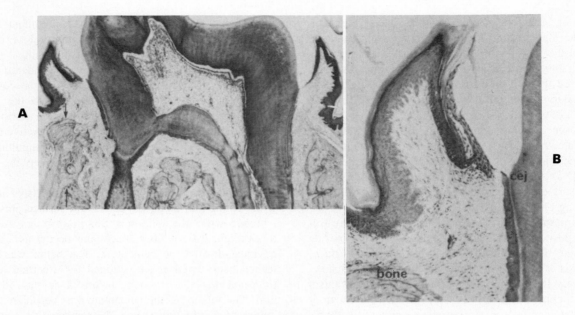

Fig. 1-40. Histologic section of mandibular rat molar after extraction of corresponding maxillary molars, allowing lower molars to move in occlusal direction. **A,** Injections with 1% lead acetate at days 0, 7, 33, and 62 show that new bone (*between arrows*) has been laid down at alveolar crest. **B,** Although tooth has moved occlusally, bottom of sulcus is still located at CEJ. (From Löe H: Unpublished data.)

The most obvious explanation for apical migration of the cells of the sulcular epithelium is that the uppermost fibers have been destroyed as a result of gingival inflammation. Indeed, histologic preparations of teeth may be encountered where the epithelium is found below the CEJ and where histologic signs of inflammation are absent. However, appearances like these do not exclude the presence of inflammatory reactions at the moment of dissolution of the fibers and apical migration of the epithelium. Histologic sections represent static pictures of the morphologic relationship at a particular moment in time. Unless the specimens are part of an experimental series, such preparations do not usually demonstrate the events that lead up to the situation that exists at the moment of examination.

Experimental results have shown that active eruption may take place without any movement of the junctional epithelium below the neck of the tooth (Figs. 1-40 and 1-41) (Karring et al., 1975). Several teeth of monkeys were ground out of occlusion so that approximately 2 mm separated the opposing teeth. In the course of 9 months, occlusal movement brought these teeth into occlusion again. New cementum and bone formed to compensate for the eruption. The most apical extension of the junctional epithelium was still located at the cervix, and the relationship between this and the margin of the alveolar bone was normal as a result of bone tissue at the alveolar margin.

In other words, occlusal movement of teeth does not necessarily imply an apical shift of the dentogingival junction. The observation that in the dentition of Eskimos the gingival margin usually covers the cervical border of the enamel even in the presence of extreme occlusal wear corroborates these experimental findings. Similar conditions may also be found in individuals who have escaped periodontal disease (Fig. 1-42).

Therefore the apical shift of the dentogingival junction, or passive eruption, does not appear to be a physiologic process. Migration of the junctional epithelium onto root cementum is possible only after dissolution of the uppermost Sharpey's fibers. This destruction is effected at the stage where the marginal inflammation has reached into the supraalveolar connective tissue. The clinical picture is characterized by recession of the gingival margin and a shallow gingival sulcus or by retention of the original level of the gingiva and a deepening of the sulcus.

It should be noted, however, that in either case the process can be arrested. If good oral hygiene is established, a normal junctional epithelium can reform at the existing level on the root surface in the same relationship that existed originally over the enamel.

CLINICAL CRITERIA OF NORMAL GINGIVA

It is widely held that clinically normal gingiva always exhibits a low degree of chronic inflammation and that the border between normal and pathologically changed gingiva is rather vague. Consequently, the term *clinically healthy*

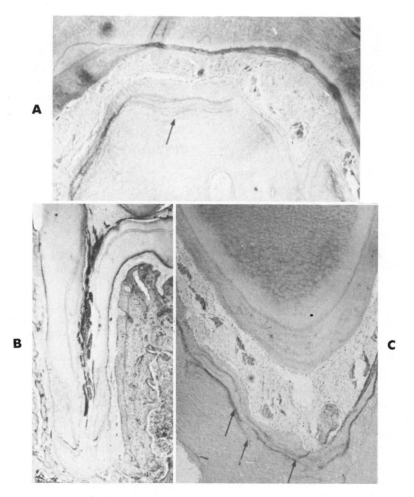

Fig. 1-41. Lower rat molar after extraction of corresponding teeth of upper jaw. Appositional lines in bone *(arrows)* are found at bifurcation area, **A,** at apical area, **C,** and in pulp cavity, **B,** according to labeling with lead acetate during experimental period. (From Löe H: Unpublished data.)

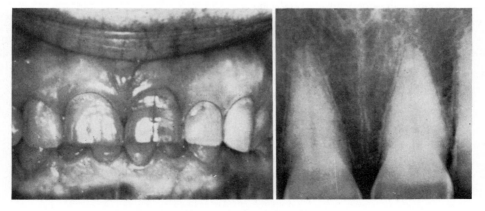

Fig. 1-42. Anterior teeth of a 78-year-old woman without periodontal disease. Although there is a great deal of occlusal wear, there is no recession of gingival margin or reduction in height of alveolar crest (i.e., passive eruption has not occurred beyond cervix of teeth).

gingiva appears to be a highly arbitrary concept, and what appears to be normal gingiva to one examiner may not fulfill the requirements of another.

Recent experimental results indicate, however, that a strictly healthy gingiva at the clinical level may also show absence of inflammation when examined in microscopic preparations (Schroeder, 1973). In such specimens the sulcular epithelium is almost entirely free of inflammatory cells, and the underlying connective tissue shows no leukocytes or other blood cells in an extravascular location. To achieve freedom of gingival inflammation such as this, an extremely regimented program of oral hygiene must be instituted. It is of interest to note that germ-free beagles raised in the complete absence of bacteria but not subject to any regimen of oral hygiene may demonstrate the presence of PMNs in junctional epithelium and the presence of lymphocytes and plasma cells in the underlying connective tissue.

The clinical counterpart to this state of induced normality is a gingiva that complies with the qualitative criteria of healthy gingiva as to color, surface, form, consistency, and gingival sulcus.

Color.   The color of healthy gingiva is usually pale pink. This pale appearance as compared with that of the redder oral mucosa is due to the thickness and keratinized state of the surface epithelium. The overall color may be modified by the presence of pigmentation in persons of dark complexion and by the blood flow through the tissues.

Surface.   The surface of dried gingiva should be matt. Ordinarily the gingiva presents an uneven, stippled surface that resembles an orange peel. However, the degree of stippling may vary considerably within the normal range.

Form.   The form of the gingiva is dependent on the shape and size of the interdental areas, which again may depend on the shape and position of the teeth. The tip of the gingival papilla is the most incisally or occlusally located part of the gingiva. The gingival margin should be thin. The gingiva may terminate against the tooth in a knife-edged fashion, although in most human teeth the gingival margin is rounded.

Consistency.   On palpation with a blunt instrument, the gingiva should be firm. The gingiva is resilient and tightly bound to the underlying hard tissues. The marginal gingiva, although slightly movable, should be closely adapted to the tooth surface.

Gingival sulcus.   The probing depth of the gingival sulcus may vary from 1 to 3 mm. Probing with a blunt probe should not cause bleeding. Normal gingiva exhibits no detectable flow of sulcular fluid.

REFERENCES

Ainamo J and Löe H: Anatomical characteristics of gingiva. I. A clinical and microscopic study of the free and attached gingiva, J Periodontol 37:5, 1966.

Becks HV: Normal and pathologic pocket formation, J Am Dent Assoc 16:2167, 1929.

Brill M and Björn H: Passage of tissue fluid into human gingival pockets, Acta Odontol Scand 17:11, 1959.

Brill N and Brönnestam R: Immuno-electrophoretic study of tissue fluid from gingival pockets, Acta Odontol Scand 18:95,1960.

Egelberg J: Blood vessels of the dento-gingival junction, J Periodontol 1:163, 1966.

Glavind L and Löe H: Capillary microscopy of the gingiva in pregnant and nonpregnant individuals, J Periodont Res 2:74, 1967.

Gottlieb B: Aetiologie und Prophylaxe der Zahne, Dtsch Msclr Stomatol 39:142, 1921.

Gottlieb B: Histologic consideration of the supporting tissues of the teeth, J Am Dent Assoc 30:1872, 1943.

Karring T, Lang NP, and Löe H: The role of gingival connective tissue in determining epithelial differentiation, J Periodont Res 10:1, 1975.

Karring T and Löe H: Blood supply to the periodontium, J Periodont Res 2:74, 1967.

Löe H: Periodontal changes in pregnancy, J Periodontol 36:209, 1965.

Löe H and Holm-Pedersen P: Absence and presence of fluid from normal and inflamed gingiva, Periodontics 3:171, 1965.

Löe H and Karring T: The three dimensional morphology of the epithelium−connective tissue interface of the gingiva as related to age and sex, Scand J Dent Res 79:315, 1971.

Löe H, Theilade E, and Jensen SB: Experimental gingivitis in man, J Periodontol 36:177, 1965.

Page R et al: Collagen fiber bundles of the normal marginal gingiva, Arch Oral Biol 19:1039, 1974.

Schroeder HE: Transmigration and infiltration of leukocytes in human junctional epithelium, Helv Odontol Acta 17:16, 1973.

Schroeder HE and Listgarten MA: Fine structure of the developing epithelial attachment of human teeth. In Wolsky A, editor: Monographs in developmental biology, vol 2, Basel, Switzerland, 1971, S Karger.

Schroeder HE and Theilade J: Electron microscopy of normal human gingival epithelium, J Periodont Res 1:95, 1966.

Waerhaug J: Current concepts concerning gingival anatomy: the dynamic epithelial cuff, Dent Clin North Am, p 715, Nov 1960.

Chapter 2

THE PERIODONTAL ATTACHMENT APPARATUS
Structure, function, and chemistry

Victor P. Terranova
Henry M. Goldman
Max A. Listgarten

Cementum
    Root cementum
    Acellular cementum
    Cellular cementum
Alveolar process
    Functional relationship of alveolar and supporting bone
    Metabolism of alveolar bone
    Microscopic appearance
    Neural supply
Periodontal ligament
Chemistry of the periodontal tissues
    Extracellular matrices
    Polypeptide growth factors
    Regenerative capacity
    Modulation of function

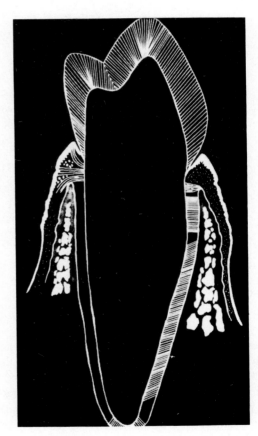

Fig. 2-1. Buccolingual aspect of periodontium: gingiva, alveolar process, and dentoalveolar unit (cementum, periodontal ligament, bone). Fibers of periodontal ligament are divided into four groups: alveolar crestal, horizontal, oblique, and apical. Difference in epithelium covering gingiva in attached, keratinized zone from epithelium of alveolar mucosa should be noted. Marginal fiber apparatus is also depicted.

The periodontal ligament, cementum, and alveolar bone constitute the periodontal attachment appartus, which anchors the tooth into the jaws. The mode of attachment of the tooth to the alveolus consists of numerous bundles of collagenous tissues (principal fibers) arranged in groups, which are separated by loose connective tissue containing blood vessels, lymph vessels, and nerves. This ligament functions as the investing and supportive mechanism for the tooth. It is termed the *periodontal ligament* (Fig. 2-1). The dentoalveolar unit comprises the *cementum*, the *periodontal ligament*, and the *alveolar bone*. The periodontal

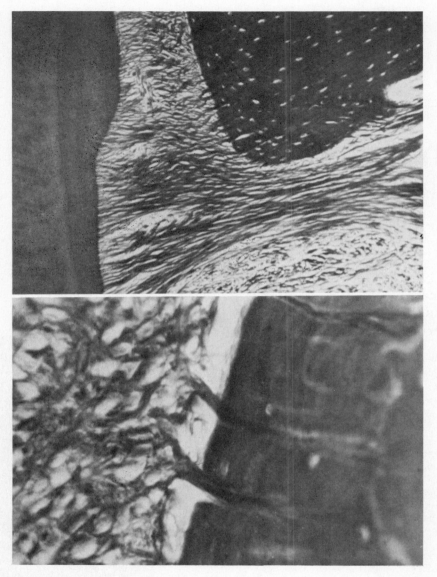

Fig. 2-2. Photomicrograph of mesiodistal section of alveolar crest, periodontal ligament, and transseptal fibers. High power shows Sharpey's fibers entering alveolar bone.

ligament is the tissue that surrounds the roots of the tooth and attaches it to the bony alveolus. Cementum is the hard bonelike tissue covering the anatomic roots of the teeth. The *alveolar bone proper* is a plate of compact bone, the radiographic image of which is termed *lamina dura*.

The main function of the dentoalveolar unit is supportive, but it also has formative, nutritive, and sensory roles. The supportive function consists of maintaining and retaining the teeth. The formative function is necessary for the replacement of tissues: cementum, periodontal ligament, and alveolar bone. Three specialized cells are associated with this function: *cementoblasts, fibroblasts,* and *osteoblasts*. The nutritive and sensory functions are accomplished by the blood vessels and nerves, respectively. Thus the attachment apparatus serves as a suspensory mechanism for the tooth, as a pericementum for the maintenance of the root covering, and as periosteum for the alveolar bone (Figs. 2-2 and 2-3).

CEMENTUM
Root cementum

Cementum is a hard tissue whose intercellular substance is calcified. It is arranged in layers around the tooth root. There are two types of root cementum: *acellular* and *cellular*. The acellular type is clear and structureless, being formed by cementoblasts that deposit the substance but do

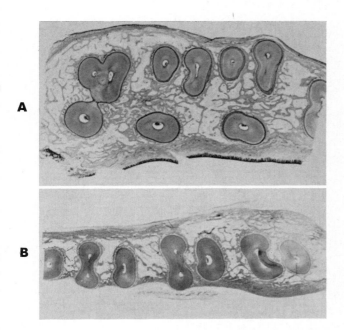

A

B

Fig. 2-3. Cross section of molar region of maxilla and mandible. **A,** Roots of molars surrounded by bone. Note contour of roots, formation of alveolar bone, and supporting bone. **B,** Roots of mandibular molars. Alveolar bone surrounding these roots is evident, and character of supporting bone is easily distinguished. These photomicrographs illustrate topography of attachment apparatus around molars.

not become embedded in it, as is the case when the cellular type is formed. During tooth formation, as the cementum is formed, collagen fibers become incorporated in it. These are known as Sharpey's fibers (Fig. 2-2). Acellular cementum always covers the cervical portion of the root, extending at times over almost all of the root except for the apical portion where cellular cementum is seen (Fig. 2-4). Cellular cementum is bonelike in character. It may later form over the acellular type. Cementocytes are found within *lacunae*. Cementum contains fewer embedded cells and fewer anastomosing canaliculi than bone tissue. It is devoid of vascular elements. Cementocyte processes anastomose with one another. Cementocytes have the same relationship to the matrix of the cementum as osteocytes have to bone. Unlike bone, cementum does not remodel, although it may continue to grow by apposition of new layers. Evidence of apposition can be determined by darkly staining lines in sections stained with hematoxylin and eosin. These lines represent periods of nonformation. However, cemental apposition is slow, since teeth in later adult life normally show only relatively few appositional layers. Electron microscopic studies of specimens from young and old mice have suggested that adult cementum formation could be described as a slow appositional mineralization of the periodontal ligament. It must be stressed, however, that changes in function will have a great influence on the activity of cemental growth. Cementoblasts lining the root surface may exhibit the cytology of cells actively synthesizing protein or may take on the appearance of resting cells.

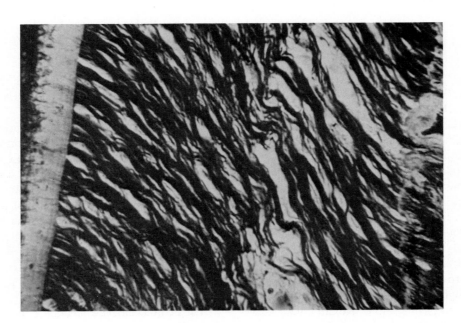

Fig. 2-4. Photomicrograph of periodontal ligament, bone, and acellular cementum. Note homogeneous appearance of acellular cementum.

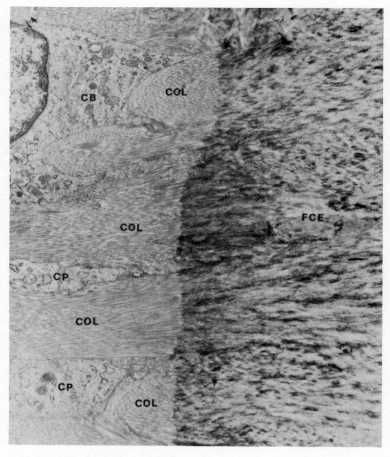

Fig. 2-5. Junction between acellular cementum *(FCE)* and periodontal ligament in which cementoblastic processes *(CP)* and collagen fiber bundles *(COL)* are visible. Collagen fiber bundles lose their identity as individual fibers after incorporation into cementum. *CB,* Cementoblast. (×5000.) (From Listgarten, M: Unpublished data, 1968.)

Acellular cementum

Acellular cementum forms a thin layer covering the dentin surface, the thickness of which varies from 20 to 50 μm near the cervix to 150 to 200 μm near the apex. In transmitted light it exhibits numerous appositional lines. In microradiographs the innermost zone nearest the dentin appears less well mineralized than the remaining cementum. Recent studies by microradiography and electron microscopy have confirmed that acellular cementum is more highly calcified than cellular cementum. Electron microscopically, the acellular cementum consists of densely packed collagen fibrils with the typical collagen bands in register between adjacent fibrils. The fibrils are continuous with the collagen fibrils of the periodontal ligament (Figs. 2-5 and 2-6). Although the periodontal ligament consists of collagen fibrils running in distinct bundles, the latter frequently lose their identity as individual bundles when they become incorporated into the acellular cementum

covering the coronal part of the root. This is particularly evident in the cementum just beneath the cervix (see Fig. 2-2).

In mineralized preparations the normal banding of the collagen fibrils is obscured by the densely packed crystals of apatite that form the mineral phase of cementum (see Fig. 2-3). The mineral component of cementum is an apatite that is deposited in the form of thin crystals (maximum size is 40 × 20 × 2 nm); the long axis is generally parallel to the collagen fibrils. The crystals at the cementum surface tend to form small projections along the insertion of individual collagen fibrils from the periodontal ligament. Near the dentinocemental junction some fibril bundles are incompletely mineralized, thereby making this region more radiolucent.

The dentinocemental junction may be identified by the different orientation and organization of the collagen fibrils. Whereas the collagen fibrils in dentin are arranged

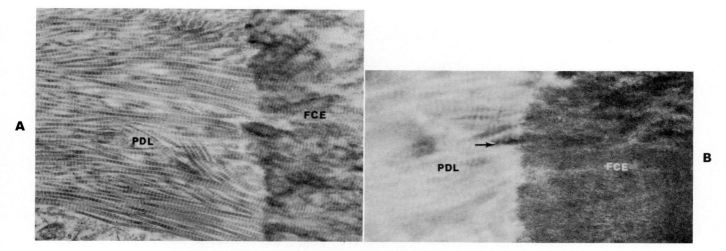

Fig. 2-6. Junction between collagen fibrils of periodontal ligament *(PDL)* and cementum *(FCE)*. **A,** Demineralized specimen. Note incorporation of periodontal ligament collagen into cementum without any alteration of natural periodicity of collagen fibrils. **B,** Mineralized specimen. Banding of collagen fibrils in cementum is obliterated by crystals of apatite. Arrow indicates mineralized portion of a single fibril that forms a small spur extending into periodontal ligament. (**A** ×16,500; **B** ×28,000.) (From Listgarten M: Unpublished data, 1968.)

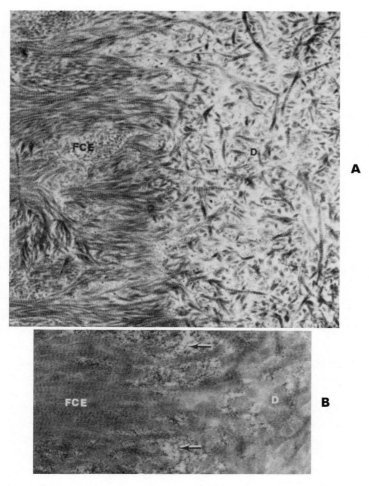

Fig. 2-7. A, Dentinocemental junction can be recognized by haphazard arrangement of collagen fibrils in dentin *(D)* bordering on relatively parallel bundles of collagen fibrils in cementum *(FCE)*. **B,** Deposits of granular, interfibrillar matrix *(arrows)* occur at junction of cementum *(FCE)* and dentin *(D)*. (**A** ×10,500; **B** ×20,000.) (From Listgarten M: Unpublished data, 1968.)

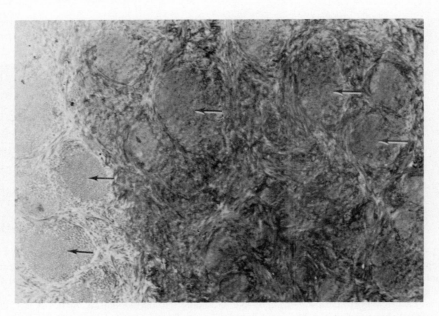

Fig. 2-8. Apical root cementum. Note that in this tangential section collagen fiber bundles *(arrows)* retain their individual organization in periodontal ligament as well as in cementum. (×5700.) (From Listgarten M: Unpublished data, 1970.)

haphazardly, with each fibril running an independent course, in acellular cementum the fibrils generally run in the same direction and more or less perpendicular to the cementum surface (Fig. 2-7).

The organic matrix of cementum consists of the collagenous component already described and an interfibrillar component that at the ultrastructural level appears finely granular. This material probably represents the mucoprotein portion of the organic matrix. It is more readily demonstrable near the dentinocemental junction.

Cellular cementum

Cellular cementum appears less regularly organized than its acellular counterpart. It may reach a thickness of 1 to several millimeters, the thickness increasing with age. The more rapid rate of formation of cellular cementum probably explains the incorporation of cementum-forming cells into typical lacunae from which canaliculi-containing cellular processes radiate through the adjacent calcified matrix. Cementocytes are usually absent from the deeper portions of the cellular cementum. With transmitted light appositional lines can also be noted in cellular cementum.

Electron microscopically the organic and inorganic components appear similar to those observed in acellular cementum. Some differences exist, however, in their organization.

Usually the periodontal fiber bundles continue within the cementum as well-defined Sharpey's fibers (Figs. 2-8 and 2-9). Although their orientation is generally perpendicular to the cementum surface, some bundles of fibers run in different directions. The central core of Sharpey's fibers may be incompletely mineralized. However, the relationship of the apatite crystals to individual collagen fibrils remains the same.

ALVEOLAR PROCESS

The tissue elements of the alveolar process are no different from those of bone elsewhere. The alveolar bone portion of the alveolar process lines the sockets into which the roots of the teeth fit. It is thin, compact bone that is pierced by many small openings through which blood vessels, lymphatics, and nerve fibers pass. The alveolar bone fuses with the cortical plates of the labial and lingual sides at the crest of the alveolar process. The alveolar bone contains the embedded ends of the connective tissue fibers of the periodontal membrane (Sharpey's fibers; Figs. 2-10 and 2-11). The cancellous portion of the process occupies the area between the cortical plates and the alveolar bone. It is continuous with the spongiosa of the body of the jaws. The spongiosa occupies most of the interdental septum but a relatively small portion of the labial or lingual plate. In these areas the incisal region has less spongiosa than it has in the molar areas. The architectural arrangement of the trabeculae and their characteristics are related to the demands of function.

Bone tissue is continually undergoing change. Characteristically, bone apposition and resorption may occur simultaneously on neighboring surfaces. In the alveolar bone, adjacent lamellae can be identified by the presence of *cementing lines*. When a bony surface is inactive for a

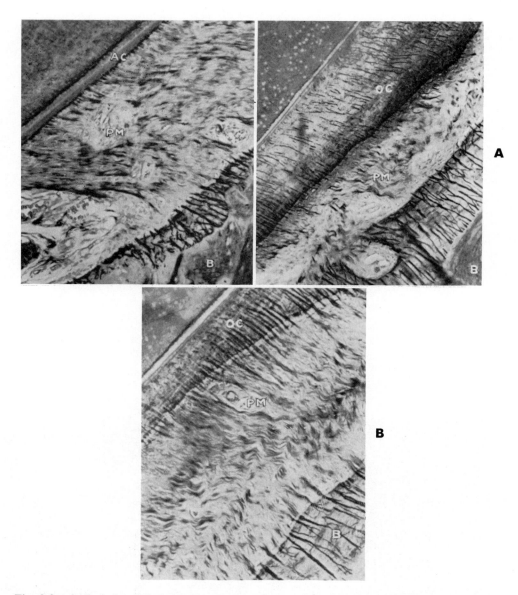

Fig. 2-9. A, Periodontal ligament fibers connected to acellular cementum *(AC) (left photomicrograph).* Sharpey's fibers are seen in osteocementum *(OC)* and bone *(B) (right photomicrograph).* **B,** Sharpey's fibers in osteocementum and bone with wavy fibers of periodontal ligament (dog material). *PM,* Periodontal ligament.

period of time, a basophilic line forms. These lines are seen over sections where apposition or resorptive phases have occurred previously. If resorption was followed by apposition, the line is known as a *reversal line* and thus reveals the changes that have taken place previously.

Thus bone is a relatively active tissue, whereas cementum is relatively inactive. This difference can easily be seen microscopically in tissues of adult individuals. Very little apposition of cementum is seen, whereas a definite remodeling of the alveolar bone is apparent. This observation is of great significance, since the periodontal ligament

unites these tissues. It can be reasoned, therefore, that there is need for some mechanism to allow for the independent behavior of these two hard tissues. This is discussed later in the chapter.

Bone is a highly specialized mesodermal tissue, consisting of organic matrix and inorganic matter. The matrix is composed of a network of osteocytes and extracellular matrix material. The inorganic portion consists chiefly of calcium, phosphate, and carbonate in the form of apatite crystals. Bone is first laid down as an open framework of spongy bone, some of which becomes compact later on.

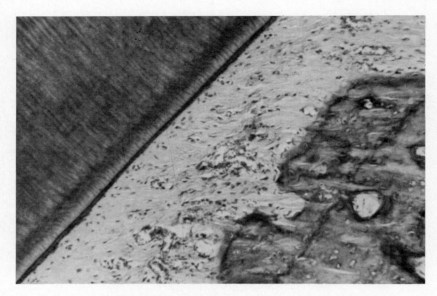

Fig. 2-10. Photomicrograph of periodontal ligament. Root is covered with a thin layer of cementum; a cementoblastic layer is evident. Note also that an osteoblastic layer is present, denoting bone formation. These findings are consistent with formative aspects of dentoalveolar unit and result from slight tension on tooth.

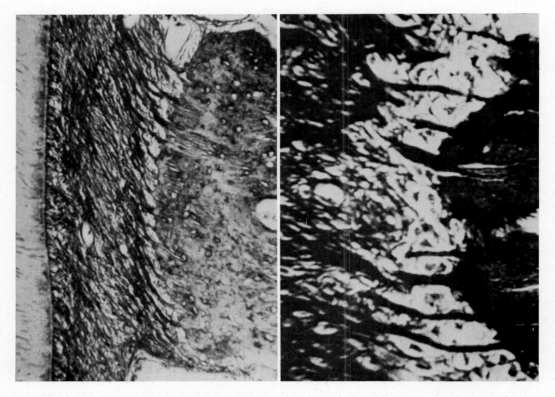

Fig. 2-11. Low- and high-power photomicrographs of a periodontal ligament, showing an active osteoblastic layer adjacent to bone. High-power view is silver stained. Note Sharpey's fibers. There is active bone formation; yet cementum is thin and no cementoid can be observed.

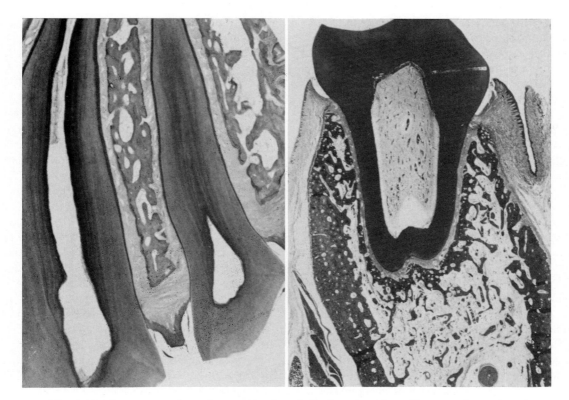

Fig. 2-12. Low-power photomicrographs of mesiodistal section of maxillary anterior teeth and buccolingual section of a mandibular molar (dog). Pictured are gingiva, alveolus, and periodontal ligament. Note openings to periodontal ligament from bone marrow.

The spaces in the spongiosa are termed *marrow spaces.* Under normal conditions bone is constantly subject to simultaneous tissue growth and resorption, which are finely coordinated. Microscopically, bone surfaces may exhibit areas of bone apposition, areas where bone is undergoing resorption, and other areas where the status quo is being maintained. Under normal conditions, as in the other portions of the skeleton, the physiologic status of the bone is dependent on age and function.

Ritchey and Orban (1953) have pointed out that in the absence of periodontal disease the configuration of the crest of the interdental alveolar septum is determined by the relative position of the adjacent cementoenamel junctions (CEJs) and also that the width of the interdental alveolar bone is determined by the tooth form present. Relatively flat approximal tooth surfaces call for narrow septa, whereas in the presence of extremely convex tooth surfaces wide interdental septa with flat crests are found.

Alveolar bone is deposited next to the periodontal ligament and is itself supported by supporting bone. One or more large arteries, veins, and nerve bundles run through the interradicular bony process, and branches from them enter the periodontal ligament through the many openings in the cribriform plates (Fig. 2-12).

Functional relationship of alveolar and supporting bone

The bone housing the tooth is dependent on the function exerted on the tooth to maintain its structure. The changes in the supporting bone and in the periodontal ligament when stress to the teeth is withdrawn, such as when antagonists are lost, attest to the dependence of these tissues on functional stimulation. In fact, after long-standing loss of function, changes in the alveolar bone may be noted. In jaws in which the teeth are subjected to intense stress, it is usual to find the spongy or supporting bone composed of thicker and more numerous trabeculae. Although bone tissue is dependent on function for the maintenance and arrangement of the trabeculae, other factors may be involved (e.g., disturbances in bone metabolism). Such an experiment has been described by Anderson et al. (1929). They have shown that the bony changes around the mandibular molars in rats after the extraction of the maxillary molars are more pronounced in rats on a low-salt diet.

Metabolism of alveolar bone

Of interest is the rate of metabolism of the alveolar bone in contrast to other bone tissue elsewhere. Rogers and Weidman (1951) have conducted a metabolic study involving the use of tracer elements with respect to the isotopes of calcium, iodine, nitrogen, and phosphorus. They have shown that not only do individual animals appear to exhibit variations in the rate of skeletal metabolism, but also that different species have different rates. It was found that the rate of metabolism of mandibular alveolar bone is slower than that of metaphyseal bone but more rapid than that of diaphyseal bone. This seems to be true for all the animals examined. Studies that have been made of dogs with renal osteodystrophy show marked changes in the alveolar and supporting bone in contrast to changes elsewhere in the skeleton. The more rapid rate of metabolism of bone tissue in the jaws than that in other skeletal areas may be a factor in those cases of periodontal disease in which local etiologic factors are at a minimum but the alveolar bone exhibits marked destructive changes.

Microscopic appearance

Bone is composed of organic and inorganic components. The organic portion is composed of cells, fibers, and amorphous cementing substance. The fibers and the cementing substance form the bone matrix. Between adjacent structural units of bone, narrow bands of fiber-free matrix are found, and these are referred to as cement lines. The inorganic component is composed of mineral salts.

Microscopically, bone is composed of osteocytes embedded in a calcified extracellular matrix, each cell within a lacuna. Extending from a lacuna are minute canals called canaliculi. These communicate with canaliculi of adjacent lacunae. Through this system of canals, nutrient material reaches the osteocyte, and the canals are also avenues for removal of waste products of metabolism.

Bone tissue of the jaws undergoes a constant exchange (as does the tissue of the entire skeleton). Bone formation and resorption are going on continually, but a physiologic equilibrium exists between the two. Bone formation is seen as a marginal layer of osteoid in relation to a layer of polyhedral osteoblasts, whereas resorptive phases are generally characterized by the presence of multinucleated osteoclasts or connective tissue cells in irregular concavities in the bone margin. This process, termed *osteoclastic resorption,* involves the participation of lysosomal enzymes.

Recently polymorphonuclear leukocytes (PMNs) have been reported to be present near osteoclasts in areas of bone resorption at the alveolar crest in periodontal disease in monkeys. It has been suggested that inflammatory cells contribute to rapid bone destruction through the release of prostaglandins, interleukin-1, and other factors that might stimulate osteoclastic activity.

Bone may be classified according to the character and pattern of the incorporated fibers and cells. Three types of bone can be distinguished on this structural basis: *woven bone, lamellar bone,* and *bundle bone.*

When numerous bundles of collagen fibers become incorporated in the bone, the term *bundle bone* is applied.

The alveolar bone adjacent to the peridontal ligament contains numerous fibers, the mineralized portion of the collagen fibers of the periodontal ligament. These are referred to as *Sharpey's fibers.* Bundle bone, because it forms the immediate bony attachment of the periodontal ligament, is of interest to the periodontist.

The changes in alveolar bone associated with age are essentially a more osteoporotic structure and a reduction in the number of periosteal cells on the bone surface. Aging osteoblasts become smaller and fusiform. Matrix production ceases.

Two types of cells that can differentiate into osteoblasts have been described: *osteogenic precursor cells* and *inductible osteogenic precursor cells.* The inductible cells normally do not differentiate but can do so with appropriate stimuli. Of clinical importance is the discovery by Melcher and Accursi (1971) that periosteum elevated from the bone of adult animals is not osteogenic, whereas periosteum adjacent to a wound and periosteum from an osteoperiosteal flap is osteogenic. Goldman (1951) has found that injury to the periosteum results in proliferation of osteoblasts.

The bone of the cranial vault and facial skeleton and the shafts of the clavicles begin to ossify directly in mesenchyme without any preceding cartilaginous stage. Clusters of osteoblasts differentiate from mesenchymal precursor cells. The osteoblasts begin the formation of bone matrix, which soon calcifies. Some of the mesenchymal cells remain undifferentiated to form a reservoir of cells from which osteoblasts can later arise. In the jaws there is a covering periosteum.

Oxytalan fibers.   The oxytalan fiber, a distinct type of connective tissue fiber, was initially described by Fullmer (1959) and Fullmer and Lillie (1958). This fiber has been demonstrated to be a normal constituent of the periodontal ligament. Oxytalan fibers generally follow the course of the collagen fibers and seemingly are related to the amount of stress placed on the ligament. They are found in increased numbers in the ligament of teeth used for bridge abutments and less frequently around nonfunctioning teeth. Interestingly, they are found in the ligament adjacent to the cementum in greater numbers than on the bone side.

Neural supply

The neural control of the muscles of mastication is derived primarily from the motor centers within the brain. However, this activity is modified by proprioceptive impulses originating within the muscles themselves, within the temporomandibular joints, and within the gingiva and periodontal ligament. The proprioceptive nerves within the periodontal ligament have been shown to be directional. It is in this way that under normal circumstances the dentoalveolar unit is protected from damage from excessive forces being brought into play by the muscles of mastication. The neural density in humans is said to be much higher in the intermediate region than in the apical region of the root; however, there is great dispute about this, with some investigators reporting the apical portion to contain more nerve endings. Also, the morphology of the neural endings varies from animal to animal according to different investigators.

Gingival innervation. The innervation of the gingiva is derived from fibers of the labial or lingual branches of the second and third divisions of the trigeminal nerve and to a much lesser extent from anastomosing fibers from the periodontal ligament. The major nerves, coursing with the blood vessels in the supraperiosteal area of the alveolar plate, form a rete, which has been termed the *deep plexus.* As these fibers pass through the connective tissue of the gingiva, branches are given off to terminate as a "superficial plexus" in the lamina propria of the dermal papillae and on occasion continue into the epithelium as fine ultraterminal fibers. The interproximal gingiva is innervated by coronal extensions of the nerve plexuses of the periodontal ligament, as well as from supracrestal ramifications of the interdental nerves terminating in the transseptal fiber systems of adjacent teeth. Bernick (1957, 1959) has reported that he did not observe specialized endings such as Krause's or Meissner's corpuscles in his 1% pepsin preparations of the gingiva. Simpson (1966) has also noted this negative observation. Other writers (Dixon, 1963), however, have reported observing these corpuscles and other complex end organs in the gingival tissues. Such absence or sparsity of organized and specialized nerve endings is not unusual, since it has also been observed in areas of skin and mucous membrane that exhibit varying degrees of sensitivity.

Innervation of the periodontal ligament. The function of the periodontal ligament nerves is to transmit impulses of resultant forces of occlusion and mastication (touch, pressure, and pain) to high neurologic centers where appropriate responses can be transmitted to the effector muscle groupings to elicit protective reactions. The prime sources of this afferent innervation are periodontal branches of the dental nerve after it perforates the alveolar plate before entering the tooth, and the intraalveolar nerve as it courses crestally and its lateral branches perforate the cribriform plate. In the alveolar phase of the periodontal ligament, the two groups anastomose and send branches both apically and occlusally to form a complex rete parallel to the long axis of the tooth. From this network branches are given off to terminate in the connective tissue. Rapp et al. (1957a, 1957b) have suggested that the larger neural branches run in association with the blood vessels, whereas the smaller nerve fibers may not. The intraseptal nerves provide the major portion of the ligament innervation, and as a consequence surgery at the apical area of the tooth or inflammatory destruction of the tissue of this region does not greatly compromise the nerve sup-

ply of the rest of the periodontal ligament. The nerves may pass close to the cementum and alveolar bone, and their peripheral endings may form fine arborizations. Sicher (1966) has described three types of observed endings: knoblike structures, rings or loops around principal fiber bundles, and free nerve endings. Simpson (1966) has commented that definite end organs are seldom seen in the periodontal ligament and that fine endings are the predominating terminal feature. Studies by Bernick (1959) also have reported the finding that Meissner's, Ruffini's, or Pacini's corpuscles are not observed. In the apical third of the periodontium of a human tooth, myelinated nerves have been seen to lose their sheath and terminate as spindlelike structures. Brashear (1936) suggested that as the coarse nerve fibers travel occlusally in the alveolar phase, sensations are mediated by the varying caliber of myelinated and nonmyelinated fibers present: pain conducted by small-diameter nerves of both types; temperature by intermediate medullated fibers; and toughness by the large myelinated nerves. Nerves may form rings or loops around principal fiber bundles or may terminate between them so as to function in proprioception and localization. In the cemental phase Rapp et al. (1957a) have observed that most neurofibrils approach the cementum to form loops and then turn back toward the midportion of the ligament. Berkelbach van der Sprenkle (1936) has described a rete of nonmedullated fibers coursing radially from the central area of the periodontal ligament to penetrate the cementum.

The coronal termination of the nerve fibers of the periodontal ligament has been reported in the circular fiber group of the gingiva where they anastomose with nerve fibers of adjacent teeth to contribute to the total innervation of the area.

PERIODONTAL LIGAMENT

The fibers of the periodontal ligament proper, attaching the tooth to the alveolar housing, are arranged in the following groups: (1) the *alveolar crestal group,* extending from the cervical area of the root to the alveolar crest; (2) the *horizontal group,* running perpendicularly from the tooth to the alveolar bone; (3) the *oblique group,* oriented obliquely with insertions in the cementum and extending more occlusally in the alveolus (approximately two thirds of the fibers fall into this group); and (4) the *apical group,* radiating apically from tooth to bone. The arrangement of the groups of fiber bundles is designed to sustain the tooth against forces to which it is subjected. The structure of the periodontal ligament, however, continuously changes as a result of functional requirements. Crumley (1964) has reported that the periodontal ligament of rat molars normally demonstrates a remarkably high rate of collagen production.

The periodontal ligament is composed primarily of collagen fibrils generally arranged in bundles (Fig. 2-13). The

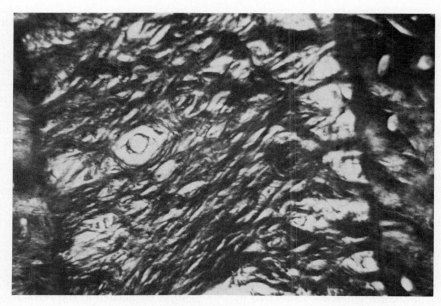

Fig. 2-13. High-power photomicrograph of periodontal ligament. Course and arrangement of prinicipal fibers and their insertion into cementum and bone, as well as small blood vessels, should be noted. Fibers on cementum side are relatively more numerous and thin, whereas on bone side they are fewer in number and of greater diameter.

fibrillar bundles unite the cementum to the alveolar bone surface. Collagen accounts for approximately 50% of the dry weight of the whole periodontal ligament; approximately 90% of the collagen of the ligament in fully erupted teeth is insoluble. The finding of collagenase and the fact that there are marked changes in the fibers of the periodontal ligament in animals maintained on diets deficient in protein suggest that there is a rapid turnover of collagen.

The course and arrangement of the principal fibers of the periodontal ligament show insertion of these fibers in the cementum and bone. It has been demonstrated that in the mouse, hamster, and marmoset the cementoalveolar fibers pass through the interdental septum and are continuous with similar fibers of adjacent teeth. The perforating fibers show frequent branching anastomoses. In humans, however, the interdental septa contain marrow spaces, and this arrangement of fibers has not been demonstrated. Selvig (1963, 1964) has demonstrated that Sharpey's fibers in both alveolar bone and cellular cementum are composed of an uncalcified core surrounded by a calcified sheath.

Bernick et al. (1977) reported findings of the course of the fibers of the periodontal ligament of one tooth to its adjacent neighbor. Sections of jaws from marmosets were stained with silver nitrate to demonstrate the intrabony course of the alveolar fibers of the periodontal ligament. They found that as the interseptal bone underwent a period of resorption and apposition, the intrabony alveolar fibers were also lost, and then re-formed. A continuum of fibers traversing the alveolar septum could not be determined. In one illustration showing the crest area of the interdental bone, the mesial and distal alveolar fibers terminated in the midregion of the bone where the ends formed an intermeshing network. In another illustration the interdental region between a first premolar and a canine from a mature marmoset was shown. The distal periodontal ligament was wider than that of the mesial surface. A serpentine resting line was seen traversing the length of the bone. The mesial and distal alveolar fibers within the bone terminated at the resting line. With advancing age there was a marked change in the depth of bony penetration of the alveolar fibers of the periodontal ligament. In these old animals the alveolar bone proper in both maxilla and mandible was reduced to a thin layer of darkly stained acellular calcification directly adjacent to the osteons filling the spongiosa. Insertion of the alveolar fibers within the alveolar bone proper was limited to this narrow area and did not extend into the haversian systems.

The periodontal fibers originate on the cementum side as numerous relatively thin bundles separated by the cellular elements of the cementoblastic layer. These bundles spread out, and the individual fibers of adjacent bundles become interwoven into a network that occupies the greatest width of the ligament. On the bone side, the origin of the fibrils from bone is similar to that noted on the cementum side, except that individual fiber bundles are fewer in number and of greater diameter than on the cementum side. These fiber bundles spread out, and their fibrillar elements become part of the network of fibers that course through the ligament.

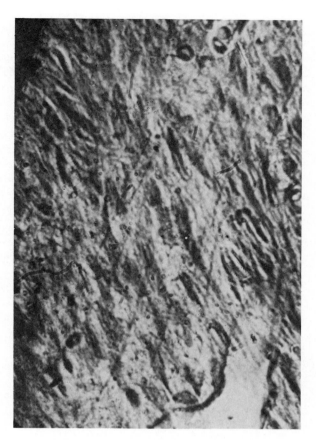

Fig. 2-14. Neural elements in periodontal ligament.

The ligament is traversed by channels of loose connective tissue that contain blood and lymph vessels as well as nerve bundles (Fig. 2-14). These channels are located approximately in the midportion of the ligament.

The blood vessels found in the periodontal ligament arise mainly from the bone marrow of the supporting bone through lateral perforations of the alveolar bone and to some extent from the periapical vessels. They form an elaborate anastomosing network (Figs. 2-15 and 2-16). These vessels are supplied with their own sympathetic nervous system. The lymphatics form a complicated pattern. The nerves are both myelinated and naked. Their endings have been described as knoblike swellings, rings, or loops around fiber bundles, and as free endings between fibers. Free endings are sensitive to pain. Some endings are proprioceptive in nature. They permit localization of masticatory stimuli and control masticatory muscle function.

In addition to the fibrous portion of the ligament and the neurovascular channels, certain cellular elements are regularly found in the ligament structure. These include cementoblasts, fibroblasts, osteoblasts, osteoclasts, and epithelial cell rests. Ultrastructurally, epithelial rests are readily identified by the presence of prominent tonofibrils in their cytoplasm, desmosomes connecting adjacent cells, and hemidesmosomes and a basement membrane surrounding the entire cell rest. These characteristics help to distinguish epithelial cells from vascular elements, the cells of which do not contain such well-defined tonofibrils, and the intercellular junctions of which consist primarily of close or tight junctions. Furthermore, the pinocytotic

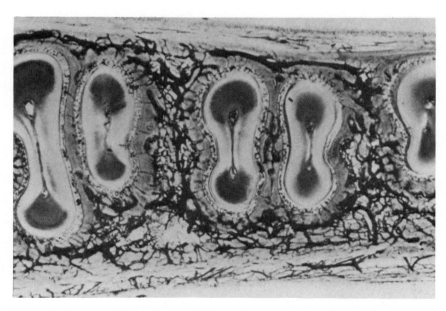

Fig. 2-15. Lower-power photomicrograph of mandibular occlusal section of a dog, showing vascularity of alveolus. Note large blood vessels feeding into periodontal ligament through nutrient canals.

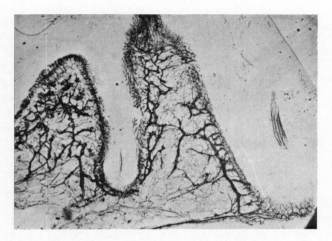

Fig. 2-16. Vascular network of periodontal ligament in a perfused dog. Note large vessel running parallel to periodontal ligament, from which are leadoffs to smaller vessels of periodontal ligament.

vesicles characteristically observed in endothelial cells are not nearly as prominent in epithelial cell rests.

The osteoblasts frequently demonstrate well-developed Golgi regions and a densely arranged rough-surfaced endoplasmic reticulum, characteristic of cells actively engaged in protein synthesis for extracellular use. The cementoblasts, on the other hand, seldom contain these organelles in such a well-developed manner (Fig. 2-17). These observations fit the autoradiographic data that indicate a greater degree of protein-synthesizing activity on the bone side of the periodontal ligament, with little activity on the cementum side. Osteoclasts, when noted, are characterized by one or more nuclei, a cytoplasm containing numerous vesicles and mitochondria, with interspersed strands of rough-surfaced endoplasmic reticulum, and a markedly convoluted cell surface on the side of the cell facing the bone surface.

Fibroblasts morphologically resemble osteoblasts and

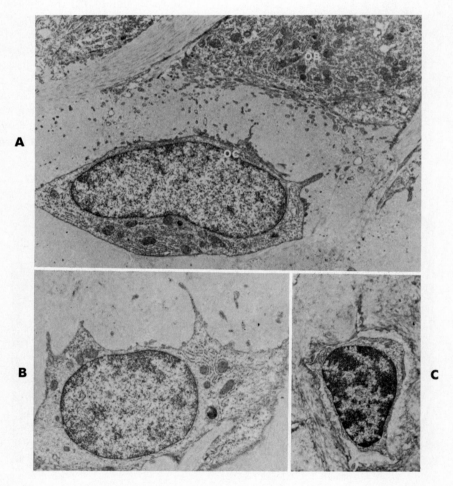

Fig. 2-17. **A,** Osteoblast *(OB)* and cell about to become an osteocyte *(OC),* with relatively high concentrations of mitochondria and rough-surfaced endoplasmic reticulum in cytoplasm. **B,** Cementoblast with relatively few cytoplasmic organelles. **C,** Cementocyte within a lacuna demonstrating cytoplasmic shrinkage and loss of most cytoplasmic organelles. (**A** ×6400; **B** ×8000; **C** ×4600.) (From Listgarten M: Unpublished data, 1969.)

cementoblasts. These cells can be distinguished from one another with any degree of certainty only because of their location in relation to the mineralized tissue surfaces. Fibroblasts usually possess thin cytoplasmic extensions that course between fiber bundles. The long axis of the cell usually extends in a plane parallel to the general direction of the fiber bundles.

The fibroblasts of the periodontal ligament frequently contain intracytoplasmic vacuoles that enclose one or more collagen fibrils. The vacuoles may demonstrate lysosomal enzyme activity, which suggests that fibroblasts contribute to collagen removal by endocytosis of fibrils. Thus fibroblasts may serve not only as a source of new collagen, but also in the destruction of already formed collagenous fibrils.

To explain relative movements of the tooth in relation to the alveolar bone (e.g., during rapid eruption), the concept of an "intermediate plexus" was introduced by Sicher [1966]). This concept provided for a zone in the periodontal ligament where fibers originating from bone could mesh with fibers originating from cementum. The essentially mechanical nature of the concept underlying the function of the intermediate plexus should be integrated with the results of autoradiographic studies, which have demonstrated regions of high collagen turnover in association with the bone side of the ligament. A number of investigators, using ^{3}H-proline as a label, have offered evidence to support the concept of differential rates of fiber formation (Grant and Bernick, 1972; Kameyama, 1975; Orlowski, 1976). The fibers in the middle of the ligament and those on the alveolar side appeared to be labeled more heavily than those on the cemental side. Carneiro (1965) showed that the periodontal ligament is the site of a high rate of synthesis and rapid turnover of collagen, particularly in the crestal and apical fibers. It is likely that turnover and remodeling occur at a molecular level. Such a state of events would not necessarily be reflected in a morphologically distinct zone (i.e., the intermediate plexus). Deporter and Ten Cate (1980) reported that examination at the hard surfaces adjacent to the periodontal ligament revealed fibroblast-like cells engaged in phagocytosis of anchored ligament fibrils. It has been suggested that in this way there can be organization of the ligament.

CHEMISTRY OF THE PERIODONTAL TISSUES

The growth, form, and function of cells are modulated by highly specific interactions between the cells and their extracellular matrices and by polypeptide growth factors. This section summarizes recent information on the characterization of extracellular matrices and their cellular interactions. Also, the biologic roles of another class of molecules, the polypeptide growth factors, are discussed. Finally, the effects of the extracellular matrices and the polypeptide growth factors on the function of cells of the periodontium are presented.

Extracellular matrices

Recent studies have suggested that specific interactions between cells and their extracellular matrices are important to the cells' growth, morphology, and function (Terranova et al., 1986b). Such studies show that extracellular matrices are cell and tissue specific, and progress has been made in characterizing these components and their specific functions (Table 2-1). In addition, these molecules have important effects on the cells in adjoining tissues and may regulate the interactions of different cell types and tissues.

Fibroblast extracellular matrix. Fibroblasts usually exist in a fibrous matrix composed of collagen types I and III, a small (Mr = 30,000) chondroitin sulfate proteoglycan, and fibronectin (Mr = 440,000). Type I collagen forms large-ordered fibers with high tensile strength. The function of the chondroitin sulfate proteoglycan is not clearly defined. Fibronectin is a large glycoprotein that binds the fibroblasts to the matrix and may have a role in fibrilogenesis. Fibronectin is distributed in tissues and blood and is known to bind to many different collagen types, to heparan sulfate, to fibrin, and to most other glycoproteins of the extracellular matrix. Recently several reports have indicated that the shape of fibronectin molecules may vary from globular to extended forms depending on the ionic strength and pH of the extracellular environment (Williams et al., 1982; Erickson and Carrell, 1983; Tooney et al., 1983.) More recently, the fibronectin receptor (Mr = 140,000) has been identified (Pytela et al., 1985).

Cartilage extracellular matrix. Another example of tissue-specific extracellular matrices with biologic specificity is cartilage. Chondrocytes exist in a homogeneous matrix containing type II collagen, a large (Mr = 10^6) chondroitin sulfate proteoglycan, link protein, hyaluronic acid and the cartilage-specific glycoprotein chondronectin (Mr = 180,000). The collagen fibers in this matrix are small and widely spaced. The proteoglycan molecules are bound along strands of hyaluronic acid, along with the link protein, and exist as large aggregates filling the space between the collagen fibers. The interaction between the collagen fibers and the proteoglycan system are not well defined. The chondrocytes bind to the matrix through chondronectin, which attaches to the proteoglycan, to the collagen, and to receptors on the cell surfaces. Removal of chondronectin from cultures of chondrocytes reverts the cultures to fibroblast-like phenotypes.

Epithelial cell extracellular matrix. The extracellular matrix of epithelial cells is also unique. Epithelial cells abut on a matrix of basement membrane that contains type IV collagen, a large (Mr = 750,000) heparan sulfate proteoglycan, and the glycoprotein laminin (Mr = 10^6) (Terranova et al., 1980). These three components are found in all basement membranes and probably interact to form a defined supramolecular structure. Fibronectin is a prominent constituent in the basement membranes of embryonic

Table 2-1. Extracellular matrix components and their major distribution

Component	Structure	Tissue distribution
Collagens and glycoproteins		
Type 1 collagen	$[\alpha1(I)]_2 \ \alpha2(I)$	Bone, cornea, dermis, dentin, ligament, tendon, heart valves, large vessel and uterine walls.
Type II collagen	$[\alpha1(II)]_3$	Hyaline cartilage, vitreous body, nucleus pulposus
Type III collagen	$[\alpha1(III)]_3$	Dermis, gingiva, heart valves, large vessel and uterine walls
Type IV collagen	$[\alpha1(IV)]_2 \ \alpha2(IV)$	Basement membrane
Type V collagen	$[\alpha1(V)]_2\alpha2(V)$ or $[a1(V)]_3$ or $[\alpha2(V)]_3$ or $[\alpha3(V)]_3$	Bone, cornea, fetal membranes, large vessel walls, heart valves, hyaline cartilage
Type VI collagen	Unknown	Blood vessels
Type VII collagen	$\alpha1(VII)$	Epithelial/mesenchymal border
Type VIII collagen	Unknown	Endothelium/mesenchymal border
Type IX collagen	Unknown	Cartilage
Type X collagen	Unknown	Cartilage
Elastin	$Mr = 72,000$	Dermis, lung, ligaments, large arteries
Fibronectin	2 chains $Mr = 210,000$ $Mr = 250,000$	Dermis, tendon, vessel walls, bone, plasma
Laminin	A-B1-B2	Basement membrane
Osteonectin	$Mr = 32,000$	Bone, plasma
Entactin (nidogen)	Unknown	Basement membrane
Chondronectin	$Mr = 180,000$	Cartilage
Proteoglycans		
Chondroitin sulfate	$Mr = 2.5 \times 10^6$	Cartilage
Large aggregating	$Mr = 200,000$ (Core protein)	Aorta Tendon
Large nonaggregating	$Mr = 10^6$ $Mr = 50,000$ or $Mr = 200,000$ (Core protein)	Skin Metaphysis Muscle
Small nonaggregating	$Mr = 70,000$ to $120,000$ $Mr = 40,000$ (Core protein)	Bone Cartilage
Dermatan sulfate	$Mr = (0.7 \text{ to } 2.5) \times 10^6$ $Mr = 4 \times 10^4$ to 5×10^5 (Core protein)	Aorta, dermis, sclera, cornea, tendon, joint capsule
Heparan sulfate	$Mr = 2.3 \times 10^5$ to 5.5×10^5 $Mr = 1.3 \times 10^5$ or 3.5×10^5 (Core protein)	Basement membrane
Hyaluronic acid	$Mr = 0.5 \times 10^6$ to 5×10^6	Cartilage Vitreous body, umbilical cord
Keratan sulfate	$Mr = ?$ 3×10^4 to 4×10^4 (Core protein)	Hyaline cartilage, cornea
Heparan	$Mr = 7.5 \times 10^4$ to 3.5×10^5 $Mr = 3 \times 10^4$ to 10^5 (Core protein)	Lung, liver

or developing tissues but is often lost from the basement membranes as the tissues mature. Type IV collagen forms the key structural element of the basement membrane. The collagen molecules are joined at their ends with disulfide bonds and with lysine-derived cross-links to form a continuous open network. This structure creates a strong extensile sheet allowing for the ready passage of fluids. Laminin binds to type IV collagen and also to receptors on the surface of epithelial and endothelial cells, thus mediating their attachment to the basement membrane. Fibronectin binds to another site on type IV collagen and could mediate fibroblast attachment. Heparan sulfate proteoglycan binds to laminin, to type IV collagen, to fibronectin, and to the surface of cells. Heparan sulfate forms a charged

Table 2-2.   Matrix sets

Cell type	Collagens	Glycoprotein	Proteoglycan
Fibroblast	Types I, III, VII	Fibronectin	Chondroitin sulfate (small)
Chondrocyte	Types II, IX, X	Chondronectin, link protein	Chondroitin sulfate (large)
Osteoblast	Types I, V	Osteonectin, fibronectin	Chondroitin sulfate (small)
Smooth muscle	Types I, III, V, VI	Fibronectin, laminin	Chondroitin sulfate (large and small)
Endothelial	Types I, III, IV, VIII	Fibronectin, laminin	Heparan sulfate
Nerve	Types I, III, IV, V	Fibronectin, laminin	Heparan sulfate
Epithelial	Type IV	Laminin	Heparan sulfate

barrier in basement membrane that prevents the passage of proteins.

The interactions of the basement membrane components in vitro are highly specific and for this reason could reflect their role in situ. Laminin and type IV collagen precipitate from solution in an equimolar complex, and only a limited amount of heparan sulfate proteoglycan binds to the laminin-type IV collagen complex.

Laminin is a major constituent of basement membranes, constituting 30% to 50% of the total protein. Laminin is localized exclusively in basement membranes and is synthesized by cells that normally reside on basement membranes. In vitro, laminin exists as a cross-shaped molecule with three short arms and one long arm. Each of the four arms has a globular end region; however, the long arm end region differs from the end regions of the short arms. One or more of the short arms' globular end regions promote cell spreading and also bind to type IV collagen. The long arm of laminin contains a heparan-binding site. The carbohydrate composition of the globular end regions of laminin is different from that of the rod-shaped regions. The long arm has recently been shown to stimulate neurite outgrowth. The intersection of the short arms contains numerous disulfide bonds and is relatively protease resistant. The protease-resistant central region of the laminin molecule binds to a specific cell surface receptor for laminin. Certain types of normal cells contain high-affinity cell surface binding sites for laminin. Recently, specific laminin binding to sulfated cell surface glycolipids of erythrocytes has been reported. In addition, some controversy exists as to which component(s) link laminin to the basement membrane. It has been found that laminin binds to native type IV collagen in a saturable manner with a dissociation constant of 5×10^{-7} M. This suggests that there is a single class of binding sites. However, since laminin also binds to heparan sulfate proteoglycan, multiple interactions probably account for the localization of laminin to basement membranes.

Cell specificity as modulated by extracellular matrices.   As outlined above, fibroblasts, chondrocytes, and epithelial cells produce and use different attachment factors (Table 2-1). Furthermore, these factors are cell spe-

Table 2-3.   Biologic activities of fibronectin and laminin

Substance	Activity
Fibronectin	Promotes mesenchymal cell adhesion
	Promotes mesenchymal cell chemotaxis
	Promotes mesenchymal cell growth
	Promotes neurite outgrowth
	Promotes phagocytosis
	Inhibits epithelial cell adhesion
	Inhibits epithelial cell growth
	Inhibits chondrogenesis
	Inhibits myotube formation
	Stimulates matrix synthesis
Laminin	Promotes epithelial and endothelial cell adhesion
	Promotes epithelial cell chemotaxis
	Promotes epithelial cell growth
	Promotes neurite outgrowth
	Inhibits adult fibroblast adhesion
	Inhibits adult fibroblast growth
	Binds to native type IV collagen
	Binds to native dentin and enamel
	Stimulates matrix synthesis

cific (Table 2-2). Laminin does not support the attachment of fibroblasts, and fibronectin does not allow epithelial cells to attach. Some specificity is also observed in the interaction between attachment factors in their binding to collagen. Laminin and epithelial cells attach to type IV collagen but not to other collagen types. These effects are not unexpected, since these are the natural associations in the tissue. Fibronectin and fibroblasts bind to all the collagens. These interactions in vitro undoubtedly reflect the mechanisms that govern the distribution and functions of cells in tissues.

Cells in culture grow better on extracellular matrices than on plastic or glass surfaces. In fact, growth on plastic or glass surfaces probably depends on the adsorption of matrix proteins that are produced by the cells or are present in serum. For example, the matrix deposited by corneal endothelial cells is a better substrate for cell growth than individual components, suggesting that more than one matrix component is involved.

Individual matrix components also stimulate growth, survival, and differentiation of cultured cells (Table 2-3).

For example, growth of fibroblasts and epithelial cells in culture is stimulated by the specific attachment factor each cell produces. In part, this may be due to more efficient attachment, but other direct effects on cell proliferation probably also contribute to growth stimulation.

A role in the differentiation of myoblasts has also been suggested for fibronectin and laminin. Myoblasts require a collagen substrate and fibronectin for attachment. Myoblasts also have fibronectin on their surface, but this is lost with fusion, and laminin appears on the surface of the myotubes. Thus the attachment proteins produced and retained by the cells change as they differentiate. Addition of exogenous fibronectin to the media prevents the myoblasts from forming myotubes. Apparently the change in cell surface proteins is necessary for, and may even initiate, differentiation.

Attachment factors specific for one cell type can alter the phenotypic properties of other cells once attached (Table 2-4). For example, chondrocytes bound to a substrate with chondronectin are then able to bind fibronectin and flatten to a fibroblastic phenotype. The bound fibronectin modifies some of the biosynthetic activities of cells. Under these conditions the cells stop synthesizing the cartilage-specific proteoglycan and begin to produce fibronectin. Apparently, the attachment of the cells unmasks receptors for fibronectin that were previously cryptic.

Interesting effects are observed when fibroblasts are exposed to laminin. When added to culture media, laminin (50 µg/ml) suppresses the growth of fibroblasts. Presumably, it is reacting with receptors on the fibroblast surface or with an essential matrix component that blocks their growth. The significance of this observation is not known but could represent a mechanism for suppressing the invasion of fibroblasts into epithelial tissues. An interaction like this would aid in the segregation of these cell types during development, as well as in stabilizing morphogenesis.

Fibronectin suppresses the growth of epithelial cells and stimulates the growth of fibroblasts and some other cells. Similar mechanisms to those postulated for the effects of

laminin on fibroblasts may be operative. In vivo fibronectin has been shown to stimulate wound repair and scar formation probably by preferentially stimulating the attachment, growth, and matrix production of fibroblasts. In some tissues, repeated stimulation by fibronectin due to persistent injury could lead to an excess of matrix, which may be manifested as fibrosis.

Endothelial cells and hepatocytes are able to use both fibronectin and laminin for attachment in vitro, and these factors influence the phenotype of the cells. Capillary endothelial cells in culture proliferate on a substrate formed from type I or III collagen and form confluent sheets. When placed on type IV collagen, these cells stop dividing and form tubes resembling capillaries. Probably the attachment factors also differ under these conditions and may regulate the different responses of the cells. Hepatocytes also bind to laminin and fibronectin but become much more fibroblastic in the presence of fibronectin. This could relate to chronic injury in the liver causing a shift to fibroblastic activities.

The studies reviewed here help to explain the interaction of specific cells with their matrices and the relationship of the extracellular matrix to tissue structure. Key effectors in these processes are the glycoprotein attachment factors (Tables 2-3 and 2-4). These bind specific cell types to matrix. In doing so, they uncover cell surface receptors for other attachment proteins. Under these conditions other factors are able to alter the phenotype of the cell. Such processes may be active in development and in repair.

Table 2-4. Specificity of laminin and fibronectin

Phenotypic characteristics	Effect of exposure of cells in culture to	
	Laminin	Fibronectin
Affinity for fibronectin	Decreases	Increases
Affinity for laminin	Increases	Decreases
Fibronectin receptors	Decreases	Increases
Laminin receptors	Increases	Decreases
Melanogenisis	Increases	Decreases
Invasiveness	Increases	Decreases
Epithelial cell growth	Increases	Decreases
Mesenchymal cell growth	Decreases	Increases

Polypeptide growth factors

Epidermal growth factor (EGF)
Platelet-derived growth factor (PDGF)
Endothelial cell growth factor (really FGFs) (ECGF)
Nerve growth factor (NGF)
Fibroblast growth factors (acidic and basic) (FGFs)
Transforming growth factors (α and β TGFs)
Insulin-like growth factors (IGF I and II)
T-cell growth factor (interleukin-2) (Il-2)
Colony-stimulating factors (CSFs)
Eye-derived growth factors (EDGFs)
Fibroblast-derived growth factor (FDGF)
Placenta-derived growth factor
Cartilage-derived growth factor (really TGF-β)
Erythropoietin
Thymosin
Bone-derived growth factor (osteonectin?)
Osteosarcoma-derived growth factor
Macrophage-derived growth factor
Neurotrophic growth factor
Periodontal ligament cell growth factor (PDL-CTX)

NOTE: Structural similarity of many of the growth factors exists.

This suggests that a cascade of reactions at the cell surface occurs that can direct the differentiation of similar cells along different paths.

Polypeptide growth factors

In addition to the extracellular matrix another class of biologic response modifiers, the polypeptide growth factors (PGFs) have recently generated great interest (see box on opposite page). The fundamental and often critical importance of PGFs in stimulating growth and maintaining viability in a broad variety of cell types has become a generally accepted principle of developmental biology. The PGFs are hormonelike in structure and function. However, recent studies have indicated that their sites of synthesis and means of transport to specific target cells are more variable than their true hormonal analogues. Most of these factors are not stored in vesicles in their synthesizing cells but are released in a continuous manner to diffuse to the target cells (this could be endocrine, paracrine, or autocrine).

This is in contrast to the bolus release into the circulation characteristic of the endocrine system. The biochemical mechanisms by which synthesis and release of the PGFs are regulated are unknown. It is believed, however, that signal transduction of the factor-induced proliferative response is mediated by high-affinity receptors present on the target cell surface.

In the past several years, major progress in definition and characterization of the PGFs has been achieved in three specific areas: identification and isolation of a large number of PGFs; structural analyses including the mRNA and gene sequences; and receptor characterization for several PGFs in terms of both structure and function. Thus it is commonly thought that the PGFs represent a large family of regulatory factors, that there are many subgroups characterized by structural similarities suggesting common ancestries (see box above), and that some PGFs are synthesized as part of large precursors that presumably are released by limited proteolysis of the prefactor.

Growth is a fundamental process that is a unique characteristic of all living organisms. Although growth is usually associated with the early stages of development (i.e., in the embryo and the newborn), it often remains a general feature of many tissues throughout adult life. This is especially evident when one considers, in wound healing, for example, the regenerative capabilities and the programmed replacement of many cell types. Although some of these processes in normal tissue, as opposed to healing tissue, are maintenance activities because there is no net increase in tissue size or mass, growth is normally accompanied by tissue or cell changes that result from an increase in either cell size (hypertrophism) or cell number (hyperplasticity). Hypertrophic responses, which result in increased production of extracellular matrix material such as bone and connective tissue, as well as increases in cell volume, are particularly well illustrated by axonal growth and synapse formation of developing neurons. In contrast, hyperplasticity provides the means for the production and maintenance of terminally differentiated tissues from pluripotent stem cells in addition to the proliferation required to achieve sufficient cell numbers to form adult tissues. At any stage of development, the mitogenic response of the cellular population of an organism can be divided into three categories: (1) cells that are postmitotic and therefore unable to undergo division, (2) cells that are constantly undergoing division, and (3) cells that are resting but are capable of reentering the cell cycle and undergoing division given the appropriate stimulus. Most cells can be stimulated to increase their size regardless of their mitotic status.

A variety of factors contribute to both stimulation and control of growth processes; hormones, PGFs, neural elements, proximal contacts by both heterologous and homologous cells, and interaction with extracellular matrix material seem to be among the most important. Each factor can signal the target cell usually through the formation of a factor complex at the exterior of the plasma membrane. Although the end results of these information transfers have been well documented, relatively little is known about the nature of the molecular signals and how they are propagated. In addition, their identification has been made more difficult by the complex nature of the growth response and the expanded period of time over which it can occur. It is likely that no single mechanism can account for all of the growth-stimulating substances; thus each factor may have to be studied individually. In addition to their growth-promoting action, some PGFs have recently been implicated in evolving a chemotactic response in the cells to which they are targeted. Thus the overall net effect could be directed cell movement accompanied by subsequent proliferation.

Chemotactic behavior is a property of a variety of cell types engaged in many biologic processes, including organ development, wound repair, neurite outgrowth, tumor invasion, and inflammation. Factors that modulate cell chemotaxis have recently been implicated in cellular growth and differentiation. The extracellular matrix proteins, laminin and fibronectin, have been shown to stimulate mammalian cell motility in a variety of cell types, including nerve cells, PMNs, fibroblasts, epithelial cells, Schwann cells, and various cells of tumorigenic origin (see Table 2-3). In addition, endothelial cell growth factor has been shown to be a potent chemoattractant for human endothelial cells, whereas platelet-derived growth factor has been shown to be a chemoattractant for smooth muscle cells and fibroblasts. Nerve growth factor and laminin have been implicated in neurite proliferation and migration.

Thus both PGFs and isolated components of the extracellular matrix appear to play an increasingly important role in our understanding of tissue definition.

Regenerative capacity

The native connective tissue attachment of the periodontium is known to be a complex consisting of fibroblasts (of various types including gingival fibroblasts and periodontal ligament cells), epithelial cells (gingival epithelium), vascular endothelial cells, nerve cell processes, cementum (cementoblasts with associated extracellular matrix), alveolar bone (various bone cell types), and extensive extracellular matrix (collagen, glycoproteins, and proteoglycans). The regeneration of this complex following periodontal disease has been a major area of recent investigation and is one ultimate goal of clinical periodontal therapy. Many clinical approaches have been attempted to obtain regeneration of the periodontal attachment. Citric acid conditioning and insertion of synthetic membranes, allowing for selective cell recolonization of the tooth root surface by cells of mesenchymal origin, have been advocated as possible adjunctive procedures to periodontal surgery.

Citric acid conditioning of the instrumental root surface during periodontal surgery has been demonstrated as a promising adjunct in attempts to generate a new connective tissue attachment in humans and in experimental animals as compared with periodontal surgery alone.

The biologic significance of citric acid utilization has been studied in several laboratories (Boyko et al., 1980). It has been demonstrated in vitro that partial surface demineralization of the root surface dentin enhances migration to and attachment of fibroblast-like cells from the periodontal ligament or human gingival fibroblasts. These data suggest that acid demineralization by exposure of the dentin collagen provides a suitable matrix for connective tissue cell adherence. In the squirrel monkey, a connective tissue reattachment did not occur on reimplantation of roots that had been surgically denuded of part of their periodontal ligament. The instrumented root surface served as a substrate for apical migration of gingival epithelial cells. When partial surface demineralization by citric acid etching followed the surgical denudation, this experimental model provided further evidence that this limited matrix modulation enhances a connective tissue attachment to the root. A fibrin network appeared to be attached to the root surface of the acid-treated specimens, and the apical termination of the epithelium was located at the coronal extent of this network. In these experiments it is conceivable that rapid attachment to the root surface of nonspecified connective tissue extracellular matrix components was promoted by the exposed collagen fibers. Such matrix components then promoted mesenchymal cell adherence. This mesenchymal cell barrier could then act as an effective circumferential seal preventing epithelial cell apical migration.

Transmission electron microscopy of surgically exposed and periodontally involved root surfaces in dogs has shown that the exposed collagen fibrils of the demineralized root surfaces retain their periodicity (Selvig et al., 1981). These studies have further demonstrated that a connective tissue attachment can be achieved on the surface of the demineralized root regardless of whether it is surgically denuded or has been exposed to the environment of an experimental periodontal pocket. Furthermore, adjunctive citric acid conditioning of instrumented root surfaces that were previously exposed to natural periodontal pockets in beagle dogs also resulted in gain of a new connective tissue attachment following periodontal surgery (Renver and Egelberg, 1981). New attachment in several circumferential locations up to the CEJ was demonstrated. The mode of wound closure in addition to the root surface exposure of a collagen matrix appears to be important for successful healing of these periodontal defects.

The gain of clinical attachment following partial surface demineralization with citric acid in conjunction with periodontal surgery in humans is limited (1 to 2 mm gain in probing attachment). Results from studies in the experimental animals indicate that the flap design (a replaced flap procedure) may have limited the amount of attachment achieved (Cole et al., 1981).

In a study on reimplanted roots in dogs, it was concluded that only partial surface-demineralized roots bearing cultured periodontal ligament cells exhibited fragments of a new fibrous tissue attachment identified as periodontal ligament. Root areas without fibrous attachment presented with ankylosis and resorption, as did roots covered with cultured gingival fibroblasts or unrecovered controls (Boyko et al., 1981). Studies addressing connective tissue healing to root surfaces partially denuded of their periodontal ligament have used implanted roots partially submerged in alveolar bone. Only root surfaces retaining their periodontal ligament exhibited a fibrous attachment to the root after reimplantation, whereas replacement healing such as ankylosis and root resorption followed implantation of denuded roots. Thus it has been proposed that a prerequisite for successful healing following periodontal regeneration procedures is that cells from the periodontal ligament are allowed to selectively colonize the instrumented root surface rather than gingival epithelial cells, gingival fibroblasts, and osteoblasts.

Insertion of semiporous membranes under the soft tissue flap during periodontal surgery is thought to mechanically exclude (1) epithelial cell apical migration along the root surface and (2) recolonization of the root surface by gingival fibroblasts. It has been suggested that this partial cell exclusion technique selectively allows for repopulation by cells from the periodontal ligament on the root surface (Nyman et al., 1982).

Studies in monkeys and dogs, however, indicate that root resorption and ankylosis frequently hamper the initially successful outcome following the use of partial root surface demineralization or insertion of synthetic barrier membranes. In humans, root resorption and ankylosis have been observed following reconstructive periodontal surgery including the use of bone grafts (Dragoo and Sullivan, 1973). In contrast, when citric acid conditioning or synthetic barrier membranes have been used in humans, root resorption and ankylosis have not been reported. This may be due to the relatively short observation periods of these cases, to lack of systematic histologic evaluation, or to true differences between experimental animal models and humans.

Apical migration of epithelial tissue or connective tissue healing, including root resorption or ankylosis, seems to induce present regeneration attempts of the periodontal ligament irrespectively of the treatment approach. Inclusion of tools of cellular biology in reconstructive periodontal therapy may alter these aberrant healing events. A limited manipulation of the periodontal wound matrix may alter the healing events by selective recruitment of specific periodontal ligament cells or by selection for specific cell phenotypes at the dentin connective tissue interface.

Modulation of function

In a study of the attachment of fibroblasts and epithelial cells to root surfaces from extracted human teeth, it was demonstrated that the attachment of fibroblasts was enhanced by fibronectin, whereas the attachment of epithelial cells was enhanced by laminin (Terranova and Martin, 1982). Thus it was postulated that specific cell types can be directed to attach to different areas on the root surface through the localized use of these extracellular matrix proteins.

When the growth of fibroblasts and epithelial cells on root surfaces from extracted human teeth was studied in culture, it was found that epithelial cells grew ten times faster than fibroblasts. After citric acid treatment of the root surface to expose type I collagen fibers and the addition of exogenous fibronectin, the growth pattern was reversed, with the fibroblasts showing a tenfold increase in growth over the epithelial cells (Terranova and Martin, 1982). Thus it appears to be possible to alter cell attachment and growth to and on surfaces of teeth.

Previously it has been difficult to produce an environment that promoted new connective tissue attachment to tooth root surfaces exposed to the oral environment. It seems likely that the epithelium has a selective advantage in growth because of its ability to bind to the mechanically treated mineralized surface and subsequently rapidly migrate along these root surfaces. As in all connective tissues, once epithelium separates the root surface from the adjacent connective tissue, attachment of fibroblasts to the root surface is precluded. This could be explained partly by the delineating basement membrane and its components being epithelial cell specific. It is possible that the attachment of connective tissue could be promoted by the local application of exogenous extracellular matrix material, and

appropriate PGFs to properly prepared root surfaces would confer a selective advantage to gingival fibroblasts, osteoblasts, and/or cells originating from the periodontal ligament.

Recent studies have shown that tetracycline hydrochloride effectively demineralizes root surface dentin in vitro (Wikesjö et al., 1986). In addition, it has been found that tetracycline hydrochloride adsorbs to enamel and dentin and desorbs in active form. Thus the dentin may act as a local delivery system for the antimicrobial compound. Tetracycline hydrochloride has been shown in vitro to inhibit collagenolytic enzyme activity and to inhibit bone resorption. In other experiments it was demonstrated that the binding of fibronectin and of fibroblasts to the tetracycline hydrochloride–treated root surfaces was markedly enhanced over that seen on root surfaces conditioned with citric acid. Furthermore, it was shown that the binding of laminin and subsequent attachment of epithelial cells was inhibited by pretreatment of root surfaces with tetracycline hydrochloride. Tetracycline hydrochloride preconditioning of the root surface not only will selectively remove the surface smear layer, but may also act favorably by inhibition of collagenase activity and bone resorption, and by its local antimicrobial effects to support these events. This combination of events (i.e., the biologic effects of local tetracycline hydrochloride application, the enhancement of fibroblast adhesion, and the reduction of epithelial cell adhesion) marks the beginning of our understanding of the molecular events necessary to mediate a new connective tissue attachment.

Recently it has been demonstrated that migration to, proliferation on, and movement on dentin surfaces of periodontal ligament cells is enhanced when the surface is preconditioned with tetracycline hydrochloride and treated with fibronectin and endothelial cell growth factor. These studies have now begun to address the fundamental question of which combination of extracellular matrix material coupled to which PGF will appropriately condition the dentin surface to make the surface receptive to mesenchymal cell adhesion and proliferation. In similar experiments laminin was shown to enhance gingival epithelial cell chemotaxis, proliferation, and movement (Terranova et al., 1986a).

Hence it is feasible that tetracycline hydrochloride and/or citric acid preconditioning of the root surface and subsequent application of biologic response modifiers may promote a connective tissue healing at the dentin–soft tissue interface by enhancement of selective cell attachment, proliferation, and migration. This cascade of events should not be limited to cells of fibroblastic origin but should also include cells of endothelial origin, cells of nervous tissue origin, smooth muscle cells, and undifferentiated precementoblast cells. Thus a series of these and other biologic response modifiers acting synergistically may be used to establish a new periodontal ligament.

REFERENCES

Anderson BJ et al: Changes in molar teeth and their supporting structures following extraction of the upper right first and second molars, Yale J Biol Med 49:145, 1929.

Berkelbach van der Sprenkel H: Microscopical investigations of the innervation of the tooth and its surroundings, J Anat 70:233, 1936.

Bernick S: Innervation of teeth and periodontium after enzymatic removal of collagenous elements, Oral Surg 10:323, 1957.

Bernick S: Innervation of the teeth and periodontium, Dent Clin North Am, p 503, July 1959.

Bernick S et al: Course of alveolar fibers on periodontal ligament, J Dent Res 56:1409, 1977.

Boyko GA, Brunette DM, and Melcher AH: Cell attachment to demineralized root surfaces in vitro, J Periodont Res 15:297, 1980.

Boyko GA, Melcher AH, and Brunette DM: Formation of new periodontal ligament by periodontal ligament cells implanted in vivo after culture in vitro, J Periodont Res 16:73, 1981.

Brashear AD: The innervation of the teeth, J Comp Neurol 64:169, 1936.

Carneiro J: Synthesis and turnover of collagen in periodontal tissues: use of radioautography investigation of protein synthesis, New York, 1965, Academic Press, Inc.

Cole R et al: Pilot clinical studies on the effects of topical citric acid application on healing after replaced periodontal flap surgery, J Periodont Res 16:117, 1981.

Crumley PJ: Collagen formation in the normal and stressed periodontium, Periodontics 2:53, 1964.

Deporter DA and Ten Cate AR: Collagen resorption by periodontal ligament fibroblasts at the hard tissue–ligament interfaces of the mouse periodontium, J Periodontol 51(8):429, 1980.

Dixon AD: Nerve plexuses in the oral mucosa, Arch Oral Biol 8:435, 1963.

Dragoo MR and Sullivan HC: A clinical and histological evaluation of autogenous iliac bone grafts in humans. II. External root resorption, J Periodontol 44:614, 1973.

Erickson HP and Carrell NA: Fibronectin in extended compact conformations: electron microscopy and sedimentation analysis, J Biol Chem 258:14539, 1983.

Fullmer HM: Observations on the development of oxytalan fibers in the periodontium of man, J Dent Res 38:510, 1959.

Fullmer HM and Lillie RD: The oxytalan fiber; a previously undescribed connective tissue fiber, J Histochem Cytochem 6:425, 1958.

Goldman HM: The topography and role of the gingival fibers, J Periodont Res 30:331, 1951.

Grant D and Bernick S: The periodontium of aging humans, J Periodont Res 43:660, 1972.

Kameyama Y: Autoradiographic study of ^{3}H-proline incorporation by rat periodontal ligament, gingival connective tissue, and dental pulp, J Periodont Res 10:98, 1975.

Melcher AH and Accursi GE: Osteogenic capacity of periosteal and osteoperiosteal flaps elevated from the parietal bone of the rat, Arch Oral Biol 16:573, 1971.

Nyman S et al: New attachment following surgical treatment of human periodontal disease, J Clin Periodontol 9:290, 1982.

Orlowski WA: The incorporation of H^3-proline into the collagen of the periodontium of a rat, J Periodont Res 11:96, 1976.

Pytela R, Pierschbacher MD, and Rouslahti E: Identification and isolation of a 140 kD cell surface glycoprotein with properties expected of a fibronectin receptor, Cell 40:191, 1985.

Rapp R, Avery JK, and Rector RA: A study of the distribution of nerves in human teeth, J Can Dent Assoc 23:447, 1957a.

Rapp R, Kirstine WD, and Avery JK: A study of neural endings in the human gingiva and periodontal membrane, J Can Dent Assoc 23:637, 1957b.

Renvert S and Egelberg J: Healing after treatment of periodontal intraosseous defects. II. Effect of citric acid conditioning of the root surface, J Clin Periodontol 8:459, 1981.

Ritchey B and Orban B: The crests of the interdental alveolar septa, J Periodontol 24:75, 1953.

Rogers HJ and Weidman SM: Metabolism of alveolar bone, Br Dent J 90:7, 1951.

Selvig KA: Electron microscopy of Hertwig's epithelial sheath and of early dentin and cementum formation in the mouse incisor, Acta Odontol Scand 21:175, 1963.

Selvig KA: An ultrastructural study of cementum formation, Acta Odontol Scand 22:105, 1964.

Selvig KA et al: Fine structure of new connective tissue attachment following acid treatment of experimental furcation pockets in dogs, J Periodont Res 16:123, 1981.

Sicher H: Orban's oral histology and embryology, ed 6, St Louis, 1966, The CV Mosby Co.

Simpson HE: The innervation of the periodontal membrane as observed by the apoxestic technique, J Periodontol 37:374, 1966.

Terranova VP and Martin GR: Molecular factors determining gingival tissue interaction with tooth structure, J Periodont Res 17:530, 1982.

Terranova VP, Rohrbach DH, and Martin GR: Role of laminin in the attachment of PAM 212 (epithelial) cells to basement membrane collagen, Cell 22:719, 1980.

Terranova VP et al: Laminin promotes rabbit neutrophil motility and attachment, J Clin Invest 77:1180, 1986a.

Terranova VP et al: Regulation of cell attachment and number by laminin and fibronectin, J Cell Physiol 127:473, 1986b.

Tooney NM et al: Solution and surface effects on plasma fibronectin structure, J Cell Biol 97:1686, 1983.

Wikesjö UME: A biochemical approach to periodontal regeneration: tetracycline treatment conditions dentin surfaces, J Periodont Res 21:322, 1986.

Williams EC et al: Conformational states of fibronectin: effects of pH, ionic strength and collagen binding, J Biol Chem 257:14973, 1982.

Chapter 3

FORMATION AND SUBSEQUENT CHANGES OF THE PERIODONTIUM

Ian C. Mackenzie

The life history of the supporting structures of a mammalian tooth may be arbitrarily divided into several phases. The developmental phase is characterized by rapid coordinated cellular activity leading to the establishment of a functioning periodontium. During the long phase of function that typically follows, the structure of the periodontium appears to be essentially stable. A state of dynamic equilibrium exists, and the continuing formation of cells and other tissue components is balanced by their removal. Such processes appear to be essential to maintain the normal structure of the periodontium to permit adaptive change; for example, tooth movement is associated with both catabolic and synthetic events (i.e., bone resorption to one side of the tooth and deposition at the other). Eventually, various changes in the periodontal tissues can be detected; these are thought to be associated with senescence.

The unfolding of the genetic program during progression from the egg to the adult depends on signals exchanged locally between cells of differing origins. Increasingly, evidence shows that such interactions, generally termed *epithelial-mesenchymal interactions,* do not completely cease when normal function of the organ or tissue is established; they seem to persist and play significant roles in maintaining structure during normal tissue turnover and may be especially important during periods of adaptation and regeneration. Periodontal disease is associated with cell proliferation and with breakdown and reorganization of the hard and soft tissues surrounding the teeth. Understanding such processes and the role of surgical therapy in regeneration of structure lost during disease ultimately rests on comprehension of the normal coordinating mechanisms by which structure is established and maintained.

DEVELOPMENT OF THE PERIODONTIUM
Tissue interactions

Tissue interactions are essential processes during fetal development, but little is known of their molecular basis. Most of the information available about their nature is based on the interpretation of experiments in which components of developing tissues are separated, variously recombined, and then maintained in conditions expected to permit their continuing development. The literature on this subject is extensive, and the following provides only the briefest outline of concepts; a more detailed introduction may be found elsewhere (e.g., Sengel, 1976; Wessells, 1977).

As indicated by the arrows entering and exiting the simplified scheme in Fig. 3-1, the interactions occurring during development are sequential. The final adult tissue is the outcome of several series of interactions, and the general pattern is that with each set of interactions the responding tissue becomes more committed (limited) to a particular type. Three types of effects can be inferred to

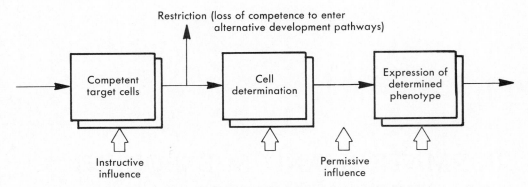

Fig. 3-1. Simplified scheme of cell interactions during development.

take place during tissue interactions. A cell population may respond to an *instructive influence* in a specific way. For example, during tooth development, foci of mesenchyme along the dental arches instruct the overlying oral epithelium to become tooth buds. Evidence for the specificity of this instruction is derived from the observations that (1) if the epithelium of this region is recombined with other mesenchyme, it fails to progress to tooth formation and (2) tooth buds may form if epithelium from a region that does not normally form tooth buds is recombined with mesenchyme from the dental arch (Kollar and Fisher, 1980).

Such instructive influences appear to be associated with selective potentiation of a particular set, or sequence, of genes and with the closing off of alternative sets that could have been expressed in other circumstances. Hence the concept of *restriction:* once a cell has responded to an instructive influence, it loses, to a greater or lesser extent, its ability to enter other pathways of development that might have been previously open to it. Cell determination (i.e., commitment to a particular pathway of subsequent development) presumably has its basis in changes at a molecular level, but at present the usual experimental test is the ability of a tissue to continue to develop along the determined pathway when removed from the environment of the instructing influence.

For differentiation to continue, the environment in which the developing tissue is placed must support growth and differentiation; in addition, it is clear that certain minimal conditions concerning temperature, nutrients, etc., are essential. However, the requirements for continued differentiation are usually more exacting, and it is in relation to these conditions that the concept of *permissive influences* arises. For example, if a developing epithelium is separated from its mesenchyme and maintained in (apparently) optimal tissue culture conditions, it usually fails to develop further. However, in the same culture conditions the presence of mesenchyme, even from another region, may permit growth and differentiation, indicating some

necessary permissive property of mesenchyme. For different tissues permissive requirements may be more or less stringent and may be provided only by certain types of mesenchyme. An exchange of signals can be inferred from the type of experiments outlined above, but the actual nature of such signals and their mechanism of transmission remain to be determined. Among the possibilities to be considered are the production of effector molecules that diffuse between cells, an influence of the matrix synthesized by the instructive population, and direct contact between the interacting cells, with the response mediated via cell surface receptors or intercellular exchange of macromolecules.

Specific developmental events

Morphologic changes associated with tooth formation occur early in embryonic life (at about 6 weeks in human embryos), with thickening of ectoderm overlying the maxillary and mandibular processes. Apparently under the influence of the underlying neural crest mesoderm (Grant and Miles, 1967), focal downgrowth of regions of epithelium into the mesenchyme leads to the formation of recognizable tooth buds. This occurs sequentially along an anteroposterior gradient and slightly earlier in the mandibular than in the maxillary arch. Under the influence of inductive interactions (Kollar and Baird, 1970a, 1970b), the epithelium of the tooth bud becomes further differentiated into inner and outer enamel epithelia and then forms a cap- and subsequently a bell-shaped structure enclosing a condensation of mesenchyme, termed the *dental papilla*. Of particular relevance to development of the periodontium, a thin layer of mesenchyme, the dental follicle, surrounds the entire developing tooth and is continuous with the dental papilla at the epithelial rim (Ten Cate et al., 1971).

Sequential reciprocal interactions between the inner enamel epithelium and the mesenchyme of the dental papilla lead to the formation of odontoblasts from dental papilla cells, ameloblasts from the inner enamel epithelium, and the production of dentine and then of enamel. Such processes continue as proliferation of the epithelium at the rim of the bell progresses to define and enlarge the morphology of the crown of the tooth.

When downgrowth of the epithelium has progressed to the region of the future cementoenamel junction (CEJ), an important change in its behavior occurs. The downgrowing epithelium continues to induce the formation of odontoblasts, but the epithelium itself is no longer subsequently induced to form ameloblasts. Instead, the advancing edge forms a cylinder of bilaminar epithelium that defines the outline of the future root of the tooth; downgrowth of this epithelium, now termed *Hertwig's epithelial root sheath,* is accompanied by extension of the dental papilla, which it encloses, and of the dental follicle, which is continuous with the dental papilla around the advancing cervical loop of epithelium.

The cellular events associated with development of the tooth root and the periodontium have been studied (Lester, 1969; Freeman and Ten Cate, 1971; Ten Cate and Mills, 1971; Ten Cate et al., 1971; Atkinson, 1972; Grant and Bernick, 1972; Palmer and Lumsden, 1987), but these processes have received less attention than those associated with the earlier phases of development of the crown of the tooth. However, apparently after inducing dentinogenesis, Hertwig's epithelial root sheath becomes fenestrated, and the surrounding mesenchymal cells of the dental follicle contact the dentine surface, differentiate into cementoblasts, and deposit cementum on it. Although the types of cellular interactions occurring during ligament formation are uncertain, it seems probable that the development of cementoblasts is associated with instructive influences from the epithelial root sheath or the newly formed dentine. Ultrastructural studies (Freeman and Ten Cate, 1971) indicate that individual cells of the investing mesenchymal follicle, considered precementoblasts, initially insinuate themselves between the epithelial cells of the root sheath to abut against the newly formed dentine. The extracellular environment of these cells contains numerous collagen fibrils. At this stage the fibers inserted into the cementum and those emerging from the developing alveolar bone are aligned perpendicular to the root surface but are separated by a zone of longitudinally aligned fibers. In rodents the epithelial remnants of the root sheath degenerate and become trapped in the forming cementum (Lester, 1969), whereas in primates they remain as strands and nests of cells, the rests of Malassez, close to the cementum surface. The cells and fibers surrounding the tooth became organized into the oblique orientation characteristic of the mature ligament at about the time of eruption. Blood vessels in the developing ligament form a plexus close to the bone surface in continuity with vessels emerging from the alveolar bone.

Following transplantation of tooth germs to subcutaneous sites (Ten Cate et al., 1971) there is formation of cementum, periodontal ligament, and a surrounding shell of bone, suggesting that the precursor cells for cementoblasts, periodontal fibroblasts, and osteogenic cells are all derived from cells of the transplanted dental follicle. The follicle of the developing tooth consists of an inner tooth-related zone termed the *investing layer,* an intermediate zone, and an outer alveolar bone–related zone (Ten Cate, 1969). Recent experiments suggest that bone formation is restricted to the outer zone cells and that the investing layer forms cementum and ligament (Palmer and Lumsden, 1987).

Development of the epithelial attachment

Fig. 3-2 schematically illustrates the sequence of relationships that exist between a tooth and the gingival epithelia. Before eruption, the crown of the tooth is covered by the reduced enamel epithelium, derived from the epithelium of the enamel organ. As the erupting tooth approaches the oral cavity, this previously quiescent epithelium begins to proliferate and fuses with the epithelium of the overlying oral mucosa. Degeneration of the inner layer of the reduced enamel epithelium is associated with migration of proliferating stratified epithelium along the enamel surface to the level of the CEJ, but this process may not be completed until several years after eruption (McHugh, 1963). At that time, three types of epithelium can be distinguished: the oral gingival, the oral sulcular, and the junctional epithelia. The origin of the cells constituting the junctional epithelium is not entirely certain. It is likely that they arise from the activated cells of the reduced enamel epithelium, but following its surgical removal, junctional epithelium can also be reformed from oral epithelium (Schroeder and Listgarten, 1977).

MAINTENANCE OF THE LIGAMENTOUS STRUCTURE

Despite its stable histologic appearance, many studies indicate that the structure of the periodontal ligament is maintained by a relatively rapid rate of formation and loss of cellular and extracellular components. The exception to this is cementum, which, despite its important role as the matrix into which Sharpey's fibers are inserted, is subject to slow accretion but not normally to resorption.

Isotope studies indicate that the mature type I and type III collagen constituting the normal ligament may have a half-life of only a few days and that the turnover of noncollagenous proteins is also rapid (Sodek, 1978). It is unclear how continuity of the fibers spanning from cementum to bone is maintained during remodeling, but the concept of a more metabolically active central intermediate plexus where fiber detachment and reattachment occur has not been supported by autoradiographic studies of the fiber turnover rates. The cells within the ligament also appear to have a high rate of turnover. Labeling studies of rodents suggest that two functionally different populations of fibroblasts may exist in the ligament: a proliferative progen-

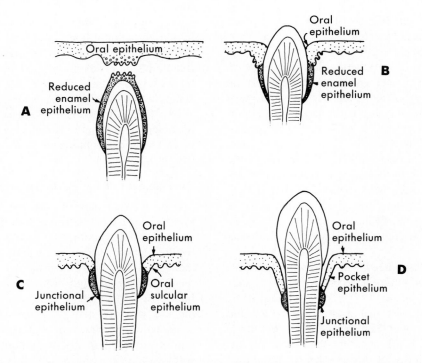

Fig. 3-2. Various stages of relationships of a tooth to gingival epithelia. As erupting tooth approaches oral cavity, **A,** proliferation of reduced enamel epithelium and oral epithelium leads to fusion of these epithelia. As tooth emerges into oral cavity, **B,** apical part of enamel initially remains covered by reduced enamel epithelium. With continuing downgrowth of proliferating epithelium to CEJ, **C,** three types of gingival epithelium (oral gingival, oral sulcular, and junctional) become distinguishable. This "ideal" situation is often disturbed by further epithelial downgrowth (e.g., in periodontal disease), which leads to formation of a pocket lined with epithelium, **D,** the characteristics of which have not been well defined. Even so, there appears to be persistence of a region of epithelium with junctional characteristics at apex of such downgrowth.

itor population, located perivascularly, which produces functionally mature cells with a life span of only about 25 days (Davidson and McCulloch, 1986), and the cells and calcified matrix of the alveolar bone, which also have a rapid turnover. It is clear that rates of resorption and deposition of bone vary in response to appropriately altered function. For example, despite bodily movement of the tooth through bone during tooth movement, ligament width (the distance between bone and cementum), returns to a relatively constant value. The factors continuously controlling such spatial organization of the component tissues of the periodontium are as yet unknown.

MAINTENANCE OF STABILITY OF THE GINGIVAL EPITHELIA

The stratified epithelia lining the oral cavity continuously proliferate, renewing their structure every few days, and act as a barrier to the entry of substances and organisms into the deeper tissues. When the continuity of an epithelium is breached, there is usually a rapid wound-healing response, with cell proliferation and migration,

which leads to restoration of structure. A tooth breaches the continuity of the oral epithelium, and there is, in some sense, a "free-edge" of epithelium at the cementoenamel margin (Fig. 3-3). This is usually a stable situation, and movement of the gingival epithelium along the root surface normally does not occur. Because this represents an important feature of periodontal disease, the mechanism that normally prevents such epithelial downgrowth must be ascertained. The presence of the dense collagenous bundles of ligament fibers inserted into the cementum has been suggested as a physical barrier to downgrowth, but epithelia are able to migrate through connective tissues (e.g., during development and wound healing), and it has now been shown that oral epithelial cells are able to produce a collagenase (Lin et al., 1987). A simple mechanical explanation for epithelial stability may therefore not be sufficient. Ultrastructural (Schroeder and Listgarten, 1977) and monoclonal antibody (Fig. 3-4) studies have shown that the phenotype of the junctional epithelium is quite different from that of other oral epithelia. It forms a cuff around the tooth, to which it is attached by hemidesmo-

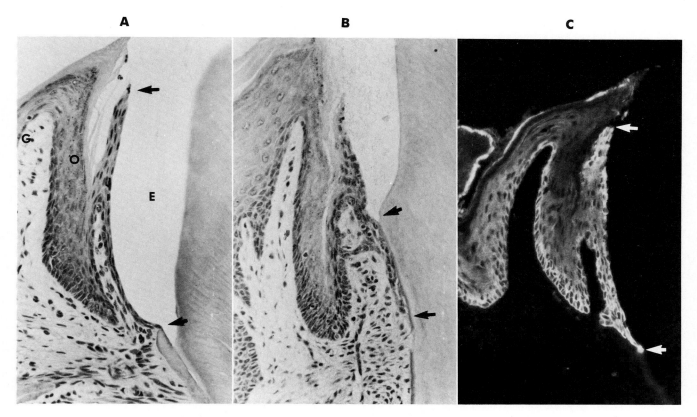

Fig. 3-3. Stained sections of decalcified specimens of buccal aspect of a normal mouse molar tooth shows, **A,** arrangement of oral *(G)*, oral sulcular *(O)*, and junctional *(J)* epithelia and extent of attachment of junctional epithelium to enamel *(E)*, indicated by arrows. **B,** Three weeks after surgical removal of gingival region, epithelial anatomy is restored, but part of junctional epithelium *(between arrows)* now lies on cementum. **C,** Frozen section of specimen of mouse gingiva dissected from tooth and stained with immunofluorescent technique using an antibody with broad reactivity against keratins shows epithelial component of gingiva and extent of junctional epithelium *(arrows)*. (Hematoxylin and eosin.)

somes, but does not seem to be designed as a particularly effective barrier; unlike other surface epithelia, it is mechanically weak and has a large proportion of extracellular space that allows free passage of fluids and macromolecules. It is possible that an important property of the junctional epithelial phenotype is its nonmigratory character. If this is so, the mechanisms determining this phenotype will be of consequence to the progression of periodontal disease (Mackenzie, 1984, 1987).

There is evidence that even in the adult, subepithelial connective tissues influence an associated epithelium by directive and permissive influences similar to those active during embryogenesis; they can redirect the type of keratin polypeptides and cell surface macromolecules synthesized by an epithelium (Schweizer et al., 1984; Mackenzie and Dabelsteen, 1987) and provide factors necessary for normal epithelial growth and differentiation (Hill and Mackenzie, 1984). The connective tissues of the periodontal lig-

ament and of the lamina propria of the gingiva have different developmental histories and, hence, potentially different influences on an adjacent epithelium. As illustrated in Fig. 3-5, the influence of periodontal connective tissue on an associated epithelium could be directive in nature, inducing formation of the regionally specific phenotype of junctional epithelium. Alternatively, the passive junctional phenotype could result from the connective tissue of the periodontal ligament lacking permissive influences necessary for migration and differentiation of epithelium to occur (Mackenzie, 1987). Either mechanism could lead to a stable relationship, but distinction between these two possible mechanisms appears to be of significance. If the junctional phenotype results from a specific directive influence, then damage by microbial or inflammatory factors could lead to loss of the influences necessary for its stability. If, however, its phenotype results from the lack of a permissive factor, apical migration would require genera-

A   **B**   **C**

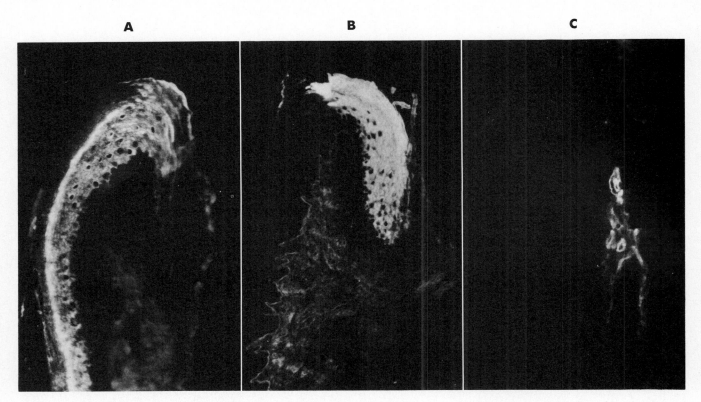

Fig. 3-4. Frozen sections of gingiva similar to those shown in Fig. 3-3 stained with three antibodies directed against different keratin polypeptides to show presence of different keratins in **A,** oral gingival epithelium, **B,** oral sulcular epithelium, and **C,** junctional epithelium.

A   **B**   **C**   **D**   **E**   **F**

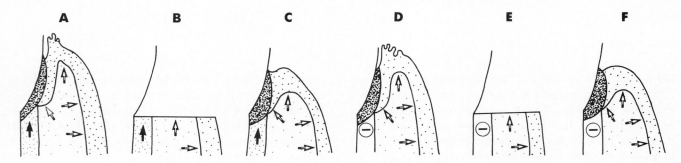

Fig. 3-5. Interactions between gingival and periodontal connective tissues that may influence overlying epithelia and be associated with development of junctional epithelial phenotype. Views **A** to **C** assume different directive influences of gingival *(open arrows)* and periodontal *(solid arrow)* connective tissues on epithelial differentiation. It is assumed that in normal gingiva, **A,** the differing phenotypes of junctional and gingival epithelia are established and maintained by these influences. After surgical removal of sulcular region, **B,** inductive influences of connective tissues remain and, with migration from cut edge of oral gingival epithelium, reestablish regionally appropriate epithelial phenotypes. Views **D** to **F** assume similar properties of gingival connective tissue but lack directive and permissive influences of periodontal connective tissue. Here junctional phenotype is conceived as that of epithelium lacking permissive connective tissue influences necessary for full differentiation. Following surgical removal, a similar pattern of migration and regeneration of gingival epithelia ensues, but junctional phenotype is conceived as that of epithelium lacking permissive connective tissue influences required for normal differentiation or further migration.

tion of a permissive stimulus. Many factors, such as interleukins, lymphokines, and growth factors, are generated during the inflammatory response and could stimulate such epithelial growth.

AGE CHANGES

Most cells and tissues of the body demonstrate functional and structural differences between the young and the aged. Usually, however, no clear causative relationship can be established for such age-associated changes, nor can it be determined whether the changes detected are (1) primary age changes intrinsic to the cells and tissues examined, (2) secondary to changes in other tissues (e.g., hormonal alterations, reduced vascularity), or (3) representative of the accumulated, unrepaired damage of minor disease or functional "wear and tear."

Many studies of human and animal periodontal tissues describe differences in structure, metabolism, or regenerative abilities associated with aging (Mackenzie et al., 1986). The types of changes described include decreased cellularity and number of fiber bundles, tendency toward thickening, irregularity of arrangement and calcification of fiber bundles, and increased cross-linking, as well as a decreased soluble fraction of the collagen composing them (Tonna, 1973; Holm-Pedersen and Viidik, 1974; Severson et al., 1978). The ultimate causes of such changes are uncertain. A decreased ligament width, possibly a secondary effect of reduced functional loading, has been described. There is no mechanism to repair occlusal wear on teeth, and continuing deposition of cementum, which leads to increased cemental thickness, particularly in the apical region, may be associated with continuing adaptive eruption. Similarly, the common finding of apical movement of the gingival attachment, with migration of the junctional epithelium onto cementum and apical repositioning of the gingival crest, has been associated with occlusal wear and passive eruption, although episodes of inflammation and local trauma may also be significant in such changes.

TISSUE INTERACTIONS AND REGENERATIVE CAPACITIES

The observation that the diversity of specialized cells and tissues in an adult organism results from a history of sequential interactions during development may have practical significance in therapeutic procedures directed toward regeneration of periodontal structure lost through disease. Questions to be resolved are as follows:

1. To what extent are the cells of specialized periodontal tissues, such as cementum and ligament, restricted to their specialized phenotype as a result of their developmental history?
2. Under what circumstances can one adult cell type be induced to acquire the properties of another? For example, transplanting a piece of liver in the expectation of regenerating thyroid seems unreasonable;

how reasonable is it to expect nonperiodontal connective tissues to regenerate periodontium?

The cells of tissues that are continuously renewed (e.g., epithelial cells [Mackenzie, 1984] and perhaps periodontal fibroblasts [Bordin et al., 1984; Davidson and McCulloch, 1986]) are heterogeneous and contain a relatively undifferentiated progenitor population, which divides to produce the fully differentiated functional cells. The undifferentiated cells, often referred to as *stem cells,* appear to possess some degree of plasticity, and there are reports of experiments in which epithelial or mesenchymal cells have been induced by various conditions to express a phenotype differing from that of the population of origin (Schweizer et al., 1984). The extent to which cells such as cementoblasts, ligament fibroblasts, and osteocytes can be derived from a common precursor during periodontal regeneration needs to be elucidated. Several observations suggest that these individual cell lineages are of importance. For example, experiments recombining various components of developing teeth suggest that the potential for odontogenic tissues to interact to reform new structure is lost quite early as development progresses (Palmer and Lumsden, 1987), and experiments with fully formed periodontium indicate that precursor cells able to regenerate cementum lie adjacent to the tooth and those forming osteoblasts lie adjacent to the bone (Gould et al., 1977; Karring et al., 1980, 1985). At present, markers for the various subpopulations of periodontal cells are lacking, but the development of various in vivo and in vitro techniques to allow selective identification and augmentation of the appropriate progenitor cell population appears to offer exciting opportunities for clinical periodontal regeneration.

REFERENCES

Atkinson ME: The development of the mouse molar periodontium, J Periodont Res 7:255, 1972.

Bordin S et al: Fibroblast subtypes in the periodontium, J Periodont Res 19:642, 1984.

Davidson D and McCulloch CAG: Proliferative behavior of periodontal ligament cell populations, J Periodont Res 21:414, 1986.

Freeman E and Ten Cate AR: Development of the periodontium: an electron microscopic study, J Periodontol 42:387, 1971.

Gould TRL, Melcher AH, and Brunette DM: Location of progenitor cells in periodontal ligament of mouse molar stimulated by wounding, Anat Rec 188:133, 1977.

Grant D and Bernick S: The formation of the periodontal ligament, J Periodontol 43:17, 1972.

Grant WA and Miles AEW: In Miles AEW, editor: Structural and chemical organization of teeth, vol 1, New York, 1967, Academic Press, Inc.

Hill MW and Mackenzie IC: The influences of differing connective tissue substrates on the maintenance of adult stratified squamous epithelia, Cell Tissue Res 237:473, 1984.

Holm-Pedersen P and Viidik A: Changes in regeneration pattern of connective tissue with age, Scand J Clin Lab Invest Suppl 141:55, 1974.

Karring T, Nyman S, and Lindhe J: Healing following implantation of periodontitis affected roots into bone tissue, J Clin Periodontol 7:96, 1980.

Karring T et al: New attachment formation on teeth with a reduced but healthy periodontal ligament, J Clin Periodontol 12:51, 1985.

Kollar EJ and Baird GR: Tissue interactions in embryonic mouse tooth germs. I. Reorganization of the dental epithelium during tooth-germ reconstruction, J Embryol Exp Morphol 24:159, 1970a.

Kollar EJ and Baird GR: Tissue interactions in embryonic mouse tooth germs. II. The inductive role of the dental papilla, J Embryol Exp Morphol 24:173, 1970b.

Kollar EJ and Fisher C: Tooth induction in cheek epithelium, Science 207:993, 1980.

Lester KS: The unusual nature of root formation in molar teeth of the laboratory rat, J Ultrastruct Res 5:135, 1969.

Lin HY et al: Degradation of type I collagen by rat mucosal keratinocytes, J Biol Chem 262:6823, 1987.

Mackenzie IC: Epithelial-connective tissue relationships and the development and maintenance of structure. In Meyer J, Squier CA, and Gerson SJ, editors: The structure and function of the oral mucosa, Oxford, 1984, Pergamon Press, Ltd..

Mackenzie IC: Nature and mechanisms of regeneration of the junctional epithelial phenotype, J Periodont Res 22:243, 1987.

Mackenzie IC and Dabelsteen E: Connective tissue influences on the expression of epithelial cell-surface antigens, Cell Tissue Res 248:137, 1987.

Mackenzie IC, Holm-Pedersen P, and Karring T: Age changes in the oral mucous membranes and periodontium. In Holm-Pedersen P and Löe H, editors: Geriatric dentistry: a textbook of oral gerontology, Copenhagen, 1986, Munksgaard.

McHugh WD: Some aspects of the development of gingival epithelium, Periodontics 1:239, 1963.

Palmer RM and Lumsden AGS: Development of periodontal ligament and alveolar bone in homografted recombinations of enamel organs and papillary, pulpal and follicular mesenchyme in the mouse, Arch Oral Biol 32:281, 1987.

Schroeder HE and Listgarten MA: Fine structure of the developing epithelial attachment of human teeth: monographs in developmental biology, vol 2, Basel, Switzerland, 1977, S Karger.

Schweizer J, Hill MW, and Mackenzie IC: The keratin polypeptide patterns in heterotypically recombined epithelia of skin and mucosa of the adult mouse, Differentiation 26:144, 1984.

Sengel P: Morphogenesis of skin, Cambridge, 1976, Cambridge University Press.

Severson JA et al: A histological study of age changes in the adult human periodontal joint (ligament), J Periodontol 49:189, 1978.

Sodek J: A comparison of collagen and non-collagenous protein metabolism in rat molar and incisor periodontal ligaments, Arch Oral Biol 23:977, 1978.

Ten Cate AR: The development of the periodontium. In Melcher AH and Bowen WH, editors: Biology of the periodontium, London, 1969, Academic Press, Ltd.

Ten Cate AR and Mills C: The development of the periodontium: the origin of alveolar bone, Anat Rec 173:69, 1971.

Ten Cate AR, Mills C, and Solomon G: The development of the periodontium: an autoradiographic and transplantation study, Anat Rec 170:365, 1971.

Tonna EA: Histological age changes associated with mouse-periodontal tissues, J Gerontol 28:1, 1973.

Wessells NK: Tissue interactions and development, Menlo Park, Calif, 1977, WA Benjamin, Inc.

Chapter 4

CLASSIFICATION AND CLINICAL AND RADIOGRAPHIC FEATURES OF PERIODONTAL DISEASE

Robert J. Genco

The most common diseases of the periodontal tissues are inflammatory processes of the gingiva and attachment apparatus of the tooth. These common periodontal diseases are microbial infections associated with local accumulation of dental plaques, a subgingival pathogenic periodontal flora, and calculus. There are other diseases of the gingiva and periodontal attachment apparatus that are not infections but are caused by traumatic, cystic, granulomatous, neoplastic, or degenerative processes. In this chapter a comprehensive classification of diseases or conditions affecting the periodontal tissues is presented, followed by a discussion of the clinical and histologic features of the common infectious forms of periodontal diseases in adults and juveniles.

CLASSIFICATION

Over the years a number of classification systems have been developed to organize and name various disease entities or conditions affecting the periodontium. The present classifications, although they reflect current knowledge and information about the clinical, radiographic, microbiologic, and systemic host response description of the disease, are likely to be supplanted by more definitive classifications once the etiologies of each of the various diseases or conditions are fully understood. For example, localized juvenile periodontitis may be called "actinobacillary periodontitis" after a major pathogenic bacteria associated with the disease—*Actinobacillus actinomycetemcomitans*. In the future, some forms of adult periodontitis associated with the black-pigmented *Bacteroides*—*Bacteroides gingivalis* or *Bacteroides intermedius*—may be called "*Bacteroides* periodontitis." This nomenclature for infectious forms of periodontal diseases is likely to follow that used for infections that are classified on the basis of the causative agent (i.e., streptoccal or pneumococcal pneumonia or streptococcal pharyngitis). Presently, however, a classification system for periodontal diseases based mainly on their clinical and radiographic appearance, as well as on the systemic health or disease states of the patient, is useful.

By far the most common periodontal pathologic conditions are gingivitis and periodontitis—diseases that occur in otherwise healthy persons. Gingivitis is an inflammatory process of the gingiva in which the junctional epithelium, although altered by the disease, is attached to the tooth at its original level. In *gingivitis* the most apical portion of the junctional epithelium is on the enamel, at or near the cementoenamel junction (CEJ). *Periodontitis* occurs when the periodontal ligament attachment and alveolar bony support of the tooth have been lost. This is associated with apical migration of the junctional epithelium onto the root surface; hence, by definition, periodontitis occurs when the junctional epithelium migrates apically to the CEJ.

Periodontal diseases have been given a variety of names in the past. For example, they have been called paradentosis (Weski, 1937), diffuse alveolar atrophy, Schmutz pyorrhea (Gottlieb, 1928), and periodontitis complex (McCall and Box, 1925), and are still called pyorrhea by many. The term *pyorrhea,* although quite descriptive, indicating pus coming from the periodontal pockets, is not generally used by the profession; the synonymous term *periodontitis* is preferred. Other terms no longer in use for periodontitis include periodontoclasia, pericementitis, alveoloclasia, Rigg's disease, and chronic suppurative periodontitis. The classification presented in the boxes on these two pages represents an effort to simplify, yet be complete in providing a set of terms that are useful in describing definitive

---

Diseases and other abnormalities of the periodontal tissues

I. Gingival diseases and conditions
   A. Gingivitis (no systemic involvement)
   B. Gingivitis and gingival changes with systemic involvement
   C. Miscellaneous gingival conditions
II. Periodontal diseases and conditions
   A. Periodontitis in adults (no systemic involvement)
   B. Periodontitis in juveniles
   C. Periodontitis with systemic involvement
   D. Miscellaneous conditions affecting the periodontium
III. Periodontal changes associated with occlusal trauma
   A. *Primary occlusal trauma:* Mobility and other periodontal changes associated with bruxism or other parafunctional habits
   B. *Secondary occlusal trauma:* Mobility and other periodontal changes associated with normal forces in the severely compromised periodontium

---

Gingival diseases and conditions

A. Gingivitis
   1. Marginal gingivitis
   2. Acute necrotizing ulcerative gingivitis (ANUG)
B. Gingivitis and other gingival changes with systemic involvement
   1. Gingival changes associated with sex hormones
      a. "Pregnancy" gingivitis
      b. Gingivitis associated with oral contraceptives
      c. Gingivitis associated with other hormonal alterations (e.g., polycystic ovaries, puberty, and menopause)
   2. Gingival changes associated with diseases of the skin and mucous membranes
      a. Pemphigus
      b. Cicatrical pemphigoid
      c. Bullous pemphigoid
      d. Lichen planus
      e. Psoriasis
      f. Desquamative gingivitis
      g. Lupus erythematosus
      h. Erythema multiforme
      i. Idiopathic gingival fibromatosis
      j. Recurrent aphthous stomatitis
   3. Gingivitis in generalized systemic diseases
      a. Acute leukemia
      b. Thrombocytopenia
      c. Hemophilia
      d. Sturge-Weber syndrome
      e. Wegener's granulomatosis
      f. Sclerosis
      g. Hypoadrenocorticism
      h. Vitamin C deficiency
      i. AIDS
      j. Sarcoidosis
   4. Infective gingivostomatitis
      a. Herpetic gingivostomatitis
      b. Herpes zoster
      c. Herpangina
      d. Syphilis
      e. Candidiasis
      f. Actinomycosis
      g. Histoplasmosis
   5. Drug-associated gingival changes
      a. Systemic medications
         i. Phenytoin (Dilantin)
         ii. Sodium valproate
         iii. Cyclosporine
         iv. The dihydropyridines: nifedipine (Procardia) and nitrendipine
      b. Compounds with local effects
         i. Caustic compounds
         ii. Heavy metals
C. Miscellaneous gingival conditions
   1. Gingival cysts
   2. Gingival fistulas
   3. Neoplasms
   4. Gingival clefts
   5. Gingival recession
   6. Aberrant frena or muscle attachments
   7. Epulis or gingival pyogenic granuloma
   8. Gingival abscesses

Periodontal diseases and conditions

A. Periodontitis in adults
  1. AAP Classification I, II, III, IV
  2. Epidemiologic: moderately and rapidly progressing periodontitis
  3. Clinical based on treatment: refractory and recurrent
  4. Clinical based on history: recurrent acute necrotizing ulcerative periodontitis and postlocalized juvenile periodontitis
B. Periodontitis in juveniles
  1. Localized juvenile periodontitis ("periodontosis")
  2. Generalized juvenile periodontitis
C. Periodontitis with systemic involvement
  1. Periodontitis in primary neutrophil disorders
    a. Agranulocytosis
    b. Cyclic neutropenia
    c. Chédiak-Higashi syndrome
    d. Neutrophil adherence abnormalities
    e. Job's syndrome
    f. "Lazy leukocyte" syndrome
    g. Neutrophil functional abnormalities
  2. Periodontitis in systemic diseases with secondary or associated neutrophil impairment
    a. Diabetes mellitus type I
    b. Diabetes mellitus type II
    c. Papillon-LeFèvre syndrome
    d. Down's syndrome
    e. Inflammatory bowel disease: Crohn's disease
    f. Preleukemic syndrome
    g. Addison's disease
    h. AIDS
  3. Other systemic diseases associated with changes in the structures of the periodontal attachment apparatus
    a. Ehlers-Danlos syndrome (VIII)
    b. Histiocytosis (eosinophilic granuloma)
    c. Sarcoidosis
    d. Scleroderma
    e. Hypophosphatasia
    f. Hypoadrenocorticism
    g. Hyperthyroidism
D. Miscellaneous conditions affecting the periodontium
  1. Periodontal abscesses
  2. Periodontal cysts
  3. Ankylosis
  4. Root resorption
  5. Periodontal-pulpal communicating lesions
  6. Pericoronal abscesses
  7. Dentinal hypersensitivity
  8. Retained roots
  9. Bony sequestration
  10. Infections associated with fractured roots, or anatomic defects
  11. Neoplasms of the attachment apparatus

disease entities or conditions affecting the periodontal tissues that are encountered in dental practice.

The classification presented on p. 64 (right) is based on that of the American Academy of Periodontology (AAP; 1986), and the terminology is in general use in the English literature. The expanded versions on p. 64 (bottom) and at left are comprehensive, listing common as well as rare conditions that may be seen in a dental practice. This classification is intended to provide a current basis of terminology that is useful for communication among practitioners, patients, and third parties involved in practice.

Subtypes of adult periodontitis

Various classification schemes have been applied to periodontitis in otherwise healthy adults. This oftentimes bewildering terminology exists because periodontitis in adults is heterogeneous, manifesting variations in clinical and radiographic appearance.

The AAP has proposed a periodontal diagnosis scheme that is useful, especially for reporting cases to third parties for reimbursement. They describe *gingivitis* as inflammation of the gingiva characterized clinically by changes in color, gingival form, position, surface appearance, and the presence of bleeding and/or exudate. The next category is *slight periodontitis,* which is described as progression of gingival inflammation into the deeper periodontal tissues and alveolar bony crest with slight bone loss. The periodontal pocket depth is 3 to 4 mm, and there is slight loss of connective attachment and slight loss of alveolar bone. Next is *moderate periodontitis,* which is a more advanced stage of slight periodontitis. It is exemplified by increased destruction of periodontal structures with noticeable loss of bony support, sometimes accompanied by increased tooth mobility. There also may be furcation involvement in multirooted teeth. *Advanced periodontitis* is further progression of periodontitis with major loss of alveolar bony support, usually accompanied by increased tooth mobility. Furcation involvement in multirooted teeth is likely.

RECOGNITION OF DISEASES OF THE PERIODONTIUM

Gingivitis and periodontitis can occur with or without systemic involvement. In most instances the inflammatory periodontal diseases are of local origin; however, they are markedly modified by the systemic conditions of the patient. There is no clear-cut example of pure systemically caused periodontitis. On the other hand, gingival disease can be primarily associated with systemic conditions, since the gingiva may be a target organ for metabolic and genetic abnormalities and drug effects. Hence a thorough medical history and systemic evaluation of the patient are essential to periodontal diagnosis. Not only are the course and nature of the periodontal disease altered by systemic involvement, but also the course of therapy may have to be modified by systemic disease or drug intake.

The examination of the patient should begin with a careful evaluation of the total oral cavity and the head, neck, and face. The dentist is in an excellent position to detect life-threatening diseases of the head and neck, such as intraoral cancer and facial basal cell carcinomas or swellings in the neck region, during the head and neck examination.

The periodontal examination includes an assessment of the gingiva and attachment apparatus. The elements in a thorough periodontal examination involve complete examination of the oral cavity, including charting of all teeth and often multiple surfaces of each tooth and adjacent periodontal tissues for the following:

1. Signs of gingival inflammation, including spontaneous bleeding, swelling, loss or detachment of papillae, redness and changes in the contour of the gingiva, and the presence and characteristics of exudates from the gingiva
2. Periodontal probing in which pocket depths and attachment levels are measured in millimeters
3. Gingival bleeding assessed 30 to 60 seconds after deep probing
4. Assessment of furcation involvements on multirooted teeth with periodontal probes, by direct visual assessment, and on radiographs
5. Evaluation of mucogingival conditions, including gingival clefts, loss of attached gingiva, and aberrant frena that may retract or otherwise alter the gingival margins
6. Measurement of tooth mobility and fremitus (mobility during occlusal function)
7. Assessment of interproximal, interradicular, and other alveolar bony changes by radiographic analysis
8. When necessary, "bone sounding" or probing the bone with the patient under local anesthesia, to better define altered bony architecture (e.g., extent and number of bony walls of an infrabony pocket)
9. Evaluation of the subgingival and oral microflora for the presence of pathogenic organisms

Periodontal charting with specific details of the clinical, radiographic, and microbiologic evaluation are discussed in later chapters. In the future, evaluation of abnormalities in the host response, including neutrophil and lymphocyte function, immunoglobulins, and antibodies, is likely to play a major role in evaluation of the patient.

Various indices have been developed to measure periodontal disease in epidemiologic surveys and in clinical studies, and these are described in Chapters 6 and 7. These indices, although useful for epidemiologic studies, are usually not adequate to determine a specific clinical diagnosis for an individual with periodontal disease.

Details of medical history taking are covered in Chapter 24, general oral examination in Chapter 27, radiographic interpretation in Chapter 25, clinical examination in Chapter 26, and occlusal analysis in Chapters 15 and 42.

GINGIVAL DISEASES AND CONDITIONS
Marginal gingivitis

Gingivitis, the most common of the periodontal diseases, can occur in any individual if sufficient plaque accumulates at the gingival margin. Gingivitis is an inflammatory disease of the gingiva characterized by the following: (1) changes in *color* from coral pink to red to bluish red; (2) changes in *form,* which normally is thin with a knife-edged margin, to edematous, often with swollen interdental papillae; (3) changes in *gingival position,* with the swollen gingival margin near or at the bulge of the crown; (4) changes in *surface texture,* often with a glossy surface and loss or reduction of gingival stippling and often with loss of interdental grooves and free marginal grooves; and (5) *bleeding,* spontaneous or with slight pressure, or the presence of suppurative exudates coming from the gingival orifice. Gingivitis is most often painless; however, patients are often aware of the swollen, red, bleeding gingiva. Gingivitis is almost always associated with plaque accumulation at or near the gingival margin.

The key histologic features of gingivitis indicate that it is inflammatory in nature, characterized by infiltration of the gingival connective tissue with (round) inflammatory cells and epithelial changes, including increased widening of the intercellular spaces and inflammatory cell infiltration of the junctional epithelium. There may be edema with gingival swelling, resulting in gingival or pseudopocket formation. However, since there is no loss of periodontal connective attachment and the apical extent of the junctional epithelium is in its original position at or near the CEJ (Figs. 4-1, *A,* 4-2, and 4-3), these gingival or pseudopockets can be distinguished from true periodontal pockets in which the apical border of the junctional epithelium has migrated apically to the CEJ. Histologic assessment cannot

Fig. 4-1. A, Marginal gingivitis. **B,** Acute necrotizing ulcerative gingivitis (ANUG) in a 25-year-old man (first episode). Note enlargement of tissue with blunting and necrosis of gingival margins, especially in interdental areas. **C,** Necrotizing ulcerative periodontitis (NUP) in a 27-year-old woman who suffered from 10 known episodes of necrotizing ulcerative gingivitis and now manifests periodontitis. **D,** Biafran child suffering from necrotizing ulcerative gingivitis. **E,** NUP in a 28-year-old man with HIV infection. **F,** Pregnancy "tumor" in a 24-year-old woman during last trimester of pregnancy. **G,** Gingival overgrowth in a 34-year-old amenorrheic woman with polycystic ovaries. **H,** Gingival overgrowth in a 16-year-old male heart transplant patient taking cyclosporine, nifedipine (Procardia), and prednisone. (**D** courtesy Dr. Aubrey Sheiham; **E** courtesy Dr. John Greenspan; **H** courtesy Dr. Thomas Van Dyke.) (See also Color Plate 1.)

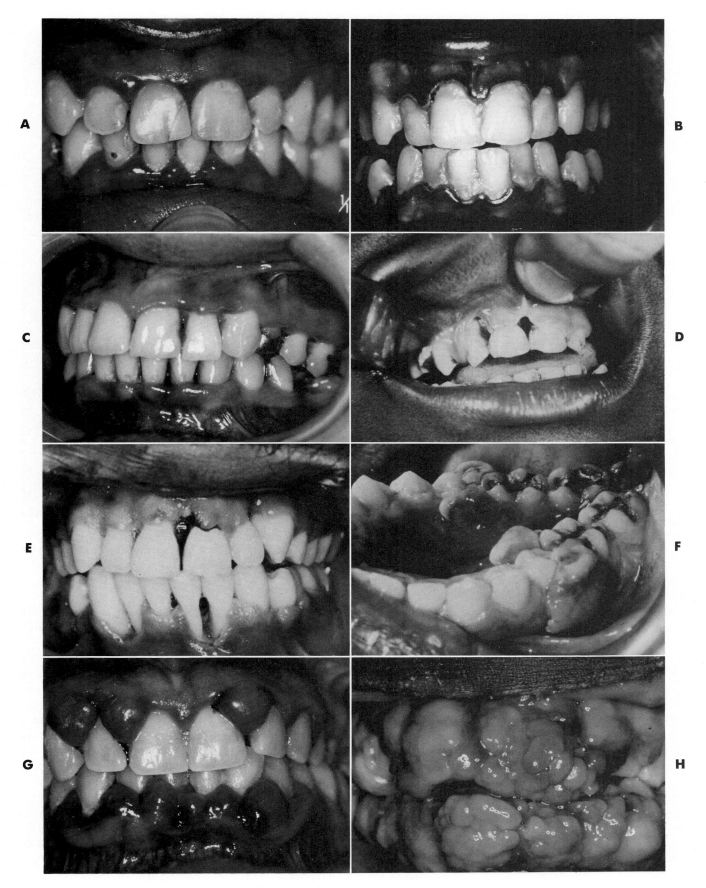

Fig. 4-1. For legend see opposite page.

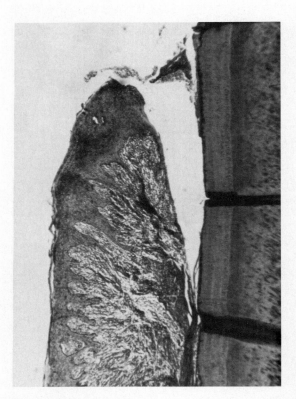

Fig. 4-2. Inflammatory infiltrate has almost completely replaced gingival connective tissue.

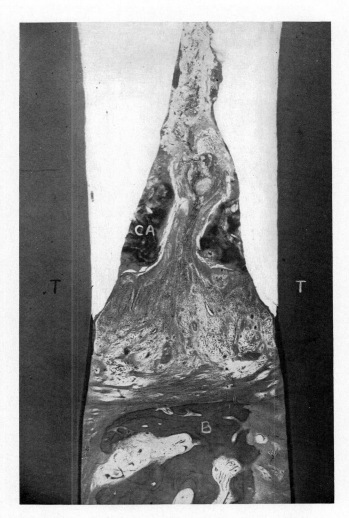

Fig. 4-3. Interdental tissue between mandibular central incisors. Junctional epithelium is still on enamel. Calculus is adherent to teeth. *T,* Tooth; *CA,* calculus; *B,* bone.

be used routinely for diagnosis; hence the clinical assessment of loss of attachment is based on periodontal probing. If periodontal attachment loss can be detected by probing (i.e., the tip of the probe is apical to the CEJ), the site is considered to have suffered from periodontitis. Periodontitis is often, but not always, associated with radiographic evidence of loss of the alveolar crest, but this is never found in gingivitis not complicated by periodontitis. The common form of gingivitis is caused by accumulation of supragingival plaque at the gingival margin; hence it is called marginal or plaque-induced gingivitis.

Acute necrotizing ulcerative gingivitis

Another, much less common, form of gingivitis is acute necrotizing ulcerative gingivitis (ANUG). It mainly affects teenagers and young adults who are often suffering from stress-related conditions. It is one of the few painful conditions of the gingiva and is also characterized by a sudden onset, with symptoms appearing in 1 or 2 days. ANUG is often seen as an ulcerated lesion covered with a white pseudomembrane, beginning at the tips of the interdental papillae and spreading laterally to involve the marginal gingiva and the base of the col (Fig. 4-1, *B*). ANUG has also been called trench mouth, fusospirochetal gingivitis, Vincent's gingivitis, and Plaut-Vincenti infection. There is a *lateral form of ANUG* affecting the lateral border of the

interdental papillae. The common form, however, begins at the tips of the interdental papillae and extends into the col and along the margin of the gingiva.

Similarities between ANUG and other acute necrotizing lesions. ANUG has a marked tendency to recur, and multiple episodes of recurrence may affect the underlying alveolar process and exhibit a characteristic form of periodontitis called *necrotizing ulcerative periodontitis (NUP)*. In NUP, there is loss of interdental alveolar bone and ulceration of the interdental gingival tissue (Fig. 4-1, *C*). This tissue loss is often irreversible, with "punched-out" interdental areas resulting. The above forms of ANUG are not associated with overt systemic disease; however, the gingival lesions seen in children suffering from severe malnutrition resemble ANUG in that they are often manifested as acute, painful, ulcerative lesions of the gingiva (Fig. 4-1, *D*). The gingival lesions seen in patients with acquired immunodeficiency disease (AIDS) may also resemble those seen in ANUG (Fig. 4-1, *E*), with ulcerative necrotic lesions present, especially in the interdental regions, in about 20% of AIDS patients.

Gingivitis with systemic involvement

Gingivitis and other gingival changes are markedly affected by a number of systemic conditions. Gingivitis associated with systemic conditions is relatively uncommon as compared with the common form of gingivitis that can occur in any healthy individual. The forms of gingivitis found with systemic involvement sometimes produce very dramatic changes, such as blood abnormalities, which are often the first indication of systemic disease. Gingivitis and gingival changes associated with systemic involvement are listed on p. 64.

The gingiva is markedly affected by sex hormones, with the development of enlargements and tumorlike projections during pregnancy (Fig. 4-1, *F*). Also, gingival enlargement is seen in diseases or conditions with altered female sex hormones. For example, the levels of luteinizing hormone and estradiol were elevated for several years in the 34-year-old amenorrheic woman suffering from polycystic ovaries shown in Fig. 4-1, *G*. Gingival changes are also seen in skin and mucous membrane diseases such as cicatricial pemphigoid and pemphigus (see Chapter 18). Gingival conditions seen in mucous membrane or skin diseases are often painful and are included in the category of *chronic desquamative gingivitis,* also called gingivosis. These painful lesions are distinct from inflammatory gingivitis lesions, although a patient most often exhibits both types of gingival lesions. Gingival changes are often early indicators of serious conditions such as acute leukemia, wherein gingival inflammation and bleeding are often seen. Granulomatous changes of the gingiva as seen in Wegener's granulomatosis and sarcoidosis also occur, and these are described in Chapter 20.

The gingiva may also be the target organ for infections with viruses such as herpes hominus. The gingiva may also be infected with *Candida albicans.* Various types of infective gingivostomatitis are described in Chapter 19.

The gingiva is remarkably sensitive to certain drugs, often responding with enlargement and overgrowth. Sometimes the overgrowth is so great that it covers the crowns of the teeth and interferes with mastication or results in tooth displacement. Phenytoin, a drug used commonly in treatment of epilepsy, has long been known to cause such gingival overgrowth. The dihydropyridines, including nifedipine (Procardia), used in the treatment of heart patients, have been shown to cause gingival changes and enlargement. Cyclosporine, an immunosuppressive drug used in transplantation, also has been shown to cause gingival enlargement (Fig. 4-1, *H*).

Other diseases can affect the gingiva, including gingival cysts, gingival fistulas, and neoplasms, and these are described in Chapter 22. There may be alterations of gingival architecture associated with trauma or muscle pull, resulting in gingival recession or gingival clefts. These aberrant frena or muscle attachments may also pull the gingival margin away from the tooth, leading to plaque accumulation and subsequent gingivitis and localized recession. The gingiva is also subject to granuloma or epulis formation and to abscess formation.

PERIODONTAL DISEASES AND CONDITIONS

The box on p. 65 shows a comprehensive list of diseases and conditions that affect the periodontal attachment apparatus, which comprises the alveolar process, the connective tissue attachment of the tooth to the bone, and the cementum. By far the most common form of periodontal disease is periodontitis in otherwise healthy adults, referred to simply as periodontitis or adult periodontitis. Periodontitis also occurs in juveniles, and localized juvenile periodontitis (LJP) or periodontosis represents a well-defined clinical entity occurring in teenagers and young adults. Periodontitis is often severe and of early onset in most patients with primary or secondary neutrophil disorders and other diseases in which neutrophil function is abnormal. Periodontitis is more severe and of higher prevalence in patients with diabetes mellitus and may be an infectious complication of that disease. Periodontitis also occurs in patients with other systemic diseases such as Ehlers-Danlos syndrome, Down's syndrome, histiocytosis, and sarcoidosis. Changes in the periodontal attachment apparatus may also occur in hypophosphatasia, hypoadrenocorticism, and hyperthroidism; however, these periodontal diseases are not often forms of true infectious periodontitis.

A series of conditions, including periodontal abscesses, periodontal cysts, root resorption, ankylosis, periodontal-pulpal communicating lesions, and infections associated with trauma can affect the periodontium. Detailed descriptions of neoplasms, systemic neutrophil disorders, and periodontal diseases in AIDS patients are given in Chapters 22, 16, and 23, respectively.

Periodontitis

The most common form of periodontitis occurs in adults. It may have an early onset; however, although it can occur in the first two decades of life, periodontitis is not as common in teenagers and young adults. A significant increase in prevalence occurs in the third to fourth decade of life. The absolute prevalence is dependent, however, on the criteria selected to define the disease. For example, using attachment loss as a criterion, over 75% of adults in a recent national survey in the United States suffered from periodontitis on the basis of having one or more sites of 4 mm or greater probing attachment loss. In this same survey 8% of adults suffered from severe periodontal disease, which was defined as one or more sites of 7 mm or greater attachment loss. Hence it can be seen that most of the adult population suffers from at least moderate periodontitis, whereas a smaller but significant portion of the population suffers from severe forms of periodontal disease. In contrast, LJP affects less than 1% of teenagers and young adults.

Moderately and rapidly progressing forms of periodontitis. From longitudinal studies of the natural history of periodontitis, two types of periodontal destruction have been described: a *moderately progressing periodontitis* and a *rapidly progressing periodontitis*. In a longitudinal study of untreated periodontitis in tea workers (Löe et al., 1986), subgroups were described that suffered from different rates of periodontal destruction. The bulk of the population (80%) experienced moderately progressing periodontitis; however, they did eventually suffer from loss of attachment ranging from 5 to 10 mm. In contrast, about 10% of the population suffered from the rapidly progressing form of periodontitis, which was initially more severe on the incisors and first molars but in the later stages occurred around all teeth, often leading to loss of teeth. The third group of about 10% were free of periodontal disease.

Rapidly progressing periodontitis was also observed in less than 10% of treated cases in the Hirschfeld and Wasserman study (1978) called "extreme downhill."

Application of the term *moderately* or *rapidly progressing periodontitis* to patients seen only once is not appropriate, since the rate of progression of disease over time must be measured to classify a patient on the basis of rate of progression of disease. This usually requires measurement at least two and preferably three or more times separated by several months to a year in order to obtain an assessment of the rate of periodontal progression with reasonable accuracy with present technology. New technologies with automated probes capable of measuring probing attachment levels in tenths of a millimeter and computer-assisted periodontal charting or sensitive quantitative computer-based radiographic techniques are used in clinical research and may soon be available for clinical practice to aid in the identification of patients with differing rates of periodontal breakdown. Identification of individual patients with rapidly progressing periodontitis will be of major importance in the clinical management of periodontitis. An example of a patient with rapidly progressing periodontitis is shown in Fig. 4-4.

Recurrent and refractory periodontitis. Periodontal disease diagnosis also can be based on the response to therapy. *Recurrent periodontitis* is defined as destruction of the attachment apparatus that occurs in a patient who was documented to have been successfully treated. *Recurrent periodontitis* in a patient represents a new episode of disease occurring some months or years after completion of successful therapy. This is a well-defined clinical condition and often results from inadequate maintenance with reinfection of patients after therapy. It should be noted that the prevalence of recurrence of periodontitis is unknown, but it appears to be relatively common and is likely to oc-

cur if adequate periodontal maintenance, both professionally and personally applied, is not achieved. It also appears to occur in localized areas, although in patients with lowered resistance to periodontal infections such as diabetics, it may be generalized. Recurrent periodontitis and progression of periodontitis after treatment are described in detail in Chapter 41.

Refractory periodontitis is defined as periodontitis that does not respond to conventional therapy. This term often refers to a patient in whom a single lesion or a few lesions do not respond to therapy. It is rare that most or all sites in a patient do not respond to therapy, although this can happen, especially if there is an underlying host susceptibility to periodontal infection as seen in uncontrolled diabetes. The difficulty with the definition of refractory periodontitis is that the thoroughness and adequacy of therapy are difficult to establish. For example, retained calculus is often found on teeth with persistent periodontal lesions that are eventually extracted. Hence what appears as refractory periodontitis may often result from incomplete therapy. However, in practice, individuals with refractory periodontitis can be defined as those who do not respond to well-documented, completed therapy that follows all of the principles of infection elimination, root preparation, elimination of all plaque retention areas, and motivation and demonstrated success of the patient in the practice of adequate plaque control. Haffajee et al. (1988) found that subjects with refractory periodontitis had deeper pockets and more attachment loss than those who responded well to treatment. The refractory patients also exhibited combinations of periodontal pathogens, including *B. gingivalis, B. intermedius, A. actinomycetemcomitans,* and *Fusobacterium nucleatum,* and elevated antibody responses to a wide range of gram-negative species, including *B. intermedius, F. nucleatum,* and *A. actinomycetemcomitans.*

Various combinations of the above terms have been used to describe periodontal diseases; however, this causes confusion. For example, the literature is replete with terms such as *refractory progressing periodontitis, generalized progressing periodontitis, refractory rapidly progressing periodontitis,* and various other combinations. These are all used with good intent; however, the definition of these conditions is oftentimes lacking, and their use is confusing. The terms *refractory, recurrent,* and *rapidly progressing* to describe periodontitis are best used for very *well defined patients* or groups who are clearly described and documented according to the guidelines given above. Unfortunately, these forms of the disease are diagnosed retrospectively at the present time. It is anticipated that the methodologies will become available to make a prospective diagnosis.

Other terminology

There is another definition of periodontitis that is often used in adults: *postlocalized juvenile periodontitis,* or *postperiodontosis.* A patient suffering from this condition is

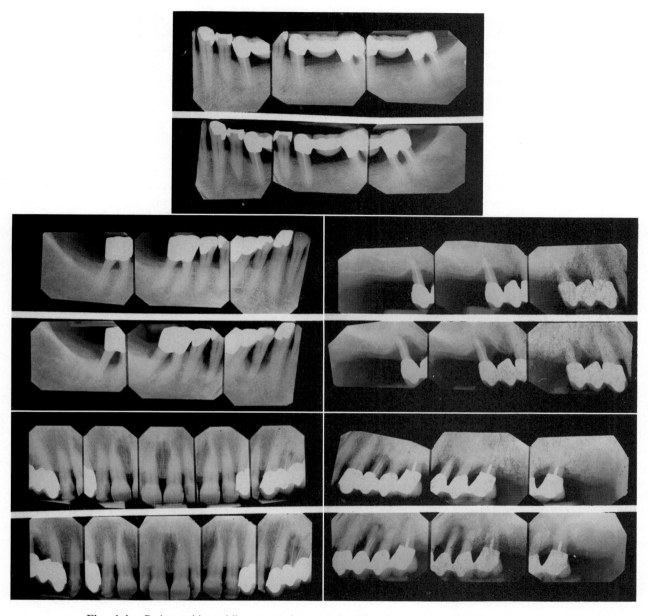

Fig. 4-4. Patient with rapidly progressing periodontitis. Upper radiographs in each set were taken 11 months earlier than lower radiographs of same area. (From Cohen DW: J Clin Periodontol 10:542, 1983. © 1983 Munksgaard International Publishers, Ltd., Copenhagen, Denmark.)

one who is documented as having suffered from juvenile periodontitis as a teenager or young adult. In later life, periodontitis may occur in such a patient either as recurrent disease or as a continuation of the original process. Although there is little evidence, it is strongly suggested that these patients are infected with *A. actinomycetemcomitans* and are often refractory to conventional therapy.

Another form of periodontal disease, which is based on history, is recurrent acute necrotizing ulcerative periodontitis, or necrotizing ulcerative periodontitis (NUP). These patients have a long history of several episodes of ANUG as young adults or teenagers and often as mature adults

suffer from periodontitis that is often characterized by loss of the interdental tissues. An example of such a patient is shown in Fig. 4-1, *E*.

Adult periodontitis

Clinical features. Periodontal disease is associated with the development of periodontal pocket depths and attachment loss apical to the CEJ. The attachment loss and periodontal pocket depths may be found on any surface of single-rooted or multirooted teeth and in furcations of multirooted teeth. The teeth with more advanced stages of disease are mobile, and they may exhibit "pathologic migration" or "wandering," with spaces developing between the teeth as they migrate out of their original position. Usually the maxillary or mandibular anterior teeth move labially. The pockets may bleed on probing, and there may be exudate coming from the pockets, which is either hemorrhagic, suppurative, or clear and watery. The gingiva may show a variety of changes; however, most commonly the gingiva exhibits redness, swelling, and inflammation, typical signs of gingivitis. The gingival connective tissue is often heavily infiltrated with round cells (see Fig. 4-2). In other patients or in other sites in patients suffering from periodontitis, the gingiva may show signs of fibrosis or recession, or may appear superficially healthy. At or near the gingival margin, supragingival and subgingival calculus and plaque accumulations are usually seen, particularly in those patients who have not had a recent dental prophylaxis.

Characteristic radiographic changes are also seen in periodontitis. On periapical and bitewing radiographs taken with good parallel technique, early lesions of the bone include development of cuplike lesions interproximally, with bone loss seen at the crest of the interproximal alveolar process, not yet involving the lamina dura. In more advanced cases reduced crestal height and loss of lamina dura occur (Fig. 4-5). If the bone loss involves most of the teeth at the same rate, *generalized,* or *horizontal,* bone loss will be seen (Fig. 4-6). Histopathologic changes associated with trauma from occlusion, including hemorrhage into a widened periodontal ligament and frontal resorption of bone, are shown in Fig. 4-6.

If alveolar bone loss progresses more rapidly in one site than in another, vertical bone loss will be seen (Fig. 4-7). Bone loss also can be seen between roots in furcations. In patients with advanced periodontitis, bone loss can extend to the apex of the teeth, in which case the prognosis is often poor. There may be a widened periodontal ligament space, areas of root resorption, and loss of lamina dura associated with infectious periodontitis; however, these changes are also seen in patients with adult periodontitis who are suffering from occlusal traumatism.

Histopathology.   Fig. 4-8 shows marginal periodontitis in the interdental area. It can be seen that the gingival subepithelial connective tissue contains a round cell infiltrate and that the junctional epithelium has lost its characteristic structure, with only the epithelial attachment intact. The remainder now appears as an irregular microulcerated structure with rete pegs, which is now termed the *pocket epithelium*. The base of the epithelial attachment is apical to the CEJ and is on the root surface. There is loss of connective tissue at or near the crest of the alveolar bone, often with crestal resorption (Fig. 4-8, *B*). In Fig. 4-9 inflammatory cells in and around the connective tissue forming the attachment can be seen in association with resorption of the alveolar process. Deep pocket formation extending apically along the root occurs with more severe loss. There is also associated loss of bony support. This is illustrated on the distal surface of the whole tooth sectioned in Fig. 4-10.

Periodontitis involving the furcation is illustrated in Fig. 4-11, where it can be seen that calculus is attached to the root surface in the furcation. Inflammatory cells are seen in the gingiva with evidence of bone resorption in the furcations. In severe deep pockets, histologic and radiographic evidence of root resorption is sometimes seen (Fig. 4-12). Buttressing bone is often formed in patients with chronic periodontal disease and can be observed on the external surface of the alveolar process, particularly in the maxillary and mandibular posterior regions, leading to ledgelike formations or lipping.

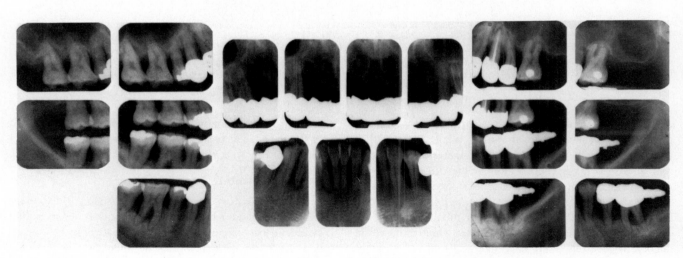

Fig. 4-5.   Periodontitis in a 49-year-old man. These radiographs illustrate both horizontal and vertical bone loss, as well as loss in furcation areas.

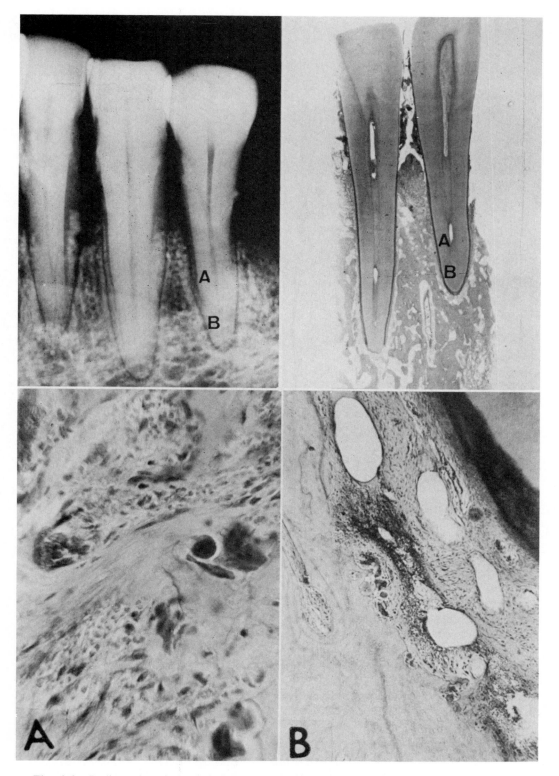

Fig. 4-6. Radiograph and photomicrographs illustrating changes in periodontal ligament histologically. Widening of periodontal ligament (*A* and *B)* is often radiographically diagnostic of occlusal trauma. Upper right photomicrograph can be used to orient higher-power photomicrographs, **A** and **B. A,** Osteoclasts can be seen in Howship's lacunae. **B,** Hemorrhage in periodontal ligament can be seen. Frontal resorption of bone is also prominent. (See Chapter 18 for description of trauma from occlusion.)

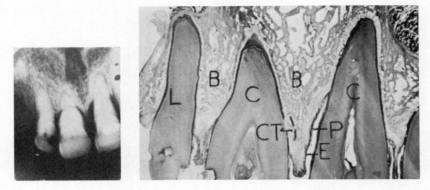

Fig. 4-7. Infrabony pocket on mesial aspect of left central incisor. *L,* Lateral incisor; *C,* central incisor; *B,* bone; *CT,* cemental tear; *P,* pocket; *E,* epithelium.

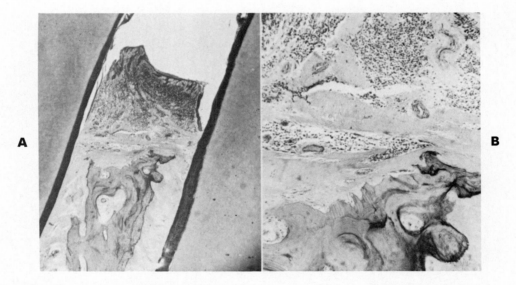

Fig. 4-8. Marginal periodontitis in interdental tissues. **A,** Gingival epithelium has migrated apically and is now situated on root surfaces of teeth. Note dense inflammatory infiltrate and thinned epithelial covering of gingiva. **B,** Crestal area of alveolar process is undergoing resorption. Note set of transseptal fibers above alveolar crest. Inflammatory infiltrate is interspersed between bundles of transseptal fiber group.

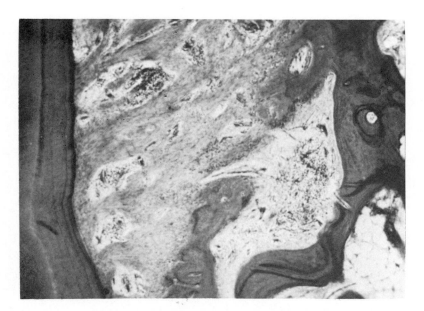

Fig. 4-9. Presence of inflammation throughout transseptal fiber bundles spreading into crestal bone. At periodontal surfaces of this alveolar septum, active remodeling is taking place, including osteogenesis.

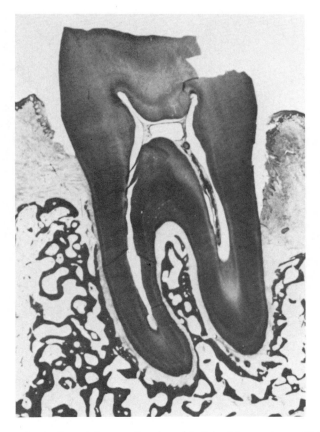

Fig. 4-10. More advanced crestal resorption is evident in this specimen. Note also, widened periodontal ligament, probably associated with trauma from occlusion.

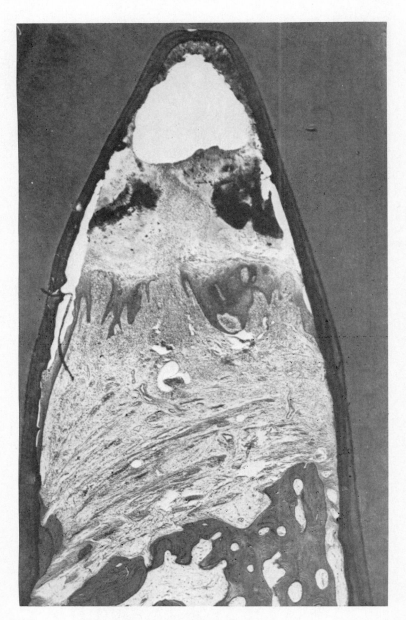

Fig. 4-11.   Bifurcation involvement in mandibular molar. Note calculus adjacent to gingival tissue and adherent to tooth surface. Gingival inflammation is evident.

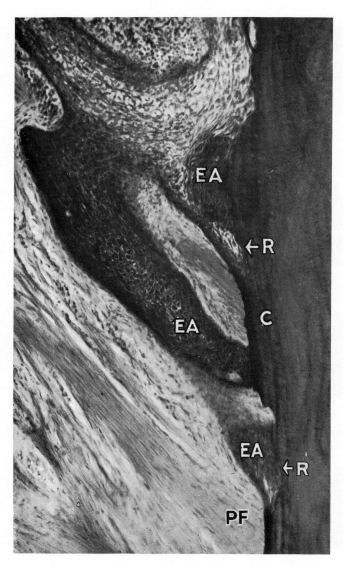

Fig. 4-12. Junctional epithelium proliferating over resorptive areas of cementum. An area of principal fibers of periodontal ligament can be seen at *C*. These bundles are bypassed by lateral ingrowths of epithelial attachment where there are no principal fibers present. *C*, Cementum; *EA*, epithelial attachment; *PF*, principal fibers; *R*, resorption.

Periodontitis in juveniles

Periodontitis is rare in humans in the first decade of life; however, when it does occur, it is often associated with severe systemic disease, including neutrophil adherence abnormalities, cyclic neutropenia, and agranulocytosis, or with other conditions such as the Papillon-LeFèvre syndrome (see Chapter 16). Periodontitis may also occur in prepubertal children who do not have overt systemic disease, but it is rare and, when seen, often occurs in families with other siblings affected with LJP. Noninflammatory periodontal attachment apparatus disease is also seen in children who suffer from hypophosphatasia (see Chapter 20).

Localized juvenile periodontitis. LJP occurs most often in teenagers and young adults. In this age group the overall prevalence of LJP is 0.1%, with a prevalence of 0.8% in blacks, 0.2% in Asians, and 0.02% in whites (Saxby, 1984).

LJP is characterized by pocket formation, connective tissue attachment loss, and alveolar bone loss affecting mainly first molars and incisors. It may occasionally include premolars and second molars. As a result of recent research, LJP is one of the best understood forms of periodontal disease, with a clear delineation of the important bacterial and host-bacterial interactions. Probably because of our understanding of the disease, it can often be treated successfully with remarkable bone growth in pockets (Zambon et al., 1986). Hørmand and Frandsen (1979) described over 150 cases of juvenile periodontitis, and they have distinguished LJP from generalized periodontitis (GJP). They have proposed that these two forms of juvenile periodontitis are discrete, with the localized variety often seen in younger individuals. The localized form is self-limiting, whereas the generalized form may continue to include severe destruction of the entire periodontium. It appears, then, that the two entities, LJP and GJP, are clinically and radiographically distinct, and there is evidence accumulating that they are associated with different bacteria: *A. actinomycetemcomitans* in LJP and *B. gingivalis* and others in GJP.

LJP has a familial tendency (Cohen and Goldman, 1960). Fig. 4-13 shows three sisters suffering from LJP in a family of eight children and illustrates the localization and familial patterns of LJP. Numerous studies have documented the familial tendency of the disease. For example, in a large study by Van Dyke et al. (1985), 22 families were evaluated. All families were enrolled by a proband who suffered from LJP. There is a marked tendency for juvenile periodontitis to occur in these families, with a prevalence of periodontitis in the siblings of these families of approximately 50%, as compared with the less than 1% prevalence that would be expected for a random nonrelated population in this age range (Fig. 4-14, *A*).

Neutrophil chemotactic disorders (reduced migration of

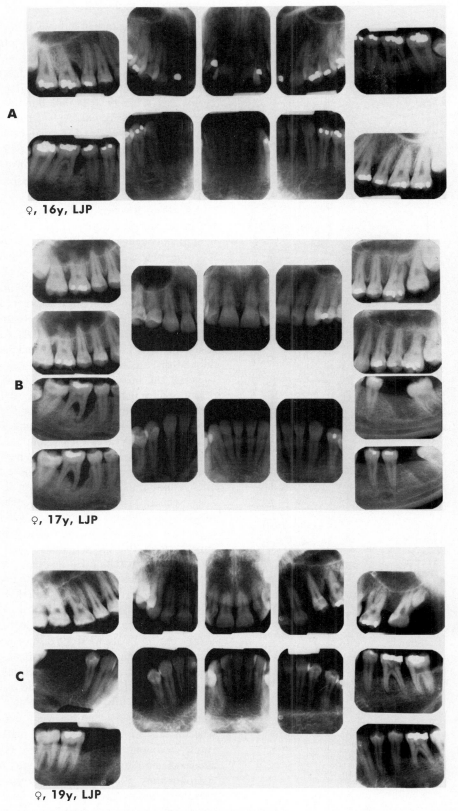

Fig. 4-13. Three sisters in a family suffering from LJP: **A,** 16-year-old; **B,** 17-year-old; and **C,** 19-year-old. Note molar and incisor bone loss characteristic of LJP. All three sisters were infected with *A. actinomycetemcomitans* and had neutrophil chemotactic defects.

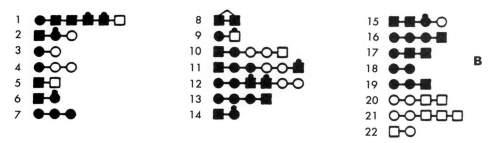

Fig. 4-14. **A,** Patients suffering from LJP in 22 families are represented by solid black figures. Proband in each family is at left. **B,** Diagrammatic representation of sibships involved in study group. In each family, proband is at extreme left. Solid black figures represent patients exhibiting depressed neutrophil chemotaxis. In this group, without correcting for sampling bias, incidence of neutrophil defects is 65.3%. Number of each family (1 to 22) corresponds to number in Fig. 4-13, *A*. ⬛ Identical twins. (From Van Dyke TE et al.: J Periodont Res 20:503, 1985. © 1985 Munksgaard International Publishers, Ltd., Copenhagen, Denmark.)

neutrophils to a chemotactic agent) are also found in about 70% of patients with LJP. The defects in chemotaxis are also found in nondiseased siblings in families with LJP (Fig. 4-14, *B),* suggesting that the reduced neutrophil function precedes the disease and may be related to the increased susceptibility of patients to LJP (Van Dyke et al., 1985).

Clinically, LJP patients rarely show calculus or plaque formation and often exhibit little or no gingivitis. However, bleeding on deep probing is almost always seen in sites where pocket depth, attachment loss, and radio-graphic bone loss are seen, suggesting that there is inflammation deep in the tissue. This is confirmed by the histologic finding of inflammatory cell accumulation in the connective tissue and widening of the intercellular spaces in the epithelium adjacent to lesion sites of LJP patients. Radiographically, the affected first molars and incisors show mesial and distal bone loss, which often exhibits bilateral symmetry. The bone loss sometimes involves furcations but often does not. Deep interproximal vertical bone loss on first molars and incisors is characteristic of LJP (see Fig. 4-13).

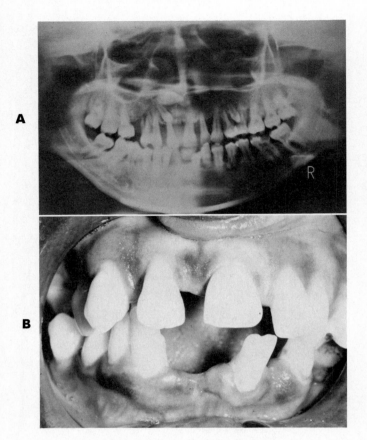

Fig. 4-15. A, Panoramic radiograph of a 13-year-old patient with severely generalized periodontitis. **B,** Clinical photograph of same 13-year-old patient. This patient was infected with *B. gingivalis, A. actinomycetemcomitans,* and *B. intermedius.* She also suffered from a neutrophil chemotactic defect. (From Wilson et al: J Periodontol 56:457, 1985.)

60% of the structures are noncellular, with about 15% composed of collagen and the rest residual tissue. Another qualitative difference is the infiltration by organisms seen in juvenile periodontitis. Here, infiltrating *A. actinomycetemcomitans* is commonly seen in the epithelium and in the deep connective tissue of the gingiva. These cells appear to be viable, since they can be cultured from the tissue biopsy specimens. The *A. actinomycetemcomitans* organisms are seen as small groups or clumps of bacteria and also appear within cells that appear to be phagocytes (Christersson et al., 1987a, 1987b).

Generalized juvenile periodontitis. This condition affects older teenagers and young adults. The mean age of GJP patients is slightly greater than that of LJP patients. The prevalence is unknown but is probably much less than that of LJP. It may represent two or more types of periodontal diseases affecting juveniles, including patients who have early-onset adult periodontitis and others who have had LJP that has progressed to a more generalized form. There is often severe gingival inflammation with extensive plaque and calculus formation and associated gingival inflammation. This gingival inflammation differentiates it from localized juvenile periodontitis. In GJP the gingiva has been described as sometimes being bright red, or "angry looking," with suppurative pockets and generalized bone loss affecting most of the teeth. In Fig. 4-15 a 13-year-old suffering from GJP is depicted (Wilson et al., 1985). As can be seen, there has been tooth loss and bone loss, both generalized and vertical. Like many others who have been studied, this GJP patient suffers from a neutrophil chemotactic disorder, and often the prognosis for long-term retention of the teeth is poor.

Histopathologically, the lesions of LJP resemble those found in adult periodontitis. There is widening of intercellular spaces in the epithelium and migration of the junctional epithelium apical to the CEJ, with conversion of the juctional epithelium to inflamed pocket epithelium with multiple rete peg formation. The subjacent connective tissue is infiltrated with inflammatory cells, with plasma cells and blast cells constititing about 70% of the volume of the lesion. In contrast, in adult periodontitis the blast cell and plasma cell population constitutes about 35% of the inflammatory lesion (Lindhe, 1982). There is a report of aplastic or hypoplastic cementum in juvenile periodontitis, and, if substantiated in most patients, this may explain some of the localization of the lesion.

Another difference between the infiltrated connective tissue in juvenile periodontitis as compared with adult periodontitis is that in juvenile periodontitis lesions about 20% of the structures are noncellular (i.e., collagen or residual tissue). In contrast, in adult periodontitis 50% to

REFERENCES

American Academy of Periodontology: Current procedural terminology for periodontics, ed 5, 1986.

Christersson LA et al: Tissue localization of *Actinobacillus actinomycetemcomitans* in human periodontitis. I. Light, immunofluorescence and electron microscopic studies, J Periodontol 58:529, 1987a.

Christersson LA et al: Tissue localization of *Actinobacillus actinomycetemcomitans* in human periodontitis. II. Correlation between immunofluorescence and culture techniques, J Periodontol 58:540, 1987b.

Cohen DW and Goldman HM: Clinical observation on the modification of human oral tissue metabolism by local intraoral factors, NY Acad Sci 85:68, 1960.

Gottlieb B: Periodontal pyorrhea and alveolar atrophy, J Am Dent Assoc 15:2196. 1928.

Haffajee AD et al: Clinical and microbiologic features of subjects with refractory periodontal diseases, J Clin Periodontol 15:390, 1988.

Hirschfeld L and Wasserman B: A long-term survey of tooth loss in 600 treated periodontal patients, J Periodontol 49:225, 1978.

Hørmand J and Frandsen A: Juvenile periodontitis: localization of bone loss in relation to age, sex, and teeth, J Clin Periodontol 6:407, 1979.

Lindhe J: Treatment of localized juvenile periodontitis. In Mergenhagen SE and Genco RJ, editors: Host-parasite interactions in periodontal diseases, Washington, DC, 1982, ASM Publications.

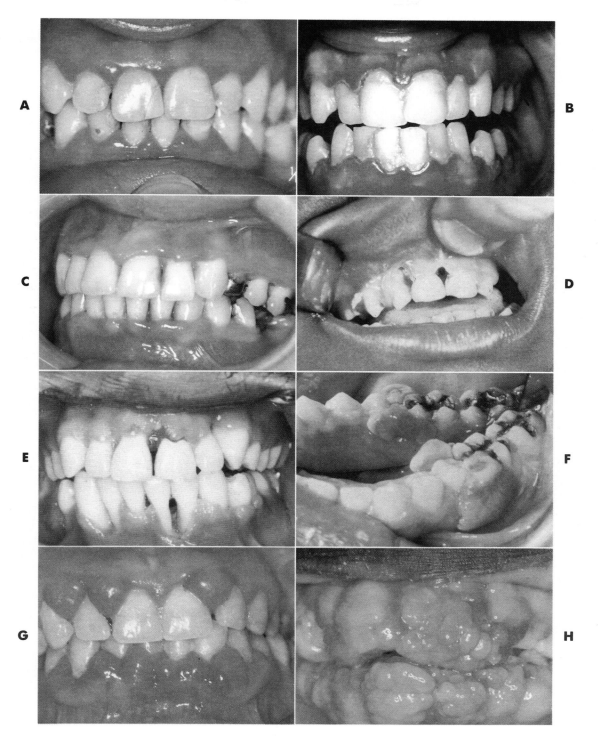

Plate 1. **A,** Marginal gingivitis. **B,** Acute necrotizing ulcerative gingivitis (ANUG) in a 25-year-old man (first episode). Note enlargement of tissue with blunting and necrosis of gingival margins, especially in interdental areas. **C,** Necrotizing ulcerative periodontitis (NUP) in a 27-year-old woman who suffered from 10 known episodes of necrotizing ulcerative gingivitis and now manifests periodontitis. **D,** Biafran child suffering from necrotizing ulcerative gingivitis. **E,** NUP in a 28-year-old man with HIV infection. **F,** Pregnancy "tumor" in a 24-year-old woman during last trimester of pregnancy. **G,** Gingival overgrowth in a 34-year-old amenorrheic woman with polycystic ovaries. **H,** Gingival overgrowth in a 16-year-old male heart transplant patient taking cyclosporine, nifedipine (Procardia), and prednisone. (**D** courtesy Dr. Aubrey Sheiham; **E** courtesy Dr. John Greenspan; **H** courtesy Dr. Thomas Van Dyke.) (See also Fig. 4-1.)

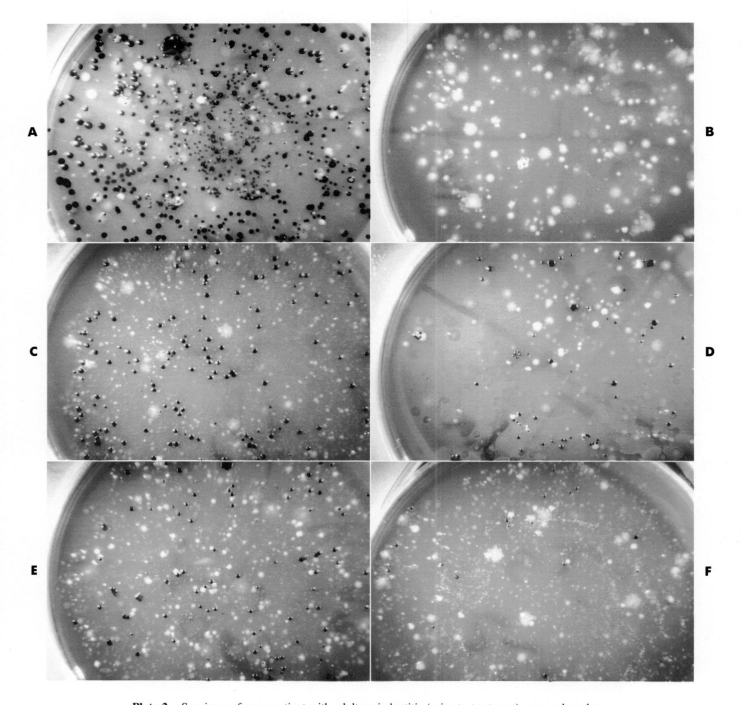

Plate 2. Specimens from a patient with adult periodontitis (prior to treatment) were cultured under anaerobic conditions using media supporting the growth of black-pigmented *Bacteroides*. Subgingival plaque was cultured; *B. gingivalis* and *B. intermedius* were present. *B. gingivalis* colonies are brown, and those of *B. intermedius* are black. Both types were also cultivated in specimens from gingival surface cultured at 10^{-2}, from saliva cultured at 10^{-4}, from tongue cultured at 10^{-3}, and from tonsil cultured at 10^{-2}. **A,** Subgingival plaque at 10^{-3} dilution. **B,** Supragingival plaque at 10^{-3} dilution was cultured, and no detectable black-pigmented *Bacteroides* were seen. **C,** Gingiva. **D,** Saliva. **E,** Tongue. **F,** Tonsil. (See also Fig. 11-1.)

Löe H et al: Natural history of periodontal disease in man: rapid, moderate and no loss of attachment in Sri Lankan laborers 14 to 46 years of age, J Clin Periodontol 13:431, 1986.

McCall JO and Box HK: Chronic periodontitis, J Am Dent Assoc 12:1300, 1925.

Saxby M: Prevalence of juvenile periodontitis in a British school population, Commun Dent Oral Epidemiol 12:185, 1984.

Van Dyke TE et al: Neutrophil chemotaxis in families with localized juvenile periodontitis, J Periodont Res 20:503, 1985.

Weski O: Paradentopathia and paradentosis, Paradentium 8:169, 1937.

Wilson M et al: Generalized juvenile periodontitis, defective neutrophil chemotaxis and *Bacteroides gingivalis* in a 13-year-old female, J Periodontol 56:457, 1985.

Zambon JJ, Christersson LA, and Genco RJ: Diagnosis and treatment of localized juvenile periodontitis, J Am Dent Assoc 113:295, 1986.

Chapter 5

ULTRASTRUCTURAL CHANGES IN PERIODONTAL DISEASES

Knut A. Selvig

Developing gingivitis
Chronic gingivitis
Periodontitis
Acute necrotizing ulcerative gingivitis
Localized juvenile periodontitis
Collagen degradation in periodontal diseases
Dental cuticle
Exposed cementum

Studies of periodontal tissues in health and disease by electron microscopy and other ultrastructural techniques have contributed to a more complete understanding of the tissue reactions involved and have helped bridge the gap between the classic, histologic approach to the study of pathology on the one hand, and the biochemistry and immunology of the disease process on the other. Ultrastructural analysis has permitted a more precise identification of the various cell types present in gingival tissues, an evaluation of their functional state, and an estimation of the volume fraction occupied by cells and intercellular components during different stages of an inflammatory reaction in the gingiva. The exact figures derived from such morphometric analyses may show great individual variations; however, the trends that they reveal have been helpful in supplementing the concepts of pathogenesis of periodontal diseases that have evolved from microbiologic and immunologic studies.

For didactic reasons, it is convenient to describe ultrastructural changes as they gradually appear when an inflammatory reaction is initiated by allowing bacterial plaque to accumulate in contact with previously healthy gingival tissues. Early stages of naturally developing gingivitis have been examined ultrastructurally in the gingiva of recently erupted temporary and permanent teeth. In addition, the acute inflammatory response and the establishment of a chronic inflammatory lesion have been studied experimentally both in humans and in laboratory animals.

DEVELOPING GINGIVITIS

Biopsy specimens of clinically healthy gingival tissues always show the presence of a small number of inflammatory cells. This is not considered to represent pathologic change but indicates the constant readiness of the host defense systems as a result of continuous exposure to a commensal oral bacterial flora. Moreover, neutrophils, macrophages, lymphocytes, and plasma cells are present in gingival tissues of germ-free experimental animals as well, indicating that in addition to bacterial products, various antigens originating in the oral cavity are capable of penetrating the epithelial barrier and give rise to a complex reaction in the adjacent connective tissue (Listgarten and Heneghan, 1971; Garant, 1976).

The acute inflammatory response in the connective tissue corresponding to the base of the gingival sulcus, which occurs within 2 to 4 days if bacterial plaque is allowed to accumulate in contact with the gingival epithelium, can be detected histologically and ultrastructurally before any signs of developing gingivitis can be seen clinically (Payne et al., 1975). Large numbers of neutrophils appear extravascularly in response to the generation of chemotactic substances by the plaque bacteria. Exudation of serum and serum proteins results in the formation of edematous spaces and deposition of fibrin in the connective tissue.

Within the junctional epithelium and the deepest part of the sulcular epithelium, the volume fraction of leukocytes may increase from 2% to 3% in the strictly healthy gingiva to 6% to 7% at this stage (Schroeder et al., 1975). Initially, the major portion of these cells are neutrophils (Fig. 5-1), although lymphocytes and other mononuclear cells are also present (Payne et al., 1975). Intercellular spaces appear dilated while the epithelial cells maintain contact at desmosomal attachments. The leukocytes within the epithelium do not have desmosomal attachment to surrounding epithelial cells.

Ultrastructurally, the neutrophils are readily identifiable by their deeply lobated nucleus and numerous cytoplasmic granules. The lymphocytes have an oval or indented nucleus with peripheral chromatin, a small amount of cyto-

plasm, and a relatively sparse distribution of rough endoplasmic reticulum and other organelles (Fig. 5-1).

With continued plaque accumulation, more extensive alterations, recognized as the *early lesion,* develop within 4 to 7 days (Payne et al., 1975). A dense cellular infiltrate is formed adjacent to the deepest portion of the sulcular epithelium, consisting predominantly of lymphocytes with a few plasma cells and macrophages. The lymphoid character of the infiltrate is a reflection of the cell-mediated immunologic reaction that is initiated at this stage of the disease. In addition, signs of acute inflammatory reaction persist. Thus extravascular neutrophils may also be increased in number and tend to aggregate immediately subjacent to the epithelial basement lamina.

While the density of cells in the infiltrated portion of the connective tissue increases, the amount of collagen is correspondingly reduced. Up to 70% of the collagen fraction may be lost within the first 4 days of an experimentally induced gingivitis (Payne et al., 1975; Schroeder et al., 1975). Also, the number of fibroblasts residing within the infiltrated region is decreased, and the remaining cells may show characteristic cytotoxic alterations (Fig. 5-2). These include enlargement and dilation of mitochondria, swelling and vacuolization of the rough endoplasmic reticulum, decreased density of nuclear chromatin, and an up to threefold increase in cell size (Schroeder et al., 1973; Simpson and Avery, 1973, 1974). Despite their increased size, the altered fibroblasts have a reduced rather than an increased capacity for collagen biosynthesis. Frequently a direct contact between lymphoid cells and altered fibroblasts can be seen, suggesting that the cell injury is effected by sensitized lymphocytes (Schroeder and Page, 1972; Simpson and Avery, 1973).

Within the junctional and sulcular epithelium, the number of neutrophils and various mononuclear leukocytes is greatly increased in the early lesion and may constitute more than 50% of the volume of these epithelia (Schroeder, 1970). When this is the case, the junctional continuity between the epithelial cells may be lost and the integrity of the epithelial barrier is altered. The neutrophils migrate through the epithelium toward the gingival sulcus where they function by phagocytosing bacteria. In this process the bacteria are engulfed in phagocytic vacuoles (Brecx and Patters, 1985) (Fig. 5-3). Subsequently, the neutrophil granules, which contain enzymes capable of catabolizing most cellular macromolecules, are released into the phagocytic vacuole. Free lysosomal bodies indicative of neutrophil degranulation and cell death may, however, also be seen. In contrast to the neutrophils, most of the lymphoid cells, which are important in antigen recognition, find their way back into the connective tissue. Thus, although the lymphocytes may make up a majority of the leukocytes residing within the epithelium at this stage, they contribute only 1% to 4% of the leukocytes that can be harvested from the gingival sulcus.

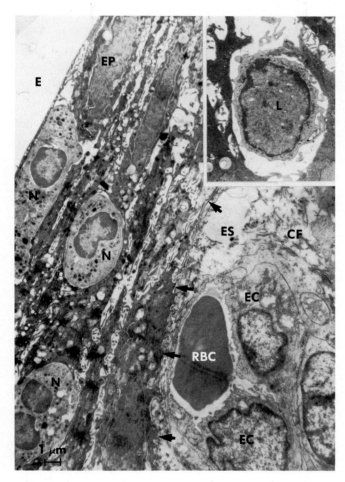

Fig. 5-1. Neutrophils *(N)* infiltrating junctional epithelium in initial stage of gingival inflammation. A capillary containing a red blood cell *(RBC)* is located very close to epithelial basement lamina *(arrows).* Two endothelial cells *(EC)* have been sectioned through nucleus. Note edematous spaces *(ES)* and scattered collagen fibrils *(CF)* in connective tissue. *Inset:* Lymphocyte *(L)* within sulcular epithelium. Inflammatory cells do not have desmosomal attachments to epithelial cells. *E,* Space left after demineralization of enamel; *EP,* epithelial cell.

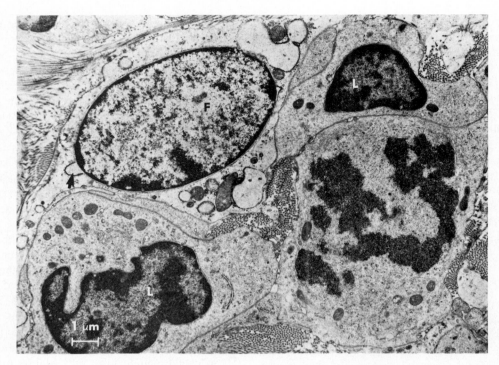

Fig. 5-2.   Gingival fibroblast *(F)* in intimate relationship to group of large lymphocytes *(L)* in early inflammatory lesion. Cell at right of field is in mitosis and also appears to be a lymphocyte. Fibroblast shows early ultrastructural alterations that may affect its capacity for collagen biosynthesis: decreased density of nuclear chromatin and dilation of rough endoplasmic reticulum and perinuclear space *(arrow)*. (From Simpson DE and Avery BE: J Periodontol 45:500, 1974.)

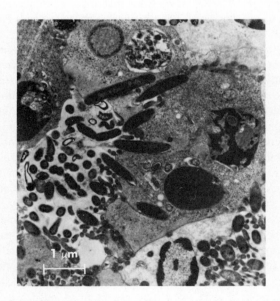

Fig. 5-3.   Phagocytosis of bacteria by neutrophils in gingival sulcus. (From Brecx M and Patters MR: J Clin Periodontol 12:591, 1985. © 1985 Munksgaard International Publishers, Ltd., Copenhagen, Denmark.)

CHRONIC GINGIVITIS

Provided that the inflammatory agent—the bacterial plaque—continues to be present, further accumulation of inflammatory cells occurs, resulting in an expansion of the cellular infiltrate laterally and apically until a balance is established between the intensity of chemotactic and antigenic stimulation on the one hand and the amount of defense forces mounted by the host organism on the other. Under experimental conditions, chronic gingivitis may develop after several weeks of plaque accumulation (Zachrisson, 1968; Page and Schroeder, 1976). When gingivitis develops naturally following eruption of temporary or permanent teeth, however, ultrastructural features intermediate between those of the early and established lesion may persist for an extended period of time (Schroeder et al., 1973; Longhurst et al., 1980).

Although the chronic gingivitis shows features characteristic of chronic inflammation, the continuous presence of the infectious agent results in the persistence of signs of acute inflammatory reaction superimposed on the chronic reaction. In a biopsy specimen these combined factors result in a characteristic layered distribution of the inflammatory cells within the infiltrated connective tissue. Neutrophils tend to form a more or less continuous layer near the basement lamina, overlying a zone of lymphoid cells

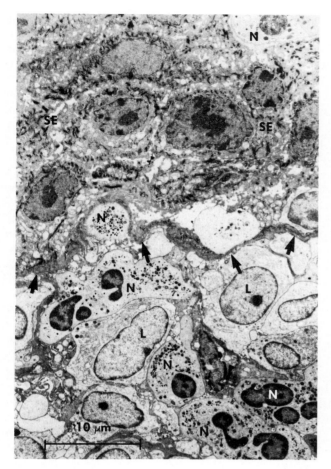

Fig. 5-4. Sulcular epithelium *(SE)* and connective tissue infiltrate in established inflammatory lesion. Numerous neutrophils *(N)* and lymphocytes *(L)* have aggregated near base of epithelium *(arrows)*. Some inflammatory cells are in process of migrating into epithelium. Deeper levels of same biopsy specimen are illustrated in Figs. 5-5 and 5-6.

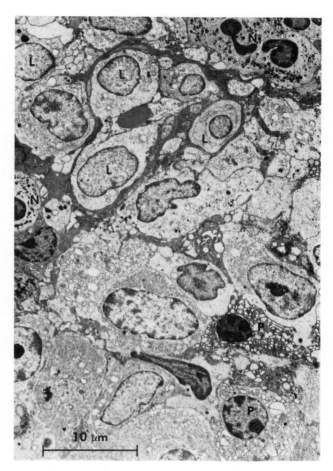

Fig. 5-5. Cellular distribution in infiltrate immediately deep to area seen in Fig. 5-4. Lymphocyte *(L)* is predominating cell at this level. Note dense packing of inflammatory cells and almost complete absence of intercellular spaces. *N,* Neutrophil; *P,* plasma cell.

(Figs. 5-4 and 5-5). Neutrophils are also present deeper in the lesion where they may show phagocytic activity, as well as discharge of lysosomal granules. The chronic nature of the lesion is demonstrated, however, by the large number of plasma cells that predominate in the body of the lesion and may now constitute up to 90% of the total cellular infiltrate (Fig. 5-6). The plasma cell is identified in both the light and electron microscopes primarily by its round or oval nucleus and characteristic clumping of chromatin along the nuclear periphery. Ultrastructurally, the plasma cell also shows a distinct Golgi apparatus and a regular arrangement of densely packed lamellae of rough endoplasmic reticulum in the cytoplasm. These features are consistent with the high protein-synthesizing activity of this cell. Since plasma cells may form locally from lymphocytes within the gingival connective tissue and perform their function within this region, lymphocytes in mitosis,

cells with ultrastructural detail intermediate between lymphocytes and plasma cells (blast cells), and both young and old plasma cells are seen. Older or injured plasma cells show dilated cisternae of rough endoplasmic reticulum and rupture of the cell membrane (Freedman et al., 1968) (Fig. 5-6).

In addition, a small number of macrophages and mast cells continue to be present (Figs. 5-7 and 5-8). Mast cell degranulation results in the release of histamine, proteases, and other substances that may enhance the inflammatory reaction.

A striking observation when the cellular infiltrate is examined by electron microscopy is the dense clumping of the various cells and vascular elements in some areas, with the intercellular compartment constituting only a very small fraction of the tissue volume (see Figs. 5-4 to 5-6). Close cell contact may be an important feature of the cel-

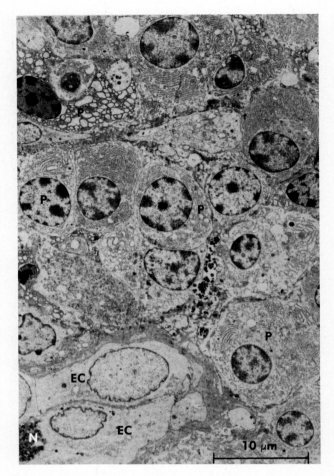

Fig. 5-6. Cellular distribution in connective tissue infiltrate approximately 100 μm deep to area seen in Fig. 5-5. Body of lesion consists almost exclusively of plasma cells *(P)*. One of these cells *(upper left-hand corner)* shows degenerative changes, including pyknotic nucleus and distended cisternae of rough endoplasmic reticulum. In lower left-hand corner is a capillary containing a neutrophil *(N)*. *EC,* Endothelial cell.

lular infiltrate, since the development of an adequate immune response requires that biologically active substances released by one cell are received by another, a process that presumably is effective only over very short distances. Collagen may be virtually absent within the body of the infiltrate in the lesion of chronic gingivitis.

Other portions of infiltrated connective tissue may show wider intercellular spaces containing large amounts of free lysosomal bodies and other granular and membranous particles that are evidence of cell degradation and death (Fig. 5-8). In particular, neutrophils, which have a very short life span after degranulation, and plasma cells, which are end cells, contribute to the accumulation of large amounts of cell debris.

Epithelial alterations associated with the inflammatory lesion of chronic gingivitis include extensive rete peg for-

mation in the sulcular and junctional epithelium, resulting in an increase in the total amount of epithelium present. Paradoxically, however, areas of epithelial proliferation may alternate with areas where the epithelial lining is extremely thin (Fig. 5-9) or even discontinuous.

The number of leukocytes within the sulcular and junctional epithelium at any one time shows large individual and local variations and is not necessarily related to the extension of the connective tissue infiltrate or to gingival health as determined by clinical indices.

Despite the close proximity of microbial plaque to a structurally compromised sulcular and junctional epithelium, bacterial cells do not generally penetrate the epithelial barrier in nonspecific, chronic gingivitis. Most often, the bacterial plaque is separated from the epithelial surface by a layer of neutrophils showing signs of active phagocytosis. In localized areas, however, bacterial aggregations may occur in direct contact with the epithelial surface, and bacterial cells may be seen invading the intercellular space as well as within degenerating epithelial cells (Fig. 5-9). More extensive bacterial invasion occurs in acute necrotizing ulcerative gingivitis and in localized juvenile periodontitis.

The basement lamina of the sulcular and junctional epithelium generally remains intact but may show a number of localized alterations, including interruptions and thinning, as well as thickening, duplication, and the presence of detached basement lamina material in the subjacent connective tissue (Freedman et al., 1968; Levy et al., 1969; Takarada et al., 1974a, 1974b). Such changes have been described in a number of other epithelia in different disease states and appear to represent a nonspecific response to the inflammatory process. The basement lamina surrounding capillaries and venules in the infiltrated region may show similar alterations (Freedman et al., 1968; Gavin, 1970).

PERIODONTITIS

In periodontitis, the connective tissue alterations seen in the established lesion have spread in an apical direction, so that the dentogingival and dentoalveolar collagen fibers are affected. The cellular infiltrate and the process of collagen degradation tend to progress apically at a distance from the root surface rather than close to the cementum. Characteristically, osteoclastic resorption at the crest of the alveolar bone results in loss of anchorage of the principal fibers of the periodontal ligament, whereas the cementum surface is relatively resistant to resorption. Eventually, however, the inflammatory process results in complete breakdown of the collagen fibers, as well as of individual fibrils along the root surface (Figs. 5-10 to 5-12). These events occur within 0.5 to 1 mm apical to the base of the pocket epithelium (Selvig, 1966, 1968; Deporter and Brown, 1980). Further apically, fiber attachment to the cementum appears normal.

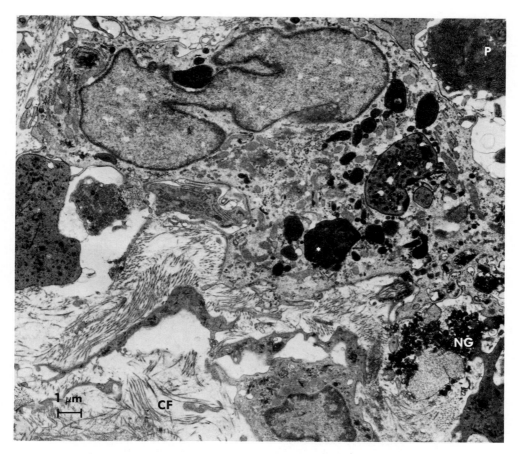

Fig. 5-7. Macrophage engaged in phagocytosis of a degenerated neutrophil. Fragments of neutrophil cytoplasm are contained within phagosomes. Aggregates of neutrophil granules *(NG)* are present extracellularly. *CF*, Collagen fibrils; *P*, plasma cell.

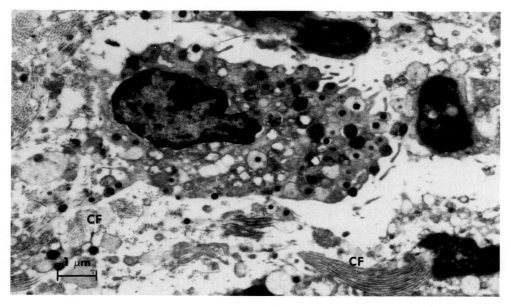

Fig. 5-8. Mast cell in process of degranulation. Several other degenerating, unidentified cells with pyknotic nuclei can also be seen. Intercellular space contains a variety of granular and membranous particles as a result of cell death. *CF*, Collagen fibrils.

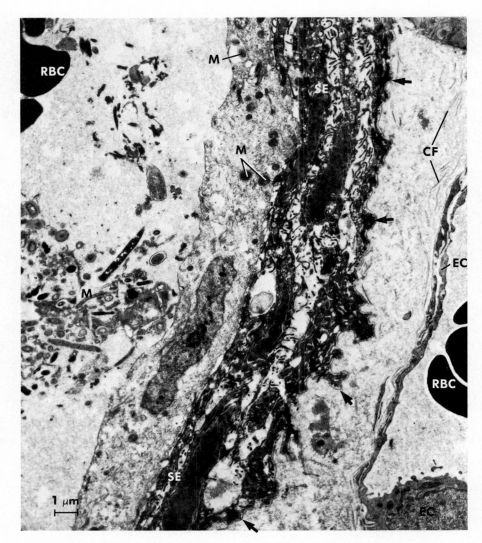

Fig. 5-9. Extremely thin sulcular epithelium *(SE),* consisting of only three to four cells, in contact with subgingival bacterial plaque. Despite enlarged intercellular spaces, microbial invasion in this instance is limited to outermost, degenerating epithelial cell layer. Epithelium-connective tissue interface is marked by arrows. Red blood cells *(RBC)* and granular precipitate are present within a small blood vessel *(right),* as well as in sulcus *(left).* CF, Collagen fibrils; EC, endothelial cell; M, microrganism.

The reasons for the relative immunity of the cementum surface to resorption in marginal periodontitis as compared with bone tissue have been a subject of much speculation. A similar difference is seen apically during the development of apical granulomas and cysts. Since cementum is formed very slowly and generally is not subject to remodeling, its organic and inorganic constituents become more stable at the molecular level and more resistant to subtle environmental changes. Similarly, collagen fibers near the cementum have a low metabolic turnover rate and presumably are more highly cross-linked than those located more peripherally. The surface layer of the cementum contains more fluoride than does bone tissue (Yoon et al., 1960), resulting in greater stability of its mineral crystals against dissolution in acids produced by clast cells. Most important, there are no blood vessels in the cementum and far less vascularization of the connective tissue occurs near the root surface than occurs near the alveolar bone. Because of these factors, cementum is normally excluded to a great extent from metabolic processes and consequently remains largely unaffected by pathologic conditions that involve bone tissue.

However, the cementum surface is not totally immune to ultrastructural alteration adjacent to an inflammatory

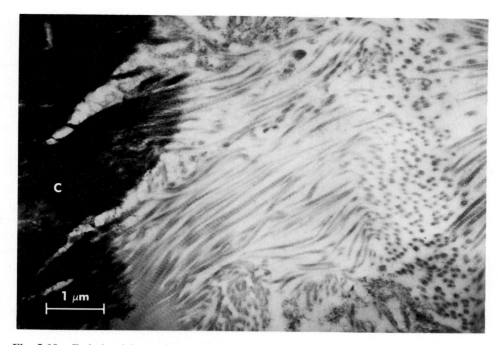

Fig. 5-10. Early breakdown of dentogingival fiber in periodontitis. Width of component collagen fibrils (50 to 70 nm) is within normal range, but bonds between them are relaxed. *C,* Cementum. (From Selvig KA: J Periodont Res 3:169, 1968. © 1968 Munksgaard International Publishers, Ltd., Copenhagen, Denmark.)

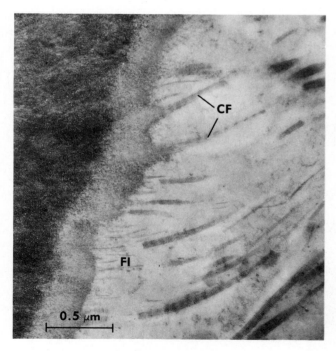

Fig. 5-11. Advanced degradation of connective tissue fiber attachment to root surface. A few cross-banded fibrils *(CF)* remain attached to cementum, together with some finer, nonbanded filaments *(FI).* Surface layer of cementum appears partially decalcified, presumably as a result of prolonged period of increased acidity in adjacent inflammatory infiltrate. (From Selvig KA: Acta Odontol Scand 24:459, 1966.)

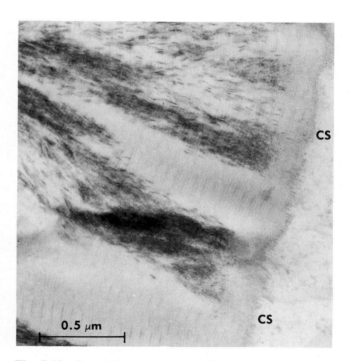

Fig. 5-12. Denuded cementum immediately apical to periodontal pocket. Dissolution of collagen fibrils has ended abruptly at cementum surface *(CS),* which has brushlike appearance. Cementum matrix contains collagen fibrils arranged at right angles to surface. Collagen cross-banding and presence of fine mineral crystals (dark, electron-dense profiles) are clearly seen. (From Selvig KA: Acta Odontol Scand 24:459, 1966.)

process. Partial decalcification and degradation of collagen fibrils in the cementum matrix (Selvig, 1966, 1968) (see Fig. 5-11) and even phagocytosis of hard tissue fragments by gingival fibroblasts (Deporter and Brown, 1980) may occur. These changes are limited to a fine surface layer within a narrow zone immediately apical to the pocket epithelium and therefore are not detectable by optical microscopy. Their frequency and clinical significance are unknown.

ACUTE NECROTIZING ULCERATIVE GINGIVITIS

Acute necrotizing ulcerative gingivitis differs dramatically from nonspecific gingivitis in clinical and histologic manifestations. Ultrastructurally, characteristic features are an extensive necrosis of epithelial and connective tissue elements and invasion of the ulcerated region by bacteria, primarily spirochetes and fusobacteria (Listgarten, 1965; Heylings, 1967). The surface of the gingival lesion consists of disintegrating cells and other necrotic tissue debris, fibrin, and large numbers of neutrophils and bacteria. Deep to this layer, clumps of spirochetes may be present within relatively well-preserved connective tissue (Fig. 5-13). Bacterial penetration may occur up to 300 μm beneath the necrotic surface layer. Phagocytosis of bacteria by neutrophils and macrophages occurs in all layers of the lesion.

LOCALIZED JUVENILE PERIODONTITIS

The rapidly progressing tissue damage seen in localized juvenile periodontitis (LJP) is associated with a bacterial flora capable of invading gingival epithelium and connective tissue. Thus microcolonies and single bacterial cells may be present between collagen fibers, inside phagocytic cells, and even in direct contact with alveolar bone (Gillett and Johnson, 1982; Carranza et al., 1983; Christersson et al., 1987a). Gram-negative, short rods compatible with the size and shape of *Actinobacillus actinomycetemcomitans* have been described in the epithelium and gingival connective tissues of LJP patients.

In a combined light, immunofluorescence, and ultrastructural study Christersson et al. (1987a) found that the gingival connective tissues in LJP patients harbor *A. actinomycetemcomitans,* an organism strongly associated with LJP. The *A. actinomycetemcomitans* antigens were detected in the connective tissue by immunofluorescence in 80% of the gingival biopsy specimens taken from sites of destruction. These sites also harbored *A. actinomycetemcomitans* subgingivally (Fig. 5-14). Transmission electron microscopic evaluation of these biopsy specimens demonstrated bacteria-like structures in clusters or as single microbes in the connective tissue. Often the bacteria were adjacent to partially destroyed collagen fibrils (Fig. 5-15). In a further study of *A. actinomycetemcomitans* in LJP, Christersson et al. (1987b) were able to culture *A. actinomycetemcomitans* from about three fourths of the gingival biopsy specimens taken from lesion areas of LJP patients. These studies suggest that *A. actinomycetemcomitans,* a prominent pathogen in LJP, can invade the gingival tissue adjacent to periodontal lesions in LJP patients and that some of the cells are viable and hence may be able to reinfect the subgingival area after scaling and root planing.

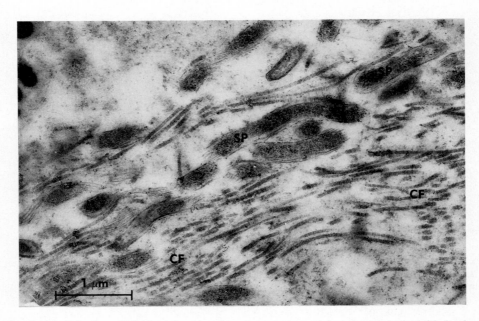

Fig. 5-13. Spirochetes *(SP)* in connective tissue in acute necrotizing ulcerative gingivitis in close relationship to bundles of collagen fibrils *(CF)*. (Courtesy Dr. Tryggve Lie.)

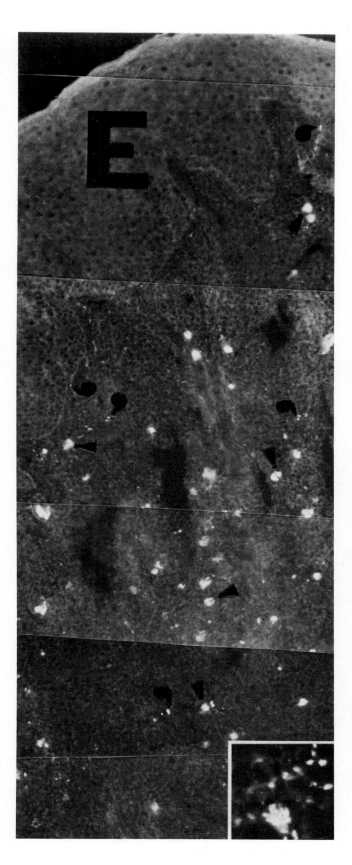

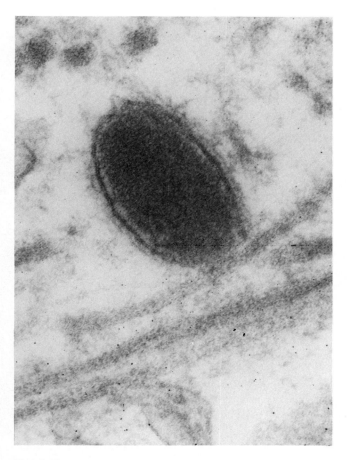

Fig. 5-14. Composite of six micrographs. Immunofluorescent staining after reaction with antisera to *A. actinomycetemcomitans. E,* Epithelium; *arrowheads,* intracellular staining; *(')* extracellular staining. (×80.) *Inset:* Granular staining of cells. (×200.) (From Christersson LA et al: J Periodontol 58:529, 1987.)

Fig. 5-15. Gram-negative bacteria in close position to collagen fibrils. (×120,000.) (From Christersson LA et al: J Periodontol 58:529, 1987.)

COLLAGEN DEGRADATION IN PERIODONTAL DISEASES

Gradual extension of the inflammatory cell infiltrate results in a net loss of collagen and ground substance components of the gingival connective tissue. Several pathways of collagen breakdown have been described, although the underlying biochemical mechanisms may be the same.

Initial degradation of collagen includes, first, severance of those cross-links that stabilize the fibrils within each fiber (see Fig. 5-10) and, second, longitudinal cleavage of the fibrils into finer elements: microfibrils or filaments (see Fig. 5-11). When the fibrils have been reduced to less than approximately 10 nm in diameter, they no longer show cross-banding, because an insufficient number of molecules remain in the staggered molecular arrangement. These changes may be caused by specific enzymes released from neutrophils, macrophages, and other cells in the area that attack the proteoglycans associated with the collagen fibers and subsequently the collagen itself. Other factors that are a consequence of the inflammatory reaction, such as increased tissue temperature, accumulation of acidic metabolic products, and changes in oxygen tension, may also contribute to the disruption of the fiber structure.

The partially degraded collagen fragments may then be phagocytosed by macrophages and completely digested intracellularly by lysosomal, proteolytic enzymes (Perez-Tamayo, 1973; Barbanell et al., 1976).

Alternatively, the entire process of collagen degradation may occur intracellularly following phagocytosis of pieces of apparently intact fibrillar collagen. While the macrophage is the cell primarily implicated in many other tissues where collagen resorption is occurring, the fibroblast seems to be the active cell in the gingiva. In both normal and inflamed gingival connective tissue, well-defined collagen fibrils are often seen in an intracellular location surrounded by a unit membrane (Ten Cate and Deporter, 1975; Deporter and Ten Cate, 1980; Melcher and Chan, 1981) (Fig. 5-16), and in vitro studies have shown that gingival fibroblasts are in fact capable of complete denaturation of collagen within phagosomes (Svoboda et al., 1979; Rose et al., 1980).

Gingival collagen is normally subject to metabolic turnover, and the maintenance of tissue integrity is dependent on a fine balance between the complementary processes of collagen biosynthesis and collagen degradation. Thus it has been pointed out that the long-term loss of collagen fibers may not necessarily result from a specific destructive process but may be accounted for by an interference by lymphoid cells with the capacity of fibroblasts to produce

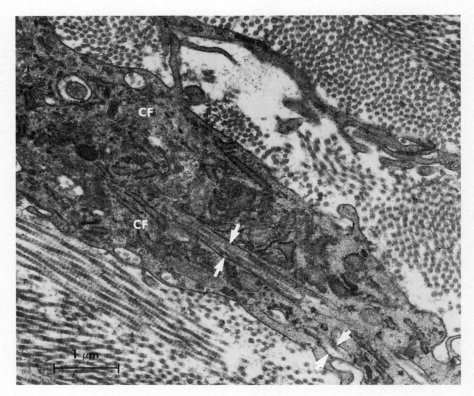

Fig. 5-16. Portion of gingival fibroblast containing ingested collagen fibrils within cytoplasmic vacuoles. Both longitudinal *(between arrows)* and cross-sectional fibrils *(CF)* can be seen. Cell is surrounded by bundles of collagen fibrils, which mainly appear in cross section.

and maintain collagen (Schroeder et al., 1973; Simpson and Avery, 1973) (see Fig. 5-2). The concept of reduced collagen biosynthetic capacity is supported by the observation that the collagen fibers immediately adjacent to the cementum surface, which normally have a very low rate of turnover, are not as rapidly affected as those located at a distance from the root surface (Selvig, 1966). Also, in the case of interference with collagen biosynthesis due to experimental C avitaminosis (Waerhaug, 1958; Glickman, 1963) or protein deficiency (Goldman, 1962), the cementum and cementum-related fibers are relatively unaffected while the more peripheral collagen fibers and the alveolar bone are gradually resorbed.

DENTAL CUTICLE

The mineral component of dental hard tissues, hydroxyapatite, has a high affinity for proteins and other electrostatically charged organic molecules, a property that has led to the routine use of hydroxyapatite in column chromatography for the separation of various organic materials. On an enamel or cementum surface adjacent to junctional epithelium or to a connective tissue inflammatory infiltrate, serum proteins and other components of the exudative process may become adsorbed and form a structureless layer identifiable by electron microscopy (Fig. 5-17). In some instances this cuticular structure may attain a thickness of several μm and become visible by optical microscopy as a distinct, clear layer interposed between the junctional epithelium and the tooth surface. When observed with the scanning electron microscope, the cuticle obscures the topography of the tooth surface (Fig. 5-18).

Adsorption of amorphous, organic material may start within the zone of collagen fiber destruction immediately below the apical extension of the epithelium (Selvig, 1966). With time, the cuticle may calcify (Jones, 1972; Eide et al. 1984).

The greater volume of rough endoplasmic reticulum and Golgi apparatus in junctional epithelial cells than in the oral gingival epithelium may indicate that these cells have a specific function and that secretory activity may contribute to the formation of a cuticle (Schroeder and Münzel-Pedrazzoli, 1970; Schroeder and Listgarten, 1971) (see Fig. 5-17). Although the origin of the dental cuticle is still

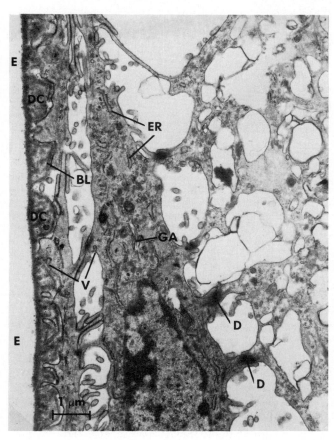

Fig. 5-17. Formation of a dental cuticle. In addition to epithelial basement lamina *(BL)*, there is accumulation of organic material *(DC)* on enamel surface *(E)* adjacent to altered junctional epithelium. Cuticular structure may consist of serum proteins and other components of gingival exudate. Note, however, well-developed Golgi apparatus *(GA)*, rough endoplasmic reticulum *(ER)*, and secretory vesicles *(V)*, which indicate a synthesizing function of epithelial cells. *D*, Desmosome.

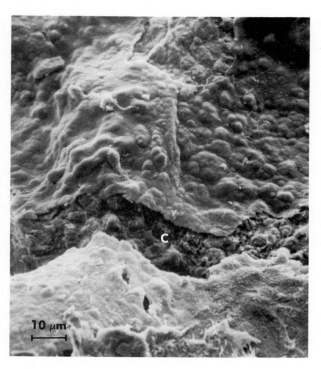

Fig. 5-18. Scanning electron micrograph of cuticular root surface coating. Through an occasional crack, underlying cementum surface proper *(C)* is visible. (From Eide B, Lie T, and Selvig KA: J Clin Periodontol 10:157, 1983. © 1983 Munksgaard International Publishers, Ltd., Copenhagen, Denmark.)

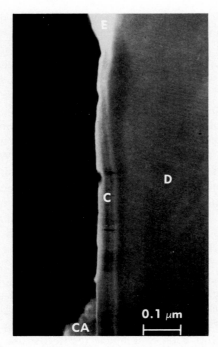

Fig. 5-19. Microradiograph of longitudinal section through a periodontally diseased tooth showing hypercalcified root surface. Relatively radiopaque surface zone decreases in thickness apically. It continues underneath calcified concrement but disappears as subgingival level is approached. *C,* Cementum; *CA,* calculus; *D,* dentin; *E,* enamel. (From Selvig KA: J Dent Res 48:846, 1969.)

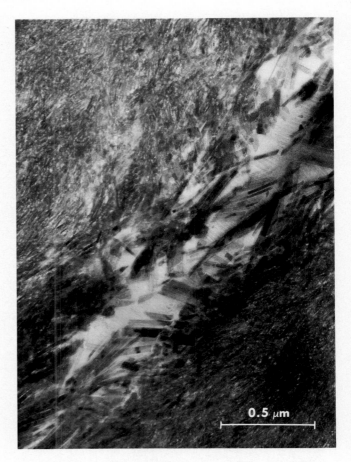

Fig. 5-21. Large, atypical mineral crystals in exposed cementum. Collagen fibrils in previously uncalcified core of Sharpey's fiber run obliquely across electron micrograph, as evidenced by cross-banding that is weakly present near upper right-hand corner. In contrast to normal calcification process in cementum, orientation of large crystals does not seem to have been determined by orientation of matrix fibrils. (From Selvig KA: J Dent Res 48:846, 1969.)

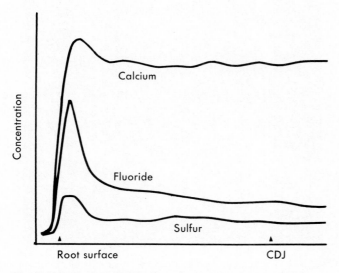

Fig. 5-20. Typical distribution of mineral and organic matter in cementum that has been exposed to environment of oral cavity for a period of time, as analyzed with electron microprobe. Surface layer of cementum has more mineral (as shown by peak of distribution curve for calcium) and organic matter (represented by sulfur) than deeper layers, as well as markedly elevated fluoride content. *CDJ,* Cementodentinal junction.

disputed, its inconsistent presence and variable thickness indicate that it is not part of the normal histology of the gingival region (Frank and Cimasoni, 1970; Lie and Selvig, 1975).

EXPOSED CEMENTUM

As the root surface in the course of periodontitis becomes exposed to the environment of the periodontal pocket and the oral cavity, alterations may occur within the exposed hard tissue (Selvig and Zander, 1962; Selvig, 1969; Selvig and Hals, 1977; Wirthlin et al., 1979). If surrounded by a predominantly acidic environment, root caries may develop; however, this process will not be described further here.

Alternatively, the oral environment may favor calcification processes, as evidenced by a tendency toward formation of dental calculus on the root surface (Fig. 5-19). Calcium, phosphate, and fluoride ions may then diffuse into the exposed cementum (Fig. 5-20). This results in an increased size of the hydroxyapatite crystals in a surface layer of the cementum, as well as deposition of additional mineral crystals in submicroscopic spaces (Fig. 5-21). Thus the mineral content of the outermost 10 to 30 μm of the cementum may increase by up to 10% as compared with normal cementum, and it appears that such a hypercalcified surface layer increases the resistance of the cementum to a subsequent caries attack (Furseth and Johansen, 1968; Hals and Selvig, 1977; Selvig, 1979).

An equally important but less studied process is the diffusion of organic substances of both salivary and bacterial origin into the surface layer of the exposed hard tissue (Selvig, 1969; Selvig and Hals, 1977; Daly et al., 1982) (see Fig. 5-20). The absorbed organic material may include lipopolysaccharide endotoxin and other cytotoxic substances that may have to be removed mechanically or chemically in the course of periodontal therapy (Jones and O'Leary, 1978; Fine et al., 1980; Moore et al., 1986).

It should be added that when a fresh surface of cementum or dentin is created by root planing of the exposed root surface, the processes described above will start again. An uptake of exogenous mineral and organic substances sufficient to be detected by microradiography and electron microscopy may then occur within a few weeks (Selvig, 1969, 1979).

REFERENCES

Barbanell RL, Lian JB, and Keith DA: A review of collagen degradation with particular emphasis upon that which occurs during inflammatory periodontal disease, Periodont Abstr 24:43, 1976.

Brecx M and Patters MR: Morphology of polymorphonuclear neutrophils during periodontal disease in the cynomolgus monkey, J Clin Periodontol 12:591, 1985.

Carranza FA Jr et al: Scanning and transmission electron microscopic study of tissue-invading microorganisms in localized juvenile periodontitis, J Periodontol 54:598, 1983.

Christersson LA et al: Tissue localization of *Actinobacillus actinomycetemcomitans* in human periodontitis. I. Light, immunofluorescence and electron microscopic studies, J Periodontol 58:529, 1987a.

Christersson LA et al: Tissue localization of *Actinobacillus actinomycetemcomitans* in human periodontitis. II. Correlation between immunofluorescence and culture techniques, J Periodontol 58(2):540, 1987b.

Daly CG et al: Histological assessment of periodontally involved cementum, J Clin Periodontol 9:266, 1982.

Deporter DA and Brown DY: Fine structural observations on the mechanism of loss of attachment during experimental periodontal disease in the rat, J Periodont Res 15:304, 1980.

Deporter DA and Ten Cate AR: Collagen resorption by periodontal-ligament interfaces of the mouse periodontium, J Periodontol 51:429, 1980.

Eide B, Lie T, and Selvig KA: Surface coatings on dental cementum incident to periodontal disease. II. Scanning electron microscopic confirmation of a mineralized cuticle, J Clin Periodontol 11:565, 1984.

Fine DH et al: Preliminary characterization of material eluted from the roots of periodontally diseased teeth, J Periodont Res 15:10, 1980.

Frank R and Cimasoni G: Ultrastructure de l'epithelium cliniquement normal du sillon et de la jonction gingivodentaires, Z Zellforsch Mikr Anat 109:356, 1970.

Freedman HL, Listgarten MA, and Taichman NS: Electron microscopic features of chronically inflamed human gingiva, J Periodont Res 3:313, 1968.

Furseth R and Johansen E: A microradiographic comparison of sound and carious human dental cementum, Arch Oral Biol 13:1197, 1968.

Garant RP: An electron microscopic study of the periodontal tissue of germfree rats and rats monoinfected with *Actinomyces naeslundii*, J Periodont Res 15:1, 1976.

Gavin JB: Ultrastructural features of chronic marginal gingivitis, J Periodont Res 5:19, 1970.

Gillett R and Johnson NW: Bacterial invasion of the periodontium in a case of juvenile periodontitis, J Clin Periodontol 9:93, 1982.

Glickman I: Acute vitamin C deficiency and periodontal disease. I. The periodontal tissues of the guinea pig in acute vitamin C deficiency, J Dent Res 27:9, 1963.

Goldman HM: Discussion of connective tissues of the periodontium, J Dent Res 41:230, 1962.

Hals E and Selvig KA: Correlated electron probe microanalysis and microradiography of carious and normal dental cementum, Caries Res 11:62, 1977.

Heylings RT: Electron microscopy of acute ulcerative gingivitis (Vincent's type), Br Dent J 122:51, 1967.

Jones SJ: The tooth surface in periodontal disease, Dent Pract 22:462, 1972.

Jones WA and O'Leary TJ: The effectiveness of in vivo root planing in removing bacterial endotoxin from the roots of periodontally involved teeth, J Periodontol 49:337, 1978.

Levy BM, Taylor AC, and Bernick S: Relationship between epithelium and connective tissue in gingival inflammation, J Dent Res 48:625, 1969.

Lie T and Selvig KA: Formation of an experimental dental cuticle, Scand J Dent Res 83:145, 1975.

Listgarten MA: Electron microscopic observations on the bacterial flora of acute necrotizing ulcerative gingivitis, J Periodont Res 36:328, 1965.

Listgarten MA and Heneghan, JB: Chronic inflammation in the gingival tissue of germ-free dogs, Arch Oral Biol 16:1207, 1971.

Longhurst P, Gillett R, and Johnson NW: Electron microscope quantitation of inflammatory infiltrates in childhood gingivitis, J Periodont Res 15:225, 1980.

Melcher AH and Chan J: Phagocytosis and digestion of collagen by gingival fibroblasts in vivo: a study of serial sections, J Ultrastruct Res 77:1, 1981.

Moore J, Wilson M, and Kieser JB: The distribution of bacterial lipopolysaccharide (endotoxin) in relation to periodontally involved root surfaces, J Clin Periodontol 13:748, 1986.

Page RC and Schroeder HE: Pathogenesis of inflammatory periodontal disease: a summary of current work, Lab Invest 34:235, 1976.

Payne WA et al: Histopathologic features of the initial and early stages of experimental gingivitis in man, J Periodont Res 10:51, 1975.

Perez-Tamayo R: Collagen degradation and resorption: physiology and pathology. In Perez-Tamayo R and Rojkind M, editors: Molecular pathology of connective tissues, New York, 1973, Marcel Dekker, Inc.

Rose GG, Toshihiko Y, and Mahan CJ: Human gingival fibroblast cell lines in vitro. I. Electron microscopic studies of collagenolysis, J Periodont Res 15:53, 1980.

Schroeder HE: Quantitative parameters of early human gingival inflammation, Arch Oral Biol 15:383, 1970.

Schroeder HE, Graf-De Beer M, and Attström R: Initial gingivitis in dogs, J Periodont Res 10:128, 1975.

Schroeder HE and Listgarten MA: Monographs in developmental biology, vol 2, Fine structure of the developing epithelial attachment of human teeth, Basel, Switzerland, 1971, S Karger.

Schroeder HE and Münzel-Pedrazzoli S: Morphometric analysis comparing junctional and oral epithelium of normal human gingiva, Helv Odontol Acta 14:53, 1970.

Schroeder HE and Page RC: Lymphocyte-fibroblast interaction in the pathogenesis of inflammatory gingival disease, Experientia 28:1228, 1972.

Schroeder HE et al: Structural constituents of clinically normal and slightly inflamed dog gingiva: a morphometric study, Helv Odontol Acta 17:70, 1973.

Selvig KA: Ultrastructural changes in cementum and adjacent connective tissue in periodontal disease, Acta Odontol Scand 24:459, 1966.

Selvig KA: Nonbanded fibrils of collagenous nature in human periodontal connective tissue, J Periodont Res 3:169, 1968.

Selvig KA: Biological changes at the tooth-saliva interface in periodontal disease, J Dent Res 48:846, 1969.

Selvig KA: Root surface alterations in periodontal disease, Am Inst Oral Biol 36:55, 1979.

Selvig KA and Hals E: Periodontally diseased cementum studied by correlated microradiography, electron probe analysis and electron microscopy, J Periodont Res 12:419, 1977.

Selvig KA and Zander HA: Chemical analysis and microradiography of cementum and dentin from periodontally diseased human teeth, J Periodontol 33:303, 1962.

Simpson DM and Avery BE: Pathologically altered fibroblasts within lymphoid cell infiltrates in early gingivitis, J Dent Res 52:1156, 1973.

Simpson DM and Avery BE: Histopathologic and ultrastructural features of inflamed gingiva in the baboon, J Periodontol 45:500, 1974.

Svoboda ELA, Melcher AH, and Brunette DM: Stereological study of collagen phagocytosis by cultured periodontal ligament fibroblasts: time course and effect of deficient culture medium, J Ultrastruct Res 68:195, 1979.

Takarada H et al: Ultrastructural studies of human gingiva. III. Changes of basal lamina in chronic periodontitis, J Periodontol 45:288, 1974a.

Takarada H et al: Ultrastructural studies of human gingiva. IV. Anchoring fibrils and perforations of the basal lamina in chronic periodontitis, J Periodontol 45:809, 1974b.

Ten Cate AR and Deporter DA: The degradative role of the fibroblast in the remodelling and turnover of collagen in soft connective tissue, Anat Rec 182:1, 1975.

Waerhaug J: Effect of C-avitaminosis on the supporting structures of the teeth, J Periodontol 29:87, 1958.

Wirthlin MR et al: The hypermineralization of diseased root surfaces, J Periodontol 50:125, 1979.

Yoon SH et al: Distribution of fluorine in teeth and alveolar bone, J Am Dent Assoc 61:565, 1960.

Zachrisson BU: A histological study of experimental gingivitis in man, J Periodont Res 3:293, 1968.

Chapter 6

GENERAL PRINCIPLES OF EPIDEMIOLOGY AND METHODS FOR MEASURING PREVALENCE AND SEVERITY OF PERIODONTAL DISEASE

John C. Greene

Epidemiology initially was concerned with the study and control of epidemics, as exemplified by John Snow's famous work (1936) on cholera. But today the discipline has broadened in scope to include the study of health and illness and associated factors in human populations. In studying human populations, the epidemiologist focuses on groups of people instead of individuals, as is done in clinical medicine or dentistry. There are three types of epidemiologic research: descriptive, analytic, and experimental.

Descriptive studies are used to observe and document the occurrence, progression, and distribution of a disease or condition in populations in relation to host, environmental, and agent factors. These studies are usually conducted when little is known about the natural history, prevalence, or determinants of a disease or condition and are especially useful in providing leads for further analysis and in constructing hypotheses for testing. A good example of this type of study is the early epidemiologic studies of Colorado brown stain conducted by McKay (1925), which led to the hypothesis that excess fluoride in the drinking water during tooth formation caused the observed enamel defects.

Analytic studies are used to investigate hypotheses derived from descriptive epidemiologic studies or other data sources such as clinical observations or National Center for Health Statistics publications. An example is the exploration by Douglass et al. (1983) of existing data from the National Center for Health Statistics to determine whether periodontal health in the United States was improving.

Experimental epidemiology is used to test hypotheses further by introducing a preventive or therapeutic agent or measure and comparing the outcome in test subjects with concurrent observations in control groups. The objective is to investigate the role of possible determinants of disease or the efficacy of therapeutic or preventive agents or procedures.

When original data are to be gathered, whether for descriptive, analytic, or experimental epidemiology of periodontal disease, some clinical assessment measure is essential. Because of the high prevalence and range of severity of periodontal disease, the investigator usually resorts to the use of indices for gingivitis, periodontitis, and associated dental plaque. No universally acceptable or usable indices for the study of periodontal disease have yet been developed. Thus investigators are faced with the problem of selecting indices from among the many that have been published. The research question and the design of the study will determine the data needs and help to narrow the choices of appropriate indices.

CLINICAL ASSESSMENT OF PERIODONTAL DISEASES
Evolution of current methods

Periodontal research has been hampered by difficulties in describing, diagnosing, counting, or assigning weights to the clinical manifestations of the periodontal diseases. Whether the study is descriptive, analytic, or experimental, the clinical entity being investigated must be clearly defined so that patients or sites can be consistently categorized as either having or not having the disease or condition. For example, when Legionnaire's disease first came to light, investigators had to decide what criteria could be used to categorize potential individuals as having bona fide cases. Only then could they begin to determine the extent of the epidemic and search for associated factors that might provide clues of causation. Without a clear definition of the disease entity, little progress can be made in studying its distribution pattern or in identifying possible causative agents.

The evolution of simple, valid, and reproducible clinical measures of periodontal disease has been painfully slow. The difficulties arise from the high prevalence, variety of clinical manifestations, gradations of severity, and episodic nature of the disease and the absence of a simple diagnostic laboratory test. In spite of these difficulties, methods for clinical assessment of periodontal disease continue to evolve, albeit very slowly, and several promising new measures are being explored (Kornman, 1987).

Periodontal disease, especially periodontitis in adults, generally is hard to define clearly in its early stages. It generally is agreed that periodontitis occurs when the junctional epithelium migrates onto the root surface apical to the cementoenamel junction (CEJ). This is difficult to measure; however, probing attachment loss is an acceptable clinical indication of early periodontitis. In epidemiologic studies, however, some probing attachment loss may be due to recession associated with abrasion, further confounding definitions of early periodontal disease. Hence, in the description of periodontal disease in a population, three features should be described: prevalence, severity, and extent of periodontal destruction. *Prevalence* requires setting a minimum level for designating an individual as suffering from periodontitis. For example, it may be set at one or more sites of 2 mm probing attachment loss (or 4 or 7 mm). Once set, the percentage of the population suffering from this level of disease is given. This is prevalence.

Severity is defined as the amount of destruction occurring, and this can usually be expressed as a mean score of, for example, probing attachment loss, or mean percent of bone loss as shown on radiographs.

Extent of disease is an indication of how many individual teeth or sites in an individual or a population suffer from a certain level of disease. For example, the extent of periodontitis in an individual may be expressed as the percent of interproximal sites suffering from 7 mm or greater attachment loss. It is clear that prevalence and extent depend very much on the limits chosen, so that absolute prevalence or extent in a population are arbitrarily defined. However, if the same definition of disease is applied to populations under study, then comparisons are possible. For example, if a normal group is compared with a diabetic group, the percentage of each group suffering from one or more sites with 7 mm probing attachment loss may show differences that have biologic meaning.

The following discussion of specific measures for assessing periodontal diseases includes only a few of the more widely used indices. These and other indices are extensively discussed in the published proceedings of conferences held in 1967 (Cohen and Ship), 1974 (Chilton), and 1986 (Chilton). For the convenience of the investigator, methods for assessing the two major components of periodontal disease, gingivitis and periodontitis, are discussed separately in the sections that follow. Thus indices that incorporate both gingivitis and periodontitis are discussed in both sections. Also, it should be noted that though there are several forms of gingivitis and periodontitis, these terms are treated generically in the following discussion.

Assessment of gingivitis

Several methods for diagnosing, categorizing, and quantifying the severity of gingivitis have been published. Most of these were developed by dental researchers to meet a specific purpose in connection with a particular study, and all have relied on one or more of the following: gingival color, contour, bleeding, extent of involvement, and gingival crevicular fluid flow (Ciancio, 1986).

The original version of the PMA Index by Schour and Massler (1947) was designed to measure the prevalence of gingivitis among Italian children after World War II. It was based on a count of the number of facial interdental papillae and marginal and attached gingival units that were affected by gingivitis. The sum of these scores was used to determine the PMA score per person.

The value of the original index lay in its simplicity and ease of use in large descriptive epidemiologic studies. The later versions of the PMA, which included severity dimensions, proved useful in clinical trials designed to document relatively small changes in short periods of time (Massler, 1967). However, criteria for assigning the range of scores were not as precise or as easy to follow as desired, and the assessments took considerable time.

Russell (1956) found the PMA index inadequate for

Table 6-1. Criteria for the Periodontal Index (PI) of Russell (1956)

Score	Criteria
0	*Negative.* There is neither overt inflammation in the investing tissues nor loss of function due to destruction of supporting tissues.
1	*Mild gingivitis.* There is an overt area of inflammation in the free gingivae, but this area does not circumscribe the tooth.
2	*Gingivitis.* Inflammation completely circumscribes the tooth, but there is no apparent break in the epithelial attachment.
6	*Gingivitis with pocket formation.* The epithelial attachment has been broken and there is a pocket (not merely a deepened gingival crevice due to swellng in the free gingivae). There is no interference with normal masticatory function.
8	*Advanced destruction with loss of masticatory function.* The tooth may be loose; may have drifted; may sound dull on percussion with a metallic instrument; may be depressible in its socket.

Table 6-2. Criteria for the Sulcus Bleeding Index (SBI) of Mühlemann and Mazor (1958)

Score	Criteria
0	No inflammation; no bleeding on probing
1	Bleeding from gingival sulcus on gentle probing; tissue otherwise appears normal
2	Bleeding on probing plus change in color due to inflammation
3	Bleeding on probing plus change in color and slight edema
4*	Bleeding on probing, color change, and obvious edema
5*	Bleeding on probing and spontaneous bleeding, color change, and marked edema with or without ulceration

*Original score 4 was subdivided into 4 and 5 (Mühlemann and Son, 1971).

large-scale descriptive epidemiologic studies of periodontal disease and developed the Periodontal Index (PI). The PI was designed to provide a quick and simple assessment of the absence or presence and severity of gingival inflammation, pocket formation, and loss of masticatory function. The PI combines gingival and periodontal assessments in a continuum, but some investigators have chosen to use only the gingivitis portion of the index for certain population studies; thus that portion only is included here (Table 6-1).

Russell reserved the score of 4 for those situations in which clinical investigators wished to detect early notch-like resorption of the alveolar crest by the use of radiographs. However, neither this score nor radiographs are a part of the basic index in practice.

When doubt arises in using the PI, the examiner is advised to assign the lesser score. Mean scores for the individual and for the group of individuals being studied, as well as the percentage of persons with periodontal disease who have destructive periodontitis, are usually reported.

The fact that only a mouth mirror and dental explorer (and no radiographs or periodontal probes) are usually used makes the PI convenient for use in large-scale population studies. It has proved useful in identifying relative differences in the state of periodontal health among population groups. In designing the index, Russell did not intend to develop a system that was sensitive enough to determine a total inventory of periodontal disease; rather, he wanted a simple, reproducible system that could detect significant differences in periodontal health within and between populations. Once populations or segments of populations are categorized according to levels of periodontal

health, then possible correlates such as age, sex, ethnicity, diet, education, income, and location can be compared. The PI has been used worldwide, and probably more data have been collected with this system than with any other index of gingivitis or periodontitis. Its utility is primarily for descriptive epidemiology and not for clinical trials, because of its insensitivity to small differences. Recent epidemiologic surveys, however, are using probing attachment measurements and various gingival indices to assess periodontal disease.

Mühlemann and Mazor (1958) used an approach similar to the PMA, called the Sulcus Bleeding Index (SBI), in their study of schoolchildren. They assessed papillae and marginal gingival units, dropped the attachment score because it was so seldom used, and added bleeding on probing as an indication of gingivitis (Table 6-2). A close relationship between bleeding on probing and inflammation has been shown (Zacchrisson, 1968; Oliver et al., 1969; Appelgren et al., 1979; Greenstein et al., 1981). The SBI is determined by averaging all of the scores for the individual.

A still different approach to assessing gingival and periodontal health for research purposes was introduced by Ramfjord (1959). The Ramfjord Periodontal Disease Index (PDI), like Russell's PI, is used to measure the presence and severity of periodontal disease in groups of people. Like the PI, the PDI includes both gingivitis and periodontitis and calls for assigning greater weight to gingivitis when it completely encircles the tooth than when it does not. In addition, the PDI gives still greater weight to severe gingivitis. The most significant feature is the concept of assessing periodontitis by using a periodontal probe to locate the bottom of the gingival sulcus in relation to the CEJ at specific sites on the tooth. To make this approach more practical, a subset of six teeth representing the entire dentition was selected for study. In the PDI, assessments of gingivitis and gingival sulcus depths in relation to the CEJ on the six selected teeth are combined to make up the Periodontal Disease Index for an individual.

The selected teeth are the upper right first molar, upper left central, upper left first premolar, lower left first molar, lower right central, and lower right first premolar. These teeth have been shown to be representative of the whole dentition (Gettinger et al., 1983).

The Gingival Index (GI) developed by Löe and Silness (1963) is a further refinement of earlier gingivitis assessment systems. Like Mühlemann and Mazor's index, it includes the dimension of bleeding on probing.

The gingival tissues surrounding each selected tooth are divided into four areas for scoring: distofacial papilla, facial margin, mesiofacial papilla, and the entire lingual margin. Each of these units is scored for gingivitis according to the criteria described in Table 6-3.

A periodontal probe is used to determine the bleeding tendency of the tissues. The scores from the four gingival units are averaged to obtain a score for each tooth, and these are combined and averaged to determine a GI score for each individual. While the original version of the index was developed and used to assess gingival tissue surrounding all teeth, in a later publication Löe (1967) suggested that the GI could be used on groups of teeth, as well as on the entire dentition.

The GI has proved useful in descriptive epidemiologic surveys, as well as in experimental epidemiology. Because it is fairly sensitive to small changes, is simple to administer, and permits calibration of examiners to minimize interexaminer and intraexaminer error, the GI is a frequent choice for use in controlled clinical trials of preventive or therapeutic agents (Ciancio, 1986).

The Papilla Bleeding Index published by Mühlemann (1977) is based on the bleeding tendency of the gingival papilla on gentle probing. In this index a periodontal probe is inserted gently into the interdental sulcus and moved occlusally along the line angle until it reaches the contact point. The same is done on the opposite side of the papilla, and if bleeding occurs in 15 seconds, the papilla is

recorded as positive. Engelberger et al. (1983) have demonstrated a direct correlation between PBI scores and inflammatory infiltrate in the papillae examined.

Assessment of periodontitis

Early studies of the epidemiology of periodontitis relied on radiographic evidence of bone loss as the primary method of determining who was affected and who was not. In contemporary studies of periodontitis, less reliance is placed on radiographs and more on attachment levels determined by direct periodontal probing of selected sites. However, the PI developed by Russell (1956) usually uses neither radiographs nor the periodontal probe, thereby gaining simplicity and ease of application in large population studies. To compensate for the amount of moderately advanced periodontitis that is undetected by the direct observational approach used in the PI, heavy numerical weights are applied to the advanced stages of destructive periodontitis. Whereas the highest score for gingivitis surrounding the whole tooth is 2, the lowest score assigned for clinically obvious destructive periodontitis is 6 and the highest is 8. The percentage of persons with destructive periodontal disease (those with scores of 6 or 8) is usually reported along with the PI for the population or for subgroups. The system has been used extensively in descriptive epidemiologic studies of the relative severity of periodontal disease in large population groups in relation to a variety of variables. However, the PI assessments are too insensitive and inaccurate to detect the small differences or small changes usually found in short-term prospective studies or in experimental or clinical epidemiology. Because of its insensitivity and because other, more sensitive measures are available, the periodontitis portion of the index is used much less frequently today. For these reasons and in view of new information about the episodic nature of disease activity, some have questioned the validity of conclusions drawn from studies that have used it in the past (Page and Schroeder, 1982).

Ramfjord (1959, 1967) proposed an approach different from that published by Russell for assessing periodontitis. In the PDI an indication of periodontal support is derived by using a thin periodontal probe with a graded millimeter scale to record distances from the bottom of the gingival sulcus to the CEJ. These measurements are made on the four areas of the same six teeth selected for the gingivitis examination (see earlier discussion). The probe measurements are integrated with those for gingivitis by using a continuous scale that goes from 0 to 3 for gingivitis and from 4 to 6 for sulcular measurements. A score of 4 is assigned when the attachment level is up to but not more than 3 mm apical to the CEJ; a score of 5 is assigned when the attachment level is 4 to 6 mm apical to the CEJ; and a score of 6 is used when the bottom of the sulcus is more than 6 mm apical to the CEJ.

Locating the bottom of the gingival sulcus in relation to

Table 6-3. Criteria for the Gingival Index (GI) of Löe and Silness (1963)

Score	Criteria
0	Normal gingiva
1	Mild inflammation, slight change in color, slight edema, no bleeding on probing
2	Moderate inflammation, redness, edema and glazing, bleeding on probing
3	Severe inflammation, marked redness and edema, ulcerations; tendency toward spontaneous bleeding

a fixed point, the CEJ, is a very significant feature of the PDI. The position of the attachment in relation to the CEJ can indicate past disease, but it cannot confirm that the disease is active. Demonstrating that there has been an increase in the distance from the CEJ to the bottom of the sulcus between two examination periods is the most practical means of confirming that the disease has been active (Goodson, 1986).

Use of the periodontal probe to determine attachment levels is not without its problems (Armitage et al., 1977). Variability in repeated probing measurements results from such factors as variations in the position of the probe, the presence or absence of calculus, variations in probing pressure, and patient cooperation. Because of this inherent variability, a change of 2 mm or more in probing depth over time appears to be necessary to determine with confidence that change has actually occurred (Listgarten, 1980; Haffajee et al., 1983; Kornman, 1987). This threshold was derived by making repeated measures on the same individuals. In studies with trained, experienced examiners where intraexaminer and interexaminer error is very low, the threshold could be lower. Using a threshold of 2 mm to define true change in repeated measurements makes the approach less sensitive in that some real change is missed, but it avoids the majority of troublesome false positive recordings. Even with its problems, for most clinical studies and trials that are concerned with the loss or gain of periodontal support, clinical probing in relation to the fixed landmark, the CEJ, is still the best available means of estimating the level of periodontal attachment (Haffajee and Socransky, 1986).

Variations in the probing approach used in the PDI, such as making fewer measurements on the selected teeth, can make the system easily usable in large population studies, and assessing additional sites or teeth may be useful in some clinical studies.

It would seem logical that since radiographs are so essential in clinical practice, they would provide valuable, unchangeable, objective data for clinical studies. However, while radiographs do provide a permanent record, the problems of angulation, superimposition, exposure, and interpretation are so great and so serious that current radiographic methods can provide only supportive or confirmatory information at best. If radiographs are to be used, long-cone paralleling techniques or identical positioning devices and standardized film interpretation should always be employed to minimize some of these problems. The use of the multienergetic x-ray beam has made it possible to capture great detail with good sensitivity, but the problem of interpreting the resulting material still produces an inability to detect all but rather extensive bone changes (Kornman, 1987).

Newer imaging techniques that have been developed for use in medical diagnosis are now being investigated for possible use in dentistry. Probably the most promising at this time is computer-assisted subtraction radiography (Bender, 1982; Ortman et al., 1982; Gröndahl and Gröndahl, 1983; Kornman, 1987). The few clinical studies in which these techniques have been used indicate that they show exciting promise.

Carlos et al. (1986) have introduced another approach for collecting data for descriptive and analytic epidemiologic studies of periodontal disease. Like the PDI, the Extent and Severity Index (ESI) focuses on loss of attachment level as determined by measurement with calibrated peridontal probes but does not take into account gingivitis.

Extensive efforts are underway to develop a simple, quick method for assessing periodontal health by analyzing the gingival crevicular fluid (GCF). Recent reports of such efforts include those of Oshrain et al. (1984), Lamster et al. (1985), Niekrash and Patters (1986), Offenbacher et al. (1986), and Sandholm (1986). Qualitative and quantitative analysis of the GCF holds considerable promise for a sensitive and accurate method of detecting the presence of periodontal disease and predicting its progression.

Application in assessment of treatment needs

All of these epidemiologic indices used to describe the extent and severity of gingivitis and periodontitis were designed for estimating the relative health status of the periodontium, not treatment needs. However, planners and administrators sometimes attempt to translate epidemiologic data into treatment and manpower needs. This type of data transformation should be performed and used with caution, particularly when the predictive value (i.e., the combined percentage of true positive and true negative assessments) of the system being used is low. A low predictive value means the assessment has a low probability of agreeing with the true disease state. Making decisions about treatment needs and manpower requirements based on data derived for another purpose, or on data not consistent with the current disease state, is very risky. Because of this concern, investigators have attempted to develop specific measures to assess a population's periodontal treatment needs. An example of this is the Community Periodontal Index of Treatment Needs (CPITN) (Ainamo et al., 1982). This index is proposed as a simple, rapid method for determining treatment needs in a population and is being promoted by the World Health Organization and the British Society of Periodontology. The protocol for the CPITN calls for recording only the worst score in each of six segments of the mouth, and treatment needs are estimated from these measurements.

Plaque measurements

Because plaque has been so closely associated with the occurrence and severity of periodontal disease, it is almost a given that any study of the epidemiology of periodontal disease, whether descriptive, analytic, or experimental, must take into account the extent and/or character of plaque accumulation. Several different approaches to measuring plaque accumulation have been published and are in use today. The most common approaches have involved assessing the tooth surface area covered by plaque; some include assessing plaque thickness as well.

One of the earliest systematic plaque measurement techniques to appear in the literature was devised by Ramfjord (1959) as part of the PDI. The same six teeth are assessed for plaque as are measured for gingivitis. This technique was later modified by Schick and Ash (1961) to restrict the screening to the gingival half of the tooth surfaces. Plaque accumulation on interproximal, facial, and lingual surfaces is scored after staining with Bismarck brown solution.

Vermillion and I introduced a similar approach that used the facial and lingual surfaces of all of the teeth, used the term *oral debris* instead of *plaque,* and included measurements of calculus to arrive at an oral hygiene index for an individual (Greene and Vermillion, 1960). We used the nonspecific term *oral debris* because we considered it impractical to use stains or a microscope in large population studies to detect subtle differences between plaque and similar substances on the teeth. We later simplified the index by demonstrating that six teeth could be used to represent the whole mouth (Greene and Vermillion, 1964). This version became known as the Oral Hygiene Index – Simplified (OHI-S).

The six surfaces used in the OHI-S are the facial surfaces of the upper right and left first molars, the lingual surfaces of the lower right and left first molars, and the labial surfaces of the upper right central and lower left central incisors. The criteria used to arrive at a debris score are shown in Table 6-4.

Scores for the selected teeth are added and divided by the number of surfaces scored to determine the debris index (DI-S) for the individual. The calculus portion (CI-S) of the index is combined with the debris portion to determine the OHI-S.

The OHI-S has been used widely around the world and usually in conjunction with Russell's PI. The main use of the OHI-S is in descriptive epidemiologic studies of large groups of people where oral hygiene practices are limited and large deposits of debris and calculus are common. The index is simple to use, and examiners can be calibrated so that the interexaminer and intraexaminer error is small. However, because the measurements are gross, the OHI-S has limited value in clinical trials where small changes need to be detected to determine treatment effect. There now are other, more sensitive systems for use in experimental epidemiology studies involving plaque assessment (Fischman, 1986). The plaque index developed by Quigley and Hein (1962) and modified by Turesky et al. (1970) has received considerable use in studies evaluating antiplaque measures such as toothbrushing, flossing, mouth rinsing, and chemical agents. In this approach the first category of the OHI-S was subdivided into three parts, giving it more sensitivity, particularly in the area adjacent to the gingiva.

Probably the system most used today for assessing plaque in clinical trials or experimental epidemiology is the Plaque Index (PlI) developed by Silness and Löe (1964) and further described by Löe in 1967. The PlI was developed as a companion to the Gingival Index of Löe and Silness, and assessments are made at the same sites as in the GI. The mesial and distal as well as the facial and lingual surfaces are scored for each selected tooth. The mean of the four scores is the tooth score, and the mean of the tooth scores is the individual's PlI (Table 6-5).

The value of the PlI is in its sensitivity to small change, and yet its upper limits include a wide range of plaque accumulation, thus making it very useful in clinical trials and longitudinal studies. The most significant problem with the index is that because the criteria are somewhat subjective, it requires well-trained and experienced examiners to obtain reliable data (Mandel, 1974).

Table 6-4. Criteria for the debris (plaque) portion of the Oral Hygiene Index – Simplified (OHI-S) of Greene and Vermillion (1964)

Score	Criteria
0	No debris or stain present
1	Soft debris covering not more than one third of tooth surface being examined, or presence of extrinsic stains without debris regardless of surface area covered
2	Soft debris covering more than one third but not more than two thirds of exposed tooth surface
3	Soft debris covering more than two thirds of exposed tooth surface

Table 6-5. Criteria for the Plaque Index (PlI) of Silness and Löe

Score	Criteria
0	No plaque in gingival area
1	No plaque visible by the unaided eye, but plaque is made visible on the point of the probe after it has been moved across surface at entrance of gingival crevice
2	Gingival area is covered with a thin to moderately thick layer of plaque; deposit is visible to the naked eye
3	Heavy accumulation of soft matter, the thickness of which fills out niche produced by gingival margin and tooth surface; interdental area is stuffed with soft debris

CLINICAL TRIALS

As our understanding of the natural history of periodontal disease continues to expand and new scientific techniques and instrumentation become available for delving still further into the mysteries of this ubiquitous malady, the already considerable interest in conducting clinical trials will increase. Future clinical trials will need to address not only whether agents are effective against plaque or gingivitis, but also whether they are effective in preventing the initiation or progression of periodontitis. To make such investigations worth the effort, new practical techniques that accurately determine the presence of active disease must be developed and the studies must be properly designed. Unfortunately, the literature contains too many reports of results of poorly designed clinical trials that show agents to be more or less effective than is the fact.

The design of the study, data needs, and types of analyses are determined by the questions the investigator is seeking to answer. Thus, before launching a clinical trial, the investigator should seek the assistance of someone who is experienced in research design and in data analysis. Design and analysis experience is necessary to address such issues as sharpening the question being asked and deciding on the population to be sampled, the sample size, the outcome variables to be measured, the selection and composition of the control group or groups, the specific clinical assessment or indices to be used, and the statistical tests to be performed to estimate the outcome of the trials. The research protocol should deal thoroughly with all of these important matters before the study gets underway (Chilton and Fleiss, 1986). As Lindhe et al. (1986) have stated, there are certain minimal requirements for the design of acceptable clinical trials: (1) a testable hypothesis, (2) an adequate number of subjects, (3) test and control groups, (4) random assignment of subjects to these groups, (5) appropriate and reproducible measurements to assess effects of therapy, (6) well-trained examiners with known intraexaminer and interexaminer error making "blind" measurements, and (7) appropriate statistical methods to test the hypothesis.

New information about the pathophysiology of periodontal disease has posed questions about the appropriate unit for statistical analysis. For years it has been customary to consider the correct unit of analysis to be the individual rather than specific sites within the individual. There is considerable logic in support of this custom. The various sites in the mouth share a common host, the same oral hygiene practices, and the same nutritional and immunologic factors and thus are not independent samples. In addition, they have been thought to share the same microbiota. However, it is now clear that different sites in the same individual progress in asynchronous episodes and that lesional morphology differs. Also, we now know that there are differences in microflora composition among diseased sites in the same mouth. This new information suggests that there is considerable independence between different periodontal sites in the same person and that data analysis should make full use of data on individual sites, as well as on individual persons. Thus, in order not to lose the value of individual site data, it is useful at least to analyze and report frequency distribution data by site as well as report composite data for persons. Haffajee et al. (1983) have suggested that in therapeutic trials, survival analysis of periodontal sites before and after surgery should be conducted.

For excellent discussions of the design and analysis of clinical trials relating to plaque and gingivitis and of the design of clinical trials of traditional therapies for periodontitis, readers are encouraged to study the proceedings of the 1986 Conference on Clinical Trials in Periodontal Diseases (Chilton and Fleiss, 1986; Lindhe et al., 1986).

Data obtained in epidemiologic studies of adult population groups show a pattern of continuous progression of chronic destructive periodontal disease with advancing age. The pattern of continuous progression, which arises from the analysis of mean values of populations, has been assumed to apply to individuals as well. This assumption is being reexamined today in view of the "burst" hypothesis that derives from data demonstrating that the progression of disease in individuals at different sites is episodic rather than continuous (Socransky et al., 1984). It is also clear that attachment level measurements and bone loss reflect the effects of prior disease activity but not necessarily current destruction and that they do not indicate what destruction will occur in the future. The only practical way to determine whether the disease has been active during a time period is to determine whether there has been attachment or bone loss during that period. Current periodontal indices do not measure current disease activity, but considerable work is underway to develop assays that will do so.

Indices developed for epidemiologic purposes should not be relied on for diagnosing and planning treatment for individual patients. Clinicians should find it unacceptable to depend on measures that fail to detect existing disease. But the epidemiologist can accept this to a degree, for his concern is not with the detection of all pathology in all individuals but with the application of standardized techniques of observation to groups of people to detect differences and determine explanations for these differences. Some components of epidemiologic indices, however, are of direct benefit to the clinician; for example, determination of bleeding on probing and changes in probing depth, particularly in relation to the CEJ, is of vital importance in assessing the current and changing status of the periodontal health of patients.

SUMMARY

Epidemiology is the study of health and disease in human populations. To study the prevalence or severity of a disease or identify its determinants, the investigator must be able to define and diagnose it. For gingivitis, periodontitis, and dental plaque, numerous approaches to systematic assessment have been developed. The selection of the most appropriate approach is determined by the research question and the study design.

Currently the most important assessments in experimental studies of periodontal disease are as follows: for gingivitis—overt signs of inflammation and bleeding on probing, as in the Gingival Index of Löe and Silness; for periodontitis—the probing attachment level in relation to the CEJ, as in the PDI of Ramfjord; and for plaque—the surface area covered in close proximity to the gingiva, as in Turesky's modification of the Quigley and Hein index or the Silness and Löe index.

Other assessment approaches, such as computer-assisted subtraction radiography (Ortman et al., 1982) and gingival crevicular fluid assessments, look very promising as possible future sources of quick, accurate diagnostic measures of active periodontal pathology.

REFERENCES

Ainamo J et al: Development of the World Health Organization (WHO) community periodontal index of treatment needs (CPITN), Int Dent J 32:281, 1982.

Appelgren R et al: Clinical and histologic correlation of gingivitis, J Periodontol 50:540, 1979.

Armitage GC et al: Microscopic evaluation of clinical measurements of corrective time attachment levels, J Clin Periodontol 4:173, 1977.

Bender IB: Factors influencing the radiographic appearance of bony lesions, J Endod 8:161, 1982.

Carlos JP et al: The Extent and Severity Index; a simple method for use in epidemiologic studies of periodontol disease, J Clin Periodontol 13:500, 1986.

Chilton NW, editor: International conference on clinical trials of agents used in the prevention/treatment of periodontal diseases, J Periodont Res 9(suppl 14):7, 1974.

Chilton NW, editor: Conference on clinical trials in periodontal diseases, J Clin Periodontol 13:344, 1986.

Chilton NW and Fleiss JL: Design and analysis of plaque and gingivitis clinical trials, J Clin Periodontol 13:400, 1986.

Ciancio SG: Current status of indices of gingivitis, J Clin Periodontol 13:500, 1986.

Cohen DW and Ship II, editors: Clinical methods in periodontal diseases based on a conference held on May 20-23, 1967, J Periodontol 38:1967.

Douglass CW et al: National trends in prevalence and severity of the periodontal diseases, J Am Dent Assoc 107:403, 1983.

Engelberger T et al: Correlations among Papilla Bleeding Index, other clinical indices and histologically determined inflammation of gingival papilla, J Clin Periodontol 10:579, 1983.

Fischman SL: Current status of indices of plaque, J Clin Periodontol 13:371, 1986.

Gettinger G et al: The use of six selected teeth in population measures of periodontal status, J Periodontol 54:155, 1983.

Goodson JC: Clinical measurements of periodontitis, J Clin Periodontol 13:446, 1986.

Greene JC and Vermillion JR: The Oral Hygiene Index: a method for classifying oral hygiene status, J Am Dent Assoc 61:172, 1960.

Greene JC and Vermillion JR: The Simplified Oral Hygiene Index, J Am Dent Assoc 68:7, 1964.

Greenstein G et al: Histologic characteristics associated with bleeding after probing and visual signs of inflammation, J Periodontol 52:420, 1981.

Gröndahl HG and Gröndahl K: Subtraction radiography for the diagnosis of periodontal bone lesions, Oral Surg 55:208, 1983.

Haffajee AD and Socransky SS: Attachment level changes in destructive periodontal disease, J Clin Periodontol 13:461, 1986.

Haffajee AD et al: Clinical parameters as predictor of destructive periodontal disease activity, J Clin Periodontol 10:257, 1983.

Kornman KS: Nature of periodontal diseases: assessment and diagnosis, J Periodont Res 22:192, 1987.

Lamster IB et al: Development of a biochemical profile for gingival crevicular fluid: methodological considerations and evaluation of collagen-degrading and ground substance–degrading enzyme activity during experimental gingivitis, J Periodontol (suppl), 1985.

Lindhe J et al: Design of clinical trials of traditional therapies of periodontitis, J Clin Periodontol 13:488, 1986.

Listgarten MA: Periodontal probing: what does it mean? J Clin Periodontol 7:165, 1980.

Löe H: The gingival index, the plaque index and the retention index systems, J Periodontol 38:610, 1967.

Löe H and Silness J.: Periodontal disease in pregnancy. I. Prevalence and severity, Acta Odontol Scand 21:533, 1963.

McKay FS: Mottled enamel: a fundamental problem in dentistry, Dent Cosmos 67:847, 1925.

Mandel ID: Indices for measurement of soft accumulations in clinical studies of oral hygiene and periodontal disease, J Periodont Res 9(suppl 14):7, 1974.

Massler M: The P-M-A index for the assessment of gingivitis, J Periodontol 38:592, 1967.

Mühlemann HR: Psychological and chemical mediators of gingival health, J Prev Dent 4:6, 1977.

Mühlemann HR and Mazor ZS: Gingivitis in Zurich school children, Helv Odontol Acta 2:3, 1958.

Mühlemann HR and Son S: Gingival sulcus bleeding: a leading symptom in initial gingivitis, Helv Odontol Acta 15:107, 1971.

Niekrash CE and Patters MR: Assessment of complement cleavage in gingival fluid in humans with and without periodontal disease, J Periodont Res 21:233, 1986.

Offenbacher S et al: The use of crevicular fluid prostaglandin E_2 levels as a predictor of periodontal attachment loss, J Periodont Res 21:101, 1986.

Oliver RC et al: The correlation between clinical scoring, exudate measurements and microscopic evaluation of inflammation in the gingiva, J Periodontol 40:201, 1969.

Ortman LF et al: Relationship between alveolar bone measured by ^{125}I absorptiometry with analysis of standardized radiographs, J Periodontol 53:311, 1982.

Oshrain RL et al: Arylsulphatase activity in human gingival crevicular fluid, Arch Oral Biol 29:399, 1984.

Page RC and Schroeder HE: Periodontitis in man and other animals, New York, 1982, S Karger.

Quigley G and Hein J: Comparative cleansing efficiency of manual and power brushing, J Am Dent Assoc 65:26, 1962.

Ramfjord SP: Indices for prevalence and incidence of periodontal disease, J Periodontol 30:57, 1959.

Ramfjord SP: The Periodontal Index (PDI), J Periodontol 38:602, 1967.

Russell AL: A system of classification and scoring for prevalence surveys of periodontal disease, J Dent Res 35:350, 1956.

Sandholm L: Proteases and their inhibitors in chronic inflammatory periodontal disease, J Clin Periodontol 13:19, 1986.

Schick RA and Ash MM: Evaluation of the vertical method of toothbrushing, J Periodontol 32:346, 1961.

Schour I and Massler M: Gingival disease in postwar Italy (1945). I. Prevalence of gingivitis in various age groups, J Am Dent Assoc 35:475, 1947.

Silness P and Löe H: Periodontal disease in pregnancy, Acta Odontol Scand 22:121, 1964.

Snow J: Snow on cholera: a reprint of two papers, New York, 1936, The Commonwealth Fund, pp 1-175.

Socransky SS et al: New concepts of destructive periodontal disease, J Clin Periodontol 11:21, 1984.

Turesky S et al: Reduced plaque formation by the chloromethyl analogue of vitamin C, J Periodontol 41:41, 1970.

Zacchrisson BU: A histological study of experimental gingivitis in man, J Periodont Res 3:293, 1968.

EPIDEMIOLOGY OF PERIODONTAL DISEASE

Harald Löe
Edith Morrison

Epidemiology, as defined in Chapter 6, deals with the factors that influence the distribution and frequency of health, disease, and mortality in human populations. The prevalence, severity, and incidence of disease and related factors are studied to aid in developing research strategies, planning prevention and treatment programs, and assessing manpower needs. Although cross-sectional studies of these factors can allow meaningful comparison of data, longitudinal studies (identical assessments in the same individuals over time) are needed to study the natural history of a disease and its determinants. Knowledge of the natural history allows analysis of potential factors and conditions that may have an impact on the disease process, possibly resulting in the development of effective control measures. However, it should be noted that close associations or statistically significant correlations between putative etiologic factors and disease occurrence as established on the basis of epidemiologic surveys cannot decide cause and effect. Studies of such causal relationships require more precision than population studies offer.

Although much information has been obtained about the different forms of periodontal disease, evaluations of prevalence have been severely hampered by differences in the criteria and index systems used to record periodontal diseases at population levels. Nevertheless, the data collected over the last decades, and especially those from recent cross-sectional national surveys and longitudinal investigations, can serve as a basis for discussing the current prevalence and severity of these diseases, their initiation, their pattern and rate of progression under different circumstances, and their relative importance in tooth mortality.

CHRONIC GINGIVITIS

Early reports on gingival health and disease during childhood and adolescence were highly inconsistent. As an example, Messner et al. (1936) found that gingivitis occurred in 3.6% to 8.6% of approximately 1 million American schoolchildren examined, whereas a comparable Swedish study (Westin et al., 1937) reported that 86.5% of the children exhibited gingivitis. There appears to be no reasonable explanation for such a vast difference in the gingival health of U.S. and Scandinavian children during the prewar era, and the apparent discrepancy probably reflects a difference in assessment criteria rather than actual disease prevalence.

During the past 40 years, index systems were developed (Schour and Massler, 1947; Russell, 1956; Ramfjord, 1959; Löe and Silness, 1963) with criteria that established some uniformity in the classification of gingival states. More recent investigations have confirmed the utility of such systems and have yielded more consistent results.

Mühlemann and Mazor (1958) found that the prevalence of gingivitis in 13-year-old Swiss children was 93%. McHugh et al. (1964) reported that 99% of the 13-year-olds in Dundee, Scotland, exhibited gingivitis. Björby and Löe (1969) confirmed that gingivitis (GI ≥ 1) occurred in virtually all children and adolescents: of 1038 Swedish children between 9 and 16 years of age, only 4 exhibited a dentition in which no gingival units were inflamed. Similar figures were reported from Israel (Rosenzweig, 1960) and are in keeping with findings in India, where practically 100% of examined boys under 17 years of age had gingivitis (Marshall-Day and Shourie, 1949; Ramfjord, 1961).

Even if gingivitis seemed almost universal, however, there were some variations in severity (King, 1944, 1945). Parfitt (1957) suggested that gingivitis in both sexes occurred at the time of puberty, peaked in severity at 14 or 15 years of age, and gradually improved throughout the remainder of the teens. On the basis of such a clinical survey, it is impossible to decide if increases in severity result from morphologic changes produced by exfoliation and eruption of teeth, from altered hormonal situations in puberty, or both. Based on the known influence of sexual hormones on tissue physiology in general and the gingival inflammatory process in particular, an already existing gingivitis could be exacerbated during this period of hormonal alteration (Löe and Silness, 1963).

Studies in areas where adolescent populations have access to and use well-developed preventive and curative dental services generally show improved oral hygiene and gingival status as the subjects approach 20 years of age. Under such conditions Anerud et al. (1979, 1983) found that more than 90% of all tooth surfaces in individuals between 17 and 20 years of age showed a high level of gingival health and did not bleed on probing. In addition, the level of gingival health attained by age 17 was maintained through mature adulthood (Anerud et al., 1979). When it was present, overt gingivitis occurred mostly in the interdental areas of posterior teeth (Lang et al., 1977; Anerud et al., 1979, 1983; Hugoson et al., 1980; Hansen et al., 1984).

Data from national surveys in Denmark in 1981 (Kirkegaard et al., 1986) and the United States in 1981 and 1986 suggested that gingival health was improving and that approximately 50% of the adult population had clinically healthy gingiva. Among the other 50% who showed gingival tissues that bled on probing (GI = 2), an average of 5% to 6% of the total number of gingival units were inflamed. Among elderly persons (over 65 years of age) overt gingivitis occurred in 60% and affected an average of 12% to 13% of the gingival units. Both in mature adults and in older groups, women tended to have less gingivitis than men, which is attributed to better oral hygiene habits and practices among women.

Studies of populations who have no active oral hygiene programs or dental health care show overt gingivitis in all individuals and in almost all areas of the dentition by the age of 14 years. The distribution and the severity of gingivitis reach a maximum before 20 years of age and are maintained with very little fluctuation in severity throughout the life of the dentition (Anerud et al., 1979).

Causal relationship between oral hygiene and gingivitis

In a crude sense, the notion that debris on teeth plays a role in the destruction of the periodontal tissues is centuries old. On the other hand, the scientific evidence to accept or reject the idea had been lacking. The etiology of periodontal disease was poorly understood; consequently, the management of this disease was ineffective.

During the 1950s considerable clinical and histologic data (Waerhaug, 1952), as well as information from epidemiologic studies (Russell, 1957a, 1957b; Greene, 1963; Waerhaug, 1967), indicated a close relationship between mineralized and nonmineralized deposits on teeth and the prevalence and severity of periodontal disease.

Supragingival and subgingival calculus is often found on tooth surfaces that are not accessible to toothbrushing or that are regularly overlooked during brushing. Where hygiene is ordinarily satisfactory (i.e., the buccal surfaces), calculus is rare (Lövdal et al., 1958). Among populations who do not perform any active mechanical oral hygiene, the accumulation of supragingival and subgingival calculus starts early in life and, if left undisturbed, will reach monstrous amounts before 40 years of age (Löe et al., 1978b).

Although the distribution of calculus and periodontal disease is closely related, periodontal disease is more prevalent than calculus (Lövdal et al., 1958). Microscopic investigations of the calculus-gingival tissue relationship (Waerhaug, 1952; Theilade, 1960) indicated that supragingival and subgingival calculus, inadequate margins of fillings and crowns, and untreated cavities are always covered by an uncalcified layer of bacterial plaque; the mineralized deposit plays only a secondary role.

The hypothesis that dental plaque was responsible for the initiation and maintenance of chronic gingivitis was tested in the so-called experimental gingivitis model (Löe et al., 1965; Theilade et al., 1966). Young, healthy individuals with clean dentition and normal gingiva were asked to refrain from any oral hygiene for 3 weeks. It appeared that all individuals showed a rapid accumulation of bacterial plaque that elicited an inflammatory reaction in the gingiva, which clinically was described as gingivitis. The time necessary to develop gingivitis varied from 10 to 21 days of plaque accumulation (Fig. 7-1). Concurrent microbiologic examinations showed that the number of bacteria colonizing the tooth surfaces increased dramatically and that distinct changes in the composition of the flora occurred. When good oral hygiene was reinstituted, the

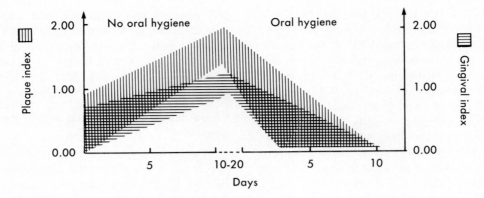

Fig. 7-1. Relationships between plaque and gingival indices during periods of no oral hygiene and good oral hygiene as monitored in experimental gingivitis system. (Modified from Löe H et al: J Periodontol 36:177, 1965.)

original sparse microflora was reestablished and the inflamed gingiva reverted to normal.

Over the years the validity of these observations has been confirmed by studies in children (Mackler and Crawford, 1973) and the aged (Holm-Pedersen et al., 1975). Also, virtually all population studies in which the association was examined have shown that the prevalence and severity of gingivitis were closely correlated with the presence and amount of supragingival plaque. In fact, the association between gingivitis and plaque is so strong that in order to investigate the role of any other local or systemic factor, the data must be balanced for oral hygiene, oral debris, or supragingival plaque before any analysis can be made.

SLOWLY PROGRESSING PERIODONTITIS

Both early and recent studies have clearly shown that slowly developing periodontitis (adult periodontitis) begins before the age of 20 based on measurements of alveolar bone loss in radiographs (Marshall-Day and Shourie, 1949; Marshall-Day et al., 1955), on the presence of periodontal pockets (Greene, 1963; Russell, 1971), and on clinical measurement of periodontal attachment loss (Ramfjord, 1960; Löe et al., 1978a).

A 1985 to 1986 study of the employed U.S. population (Miller et al., 1987) showed that approximately 50% of individuals 18 to 19 years of age had one or more sites with at least 2 mm *loss of attachment* (Table 7-1). The prevalence of attachment loss increased with age, and by 65 years approximately 90% showed one or more sites with loss of attachment. More severe periodontal destruction (4 mm or more attachment loss) was found in 24% of adults (Fig. 7-2).

A 1981 study of U.S. adults (Brown et al., 1988) showed that approximately 65% of individuals between 19

Table 7-1. Percentage of employed dentate Americans with at least one site with attachment loss of 2 mm or more by age and sex in 1985-1986

Age group (years)	Male (%)	Female (%)	Both (%)
18-19	52.71	50.30	51.53
20-24	64.55	55.07	59.97
25-29	70.89	62.54	67.14
30-34	77.22	74.32	75.95
35-39	83.85	76.59	80.67
40-44	82.92	80.89	82.02
45-49	89.34	83.69	86.94
50-54	96.58	88.51	93.24
55-59	97.36	86.41	92.74
60+	95.70	89.10	92.90
All ages	79.97	72.56	76.68

From Miller AJ et al: The national survey of oral health in U.S. employed adults and seniors: 1985-1986, NIH Pub No 87-2868, Aug 1987.

Table 7-2. Percentage of persons by deepest pocket and by age in the U.S. population in 1981

Age	All pockets < 4mm	1 or more pockets 4-6 mm	1 or more pockets > 6 mm
19-44	71.2	25.4	3.4
45-64	52.5	31.3	16.3
	*	*	*
65+	51.8	34.2	14.0
	*	*	*
All ages	64.0	28.0	8.0

From Brown LJ et al: J Periodontol 60:363, 1989.
*Between the rows indicates that the difference in percentages between the age groups is statistically significant at the 1% level.

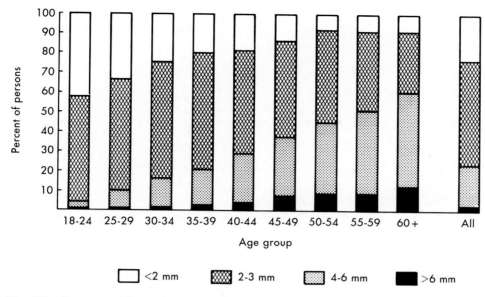

Fig. 7-2. Percentage of employed dentate Americans between 18 and 65 years of age by most severe loss of attachment. (From Miller AJ: The national survey of oral health in U.S. employed adults and seniors: 1985-1986, NIH Pub No 87-2868, Aug 1987.)

and 65 years of age had a maximum *pocket depth* of 3 mm or less; maximum pocket depths between 4 and 6 mm occurred in 28% of individuals, and 8% had one or more pockets deeper than 6 mm (Table 7-2). A national sample of the Danish adult population examined in 1981 showed similar levels of periodontal destruction. Approximately 50% of Danes between 16 and 80 years had a healthy periodontium; the other half of the population had gingivitis or periodontitis to varying degrees: 60% had two or more pockets between 3.5 and 5.5 mm, and approximately 10% had two or more pockets deeper than 5.5 mm.

In Americans 65 years of age and older, 95% had at least one site in the mouth with periodontal attachment loss (see Table 7-1) and more than 65% had attachment loss measuring 4 mm or more (Miller et al., 1987). Among Americans of all age groups, males had a higher rate of periodontal destruction than females (Table 7-3).

One of the interesting features in the assessment of attachment loss and pocket depth in these populations is the indirect evidence of a high prevalence of gingival recession (Table 7-4). To what extent recession is a component of periodontal pathogenesis or the result of personal and/or professional initiative is not entirely clear.

In adults the deepest pockets are more frequently found in the posterior teeth, and more often in interdental areas than in buccal or lingual sites (Lövdal et al., 1958). The distribution of the periodontal pockets (Schei et al., 1959) and loss of attachment (Löe et al., 1978a) appears to be symmetric in both jaws (Figs. 7-3 and 7-4).

Longitudinal studies (Löe et al., 1978a) have shown that for middle-class populations living in industrialized countries in which personal and professional dental care is optimal, the adult periodontitis lesion progresses very slowly (individual mean between 0.05 and 0.1 mm per year) (Table 7-3). Among some populations of the developing world (Löe et al., 1986) who do not practice oral hygiene and who have no access to dental care services, the mean rate of progression is three to four times greater (individual mean between 0.1 and 0.3 mm per year) (Table 7-4).

Table 7-3. Percentage of employed dentate Americans between 18 and 65 years of age by most severe site of attachment loss in 1985-1986

Severity of attachment loss (mm)	Male (%)	Female (%)	Both %	Both Cum %
2	30.54	33.91	32.04	76.68
3	21.40	19.49	20.55	44.64
4	11.33	9.41	10.48	24.09
5	7.24	4.57	6.05	13.65
6	4.30	2.66	3.57	7.56
7	2.16	1.01	1.65	3.99
8	1.45	0.66	1.10	2.34
9	0.68	0.34	0.53	1.24
10	0.41	0.11	0.27	0.71
11	0.23	0.17	0.20	0.44
12+	0.24	0.23	0.24	—

From Miller AJ et al: The national survey of oral health in U.S. employed adults and seniors: 1985-1986, NIH Pub No 87-2868, Aug 1987.

Table 7-4. Annual rate of attachment loss (LA) on mesial and buccal tooth surfaces during various age periods based on mean increments in those who participated in all surveys in Norway and Sri Lanka

	Norway			Sri Lanka	
		Mean annual LA rate			Mean annual LA rate
Age period (years)	Mesial	Buccal	Age period (years)	Mesial	Buccal
			15-21	0.18	0.18
17-23	0.09	0.14	17-23	0.22	0.21
19-25	0.10	0.13	19-25	0.23	0.23
21-27	0.06	0.11	21-27	0.24	0.24
23-29	0.05	0.09	23-29	0.25	0.22
25-31	0.07	0.09	25-31	0.26	0.21
27-33	0.07	0.08	27-33	0.24	0.23
29-25	0.08	0.11	29-35	0.28	0.25
31-37+	0.08	0.12	31-37+	0.29	0.21

From Löe H et al: J Periodontol 49:607, 1978.

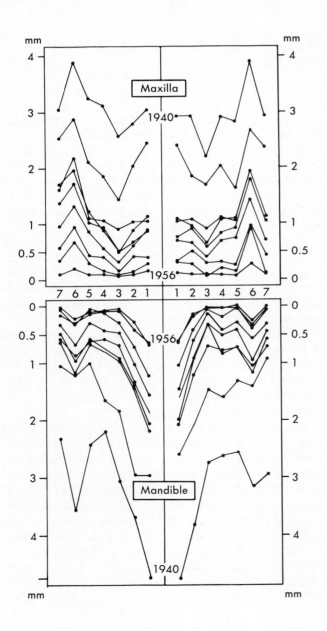

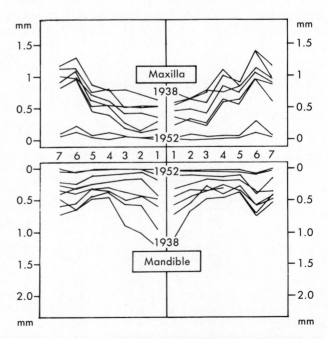

Fig. 7-3. Mean loss of attachment in different teeth (1 to 7) of Sri Lankan tea laborers between 15 and 30+ years of age. (From Löe H et al: J Periodontol 49:607, 1978.)

Fig. 7-4. Mean loss of attachment in different teeth (1 to 7) of a Norwegian middle-class population between 16 and 30+ years of age. (From Löe H et al: J Periodontol 49:607, 1978.)

Mechanism of initiation and progession of adult periodontitis

Slowly developing periodontitis in the young is first seen in the interdental areas of posterior teeth in both jaws, where plaque and gingivitis most frequently form. Early epidemiologic reviews (Löe 1963; Scherp, 1963; Waerhaug, 1966) suggested that chronic gingivitis leads to adult periodontitis. However, during the last few years the relationship between the prevalence and severity of gingivitis and the onset of adult periodontitis has been questioned. At the heart of this discussion lies a concept that gingivitis is a pathologic entity of its own, distinctly different from periodontitis (Page and Schroeder, 1982) and that evidence that untreated gingivitis progresses to periodontitis is non-existent (Goodson, 1986).

Not all gingivitis proceeds to periodontitis, as shown in population groups and for individual teeth in human patients, as well as in laboratory animals who otherwise develop periodontitis. However, showing that untreated gingivitis does not advance to periodontitis in a few populations around the world or in a few teeth in beagles may not justify abandoning the existing paradigm that gingivitis precedes periodontitis. Not *all* gingivitis leads to periodontitis. However, if periodontitis develops, it has been *preceded* by gingivitis. At this time no data suggest that periodontitis develops *in the absence* of gingivitis. Since we are presently unable to predict which gingivitis lesion will proceed to periodontitis and which will not, current concepts hold that only control of gingivitis can prevent the development of the advanced lesion. Similar principles form the basis for maintenance programs intended to prevent recurrence of the disease in patients treated for periodontal destruction.

All available data from cross-sectional and longitudinal studies suggest that the prevalence of adult periodontitis increases with age and that the periodontal lesion as measured by attachment loss and/or pocket depth progresses slowly throughout adult life, although the rates of progression differ among populations, individuals, and different teeth within the same individual (Schei et al., 1959; Löe et al., 1978a, 1986). Recently a cyclic pattern of progression has been suggested that is characterized by bursts in disease activity, followed by periods of remission or even gains in periodontal attachment (Goodson et al., 1982; Socransky et al., 1982; Hafajee et al., 1982, 1983). This concept was derived from repeated clinical measurements, computer simulations, and statistical modeling of periodontal lesions that suggested that at any one time only a few lesions (perhaps 1% to 2%) in any given patient are active sites of progressive disease. The remaining lesions are allegedly inactive and nonprogressing. This view of periodontal pathogenesis is still only a hypothesis and will require further experimentation and evidence before acceptance.

Longitudinal studies of *untreated* periodontal disease in animals (Saxe et al., 1965; Lindhe et al., 1975) and in humans (Löe et al., 1978c) show that the most conspicuous characteristic of the untreated periodontal lesion is that it continues, with more and more periodontium lost over the years. This process may be slow at times and accelerated at others, but as documented in both rapidly and moderately progressing disease groups in Sri Lanka, without intervention the disease process continues until the entire periodontium is affected. The results are loss of a tooth, multiple teeth, or the entire dentition (Löe et al., 1986).

Another important implication of the "episodic disease activity concept" is that remission of the advanced lesion or even regained attachment is common. To what extent this is true for populations in industrialized countries is unclear. However, regained attachment and spontaneous remission are not prominent pathogenic features of *untreated* periodontal disease (Löe et al., 1986).

The continuous progression of untreated periodontal lesions over a lifetime does not rule out discrete local exacerbations as possible mechanisms of disease progress. Linear decay and linear increase in severity are rare phenomena in any chronic disease.

Currently, study of the natural history of this disease suggests that over time, if periodontal disease in humans is not subjected to optimal personal or professional intervention, irrespective of possible short periods of activity and inactivity, continuous progress is seen.

Significant etiologic factors

Although the prevalence and the severity of periodontitis usually increase from adolescence through adulthood to old age, it is not likely that *age per se* is a significant factor (Abdellatif and Burt, 1987). Both gingivitis and periodontitis are consistently associated with poorer levels of oral hygiene, regardless of age (Suomi et al., 1971). Also, longitudinal studies suggest that periodontal disease development is virtually halted when adults maintain a high degree of oral cleanliness (Löe et al., 1978a; Anerud et al., 1979).

Populations of industrialized countries show a significantly lower prevalence and severity of periodontitis in women than in men. The difference is seen at an early age and persists throughout life (Tables 7-5 to 7-7; see also Table 7-1). This association tends to disappear and even reverse in developing nations (Waerhaug, 1966). Therefore whether these are genuine *sex differences* is not clear at this time. The phenomenon may have less to do with gender than with local or cultural factors.

The *geographic* distribution of periodontal disease varies widely. For instance, some populations on the Indian subcontinent and in other parts of Asia seem to be more susceptible to periodontal disease than are North Americans or Europeans. The highest incidence and degree of severity ever seen was found in South Vietnam (Russell, 1960), where advanced disease with loosening of the teeth

Table 7-5. Percentage and cumulative percentage by most severe pocket depth of employed dentate Americans between 18 and 65 years of age in 1985-1986

Pocket depth (mm)	Male		Female		Both	
	%	Cum %	%	Cum %	%	Cum %
2	50.52	96.36	56.51	93.69	53.18	95.18
3	28.76	45.85	26.47	37.18	27.74	42.00
4	11.86	17.09	7.58	10.71	9.96	14.26
5	3.05	5.23	2.05	3.14	2.61	4.30
6	1.39	2.18	0.72	1.08	1.09	1.70
7	0.53	0.80	0.30	0.37	0.43	0.61
8	0.11	0.27	0.05	0.06	0.08	0.18
9	0.06	0.16	0.01	0.01	0.04	0.09
10	0.07	0.10	0.01	0.01	0.04	0.06
11	0.00	0.03	0.00	0.00	0.00	0.01
12+	0.02	0.02	0.00	0.00	0.01	0.01

From Miller AJ et al: The national survey of oral health of U.S. employed adults and seniors: 1985-1986, NIH Pub No 87-2868, Aug 1987.

Table 7-6. Percentage of dentate senior Americans with at least one site with attachment loss of 2 mm or more by age and sex in 1985-1986

Age group (years)	Male (%)	Female (%)	Both (%)
65-69	98.13	94.10	95.47
70-74	98.63	93.23	95.24
75-79	97.19	93.81	94.89
80+	96.56	93.48	94.32
All ages	97.91	93.68	95.10

From Miller AJ et al: The national survey of oral health in U.S. employed adults and seniors: 1985-1986, NIH Pub No 87-2868, Aug 1987.

Table 7-7. Percentage and cumulative percentage of dentate senior Americans by most severe pocket depth in 1985-1986

Pocket depth (mm)	Male		Female		Both	
	%	Cum %	%	Cum %	%	Cum %
2	37.29	94.91	48.60	91.44	44.81	92.60
3	27.84	57.62	24.46	42.85	25.60	47.79
4	17.72	29.78	13.07	18.38	14.62	22.20
5	4.79	12.06	2.85	5.31	3.50	7.57
6	4.97	7.27	1.33	2.46	2.55	4.07
7	0.81	2.30	0.54	1.13	0.63	1.52
8	0.37	1.49	0.26	0.60	0.30	0.89
9	0.26	1.12	0.16	0.33	0.19	0.60
10	0.82	0.86	0.00	0.18	0.28	0.41
11	0.00	0.03	0.00	0.18	0.00	0.13
12	0.03	0.03	0.18	0.18	0.13	0.13

From Miller AJ et al: The national survey of oral health of U.S. employed adults and seniors: 1985-1986, NIH Pub No 87-2868, Aug 1987.

was common in teenagers. Studies of natives in the Pacific area (Davies, 1956), Africa, (Olsson, 1976), and South America (Russell, 1960) indicate that the prevalence in some populations is conspicuously high and that the severity may vary considerably within subpopulations.

At first glance *racial factors* were thought to be responsible for these variations, a notion initially supported by the finding that black Americans had more periodontal disease than white Americans. However, when comparison of periodontal disease status was made between blacks and whites of the same socioeconomic group, the differences in occurrence and severity disappeared (Russell and Ayers, 1960).

In industrialized nations children and youth from *rural* areas have more gingivitis than age mates from *urban* and metropolitan centers (Benjamin et al., 1957; Russell et al., 1957a, 1957b). A study of the *socioeconomic* groupings showed that among Danish men (Pindborg, 1951), office clerks and teachers had a healthier periodontium than skilled blue collar workers, who, again, showed better periodontal status than unskilled laborers. Similar correlations between socioeconomic and periodontal status have been observed in adult white Americans (Russell and Ayers, 1960).

These variations in periodontal health could be attributed to differing economic capabilities and a subsequent inability to pay for routine examination and care. However, a study of U.S. occupational and income characteristics suggested that *educational level* had more significant impact on periodontal status than did economic level (Russell and Ayers, 1960). Generally, this is also true for Scandinavians (Lövdal et al., 1958), Indians (Marshall-Day and Shourie, 1949), and Sri Lankans (Waerhaug, 1967).

It is tempting to ascribe the higher frequency and degree of severity of periodontal disease among developing countries and lower socioeconomic groups to general *malnutrition*, lack of specific nutritional components, and/or special *systemic diseases* caused by factors related to poor living conditions. General health and nutrition have long been considered important to periodontal health. The role of nutrition in periodontal disease was studied as part of a major nutritional survey in Alaska (Russell et al., 1961); results suggested that periodontal disease in individuals with a clear deficiency of one or more nutritional components showed little or no difference from the condition in patients with no diagnosed deficiency. Similar studies in Asia and Africa (Waerhaug, 1967; Russell, 1962) concluded that no relationship could be established between group periodontal status and group nutritional status or group serum or urinary vitamin levels.

Similarly, insufficient epidemiologic evidence exists to suggest that general health status plays a major role in periodontal disease. This does not mean that general health, including nutritional status, is of no significance. Individuals suffering from insulin-dependent diabetes (juvenile diabetes or type I diabetes) generally show increased susceptibility to periodontitis (Glavind et al., 1968; Cianciola et al., 1982). Probably all diseases that affect the general condition of the patient will affect the course of the periodontal disease. The fact that epidemiologic research has been unable to disclose the precise relationships probably reflects the critical shortage of analytic epidemiologic studies and/or inadequate methodology rather than the actual unimportance of health and nutrition in the development and progression of adult periodontitis. On the other hand, adequate nutrition in industrialized nations and good general health are not necessarily synonymous with periodontal health.

RAPIDLY PROGRESSING PERIODONTITIS

Rapidly progressing periodontitis in the young is characterized by minimal gingival inflammation and by loss of connective tissue attachment and bone in the regions of the incisors and first molars, a condition known as localized juvenile periodontitis. A more generalized pattern of destruction involving all groups of teeth has also been described, although the localized pattern may occur more frequently in teenagers (Hørmand and Frandsen, 1979). In contrast to earlier reports, advanced periodontitis lesions in young people may be significantly associated with dental plaque and gingivitis (Burmeister et al., 1984; Löe et al., 1986). The most conspicuous feature of this form of periodontal disease is the rate at which the periodontium is destroyed (Löe et al., 1986) (Fig. 7-5). Loss of the involved teeth before the age of 20 years is not uncommon.

Estimates of the prevalence of rapidly progressing periodontitis in juveniles vary greatly, possibly because of differences in examination procedures and criteria, and the use of clinical studies of select population groups rather than random sampling in epidemiologic studies. In general, rapidly progressing periodontitis is relatively rare. Studies based on a combination of radiographic and probing assessments report prevalence values of 0.2% for Norway (Gjermo et al., 1984), 0.1% for Finland (Saxen, 1980), 0.5% for Brazil (Hansen et al., 1984), and 0.75% for Nigeria (MacGregor, 1980). In 1979 Hørmand and Frandsen reported a male-to-female ratio of 1:2.5, with some variation associated with age. Barnett et al. (1982) recorded a male-to-female ratio of approximately 1:2 in patients attending a dental clinic for treatment. However, such marked differences in the sex ratio have not been confirmed in studies with well-defined diagnostic criteria carried out in random samples (Saxby, 1984).

Historically, a racial association has been observed in population studies. In a recent survey of 7266 children (14 to 19 years) in England, the prevalence of juvenile periodontitis was found to be 0.1% (Saxby, 1984). In the same group the prevalences were 0.02% for whites, 0.2% for Asians, and 0.8% for blacks. Thus blacks and Asians appear to be at greater risk for the development of rapidly progressing periodontitis. Limited evidence suggests that

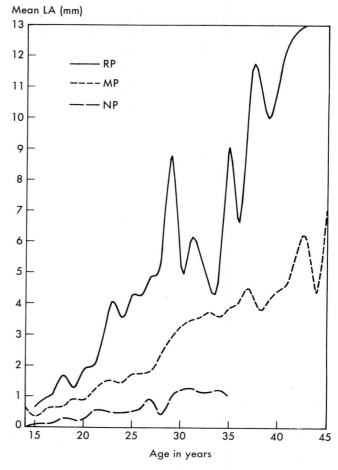

Fig. 7-5. Mean loss of attachment in three subgroups of Sri Lankan tea laborers between 15 and 45 years of age showing rapid progression *(RP)*, moderate progression *(MP)*, and no progression *(NP)* of attachment loss. (From Löe et al: J Clin Periodontol 13:431, 1986. © 1986 Munksgaard International Publishers, Ltd., Copenhagen, Denmark.)

juvenile periodontitis shows a familial distribution or is genetically determined, with the disease being transmitted either as an autosomal recessive or as an x-linked dominant trait (Saxen, 1980; Saxen and Nevanlinna, 1984; Lang et al., 1987).

PERIODONTITIS AND TOOTH LOSS

During the 1960s almost 10% of U.S. adults aged 35 to 44 years had lost all their teeth (Fig. 7-6); approximately 20% of those aged 45 to 54 years were edentulous; more than 35% of the 55- to 64-year-olds were without teeth; and at 65 years of age and beyond almost 50% were edentulous. The percentage of edentulous persons increased almost linearly with age (Fig. 7-6).

The most recent data (1985 to 1986) revealed that only 4% of the U.S. population under 65 years of age were edentulous and that for the 35- to 64-year age group, edentulism had been reduced by 50% to 60% as compared with that of their age mates 15 years ago (Fig. 7-6). In contrast,

Table 7-8. Average number of teeth by age group for total sample and dentate employed Americans between 18 and 65 years of age in 1985-1986

Age groups (years)	Total sample	Dentate persons
18-19	26.96	26.96
20-24	26.93	26.93
25-29	26.54	26.60
30-34	26.02	26.08
35-39	24.35	24.88
40-44	23.16	24.01
45-49	20.84	22.41
50-54	19.14	21.55
55-59	17.55	20.69
60-64	17.92	20.76
65+	13.97	17.52
All ages	23.60	24.63

From Miller AJ et al: The national survey of oral health in U.S. employed adults and seniors: 1985-1986, NIH Pub No 87-2868, Aug 1987.

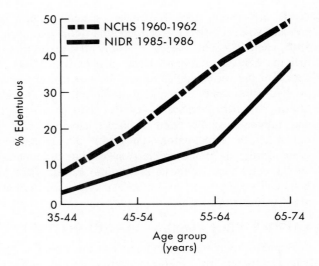

Fig. 7-6. Percentage of toothless persons among adult U.S. populations surveyed in 1960 to 1962 and in 1985 to 1986. (From Miller AJ et al: The national survey of oral health in U.S. employed adults and seniors: 1985-1986, NIH Pub No 87-2868, Aug 1987.)

Table 7-9. Average number of teeth by age group for total sample and dentate employed Americans 65 years of age and beyond in 1985-1986

Age groups (years)	Total sample	Dentate persons
65-69	13.30	19.57
70-74	11.37	19.44
75-79	10.25	18.66
80-84	8.95	17.25
85+	8.10	16.70
All ages	11.14	18.93

From Miller AJ et al: The national survey of oral health of U.S. employed adults and seniors: 1985-1986, NIH Pub No 87-2868, Aug 1987.

Table 7-10. Percentage of persons in U.S. population by age and by number of teeth indicated for extraction due to periodontal disease in 1981

No. of teeth	Age groups						
	19-44 years		45-64 years		65+ years		All ages
0	98.8	*	91.4	*	89.9		95.8
1	0.4	*	1.8	*	2.9		1.1
2	0.3	*	1.6	*	1.5		0.7
3+	0.5	*	5.2	*	5.7		2.4

From Brown LJ et al: J Periodontol 60:363, 1989.
*Between columns indicates that the difference in percentages between the age groups is statistically significant at the 1% level.

42% of persons 65 years of age and older had lost all their teeth. Although this also represents a decrease when compared with similar age groups studied earlier, the percentage of reduction is less than for younger adults. Recent national data from Denmark (1986) tend to confirm that in industrialized countries total loss of the natural dentition before 45 years of age is becoming rare, but also that edentulism is still conspicuous in mature and older adults.

Dentate Americans between 18 and 65 years of age had an average of approximately 24.6 teeth (third molars excluded). As Table 7-8 shows, there was a gradual decrease in the number of teeth with age. However, between 65 and 80 years of age and beyond, there was still an average of 18 to 19 teeth present (Table 7-9).

The relative contribution of the various oral and dental diseases to tooth loss has never been examined with any degree of precision. Early data (Brekhus, 1929) suggested that caries and periodontal disease were jointly responsible for 97% of tooth extractions. At that time, tooth loss caused by caries was greatest during childhood and adolescence, whereas periodontal disease was considered to be the major cause of tooth mortality during adult life. In 1952 the American Dental Association published a review based on reports of 4000 dentists, in which the needs of 39,000 patients were analyzed. It was found that in patients 35 to 40 years of age, extractions due to periodontal disease were three times more frequent than those for caries.

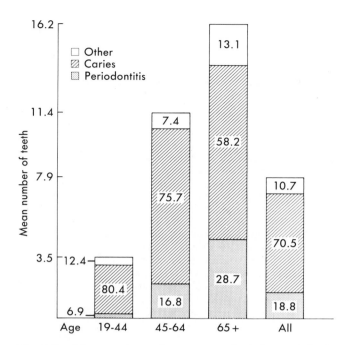

Fig. 7-7. Mean number and percentage of missing teeth in the United States by cause and age. (From Brown LJ et al: J Periodontol 60:363, 1989.)

orthodontic, and other causes had led to the loss of approximately 11%. Slightly less than 20% of the teeth were lost because of periodontal disease. The mean number of teeth lost because of periodontal reasons increased from 0.2 for the 19- to 44-year age group to 1.9 for the 45- to 64-year age group, reaching a high of 4.7 in the elderly. Even with the elderly, only 29% of missing teeth were due to periodontal disease (Fig. 7-7).

REFERENCES

Abdellatif HM and Burt BA: An epidemiological investigation into the relative importance of age and oral hygiene status as determinants of periodontitis, J Periodont Res 66:13, 1987.

Anerud A et al: The natural history of periodontal disease in man: changes in gingival health and oral hygiene before 40 years of age, J Periodont Res 14:526, 1979.

Anerud KE et al: Periodontal disease in three young adult populations, J Periodont Res 18:655, 1983.

Barnett ML et al: The prevalence of juvenile periodontitis ("periodontosis") in a dental school patient population, J Dent Res 61:391, 1982.

Benjamin EM et al: Periodontal disease in rural children of 25 Indiana counties, J Periodontol 28:294, 1957.

Björby A and Löe H: Gingival and oral hygiene conditions in school children in Gothenburg, Sweden, Sverig Tandlak T 61:561, 1969.

Brekhus PJ: Dental disease and its relation to the loss of human teeth, J Am Dent Assoc 16:2237, 1929.

Brown LJ et al: Periodontal disease in the U.S. in 1981: prevalence, severity, extent and role in tooth mortality, J Periodontol 60:363, 1989.

Burmeister JA et al: Localized juvenile periodontitis and general severe periodontitis: clinical findings, J Clin Periodontol 11:181, 1984.

Cianciola LJ et al: Prevalence of periodontal disease in insulin-dependent diabetes mellitus (juvenile diabetes), J Am Dent Assoc 104:653, 1982.

Davies GN: Dental conditions among the Polynesians of Pakapuka (Danger Island). II. The prevalence of periodontal disease, J Dent Res 35:734, 1956.

Gjermo P et al: Prevalence of bone loss in a group of Brazilian teenagers assessed on bite-wing radiographs, J Clin Periodontol 11:104, 1984.

Glavind L et al: The relationship between periodontal state and diabetes duration, insulin dosage and retinal changes, J Periodontol 39:341, 1968.

Goodson JM: Clinical measurements of periodontitis. In Chilton NW, editor: Conference on clinical trials in periodontal diseases, Chicago, 1985, J Clin Periodontol 13:549, 1986.

Goodson JM et al: Pattern of progression and regression of advanced destructive periodontal disease, J Clin Periodontol 9:472, 1982.

Greene J: Oral hygiene and periodontal disease, Am J Public Health 53:913, 1963.

Haffajee AD et al: Periodontal disease activity, J Periodont Res 17:521, 1982.

Haffajee AD et al: Clinical parameters as predictors of destructive periodontal disease activity, J Clin Periodontol 10:257, 1983.

Hansen BF et al: Periodontal bone loss in 15-year-old Norwegians, J Clin Periodontol 11:125, 1984.

Holm-Pedersen P et al: Experimental gingivitis in young and elderly individuals, J Clin Periodontol 2:14, 1975.

Hørmand J and Frandsen A: Juvenile periodontitis: localization of bone loss in relation to age, sex, and teeth, J Clin Periodontol 6:407, 1979.

Hugoson A et al: Dental health between 1973 and 1978 in individuals aged 3-20 years in the community of Jönköping, Sweden, Swed Dent J 4:217, 1980.

King JD: Gingival disease in Gibraltar evacuee children, Lancet 1:495, 1944.

Obviously, in populations who have little or no caries but are susceptible to periodontal disease, the percentage of tooth loss found to be caused by advanced periodontal disease will be high (Löe et al., 1978b). During a U.S. survey in 1981, examiners were asked to indicate which teeth currently in the mouth should be extracted and whether the extraction was required because of caries, periodontal disease, or other reasons (Brown et al., 1988). *Teeth requiring extraction* for periodontal reasons were rare. Ninety-six percent of all persons did not have any of these teeth at the time of the examination (Table 7-10). Only 1 in 100 persons 19 to 44 years old had a tooth that required extraction due to periodontal problems; this increased to 1 in 10 for persons aged 45 or older. Persons 19 to 44 years of age requiring three or more periodontally related extractions were even more rare (0.5%); not unexpectedly, the percentage increased in persons aged 45 and over to over 5%. Of course, this represents the backlog of teeth requiring extraction from advanced disease. Many of these teeth would have already been extracted, reducing the number left in the mouth at a point in time. This is a traditional problem with cross-sectional data. The *number of missing teeth* for any reason increased from 3.5 teeth in adults under age 45 to approximately 11.4 teeth in the 45- to 64-year age group and to 16 in those aged 65 and older (Fig. 7-7). The reasons for the extraction of teeth, as determined by the examiner, revealed that caries accounted for just over 70% of the extractions, whereas prosthetic,

King JD: Gingival disease in Dundee, Dent Rec 65:9, 1945.

Kirkegaard E et al: Oral health status, dental treatment need, and dental care habits in a representative sample of the adult Danish population: survey of oral health of Danish adults, Aarhus, Denmark, 1986, Odontologisk Boghandel.

Lang KP et al: Oral hygiene and gingival health in Danish dental students and faculty, Community Dent Oral Epidemiol 5:237, 1977.

Lindhe J et al: Plaque induced periodontal disease in beagle dogs: a 4-year clinical, roentgenographical and histometric study, J Periodont Res 10:243, 1975.

Löe H: Epidemiology of periodontal disease, Odontol T 71:479, 1963.

Löe H and Silness J: Periodontal disease in pregnancy. I. Prevalence and severity, Acta Odontol Scand 21:533, 1963.

Löe H, Theilade E, and Jensen SB: Experimental gingivitis in man, J Periodontol 36:177, 1965.

Löe H et al: The natural history of periodontal disease in man: the rate of periodontal destruction before 40 years of age, J Periodontol 49:607, 1978a.

Löe H et al: The natural history of periodontal disease in man: study design and baseline data, J Periodont Res 13:550, 1978b.

Löe H et al: The natural history of periodontal disease in man: tooth mortality before 40 years of age, J Periodont Res 13:563, 1978c.

Löe H et al: The natural history of periodontal disease in man: rapid, moderate and no loss of attachment in Sri Lankan laborers 15 to 45 years of age, J Clin Periodontol 13:431, 1986.

Long JC et al: Early onset periodontitis: a comparison and evaluation of two proposed modes of inheritance, Genet Inheritance 4:13, 1987.

Lövdal A et al: Incidence of clinical manifestations of periodontal disease in light of oral hygiene and calculus formation, J Am Dent Assoc 56:21, 1958.

MacGregor ID: Radiographic survey of periodontal disease in 264 adolescent school boys in Lagos, Nigeria, Community Dent Oral Epidemiol 8:56, 1980.

Mackler SB and Crawford JJ: Plaque development and gingivitis in the primary dentition, J Periodontol 48:705, 1973.

Marshall-Day CD and Shourie KL: A roentgenographic survey of periodontal disease in India, J Am Dent Assoc 39:572, 1949.

Marshall-Day CD et al: Periodontal disease: prevalence and incidence, J Periodontol 26:185, 1955.

McHugh DW et al: Dental disease and related factors in 13-year-old children in Dundee, Br Dent J 117:246, 1964.

Messner CT et al: Dental survey of school children ages 6-14 years, made in 1933-1934 in 26 states, Public Health Bull No 226, Washington DC, 1936, US Government Printing Office.

Miller AJ et al: The national survey of oral health in U.S. employed adults and seniors: 1985-1986, NIH Pub No 87-2868, Aug 1987.

Mühlemann HR and Mazor ZS: Gingivitis in Zurich school children, Helv Odontol Acta 2:3, 1958.

Olsson B: Periodontal disease and oral hygiene in Arussi province, Ethiopia, Community Dent Oral Epidemiol 6:139, 1978.

Page RC and Schroeder HE: Periodontitis in man and other animals: a comparative review, Basel, Switzerland, 1982, S Karger.

Parfitt HGJ: A five year longitudinal study of the gingival condition of a group of children in England, J Periodontol 26:26, 1957.

Pindborg JJ: Gingivitis in military personnel with special reference to ulceromembranous gingivitis, Odontol T 59:408, 1951.

Ramfjord SP: Indices for prevalence and incidence of periodontal disease, J Periodontol 30:51, 1959.

Ramfjord SP: Survey of the periodontal status of boys 11 to 17 years old in Bombay, India, J Periodontol 32:237, 1961.

Rosenzweig KA: Gingivitis in children of Israel, J Periodontol 31, 404, 1960.

Russell AL: A system of classification and scoring for prevalence surveys of periodontal disease, J Dent Res 35:350, 1956.

Russell AL: A social factor associated with the severity of periodontal disease, J Dent Res 36:922, 1957a.

Russell AL: Some epidemiological characteristics of periodontal disease in a series of urban population, J Periodontol 28:286, 1957b.

Russell AL: Geographical distribution and epidemiology of periodontal disease, WHO/BH/33/34, Geneva, 1960.

Russell AL: Periodontal disease in well and malnourished populations, Arch Environ Health 5:153, 1962.)The prevalence of periodontal disease in different populations during the circumpubertal period, J Periodontol 62:508, 1971.

Russell AL and Ayers P: Periodontal disease and socio-economic status in Birmingham, Ala., Am J Public Health 50:206, 1960.

Russell AL et al: Periodontal disease and nutrition in Eskimo scouts of the Alaska national guard, J Dent Res 40:604, 1961.

Saxby M: Prevalence of juvenile periodontitis in a British school population, Community Dent Oral Epidemiol 12:185, 1984.

Saxe SR et al: Oral debris, calculus, and periodontal disease in the beagle dog, Periodontics 5:217, 1965.

Saxen L: Heredity of juvenile periodontitis, J Clin Periodontol 7:276, 1980.

Saxen L and Nevanlinna HR: Autosomal recessive inheritance of juvenile periodontitis: test of a hypothesis, Clin Genet 25:332, 1984.

Schei O et al: Alveolar bone loss as related to oral hygiene and age, J Periodontol 30:7, 1959.

Scherp HW: Current concepts in periodontal disease research: epidemiological contributions, J Am Dent Assoc 68:667, 1963.

Schour I and Massler M: Gingival disease in Italy 1945. I. Prevalence of gingivitis in various age groups, J Am Dent Assoc 35:475, 1947.

Socransky SS et al: New concepts of destructive periodontal disease, J Clin Periodontol 11:21, 1984.

Suomi JD et al: The effect of controlled oral hygiene procedures on the progression of periodontal disease in adults: results after third and final year, J Periodontol 42:152, 1971.

Theilade E et al: Experimental gingivitis in man. II. A longitudinal clinical and bacteriological investigation, J Periodont Res 1:1, 1966.

Theilade J: The microscopic structure of dental calculus, thesis, Rochester, NY, 1960, University of Rochester.

US Health Research and Service Administration National Household Probability Study of Dental Health Outcomes Related to Prepayment, 1981.

Waerhaug J: Gingival pocket: anatomy, pathology, deepening and elimination, Odontol T 60(suppl 1), 1952.

Waerhaug J: Epidemiology of periodontal disease. In Ramfjord SP, Keer DA, and Ash MM, editors: Workshop in periodontics, Ann Arbor, 1966, University of Michigan Press.

Waerhaug J: Prevalence of periodontal disease in Ceylon: association with age, sex, oral hygiene, socio-economic factors, vitamin deficiencies, malnutrition, betel and tobacco consumption and ethnic group; final report, Acta Odontol Scand 25:205, 1967.

Westin G et al: Conditions of the teeth and dental disease in upper Norrland: an investigation into questions of social hygiene in the counties of Vasterbotten and Norrbotten, Sweden, part III, Lund, Sweden, 1937, Medicinalstyrelsen.

Chapter 8

SALIVA AND DENTAL PELLICLES

Frank A. Scannapieco
Michael J. Levine

SALIVA

Saliva has been defined as "the fluid secreted by the salivary glands that begins the digestion of foods." Saliva, however, is hardly the simple body fluid, nor does it have the limited function, implied in this definition. The functions of saliva are best appreciated by individuals having diminished salivary function, or xerostomia (Mandel, 1987). These individuals suffer from increased caries and periodontal disease; their oral mucosa is constantly irritated and sore; food is difficult to chew and swallow; and taste acuity is impaired. Collectively, these clinical observations point to the protective capacity of saliva.

Saliva is thought to function in part by forming protective tenacious films, or pellicles, on the available oral surfaces. These dental pellicles may mediate many of the interactions that occur at intraoral surfaces. For example,

□Supported in part by USHPHS Grants DE00158, DE08240, and DE07585 from the National Institute of Dental Research.

salivary pellicles can serve as the receptor(s) for initial bacterial colonization, which leads to the formation of organized communities or dental plaques. These bacterial dental plaques are responsible for initiating two of the most common human afflictions: caries and periodontal disease.

The "whole" saliva that bathes the oral cavity is primarily a mixture of secretions from the paired major (parotid, submandibular, and sublingual) glands and the numerous minor (labial, buccal, glossopalatine, palatine, and lingual) glands. While salivary glands are normally not found in the gingival tissues, atopic salivary gland tissue has been reported in gingiva (gingival salivary gland choristoma; Moskow and Baden, 1986). Whole saliva also contains bacteria (about 10^8 to 10^9/ml); their products, such as organic acids and enzymes; epithelial cells; food debris; and components from gingival crevicular fluid.

Anatomy and physiology

Salivary glands are composed of acini, ducts, and stroma. Acini are composed of two cell types: mucous cells, which secrete the viscous mucins, and serous cells, which secrete a less viscous watery fluid. The parotid glands possess exclusively serous cells; the sublingual and minor glands contain predominantly mucus-secreting cells; and the submandibular glands are mixed. Acinar cells produce the majority of macromolecules and water found in salivary secretions and are involved in salt transport. Cells that line the secretory ducts also contribute components to the secretions and help regulate the electrolyte content of saliva. Stimulation of salivary gland tissues results in the release of components contained within the secretory granules into the salivary ducts. The secretion at this point is isotonic with respect to electrolytes. As the secretion trav-

Table 8-1. Normal flow rates: whole and gland-derived saliva

Source	Unstimulated saliva	Stimulated (2% citric acid)
Whole saliva*	0.3-0.5 (ml/min)	1.0-3.0 (ml/min)
Parotid*	0.04-0.06 (ml/min/gland)	0.60-0.80 (ml/min/gland)
SM/SL*	0.15 (ml/min/gland)	0.60 (ml/min/gland)
Labial†		0.0021 (ml/min)

*Data from Sreebny and Broich (1987).
†Data from Pedersen et al. (1985).

Table 8-2. Salivary composition in normal adults

	Mean values		
	Parotid	Submandibular	Plasma
Electrolytes (mEq/L)*			
Potassium (K^+)	20	17	4
Sodium (Na^+)	23	21	140
Chloride (Cl^-)	23	20	105
Bicarbonate (HCO_3^-)	20	18	27
Calcium (Ca^{2+})	2	4	5
Magnesium (Mg^{2+})	0.2	0.2	2
Phosphorus (HPO_4^{3-})	6	5	2
Organics (mg/100 ml)†			
Protein‡	221	132	7000
Lipids‡	8	8	600
Carbohydrate§	31	15	
Sulfate§	1	3	4
Viscosity (centipoise)‖	0.9	1.8	
Lubrication (% glycerol)‖	63	64	
pH	6.8-7.2	6.8-7.2	7.4

*Data from Mandel (1988).
†Values are from citric acid–stimulated parotid and submandibular-sublingual salivas.
‡Data from Slomiany et al. (1982).
§Data from Levine et al. (1978).
‖Data from Levine et al. (1987a).

Table 8-3. Major proteins of human saliva*

Function(s)

	Formation of intraoral pellicles	Lubrication of hard and soft tissues	Selective clearance and adherence of microflora	Antimicrobial activity	Microbial substrate	Digestion and taste	Buffering capacity	Proteolytic processing	Heterotypic complexing	Remin/demin
Acinar cell families										
Mucins	+	+	+		+				+	
Proline-rich proteins and glycoproteins	+	+	+		+	+				+
Histatins and statherin	+			+			+			++
Cystatins	+			+					+	
Amylases	+		+	+	+	+			+	
Peroxidases				+			++			
Carbonic anhydrases							++			
Ductal and stromal products										
Lactoferrin	+		+	+						
Lysozyme	+		+	+					+	
Secretory IgA	+		+		+				+	
Kallikrein								+	+	
Fibronectin			+		+				+	

*The major constituents from human parotid and submandibular-sublingual salivas.

els distally, electrolytes are readsorbed from the secretion by ductal cells, resulting in a final secretion that is hypotonic with respect to plasma (Martinez, 1987).

The secretion of saliva is regulated by a complex series of neurotransmitter-mediated receptor-coupling events that are controlled by fibers of the autonomic nervous system with origins in the superior and inferior nuclei of the medulla (Baum, 1987). For example, in the rat, sympathetic stimulation via beta-adrenergic receptors leads to a rapid rise in cyclic adenosine monophosphate (cAMP). This is followed by activation of cAMP-dependent protein kinase, which then leads to protein secretion. In contrast, fluid secretion is mediated by fibers of both the sympathetic and parasympathetic system via activation of muscarinic-cholinergic and alpha-1-adrenergic receptors, respectively.

The secretion of saliva, or salivary flow, is primarily influenced by unconditioned gustatory and masticatory reflexes. In addition, salivary flow is affected by secondary factors such as the degree of body hydration, position of the body, circadian rhythms (maximal flow occurring in the afternoon, minimal flow occurring during sleep), psychic and emotional factors, numerous diseases, hormonal factors, and drugs (Dawes, 1987). The normal mean unstimulated salivary flow rate varies from 0.3 to 0.5 ml/min (Table 8-1). Unstimulated or resting saliva constitutes 10% to 20% of the daily production. When stimulation of salivary flow occurs before and during eating, the flow rate can increase to over 1 to 3 ml/min, leading to an output of 1 to 1.5 L/day (Mandel, 1988). Approximately 85% to 90% of stimulated saliva is derived from the parotid and submandibular glands, 5% from the sublingual glands, and 5% to 10% from the minor glands. During sleep, most of the secretion comes from the minor glands, since the flow from the major glands is negligible. In general, the concentration of proteins in saliva is inversely proportional to the flow rate. In addition, there is wide variation in the concentration of various components between individuals.

Composition

Each salivary gland produces a characteristic and complex secretion consisting of electrolytes, proteins, glycoproteins, and lipids, each of which differs significantly from plasma (Table 8-2). In fact, an increase in the salivary concentrations of constituents such as sodium, chloride, and serum albumin may be diagnostic for salivary gland disorders wherein the saliva-blood barrier is compromised (e.g., sialadenitis).

In general, the nonimmune and immune (secretory IgA) components of saliva provide an initial protective barrier against the invasion of foreign substances and pathogens in the oral cavity (Mandel, 1987). Over the last decade, modern technology has advanced our understanding of the molecular composition and function of saliva, and certain concepts have come forth. For example, acinar cells tend to produce groups or families of molecules, whereas ductal

and stromal cells produce single species (Table 8-3). Although each family consists of several members that share common structural and functional features, each family member may also possess distinct functional and structural features as a result of transcriptional, translational, and/or posttranslational processing. Since a family member may exhibit functions similar to, or different from, other constituents within the same family, each family may therefore have multiple functions (Table 8-3).

Acinar cell families

Mucins. These are high molecular weight glycoproteins that are more than 40% carbohydrate. The peptide backbone of mucins contains a high number of carbohydrate side chains, which vary in size, composition, and charge (Tabak et al., 1982). Two chemically distinct mucins have been identified in human submandibular-sublingual saliva and have been designated mucin-glycoprotein 1 (MG1) and mucin-glycoprotein 2 (MG2) (Levine et al., 1987b). MG1 has a molecular weight greater than 10^3 kilodaltons, whereas MG2 is considerably smaller (150 to 200 kilodaltons).

In general, the viscoelastic properties of mucins may aid in the formation of the food bolus for efficient mastication and swallowing. However, the structural differences between the two mucins indicate that they may participate in different functions. For example, MG1 may function at hard and soft tissue interfaces to provide a permeability barrier for protection against environmental insult and dessication. Commensurate with this proposed function, MG1 may also act as a glycoprotein lubricant to minimize abrasion between occluding tooth surfaces. By complexing with antimicrobial factors in saliva, MG1 may also act as a carrier to localize these protective molecules at tissue-environmental interfaces. Several studies have shown that bacterial attachment to the tooth surface is mediated by salivary mucins that coat the tooth surface as part of the acquired enamel pellicle. In contrast, the coating of unattached bacteria by salivary molecules such as mucins may inhibit their attachment to oral surfaces and thus facilitate microbial clearance from the oral cavity. These interactions appear to be selective and can be mediated, in part, by the mucin's carbohydrate chains.

Proline-rich proteins and glycoproteins. This superfamily of some 20 members comprises acidic and basic phosphoproteins and basic glycoproteins that are characterized by an amino acid content containing 75% to 80% proline, glutamine, and glycine (Bennick, 1987). Recent studies have suggested that the majority of these molecules may arise from six genes by means of differential RNA splicing and posttranslational modifications of the gene products. These molecules also exhibit genetic polymorphism manifested as differences in the number and structure of proline-rich proteins between individuals. Together, these molecules represent a substantial quantity of the total salivary protein. Proline-rich phosphoproteins can bind calcium, have a high affinity for hydroxyapatite, and make up part of the acquired enamel pellicle. In addition, acidic proline-rich phosphoproteins can inhibit the precipitation of calcium-phosphate salts and thus protect the tooth surface from demineralization and calculus formation. A negative correlation was found between the concentration of acidic proline-rich phosphoproteins in whole saliva and dental plaque, suggesting that bacteria in plaque may influence the half-life of these molecules in vivo. The proline-rich glycoproteins provide lubricating properties on the tooth surface, especially when complexed to serum albumin, a major constituent of gingival crevicular fluid (Hatton et al., 1985; Levine et al., 1987a). Both the proline-rich phosphoproteins and the glycoproteins play a role in modulating the oral flora. The peptide backbone of these molecules may mediate attachment of *Actinomyces viscosus* to the enamel surface, and the carbohydrate portion of the glycoproteins may function to mediate attachment and/or clearance of streptococci (Bergey et al., 1986; Gibbons and Hay, 1988).

Histatins and statherin. The histatins are a family of small basic peptides characterized by a high content of histidine. At least seven members, one of which is phosphorylated, have been identified; these vary in size from 3 to 5 kilodaltons. These molecules may also form part of the acquired enamel pellicle and inhibit the precipitation of calcium phosphate salts. Interestingly, these proteins have recently been shown to display bactericidal and fungicidal activities. Histatins can inhibit the development of *Candida albicans* from the noninfective vegetative state to the infective germinating form (Pollock et al., 1984; Oppenheim et al., 1988). Finally, these basic peptides help to maintain a relatively neutral pH in the oral cavity.

Statherin is a tyrosine-rich phosphopeptide containing 43 amino acid residues, which may have evolved from a common ancestral histatin gene. This molecule binds calcium, has a high affinity for hydroxyapatite, and plays a role in demineralization by inhibiting the precipitation of calcium-phosphate salts (Schlesinger and Hay, 1977).

Cystatins. These molecules constitute a diverse group of thiol protease inhibitors that are found in several tissues and body fluids, including saliva. At least seven cystatins are present in human saliva; they differ slightly in molecular weight (14 to 15 kilodaltons), charge, and degree of phosphorylation (Al-Hashimi et al., 1988). Their ability to complex with mucins may serve to target cystatins to various oral surfaces where they may play a role in remineralization/demineralization processes and suppress the growth and thiol protease activity of oral pathogens.

Alpha-amylases. This family, which represents the most abundant enzyme found in saliva, can be divided into either glycosylated or nonglycosylated groups (62 or 55 kilodaltons, respectively). Each group comprises several isoenzymes that differ on the basis of their charge properties (Zakowski and Bruns, 1985). It has long been thought that the major role of this calcium-requiring metalloenzyme was the preparation of starches for digestion by hydrolyzing $\alpha 1,4$ linkages in glucose-containing polysaccharides to end products of glucose and maltose. Recently, additional functions for this molecule have been described. Its ability to inhibit the growth of *Neisseria gonorrhoeae*, its presence in acquired enamel pellicle, and its capacity to bind *Streptococcus sanguis* suggest a role in oral microbial colonization.

Salivary peroxidases. The salivary peroxidase system consists of the peroxidase enzyme (at least two species of 78 and 80 kilodaltons), the thiocyanate ion (SCN^-), and hydrogen peroxide. The enzyme catalyzes the oxidation of SCN^- by H_2O_2, generating highly reactive, oxidized forms of thiocyanate such as $OSCN^-$ (Mansson-Rahemtulla et al., 1988). These products have a direct toxicity on a variety of microorganisms, including *Streptococcus mutans*. Salivary peroxidase also neutralizes the deleterious effects of hydrogen peroxide produced by a number of oral microorganisms, is effective in reducing acid production by glucose-stimulated dental plaque, and can inhibit glucose uptake by *S. mutans*.

Carbonic anhydrases. These zinc metalloenzymes constitute a family of at least six distinct isoenzymes and are responsible for the reversible hydration of carbon dioxide. They probably play a role in bicarbonate formation and thus contribute to the buffering capacity of saliva.

Ductal and stromal products

Lactoferrin. This 76-kilodalton glycoprotein binds two atoms of iron per molecule, with the simultaneous binding of two molecules of bicarbonate. Lactoferrin's probable function in the oral cavity is antimicrobial and may be due in part to its ability to sequester iron. In addition, lactoferrin may also possess a direct, iron-independent, bactericidal effect on various strains of streptococci mediated by an anionic target site for lactoferrin on the surface of these microorganisms (Lassiter et al., 1987).

Lysozyme (muramidase). This 14-kilodalton basic protein can lyse the cell walls of gram-positive bacteria by hydrolyzing the $\beta 1,4$ glucosidic linkages between *N*-acetylmuramic acid and *N*-acetylglucosamine peptidoglycan constituents. Lysozyme may also kill bacteria found to be insensitive to its muramidase activity by activating endogenous bacterial enzyme(s) (Pollock et al., 1987). Complexing of lysozyme to mucins provides a mechanism whereby this enzyme may implement its function at various tissue interfaces. In addition, lysozyme may also aggregate certain bacteria, thus effecting their clearance from the oral cavity.

Secretory IgA. This glycoprotein is the predominant immunoglobulin found in all mucosal secretions, including saliva (McNabb and Tomasi, 1981). It is composed of an IgA dimer (300 kilodaltons), secretory component (70 kilodaltons), and J chain (15 kilodaltons). The J chain connects two IgA molecules into a dimer while the secretory component stabilizes the molecule and lessens its susceptibility to attack by acids or proteases in the oral cavity. In general, secretory immunoglobulins participate in the local regulation of environmental antigens (i.e., soluble antigens) by providing a "first line of defense" via immunologic means in the oral cavity. The ability of sIgA to bind to antigens is a beneficial process, since local aggregation of oral microorganisms would inhibit their adherence to hard and tissue surfaces and thus hinder subsurface microbial invasion into deeper host tissues. The presence of local antibody can also play a role in viral neutralization, attenuation of viral growth and replication on oral surfaces, and neutralization and disposal of toxins and food antigens.

Kallikrein. Kallikrein is a glycoprotein of 27 to 40 kilodaltons, consisting of a single polypeptide chain. It is a serine protease that can cleave C-terminal and N-terminal peptides from proline-rich proteins and cystatins, respectively. This posttranslational processing of acinar cell products takes place in the secretory duct prior to the molecules' entry into the oral cavity. The functional significance of these events remains to be determined.

Fibronectin. Fibronectin, a high molecular weight glycoprotein (450 kilodaltons) is found at cell surfaces, in basement membranes, in extracellular matrices, and in connective tissues, as well as in a wide variety of body fluids, including serum and saliva. Fibronectin has been identified along the interface between the tooth and the gingival connective tissue, as well as along the junctional epithelium-cementum interface. Fibronectin on the epithelial cell surfaces may preclude attachment of potential pathogens such as *Pseudomonas aeruginosa* (Woods, 1987). In addition, complexing of cell surface fibronectin with salivary molecules (e.g., alpha-amylases) can inhibit the epithelial colonization of gram-negative bacteria such as *Escherichia coli* (Hasty and Simpson, 1987).

DENTAL PELLICLES

Pellicle can be defined as a thin biofilm or cuticle. In the mouth it was traditionally thought of as the salivary film that formed on a clean tooth surface and was termed the *acquired enamel pellicle*. However, several new concepts concerning the nature of dental pellicles have recently emerged (Levine et al., 1985). First, pellicles form on all oral surfaces, including enamel, cementum, mucosa (keratinized and nonkeratinized oral epithelium), and dental appliances and restorations. In addition, the surface of the adherent oral microflora can be coated with a film or pellicle derived from the fluids in which they are bathed. Second, these fluids comprise constituents from saliva,

gingival crevicular fluid, and microbial and cellular products. Third, the selective deposition of these constituents onto various oral surfaces gives rise to pellicles of differing composition.

The best-studied pellicle is the acquired enamel pellicle. Its formation has been observed by examining freshly extracted teeth or, more conveniently, by placing plastic strips or epoxy crowns into the oral cavity as analogues of the tooth (Brecx et al., 1981). Morphologically, the pellicle and dental plaque on these plastic surfaces resemble those seen on the tooth. Electron microscopic inspection of acquired enamel pellicle reveals a thin, amorphous, electron-dense layer immediately adjacent to the hard surface. The thickness of this pellicle can vary from site to site but has been reported to range from 1 to 2 μm.

Early pellicle

Numerous studies have shown that the acquired enamel pellicle forms rapidly (within 2 hours) on a cleaned tooth surface. This pellicle can be termed *early pellicle* and is characterized by an absence of bacteria and their products. Histochemical staining has suggested that this pellicle is composed of proteins and glycoproteins. The amino acid profiles of early (2-hour) in vivo acquired pellicle demonstrate a higher content of threonine, serine, and alanine but considerably less proline than saliva, indicating that a selective adsorption of salivary components onto the tooth surface has taken place (Table 8-4). The salivary molecules that have been found in acquired enamel pellicle are indicated in Table 8-3. Recent studies have suggested that only certain members of salivary protein families are involved in early enamel pellicle formation. It is noteworthy that components that are not of salivary gland origin can also be present in early-acquired enamel pellicle. These constituents, including albumin, originate from the gingival crevicular fluid.

Pellicle formation involves a combination of physical forces (ionic, hydrophobic, hydrogen bonding, and van der Waals) between oral surfaces and organic and inorganic components in the surrounding fluids. Since cleaned enamel has many more accessible phosphate groups than calcium ions, the adsorption of molecules onto this surface may involve the interaction of these phosphate groups with calcium ions in saliva to form "bridges" with negatively charged (carboxyl, phosphate, sulfate, and sialic acid) groups on salivary and crevicular fluid components (Rolla, 1983) (Fig. 8-1, *A*). In addition, positively charged groups on salivary components may interact directly with phosphate groups on the enamel surface.

The protective functions of early enamel pellicle largely coincide with those of saliva. First, they protect the underlying surfaces from dessication, since many of the pellicle components (especially mucins) are highly hydrated and thus retain water. Glycoproteins in pellicles can play a role

Table 8-4. Comparison of the amino acid composition* of early enamel pellicle (EP) with human salivas

Amino acid	2-hour in vivo EP				HSMSL†	HPS†	HWS†
	Al-Hashimi and Levine (1989)	Sonju and Rolla (1973)	Belcourt et al. (1974)	Kuboki et al. (1987)			
Asp	8.3	7.5	9.8	4.8	8.4	8.0	8.4
Thr	5.2	3.5	4.9	5.0	2.7	1.4	4.4
Ser	9.2	9.5	11.1	8.1	4.5	4.8	4.5
Glu	14.6	12.5	16.1	12.5	17.6	17.5	15.2
Pro	5.1	2.2	6.7	7.8	18.1	26.6	18.1
Gly	14.0	17.6	15.7	18.7	13.2	16.9	13.8
Ala	7.8	7.4	8.6	6.1	3.6	2.8	4.9
1/2 Cys	1.3	1.0	–	–	0.4	0.2	0.7
Val	4.9	4.0	4.3	2.7	4.2	2.5	4.4
Met	0.8	–	–	2.8	0.4	0.4	0.7
Ile	3.3	2.8	2.3	3.5	2.7	1.8	2.5
Leu	6.7	6.1	5.2	8.1	4.8	2.6	4.8
Tyr	2.9	1.8	0.9	4.6	3.6	1.4	2.5
Phe	3.6	2.6	2.3	3.6	3.2	1.7	2.6
His	2.1	4.1	1.7	2.5	3.3	1.6	2.1
Lys	4.8	13.2‡	7.4	3.4	3.9	5.1	5.0
Arg	4.7	4.1	2.8	4.9	5.4	4.7	4.5

*Residues per 100 amino acid residues.

†In vivo EP, human submandibular-sublingual (HSMSL), parotid (HPS), and whole (HWS) saliva data represent average values from three separate donors.

‡Lysine + ornithine.

in lubrication by decreasing frictional forces between opposing tooth surfaces as they glide past each other. Pellicles may selectively concentrate antimicrobial substances such as immunoglobulins, lysozyme, and cystatins at different oral surfaces. Phosphoproteins in pellicles participate in remineralization-demineralization events to control the solubility of mineralized surfaces and prevent calculus formation.

Later pellicle

With time, early pellicle undergoes a transition involving the modification of existing constitutents, as well as the layering on or acquisition of additional and/or modified salivary and gingival crevicular components and bacterial products. The conditioning of early pellicles can be due in part to processing by enzymes in whole saliva that originate from bacteria, desquamated epithelial cells, and polymorphonuclear leukocytes (PMNs) entering saliva from the crevicular fluid. The formation of later pellicle most likely involves protein-protein or protein-carbohydrate interactions, which can also be stereospecific in nature (Fig. 8-1, B). For example, A. viscosus and Streptococcus mitis produce a neuraminidase that cleaves terminal sialic acid residues on the glycoproteins in saliva or early pellicles to expose penultimate galactose residues (Costello et al., 1979; Ellen et al., 1980; Murray et al., 1984). This structural modulation leads to modified salivary components in pellicle or the deposition of modified components from saliva, which then provides receptors for attachment to ad-

hesins or binding proteins on oral bacteria such as the galactose-binding lectin on A. viscosus (Fig. 8-1, C). These findings are consistent with experimental observations that have shown that neuraminidase-treated salivary pellicles bind less Streptococcus sanguis but have more exposed galactose residues to serve as receptors for enhanced S. mutans attachment. Other bacteria such as S. sanguis produce an IgA protease that specifically cleaves this immunoglobulin at its hinge region (Kilian et al., 1983). The action of this enzyme may affect the protective role of IgA in modulating the oral flora. Recent studies have demonstrated the presence of bacterial products such as glucosyltransferases from S. mutans in later pellicle. This enzyme could serve as an adhesin to promote the attachment of S. mutans to the tooth surface (Rolla et al., 1983). Collectively, these mechanisms may be important for the initial colonization and subsequent conversion of the oral flora from one dominated by gram-positive bacteria in health to one dominated by gram-negative bacteria in plaque-mediated disease.

Dental plaque formation

The vast majority of bacteria in the oral cavity are removed, with only a small fraction able to attach and persist. This removal or clearance occurs by mechanical flushing due to physiologic movements (e.g., swallowing, chewing, speaking) and is facilitated by the binding of components in whole saliva to adhesins on the bacteria. These interactions can result in the clumping and swallow-

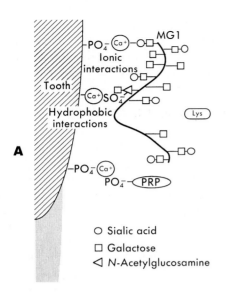

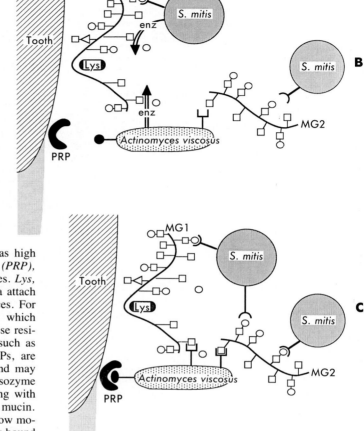

Fig. 8-1. A, Early pellicle. Salivary molecules, such as high molecular weight mucin *(MG1)* and proline-rich proteins *(PRP)*, interact with tooth surface via ionic and hydrophobic forces. *Lys,* Lysozyme. **B,** Later pellicle/early dental plaque. Bacteria attach to pellicle components by physical and stereospecific forces. For example, streptococci and *Actinomyces* possess lectins, which bind sugar residues of pellicle glycoproteins. Some of these residues are exposed by action of bacterial enzymes *(enz)* such as neuraminidases. Other pellicle components, such as PRPs, are thought to change conformation when bound to tooth and may then interact with certain bacteria. Molecules such as lysozyme *(Lys)* may be concentrated at oral surfaces by complexing with early pellicle components. *MG2,* Low molecular weight mucin. **C,** Plaque maturation. Other salivary molecules, such as low molecular weight mucin *(MG2),* may bind to bacteria already bound to tooth, which in turn leads to bacterial interactions.

ing of bacteria (saliva-mediated aggregation), which then precludes their attachment to oral surfaces. Nevertheless, there is selective adherence and colonization of some bacteria, but not others, to dental pellicles despite potent forces promoting bacterial clearance from the oral cavity.

Dental plaque formation can be divided into two stages. The first stage involves the adherence of bacteria to the tooth, and the second stage, plaque maturation, involves multiplication or growth of adherent bacteria and subsequent microbial succession (Gibbons and van Houte, 1980). Following initial random contact, bacterial attachment to enamel pellicles can occur by two different but complementary mechanisms. One mechanism involves nonspecific forces (such as ionic, hydrophobic, hydrogen bonding, and van der Waals) between the microbial surface and the pellicle. For example, ionic interactions involving calcium bridges may exist between negatively charged components on the bacterial surface and in the pellicle. Such forces cannot, however, account for the selective bacterial adherence to various oral surfaces. For instance, bacteria such as *S. sanguis, S. mitis,* and *A. visco-*

sus are found in higher numbers on teeth than on soft tissues, whereas other streptococci (e.g., *Streptococcus salivarius*) predominate on the dorsum of the tongue. Thus another mechanism involving specific or stereochemical interactions between bacterial surface adhesins and pellicle components can occur (Fig. 8-1, *C*). These interactions, analogous to those between antibody and antigen or enzyme and substrate, can be highly specific and may be superimposed on the nonspecific forces described above. For instance, mucin oligosaccharide chains terminating in sialic acid can clump strains of *S. sanguis.* This interaction is remarkably stereospecific and involves a trisaccharide sequence, Neuα1,3Galβ1,3GalNAc, of mucin binding to a specialized binding protein or adhesin on the bacterial surface (Murray et al., 1982) (Table 8-5).

The second stage of plaque formation involves the growth, multiplication, and sequestration of microorganisms on the pellicle-coated tooth surface, followed by microbial succession. Here saliva may serve as a source of nutrients as specific salivary proteins are degraded by certain bacteria to satisfy their amino acid requirements for

Table 8-5. Hemagglutination inhibition of *Streptococcus sanguis*

Inhibitor	50% inhibition [mM]			
	Strain: G9B	10556	KS32AR	10557
Sialic acid (NeuAc)	0.5	1	1	1
Colominic acid*	8	8	4	4
D-Glucuronic acid	>33	>33	>33	>33
D-Galacturonic acid	>33	>33	>33	>33
Galactose (Gal)	4	2	8	8
Lactose†	8	2	8	4
Sialyllactose‡	0.04	0.08	0.04	0.08
Mucin trisaccharide§	0.005	0.01	0.02	0.01

From Murray PA et al: Biochem Biophys Res Comm 106:390, 1982.
*NeuAcα2,8NeuAc.
†Galβ1,4Glc.
‡NeuAcα2,3Galβ1,4Glc.
§NeuAcα2,3Galβ1,3GalNAcol.

growth. Next, a complex series of interactions among dissimilar bacterial species leads to microbial succession (Fig. 8-1, *C*). These events also display a considerable degree of selectivity and are discussed further in Chapter 9.

GINGIVAL CREVICULAR FLUID

Gingival crevicular fluid is an altered serum transudate found in the gingival sulcus. The flow and composition of gingival crevicular fluid serve as a gauge or barometer of the intensity of gingival inflammation. With mild inflammation, this fluid contains all of the plasma proteins, as well as cellular elements such as PMNs. Indeed, certain proteolytic enzymes found in whole saliva originate from the lysosomal contents of these cells. With severe inflammation, the composition of crevicular fluid is characterized by the appearance of bacterial products (e.g., endotoxins), degradation products of the host immune system (e.g., C3 conversion to C3c and C3d), mediators of inflammation (e.g., leukotrienes), and by-products of connective tissue breakdown (e.g., chondroitin sulfates). Clinically, the monitoring of gingival crevicular fluid flow and the quality of its contents may be useful diagnostically to assess (1) the severity of gingival inflammation, (2) the effectiveness of oral hygiene, (3) the response of tissues to periodontal therapy, and (4) the effectiveness of pharmaceuticals such as antibiotics as adjuncts of periodontal therapy. The reader is referred to a monograph by Cimasoni (1983) for a more complete overview of this topic.

Pellicle and plaque formation

Recent studies have suggested that crevicular fluid components, including albumin and lysosomal enzymes, may inhibit the adherence of *S. sanguis* and, to a lesser extent, *Bacteroides gingivalis* to the tooth surface (Cimasoni et

al., 1987). Also, enzymes in crevicular fluid may have a potent lytic effect on oral microorganisms. Thus the organic components that contribute to the pellicles coating enamel and cementum marginal surfaces may play a role in the colonization of oral flora.

FUTURE STUDIES AND CLINICAL APPLICATIONS

The increasing body of knowledge dealing with salivary protein structure is shedding more light on the precise mechanisms by which these molecules perform their biologic functions. These studies are enhanced through the use of specific probes such as monoclonal antibodies and genetic reagents that recognize different structural elements or domains within individual salivary molecules. For example, monoclonal antibodies will enable us to determine the spatial orientation, conformation, and distribution of structural domains within salivary molecules. In addition, these reagents will permit the identification and quantitiation of defined structural domains within pellicle and plaque and thus provide information regarding the presence or accessibility of such domains on selected mucosal or hard tissue surfaces. Finally, immunologic and genetic probes will be valuable in the diagnosis of oral diseases and dysfunctions, such as Sjogren's syndrome, xerostomia, and salivary gland neoplasia, where alterations in the structural profile of salivary molecules may be manifested.

Knowledge of the precise structure and function of selected salivary molecules will also enable the purposeful design and synthesis of custom-engineered salivary molecules for use as artificial salivas. An ideal artificial saliva should be "long lasting," provide lubrication, inhibit colonization of pathogenic microflora, inhibit demineralization and/or enhance remineralization of hard tissues, and coat the oral soft tissues for protection against environmental insult and dessication. Therefore, artificial salivas of the future should be constructed from a library of defined structural domains that would combine the desired protective properties of several salivary molecules. For example, an artificial saliva could include a remineralization domain from a proline-rich protein coupled with a bactericidal domain derived from lactoferrin or salivary peroxidase. This composite or hybrid molecule could then be used as a saliva substitute for combatting the increased incidence of dental caries and gingivitis associated with xerostomia.

REFERENCES

Al-Hashimi I, Dickinson DP, and Levine MJ: Purification, molecular cloning, and sequencing of salivary cystatin SA-I, J Biol Chem 263:9381, 1988.

Al-Hashimi I and Levine MJ: Characterization of in vivo salivary derived enamel pellicle, Arch Oral Biol 34:289, 1989.

Baum BJ: Neurotransmitter control of secretion, J Dent Res 66(special issue):623, 1987.

Belcourt A, Frank RM, and Houver G: Analyse des acids amines de la pellicle exogene acquise et des proteines de l'email superficial chez l'homme, J Biol Buccale 2:161, 1974.

Bennick A: Structural and genetic aspects of proline-rich proteins, J Dent Res 66:457, 1987.

Bergey EJ et al: Use of the photoaffinity cross-linking agent, N-hydroxy-succinimidyl-4-azidosalicylic acid, to characterize salivary-glycoprotein-bacterial interactions, Biochem J 234:43, 1986.

Brecx M et al: Early formation of dental plaque on plastic films, J Periodont Res 16:213, 1981.

Cimasoni G: Crevicular fluid undated, Monogr Oral Sci 12:1, 1983.

Cimasoni G, Song M, and McBride BC: Effect of crevicular fluid and lysosomal enzymes on the adherence of streptococci and Bacteroides to hydroxyapatite, Infect Immun 55:1484, 1987.

Costello AH et al: Neuraminidase-dependent hemagglutination of human erythrocytes by strains of *Actinomyces viscosus* and *Actinomyces naeslundii*, Infect Immun 26:563, 1979.

Dawes C: Physiological factors affecting salivary flow rate, oral sugar clearance, and the sensation of dry mouth in man, J Dent Res 66(special issue):648, 1987.

Ellen RP et al: Sialidase-enhanced lectin-like mechanism for *Actinomyces viscosus* and *Actinomyces naeslundii* hemagglutination, Infect Immun 27:335, 1980.

Gibbons RJ and Hay DI: Human salivary acidic proline-rich proteins and statherin promote the attachment of *Actinomyces viscosus* LY7 to apatitic surfaces, Infect Immun 56:439, 1988.

Gibbons RJ and van Houte J: Bacterial adherence and the formation of dental plaque. In Beachey EH, editor: Bacterial adherence, New York, 1980, Chapman and Hall.

Hasty DL and Simpson WA: Effects of fibronectin and other salivary macromolecules on the adherence of *Escherichia coli* to buccal epithelium, Infect Immun 55:2103, 1987.

Hatton MN et al: Masticatory lubrication: the role of carbohydrate in the lubricating property of a salivary glycoprotein-albumin complex, Biochem J 230:817, 1985.

Kilian M et al: Occurrence and nature of bacterial IgA proteases, Ann NY Acad Sci 409:612, 1983.

Kuboki Y, Teraoka K, and Okada S: X-ray photoelectron spectroscopic studies of the adsorption of salivary constituents on enamel, J Dent Res 66:1016, 1987.

Lassiter MO et al: Characterization of lactoferrin interaction with *Streptococcus mutans*, J Dent Res 66:480, 1987.

Levine MJ et al: Biochemical and immunological comparison of monkey (Macaca arctoides) and human salivary secretions, Comp Biochem Physiol 60B:423, 1978.

Levine MJ et al: Nature of salivary pellicles in microbial adherence: role of salivary mucins. In Mergenhagen SE and Rosan B, editors: Molecular basis of oral microbial adhesion, Washington DC, 1985, American Society for Microbiology.

Levine MJ et al: Artificial salivas: present and future, J Dent Res 66(special issue):693, 1987a.

Levine MJ et al: Structural aspects of salivary glycoproteins, J Dent Res 66:436, 1987b.

Mandel ID: The functions of saliva, J Dent Res 66(special issue):623, 1987.

Mandel ID: Saliva. In Grant DA, Stern IB, and Listgarten MA, editors: Periodontics: in the tradition of Orban and Gottlieb, ed 6, St Louis, 1988, The CV Mosby Co.

Mansson-Rahemtulla B et al: Purification and characterization of human salivary peroxidase, Biochemistry 27:233, 1988.

Martinez JR: Ion transport and water movement, J Dent Res 66(special issue):638, 1987.

McNabb PC and Tomasi TB: Host defense mechanisms at mucosal surfaces, Ann Rev Microbiol 35:477, 1981.

Moskow BS and Baden E: Gingival salivary gland choristoma—a report of a case, J Clin Periodontol 13:720, 1986.

Murray PA et al: Specificity of salivary-bacterial interactions. II. Evidence for a lectin on *Streptococcus sanguis* with specificity for a NeuAcα2, 3Galβ1, 3GalNAc sequence, Biochem Biophys Res Comm 106:390, 1982.

Murray PA et al: Neuraminidase activity: a biochemical marker to distinguish *Streptococcus mitis* from *Streptococcus sanguis*, J Dent Res 63:111, 1984.

Oppenheim FG et al: Histatins, a novel family of histidine-rich proteins in human parotid secretion, J Biol Chem 263:7472, 1988.

Pedersen W et al: Age-dependent decreases in human submandibular flow rates as measured under resting and post-stimulation conditions, J Dent Res 64:1149, 1985.

Pollock JJ et al: Fungistatic and fungicidal activity of the human parotid salivary histidine-rich polypeptides on *Candida albicans*, Infect Immun 44:695, 1984.

Pollock JJ et al: Lysozyme-protease-inorganic monovalent anion lysis of oral bacterial strains in buffers and stimulated whole saliva, J Dent Res 66:467, 1987.

Rolla G: Pellicle formation. In Lazzari EP, editor: Handbook of experimental aspects of oral biochemistry, Boca Raton, Fla, 1983, CRC Press, Inc.

Rolla G, Ciardi JE, and Schultz SS: Adsorption of glucosyltransferase to saliva coated hydroxyapatite: possible mechanism for sucrose dependent bacterial colonization of the teeth, Scand J Dent Res 91:112, 1983.

Schlesinger DH and Hay DI: Human salivary statherin: a peptide inhibitor of calcium phosphate precipitation. In Wasserman RH et al, editors: Calcium binding proteins and calcium function, Amsterdam, 1977, Elsevier/North Holland.

Slomiany BL et al: Lipid composition of human parotid and submandibular saliva from caries-resistant and caries-susceptible adults, Arch Oral Biol 27:803, 1982.

Sonju T and Rolla G: Chemical analysis of the acquired pellicle formed in two hours on cleaned human teeth in vivo, Caries Res 7:30, 1973.

Sreebny LM and Broich G: Xerostomia, dry mouth. In Sreebny LM, editor: The salivary system, Boca Raton, Fla, 1987, CRC Press, Inc.

Tabak LA et al: Role of salivary mucins in the protection of the oral cavity, J Oral Pathol 11:1, 1982.

Woods DE: Role of fibronectin in the pathogenesis of gram-negative bacillary pneumonia, Rev Infect Dis 9(suppl 4):386, 1987.

Zakowski JJ and Bruns DE: Biochemistry of human alpha amylase isoenzymes, CRC Rev Clin Lab Sci 21:283, 1985.

Chapter 9

MICROBIAL DENTAL PLAQUE

Robert J. Genco

DEFINITION AND CLASSIFICATION

Dental plaques are essential for the development of periodontal diseases, and hence plaque control is critical in their management. It is important, therefore, to understand the structure, development, mechanism of formation, and inhibition and dispersion of dental plaques.

Dental plaques, bacterial plaques, or perhaps most accurately *microbial dental plaques,* may be described as aggregations of bacteria that are tenaciously attached to the teeth and other oral surfaces. Although plaques are primarily aggregates of bacterial cells, a few inflammatory and epithelial cells are also found. Plaques exhibit a definite microscopic architecture, with the bacterial cells arranged in clumps or columns of microcolonies. The spaces between these cells and the microcolonies are bridged by intercellular substances. Saliva, gingival fluid, and liquids from the diet can percolate through this structure to a variable extent, depending on the porosity. The porosity in turn depends on the specific arrangement of cells and intercellular material and the extent to which the intercellular spaces are filled with polysaccharides and other matrix substances synthesized by plaque bacteria.

Microbial dental plaques are classified as supragingival or subgingival according to location. *Supragingival plaques* refer mainly to those microbial aggregations found on the tooth surfaces; however, they may extend into the orifice of the gingival crevice where they are in immediate contact with the marginal gingiva. *Subgingival plaques* refer to those bacterial aggregations found entirely within the gingival crevice or periodontal pockets. The subgingival plaques in periodontal pockets are composed of bacteria often arranged in layers or zones with attached or adherent plaque on the tooth surface and more loosely arranged bacterial cells at the tissue interface. Some of the bacteria in subgingival plaques adhere to the epithelial lining of the pocket, thereby resisting removal by the flow of gingival fluid. There are also aggregations of bacteria that represent a form of dental plaque in the pits and fissures of the tooth crown, and it is likely that these plaques are associated with dental caries in these sites. Dental plaques accumulate in and around dental restorations and on all prosthetic devices placed in the oral cavity.

Dental plaques can be distinguished from other accumulations or accretions on the tooth surface, such as:

1. *Materia alba,* an amorphous bacterial accumulation in an unclean mouth containing bacteria, leukocytes and desquamated oral epithelial cells, and often food particles. Materia alba is easily removed with a strong water spray.
2. *Pellicle,* an organic film derived mainly from the saliva and deposited on the tooth surface. Pellicle contains few or no bacteria in its early stages; however, a few hours after its deposition, oral bacteria deposit on the pellicle, changing its composition.
3. *Calculus,* which represents calcified dental plaque. Calculus is almost always covered with a layer of uncalcified plaque.
4. *Stains.* Plaques, pellicles, and calculus stain yellow,

brown, black, or green, depending on the diet or use of plaque inhibitors, age, and smoking or other habits of the person.

CLINICAL ASSESSMENT

After reaching a certain thickness, supragingival plaques are readily detectable with the naked eye. This occurs in 1 or 2 days in areas where the plaques are not removed intentionally or by the forces of mastication and other oral functions. These plaques are yellow or whitish and are often thickest along the gingival third of the tooth and in the interproximal areas. When dental plaque is too sparse to be detected, its presence may be determined by the use of a disclosing solution such as erythrosin. Plaque can also be detected by scraping the tooth surface with a probe or scaler. Supragingival plaque is usually found at the gingival third of the crown, an area that is not naturally self-cleansing. The abrasivity of food, oral hygiene, and the action of normal mastication are often sufficient to prevent significant plaque deposits from forming on the smooth surfaces and the occlusal two thirds of the buccal and lingual surfaces of the crown. The interproximal areas often harbor plaque, since they are not self-cleansing and are difficult to reach with a toothbrush. Plaque deposits are regularly present in the fissures of the teeth, in the pits and irregularities of the occlusal surfaces, and in cracks or undulations of the smooth surfaces of the crown. Dental plaque forms readily on removable orthodontic appliances and dentures, as well as on restorations of all types.

Subgingival plaques are usually thin, contained within the periodontal pocket or gingival crevice, and hard to visualize in situ. Subgingival deposits can be detected after removal from the pocket by scraping the root surface with a probe or scaler. There are several sampling procedures for the microbial assessment of the periodontal flora that require sampling the subgingival plaques with absorbent sterile paper points or with other sampling devices. Such subgingival samples then are evaluated microbiologically for their content of periodontal pathogens by culturing or by rapid tests using specific antibodies or nucleic acid probes (see Chapter 11).

COMPOSITION AND STRUCTURE
Microbial composition

Dental plaque is composed mainly of microbial cells, with a cuticle or pellicle interposed between these masses and the tooth surface. Total microscopic counts show about 250 million organisms per milligram of wet weight of plaque, which occupies a volume of about 1 mm^3 of plaque. Since a centrifuged pellet of a pure culture of streptococcus has about the same number of cells per milligram wet weight, it is clear that most of the weight of plaque is due to bacteria. There are estimated to be 200 to 300 species of bacteria present in plaque, and it is not currently possible to culture or identify them all. There are

also microorganisms other than bacteria in plaques, including mycoplasms, small numbers of yeasts and protozoa, and viruses, including bacteriophages.

Fully formed supragingival plaque appears under the light microscope as a mass of bacterial cells with filamentous bacteria at right angles to the pellicle and the tooth surface. Closer to the periphery, the filaments curve and are irregular. In the outer, younger portion of plaque, many cocci and other small bacterial forms are found.

The ultrastructure of the microbial flora associated with the tooth and periodontal tissues in various states of health and disease show a high level of organization. There are marked differences between plaques seen in health and in disease. Examples of the ultrastructure of dental plaques found in the normal state and in gingivitis, periodontitis, or localized juvenile periodontitis are described in the following paragraphs.

In the *normal state* of periodontal health, the dental plaque microbial flora is supragingival, mostly confined to the enamel surface. The microbial flora consists of a relatively thin layer of adherent bacterial cells. The arrangement varies from isolated single cells resting on the pellicle surface, to cells that are densely packed as microcolonies, to others arranged in columns at roughly right angles to the surface of the tooth (Fig. 9-1). At the interface between the enamel surface and the plaque bacteria is an electron-dense layer, the dental pellicle. Cells of plaque associated with healthy gingiva are predominantly coccoid in shape, with a majority exhibiting cell wall features of gram-positive microorganisms. Filamentous forms and gram-negative organisms are present in small numbers, frequently on the outer surface of the microbial layer. Few flagellated cells or spirochetes are observed in microbial flora associated with the normal state.

The microbial flora found adjacent to sites exhibiting *gingivitis* is associated with the enamel surface of the tooth, since the epithelial attachment is at or near the ce-

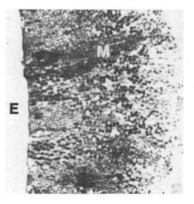

Fig. 9-1. Normal. Note coccoid flora on enamel surface. *E,* Enamel space; *M,* columnar microcolony. (×1325.) (Modified from Listgarten M: J Periodontol 47:1, 1976.)

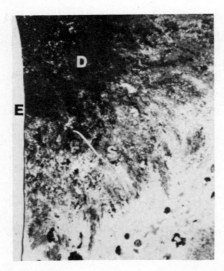

Fig. 9-2. Gingivitis. Note apical extension of microbial layer. (×400.) (Modified from Listgarten M: J Periodontol 47:1, 1976.)

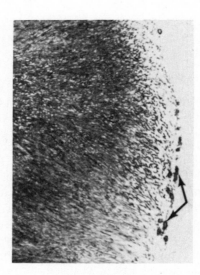

Fig. 9-3. Gingivitis. Note dense filamentous bacteria with corncob formations at surface. (×550.) (Modified from Listgarten M: J Periodontol 47:1, 1976.)

mentoenamel junction in gingivitis not associated with periodontitis. A variety of microorganisms, including coccoid and filamentous forms, and cells with gram-positive and gram-negative cell wall patterns are present (Fig. 9-2). Bacterial deposits may reach a thickness of 0.4 mm or more and are considerably thicker than those found in the normal state. The deeper layers of the adherent bacterial mass have undergone lysis, and mineralization of cells and zones in these plaques is common. Filamentous bacteria are relatively more numerous than in the normal samples, and the dense masses are occasionally covered with "corncob" formations composed of long filaments covered with cocci (Fig. 9-3). In the gingivitis samples, flagellated bacteria and spirochetes are observed in the apical portions of the plaque adjacent to the gingiva (Fig. 9-4). Epithelial cells and polymorphonuclear leukocytes are found in the most apical portion of the microbial mass at the tissue interface (Figs. 9-2 and 9-4).

In *periodontitis,* the epithelial attachment is located on the root surface, and subgingival plaques extend from the supragingival area into pockets bordered by the root surface and epithelium. The surface area occupied by the microbial deposits is greater than on teeth from persons with normal periodontal health or those with gingivitis. Filamentous forms are prominent; however, the morphologic cell types encountered in gingivitis are also observed in periodontitis (Fig. 9-5). Corncob formations are common at the surface of the supragingival deposits (Fig. 9-5 and 9-6). In the coronal to apical dimension, there is a transition zone between the predominantly filamentous supragingival plaque and the largely motile-appearing subgingival plaque (Fig. 9-7). Also in this transition zone, there is a

substantial increase in the number of flagellated bacteria.

The most distinct features of the periodontitis plaque samples are noted in the portion of the deposits that occupy the periodontal pocket (Fig. 9-8). The subgingival plaque constitutes an adherent and loosely arranged zone of motile-appearing organisms. The adherent zone is of varied thickness, is attached to the root surface, and comprises aggregations of bacteria. On the surface of this adherent layer, at the bacteria-tissue interface, there is a layer of motile microorganisms, many of which are flagellated. In this superficial layer of bacteria, there are also many "bristle brush" or "test-tube brush" formations, surrounded by spirochetes and other small motile organisms (Fig. 9-9). Also, on the tissue side of the subgingival flora are other cell types, including gram-negative bacteria with concave bodies and multiple flagella resembling the species *Selenomonas sputigena* (Fig. 9-10). There are also very narrow coccoid organisms and a variety of rods with gram-negative cell walls in this nonadherent superficial layer (Fig. 9-11).

The surface of the subgingival microbial mass closest to the pocket epithelium is generally covered with polymorphonuclear leukocytes and a few mononuclear cells. These neutrophils occasionally contain internalized bacteria and often appear degranulated. Some of the subgingival bacteria attach to and penetrate the gingival pocket epithelium.

The surfaces of teeth extracted from patients with *localized juvenile periodontitis* are remarkable for their lack of grossly detectable calculus or other surface deposits corresponding to those of the subgingival pocket sites. When examined microscopically, however, the surfaces of these teeth are frequently found to be covered with a thick cuti-

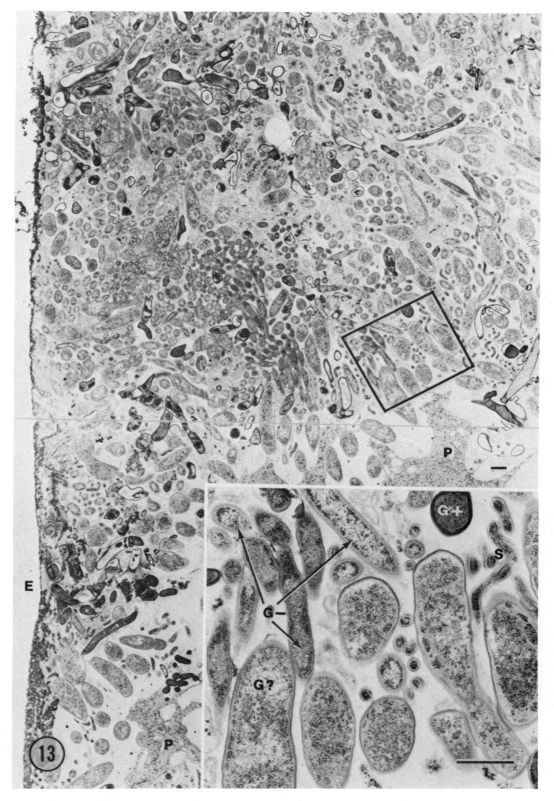

Fig. 9-4. Gingivitis sample; higher-power view of apically located microbial mass with details in inset. *E*, Enamel space; *P*, projections from adjacent polymorphonuclear leukocytes. (×4500.) In inset note presence of small spirochetes *(S)* and gram-positive *(G+)*, gram-negative *(G-)*, and atypical cells *(G?)*. (Modified from Listgarten M: J Periodontol 47:1, 1976.)

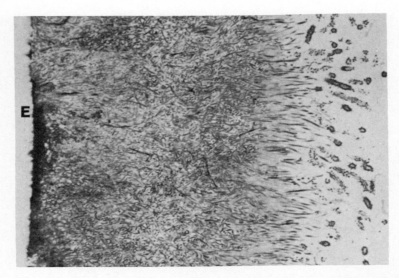

Fig. 9-5. Periodontitis: dense, predominantly filamentous bacterial mass adherent to enamel surface. Corncob formations extend from surface. *E*, Enamel space. (×850.) (Modified from Listgarten M: J Periodontol 47:1, 1976.)

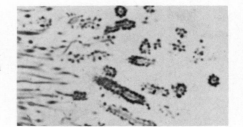

Fig. 9-6. Magnified view of corncob formations in Fig. 9-5. Corncobs consist of a central filamentous microorganism surrounded by adherent coccoid cells. (×1500.) (Modified from Listgarten M: J Periodontol 47:1, 1976.)

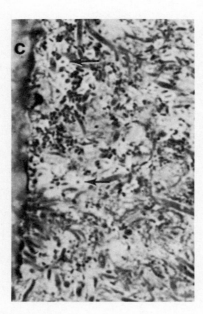

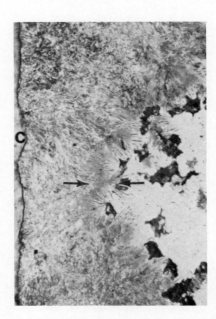

Fig. 9-7. Periodontitis: microbial layer adherent to cementum *(C)* in transitional zone between supragingival and subgingival microbial flora. Arrows point to cross sections of large filaments surrounded by a clear zone. (×3100.) (Modified from Listgarten M: J Periodontol 47:1, 1976.)

Fig. 9-8. Periodontitis: subgingival flora. Surface of adherent flora is covered by a palisading layer of test-tube brush formations and spirochetes *(between arrows)*. Adherent flora is less filamentous than supragingival flora and shows no particular orientation with respect to cementum surface *(C)*. (×600.) (Modified from Listgarten M: J Periodontol 47:1, 1976.)

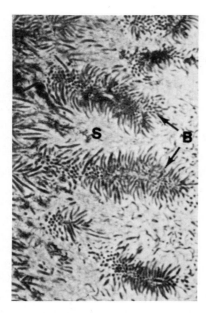

Fig. 9-9. Longitudinal section through test-tube brush formations *(B),* the base of which is surrounded by a spirochete-rich flora *(S).* (×1500.) (Modified from Listgarten M: J Periodontol 47:1, 1976.)

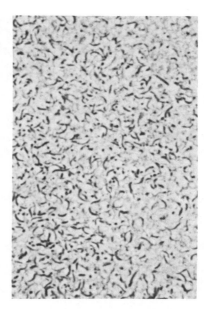

Fig. 9-10. Predominantly gram-negative flora with curved microorganisms resembling *Selenomonas sputigena.* (×1500.) (Modified from Listgarten M: J Periodontol 47:1, 1976.)

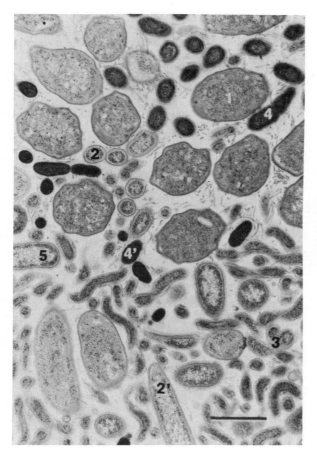

Fig. 9-11. Periodontitis: representative subgingival flora. *1,* Large, irregularly contoured filament *(shown in cross section)* with peritrichous flagellation; *2* and *2',* thin, gram-negative filaments resembling fusiforms; *3,* spirochetes; *4* and *4',* small, electron-dense coccoid bacteria; *5,* gram-negative rod. (×15,000.) (Modified from Listgarten M: J Periodontol 47:1, 1976.)

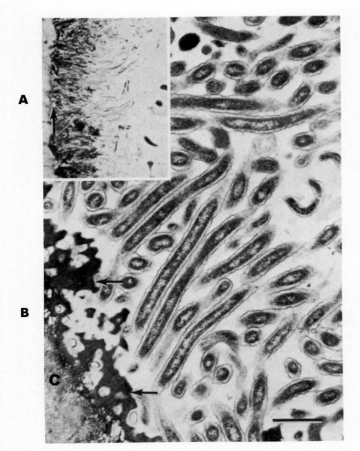

Fig. 9-12. A, Periodontosis. Relatively sparse flora is associated with cementum surface *(arrow)*. (×1100.) **B,** Electron micrograph of **A.** Thin filaments with loosely adapted gram-negative cell walls are oriented more or less perpendicular to dense cuticle *(arrows)* covering cementum surface *(C)*. (×13,000.) (Modified from Listgarten M: J Periodontol 47:1, 1976.)

cle that exhibits an irregular contour (Fig. 9-12) and bacterial plaques. Small clumps of gram-negative coccoid bacteria and polymorphonuclear leukocytes in varying stages of disintegration are intimately associated with the lobulated root surface cuticle. Thin filaments with loosely adapted gram-negative cell walls form deposits covering the cementum surface (Fig. 9-12). The bacterial population associated with these teeth is a sparse gram-negative flora that is relatively simple when compared with the populations seen in periodontitis and gingivitis.

It is quite clear from the ultrastructural studies that there are many types of microbes associated with periodontal tissues in health and in disease. In periodontitis and localized juvenile periodontitis, the subgingival plaques fill the periodontal pockets with a loosely arranged flora found at the advancing front of the lesion. The microbes at this tissue interface are likely to be of major importance in the destructive events occurring in periodontal disease. There

is also a supragingival flora, predominantly coccoid, that is compatible with periodontal health.

Chemical composition

The chemical composition of dental plaque is difficult to characterize, since it varies markedly with age and diet. In general, however, plaque is about 80% water and 20% solids. The solids include cells, mainly bacterial, which make up about 35% of the dry weight, and extracellular components, which make up the remaining 65% of the dry weight. Polysaccharides in supragingival plaques have been studied extensively, and dextran appears to be the major (95%) hexose-containing polysaccharide. Most of the remaining 5% of plaque hexose-containing polysaccharide is levan. Both dextran and levan are formed by bacterial enzymes from sucrose. Dextran is an adhesive material that plays a major role in colonization of certain plaque bacteria such as *Streptococcus mutans*. Levan, on the other hand, may function as a storage polysaccharide, providing a source of fermentable carbohydrate when hydrolyzed. There are very low levels of sialic acid and fucose in supragingival plaques, although plaques contain salivary glycoproteins, which in their native state are rich in these sugars. There is evidence of bacterial enzymatic removal of the sugars from salivary glycoproteins, and this "conditioning" of the salivary matrix may be of significance in plaque formation.

DEVELOPMENT

Dental plaque development on exposed tooth surfaces begins with the laying down of a salivary-derived pellicle. Chemical studies of human dental pellicles provide strong evidence that pellicle mainly comprises glycoproteins derived from the submandibular glands. An acquired salivary pellicle forms on artificial tooth surfaces and dentures, as well as on natural teeth. The acquired salivary pellicle is clearly distinct in composition and origin from the primary cuticle (Nasmyth's membrane), which is present as a developmental remnant on the orally exposed surfaces of newly erupted teeth.

Bacterial colonization of the surface of the acquired pellicle is the next step in plaque formation. Microbiologic studies of developing plaque formation have shown that colonization takes place very rapidly. For example, within a few minutes after the surface of a molar has been pumiced to remove existing plaque and pellicle, approximately 1 million organisms are deposited per square millimeter of enamel surface. The two major groups of organisms found in plaques in the first few hours are gram-positive facultative pleomorphic rods and strains of *Streptococcus sanguis*. Few or no gram-negative organisms are detected in these very early plaques.

Studies of plaque formation in healthy mouths over a period of 2 to 3 weeks led Löe et al. (1967) to describe microbial maturation of plaques associated with experimental gingivitis. In the experimental gingivitis model, periodontally healthy volunteers have their teeth cleaned until there is little or no detectable plaque or gingivitis. They are then asked to refrain from oral hygiene for up to 4 weeks, during which period samples of plaque are studied and the development of gingivitis is followed. Starting with a cleaned tooth surface, there are three relatively distinct phases of plaque formation, with some variations in time periods among teeth and individuals.

The *first phase* occurs within 2 days without oral hygiene. During this phase there is a proliferation of gram-positive cocci and rods and an addition of 30% gram-negative cocci and rods.

The *second phase* (1 to 4 days) is characterized by the appearance and increase in numbers of fusobacteria and filaments.

The *third phase* (4 to 9 days) is characterized by the appearance of spirilla and spirochetes. Gingivitis is clinically detectable at the time of formation of these complex, mature supragingival plaques found in 4 to 9 days.

The presence of gingivitis may increase the rate of plaque formation (Saxton, 1973; Brecx et al., 1980). In the presence of gingivitis, a more complex flora is reached earlier than in subjects with little or no gingivitis.

Studies of microbial population shifts during the formation of plaque give us insight into the nature of plaque formation and may help distinguish between organisms that are primary etiologic factors in periodontal disease and those that appear as a result of tissue damage. Similar phases of plaque maturation have been described for subgingival plaques forming on mylar strips experimentally placed into periodontal pockets.

In a culture study of bacterial plaques developing in an experimental gingivitis model in young adults (Moore et al., 1982), a very complex picture has emerged. With the use of anaerobic and aerobic cultures, 160 different bacterial taxa were found, and of these, 74 increased in proportion as plaque formation occurred over time. Significant increases in proportions over those found in the normal flora were seen for certain species of *Actinomyces, Streptococcus, Fusobacterium, Veillonella,* and *Treponema.* Also, some *Bacteroides* species were seen in the later stages of plaque formation associated with gingival bleeding.

In spite of the complexity of the developing flora of supragingival plaque left undisturbed for 7 to 10 days, the culture studies noted above show a remarkably orderly succession of organisms. Streptococci and *Actinomyces* are involved in earliest plaques. As the plaque matures, there are increases in proportions of these organisms, with the addition of others such as *Fusobacterium, Veillonella, Treponema,* and *Bacteroides* species. This latter mature plaque is often associated with gingivitis.

Similar culture studies of plaques developing in experimental gingivitis experiments were carried out in children

Table 9-1. Possible factors in the formation of microbial dental plaque

Attachment or adhesion	Multiplication and growth
Adhesion to pellicle or tooth surface mediated by extracellular polysaccharide (i.e., dextran or levan) or by "receptors" on cell surface	Availability of nutrients
	Secretion of metabolites
	Physical crowding limiting growth
	Change in oxidation-reduction potential
Cell-to-cell adhesion, either dextran induced or salivary induced	Host factors (i.e., antibodies) and phagocytotic cells may inhibit plaque formation
Interbacterial agglutination	Microbial synergisms and antagonisms

(Moore et al., 1984), and differences were found. For example, children harbor higher levels of *Capnocytophaga, Selenomonas,* and some *Bacteroides* species than adults. Children also harbor more gram-negative bacteria and motile bacteria, yet they develop gingivitis more slowly and of lesser severity than adults.

MECHANISMS OF FORMATION

"Colonization" by oral organisms describes early dental plaque formation, whereas bacterial growth is important in increasing the mass of plaques. There are at least two stages in colonization of a surface by a microbial flora: attachment and growth. Considerable attention has been given to the nature of these stages, with the hope that with better understanding of the mechanisms of dental plaque formation we may be better equipped to disperse or inhibit the formation of these deposits.

In the first stage of plaque formation, *attachment* of cells occurs, resulting in implantation of free-living microorganisms from the saliva on the surface to be colonized. In the second stage, *growth* of the attached organisms occurs by multiplication, and the organisms become residents of the plaques. Organisms that attach but fail to grow on the surface often do not become a stable part of plaques, and these are termed *transient organisms*. The possible mechanisms involved in dental plaque formation are listed in Table 9-1.

INHIBITION AND DISPERSAL

Our understanding of the essential role of dental plaque in smooth surface caries and gingivitis, the "plaque" infections, has led to the widespread realization that regular plaque dispersal or inhibition of plaque formation will lead to the prevention of these infections. Clearly, one of the most important methods of presently available plaque control involves mechanical self-removal at regular intervals with toothbrushes, dental floss, and other oral hygiene aids described in Chapter 35. Unfortunately, for many individuals the mechanical removal of dental plaques may be difficult to accomplish, and for many others sufficient motivation to carry out mechanical plaque control is lacking. In spite of these limitations, considerable success has been achieved in inhibiting or dispersing supragingival dental plaques by means of antiplaque or antimicrobial agents in mouth rinses and dentifricies. It should be noted, however, that *none* of these chemical methods is effective in *subgingival plaque* removal once pocket depths reach 4 or 5 mm.

Numerous antimicrobial agents other than true antibiotics have been used in mouthwashes. Some of these chemical disinfectants have recently been reinvestigated for their effects on plaque formation. One of the agents, chlorhexidine gluconate (Hibitane), has been shown by Löe and Schiött (1970) to be very effective in preventing the formation of dental plaque and is available in the United States as a 0.12% rinse. This formulation of chlorhexidine is very effective in plaque inhibition and has many uses as an adjunct to or a temporary replacement for mechanical plaque control. Chlorhexidine has undesirable side effects, including disturbance of taste sensation, especially salt perception, and brown or black staining of the teeth, especially around composite restorations in some patients. The staining is pronounced in individuals who drink tea or red wines.

To what extent this and similar antimicrobial or antiplaque agents can be used in long-term control of plaque will depend on studies of long-term effectiveness, as well as safety and possible adverse effects on the flora.

REFERENCES

Brecx M, Theilade J, and Attström R: Influence of optimal and excluded oral hygiene on early formation of dental plaque on plastic films: a quantitative and descriptive light and electron microscopic study, J Clin Periodontol 7:361, 1980.

Löe H and Schiött CR: The effect of suppression of the oral microflora upon the development of dental plaque and gingivitis. In McHugh WD, editor: Dental plaque, Edinburgh, 1970, E & S Livingstone, Ltd.

Loë H et al: Experimental gingivitis in man. III. The influence of antibiotics on gingival plaque development, J Periodont Res 2:282, 1967.

Moore WEC et al: Bacteriology of experimental gingivitis in young adult humans, Infect Immun 38:651, 1982.

Moore WEC et al: Bacteriology of experimental gingivitis in children, Infect Immun 46:1, 1984.

Saxton CA: Scanning electron microscopic study of formation of dental plaque, Caries Res 7:102, 1973.

Chapter 10

DENTAL CALCULUS (CALCIFIED DENTAL PLAQUE)

Irwin D. Mandel

The discovery of toothpicks of gold and silver in Sumerian tombs dating as far back as 3500 BC attests to the importance given to mouth hygiene and the removal of tooth deposits throughout the ages. Perhaps the first formal association between dental deposits and oral disease can be found in the writings of Hippocrates (460-377 BC), the Greek physician who founded modern medicine. He noted the deleterious effects on the teeth and gums of pituita

□Portions of this chapter are from Mandel ID and Gaffar A: Calculus revisited: a review, J Clin Periodontol 13:249, 1986. © 1986 Munksgaard International Publishers, Ltd., Copenhagen, Denmark.

(calculus), which insinuated itself under the roots of the teeth. It was Albucasis (936-1013), however, an Arabian physician and surgeon, who most clearly enunciated the relationship between calculus and disease and the need for thorough removal of the deposits. "There accumulates on the roots of teeth from inside and outside and between the gums, rough and ugly scales which may be black, yellow or green. As a result of this there is a corruption of the gums and suppuration around the teeth. Scrape the teeth that have the scales or the sandlike substance until nothing remains of them." He designed a set of 14 scrapers or scalers that are the progenitors of our modern instruments and described their use in the meticulous removal of deposits (Weinberger, 1948).

In 1535 Paracelsus, a Swiss-German physician and alchemist, introduced the term *tartar* as a designation for a variety of stony concretions that form in humans, noting their physical comparability to the deposits that develop at the bottom of wine casks from potassium bitartrate. He observed that these tophi could be found about the teeth, in the urinary bladder, in the gallbladder, and in gouty joints. Paracelsus looked on tartars as the principal cause of certain maladies, which he termed "tartaric diseases" (Prinz, 1921). Until very recently most dentists agreed with Paracelsus and considered periodontal disease to be appropriately placed in the category of a tartaric disease. In the past 25 years, however, calculus has been deposed by plaque in the etiologic hierarchy, and the hardened criminal has come to be viewed by many as a fossilized remnant of minor significance (Mandel, 1974a)—an unfortunate and premature relegation to the ash heap, since the calcified deposits do contribute to the development of pathologic conditions.

DEFINITION AND DESCRIPTION

In humans calculus is essentially mineralized plaque, covered on its external surface by vital, tightly adherent, nonmineralized plaque. There may also be a loosely held covering of materia alba, shed bacteria, desquamated epithelial cells, and blood cells derived from the crevicular area. In special situations, such as germ-free animals where microbial plaques do not form, some calcified tooth deposits do occur, probably as a result of mineralization of cell-free organic films such as pellicle and/or food derivatives (Baer and Newton, 1959; Theilade et al., 1964). A comparable situation could occur in humans with the use of effective antibacterial (antiplaque) agents, but virtually all calculus seen clinically results from the deposition of calcium and phosphate salts within bacterial plaques. The oral cavity is the site of a variety of abnormal calcified deposits that can form within the gingiva, tooth pulps, and salivary glands, as well as on dentures and other oral appliances (Mandel, 1963). The most common oral deposits, however, form on the teeth, and it is these, which are in close juxtaposition to the gingiva and other supporting tissues, that generate the concern in periodontal disease.

Supragingival calculus

The tightly adherent calcified deposits that form on the clinical crowns of the teeth above the free gingival margin are classified as supragingival calculus. These deposits are usually white-yellow in color as they form but can darken with age and exposure to food and tobacco. Since the salivary secretions are the main source of mineral salts, supragingival calculus is most abundant on the lingual surfaces of the lower anterior teeth (Fig. 10-1, *A*), opposite the orifices of the submandibular glands, and on the buccal surfaces of the upper molars, opposite the openings of the parotid glands. In persons with an inherent propensity for calculus deposition, however, other surfaces may be involved as well (Fig. 10-1, *B*). Poor oral hygiene, lack of adequate masticatory function, and tooth malposition can contribute to an increased rate and extent of deposition.

Subgingival calculus

As its name implies, subgingival calculus is the term used to describe the calcified deposits that form on the root surfaces below the free margin of gingiva and extend into the periodontal pocket. As is the case with supragingival

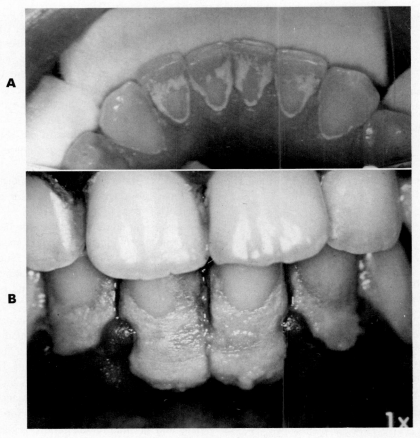

Fig. 10-1. **A,** Supragingival calculus on lingual surfaces of lower anterior teeth. **B,** Supragingival calculus on labial surfaces of lower anterior teeth. Note overlying plaque.

calculus, it is essentially mineralized plaque covered on its external surface by unmineralized plaque and loosely adherent shed bacteria and host cells derived from the crevicular lining and inflammatory exudate (Fig. 10-2). Subgingival deposits are usually dark brown to green-black in color and are harder than supragingival deposits.

For the most part, subgingival calculus does not form by direct extension of supragingival calculus but rather from mineralization of subgingival plaque that extends from, or is seeded by, supragingival plaque. The supragin-

gival and subgingival plaques are primarily responsible for inflammatory changes in the gingiva and supporting tissues, which generate the fluids (inflammatory exudate and gingival crevicular fluid) that are the source of the mineral salts. Since saliva is not involved in subgingival calculus formation, the distribution of these deposits is unrelated to supragingival deposits. Subgingival calculus can be found on any root surface with a periodontal pocket. Morphologically, subgingival calculus occurs in a variety of forms, the most common being ringlike or ledgelike formations

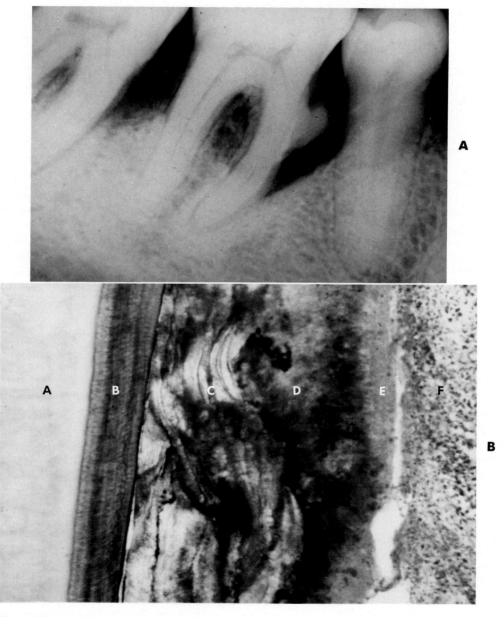

Fig. 10-2. A, Radiograph of molar with large mass of subgingival calculus on mesial root. **B,** Histologic section of tooth and calculus in **A.** *A,* Dentin; *B,* cementum; *C,* mineralized calculus; *D,* unmineralized plaque; *E,* loosely adherent bacteria and cells; *F,* inflammatory exudate. (Courtesy Dr. Bernard Moskow.)

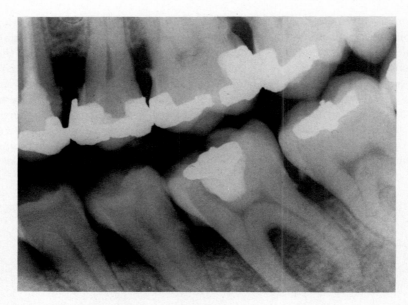

Fig. 10-3. Radiograph of teeth with deposits of subgingival calculus in a variety of forms.

and crusty, spiny, or nodular deposits clearly visible in radiographs (Fig. 10-3). Less frequently seen are fingerlike and fernlike formations, thin, smooth veneers, and individual spots or islands of calculus (Everett and Potter, 1959).

CLINICAL MEASUREMENT

In clinical practice quantitative assessments of the amount of calculus or rate of formation are rarely made. Patients are usually considered light, moderate, or heavy calculus formers on the basis of the amount of supragingival deposit they exhibit at a semiannual recall visit for scaling and prophylaxis. There are no formal guidelines, however, for the various categories. In epidemiologic surveys both prevalence (frequency of occurrence) and intensity (amount of deposit) have been reported. In a review of the worldwide data Schroeder (1969) noted that supragingival calculus is more prevalent than subgingival calculus and that both types have been found from early childhood on. However, the percentage of persons with both types rises from the eighth to the fortieth year, with reports of 40% to 95% in the 20- to 30-year age groups and peaks of 80% to 100% occurring in the over-30 category. There have been no reports of a sex difference in prevalence or intensity, but some geographic variation has been noted. It should be recognized that prevalence (as well as intensity) data are affected by the frequency and extent of dental care: hence geographic differences are difficult to interpret unless access to dental care is comparable.

Two indices have been employed for quantitating calculus deposits in epidemiologic surveys: the calculus component of the Oral Hygiene Index (Greene and Vermillion,

1960) and the calculus component of the Periodontal Disease Index (Ramfjord, 1959). Both indices use selected teeth and grade the amount of deposit from 0 to 3 (see Chapter 6).

Several indices have been developed for quantitating the effect of anticalculus agents. These include the calculus surface index (CSI) (Ennever et al., 1961) and the marginal line calculus index (MLCI) (Mühlemann and Villa, 1967), which are most applicable to short-term sudies of less than 8 weeks' duration, and the Volpe-Manhold index (VMI) (Volpe et al., 1965) which is widely used for 3- to 6-month studies but is appropriate for longer studies as well.

In the *CSI* all four surfaces of the four lower anterior teeth are examined, and the presence of calculus is determined. The total number of surfaces on which calculus is detected is considered to be the subject's score, the maximum possible score being $4 \times 4 = 16$. It is actually a prevalence rather than an intensity score. The *MLCI* scores only the supragingival calculus formed adjacent and parallel to the gingival margin on the lingual surfaces of the four lower anterior teeth. Quantitation is based on the percentage of the total lingual surface covered by calculus deposits. The means of the four teeth are averaged to give the subject's score, the maximum possible score being 100%.

The *VMI* employs a calibrated probe to measure the height and width of the calcified deposits on the lingual surfaces of the six lower anterior teeth. Measurement is made in three planes: (1) bisecting the lingual surface, (2) diagonally through the area of greatest calculus height at the mesioincisal angle of the tooth, and (3) diagonally through the distoincisal angle (Fig. 10-4). This index has been shown to have an excellent correlation with dry weight of deposits removed from the lower anterior teeth (Sharaway et al., 1966).

STRUCTURE AND ATTACHMENT TO THE TOOTH

The combination of histologic and histochemical studies of decalcified sections of teeth with adherent calculus deposits (Zander, 1953; Mandel and Levy, 1957) and transmission (Gonzales and Sognnaes, 1960; Schroeder, 1969; Selvig, 1970; Friskopp, 1983) and scanning electron microscopy (Friskopp and Hammarstrom, 1980) provides a

detailed view of the structure of mature deposits and their relationship to the tooth surface. Mineral crystals are deposited in an organic matrix composed of degraded microorganisms, which are often filamentous, embedded in a finely granular, fibrillar, or amorphous ground substance, and derived from the organisms (e.g., glucans) and the respective oral fluids (e.g., glycoproteins and lipids). The calculi are divided by structurally and histochemically recognizable stratifications, or incremental lines (similar to pellicle in appearance), which tend to follow the tooth surface, usually horizontally in supragingival calculus and vertically in subgingival calculus (see Fig. 10-2, *B*). This stratification is considered to be indicative of calculus deposits growing by apposition of new layers of calcifying plaque.

A number of different crystal types can be seen between and within the bacterial remnants, varying from small needle-shaped crystals, identified by electron diffraction as hydroxyapatite, to long ribbonlike crystals of octocalcium phosphate oriented in bundles or rosettes. In young deposits of supragingival calculus large crystalline aggregates of brushite can be seen. The matrix of subgingival calculus appears to be more homogeneous than that of supragingival deposits, which frequently exhibit areas of noncalcified material appearing at all levels. Both types of deposits are covered by a layer of unmineralized plaque. The plaque overlying supragingival calculus is composed primarily of filamentous organisms oriented perpendicularly to the underlying calcified portions. Subgingival calculus is usually covered by cocci, rods, and filaments with no distinct pat-

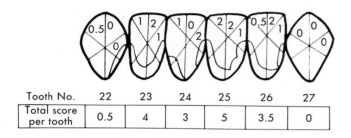

Tooth No.	22	23	24	25	26	27
Total score per tooth	0.5	4	3	5	3.5	0

Total Score_____16_____

Examiner_____

Fig. 10-4. Example of a scoring pattern with Volpe-Manhold index. (From Volpe A et al: J Periodontol 36:292, 1965.)

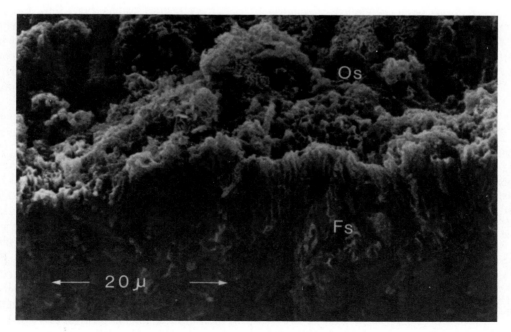

Fig. 10-5. Scanning electron microscopic view of supragingival calculus fractured and washed in sodium hypochlorite. *Os,* Rough, porous outer surface; *Fs,* channels penetrating into calculus along fracture surface. (From Friskopp J and Hammarstrom L: J Periodontol 51:553, 1980.)

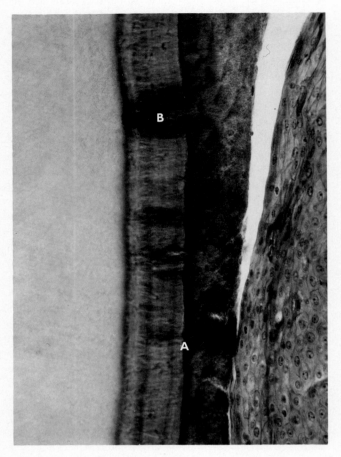

Fig. 10-6. Attachment of subgingival calculus to cementum via pellicle *(A)* and by direct extension of microorganisms into defect area *(B)*. (Courtesy Dr. Bernard Moskow.)

Table 10-1. Composition of mature supragingival calculus

Component	% of dry wt.
Inorganic	
Calcium	27-29
Phosphorus	16-18
Carbonate	2-3
Sodium	1.5-2.5
Magnesium	0.6-0.8
Fluoride	0.003-0.04
Organic	
Total matrix	15-20
% of matrix	
Protein: 50-60	
Carbohydrates: 12-20	
Lipids: 10-15	

tern of orientation. A number of investigators have noted the presence in both supragingival and subgingival calculus of empty spaces or tubular holes representing the sites of entombed and degenerating organisms or noncalcified bacteria (Fig. 10-5). Indeed, all of the recent morphologic studies attest to the relatively porous nature of the calculus deposits.

Formed residues of food, epithelial cells, and blood-derived cells occur only occasionally, usually as part of the easily detached surface coating (materia alba). They are a minor contributor to the structure of mature calculus.

Means of attachment

Since calculus is essentially calcified plaque, the same means of attachment to the tooth surfaces should apply to both types of deposits. This is clearly evident on the enamel surface where the acquired pellicle binds strongly to the tooth surface and in turn serves as the adherent layer for the developing plaque (McDougall, 1963) and the calcifying deposit (Mandel et al., 1957; Theilade, 1964). On some enamel surfaces the pellicle grows into micropore openings and forms a "dendritic" structure below the tooth surface, futher enhancing the tenacity of the pellicle attachment (Leach and Saxton, 1966).

Pellicle can also serve to anchor subgingival calculus to the cementum surface (Fig. 10-6). It has been noted (Zander, 1953; Mandel and Levy, 1957), however, that if pellicle was absent the deposit became attached by direct extension of microorganisms into irregularities in the cementum surfaces, such as spaces formerly occupied by Sharpey's fibers, defect areas, resorption lacunae, or areas of arrested caries lesions (Fig. 10-6). Electron microscopic studies (Selvig, 1970) suggested that attachment could also be enhanced by crystal growth into cemental defects and intercrystalline bonding of calculus and tooth crystals. The various attachment mechanisms for subgingival calculus result in deposits that are often very difficult to remove from the root surface.

COMPOSITION
Inorganic matter

Mature calculus is a highly mineralized deposit with an inorganic content closely resembling that of bone, dentin, and cementum (Table 10-1). In addition to calcium and phosphorus, calculus contains carbonate, sodium, magnesium, potassium, and a number of trace components, including fluoride, zinc, and strontium (Little et al., 1963, 1964; Lundberg et al., 1966; Gron et al., 1967; Schroeder, 1969). In general, subgingival calculus contains a higher concentration of calcium, magnesium, and fluoride than does supragingival calculus, reflecting the higher concentration of these ions in gingival crevicular fluid than in saliva.

In mature deposits (over 6 months of age) the major crystalline form is hydroxyapatite ($Ca_{10}[PO_4]_6 \cdot OH_2$), with lesser amounts of octocalcium phosphate ($Ca_8[HPO_4]_4$), whitlockite, a magnesium-containing tricalcium phosphate ($Ca_3[PO_4]_2$), and brushite ($Ca[HPO_4]\cdot 2H_2O$). In young deposits (up to 3 months of age) almost half of the crystals may be brushite (Rowles, 1964). Longitudinal study of developing calculus indicates that brushite appears first, then octocalcium phosphate, and, as the calculus ages, whitlockite and hydroxyapatite (Schroeder, 1969).

Organic components

The organic matrix constitutes about 15% to 20% of the dry weight of mature supragingival calculus (Table 10-1). More than half of the matrix is composed of proteins contributed by the entombed bacteria and the salivary proteins that became incorporated in the matrix as the deposit was forming. The carbohydrates are derived largely from the proteoglycans of the bacteria, the extracellular polymers (such as glucan) produced by the bacteria, and the carbohydrate moieties of the salivary glycoproteins and glycolipids from bacteria and saliva. There are a variety of carbohydrates present: hexoses (the major carbohydrates, mainly glucose, with some galactose); methylpentoses (rhamnose from bacteria and fucose from saliva); hexosamines; and sialic acid (Little et al., 1961; Mandel et al., 1962; Mandel, 1968). Small amounts of glycosaminoglycans (GAGS) have also been reported in supragingival and subgingival calculus, probably derived from the breakdown of gingival tissues (Osuoji and Rowles, 1972).

Recent studies by Slomiany et al. (1983) on the lipids of supragingival calculus have shown that the neutral lipids form the largest fraction (62%) and have a very high content of free fatty acids, with modest amounts of triglycerides, cholesterol, and cholesterol esters. Glycolipids account for 28% of the calculus lipids and are composed of simple glycosphingolipids and neutral and sulfated glyceroglucolipids. The phospholipids constitute the remaining 10% of total lipids and contain predominantly phosphatidylethanolamine and diphosphatidyl glycerol. The spectrum of lipids reflect both bacterial and salivary contributions.

FORMATION OF CALCULUS

Plastic strips wired to the teeth provide an excellent means of studying the early stages of plaque and calculus formation (Mandel et al., 1957; Schroeder, 1969) and can be used for subgingival as well as supragingival deposition (Oshrain et al., 1971). The early stages of calculus formation are identical to plaque formation—deposition of a pellicle and rapid colonization by gram-positive coccoidal organisms. Pellicle forms subgingivally as well as supragingivally and is histologically similar despite differences in the chemistry of the fluid environment. Histologically, coccoidal organisms dominate the early deposit, but by about the fifth day the plaque becomes largely filamentous in structure and resembles the matrix of decalcified mature

calculus. The microorganisms appear to be enveloped in an amorphous and/or fibrillar ground substance.

With the use of special stains for calcium, the onset and progression of mineralization can be studied histologically. Calcification can begin as early as a few days after bacterial deposition and is usually identified as a focal patch within the plaque adjacent to the pellicle. Mineralization usually proceeds by the establishment of additional foci, which enlarge and coalesce (Fig. 10-7). Only on occasion do foci of calcification appear in the outer areas of the plaque (Fig. 10-7). As calcification continues, a laminated structure becomes evident (Fig. 10-8), with alternating deep- and pale-staining bands.

The time of onset of calcification appears to vary considerably from tooth to tooth and from person to person. Supragingivally, the surfaces closest to the duct orifices of the salivary glands (e.g., lingual of lower centrals) appear to mineralize first. Subgingivally, the onset of mineralization is slower and seems to be unrelated to the pattern of calcification in the supragingival area. The mechanism of mineralization appears to be identical in the two areas even though the source of the mineral salts in the subgingival area is the gingival crevicular fluid, not saliva.

In time (as little as 1 week in some instances, as much as several months in others), the bulk of the plaque becomes calcified. There is, however, always some unmineralized plaque on the surface of the mineralized portion. Electron microscopic studies of developing calculus (Gonzales and Sognnaes, 1960; Zander et al., 1960) support the observations made with the light microscope. Mineralization usually occurs first within the interbacterial matrix, then around the walls of the bacteria, and finally within the bacterial cells. A second pattern of mineralization, probably of brushite (Schroeder, 1969), does not seem to involve an organic matrix but makes use of a preexisting mineralized fringe for its base.

Theories of mineralization

A number of theories have been offered over the past 40 years to explain the mechanisms of calcification, both the organized "programmed" calcifications such as teeth and bone and the "ectopic calcifications" such as supragingival and subgingival calculus.

Booster mechanism. According to this theory, calcification will occur in a particular locus when the local pH and calcium and phosphorus concentrations are high enough to allow for precipitation of a calcium phosphate salt. Such factors as loss of CO_2 and production of ammonia could account for an elevation in pH; acid or alkaline phosphatase activity could result in a higher phosphate concentration; liberation of bound or complexed calcium from the salivary proteins would produce increases in calcium levels.

Epitaxic concept. One of the most widely held theories has been the "epitaxic concept," which recognizes that

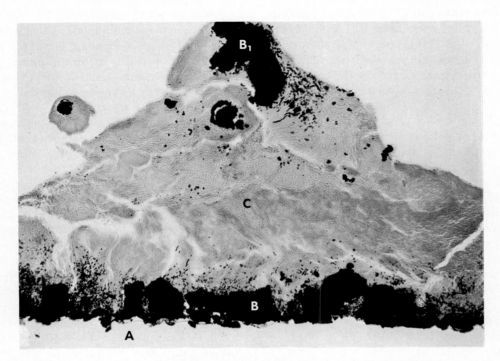

Fig. 10-7. Von Koss stain (for calcium) of 1-week-old supragingival calculus. *A*, Plastic strip; *B*, *B₁*, foci of calcification beginning to coalesce; *C*, unmineralized plaque; *B₁*, occasional focus of calcification in outer portions of plaque. (From Oshrain H et al: J Periodontol 42:31, 1971.)

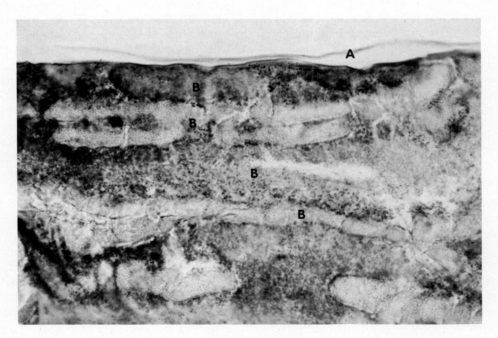

Fig. 10-8. Gram stain of developing subgingival calculus. *A*, Pellicle; *B*, laminations, alternating dark- and light-staining bands. (From Oshrain H et al: J Periodontol 42:31, 1971.)

the concentration of calcium and phosphate ions is not high enough in tissue fluids and saliva to precipitate spontaneously, but is sufficient to support growth of a hydroxyapatite crystal once an initial seed or nucleus is formed. Tissue fluids and saliva are therefore called metastable solutions. The formation of the initial crystal or nucleus is called nucleation and is thought to occur when a proper organic matrix is available on which the nucleus can crystallize in exact structural configuration. In other words, the matrix provides the architectural template or geometric configuration for the initial hydroxyapatite crystal. Crystal growth then proceeds in the presence of a metastable solution. A number of nucleating molecules have been suggested, including some types of collagen and proteoglycans (Boskey, 1981). Current evidence suggests that calcium-phospholipid-phosphate complexes are important nucleators in numerous normal and ectopic calcifications, including salivary gland stones (Boskey et al., 1981) and bacteria from salivary calculus (Ennever et al., 1976).

Inhibition theory. Another approach considers calcification as occurring only at specific sites because of the existence of an inhibiting mechanism at noncalcifying sites. Where calcification occurs, the inhibitor is apparently altered or removed. One possible inhibiting substance is thought to be pyrophosphate (and possibly other polyphosphates), and among the controlling mechanisms is the enzyme alkaline pyrophosphatase, which can hydrolyze the pyrophosphate to phosphate (Russell and Fleisch, 1970). The pyrophosphate inhibits calcification by preventing the initial nucleus from growing, possibly by "poisoning" the growth centers of the crystal.

Transformation. A most attractive hypothesis is the idea that hydroxyapatite need not arise exclusively via epitaxy and nucleation. Amorphous noncrystalline deposits and brushite can be transformed to octocalcium phosphate and then to hydroxyapatite (Eanes et al., 1970). It has been suggested that the controlling mechanism in the transformation process may be pyrophosphate (Fleisch et al., 1968).

It may well be that *all* the theories might explain some part of the calcification mechanism, especially in calculus, where calcium exists in a variety of forms. In salivary calculus brushite may develop spontaneously as a result of local elevation of pH, calcium, and phosphate and then in the maturing process be modified to crystals of higher calcium-to-phosphate ratios. Early amorphous deposits could be transformed to more crystalline material. Nucleating substances arising from the bacterial or salivary proteins and lipids could also initiate calcification and account for the hydroxyapatite in early deposits.

Role of bacteria

The role of bacteria in calculus formation is apparently a complex one. Although the formation of calculus in germ-free animals indicates that bacteria are not essential, when present they obviously play an important role; calcu-

lus is far more abundant in infected than in germ-free animals. Viability of organisms is not necessary for their participation in mineralization, however, since nonviable organisms calcify readily (Ennever, 1967). Indeed, a decrease in metabolic activity with reduced production of the organic acids that result from glycolysis may be a prerequisite before bacteria can mineralize. Calcification of the interbacterial area may require altered cell permeability and availability of nucleating substances.

Individual variation

Clinically it is possible to identify individuals who are rapid and heavy formers of supragingival calculus and others who form little or no calcified deposits over a period of many months. The plaques of heavy calculus formers exhibit significantly higher levels of calcium and phosphorus than those of light formers within a few days after a prophylaxis (Schroeder, 1969; Mandel, 1974a). The most likely basis for the marked differences in propensity to calculus formation is the salivary environment, although differences in bacterial flora (Sidaway, 1978) and dietary factors could be contributing factors. Based on our current concepts of mineralization, a tendency toward heavy salivary calculus formation could be related to elevations in (1) pH, (2) concentration of homogeneous nucleators (calcium), or (3) heterogeneous nucleators (salivary or bacterial proteins or lipids); or to low levels of inhibitors. Despite some contradictory data (see Schroeder, 1969; Mandel, 1974a, 1974b), the findings do indicate that heavy formers usually have higher values for submandibular urea and total protein (Mandel and Thompson, 1967), as well as calcium (Mandel, 1974b). Total lipids are elevated in both parotid and submandibular saliva of heavy formers (Slomiany et al., 1980, 1981). Which specific salivary proteins and lipids are involved has not been determined. Light calculus formers have been shown to have higher levels of parotid pyrophosphate (an inhibitor of calcification) than do heavy formers (Vogel and Amdur, 1967).

PATHOGENIC POTENTIAL OF SUPRAGINGIVAL AND SUBGINGIVAL CALCULUS
Supragingival calculus

Until 1960 the prevailing view was that calculus was the major etiologic factor in periodontal disease. Its pathogenicity was attributed to its rough outer surface, which mechanically irritated the adjacent tissues. The current view, enunciated by Schroeder (1969), is that the initial damage to the gingival margin in periodontal disease is due to the immunologic and enzymatic effects of the microorganisms in plaque. The process is enhanced, however, by supragingival calculus, which provides further retention and thus promotes new plaque accumulations. It is still not clear, however, whether calculus plus plaque provokes a greater reaction than plaque alone, although there is some suggestive evidence for the former (Schwartz et al., 1971). There is no question, however, that the mineralized deposit does (1) bring the bacterial overlay closer to the supporting tissues, (2) interfere with local self-cleansing mechanisms, and (3) make plaque removal more difficult for the patient. Partial inhibition of plaque mineralization can be accomplished by chemical agents, but there has been no demonstration in humans of a reduction in gingivitis (Suomi et al., 1974). It remains to be established what level of inhibition, if any, is required to have more than a cosmetic effect.

Subgingival calculus

A number of studies support the view that the presence of subgingival calculus contributes to the chronicity and progression of periodontal disease (Mandel and Gaffar, 1986). Clinical studies attest to the importance of frequent and thorough removal of root deposits by scaling and root planing to prevent attachment loss (Pihlstrom et al., 1983). Morphologic studies show that the calcified deposits are porous and could act as a reservoir for irritating substances. Experimental studies have established the permeability of subgingival calculus to endotoxin (Baumhammers and Rohrbaugh, 1970) and the presence in the deposits of high levels of toxic stimulators of bone resorption and antigens from *Bacteroides gingivalis* (Patters et al., 1982). When coupled with the increasing buildup of plaque on the surface of calculus, the combination has the potential for increasing the rate of displacement of the adjacent junctional epithelium and extending the radius of destruction of bone beyond that of plaque alone (Mandel and Gaffar, 1986). Thorough removal of the porous, bacterial retentive subgingival calculus is a key phase in periodontal therapy.

PREVENTIVE ASPECTS: CONTROL BY DENTIFRICES, MOUTH RINSES, AND ORAL HYGIENE

Until the mid-1950s virtually all of the many anticalculus agents introduced (see Schroeder, 1969, for review) were directed toward the dissolution or softening of the established deposits. Most of the substances were decalcifying, complexing, or chelating agents and unfortunately were damaging to the tooth substance, especially cementum. A few agents were aimed at affecting the calculus matrix, the scaffolding that maintained the mineralized structure. One such agent, sodium-ricinoleate, the salt of fatty acids from castor oil, showed promise in reducing early calculus deposits but suffered from an unacceptable taste.

In the following decade the emphasis changed from altering the mature deposits to a preventive approach, preventing the buildup of the early mineralized plaque. Agents employed included (1) antiseptics and antibiotics, (2) a variety of enzymes and enzyme combinations, (3) cationic surface-active compounds, and (4) high concentrations of urea (see Weinstein and Mandel, 1964, for review). Despite some initial enthusiasm, none of the agents exhibited sufficient efficacy and/or safety to warrant continued research and marketing.

The major anticalculus strategy in the 1970s was the inhibition of crystal growth of hydroxyapatite by pyrophosphates or their analogues. Preliminary studies with pyrophosphate per se indicated a breakdown in the oral cavity by bacterial pyrophosphatases, and hence an analogue was developed, diphosphonate, in which substitution of two oxygens by carbon yielded a molecule less susceptible to bacterial hydrolysis. Suomi et al. (1974) examined the effects on 200 adults over an 18-month period of uninstructed use of a dentifrice containing 3% sodium etidronate (a diphosphonate) and 0.22% sodium fluoride. At the end of the study there was a 42% reduction in the amount of supragingival calculus and a 27% reduction in subgingival deposit. There was no significant difference in gingivitis. In this study, as well as in all other studies in which the relationship between calculus and gingivitis has been examined, mean values for gingivitis have been compared with a mean calculus score. Since calculus forms on only a limited number of teeth, we cannot tell if the reduction in calculus affects the gingivitis score on specific teeth (Mandel and Gaffar, 1986). The diphosphonate dentifrice was never marketed.

After a 10-year period in which research interests were focused almost exclusively on antiplaque agents, interest in supragingival calculus as an entity resurfaced with a reexamination of pyrophosphates. A dentifrice formulation with 3.3% soluble pyrophosphate (a mixture of tetrasodium and disodium dihydrogen pyrophosphate) and 0.24% sodium fluoride appeared to be able to affect crystal growth despite bacterial pyrophosphatase in the oral cavity. In a 6-month study on 418 adults, Zacherl et al. (1985) found 37% less supragingival calculus in the pyrophosphate than in the control group when the dentifrices were used once a day in the usual manner. Another formulation containing 3.3% pyrophosphate, 5% tetrasodium pyrophosphate, a copolymer of methoxyethelene and maleic acid, and 0.24% sodium fluoride has also been shown to be effective in reducing supragingival calculus in adults, with a reduction of 44% at the end of 3 months (Lobene, 1986).

One of the potential problems with an agent that interferes with crystal growth is an interference with the protective salivary property of remineralization of early demineralized areas in enamel. Lu et al. (1985) found that a pyrophosphate-fluoride toothpaste reduced caries 39% over a 1-year period in a large group of children aged 8-15, indicating that the fluoride-augmented remineralizing effect was not compromised.

There has been considerable interest over the years in zinc salts as antiplaque and anticalculus agents. In a recent study with an experimental dentifrice containing 2% zinc chloride and 0.22% sodium fluoride, there was a 47% reduction in calculus at the end of 6 months (Lobene et al.,

1985). Other zinc salts, such as zinc citrate, are also under study.

Mouth rinses with proposed anticalculus properties are available commercially. It should be noted that chlorhexidine-containing rinses, while effective antiplaque agents, can cause an *increase* in supragingival calculus deposits (Grossman et al., 1986).

Anecdotally, it has been a common observation that good toothbrushing per se can slow the rate of calculus deposition. Using a quantitative scoring procedure, Villa (1968) was able to demonstrate that habitual toothbrushing alone could reduce calculus formation by approximately 50% on the lingual surfaces of the lower anterior teeth.

SUMMARY

Dental calculus, also termed *tartar,* is mineralized dental plaque covered on its external surface by nonmineralized plaque. Dental calculus forms by the deposition of calcium and phosphate salts within bacterial plaque. Calculus that forms above the free gingival margin is termed *supragingival calculus.* Salivary secretions are the main source of mineral for supragingival calculus. Supragingival calculus is most abundant on the lingual surfaces of the lower anterior teeth and buccal surfaces of the upper molars opposite the orifices of the salivary glands.

Subgingival calculus deposits, on the other hand, form on the root surfaces below the free margin of the gingiva and often extend to the base of periodontal pockets. Subgingival calculus is covered by nonmineralized plaque and loosely adherent bacteria. Subgingival calculus forms by mineralization of the subgingival plaque that extends from plaque at the orifice of the gingival crevice, and inflammatory exudate and gingival crevicular fluid are its main sources of mineral salts. Subgingival calculus deposits can be found on any root surfaces with periodontal pockets and may be ringlike or ledgelike or form crusty, spiny, or nodular deposits, which are often seen in radiographs. Less frequently they are fernlike formations or smooth veneers or occur as individual islands on the root surface.

Histologically, calculus is stratified, indicating that the deposits grow by apposition of new layers. Different crystal types within the bacterial remnants vary from small needle-shaped crystals identified as hydroxyapatite to long ribbonlike crystals of octocalcium phosphate oriented in bundles. In young deposits of supragingival calculus, crystalline aggregates of brushite can be seen. On enamel surfaces supragingival calculus binds to the acquired pellicle. The pellicle also serves to anchor subgingival calculus to the cementum surface. Also, subgingival calculus can form on root surfaces by direct extension and subsequent calcification of microorganisms into cemental irregularities, including spaces formerly occupied by Sharpey's fibers, resorption lacunae, or areas of arrested caries. Electron micrographic studies show crystal growth into cemental defects and intercrystalline binding of calculus and tooth crystals. These various methods of attachment result in subgingival calculus deposits that are difficult to completely remove from the root surface.

The organic matrix of supragingival calculus constitutes 15% to 20% of its dry weight. The matrix is composed of proteins contributed by bacteria and saliva, as well as carbohydrates. Recently lipids have also been shown to be present.

Calcification begins as early as a few days after bacterial deposition on the tooth surface. Additional foci then form, which enlarge and coalesce. In as little time as 1 week in some individuals and as much time as several months in others, the bulk of plaque becomes calcified if left undisturbed.

Bacteria play an important role in calculus formation. They are not essential, since calculus forms in germ-free animals. However, when present, bacteria clearly play a role, since calculus is far more abundant in infected than in germ-free animals.

Clinically, there are individuals who are rapid and heavy formers of supragingival calculus and others who form little or no calcified deposits. The salivary environment and, to a lesser extent, differences in bacterial flora and dietary factors contribute to these marked differences in the rate of calculus formation among individuals.

Assessing the role of calculus in periodontal destruction is complicated by the fact that it is always covered with unmineralized plaque. However, there is no question that the mineralized deposits (1) bring the bacterial overlay closer to the supporting tissues, (2) interfere with local self-cleansing mechanisms, and (3) make plaque removal more difficult. Subgingival calculus most likely contributes to the chronicity and progression of periodontal disease, and it is clear that frequent and thorough removal of root deposits by scaling and root planing is necessary to prevent further attachment loss and to provide an environment for periodontal healing. Therefore complete removal of subgingival calculus is a key element in periodontal therapy.

There are several agents available that in human clinical studies show a modest reduction of calculus. These and more advanced oral health products are sure to be important in the future in preventing calculus formation.

REFERENCES

Baer P and Newton WL: The occurrence of periodontal disease in germ-free mice, J Dent Res 38:1238, 1959.

Baumhammers A and Rohrbaugh EA: Permeability of human and rat dental calculus, J Periodontol 41:39, 1970.

Boskey AL: Current concepts of the physiology and biochemistry of calcification, Clin Orthop 157:225, 1981.

Boskey AL et al: Lipids associated with mineralization of human submandibular gland sialoliths, Arch Oral Biol 26:779, 1981.

Eanes ED et al: An electron microscopic study of the formation of amorphous calcium phosphate and its transformation to crystalline apatite, Calcif Tissue Res 6:32, 1970.

Ennever J: Microbiologic calcification: bone mineral and bacteria, Calcif Tissue Res 1:87, 1967.

Ennever J et al: The calculus surface index: method for scoring clinical calculus studies, J Periodontol 32:54, 1961.

Ennever J et al: Nucleation of microbiologic calcification by proteolipid, Proc Soc Exp Biol Med 152:147, 1976.

Everett FG and Potter GR: Morphology of submarginal calculus, J Periodontol 30:27, 1959.

Fleisch H et al: Influence of pyrophosphate on the transformation of amorphous to crystalline calcium phosphate, Calcif Tissue Res 2:49, 1968.

Friskopp J: Ultrastructure of nondecalcified supragingival and subgingival calculus, J Periodontol 54:542, 1983.

Friskopp J and Hammarstrom L: A comparative scanning electron microscopic study of supragingival and subgingival dental calculus, J Periodontol 51:553, 1980.

Gonzales F and Sognnaes RF: Electron microscopy of dental calculus, Science 131:156, 1960.

Greene JC and Vermillion JR: The oral hygiene index: a method for classifying oral hygiene status, J Am Dent Assoc 61:171, 1960.

Gron P et al: Human dental calculus: inorganic chemical and crystallographic composition, Arch Oral Biol 12:829, 1967.

Grossman E et al: Six month study of the effects of a chlorhexidine mouthrinse on gingivitis in adults, J Periodont Res 21(suppl 16):33, 1986.

Leach SA and Saxton CA: An electron microscopic study of the acquired pellicle and plaque formed on the enamel of human incisors, Arch Oral Biol 11:1081, 1966.

Little MF et al: The organic matrix of dental calculus, J Dent Res 40:753, 1961.

Little MF et al: Dental calculus composition. I. Supragingival calculus, J Dent Res 42:78, 1963.

Little MF et al: Dental calculus composition. II. Subgingival calculus, J Dent Res 43:645, 1964.

Lobene RA: A clinical study of the anticalculus effect of a dentifrice containing soluble pyrophosphate and sodium fluoride, Clin Prev Dent 8:5, 1986.

Lobene RA et al: The clinical effectiveness of an experimental anticalculus dentifrice, J Dent Res 64(special issue):235, 1985 (abstract 543).

Lu KH et al: The effect of a fluoride dentifrice containing an anticalculus agent on dental caries in children, J Dent Child 52:449, 1985.

Lundberg M et al: Analyses of some elements in supra and subgingival calculus, J Periodont Res 1:245, 1966.

Mandel ID: Histochemical and biochemical aspects of periodontal disease, Periodontics 1:43, 1963.

Mandel ID: Plaque and calculus, Ala J Med Sci 5:313, 1968.

Mandel ID: Biochemical aspects of calculus formation. I. Comparative studies of plaque in heavy and light calculus formers, J Periodont Res 9:10, 1974a.

Mandel ID: Biochemical aspects of calculus formation. II. Comparative studies of saliva in heavy and light calculus formers, J Periodont Res 9:211, 1974b.

Mandel ID and Gaffar A: Calculus revisited: a review, J Clin Periodontol 13:249, 1986.

Mandel ID and Levy BM: Studies on salivary calculus. I. Histochemical and chemical investigations of supra and subgingival calculus, Oral Surg 10:874, 1957.

Mandel ID and Thompson RH: Chemistry of parotid and submaxillary saliva in heavy calculus formers and non-formers, J Periodont Res 38:310, 1967.

Mandel ID et al: Histochemistry of calculus formation, J Periodontol 28:132, 1957.

Mandel ID et al: Carbohydrate components of supragingival salivary calculus, Proc Soc Exp Biol Med 110:301, 1962.

McDougall WA: Studies on the dental plaque. I. The histology of the dental plaque and its attachment, Aust Dent J 8:261, 1963.

Mühlemann HR and Villa P: The marginal line calculus index, Helv Odontol Acta 11:175, 1967.

Oshrain H et al: An histologic comparison of supra and subgingival plaque and calculus, J Periodontol 42:31, 1971.

Osuoji EI and Rowles SL: Isolation and identification of acid glycosaminoglycans in oral calculus, Arch Oral Biol 17:211, 1972.

Patters MR et al: Bacteroides gingivalis antigens and bone resorbing activity in root surface fractions of periodontally involved teeth, J Periodont Res 17:122, 1982.

Pihlstrom BL et al: Comparison of surgical and nonsurgical treatment of periodontal disease: a review of current studies and additional results after 6½ years, J Clin Periodontol 10:524, 1983.

Prinz H: The origin of salivary calculus, Dent Cosmos 63:231, 1921.

Ramfjord SP: Indices for prevalence and incidence of periodontal disease, J Periodontol 30:51, 1959.

Rowles SL: Biophysical studies on dental calculus in relation to periodontal disease, Dent Pract Dent Res 15:2, 1964.

Russell RG and Fleisch H: Inorganic pyrophosphate and pyrophosphatases in calcification and calcium homeostasis, Clin Orthop 69:101, 1970.

Schroeder HE: Formation and inhibition of dental calculus, Bern, Switzerland, 1969, Hans Huber Publishers.

Schwartz SR et al: Gingival reactions to different types of tooth accumulated materials, J Clin Periodont 42:144, 1971.

Selvig KA: Attachment of plaque and calculus to tooth surfaces, J Periodont Res 5:8, 1970.

Sharaway AM et al: A quantitative study of plaque and calculus formation in normal and periodontally involved mouths, J Periodontol 37:495, 1966.

Sidaway DA: A microbiological study of dental calculus. II. The in vitro calcification of microorganisms from dental calculus, J Periodont Res 13(4):360, 1978.

Slomiany A et al: Lipid composition of human parotid saliva from light and heavy dental calculus-formers, Arch Oral Biol 26:151, 1981.

Slomiany BL et al: Lipid composition of human submandibular gland secretion from light and heavy calculus formers, Arch Oral Biol 25:749, 1980.

Slomiany BL et al: Lipids of supragingival calculus, J Dent Res 62:862, 1983.

Suomi JD et al: A clinical trial of a calculus inhibitory dentifrice, J Periodontol 45:139, 1974.

Theilade J: Electron microscopic study of calculus attachment to smooth surfaces, Acta Odontol Scand 22:379, 1964.

Theilade J et al: Electron microscopic observations of dental calculus in germ free and conventional rats, Arch Oral Biol 9:97, 1964.

Villa P: Degree of calculus inhibition by habitual toothbrushing, Helv Odontol Acta 12:31, 1968.

Vogel JJ and Amdur BH: Inorganic pyrophosphate in the parotid saliva and its relation to calculus formation, Arch Oral Biol 12:159, 1967.

Volpe AR et al: In vivo calculus assessment. I. A method and its examiner reproducibility, J Periodontol 36:292, 1965.

Weinberger B: History of dentistry, St Louis, 1948, The CV Mosby Co.

Weinstein E and Mandel ID: The present status of anti-calculus agents, J Oral Ther 1:327, 1964.

Zacherl WA et al: The effect of soluble pyrophosphates on dental calculus in adults, J Am Dent Assoc 110:737, 1985.

Zander HA: The attachment of calculus to root surfaces, J Periodontol 24:16, 1953.

Zander HA et al: Mineralization of dental calculus, Proc Soc Exp Biol Med 103:257, 1960. Legends

Chapter 11

MICROBIOLOGY OF PERIODONTAL DISEASE

Joseph J. Zambon

HISTORICAL BACKGROUND

The history of oral microbiology parallels the history of microbiology and infectious disease in general. In the first studies of microorganisms using his newly devised microscope, Antonie van Leeuwenhoek wrote in 1772, "I took this stuff out of the hollows in the [tooth] roots, and mixed it with clean rainwater, and set it before the magnifying-glass . . . I must confess that the whole stuff seemed to me to be alive . . . the animalcules, with their strong swimming through the water, put many little particles which had no life in them into a like motion" (van Leeuwenhoek, 1941). Since van Leeuwenhoek, a number of dental research pioneers have studied oral microorganisms to determine their role in dental caries and periodontal disease. W.D. Miller (reprinted 1973) gained fame for his acidogenic theory of dental caries and also proposed that "pyorrhoea alveolaris is not caused by a specific bacterium, which occurs in every case (like the tubercle-bacillus in tuberculosis), but various bacteria may participate in it, just as in suppurative processes not only one but generally various species have been found." This is one of the first statements of what has become known as the nonspecific plaque hypothesis. According to this idea, dental plaque is a homogeneous bacterial mass that causes periodontal disease when it accumulates to the point of exceeding host defenses.

Later Bass, who developed the toothbrushing technique that bears his name (Bass and Johns, 1915), hypothesized that a specific microorganism, *"Endoameba buccalis,"* was the cause of periodontal disease and that a vaccine developed against this microorganism could be used to prevent the disease. This is one of the first suggestions of what is now called the specific plaque hypothesis. According to the specific plaque hypothesis, dental plaques from periodontally diseased sites are different from those adjacent to healthy sites. A corollary to the specific plaque hypothesis proposes that a few specific microorganisms in the subgingival flora are responsible for one or another of the different forms of periodontal disease.

The dichotomy represented in the specific and nonspecific plaque hypotheses holds a great deal of significance with regard to what constitutes appropriate therapy. It has been the focus of many investigations in the past several years.

INFECTIOUS NATURE OF PERIODONTAL DISEASE

The periodontal diseases, gingivitis and periodontitis, are caused by bacterial dental plaque. They are therefore infectious diseases, with several lines of evidence supporting their infectious nature (Socransky, 1979). First, there are both cross-sectional and longitudinal oral hygiene studies that correlate increased severity of gingivitis with increased accumulations of dental plaque. Longitudinal studies, in particular the classic experimental gingivitis studies of Löe et al. (1965), demonstrated that the development of dental plaque can be correlated with clinically demonstrable gingivitis. In these studies subjects were asked to refrain from all oral hygiene procedures. Within a period of 10 to 21 days, all subjects accumulated dental plaque and developed marginal gingivitis. Reinstitution of oral hygiene resulted in the elimination of the accumulated plaque and resolution of the marginal gingivitis; hence these studies demonstrate that dental plaque can cause gingivitis in humans.

The second line of evidence supporting the infectious nature of periodontal disease relates to the treatment of destructive periodontitis. Treatment that decreases the total number of plaque microorganisms and eliminates certain microbial species can be correlated with clinical improvement. Periodontal therapy may involve mechanical debridement of the periodontal pocket, as occurs in scaling and root planing, or debridement by chemotherapeutic agents, including antibiotics such as tetracycline or disinfectants and antiseptics such as iodine and chlorhexidine. Numerous clinical studies such as those by Rosling et al. (1976) have shown that periodontal disease can be arrested in patients maintaining meticulous plaque control after thorough debridement of subgingival lesions. Such patients do not suffer additional periodontal attachment loss; on the contrary, they can even exhibit healing in osseous defects with a gain of attachment and new bone formation.

A third line of evidence supporting the infectious nature of periodontal disease can be found in in vivo and in vitro pathogenicity studies of specific plaque bacteria. Demonstration of in vivo pathogenicity can be seen in reports of extraoral infections by plaque microorganisms and by experimental periodontitis studies in animal models. Numerous case reports have noted oral microorganisms causing severe, even life-threatening infections in extraoral sites (Pierce et al., 1984; Zambon, 1985). Many of the microorganisms found in human dental plaque can induce periodontal disease following oral implantation into germ-free and conventional animals (Holt et al., 1988). The resulting histopathology mimics many aspects of natural periodontal disease, including gingival inflammation, destruction of connective tissue, vasculitis, osteoclastic bone resorption, and apical migration of the junctional epithelium. Monoinfection of *Bacteroides gingivalis* into a rodent model, for example, leads to rapid alveolar bone loss (Chang et al.,

1988). Mixed infections with two or more bacterial species can also cause experimental periodontitis.

In vitro pathogenicity relates to the ability of plaque bacteria to produce virulence factors, including endotoxin, exotoxin, enzymes, and toxic products of bacterial metabolism. The predominance of gram-negative bacteria within periodontal pockets leads to locally high concentrations of lipopolysaccharide endotoxin. This highly toxic substance can exert cytotoxic effects on host tissues, stimulate osteoclastic bone resorption in vitro, and cause a localized Schwartzman reaction with tissue necrosis. Indirect effects include leukopenia, activation of factor XII (or Hageman factor), which can result in intravascular coagulation, and activation of the alternate complement pathway. In addition, both gram-positive and gram-negative bacteria produce toxic metabolic end products capable of tissue destruction, including fatty and organic acids such as butyric and propionic acids, amines, volatile sulfur compounds, indole, and ammonia. (For a review of the virulence mechanism of periodontal pathogens, see Slots and Genco, 1984.)

Bacterial enzymes produced by oral bacteria can increase the permeability of the epithelium lining the gingival sulcus, destroy gingival connective tissue, and promote apical proliferation of the junctional epithelium along the root surfaces. Among these enzymes is collagenase, which is produced by *B. gingivalis* and by *Actinobacillus actinomycetemcomitans* and hyaluronidase. These enzymes most likely lead to widening of the intercellular spaces and increased permeability of gingival epithelium. Other bacterial enzymes probably associated with periodontal disease include proteinase, gelatinase, aminopeptidases, phospholipase A, alkaline phosphatase, acid phosphatase, DNAse, and RNAse. Bacteria also produce factors that enable the microorganisms to evade host defense mechanisms. These include bacterial capsules, which can inhibit phagocytosis by polymorphonuclear leukocytes and macrophages, and leukotreines, which kill phagocytes.

EVIDENCE IMPLICATING SPECIFIC MICROORGANISMS IN THE ETIOLOGY OF HUMAN PERIODONTAL DISEASE

The past two decades have witnessed a revolution in our understanding of the microbial pathogenesis of human periodontal disease. Through the experimental gingivitis studies of Löe et al. (1965), the infectious nature of these diseases has become apparent. A new idea has also emerged—the concept of microbial specificity in the etiology of periodontal disease (Loesche, 1976; Socransky, 1977). Previously, it was believed that periodontal disease resulted from the gross accumulation of dental plaques that were essentially the same. The many different forms of periodontal disease are now, however, thought to be associated with qualitatively distinct dental plaques, and as an important corollary, specific bacteria are thought to be re-

Table 11-1. Subgingival microorganisms associated with periodontal diseases

Disease	Microorganism
Acute necrotizing ulcerative gingivitis	*Bacteroides intermedius* Intermediate-sized spirochetes
Adult periodontitis	*Actinobacillus actinomycetem-comitans* *Bacteroides intermedius* *Bacteroides gingivalis* *Bacteroides forsythus* *Capnocytophaga gingivalis* *Eikenella corrodens* *Eubacterium* species *Fusobacterium nucleatum* *Propionibacterium acnes* *Streptococcus intermedius* *Wolinella recta*
Localized juvenile periodontitis	*Actinobacillus actinomycetem-comitans* *Bacteroides* species
Generalized juvenile periodontitis	*Actinobacillus actinomycetem-comitans* *Bacteroides gingivalis* *Bacteroides intermedius* *Capnocytophaga* *Eikenella corrodens* *Neisseria*
Periodontal abscesses	Gram-negative anaerobic rods *Bacteroides gingivalis* *Fusobacterium* species *Capnocytophaga* *Vibrio* species
Periodontitis associated with insulin-dependent diabetes mellitus	*Actinobacillus actinomycetem-comitans* Anaerobic *vibrios* *Campylobacter* *Capnocytophaga*
Periodontitis associated with non-insulin-dependent diabetes mellitus	*Bacteroides gingivalis* *Bacteroides intermedius* *Fusobacterium* species *Wolinella recta*
Pregnancy gingivitis	*Bacteroides intermedius*
Refractory or recurrent periodontitis	*Actinobacillus actinomycetem-comitans* *Bacteroides forsythsus* *Bacteroides gingivalis* *Bacteroides intermedius* *Wolinella recta*

sponsible for the initiation and progression of periodontal diseases. Cross-sectional and longitudinal studies of the predominant cultivable microflora have revealed that of the 300 to 400 bacterial species that can inhabit the human oral cavity, only a small number are associated with human periodontal disease (Moore et al., 1983). The concept of bacterial specificity has been further supported by clinical observations, by the therapeutic effect of antiinfective therapy, and by experimental models of periodontitis in both gnotobiotic and conventionally maintained animals.

A variety of predominantly gram-negative organisms

have been implicated in the etiology of periodontal disease, including *A. actinomycetemcomitans*, *B. gingivalis*, *Bacteroides intermedius*, *Capnocytophaga* species, *Eikenella corrodens*, *Fusobacterium nucleatum*, and *Wolinella recta*, as well as certain gram-positive bacteria such as *Eubacterium* species. A list of the microbial pathogens associated with various forms of periodontal disease is given in Table 11-1.

Since periodontal disease occurs in an area normally inhabited by many bacteria, it is difficult to identify the specific microorganisms responsible for periodontal disease using the same criteria as those developed to pinpoint the causative microorganisms in monoinfections. That is, Koch's postulates, which have been used to pinpoint the cause of infectious diseases caused by single organisms infecting otherwise sterile sites, have not been useful in studies of the periodontal microflora. Alternative criteria have been proposed by Socransky (1977) to identify the key microorganisms in periodontal infections. These include the following:

1. The putative pathogen is present in proximity to the periodontal lesions and in high numbers as compared with either the absence of the microorganism or its presence in much smaller numbers (carrier state) in periodontally normal subjects or in subjects with other forms of periodontal disease. In contrast, the microorganism should either be absent or present only in small numbers in dental plaques associated with periodontally healthy sites.
2. Patients infected with these periodontal pathogens often develop high levels of antibodies in serum, saliva, and gingival crevicular fluid and may also develop a cell-mediated immune response to the putative pathogen.
3. These microorganisms can often demonstrate in vivo production of virulence factors that can be correlated with clinical histopathology.
4. Experimental implantation of the organism into the gingival crevice of an appropriate animal model should lead to the development of at least some of the characteristics of the naturally occurring disease (e.g., inflammation, connective tissue disruption, and bone loss).
5. Clinical treatment that eliminates these microorganisms from periodontal lesions should result in clinical improvement.

There are several difficulties encountered in determining the etiology of periodontal diseases, many of which have been addressed over the last 20 years. These occur in three categories:

1. Technical problems, including sample taking and difficulties in cultivation and identification of isolates.
2. Problems associated with the complexity of the microbiota. Periodontal infections are mixed infec-

tions, in which it is difficult to distinguish secondary invaders from true pathogens.

3. Problems associated with the nature of periodontal disease. Periodontal disease appears to be episodic, and differentiation between active and inactive sites sampled for microbiologic studies may be important.

Despite these difficulties, considerable progress has been made in identifying periodontal pathogens by applying multiple criteria, including the host response. As a result of intense research in periodontal microbiology and immunology in the past two decades, several specific pathogenic bacteria have emerged as candidates for causative agents in periodontal disease.

PUTATIVE PERIODONTAL PATHOGENS AND BACTERIAL VIRULENCE FACTORS

A clinically significant advance in periodontology has been the identification of specific oral microorganisms associated with lesions in different forms of human periodontal disease—research that is comparable in importance to the discovery of *Streptococcus mutans* as the main cause of dental caries. These periodontal pathogens are discussed here.

Actinobacillus actinomycetemcomitans

A. actinomycetemcomitans has been strongly implicated in the pathogenesis of localized juvenile periodontitis (LJP) (Zambon, 1985). This microorganism is also associated with cases of adult periodontitis in which alveolar bone loss occurs at an unusually rapid rate (Tanner et al., 1979) and with periodontitis that continues to progress after meticulous scaling, root planing, plaque control, and even periodontal surgery. This latter disease entity is known as refractory periodontitis.

A. actinomycetemcomitans was first isolated by the German microbiologist Klinger in 1912 from lesions of cervicofacial actinomycosis. The microorganism was isolated together with *Actinomyces israelii*. Hence the species name, *actinomycetemcomitans,* means "together with *Actinomyces*." *A. actinomycetemcomitans* colonies exhibit a star-shaped internal morphology, and the cells are gram-negative, capnophilic, nonmotile coccobacilli. Hence the genus name *Actinobacillus:* "actino" referring to the star-shaped internal morphology of the colonies and "bacillus" referring to the cell shape. The organism ferments sugars, does not require X (hemin) or V (NADH) factors, and is catalase positive. While it is closely related to bacterial species in the genus *Haemophilus,* it can be differentiated on the basis of X and V factor requirements and the production of beta-galactosidase. The primary oral ecologic niche for *A. actinomycetemcomitans* (i.e., the environment in which it is most likely to be found) is dental plaque.

Periodontal pathogens such as *A. actinomycetemcomitans* are true human pathogens, since they cause disease in extraoral sites as a result of direct extension or hematogenous spread from the oral cavity. There are, for example, over 60 reported cases of endocarditis due to *A. actinomycetemcomitans* (Table 11-2). These include at least two cases of endocarditis due to penicillin-resistant *A. actinomycetemcomitans* occurring in patients who were taking penicillin as part of the usual antibiotic prophylaxis against subacute bacterial endocarditis. *A. actinomycetemcomitans* can also cause thyroid gland abscesses, urinary tract infection, brain abscesses, vertebral osteomyelitis, and other infections. Overall, 19% of the reported cases of extraoral infection with *A. actinomycetemcomitans* in humans have been fatal (Table 11-2).

Certain *A. actinomycetemcomitans* serotypes and corresponding serotype antigens may be related to specific sites of infection. Three serotypes of *A. actinomycetemcomitans* have been identified (Zambon et al., 1983b). The serotype antigens are high molecular weight, heat-stable, primarily carbohydrate moieties. In the human oral cavity, serotypes a and b are those most commonly found, whereas serotype c makes up only approximately 10% of *A. actinomycetemcomitans* human oral isolates. In LJP, the prevalence of serotype b is significantly elevated in subgingival dental plaque, suggesting that the serotype b antigen may be particularly important in the pathogenesis of this disease. Recent studies have indicated that serotype c *A. actinomycetemcomitans* is especially important in extraoral infections.

The relationship of *A. actinomycetemcomitans* to periodontal disease begins with clinical descriptions of "periodontosis" or, as it is now known, LJP. This disease tends to occur among members of the same family and is characterized by periodontal pockets and alveolar bone loss, which mainly affects the permanent first molars and incisor teeth in teenagers and young adults. The severity of the clinical lesions is much greater than would be expected on the basis of the low plaque and calculus levels seen at the lesion sites. The increased susceptibility of families to *A. actinomycetemcomitans*–associated LJP may be in part due to the fact that they often exhibit defective neutrophil function. The clinical picture suggests an etiology other

Table 11-2. *Actinobacillus actinomycetemcomitans* in extraoral infections of humans

Disease	No. cases reported	Deaths
Infectious endocarditis	66	11
Actinomycosis	45	11
Abscesses of brain, hand, face, mediastinum, and thyroid gland	6	1
Other infections: endarteritis, endopthalmitis, meningitis, pneumonia, septicemia, urinary, vertebral osteomyelitis	7	1
TOTAL	124	24 (19%)

than simple plaque and calculus accumulation for this form of periodontal disease.

Initial studies of the microflora in LJP lesions revealed high numbers of an unknown gram-negative rod (Slots, 1976; Newman and Socransky, 1977), which was later identified as *A. actinomycetemcomitans*. Subsequent studies of LJP patients demonstrated that a large proportion of the subgingival flora was made up of *A. actinomycetemcomitans* in lesion sites, whereas adjacent periodontally healthy sites exhibited few if any *A. actinomycetemcomitans* (Slots et al., 1980). The prevalence of *A. actinomycetemcomitans*, determined in several different studies and patient groups, is given in Table 11-3. These disease associations provide evidence of *A. actinomycetemcomitans* in the pathogenesis of LJP. To briefly summarize this data (Zambon, 1985):

1. LJP patients harbor large numbers of this microorganism in lesion sites but not in adjacent periodontally healthy sites in the same patient; nor are large numbers of the organism found in periodontal pockets in other types of periodontitis (see Table 11-4 for a comparison of the presence of *A. actinomycetemcomitans* in various oral sites in normal subjects and in patients with LJP).

2. LJP patients develop high levels of serum, salivary, and gingival crevicular fluid antibodies to *A. actinomycetemcomitans* as compared with the very low levels of antibodies seen in patients with other types of periodontal disease. Table 11-4 shows the close relationship between colonization with *A. actinomycetemcomitans* and serum antibodies to this organism.

3. *A. actinomycetemcomitans* produces a number of virulence factors that may be involved in the pathogenesis of periodontitis.

4. Periodontal treatment that results in elimination of *A. actinomycetemcomitans* from subgingival sites can be correlated with clinical improvement.

Table 11-3. Prevalence of *Actinobacillus actinomycetemcomitans* in human periodontal disease

Patient group	Slots et al. (1980)	Mandell and Socransky (1981)	Zambon et al. (1983a)	Eisenmann et al. (1983)	Four-study average prevalence
Healthy juveniles	2/10				20%
Localized juvenile periodontitis	9/10	6/6	28/29	12/12	96%
Healthy adults	4/11		24/142		18%
Adult periodontitis	6/12	0/48	28/134	6/10	20%

Table 11-4. *Actinobacillus actinomycetemcomitans* on oral surfaces of normal subjects and those with LJP (percent of total bacteria)

Subject	Subgingival plaque	Saliva	Tongue	Cheek	Serum antibodies to *A. actinomycetemcomitans*
Normal					
1	—	—	—	—	—
2	—	—	—	—	—
3	—	—	—	—	—
4	—	—	—	—	—
5	—	—	—	—	—
6	—	—	—	—	—
7	—	—	—	—	—
8	0.008	—	0.002	0.06	+
Localized juvenile periodontitis					
9	7.5	0.002	—	0.02	+
10	0.3	—	—	—	+
11	1.1	0.005	—	0.01	+
12	16.0	—	0.0015	0.03	+
13	0.5	—	—	—	+
14	1.9	0.004	0.004	0.01	+
15	15.6	0.06	0.035	0.1	+
16	5.5	0.01	—	0.1	+
17	1.8	0.005	0.003	0.7	+

Serologic (Zambon et al., 1983a) and implantation studies (Christersson et al., 1985a) have suggested that *A. actinomycetemcomitans* can be transmitted among family members. However, it does not appear to be readily transmissible (i.e., the disease is not "contagious"). Multiple contacts are probably required for oral colonization to occur.

LJP patients have high levels of antibodies to *A. actinomycetemcomitans* in their serum, saliva, and gingival crevicular fluid. This compares with the very low levels of anti–*A. actinomycetemcomitans* antibodies seen in healthy individuals and in patients with other types of periodontal disease. Data from representative studies all point to the presence of elevated levels of antibodies to the organism in LJP patients as compared with much lower levels in other patient groups. A study by Genco et al. (1985), for example, showed that 96% of LJP patients had serum antibodies to *A. actinomycetemcomitans,* whereas normal subjects had low levels of serum antibody to *A. actinomycetemcomitans.* Studies by Sandholm et al. (1987) have demonstrated that 55% of patients with untreated juvenile periodontitis and 28% of patients with treated juvenile periodontitis exhibited elevated levels of salivary IgG antibody to *A. actinomycetemcomitans,* suggesting that treatment lowers the levels of *A. actinomycetemcomitans* infection, which in turn results in reduced levels of serum IgG antibody to this organism.

A. actinomycetemcomitans produces a number of virulence factors that may be involved in the pathogenesis of periodontitis. These can be classified as factors that assist the microorganism in colonizing dental plaque and/or the gingival sulcus, such as bacterial capsules and fimbriae; factors that permit the microorganism to evade host defense mechanisms, such as a leukotoxin that can destroy polymorphonuclear leukocytes (Tsai et al., 1979) and a component that inhibits polymorphonuclear leukocyte chemotaxis to the site of infection; and factors that can cause tissue destruction, including a lipopolysaccharide endotoxin that can stimulate bone resorption, a collagenase that can dissolve gingival connective tissue, and a factor that can prevent healing.

Prominent among the factors that can inhibit host immune defenses is the *A. actinomycetemcomitans* leukotoxin. This is a heat-labile factor that can destroy human and monkey polymorphonuclear leukocytes. It is neutralized by sera from LJP patients—a factor that may play a role in host resistance to infection. *A. actinomycetemcomitans* strains isolated from periodontally diseased subjects demonstrated leukotoxic activity in higher proportions than did isolates from periodontally normal subjects, providing further evidence for the role of the leukotoxin in the disease (Zambon, et al., 1983d). Also, leukotoxic strains of *A. actinomycetemcomitans* are found more often in younger patients than in older patients, suggesting that the effect of leukotoxin in the pathogenesis of *A. actinomyce-*

temcomitans–associated periodontal disease may be more important during the earlier phases of the disease (Tsai and Taichman, 1986).

Bacteriophage has also been associated with *A. actinomycetemcomitans* virulence. Preus et al. (1987) reported that phage-infected *A. actinomycetemcomitans* was found in periodontal pockets that showed bone loss during the previous 12 months. A "burned out" site became active again at the same time that *A. actinomycetemcomitans* in that site became infected with phage.

Among *A. actinomycetemcomitans* adherence factors are bacterial capsules and fimbriae. A microcapsule observable by electron microscopic examination of ruthenium red–stained bacterial cells was described by Holt et al. (1980). Subsequently, heat-stable, cell surface serotype antigens were purified and found to be carbohydrate antigens suggestive of cell surface mannans (Zambon et al., 1983c). These may contribute to the bacterial cell surface hydrophobicity noted for *A. actinomycetemcomitans.* Fimbriae, which also play a role in bacterial adherence, have been described on *A. actinomycetemcomitans.* Recent data indicate that environmental factors may play a role in the expression of *A. actinomycetemcomitans* fimbriae. Bacterial cells grown under relatively anaerobic conditions produce more fimbriae than do the same strains grown under relatively aerobic conditions (Scannapieco et al., 1987).

One additional virulence factor is the lipopolysaccharide from *A. actinomycetemcomitans.* This contains carbohydrate, lipid A, C14 and β-OH C14 fatty acids, and ketodeoxyoctonate. This lipopolysaccharide is active in biologic assays such as the Schwartzman reaction, in vitro bone resorption (Iino and Hopps, 1984), and macrophage activation.

The final line of evidence implicating *A. actinomycetemcomitans* in the etiology of certain forms of periodontal disease is the fact that periodontal treatment that results in the elimination of *A. actinomycetemcomitans* from subgingival sites can be correlated with clinical improvement. Treatment studies such as those reported by Slots and Rosling (1983) and by Christersson et al. (1985a) have shown that elimination of *A. actinomycetemcomitans* from lesions in LJP patients is associated with clinical improvement. These studies have indicated that sites that gained more than 2 mm of probing attachment level after treatment had undetectable levels of subgingival *A. actinomycetemcomitans.* On the other hand, those few treated sites that continued to harbor high numbers of *A. actinomycetemcomitans* experienced continued loss of probing attachment. Treatment studies have also indicated that conventional periodontal therapy consisting of scaling and root planing is ineffective in eliminating *A. actinomycetemcomitans* from subgingival sites. This is most likely due to the ability of this microorganism to invade the gingival connective tissue. Persistence of *A. actinomycetemcomitans* in the subgingival flora can be correlated with its presence in the tissue in a viable form (Christersson et al., 1987a, 1987b). Effective therapy for *A. actinomycetemcomitans* subgingival infection and, accordingly, for periodontal disease due to this microorganism, such as LJP, necessarily involves the use of antibiotics alone or in combination with periodontal surgery to eliminate the *A. actinomycetemcomitans*–infected tissue (Zambon et al., 1986b). In addition, microbiologic assays for the presence of *A. actinomycetemcomitans* in subgingival plaque during diagnosis and treatment and at recall examination is valuable in the clinical management of these types of infections (Bonta et al., 1985).

Black-pigmented *Bacteroides*

Bacterial species within the genus *Bacteroides* constitute one of the five major genera in the human gastrointestinal tract. While most of these microorganisms are commensal in the gut, this group also includes opportunistic pathogens such as *Bacteroides fragilis*, which can cause septicemia and abscesses in various parts of the body. Similarly, other members of the genus *Bacteroides,* especially the black-pigmented *Bacteroides,* are important residents of the human oral cavity, where they can be found inhabiting a number of distinct oral sites, including the tonsils, saliva, tongue, and buccal mucosa. These microorganisms can also cause severe medical infections in extraoral sites, including abscesses in the brain, genitourinary tract, and lungs; mediastinitis; and foot infections in diabetic patients.

The black-pigmented *Bacteroides* species were first described by Oliver and Wherry (1921) as *Bacterium melaninogenicum* (Table 11-5). Later they were assigned to the genus *Bacteroides* and named *Bacteroides melaninogenicus.* They are gram-negative, anaerobic, nonmotile bacilli that produce brown- to black-pigmented colonies when grown on medium containing blood. They were initially divided into strongly sugar-fermenting, weakly sugar-fermenting, and non-sugar-fermenting groups, which Holde-

man and Moore (1970) named *B. melaninogenicus* ssp. *melaninogenicus, B. melaninogenicus* ssp. *intermedius,* and *B. melaninogenicus* ssp. *asaccharolyticus,* respectively. In view of the significant differences in guanine-cytosine (G + C) content between groups, these subspecies were raised to species level as *B. melaninogenicus, B. intermedius,* and *B. asaccharolyticus. B. asaccharolyticus* was itself found to be genetically heterogeneous. Human oral isolates had 46.7 to 49.1 mol% G + C, whereas human nonoral isolates had 51.6 to 53.4 mol% G + C. Hybridization studies similarly revealed very low levels of DNA homology between oral and nonoral strains. Based on this data, the oral genotype was established as a new species, *B. gingivalis* (Coykendall et al., 1980).

Currently the species of black-pigmented *Bacteroides* found in humans (van Winkelhoff, 1986; see Table 11-5) include the saccharolytic (sugar-fermenting) species: (1) *B. melaninogenicus,* comprising more than one DNA homology group; (2) *Bacteroides loescheii,* formerly grouped with *B. melaninogenicus* and currently comprising more than one DNA homology group (Holdeman and Johnson, 1981); (3) *Bacteroides denticola,* a former DNA homology group within *B. melaninogenicus;* (4) *B. intermedius,* which contains two DNA homology groups and three serogroups; and (5) *Bacteroides corporis* (Johnson and Holdeman, 1983), formerly a DNA homology group and serogroup within *B. intermedius.* The asaccharolytic (nonsugar-fermenting) species include (1) *B. gingivalis,* which is genetically, phenotypically, and antigenically distinct from the nonoral species, *B. asaccharolyticus,* and (2) *Bacteroides endodontalis,* which is a recently described species of black-pigmented *Bacteroides* isolated from periapical abscesses of endodontic origin. *B. asaccharolyticus* and *B. corporis* are usually found in the intestine, whereas *B. gingivalis, B. endodontalis, B. intermedius, B. melaninogenicus, B. loescheii,* and *B. denticola* are predominantly oral species. *B. levii* and *B. macacae* are nonhuman animal species.

A number of studies have indicated that the black-pigmented *Bacteroides* species are pathogenic and participate in both mixed anaerobic infections and monoinfections in animal models. There are distinct differences among the eight species listed in Table 11-5 with regard to virulence. Subcutaneous inoculation of black-pigmented *Bacteroides* together with other gram-positive and gram-negative microorganisms such as *Veillonella parvula* can produce lesions in experimental animals. The accompanying bacteria provide growth nutrients for the *Bacteroides* species, which are the key pathogens in these mixtures. Early studies showed, however, that monoinfections caused by a black-pigmented *Bacteroides* strain, most likely *B. gingivalis* originally isolated from a patient, could be produced in guinea pigs and in conventional and germ-free mice. Similarly, Kastelein et al. (1981) demonstrated that *B. gingivalis* strain W83, a "clinical isolate," was virulent as a

Table 11-5. Black-pigmented *Bacteroides*

1939	1970	1980 to present
Nonfermenters		
	B. melaninogenicus ssp. *asaccharolyticus*	*B. gingivalis* *B. asaccharolyticus* *B. endodontalis*
Weak fermenters		
Bacteroides melaninogenicus	*B. melaninogenicus* ssp. *intermedius*	*B. intermedius* *B. corporis*
Strong fermenters		
	B. melaninogenicus ssp. *melaninogenicus*	*B. melaninogenicus* *B. loescheii* *B. denticola*

monoinfectant in guinea pigs and Swiss mice. Some *B. gingivalis* strains are highly virulent and produce localized and secondary abscesses and often death within 12 to 48 hours in mice, even when inoculated alone.

B. gingivalis has been strongly implicated in the etiology of adult forms of human periodontal disease and is found in the subgingival flora of over 90% of patients with adult periodontitis (Christersson et al., 1989). Based on criteria similar to those used for *A. actinomycetemcomitans,* *B. gingivalis* has been associated with certain cases of rapidly progressing adult periodontitis, chronic adult periodontitis, and generalized juvenile periodontitis.

B. gingivalis is found in high frequency and in high numbers, often as a major component of the subgingival flora, in adult periodontitis lesions. By contrast, it is found with much lower frequency and in much smaller numbers or not at all in subgingival dental plaque from periodontally normal subjects. Furthermore, *B. gingivalis* is not detectable in the subgingival flora of patients with gingivitis who are not affected by periodontitis (Table 11-6).

It is clear that *B. gingivalis* either is not present or is present at very low levels in the oral flora of normal subjects. It is not generally found in gingivitis patients. In marked contrast, the oral cavity of patients with adult periodontitis is often infected with black-pigmented *Bacteroides,* especially *B. gingivalis.* Fig. 11-1 illustrates the large numbers of black-pigmented *Bacteroides,* including *B. gingivalis* (brown colonies) and *B. intermedius* (black colonies), in a typical periodontitis patient. It can be seen that black-pigmented *Bacteroides* are found in several areas of the oral cavity, including the subgingival plaque, the gingival surface itself, the tongue, the tonsils, and in saliva. Interestingly, black-pigmented *Bacteroides* are not often found in the supragingival plaque from patients with adult periodontitis. Hence it appears that *B. gingivalis* colonizes the saliva and most oral mucous surfaces of periodontitis patients. Preliminary studies of the vagina, the gut, and feces have not yielded *B. gingivalis,* so it appears that the primary ecologic niche of *B. gingivalis* is the oral mucous membranes and the subgingival region of patients with adult forms of periodontitis (Fig. 11-1).

Patients with adult periodontitis have elevated levels of

serum antibody to *B. gingivalis,* whereas few normal subjects or patients with other forms of periodontitis exhibit elevated levels of serum antibody to this microorganism, further implicating *B. gingivalis* as a pathogen. *B. gingivalis* can produce a number of potential virulence factors, which may play a role in the pathogenesis of adult periodontitis. These destructive factors include collagenase, potent proteolytic activity, a "trypsin-like" activity, cell toxins, and a lipopolysaccharide that inhibits in vitro bone formation. *B. gingivalis* lipopolysaccharide also is a potent stimulator of interleukin-1 production by monocytes, which in turn is likely to be involved in osteoclast-mediated bone resorption.

Bacteroides intermedius

B. intermedius is often a dominant subgingival organism in acute necrotizing ulcerative gingivitis (ANUG), where it may account for one fifth of the flora. In ANUG there are elevated levels of antibody to one serotype (B) of *B. intermedius,* further implicating this organism in ANUG.

B. intermedius is often a major subgingival organism in patients with adult periodontitis and along with *B. gingivalis* may affect 95% of such patients, accounting for 20% to 50% of the cultivable flora (Table 11-7 and Fig. 11-1). *B. intermedius* may also be present alone as a major component of the subgingival flora in patients with adult periodontitis (Table 11-7, patient No. 8). *B. intermedius* can be found in gingivitis patients and in over one half of normal subjects. *B. intermedius* is heterogeneous. It comprises two DNA homology groups and three serogroups (Nakazawa et al., 1988). It has been hypothesized that certain *B. intermedius* strains are more virulent than others, and if this is so, the more virulent would be expected in lesions of patients. In adult periodontitis lesions the levels of *B. gingivalis* and *B. intermedius* are often related. When high levels of *B. gingivalis* occur, low levels of *B. intermedius* are found, and vice versa (Table 11-7). Further studies are needed to resolve the role of *B. intermedius* in periodontal disease.

Other black-pigmented *Bacteroides* appear not to play a major role in periodontal disease, since they are not often

Table 11-6. Comparison of *Bacteroides gingivalis* and *Bacteroides intermedius* in the subgingival flora of adults with periodontitis and adults with gingivitis only

Group	Probing attachment loss	% Sites bleeding on probing	B. gingivalis (% subjects positive)	B. intermedius (% subjects positive)
Gingivitis (n = 33)	None >2 mm over 1 year of observation	47 + 3	0	42
Periodontitis (n = 53)	Yes, many sites >2 mm PAL	88 + 2	94	88

From Christersson LA et al: Specific subgingival bacteria and diagnosis of gingivitis and periodontitis, Adv Dent Res, 1989 (in press).

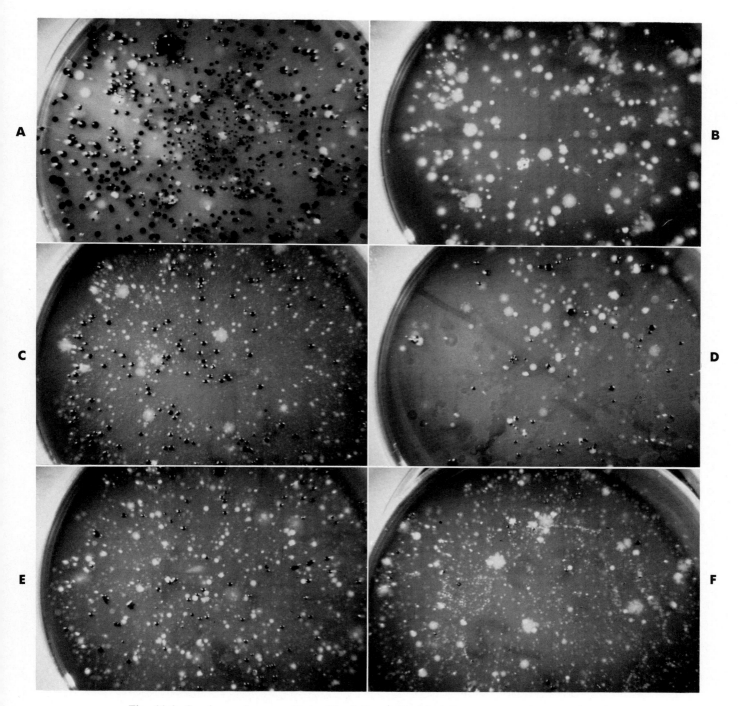

Fig. 11-1. Specimens from a patient with adult periodontitis (prior to treatment) were cultured under anaerobic conditions using media supporting the growth of black-pigmented *Bacteroides*. Subgingival plaque was cultured; *B. gingivalis* and *B. intermedius* were present. *B. gingivalis* colonies are brown, and those of *B. intermedius* are black. Both types were also cultivated in specimens from gingival surface cultured at 10^{-2}, from saliva cultured at 10^{-4}, from tongue cultured at 10^{-3}, and from tonsil cultured at 10^{-2}. **A,** Subgingival plaque at 10^{-3} dilution. **B,** Supragingival plaque at 10^{-3} dilution was cultured, and no detectable black-pigmented *Bacteroides* were seen. **C,** Gingiva. **D,** Saliva. **E,** Tongue. **F,** Tonsil. (See also Color Plate 2.)

Table 11-7. Percentages of black-pigmented *Bacteroides* species in pockets of patients with adult periodontitis

Patient	Pocket							
	A		**B**		**C**		**D**	
	B.g.	*B.i.*	*B.g.*	*B.i.*	*B.g.*	*B.i.*	*B.g.*	*B.i.*
1	58	0	32	0	21	0.01	55	0
2	45	0	40	0	53	0	75	0
3	63	0	0	4	1	1	66	1
4	5	2	1	1	1	1	37	2
5	55	0	42	0.1	7	0.1	44	0.1
6	12	1	11	1	18	0.1	0	4
7	18	0.1	27	0.1	31	1	17	0.1
8	0	0	0	30	0	20	0	11

From van Winkelhoff AJ: Black-pigmented *Bacteroides* in human oral infections, thesis, Amsterdam, 1986, Free University Press.
B.g., *Bacteroides gingivalis*; *B.i.*, *Bacteroides intermedius*.

associated with periodontal lesions. *B. endodontalis*, however, is virulent and often associated with acute abscesses of pulpal origin.

Wolinella species

Microorganisms in the genus *Wolinella* are gram-negative, motile anaerobes that can be found as helical, curved, or straight bacterial cells 0.5 to 1 μm by 2 to 6 μm with tapered or round ends. These microorganisms can be found in large numbers in the subgingival dental plaque of patients with adult periodontitis and may be involved in the pathogenesis of this form of periodontal disease. They are also found in infected root canals. The genus is part of the family Bacteroidaceae, which includes other gram-negative microorganisms found in subgingival dental plaque, including black-pigmented *Bacteroides*.

By phase-contrast microscopy, *Wolinella* organisms exhibit a rapid, darting type of bacterial motility by means of flagella located at one pole of the bacterial cell. The bacteria form three types of colonies on agar. One type is a pale, translucent, nonspreading yellow colony. Another type is a gray translucent colony that may be mistaken for a water droplet on the agar. Another colony variant can, depending on the growth medium, pit the agar surface. The microorganism grows best at 37° C in an anaerobic environment of 85% N_2, 10% H_2, and 5% CO_2.

Many of the bacteria previously referred to as *Vibrio succinogenes* are now categorized in the genus *Wolinella*. The genus exhibits 42 to 48 mol% G + C. There are currently three species of *Wolinella*, including *W. recta*, *W. succinogenes*, and *W. curva*, of which the former two have been best described. *W. succinogenes* appears as spiral or curved cells and can be distinguished from *W. recta*, which appears mainly as straight cells. *W. succinogenes*, as the name implies, also has a growth requirement for

Table 11-8. Predominant bacterial species in subgingival plaque from periodontitis patients with non-insulin-dependent diabetes mellitus

Bacterial species	% Positive patients	% Positive sites
Bacteroides intermedius	88	56.3
Wolinella recta	67	50.0
Bacteroides gingivalis	75	56.3
Streptococcus sanguis	88	75.0
Actinomyces naeslundii	88	68.8
Capnocytophaga species	67	43.8
Actinomyces odontolyticus	25	25.0
Fusobacterium nucleatum	50	37.5
Veillonella dispar	50	31.3
Actinomyces viscosus	50	37.5
Fusobacterium species	38	25.0
Actinobacillus actinomycetemcomitans	13	6.3
Eikenella corrodens	38	18.8
Propionibacterium species	67	37.5
Gram-negative anaerobic rods	11	18.8
Eubacterium species	38	31.3
Neisseria species	38	18.8
Peptostreptococcus anaerobius	12	6.3
Arachnia propionica	25	12.5
Bacteroides loescheii	12	12.5
Actinomyces meyerii	12	6.3
Selenomonas sputigena	25	12.5
Campylobacter concisus	12	6.3
Haemophilus aphrophilus	12	12.5
Staphylococcus epidermidis	25	12.5
Actinomyces israelii	12	6.3
Bacteroides buccae	12	6.3
Bacteroides corporis	12	6.3
Bacteroides denticola	12	6.3
Bacterionema matruchotti	12	6.3
Fusobacterium periodonticum	12	6.3
Veillonella parvula	12	6.3

From Zambon JJ et al: J Periodontol 59(1):23, 1988.

succinate or for compounds such as pyruvate and bicarbonate, which can be converted to succinate during bacterial metabolism. Electron microscopy demonstrates an unusual feature in *W. recta:* the outer cell membrane is covered by hexagonal subunits. The species can also be differentiated from the other *Wolinella* species on the basis of sensitivity to various dyes and antibiotics.

As previously mentioned, *W. recta* can be found in high numbers in subgingival dental plaque in patients with adult periodontitis. It is a predominant bacterial species in subgingival plaque from periodontitis patients with non-insulin-dependent diabetes mellitus (Zambon et al., 1988; Table 11-8). Of 392 bacterial isolates recovered from eight patients, *B. intermedius* was the most frequently isolated microorganism, constituting 16% of the total isolates, whereas *W. recta* and *B. gingivalis* each accounted for 13% of the total. It appears that an occasional periodontitis patient has high titers of serum antibody to *W. recta*, suggesting that this organism may be important in some patients as a cause of periodontal disease. Data such as these point to the importance of *W. recta* in the etiology of adult periodontitis.

Oral spirochetes

Human oral spirochetes are gram-negative, strict anaerobes, 5 to 20 μm long and 0.1 to 0.5 μm wide, with a cell morphology consisting of very flexible cytoplasmic cylinders surrounded by an outer sheath or envelope. Between the outer sheath and the cytoplasmic cylinder is a third cell structure unique to these microorganisms, known as the axial filament. The axial filament, also called axial fibrils, axial flagella, or periplasmic fibrils, originates at the subterminal ends of the cytoplasmic cylinders and is used in the classification of spirochetes. The light microscopic appearance of spirochetes can also be used to classify them as small, intermediate sized, or large. *Treponema denticola*, with two to three axial filaments, and *Treponema vincentii*, with four to six axial filaments, are prominent among the oral spirochetes. Spirochetes, unlike other microorganisms, do not form colonies on agar media but instead form "spirochetal haze" as they move through the agar when cultured by membrane-filter or agar-well techniques. These microorganisms are also sensitive to mechanical forces during sample dispersion or dilution and to atmospheric oxygen.

Several lines of evidence suggest the importance of spirochetes in the pathogenesis of periodontal disease. Spirochetes can be found in high numbers in subgingival plaque and exhibit an apparent affinity for host tissue. Electron microscopic studies reveal that the different bacteria in plaque are not randomly distributed but are in certain locations. Spirochetes are found in "superficial layers" of plaque near host tissues where they are actively motile, suggesting that oral spirochetes have a strong affinity for

host tissues such as gingiva. Spirochetes are also capable of invading host tissues, as in ANUG (Listgarten, 1965). This disease is characterized by four tissue zones extending from the surface to the depths of the lesions, including (1) a bacterial zone, which is the most superficial zone and which contains small, intermediate-sized, and large spirochetes; (2) a neutrophil-rich zone; (3) a zone of necrotic tissue with spirochetes and rod-shaped bacteria; and (4) a zone of spirochetal infiltration. Listgarten (1965) observed masses of "almost pure cultures" of intermediate-sized and large spirochetes between the intercellular spaces of the affected tissues.

Eikenella corrodens

E. corrodens is a gram-negative, facultatively anaerobic rod characterized by its ability to pit or corrode the agar surface on which it is growing. These corroding types of colonies may also translocate across an agar surface by means of "twitching" or "jerking" types of movements. This microorganism is often found in the human oral cavity, upper respiratory tract, and urogenital tract. It is considered to be an opportunistic pathogen, especially in immunocompromised patients, and has been found in extraoral lesions, including cervicofacial actinomycosis, and in brain abscesses secondary to dental infections. It is also found in elevated levels in subgingival plaque from young adults with advanced periodontitis lesions and from patients with juvenile periodontitis. Tanner et al. (1979) examined the former group and found two patients with advanced alveolar bone loss, severe gingival inflammation, and suppuration in whom the predominant subgingival microflora was made up of *E. corrodens, B. intermedius,* and a fusiform-shaped *Bacteroides* species that was later named *Bacteroides forsythus*.

Fusobacterium nucleatum

F. nucleatum is a gram-negative, obligately anaerobic bacillus frequently isolated from subgingival dental plaque in patients with adult periodontitis. The bacterial cells are long with tapered ends and often have intracellular granules. *F. nucleatum* represents a heterogenous group of microorganisms, many of which were formerly classified in other species. As such, *F. nucleatum* contains strains with considerable genetic and serologic diversity. Type II *F. nucleatum* is correlated with increased gingival inflammation (Vincent et al., 1985). In periodontitis, high numbers of *F. nucleatum* are often detectable in sites undergoing active periodontal destruction. However, since high numbers of *F. nucleatum* can also be found in inactive sites, the role of this species in periodontitis in not well defined.

Bacteroides forsythus

Formerly known as "fusiform" *Bacteroides, B. forsythus* is a gram-negative, nonmotile anaerobe that exhibits filament-shaped bacterial cells with tapered ends and that may have central swellings. *B. forsythus* was first isolated from the subgingival dental plaque of young adults with severe periodontitis (Tanner et al., 1979). The microorganism is often found together with *F. nucleatum* and appears in fact to utilize growth factors from this microorganism as part of its nutritional requirements. It is a slow-growing, fastidious microorganism that is difficult to culture. This microorganism is found in higher proportions in subgingival plaque from sites losing periodontal attachment as compared with sites having no loss of attachment (Dzink et al., 1988).

ROLE OF SPECIFIC MICROORGANISMS

Numerous studies over the past decade have pointed to two groups of microorganisms in the etiology of periodontal disease. The first group of pathogens probably account for the majority of cases. *A. actinomycetemcomitans* is associated with most cases of LJP (80% to 90%) and some cases of adult periodontitis. *B. gingivalis* is associated with most cases of adult periodontitis (80% to 90%), often together with *B. intermedius.*

The second group of organisms are associated with occasional cases of periodontal disease. This group includes *Wolinella, E. corrodens, F. nucleatum,* spirochetes, and *B. forsythus.* Other organisms are also likely to be found in association with occasional cases of periodontitis.

In cases treated with multiple courses of antibiotics, *Candida albicans, Escherichia coli, Pseudomonas,* and other organisms have been found in the subgingival flora. However, from a statistical point of view, most cases of adult periodontitis are associated with *B. gingivalis* and/or *B. intermedius,* and most cases of juvenile periodontitis are associated with *A. actinomycetemcomitans.*

TRANSMISSION OF PERIODONTAL PATHOGENS

As certain microorganisms have been implicated as periodontal pathogens, there has been increasing interest in the source and route of infection by these microorganisms. Currently there are two theories (Genco et al., 1988; Christersson et al., 1989). The first theory proposes that the periodontal pathogens are components of the indigenous or resident oral microflora and that they overgrow to become opportunistic pathogens causing periodontal diseases. According to this theory, dental plaque represents a microbial climax community that forms on the tooth surface and in the gingival sulcus. Development of a "mature" plaque culminates with the colonization and growth of putative pathogens. A second, alternative theory proposes that periodontal pathogens are not components of the indigenous oral microflora but, like many other medically important pathogenic microorganisms, are exogenous pathogens derived from outside sources. According to this exogenous theory, gross accumulations of dental plaque

are not in themselves sufficient to cause periodontitis. The patient must also become infected with specific periodontal pathogens that are transmitted from another source (Genco et al., 1988).

For several of the putative periodontal pathogens, there is recent evidence to support the exogenous theory. These studies have indicated that the great majority of people do not harbor putative periodontal pathogens in subgingival dental plaque. When examined by either bacterial culture or immunofluorescence microscopy, dental plaque from over 90% of healthy subjects did not demonstrate *A. actinomycetemcomitans* or *B. gingivalis,* or it harbored only trace amounts of these microorganisms, suggesting that they are not indigenous (Zambon et al., 1985; Zambon et al., 1986a).

If these microorganisms are not part of the normal flora, then they must be transmitted from other sources. Several studies have suggested that one likely source is through contact with other infected family members. For example, the source of *A. actinomycetemcomitans* in LJP patients, as well as pathogens in other periodontal diseases, has not been well studied. Some data suggest that the microorganisms involved in periodontal diseases are transmissible between patients and between sites within the same patient. It is known, for example, that much of the gastrointestinal microflora is derived from family members. Husbands and wives often harbor similar microorganisms, suggesting microbial transmission between close household contacts (Offenbacher et al., 1985). An intrafamilial route of transmission for *A. actinomycetemcomitans* has also been suggested by a study wherein it was found that family members of LJP patients all harbored the same biotype (biochemical group) and serotype (antigenic group) of *A. actinomycetemcomitans* (Zambon et al., 1983a). This may explain, in part, the familial tendency of this disease.

The low rate of *A. actinomycetemcomitans* infection among family members of LJP patients (approximately one third were infected) also suggests that *A. actinomycetemcomitans* is not easily transmissible, even among persons presumably in close daily contact. Christersson et al. (1985b) found that *A. actinomycetemcomitans* could be transferred from infected periodontal pockets to uninfected healthy sites by means of periodontal probes. However, *A. actinomycetemcomitans* inoculated into the healthy gingival sulci did not permanently colonize those sites but were eliminated within 3 weeks.

SUMMARY

Periodontal diseases are mainly caused by bacterial infections, and the causative organisms are located primarily in the gingival or periodontal pockets. The various forms of periodontal diseases, including gingivitis, ANUG, adult periodontitis, refractory periodontitis, periodontitis in diabetes, and LJP, are associated with different groups of subgingival organisms. Several subgingival organisms are common to adult forms of periodontitis, including *B. gingivalis* and *B. intermedius*. Juvenile forms of periodontitis are frequently associated with *A. actinomycetemcomitans*. These three organisms are pathogenic, possessing a host of virulence factors, and they can also evade host defenses, especially antibody-neutrophil–dependent responses. Other oral organisms often associated with periodontal lesions include *W. recta*, oral spirochetes, *E. corrodens*, *F. nucleatum*, and *B. forsythus*.

Based on our knowledge of the periodontal microflora and its causal role, prevention and treatment of periodontal diseases can be directed at these microorganisms. Antiinfective treatment directed toward reducing the mass of subgingival organisms and suppressing or eliminating the major specific pathogens such as *A. actinomycetemcomitans* and *B. gingivalis* is effective in resolving the inflammatory aspects of periodontal diseases. Preventive measures directed toward reducing the mass of supragingival plaques at the gingival margin are also effective. The future management of periodontal infections will most likely involve the elimination or suppression of specific pathogens in a long-lasting fashion.

REFERENCES

Bass CC and Johns IM: Alveolodental pyorrhea, Philadelphia, 1915, WB Saunders Co.

Bonta Y et al: Rapid identification of periodontal pathogens in subgingival dental plaque: comparison of indirect immunofluorescence microscopy with bacterial culture for detection of *Actinobacillus actinomycetemcomitans*, J Dent Res 64:793, 1985.

Chang KM et al: Infection with a gram-negative organism stimulates gingival collagenase production in non-diabetic and diabetic germfree rats, J Periodont Res 23:239, 1988.

Christersson LA et al: Microbiological and clinical effects of surgical treatment of localized juvenile periodontitis, J Clin Periodontol 12:465, 1985a.

Christersson LA et al: Transmission and colonization of *Actinobacillus actinomycetemcomitans* in localized juvenile periodontitis patients, J Periodontol 56:127, 1985b.

Christersson LA et al: Tissue localization of *Actinobacillus actinomycetemcomitans* in human periodontitis. I. Light, immunofluorescence and electron microscopic studies, J Periodontol 58:529, 1987a.

Christersson LA et al: Tissue localization of *Actinobacillus actinomycetemcomitans* in human periodontitis. II. Correlation between immunofluorescence and culture techniques, J Periodontol 58:540, 1987b.

Christersson LA et al: Specific subgingival bacteria and diagnosis of gingivitis and periodontitis, Adv Dent Res, 1989 (in press).

Coykendall AL, Kaczmarek FS, and Slots J: Genetic heterogeneity in *Bacteroides asaccharolyticus* (Holdeman and Moore, 1970; Finegold and Barnes, 1977; approved lists, 1980) and proposal of *Bacteroides gingivalis* sp. nov. and *Bacteroides macacae* (Slots and Genco) comb. nov., Int J System Bacteriol 30:559, 1980.

Dzink JL, Socransky SS, and Haffajee AD: The predominant cultivable microbiota of active and inactive periodontal lesions, J Clin Periodontol 15:316, 1988.

Eisenmann AC et al: Microbiological study of localized juvenile periodontitis in Panama, J Periodontol 54:712, 1983.

Genco RJ, Zambon JJ, and Christersson LA: The origin of periodontal infections, Adv Dent Res 2:364, 1988.

Genco RJ, Zambon, JJ, and Murray PA: Serum and gingival fluid anti-

bodies as adjuncts in the diagnosis of *Actinobacillus actinomycetemcomitans*–associated periodontal disease, J Periodontol 56:41, 1985.

Holdeman LV and Johnson JL: Description of *Bacteroides loescheii* sp. nov. and emendation of the descriptions of *Bacteroides melaninogenicus* (Oliver and Wherry; Roy and Kelly 1939) and *Bacteroides denticola* (Shah and Collins), Int J System Bacteriol 32:399, 1981.

Holt SC, Tanner AC, and Socransky SS: Morphology and ultrastructure of oral strains of *Actinobacillus actinomycetemcomitans* and *Haemophilus aphrophilus*, Infect Immun 30:588, 1980.

Holt SC et al: Implantation of *Bacteroides gingivalis* in nonhuman primates initiates progression of periodontitis, Science 239:55, 1988.

Iino Y and Hopps RM: The bone-resorbing activities in tissue culture of lipopolysaccharides from the bacteria *Actinobacillus actinomycetemcomitans*, *Bacteroides gingivalis* and *Capnocytophaga ochracea* isolated from human mouths, Arch Oral Biol 29:59, 1984.

Johnson JL and Holdeman LV: *Bacteroides intermedius* comb. nov. and descriptions of *Bacteroides corporis* and *Bacteroides levii* sp. nov., Int J System Bacteriol 33:15, 1983.

Kastelein P et al: An experimentally induced phlegmonous abscess by a strain of *Bacteroides gingivalis* in guinea pigs and mice, Antonie van Leeuwenhoek 47:1, 1981.

Klinger R: Untersuchungen uber menschliche Aktinomykase, Centralblat Bakteriol 62:191, 1912.

Listgarten MA: Electron microscopic observations on the bacterial flora of acute necrotizing ulcerative gingivitis, J Periodontol 36:328, 1965.

Löe H, Theilade E, and Jensen SB: Experimental gingivitis in man, J Periodontol 36:177, 1965.

Loesche WJ: Chemotherapy of dental plaque infections, Oral Sci Rev 9:63, 1976.

Mandell RL and Socransky SS: A selective medium for *Actinobacillus actinomycetemcomitans* and the incidence of the organism in juvenile periodontitis, J Periodontol 52:593, 1981.

Miller WD: The microorganisms of the human mouth, Basel, Switzerland, 1973, S Karger.

Moore WEC et al: Bacteriology of moderate (chronic) periodontitis in mature adult humans, Infect Immun 42:510, 1983.

Nakazawa F et al: Serological studies of oral *Bacteroides intermedius*, Infect Immun 56:1647, 1988.

Newman MG and Socransky SS: Predominant cultivable microflora in periodontosis, J Periodont Res 12:120, 1977.

Offenbacher S, Olsvik B, and Tonder A: The similarity of periodontal microorganisms between husband and wife cohabitants: association or transmission, J Periodontol 56:317, 1985.

Oliver WW and Wherry WB: Notes on some bacterial parasites of the human mucous membranes, J Infect Dis 28:341, 1921.

Pierce CS et al: Endocarditis due to *Actinobacillus actinomycetemcomitans* serotype c and patient immune response, J Infect Dis 149:479, 1984.

Preus HR, Olsen I, and Namork E: Association between bacteriophage-infected *Actinobacillus actinomycetemcomitans* and rapid periodontal destruction, J Clin Periodontol 14:245, 1987.

Rosling B, Nyman S, and Lindhe J: The effect of systematic plaque control on bone regeneration in infrabony pockets, J Clin Periodontol 3:38, 1976.

Sandholm L, Tolo K, and Olsen I: Salivary IgG, a parameter of periodontal disease activity? J Clin Periodontol 14:289, 1987.

Scannapieco F et al: Effect of anaerobiosis on the surface ultrastructure and surface proteins of *Actinobacillus actinomycetemcomitans*, Infect Immun 55:2320, 1987.

Slots J: The predominant cultivable organisms in juvenile periodontitis, Scand J Dent Res 84:1, 1976.

Slots J and Genco RJ: Black-pigmented *Bacteroides* species, *Capnocytophaga* species, and *Actinobacillus actinomycetemcomitans* in human periodontal disease: virulence factors in colonization, survival, and tissue destruction, J Dent Res 63:412, 1984.

Slots J, Reynolds HS, and Genco RJ: *Actinobacillus actinomycetemcomitans* in human periodontal disease: a cross-sectional microbiological investigation, Infect Immun 29:1013, 1980.

Slots J and Rosling BG: Suppression of the periodontopathic microflora in localized juvenile periodontitis by systemic tetracycline, J Clin Periodontol 10:465, 1983.

Socransky SS: Microbiology of periodontal disease—present status and future considerations, J Periodontol 48:497, 1977.

Socransky SS: Criteria for infectious agents in dental caries and periodontal disease, J Clin Periodontol 6:16, 1979.

Tanner ACR et al: A study of the bacteria associated with advancing periodontitis in man, J Clin Periodontol 6:278, 1979.

Tsai CC, McArthur WP, and Baehni PC: Extraction and partial characterization of a leukotoxin from a plaque-derived gram-negative microorganism, Infect Immun 24:427, 1979.

Tsai CC and Taichman N: Dynamics of infection by leukotoxic strains of *Actinobacillus actinomycetemcomitans* in juvenile periodontitis, J Clin Periodontol 13:330, 1986.

van Leeuwenhoek A: Opera omnia sive alcana naturae ope microscopiorum exactissimorum detecta, 1772. In Collected letters in eight volumes, Amsterdam, 1941, Swets en Zeitlinger.

van Winkelhoff AJ: Black-pigmented *Bacteroides* in human oral infections, thesis, Amsterdam, 1986, Free University Press.

Vincent JW et al: Biologic activity of type I and type II *Fusobacterium nucleatum* isolates from clinically characterized sites, J Periodontol 56:334, 1985.

Zambon JJ: *Actinobacillus actinomycetemcomitans* in human periodontal disease, J Clin Periodontol 12:1, 1985.

Zambon JJ, Bochacki V, and Genco RJ: Immunological assays for putative periodontal pathogens, Oral Microbiol Immunol 1:39, 1986a.

Zambon JJ, Christersson LA, and Genco RJ: Diagnosis and treatment of localized juvenile periodontitis (periodontosis), J Am Dent Assoc 113:295, 1986b.

Zambon JJ, Christersson LA, and Slots J: *Actinobacillus actinomycetemcomitans* in human periodontal disease: prevalence in patient groups and distribution of biotypes and serotypes within families, J Periodontol 54:707, 1983a.

Zambon JJ, Slots J, and Genco RJ: Serology of oral *Actinobacillus actinomycetemcomitans* and serotype distribution in human periodontal disease, Infect Immun 41:19, 1983b.

Zambon JJ et al: Purification and characterization of the serotype c antigen from *Actinobacillus actinomycetemcomitans,* Infect Immun 44:22, 1983c.

Zambon JJ et al: Studies of leukotoxin from *Actinobacillus actinomycetemcomitans* using the promyelocytic HL-60 cell line, Infect Immun 40:205, 1983d.

Zambon JJ et al: Rapid identification of periodontal pathogens in subgingival dental plaque: comparison of indirect immunofluorescence microscopy with bacterial culture for detection of *Bacteroides gingivalis,* J Periodontol 56(suppl):32, 1985.

Zambon JJ et al: Microbiological and immunological studies of adult periodontitis in patients with noninsulin-dependent diabetes mellitus, J Periodontol 59(1):23, 1988.

Chapter 12

SENSITIVITY OF PERIODONTAL ORGANISMS TO ANTIBIOTICS AND OTHER ANTIMICROBIAL AGENTS

Benjamin F. Hammond
Robert J. Genco

Bacteria are essential in the etiology of human periodontal disease; hence the use of antibiotics and antimicrobial agents as adjuncts in the therapy and prevention of periodontal disease is both logical and predictable. Moreover, the use of microbiologic culturing data in identifying suspected periodontopathic bacteria in the subgingival plaques of patients has been of great value in diagnosing periodontal disease and monitoring various therapeutic modalities. An important aspect in antiinfective therapy for periodontal disease is the determination of in vitro antibiotic sensitivities of the pathogenic periodontal flora, which allows a rational and experimentally sound basis for various therapeutic modalities to be established. It is clear that antibiotic therapy is not always indicated in routine therapy, but when it is, knowledge of the antimicrobial sensitivity of the periodontal flora is necessary. When microbiologic data are required and when antibiotic therapy is indicated (see Chapters 27, 35, 39, and 40), it is important to understand the principles, applications, and limitations of antibiotic sensitivity testing for periodontal bacteria. This chapter highlights some of the recent advances and guidelines associated with the use of antibiotic sensitivity testing and the in vitro susceptibility of periodontal microorganisms to antibiotics and other antimicrobial agents used to manage periodontal disease.

ANTIBIOTIC SENSITIVITY TESTING
General considerations of the periodontal microflora

The microbial etiology of the various periodontal diseases is dealt with in Chapter 11. Recent publications indicate that no single agent is responsible for all forms of the disease; however, a few organisms are most likely associated with most cases of periodontitis. Microbial sensitivity testing is useful in establishing the antibiotic susceptibility patterns of the common members of the pathogenic periodontal microbiota and is also useful in those cases where unusual organisms are encountered after unsuccessful antimicrobial therapy or in those cases where the common pathogens are not found.

Procedures for taking microbiologic samples for susceptibility testing

Visible supragingival plaque is carefully removed with a dental scaler or cotton pellet; bacterial samples of subgingival plaque can then be sampled. Three fine paper points are placed into the disease site (periodontal pocket) for 10 seconds, after which they are immediately placed into a tube containing 0.5 ml of prereduced dispersion medium (Moeller, 1966) and vortexed for 30 seconds. The subgingival plaque suspension is then sent to the laboratory for culture within 24 hours. In the laboratory, dilutions of the sample are plated on selective media and incubated anaerobically, aerobically, and in an atmosphere containing carbon dioxide. After growth has occurred, isolated colonies representing the putative pathogens and other predominant organisms are Gram stained and subcultured for subsequent antibiotic sensitivity testing.

Lawns of pure cultures of periodontal isolates are then seeded onto standard Mueller-Hinton (Difco) plates, again with a cotton swab of log-phase broth culture. In some instances the Mueller-Hinton medium is replaced with a different enrichment agar to allow for luxuriant growth of the test organism *(Eubacterium limosum),* or the Mueller-Hinton medium is enriched with additional yeast extract, 1% blood, or defibrinated blood (5%). Discs containing the different antibiotics are applied to the agar surfaces.

After appropriate incubation (16 to 18 hours for most organisms and 5 to 10 days for *Bacteroides* spp.) the zones of complete inhibition are recorded. The zone diameters for individual antibiotics are interpreted using standards. Fig. 12-1 shows a typical sample of a periodontal isolate being checked for sensitivity to various antibiotics.

Alternatively, the in vitro sensitivities of periodontal bacteria can be determined by the *agar dilution technique* (Walker et al., 1979a, 1979b) in which the *minimal inhibitory concentrations (MICs)* for each antibiotic are obtained. The MIC is defined as the lowest concentration of the antibiotic that results in no growth. Plates containing various concentrations of antibiotics are prepared, and the pure culture isolates (originally obtained from the clinical sample) are inoculated onto the agar surface. After incubation the minimum concentration of antibiotic that suppresses growth is recorded and reported as the MIC, usually in micrograms per milliliter. This value can then be compared with the concentration of antibiotic achieved in blood or in the gingival fluid under usual dosage conditions (the serum or gingival fluid "break point").

Antibiotic sensitivity testing is a valuable guide in choosing an antimicrobial agent. However, it may not be necessary to test for antimicrobial susceptibility when the

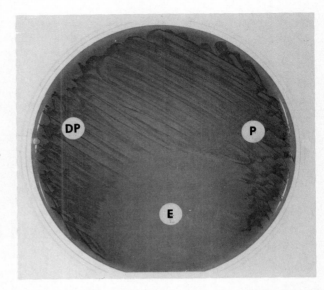

Fig. 12-1. Antibiotic sensitivity of a patient with *Bacteroides intermedius* with discs impregnated with erythromycin *(E),* methicillin *(DP),* and penicillin *(P).* Note inhibition of growth (clear zone) surrounding erythromycin disc.

known or suspected pathogens have well-established antibiotic sensitivity patterns. These patterns are presented in Table 12-1 for several of the pathogenic periodontal microorganisms. For example, the common pathogenic periodontal organisms *Actinobacillus actinomycetemcomitans* and *Bacteroides gingivalis* are susceptible to several antibiotics, including tetracycline and minocycline, which might be considered for use in cases where these organisms are identified or suspected. However, antibiotic susceptibility testing to the tetracyclines may not be necessary, since *A. actinomycetemcomitans* and *B. gingivalis* have not as yet been shown to be tetracycline resistant. *Bacteroides intermedius* is susceptible to the penicillins, clindamycin, and metronidazole, whereas some strains of *B. intermedius* are resistant to tetracycline. If tetracycline were chosen for therapy, antibiotic susceptibility testing of *B. intermedius* would be useful; however, if a penicillin, clindamycin, or metronidazole were chosen, antibiotic susceptibility testing might not be necessary. Culture and antibiotic susceptibility testing is often necessary for refractory cases treated with multiple courses of antibiotics in which unusual periodontal organisms such as *Staphylococcus aureus,* enterococci, pseudomonads, and yeasts are often found.

Limitations of in vitro antimicrobial susceptibility tests

Although in vitro susceptibility of an organism is well below the level usually achieved in the blood, the organism may not be exposed to these concentrations in the periodontal lesion for the following reasons: (1) the antibiotic may be destroyed or inactivated in the diseased site (e.g., beta-lactamase is inactivated by penicillin); (2) the

Table 12-1. In vitro antibiotic susceptibility of cultured strains of periodontal bacteria

Antibiotic	Actinobacillus actinomycetemcomitans	Bacteriodes intermedius	Bacteriodes gingivalis	Other Bacteroides	Capnocytophaga species	Eikenella corrodens	Eubacterium species	Fusobacterium nucleatum	Selenomonas sputigena	Peptostreptococcus species	Wolinella recta
Penicillins											
Benzylpenicillin	S,I	S	S	S	S	R		S	R	S	S
Ampicillin	S	S	S	S	S	R		S	R	S	S
Amoxicillin	S	S	S	S	S	S,R	S	S	R		S
Carbenicillin disodium	R	S	S	S	R	S,R		S	S		
Aminoglycosides											
Kanamycin	R	R	R		R	R		R			
Neomycin	R	R	R		R	R		R			
Streptomycin	R	R	R		R	R		R			
Tetracyclines											
Tetracycline	S	S,R	S	S	S	S	S	S	S,R	S,R	S
Chlortetracycline	I	I	I		S	I		S			
Oxytetracycline	I	I	I		S	I		I			
Doxycycline	I	S	S		S	I		S			
Minocycline	S	S	S	S	S	S		S	S,R	S,R	S
Macrolides and others											
Clindamycin	R	S	S	S	S	R	S	S	S	S	S
Erythromycin	R	S,R	S	S,R	S	R		R	R	R	S
Spiramycin	R	S	S		S	R		R			
Chloramphenicol	S	R	R		R	R		R			
Vancomycin	R	I	R		S	R		R			
Metronidazole	S,R	S	S	S	S,R	R		S	S		S

Data from Baker et al. (1985); Baker et al. (1983); Walker et al. (1981); and Mashimo et al. (1981).

S stands for susceptible (or sensitive) and implies that an infection with the species tested may be expected to respond to the usual dosage recommended for that antibiotic (i.e., the minimum inhibitory concentration for all strains tested is well below the concentration of antibiotic achieved—"break point"). R, or resistant, refers to species not completely inhibited within the usual therapeutic range. I, or intermediate, describes species for which a majority of strains are resistant to the usual levels of antibiotic achieved, but the strains may respond to higher levels achieved by increased doses or different routes of administration.

antibiotic may not reach the site in high enough concentration; or (3) patient compliance may be poor, especially when the antibiotic causes uncomfortable side effects such as the vertigo caused by systemic minocycline.

In vitro antimicrobial sensitivity testing may not always predict clinical outcome in a disease with a complex flora such as periodontal disease. For example, if a pathogen is resistant to an antibiotic in vitro, it may well be suppressed as a result of use of the antibiotic in therapy if the antibiotic suppresses other organisms in the plaque that produce substances required by the pathogen. For example, *B. gingivalis* requires vitamin K, and diptheroids in plaque may furnish this vitamin. If these diptheroids were suppressed by the antibiotic, then *B. gingivalis* might also be suppressed.

GUIDELINES FOR ANTIBIOTIC USE
Penicillin

Penicillin (benzylpenicillin, penicillin G) is a beta-lactam bactericidal compound that acts by inhibiting cell wall synthesis of sensitive organisms. It is one of the least toxic of all antibiotics and probably the most widely used antibiotic in all medicine. Patient hypersensitivity is the most serious problem with this drug and other penicillins (methicillin, oxacillin, carbenicillin, ampicillin/amoxicillin) and is known to occur in approximately 15% of adults who have allergenic tendencies, as well as in 5% of nonallergic adults. Most periodontal bacteria tested are sensitive to penicillin, and it is the most active antibiotic in suppressing the total subgingival flora, with 1 μg/ml suppressing 99.9% of the cultivable subgingival flora from

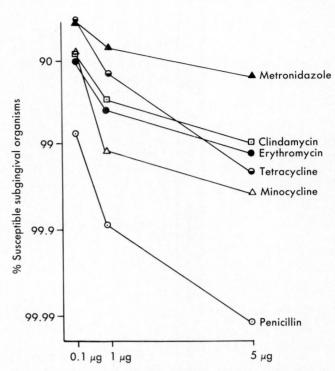

Fig. 12-2. Subgingival plaque samples from nine patients with adult periodontitis and two LJP patients were cultured anaerobically on blood agar plates, and geometric mean percent of organisms susceptible calculated from difference in numbers of colonies with and without antibiotics. (Modified from Mashimo PA et al: Pharmacol Ther Dent 6:45, 1981.)

Table 12-2. Periodontal pocket organisms that are resistant to low levels of antibiotics in vitro

Benzylpenicillin (1 μg/ml)	Minocycline (1 μg/ml)	Tetracycline (1 μg/ml)
"Anaerobic vibrios"	*Streptococcus sanguis*	*Streptococcus sanguis*
Veillonella parvula	*Streptococcus mitis*	*Veillonella parvula*
Actinobacillus actinomycetemcomitans	*Veillonella parvula*	*Streptococcus mitis*
Bacteroides fragilis	*Actinomyces viscosus*	"Anaerobic vibrios"
Staphylococcus spp.	"Anaerobic vibrios"	*Actinomyces naeslundii*
	Peptococcus magnus	
Proteus spp.	*Actinomyces naeslundii*	
Actinomyces naeslundii		*Propionibacterium* spp.
Gram-negative rod		*Actinomyces viscosus*
Streptococcus sanguis	*Streptococcus milleri*	*Peptococcus magnus*
Arachnia propionica	Gram-negative rod	Gram-negative rod
Bacteroides corrodens	*Saccharomyces cerevisiae*	*Leptotrichia buccalis*
Streptococcus milleri	*Streptococcus salivarius*	*Fusobacterium nucleatum*
Propionibacterium spp.		*Arachnia propionica*
Actinomyces viscosus		*Bacteroides corrodens*
Fusobacterium nucleatum		

Modified from Mashimo PA et al.: Pharmacol Ther Dent 6:45, 1981.

Organisms are listed in order from most prevalent among the total resistant to 1 μg/ml of each antibiotic at the top of the column to least prevalent at the bottom. Organisms listed above the line represent 5% or more of the total number of subgingival bacteria resistant to 1 μg/ml of antibiotic. Those below the line each represent less than 5% of the total resistant organisms.

periodontitis patients (Fig. 12-2). However, major resistance was noted in strains of *Eikenella corrodens* and *Selenomonas sputigena* (Table 12-1). Some strains of *Peptostreptococcus*, *Fusobacterium* species, and *A. actinomycetemcomitans* are also insensitive to penicillin. Slots et al. (1980) reported that approximately 50% of strains of *A. actinomycetemcomitans* obtained from human periodontitis patients were resistant to ampicillin G at 4 μg/ml, and *A. actinomycetemcomitans* strains are among the most common penicillin-resistant strains seen in the subgingival flora from periodontitis patients (Table 12-2). Some strains of *A. actinomycetemcomitans* are also resistant to methicillin. Amoxicillin has a greater inhibitory effect than either penicillin or ampicillin on bacterial isolates from periodontal lesions. van Osten et al (1986) showed that a single course of systemically administered amoxicillin markedly changed the composition of the subgingival microflora.

Studies on the production of *beta-lactamases* by oral bacteria were performed by Valdes et al. (1982), and these studies indicated that oral organisms positive for beta-lactamase (penicillinase) production were members of the genus *Bacteroides* (the *B. melaninogenicus*/*B. oralis* subgroup) and one species of *Veillonella parvula*.

It is not clear that in vitro data necessarily reflect the in vivo antimicrobial activity of the penicillins. For example, amoxicillin is sensitive to beta-lactamases produced by other periodontal bacteria (see above), and it is possible that some of the clinical failures associated with the adjunctive use of amoxicillin in periodontal therapy result from beta-lactamase production by subgingival flora. Amoxicillin combined with clavulanic acid, an inhibitor of beta-lactamase, may overcome in vivo resistance to amoxicillin (Yogev et al., 1981). Also, the concentrations of each of these antibiotics in the gingival crevice are likely to be different. Layton et al. (1983) showed that amoxicillin penetrates well into the crevicular fluid and has a significantly higher serum level than other penicillins. Amoxicillin and amoxicillin-clavulanic acid combinations hold promise as useful adjuncts in the antiinfective phase of periodontal therapy.

Tetracyclines

The tetracyclines are probably the most commonly used antibiotics for the adjunctive treatment of periodontitis. Tetracyclines are broad-spectrum antibiotics that inhibit protein synthesis at the level of binding of transfer–RNA–acid complexes to the ribosomes. They inhibit protein synthesis in bacteria and to a much lesser extent in eukaryotic cells. Included in the group are oxytetracycline, chlortetracycline, dimethylchlortetracycline, doxycycline, and minocycline. The last two (doxycycline and minocycline) are semisynthetics, and they are more completely absorbed from the intestine and are consequently less inhibitory to the normal gut flora. Doxycycline and minocycline, because of their lipophilic nature, are not easily deposited in

calcified tissue. The *tetracyclines are not recommended for children 9 years of age or under,* because they deposit in forming calcified tissues and interfere with development of these tissues.

Several reports have described the clinical efficacy of the tetracyclines in the treatment of periodontal disease (Ciancio, 1976; Slots and Rosling, 1983). Although there are some differences of opinion about the benefits of tetracycline therapy (see Listgarten et al., 1978; Slots et al., 1979) most studies show a beneficial effect of systemic tetracyclines beyond that achieved with scaling and root planing or surgery alone, especially in localized juvenile periodontitis (LJP) (Zambon et al., 1986; Mandell and Socransky, 1988).

Some of the reasons for the efficacy of tetracycline in periodontitis reside in its unique properties. First, most species of potential pathogenic periodontal bacteria are clearly inhibited in vitro by concentrations of tetracycline equivalent to or lower than those known to occur in the crevicular fluid at tetracycline dosages of 1 g/day (i.e., 4 to 8 μg/ml in crevicular fluid) (Fig. 12-2). Some of the organisms known to be susceptible to tetracycline are listed in Tables 12-2 and 12-3. It is indeed impressive that such

Table 12-3. Tetracycline sensitivity of crevicular bacteria

Bacteria	No. of strains	Cumulative % susceptible to concentration	
		4 μg/ml	8 μg/ml
Actinomyces israelii	13	92	92
Actinomyces odontolyticus	4	100	100
Actinomyces viscosus	12	100	100
Actinobacillus actinomycetemocomitans	24	79	
Bacteroides gingivalis	15	100	100
Bacteroides melaninogenicus	32	94	
Bacteroides gracilis	14	100	
Other *Bacteroides*	10	90	90
Campylobacter concisus	8	100	
Campylobacter species	30	100	
Eikenella corrodens	17	88	88
Eubacterium species	6	100	
Fusobacterium nucleatum	40	95	100
Other *Fusobacterium*	18	100	
Selenomonas sputigena	9	78	89
Streptococci	37	46	49
Peptostreptococci	15	87	87
Propionibacterium	4	100	
Wolinella recta	18	100	

Modified from Walker CB et al.: J Periodontol 52:613, 1981.

a broad range of periodontal organisms is sensitive to this concentration of antibiotic, including both gram-positive organisms *(Actinomyces, Peptostreptococci, Propionibacteria, Eubacteria,* and *Lactobacilli)* and essentially all of the organisms associated with periodontal disease *(A. actinomycetemcomitans, B. gingivalis, Eikenella corrodens,* and *Wolinella recta).* An exception is *B. intermedius,* where a few strains are resistant to the tetracyclines.

Second, tetracyclines concentrate in the gingival fluid. For example, a single oral dose of tetracycline or minocycline results in crevicular fluid concentrations that are 2 to 10 times higher than blood levels (Ciancio et al., 1982).

Third, it has recently been proposed that tetracycline has unique efficacy in juvenile periodontitis (Zambon et al., 1986). A likely explanation for the efficacy of tetracycline in the treatment of juvenile periodontitis comes from the finding that viable *A. actinomycetemcomitans* cells persist deep in the connective tissue in the gingiva of patients with LJP and hence are accessible to the systemic effects of tetracycline (Christersson et al., 1987).

Fourth, tetracyclines inhibit tissue and bacterial collagenases (Golub et al., 1984), an activity that seems to help healing during tetracycline therapy.

Tetracycline resistance. Resistance to both tetracycline and minocycline (>4 μg/ml) has been reported for a variety of oral bacteria; however, most of the resistant organisms appear *not* to be among the pathogenic periodontal flora. Approximately 50% of plaque streptococci such as *Streptococcus sanguis* are resistant to these concentrations, but only 5% to 15% of other species and genera are resistant to tetracycline at concentrations achievable in the crevicular fluid (Table 12-3). At 1 μg/ml the most common tetracycline-resistant cultivable pocket organisms are *S. sanguis, V. parvula, Streptococcus mitis,* "anaerobic vibrios," and *Actinomyces naeslundii* (Table 12-2).

There is greater resistance to chlortetracycline and oxytetracycline as compared with tetracycline or minocycline. From Table 12-1 it can be seen that *A. actinomycetemcomitans, B. intermedius, B. gingivalis,* and *E. corrodens* are of intermediate resistance to either chlortetracycline or oxytetracycline. Deoxycycline is somewhat more active against the periodontal microbiota; however, *A. actinomycetemcomitans and E. corrodens* show intermediate sensitivity to this tetracycline analogue.

In general, minocycline is the most active of the tetracyclines, followed closely by tetracycline.

Clindamycin

Clindamycin is the chloroderivative of lincomycin, and its bacteriostasis, antibacterial range, and clinical efficacy have made it a suitable substitute for penicillin in allergic individuals. Clindamycin blocks protein synthesis by binding to 50S bacterial ribosomes and interfering with peptidyl transfer.

Because of the importance of anaerobes in periodontitis, clindamycin has potential as a chemotherapeutic agent in periodontal disease. One of the early problems with the administration of the lincomycin/clindamycin antibiotics was the antibiotic-associated pseudomembranous ulcerative colitis. It is now clear that the colitis was the result of an overgrowth of toxin-producing *Clostridium difficile* following systemic administration of antibiotics. Proper precautions, including monitoring of the patient for gastrointestinal symptoms, especially watery diarrhea, may help reduce this sometimes fatal side effect of clindamycin. It is clear that pseudomembranous ulcerative colitis may occur after systemic use of a wide range of antibiotics; hence close monitoring of all patients receiving antibiotics for this serious side effect is necessary.

Spectrum of clindamycin and use in periodontal therapy. Clindamycin has been shown to be effective against a wide range of periodontal bacteria at concentrations easily obtainable in gingival crevicular fluid and blood. The minimal inhibitory concentration of this antibiotic is <2 μg/ml for practically all of the gram-negative bacteria, particularly strains of *Bacteroides* (pigmented and nonpigmented), *Wolinella recta, Fusobacterium* spp., and *Selenomonas* (Baker et al., 1983; Walker et al., 1983). However, almost all strains of *E. corrodens* and about two thirds of the *A. actinomycetemcomitans* strains are resistant to clindamycin at these concentrations (see Table 12-1).

Erythromycin

Erythromycin is a macrolide antibiotic that interferes with protein synthesis at the 50S ribosome site in both gram-positive and gram-negative bacteria. It is commonly used as a substitute for penicillin. Its effectiveness as an antibiotic in periodontal therapy has been evaluated by several investigators, and generally it has been demonstrated to be less effective than most of the other commonly used antibiotics. Mills et al. (1979) showed that it was considerably less effective than spiramycin in reducing the clinical signs of periodontitis, although both antibiotics possess a similar chemical structure and have a similar mechanism of action and antibacterial spectrum.

Resistance to erythromycin (MICs > 2 μg/ml) is the most widespread of antibiotics tested to date against bacterial isolates from periodontal lesions (see Table 12-1). Almost all strains of *E. corrodens, A. actinomycetemcomitans,* and *Fusobacterium* are highly resistant to this antibiotic, and 75% of *S. sputigena* and 25% of *Bacteroides* strains are resistant to 2 μg/ml of erythromycin. This level is equivalent to those achievable in body fluids with oral dosages. It has been concluded that although erythromycin is often used in the treatment of oral infections, it does not appear to be a good choice as an adjunct in the control of periodontal microorganisms (Baker et al., 1983; Walker et al., 1983).

Metronidazole

Metronidazole (Flagyl) is a nitroimidazole that is specifically active against anaerobic organisms, including the spirochetes. It was originally used in trichomoniasis *(Trichomonas vaginalis)* and amebiasis *(Endamoeba histolytica),* but it also has a marked effect against anaerobic bacteria. It was shown to be effective in the treatment of acute necrotizing ulcerative gingivitis (ANUG) (Shinn, 1962) and in the treatment of periodontitis (Loesche et al., 1981). A 1-week course of therapy with this antibiotic significantly reduced the proportions of *B. asaccharolyticus (B. gingivalis)* and spirochetes in adult periodontitis lesions and resulted in an improvement in the clinical parameters when coupled with complete root debridement.

Resistance to metronidazole has been noted. From Table 12-1 it can be seen that this antibiotic is inhibitory against the strictly anaerobic organisms such as *Bacteroides, Fusobacterium, S. sputigena, Peptostreptococcus,* and *W. recta.* However, there is widespread resistance to metronidazole among capnophilic and facultative bacteria, including *Actinomyces, A. actinomycetemcomitans, Capnocytophaga, E. corrodens,* and *Streptococcus* (Baker et al., 1983; Walker et al., 1983). Table 12-3 illustrates that the upper range of metronidazole MICs is 128 µg/ml for the *Actinomyces* and greater than 19 µg/ml for *Capnocytophaga* spp. Also from Table 12-3 it can be seen that over 20% of *A. actinomycetemcomitans* strains are resistant to 4 µg/ml of metronidazole. In general, the activity of this antibiotic apparently decreases as the degree of aerotolerance increases.

Combinations of metronidazole and spiramycin, or metronidazole and penicillin, or metronidazole and amoxicillin show promise in the treatment of periodontal infections (see Chapter 35).

Aminoglycosides

From Table 12-1 it can be seen that the pathogenic periodontal flora is relatively resistant to kanamycin, neomycin, and streptomycin; hence there is presently little interest in these antibiotics to treat common forms of periodontal infections.

Other antibiotics that may have use in periodontal therapy include ampicillin, cefoxitin, ciprofloxacin, and a combination of trimethoprim-sulfamethoxazole. These are used where indicated by culture and antibiotic sensitivity testing, especially of previously treated refractory patients.

TOPICAL USE OF ANTIMICROBIAL AGENTS

Topical use of antimicrobial agents with low toxicity in a broad antimicrobial spectrum may be important in enhancing the effects of mechanical subgingival debridement (Rosling et al., 1983, 1986). By applying antimicrobial agents such as povidone-iodine into periodontal pockets at the time of debridement, a relatively low total dose can be administered while high concentrations are achieved at the site of infection. However, effective delivery of the chemotherapeutic agent into the subgingival periodontal lesion is difficult unless it is carried out with the patient under local anesthesia at the time of surgery or time of definitive scaling and root planing. The efficacy of irrigation using different types of antimicrobial agents has been tested; some show promise, especially povidone-iodine administered throughout the subgingival debridement procedure (Rosling et al., 1986). Simple flushing of periodontal pockets with topical antimicrobial agents such as H_2O_2, chlorhexidine, and fluorides has not been shown to be more effective than scaling and root planing alone. Most likely this is because the time and thoroughness of application to the subgingival area is limited when simple short-term irrigation without access is attempted.

The resistance of the periodontal microflora to germicidal antimicrobial agents has also been evaluated, and these agents are reviewed below.

Iodine

Casimir Devains first recognized the germicidal action of iodine in 1873, and since then it has been used in various vehicles for disinfection of skin and mucous membranes. Iodine is remarkable for its strong antimicrobial action on different species of microorganisms. It is effective against gram-negative as well as gram-positive bacteria, and it acts as a fungicide and virucide and also shows sporocidal effects (Higgins et al., 1964). It appears, then, that iodine is a highly effective antimicrobial agent. The organic iodine derivatives such as povidone-iodine have overcome many of the side effects, markedly reducing sensitization and irritation of mucous membranes and skin. Rosling et al. (1986) have reported on the usefulness of 1% povidone-iodine irrigation as an adjunct to mechanical subgingival debridement with the patient under local anesthesia in the treatment of adult periodontitis. Under these conditions, adjunctive use of iodine irrigation resulted in a 50% increase in attachment gain in deep pockets over that achieved with mechanical therapy alone.

Chlorhexidine and supragingival plaque control

Chlorhexidine (Hibitane) is clearly the front-runner and "bench mark" against which most of the other topical supragingival antiplaque agents have been compared. Chemically, it is a cationic *bis*-biguanide usually marketed as a gluconate salt. For example, a commercially available oral rinse contains 0.12% chlorhexidine gluconate in a base containing water, 11.6% alcohol, glycerine, flavoring agents, and saccharin. Chlorhexidine at concentrations of 0.1% to 2% has well-established supragingival plaque-inhibiting properties. Approximately 30% of the active ingredient is retained in the oral cavity after rinsing and is slowly released into the oral fluids.

The bactericidal nature of chlorhexidine at concentrations of 100 µg/ml is due, in part, to its ability to orient itself in the lipid portion of the cytoplasmic membrane so as to alter membrane permeability and allow leakage of intracellular components. However, the critical feature of its bactericidal nature is its ability to bind to proteins via carboxyl groups and other intracellular molecules, with similarly charged groups (phosphate) inactivating the associated biologic functions. This mechanism would be expected to affect most types of bacteria in varying degrees (see Kornman, 1986, for a review).

Gram-positive bacteria are inhibited by chlorhexidine and several of its analogues at concentrations at or below the 10 μg/ml level, although there are differences. For example, *S. sanguis* is less sensitive than *S. mutans* to inhibition by chlorhexidine. Gram-negative bacteria show a much wider range of variation, with some (*Proteus* species) having a minimal inhibitory concentration of >100 μg/ml. It is not clear whether the decreased effectiveness of chlorhexidine as a topical antimicrobial on a long-term basis is a reflection of this variation or of the emergence of resistant mutants.

Its effectiveness in subgingival treatment of periodontitis is not demonstrated, since most studies show little or no benefit over scaling and root planing alone. However, its use as a supragingival plaque inhibitor in the control of gingivitis is well established (Fardal and Turnbull, 1986; Kornman, 1986). Chlorhexidine oral rinse is indicated for use between dental visits for supragingival plaque and gingivitis control. It has not been tested in ANUG patients. In patients having coexisting gingivitis and periodontitis, the presence or absence of gingival inflammation following chlorhexidine use is not useful as an indicator of underlying periodontitis.

Chlorhexidine is contraindicated in persons known to be hypersensitive to chlorhexidine gluconate (Wahlberg and Wennersten, 1971; Ljunggren and Möller, 1972; Okano et al., 1989). Precautions are advised for usage in pregnancy, nursing mothers, and in children under 18, since safety and efficacy have not been established in these groups.

In vivo resistance to chlorhexidine. Although the development of resistance to antibacterial compounds is common among bacteria, there appear to be few oral organisms that develop resistance to chlorhexidine when used for supragingival plaque control. The report of Emilson and Fornell (1976) showed that while 0.002% of *S. sanguis* isolates were resistant to chlorhexidine, 50 μg/ml) before the agent was used, 34% of the *S. sanguis* isolates were resistant to that level after therapy.

Alexidine and octenidine

Alexidine and octenidine are structurally similar to chlorhexidine, and both show effectiveness as antiplaque/antigingivitis agents in short-term studies.

Sanguinarine

Sanguinarine, a benzophenanthridine alkaloid, is an herbal extract that has been used in homeopathic medicine for many years. It has been evaluated recently and shown to be variably effective as an inhibitor of supragingival plaque formation and gingivitis. It has also been shown to be effective against many periodontal bacteria. Subgingival therapy with sanguinarine has yet to be evaluated.

Peroxide

Hydrogen peroxide is a well-known antiseptic agent that is toxic to many bacteria because of its strongly oxidizing properties. The critical factor in peroxide activity is the fact that hydrogen peroxide and other reduction products of oxygen (e.g., superoxide anions) can generate the more toxic hydroxyl radicals. Many of these reactive oxygen species damage cell membranes, inactivate bacterial enzymes via oxidation of sulfhydryl groups, and disrupt the bacterial chromosome. In addition, hydrogen peroxide is also required for the potent bactericidal action of myeloperoxidase, a lysosomal phagocytic enzyme.

Peroxides are toxic to the host, causing peroxidation of lipids in cell membranes and certain chromosomal changes, depending on the concentration of the agent and the duration of usage. It has even been suggested that chronic treatment with hydrogen peroxide may have long-term toxicity for humans (Weitzman et al., 1984), although there is no direct demonstration of such effects.

Bacteria vary markedly in their susceptibility to peroxide, and the basis of this resistance is often the production of catalase. However, other mechanisms of resistance to peroxides occur.

It appears that peroxide alone used subgingivally has little or no benefit beyond that achieved with complete scaling and root planing alone in the management of adult periodontitis (Christerson et al., 1988).

Stannous fluoride

Stannous fluoride (SnF_2) has also been used subgingivally (Mazza et al., 1981). Stannous fluoride at 600 to 1000 parts/million was found by Yoon and Newman (1980) to kill candidate periodontopathic organisms. It produces a beneficial but marginal adjunctive effect on healing beyond that achieved with complete scaling and root planing alone.

ANTIBIOTICS USED TOPICALLY

Systematic study of the antibacterial activity of antimicrobials that might have topical use in the body has been evaluated by Baker et al. (1983). Each antibiotic manifests a spectrum of resistance and susceptibility in vitro that might also be expected to be reflected in vivo.

Topical use of the tetracyclines has been shown to result in attachment gain significantly greater than that achieved with complete scaling and root planing alone (Puchalsky et al., 1988) when the tetracycline is applied as a concentrated solution for 5 minutes to the exposed root surface. Under these conditions, aqueous tetracycline is acidic; it etches the root surface, binds, and is released in active form (Terranova et al., 1986).

Other methods of topical application of tetracyclines using impregnated threads (Goodson et al., 1983) and slow-release beads are presently under investigation.

SUMMARY

In summary, based on the susceptibility of periodontic pathogens, antibiotics, especially systemic tetracyclines, the penicillins, and metronidazole, are useful adjuncts in the treatment of some cases of periodontitis. Topical use of povidone-iodine has an adjunctive effect on healing when used at the time of surgical debridement of periodontal lesions in adult periodontitis. Aqueous solutions of concentrated tetracycline used to etch exposed root surfaces also have adjunctive effects when used in conjunction with scaling and root planing. Finally, chlorhexidine oral rinses are effective in supragingival plaque and gingivitis control. None of the above-mentioned antibiotics, povidone-iodine, or chlorhexidine leads to the emergence of significant resistant flora when used under carefully controlled conditions. There are other antimicrobial agents under development for the management of periodontal disease; however, even the existing agents offer a choice among remarkably effective agents for prevention and management of various periodontal diseases.

REFERENCES

Baker PJ et al: Minimal inhibitory concentrations of various antimicrobial agents for human oral anaerobic bacteria, Antimicrob Agents Chemother 24:420, 1983.

Baker PJ et al: Susceptibility of human oral anaerobic bacteria to antibiotics suitable for topical use, J Clin Periodontol 12:201, 1985.

Christersson LA et al: Tissue localization of Actinobacillus actinomycetemcomitans in human periodontitis. I. Light, immunofluorescence and electron microscopic studies, J Periodontol 58(8):529, 1987.

Christersson LA et al: Monitoring of subgingival Bacteroides gingivalis and Actinobacillus actinomycetemcomitans in the management of advanced periodontitis Adv Dent Res 2(2):382, 1988.

Ciancio SG: Tetracyclines and periodontal therapy, J Periodontol 47:155, 1976.

Ciancio SG et al: An evaluation of minocycline in patients with periodontal disease, J Periodontol 51:557, 1982.

Emilson CG and Fornell J: The effect of tooth brushing with chlorhexidine gel on salivary microflora, oral hygiene and caries, Scand J Dent Res 84:308, 1976.

Fardal O and Turnbull RS: A review of the literature on use of chlorhexidine in dentistry, J Am Dent Assoc 112:863, 1986.

Golub L et al: Tetracyclines inhibit tissue collagenolytic enzyme activity: a new concept in the treatment of periodontal disease, J Periodont Res 19:651, 1984.

Goodson JM et al: Monolithic tetracycline-containing fibers for controlled delivery to periodontal pockets, J Periodontol 54:575, 1983.

Higgins HB et al: The effect of povidone-iodine (Betadine) on serum protein bound iodine when used as surgical preparation on intact skin, Can Med Assoc J 90:1298, 1964.

Kornman KS: Antimicrobial agents—state of the science review. In Löe H and Kleinman D, editors: Dental plaque control measures and oral hygiene practices, Oxford, 1986, IRL Press.

Layton JM et al: Gingival fluid levels of amoxicillin and its MICs for periodontal bacteria, J Dent Res 62(abstr 1086):290, 1983.

Listgarten M et al: The effect of tetracycline and/or scaling on human periodontal disease—clinical, microbiological and histological observations, J Clin Periodontol 5:246, 1978.

Ljunggren B and Möller H: Eczematous contact allergy to chorhexidine, Acta Derm Venereol 52:308, 1972.

Loesche WJ et al: Treatment of periodontal infections with metronidazole: case reports of 5 patients, J Clin Periodontol 8:29, 1981.

Mandell RL and Socransky SS: Microbiological and clinical effects of surgery plus doxycycline on juvenile periodontitis, J Periodontol 59:373, 1988.

Mashimo PA et al: In vitro evaluation of antibiotics in the treatment of periodontal disease, Pharmacol Ther Dent 6:45, 1981.

Mazza JE et al: Clinical and antimicrobial effects of stannous fluoride on periodontitis, J Clin Periodontol 8:203, 1981.

Mills WH et al: Clinical evaluation of spiramycin and erythromycin in control of periodontal disease, J Clin Periodontol 6:308, 1979.

Moeller AJR: Microbiological examination of root canals of periapical tissues of human teeth, Odontol T 74:1, 1966.

Okano M et al: Anaphylactic symptoms due to chlorhexidine gluconate, Arch Dermatol 125:50, 1989.

Puchalsky CS et al: Topical application of tetracycline-HCl in human periodontitis, J Dent Res 67(special issue, abstr 766), 1988.

Rosling BG et al: Microbiological and clinical effects of topical subgingival antimicrobial treatment on human periodontal disease, J Clin Periodontol 10:487, 1983.

Rosling BG et al: Topical antimicrobial therapy and diagnosis of subgingival bacteria in the management of inflammatory periodontal disease, J Clin Periodontol 13:975, 1986.

Shinn DLS: Metronidazole in acute ulcerative gingivitis (correspondence), Lancet 1:1191, 1962.

Slots J and Rosling BG: Suppression of the periodontopathic microflora in localized juvenile periodontitis by systemic tetracycline, J Clin Periodontol 10:465, 1983.

Slots J et al: Periodontal therapy in humans. I. Microbiological and clinical effects of a single course of periodontal scaling and root planing, and of adjunctive tetracycline therapy, J Periodontol 50(10):495, 1979.

Slots J et al: In vitro antimicrobial susceptibility of Actinobacillus actinomycetemcomitans, Antimicrob Agents Chemother 18(1):9, 1980.

Terranova VP et al: A biochemical approach to periodontal regeneration: tetracycline treatment of dentin promotes fibroblast adhesion and growth, J Periodont Res 21:330, 1986.

Valdes MV et al: Beta-lactamase producing bacteria in the human oral cavity, J Oral Pathol 11:58, 1982.

van Osten et al: The effect of amoxicillin on destructive periodontitis, J Periodontol 57:613, 1986.

Wahlberg JE and Wennersten G: Hypersensitivity and photosensitivity to chlorhexidine, Dermatologica 143:376, 1971.

Walker CB et al: Agar medium for use in susceptibility testing of bacteria from human periodontal pockets, Antimicrob Agents Chemother 16:452, 1979a.

Walker CB et al: Medium for selective isolation of Fusobacterium nucleatum from human periodontal pockets, J Clin Microbiol 10:844, 1979b.

Walker CB et al: Gingival crevicular fluid levels of tetracycline and the in vitro effect on periodontal bacteria. II. Susceptibilities of periodontal bacteria, J Periodontol 52:613, 1981.

Walker CB et al: Antibiotic susceptibility testing of subgingival plaque samples, J Clin Periodontol 10:422, 1983.

Weitzman SA et al: Chronic treatment with hydrogen peroxide: is it safe? J Periodontol 55:510, 1984.

Yogev R et al: In vitro and in vivo synergism between amoxicillin and clavulanic acid against ampicillin-resistant Haemophilus influenzae, Antimicrob Agents Chemother 19:993, 1981.

Yoon AN and Newman MG: Antimicrobial effect of fluorides of Bacteroides melaninogenicus subspecies and Bacteroides asaccharolyticus, J Clin Periodontol 7:489, 1980.

Zambon JJ et al: Diagnosis and treatment of localized juvenile periodontitis, J Am Dent Assoc 113:295, 1986.

Chapter 13

MECHANICAL PLAQUE RETENTION FACTORS

Niklaus P. Lang
Beatrice E. Siegrist

In this chapter mechanical factors that favor the retention and growth of dental plaques and therefore act as secondary etiologic factors are considered. They are of two types: those associated with restorative dentistry and those resulting from abnormal anatomic features of the crown or roots. According to the historical principles of reconstructive dentistry, even the smallest cavity must be excavated to a more or less standardized size to prevent the development of secondary caries. The concept of "extension for prevention" dates back to G.V. Black (1908) and demands that the margin of a restoration be placed in a region that is self-cleansing as a result of the friction associated with mastication. Furthermore, it was postulated that the cervical margins of all smooth-surface (Class V) restorations should be located subgingivally. The reasoning on which this concept was based was that an initial carious lesion could never occur on enamel that was covered by gingiva (Black, 1908).

As a result of Black's postulate, the idea of "extension for prevention" still occupies a prominent position as a fundamental principle in prophylactic therapy for dental caries. Without doubt, the application of this concept has dominated reconstructive dentistry for the last 80 years. Our current knowledge concerning the pathogenesis and etiology of caries and periodontal diseases, as well as the accepted principles of preventive dentistry, have made it abundantly clear, however, that the concept of "extension for prevention" has become untenable and should therefore be revised (Löe, 1968). Adherence to the outdated concept has led to the unreasonable situation wherein both vertical and horizontal extension of a cavity in the course of treatment may significantly affect the destruction of periodontal tissues.

PREPARATION MARGINS IN RECONSTRUCTIVE DENTISTRY

It has been demonstrated again and again that without effective oral hygiene, healthy patients with a complete dentition and normal occlusion will experience massive plaque accumulation (Löe et al., 1965). Plaque buildup, especially on the cervical half of the clinical tooth crown, is hardly ever susceptible to the self-cleansing effect of chewing, even when extremely fibrous foods are consumed. For this reason, and because of the eating habits of most people today, self-cleansing is, practically speaking, nonexistent. Furthermore, the concept of "extension for prevention" is based on the assumption that restorations whose margins extend into the gingival sulcus are covered by healthy gingiva. However, it has been pointed out that all subgingivally placed margins of dental restorations are associated with pathologic alteration of the adjacent gingiva (Waerhaug, 1960). Thus all subgingival restoration margins of inlays, crowns, and fillings are in fact covered by pathologically altered gingiva, because the margin itself represents an area of increased plaque accumulation. Since it is technically quite difficult to achieve a perfect marginal adaptation of the restoration, a more or less extensive crevice exists between the prepared tooth margin and the edge of the reconstruction. This crevice may be 20 to 60 μm if the best possible laboratory procedures are used. However, quite often marginal crevices of 100 μm or more are encountered. These gaps quickly become filled with bacterial plaque and will elicit or enhance a gingival lesion (Waerhaug 1960) (Fig. 13-1).

Follow-up examinations of fixed reconstructions have demonstrated that the position of the preparation in relation to the gingivae may have a significant influence on the Gingival Index (GI) value, as well as on the depth of the gingival sulcus or pocket and the level of probing attachment (Silness, 1970, 1974; Valderhaug, 1972; Silness and Ohm, 1974; Valderhaug and Birkeland, 1976). It has been shown that crown margins positioned subgingivally are associated with the highest GI values, whereas supragingivally located crown margins are associated with the lowest GI values. Crown margins that are located directly at the height of the free gingival margin are associated with GI values intermediate between the highest and lowest (Valderhaug, 1972; Valderhaug and Birkeland, 1976). It has also been ascertained that the severity of the GI is related to the depth of the crown margin in the gingival sulcus. Thus Newcomb (1974) published data that would lead one to suspect that a positive correlation exists between the depth of the crown margin in a gingival sulcus and the severity of the inflammatory reactions within the gingiva.

The results of these epidemiologic studies agree with and support additional clinical investigations. Mannerberg (1971) used measurements of gingival exudate and leukocyte emigration from the sulcus of teeth treated with porcelain jacket crowns to demonstrate that the gingival condition of these crowned teeth was significantly poorer than that of contralateral control teeth that had never been crowned. Renggli and Regolati (1972) and Moermann et al. (1974) came to the conclusion that during cavity or crown preparation supragingival margins should be chosen whenever possible. In a 5-year longitudinal study of 335 crowned teeth, Valderhaug and Birkeland (1976) found that the loss of periodontal attachment was significantly greater around teeth with subgingivally located crown mar-

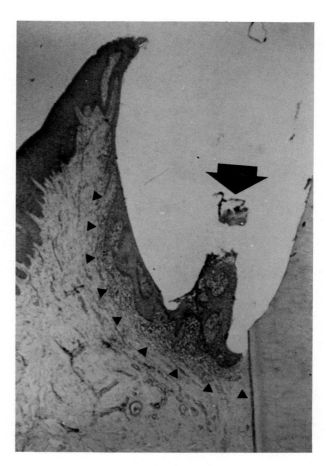

Fig. 13-1. Photomicrograph of marginal gingiva around a tooth whose gold crown extended far into gingival sulcus. Crown margin was opened by about 150 μm. Note epithelial proliferation that penetrated into this open marginal area when cement had washed away. Heavy inflammatory infiltrate in region of preparation margin *(small arrows)* was elicited by bacterial plaque within open margin *(large arrow)*. (From Waerhaug J: Dent Clin North Am, p 161, 1960.)

gins when compared with similar teeth with crown margins located supragingivally (Fig. 13-2). Furthermore, 5 years after cementation the subgingivally prepared teeth exhibited deeper pockets than teeth that had been prepared with the margin at the height of the gingiva or supragingivally (Fig. 13-3). The same study showed that 5 years after cementation 30% of the subgingivally located crown margins were associated with gingival recession, which was assumed to be the result of constant irritation.

With regard to the question of secondary caries in crowned teeth and the relationship of its incidence to the location of the preparation margin, there have been very few well-controlled clinical studies. Valderhaug and Helöe (1977) found a secondary caries incidence of 3.5% in all of the crowned teeth that they studied. Hammer and Hotz (1979) reported that significantly more secondary carious lesions were found around subgingivally located margins

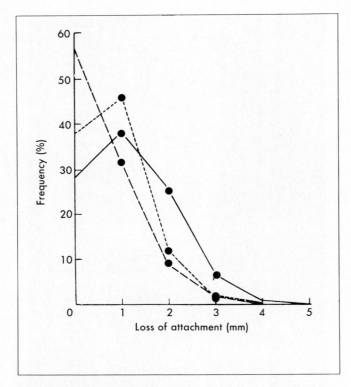

Fig. 13-2. Frequency distribution of loss of periodontal attachment in 335 crowned teeth 5 years after cementing. Subgingivally located surfaces exhibit obviously more attachment loss when compared with supragingival margins. ——— Subgingivally, 1.2 ± 0.92; ------ at gingiva, 0.8 ± 0.86; ---- supragingivally, 0.6 ± 0.72. (From Valderhaug J and Birkeland JM: J Oral Rehabil 3:237, 1976.)

than around supragingival ones. While 15.4% of the supragingivally located amalgam restoration margins exhibited secondary caries after 5 years, this figure was 30.4% for subgingivally located amalgam restoration margins.

Several conclusions may be drawn from clinical epidemiologic and histologic investigations:

1. Periodontal injury caused by crown margins may be most severe if the margin of the crown is located subgingivally.
2. The deeper a crown margin intrudes into the gingival sulcus, the greater may be the degree of periodontal injury.
3. Supragingivally positioned crown margins may not adversely affect the periodontal tissues.
4. 4.The incidence of secondary caries is higher than or at least as high in subgingivally prepared teeth as in restorations with supragingivally positioned crown margins (Fig. 13-4).

Clinical implications

There is adequate proof from scientific research, as well as from clinical practice, that all dental restorations (re-

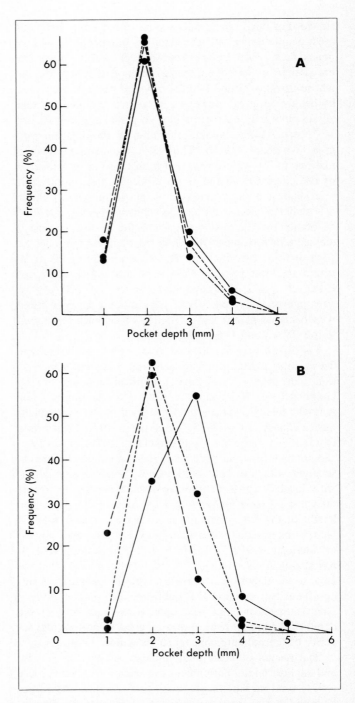

Fig. 13-3. Frequency distribution of pocket probing depths around crowned teeth. **A,** At time of cementation, distribution curves for all 389 teeth were identical regardless of position of preparation margins. ——— Subgingivally; ------ at gingiva; ---- supragingivally. **B,** Five years later, clearly deepened periodontal probing depths were apparent in the 335 crowned teeth when preparation margins were located subgingivally. In cases of supragingival preparation margins, pocket depths were practically identical to those measured 5 years previously. In teeth where preparation margins were located directly at margin of gingiva, a slight deepening of pockets was apparent. ——— Subgingivally; ------ at gingiva; ---- supragingivally. (From Valderhaug J and Birkeland JM: J Oral Rehabil 13:327, 1976.)

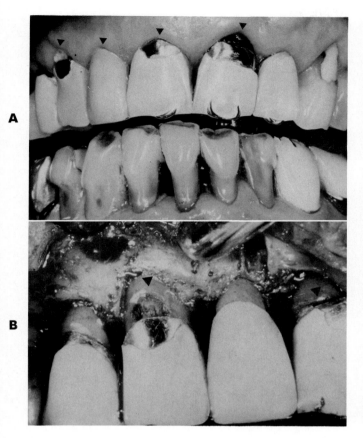

Fig. 13-4. Secondary caries may be detected on teeth whose crowns extend into gingival sulcus. **A,** Carious lesions were found on every buccal margin (*arrows:* teeth Nos. 6, 7, 8, and 9. **B,** These lesions were especially obvious during a flap operation.

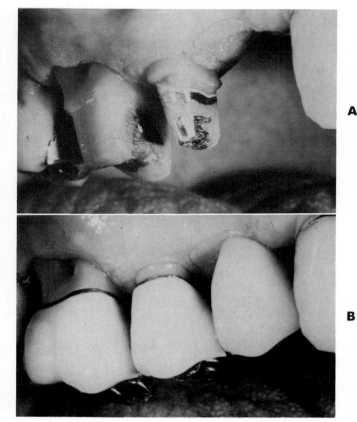

Fig. 13-5. Filling and crown margins should be located in regions that are accessible for mechanical plaque removal. It appears reasonable to avoid subgingival preparations whenever possible. **A,** After periodontal treatment, margins of abutment crowns on teeth Nos. 15 and 16 are located supragingivally. **B,** Same abutment teeth 3½ years later. Gingivae are still clinically healthy. Recall interval for this patient was 4 months.

gardless of the material employed) that extend into the subgingival region can and will injure periodontal tissues. This injury occurs either through direct irritation by the materials used or by the creation of a retention area for bacteria, a zone that enhances subgingival plaque accumulation.

It therefore appears reasonable to avoid tooth preparations extending into the gingival sulcus (Fig. 13-5). Exceptions to this rule may include:

1. Esthetics in the maxillary anterior region
2. Problems of retention (Fig. 13-6)
3. Expansive carious lesions
4. Replacement of defective, extensive restorations
5. Patient's resistance to periodontal disease

The concept of "extension for prevention" must therefore be modified to place the margins of preparation in regions accessible to the currently used oral hygiene techniques and material.

RETENTION AREAS
Overhanging restoration margins

The transition zone that encompasses the crown margin, the cement, and the prepared tooth achieves great significance if the crown margin is located subgingivally. In this zone a crevice is almost always found, since no commercially available cement provides a perfect closure (seal). The surface of the cement is always rough and porous. It has been demonstrated that the surface of this "cement line" associated with seated crowns may approach several square millimeters (Silness and Hegedahl, 1970). Histologic studies (Waerhaug, 1956) have also documented that this subgingival cement roughness enhances plaque accumulation in the gingival sulcus or pocket. The significance of the cement line in the transition zone with regard to periodontal injury is all the more important because too often the clinician observes ill-fitting crowns with obviously overhanging and open margins. Björn et al. (1969, 1970)

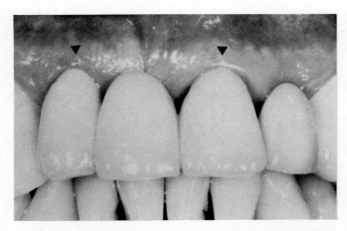

Fig. 13-6. In maxillary anterior region it is often necessary to make some compromises for esthetic considerations. In this particular case, preparation margins are located at gingival margin. An extremely fine band of metal is therefore all that remains visible. This compromise can be very satisfactory, as indicated in case depicted here, in which crowns on Nos. 7 and 9 have already been in situ for 7 years.

showed that the fit and precision in crown and bridge elements are, as a rule, poor. Eighty percent of the radiographically studied reconstructions exhibited marginal defects on the proximal surfaces. Margins that were open by more than 0.2 mm were always associated with alveolar bone loss. Also, a more recent publication from Germany (Lange 1984) showed that 69% of fillings and 82% of bridge retainers in 35-year-old subjects from Münster yielded ill-fitting margins.

The close association between restorations with overhanging margins and chronic destructive periodontitis has been known for many years. However, the mechanisms by which overhanging restorations will interact in the pathogenesis of periodontal disease are still unknown. Generally, it is accepted that overhanging restorations contribute to the promotion of the disease process by virtue of their capacity to retain bacterial plaque. In an experimental study (Lang et al., 1983), an attempt was made to determine if the placement of subgingival restorations with overhanging margins resulted in changes in the subgingival microbiota. In this study five MOD cast gold onlays with 0.5 to 1 mm proximal overhanging margins were placed in mandibular molars for 19 to 27 weeks. They were replaced in a crossover design by similar onlays with clinically perfect margins, which served as controls. Another five onlays were placed in reverse order in the remaining four of the eight dental students participating (Fig. 13-7).

Prior to and every 2 to 3 weeks after insertion, subgingival microbiologic samples were obtained by inserting a fine sterile paper point for 30 seconds into the gingival sul-

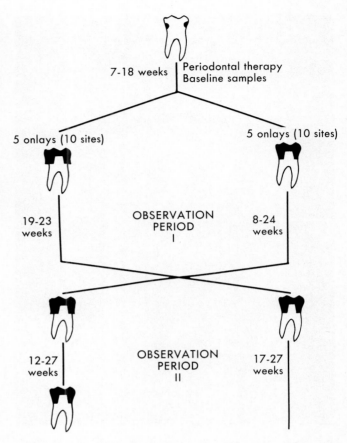

Fig. 13-7. Experimental protocol for a clinical crossover study of effects of overhanging margins on periodontium. (From Lang NP et al: J Clin Periodontol 10:563, 1983. © 1983 Munksgaard International Publishers, Ltd., Copenhagen, Denmark.)

cus subjacent to the restoration. The predominant cultivable flora was determined using continuous anaerobic culturing techniques. Following the placement of the restorations with overhanging margins, a subgingival flora was detected that closely resembled that of chronic periodontitis. Increased proportions of gram-negative anaerobic bacteria (black-pigmented *Bacteroides* of up to 18% to 23%) and an increased anaerobe–to–facultative bacteria ratio were noted. Following the placement of the restorations with clinically perfect margins, a microflora characteristic of gingival health or initial gingivitis was observed (Fig. 13-8). At that time, black-pigmented *Bacteroides* organisms were detected in very low proportions (1.6% to 3.8%). These changes in the subgingival microflora were obvious irrespective of whether the restorations with the overhanging margins were placed in the first period of the experiment or following the crossover. Clinically, increasing gingival indices were detected at the sites where overhanging margins were placed. Bleeding on gentle probing always preceded the peak level of black-pigmented *Bac-*

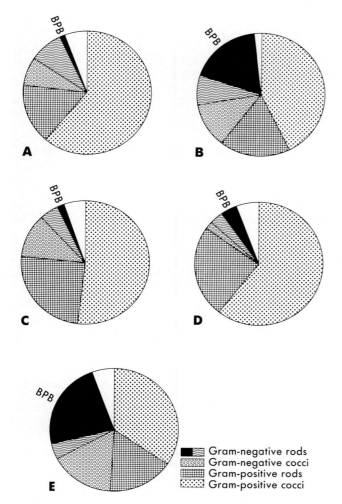

Fig. 13-8. Total cultivable subgingival microbiota: proportions of gram-positive and gram-negative cocci and rods. *BPB,* Black-pigmented *Bacteroides.* **A,** Preexperimental percentages. **B,** Subgingival microbiota following incorporation of an overlay with an overhanging margin. **C,** Replacement of overlay of **B** with a clinically perfect overlay. **D,** Subgingival microbiota in second group at site of clinically perfect overlay. **E,** Changes in subgingival microbiota in second group following replacement of overlay of **D** with an overhanging overlay. (From Lang NP et al. J Clin Periodontol 10:563, 1983. © 1983 Munksgaard International Publishers, Ltd., Copenhagen, Denmark.)

teroides. Loss of attachment was not detected in any site.

In conclusion, this study demonstrated that the placement of restorations with overhanging subgingival margins resulted in a change in the composition of the subgingival microbiota at that site to one that may be associated with periodontitis, rather than simply harboring increased amounts of plaque. The obvious potential for iatrogenic initiation of periodontal disease because of an environment favoring growth of periodontal pathogens is clearly a result of subgingival margins with overhangs.

Orthodontic bands

During orthodontic therapy, inflammation of the gingival tissues is often observed (Rateitschak et al., 1968; Zachrisson and Zachrisson, 1972). Lack of adequate oral hygiene in conjunction with the placement of fixed orthodontic appliances is considered a major factor for an accentuated accumulation of bacterial plaque and the subsequent inflammatory response (Zachrisson, 1976). However, in many incidences only minor or no permanent damage of the periodontal tissues will result, even though adequate plaque control is not assured (Zachrisson and Alnaes, 1973, 1974; Kloehn and Pfeifer, 1974; Zachrisson, 1976; Trossello and Gianelly, 1979; Sadowsky and Begole, 1981; Polson and Reed, 1984).

Although the host response of the periodontal tissues may be able to cope with some of the more aggressive factors of bacterial plaque during orthodontic therapy, the importance of prophylactic or curative measures should not be underestimated. Severe gingivitis and irreversible periodontal damages have been documented in animals (Ericsson et al., 1977), as well as in some individuals (Zachrisson and Alnaes, 1973), as a result of orthodontic treatment. Quite frequently, an increase in gingival inflammation is noted with the concomitant placement of fixed orthodontic appliances. These pathogenic changes may well reflect the start of a destructive process in the periodontium.

A recently published clinical experiment studied the changes occurring in the subgingival plaque in children following the placement of orthodontic bands in the absence of a specific prophylactic oral hygiene program (Diamanti-Kipioti et al., 1987). Furthermore, the correlation between the growth of bacterial plaque and the increase in the percentages of specific bacterial species with clinical parameters was evaluated. Twelve children aged 10 to 15 years were selected for the study. The experimental group consisted of six subjects scheduled for orthodontic treatment including the placement of fixed appliances. They were seen 1 week before and just prior to the placement of orthodontic bands. The control group involved six children in the maintenance phase of orthodontic therapy in which removable retainers were used. All subjects were examined at 3- to 5-week intervals for a period of 4 months. At each examination, microbiologic subgingival plaque samples were collected by means of sterile paper points. Plaque index (PlI) and GI scores, as well as pocket probing depths at the site of sampling, were determined. The microbiologic samples were processed using continuous anaerobic culturing techniques.

Following tooth banding, an increase in pocket probing depth was observed while the PlI and GI scores remained unaffected. A statistically significant increase from baseline values (p < .01) was found for the percentages of black-pigmented *Bacteroides, Bacteroides intermedius*

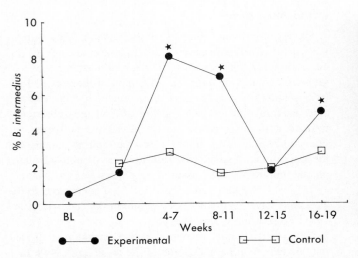

Fig. 13-9. Changes in mean percentage of *Bacteroides intermedius* in relation to total cultivable subgingival microbiota: statistically significant (*) increase (p < .01) in experimental group following placement of orthodontic bands. (From Diamanti-Kipioti A, Gusberti FA, and Lang NP: J Clin Periodontol 14:326, 1987. © 1987 Munksgaard International Publishers, Ltd., Copenhagen, Denmark.)

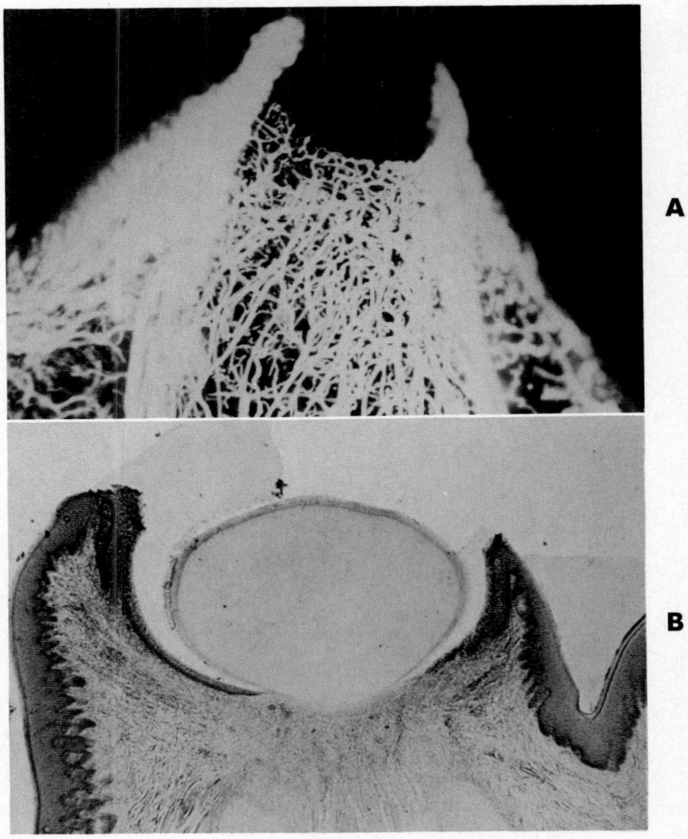

Fig. 13-10. Morphologic features of interdental area: cross sections through contact area of col region. **A,** Gingival blood supply with delicate network of capillaries. **B,** Buccal and lingual papillae of col region between molars: junctional epithelium lining entire col. (**A** from Hock J: J Periodont Res 9:298, 1974. © 1974 Munksgaard International Publishers, Ltd., Copenhagen, Denmark.)

(Fig. 13-9), and *Actinomyces odontolyticus* species concomitantly with a decrease of the anaerobe–to–facultative bacteria ratio in the experimental but not the control group.

These results document the potential of subgingivally placed orthodontic bands for changing the subgingival ecosystem, favoring the dominance of periodontopathic microorganisms, in subjects not given special oral hygiene instructions.

Clinical implications

The experimental clinical studies (Lang et al., 1983; Diamanti-Kipioti et al., 1987) have clearly demonstrated that iatrogenic retentive factors may not only nonspecifically increase the plaque biomass in the subgingival compartment, but may also selectively alter the composition of the subgingival microbiota. Retention areas such as overhanging margins and/or subgingivally placed orthodontic bands may provide an opportunity for presumptive periodontopathic microorganisms to colonize the subgingival area and hence increase the chance for the progression of gingivitis into periodontitis.

CROWN CONTOURS

Overcontouring elicits effects similar to those of overhanging margins of restorations and that may be detrimental to the periodontal tissues. Although controlled research data on this aspect of reconstructive dentistry are scarce, it is generally agreed that gingival irritation often results from unsatisfactory crown contours (Morris, 1962; Wheeler, 1962; Yuodelis et al., 1973), since there is practically no self-cleansing effect in the area of the gingival third of the teeth (Lindhe and Wicén, 1968). Overcontouring of reconstructions provides additional retentive areas for plaque accumulation. On the other hand, undercontouring has not been shown to be detrimental to the gingival tissues in controlled studies.

Overcontouring may occur in several dimensions: interdental areas, buccolingual aspects, and furcation aspects.

Interdental areas

Quite often interproximal contact areas of reconstructions are grossly overcontoured. This will not only impinge on the tissues of the interdental area, which represent a delicate network of gingival blood vessels within a fine connective tissue of the col area (Fig. 13-10, *A*), but also jeopardizes the possibility of effectively cleaning this area using special aids for oral hygiene (Fig. 13-10, *B*).

Studies (Stolk, 1977) have shown that the interdental papilla experiences a remodeling process following the preparation of the adjacent tooth that lasts at least 6 months. However, even after a period of 18 months, the original morphology of the papillary region may not be obtained.

The approximal surfaces of natural teeth present with a flat or even concave outline (Wheeler, 1962). Nevertheless, this anatomic feature is continuously being neglected in reconstructive dentistry. Quite often the interproximal contours of fillings and restorations are made too wide and hence close the interproximal space (Fig. 13-11). Plaque control is more difficult, and a hyperplastic gingivitis will completely close the col region (Fig. 13-11, *A*). This again will enlarge the buccal and lingual papillae and hence favor the accumulation of plaque.

On the other hand, interproximal spaces that are widely open do not provide a hazard to the gingival tissues (Fig. 13-11, *C*). Special aids including interdental brushes, wide balsa toothpicks, and thick floss have been designed to effectively remove bacterial plaque in these areas. It is therefore preferable to undercontour rather than overcontour an artificial crown.

Buccolingual aspects

The main reason for overcontouring in the buccolingual dimension lies with the fact that not enough tooth substance is cut on the labial aspect of prepared teeth to provide sufficient space for the placement of the material of an artificial crown (metal frame and porcelain) (Fig. 13-12). Such overcontouring inhibits the close adaptation of the gingival tissues to the tooth and hence impinges on the "sealing" effect of the dentogingival junction. Enhanced plaque accumulation will continuously trigger gingival inflammation and may lead to attachment loss and loss of alveolar support.

Furcation aspects

Teeth with beginning furcation involvements and open furcations deserve special attention during tooth preparation. To provide sufficient space for the dental materials of an artificial crown, the contours of the furcations have to be accentuated (Fig. 13-13). If not enough space is provided, overcontouring of the furcation region is inevitable, providing conditions that will favor the accumulation of plaque in this most critical area.

Clinical implications

On the basis of histologic and clinical-experimental studies on the epidemiology (Cumming and Löe, 1973) and pathogenesis of periodontal diseases (Löe et al., 1978) and root surface caries, it must be concluded that the cleansing of the interdental area plays a central role in preventing dental plaque infections. Because of this, prosthetic reconstructions must never interfere with the patient's ability to perform optimal interdental cleansing. Overcontouring of crown margins, especially in the interdental area or at the orifice of furcations, must be avoided.

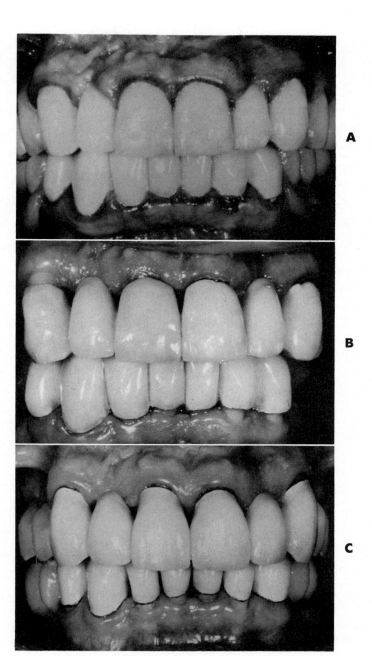

Fig. 13-11. Plaque retention area iatrogenically created by closing interdental spaces of bridge retainers. **A,** Reconstruction with overcontoured retainers resulting in severe chronic gingivitis. **B,** Overcontouring visible following successful periodontal therapy. **C,** Replacement of reconstruction with contours compatible with periodontal health (open interproximal spaces, concave contours of crowns at cementoenamel junctions, and well-fitting margins).

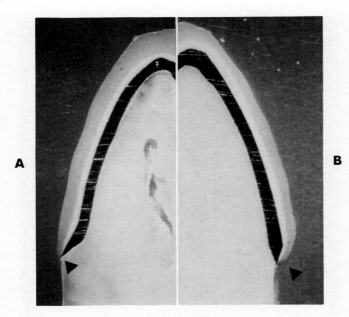

Fig. 13-12. Correct cutting of tooth preparations provide adequate space for dental materials in artificial crowns. Cross section of crown preparation gold *(black area)* and porcelain overlay. **A,** No overcontouring. **B,** Inadequate space for metal and porcelain leads to overcontouring.

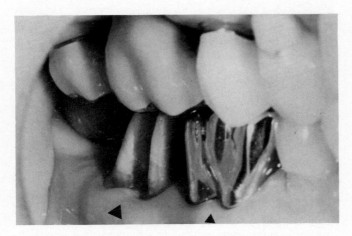

Fig. 13-13. Furcation aspects of two lower molars with beginning furcation Class I involvement. Accentuated preparations in furcation area of second molar allow for proper contouring and provide access for oral hygiene.

If crowns are undercontoured, aids for oral hygiene procedures should be adequate to prevent reinfection of these areas, which are at risk for root caries and periodontal diseases. Whenever possible, the interdental space of prosthetic reconstructions should be sufficiently large to provide adequate space for interdental brushes (Waerhaug, 1976).

PONTIC DESIGN

When lost teeth are replaced with fixed prosthetic reconstructions, new hard surfaces susceptible to plaque formation are introduced in the oral cavity. Inflammatory tissue reactions of the mucosa covering the alveolar ridge have repeatedly been reported in close association with bridge pontics (Silness, 1980), and histologic studies have documented that these changes may be noticed after a relatively short period of time (Reichenbach, 1931; Henry et al., 1966; Stein, 1966; Podshadley, 1968). This mucosal inflammation may be caused primarily by the bacterial deposits underneath the pontics with or without concomitant recontouring of the pontic body (Stein, 1966; Silness et al., 1982).

In a clinical experimental study, plaque accumulation on the gingival surface of bridge pontics was examined in vivo (Gusberti et al., 1985). Four different pontic designs were constructed (Fig. 13-14):

1. Modified ridge lap pontic with concave gingival surface and open interproximal spaces
2. Lap-facing pinpoint contact pontic with open interproximal spaces
3. Lap-facing pinpoint contact pontic with closed interproximal spaces
4. Sanitary pontic

A total of eight bridges were prepared that had an exchangeable gingival part of the pontic. For each patient and bridge, plaque was allowed to accumulate successively on the four pontics with different designs. After 48 hours in situ, each pontic, along with the adherent dental plaque, was prepared for scanning electron microscopy. The results show that plaque formation was highly variable among patients. On all pontics with different designs, plaque formation was predominant at specific locations (i.e., in interproximal spaces, at the borderlines [line angles] between buccal or lingual surfaces and the gingival surface, and also in surface concavities).

Retention areas such as open interdental spaces and gingival surfaces facing the alveolar mucosa (sanitary pontics) allowed more pronounced development of bacterial plaque. However, the clinical closure of these spaces by the lap-facing pontic body did not suppress bacterial colonization. Failures in preventing plaque formation by placing the gingival surface of the pontic in contact with the adjacent alveolar mucosa have been well documented; this approach may later favor mucosal inflammation (Henry et al., 1966; Stein, 1966; Silness, 1980).

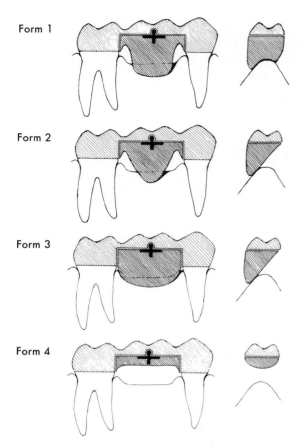

Form 1

Form 2

Form 3

Form 4

Fig. 13-14. Shapes of four different experimental pontics: mesiodistal and buccolingual sections. (From Gusberti FA, Finger M, and Lang NP: Schweiz Monatsschr Zahnmed 95:539, 1985.)

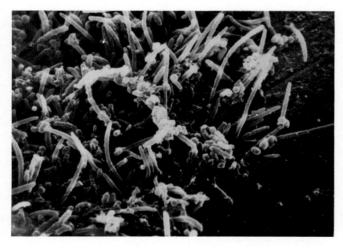

Fig. 13-15. High magnification of area with concavity (gingival part) of pontic demonstrating a more mature plaque characterized by rods and filaments. (×2800.) (From Gusberti FA, Finger M, and Lang NP: Schweiz Monatsschr Zahnmed 95:539, 1985.)

In individuals with light plaque formation, coccoid bacteria were predominantly observed, whereas those who showed heavy plaque accumulation after 48 hours harbored a more complex microbiota. The accentuated bacterial colonization of the pontic surface in these latter individuals may have been responsible for the establishment of suitable conditions for specific changes in the composition of bacterial plaque. Of special interest were observations on initial colonization of the gingival surface of pontics by rods and filaments, which were found only in the heavy plaque formers. These findings suggest that early colonization of hard surfaces is not restricted to coccal bacterial forms. Furthermore, in individuals with accentuated plaque formation, the rapid establishment of a complex flora was also dependent on the location of the surfaces on which plaque developed. Hence the gingival part of buccal surfaces (Lie, 1979) and other retention sites, such as gingival surfaces of pontics, may be more suitable for the establishment of a more mature and eventually more pathogenic microbiota (Fig. 13-15).

The relationship between bacterial accumulation on pontics and inflammation of the underlying alveolar mucosa has been sufficiently described (Silness, 1980). Contact between pontics and alveolar mucosa should be avoided or restricted to a minimal pinpoint area that can be maintained free of plaque (Fig. 13-16). Sanitary pontics with complete separation of their gingival surface from the alveolar mucosa will not prevent inflammation in the absence of adequate plaque control (Silness et al., 1982).

Clinical implications

Since pontic design per se is not preventing dental plaque accumulation and subsequent inflammation, priority has to be given to the feasibility of mechanical plaque removal. Only the removal of bacterial plaque and the establishment of an anatomic relationship to allow proper hygiene will result in maintenance of periodontal health in close proximity to bridge pontics.

TOOTH POSITION

For a long time tooth malposition without or in conjunction with missing teeth was thought to be of primary importance in the etiology of periodontal diseases (Wachsman, 1951; Ditto and Hall, 1954; McCombie and Stothard, 1964). However, no controlled clinical studies were able to confirm such a hypothesis. Even though there is evidence that (especially in children) incisor crowding may be associated with an increased incidence of gingivitis (Gould and Picton, 1966; Sutcliffe, 1968), this association has been explained solely on the basis that crowding of teeth may enhance plaque accumulation (Geiger, 1962; Ainamo, 1972; Jacobson and Linder-Aronson, 1972). Hence no increased susceptibility to periodontal disease has to be expected if effective oral hygiene is performed.

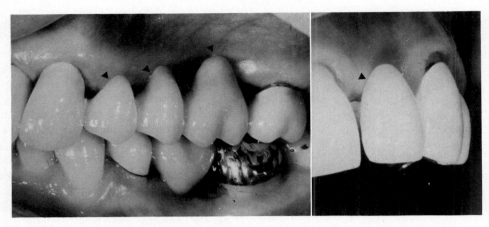

Fig. 13-16. Ideally, pontics should not have concave surfaces. This "egg-shaped" outline provides a pinpoint contact with underlying mucosa.

A series of studies by Silness and Röynstrand (1984, 1985) examined the relationship between tooth alignment, overbite and overjet, anterior spacing of teeth, and dental health. These studies demonstrated associations between none or few nonaligned teeth and a more favorable periodontal state than in anterior segments with an increased number of nonaligned teeth. Also, subjects with a higher overbite-to-overjet ratio yielded more favorable periodontal conditions than subjects with ratios of less than 1:2. Furthermore, in 15-year-old adolescents a relationship between visible spaces (missing contacts) in the anterior segment and gingival health was established. On the other hand, no correlation between crowding of anterior teeth and the periodontal condition has been established in a group of subjects performing average oral hygiene (Ingervall et al., 1977).

Clinical implications

There is no evidence that tooth position per se may cause gingivitis or periodontal disease. However, extreme crowding of teeth may lead to increased plaque accumulation or to difficulty in efficiently removing bacterial plaque. This in turn may aggravate gingivitis but hardly ever leads to periodontal disease. Therefore special instruction in oral hygiene is a prerequisite for the prevention and therapy of dental plaque infections in dentitions with multiple areas of plaque retention resulting from tooth malposition.

ANATOMIC ABNORMALITIES THAT LEAD TO LOCALIZED AREAS OF PERIODONTAL DISEASE
Enamel on the root surface

When enamel forms on the root surface apical to the level of the normal cementoenamel junction (CEJ), connective tissue attachment of the gingiva and periodontium is precluded, since only epithelial attachment can occur to enamel. Often these ectopic deposits of enamel extend into root furcations, in which case they are called *enamel projections*. In other areas they exist as round islands of enamel on the root surface called *enamel pearls*. It has been observed clinically that sites where enamel projection occur often exhibit localized severe periodontal pockets. Masters and Hoskins (1964) classified enamel projections into three classes: I, II, and III. These enamel furcation projections have been associated with periodontal lesions (Simon et al., 1971; Bissada and Abdelmalek, 1973) (Fig. 13-17).

Enamel pearls have been seen in periodontal lesions, and it is likely that they may contribute to the development of the periodontal lesion by encouraging plaque formation once the pocket has extended apically to the pearl (Fig. 13-18).

Distolingual grooves

The aberrant formation of distolingual grooves (also called palatal-gingival grooves) on the root is an invagination resulting from incorrect formation of the root. Maxillary lateral incisors are involved most often, but other incisors, especially the maxillary, may also be affected (Everett and Kramer, 1972). The grooves often begin at the cingulum and extend a variable distance apically on the root surface between the midpalatal line and the line angle. The common finding of a localized periodontal pocket following the course of these grooves supports their role in accumulation of plaque, which in turn leads to the development of a localized periodontal pocket.

Aberrant root anatomy

Once periodontal attachment loss has occurred, root topography plays a major role in providing areas of plaque retention. For example, enamel or cervical projections at

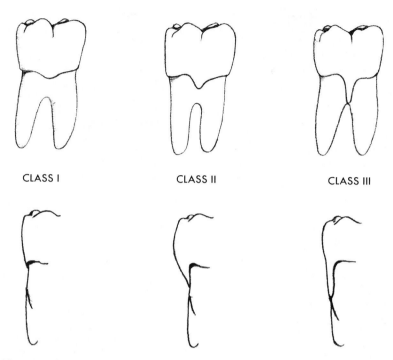

CLASS I   CLASS II   CLASS III

Fig. 13-17. Enamel projections as classified by Masters and Hoskins. (From Masters D and Hoskins S: J Periodontol 35:49, 1964.)

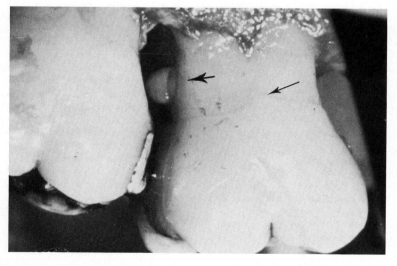

Fig. 13-18. Enamel pearl apical to CEJ. Also note Class I enamel projection. (Courtesy Dr. A. Goldstein, SUNY at Buffalo.)

the CEJ, root concavities, and coronally placed furcation openings may all be plaque retention areas.

The furcation opening may be close to the CEJ, as often occurs on the mesial surface of the maxillary first premolar and in the buccal furcations of the maxillary and mandibular first molars. If this occurs, a few millimeters of attachment loss from the CEJ may lead to a furcation area that is difficult to keep free of plaque and hard to professionally debride.

REFERENCES

Ainamo J: Relationship between malalignment of teeth and periodontal disease, Scand J Dent Res 80:104, 1972.

Bissada NF and Abdelmalek RG: Incidence of cervical enamel projections and its relationship to furcation involvements in Egyptian skulls, J Periodontol 44:583, 1973.

Björn A, Björn H, and Grkovic B: Marginal fit of restorations and its relation to periodontal bone level. I. Metal fillings, Odontol Revy 20:311, 1969.

Björn A, Björn H, and Grkovic B: Marginal fit of restorations and its relation to periodontal bone level. II. Crowns, Odontol Revy 21:337, 1970.

Black GV: Operative dentistry: pathology of the hard tissues of the teeth, vol 1, Chicago, 1908, Medico-Dental Publishing Co.

Cumming BR and Löe H: Consistency of plaque distribution in individuals without special home care instruction, J Periodont Res 8:94, 1973.

Diamanti-Kipioti A, Gusberti FA, and Lang NP: Clinical and microbiological effects of fixed orthodontic appliances, J Clin Periodontol 14:326, 1987.

Ditto WM and Hall DC: A survey of 143 periodontal cases in terms of age and malocclusion, Am J Orthod 40:234, 1954.

Ericsson I et al: The effect of orthodontic tilting movements on the periodontal tissues of infected and non-infected dentitions in dogs, J Clin Periodontol 4:278, 1977.

Everett FG and Kramer GM: The disto-lingual groove in the maxillary lateral incisor: a periodontal hazard, J Periodontol 43:352, 1972.

Geiger AM: Occlusal studies in 188 consecutive cases of periodontal disease, Am J Orthod 48:330, 1962.

Gould MSE and Picton DCA: The relation between irregularities of teeth and periodontal disease, Br Dent J 121:20, 1966.

Gusberti FA, Finger M, and Lang NP: Scanning electron microscope study of 48-hour plaque on different bridge pontics designs, Schweiz Monatsschr Zahnmed 95:539, 1985.

Hammer B and Hotz PR: Nachkontrolle von 1- bis 5 jährigen Amalgam-, Komposit- und Goldgussfüllungen, Schweiz Monatsschr Zahnmed 89:301, 1979.

Henry PJ, Johnston JF, and Mitchell DF: Tissue changes beneath fixed partial dentures, J Prosthet Dent 16:937, 1966.

Hock J: The formation of the vasculature of free gingiva in deciduous teeth of cats and dogs, J Periodont Res 9:298, 1974.

Ingervall B, Jacobsson U, and Nyman S: A clinical study of the relationship between crowding of teeth, plaque and gingival condition, J Clin Periodontol 4:214, 1977.

Jacobson L and Linder-Aronson S: Crowding and gingivitis: a comparison between mouthbreathers and nosebreathers, Scand J Dent Res 80:500, 1972.

Kloehn JS and Pfeifer JS: The effect of orthodontic treatment on the periodontium, Angle Orthod 44:127, 1974.

Lang NP, Kiel RA, and Anderhalden K: Clinical and microbiological effects of subgingival restorations with overhanging or clinically perfect margins, J Clin Periodontol 10:563, 1983.

Lange DE: Attitudes and behaviour with respect to oral hygiene and periodontal treatment needs in selected groups in West Germany. In Fraud-sen A, editor: Public health aspects of periodontal disease, Chicago, 1984, Quintessence Publishing Co, Inc.

Lie T: Morphologic studies on dental plaque formation, Acta Odontol Scand 37:73, 1979.

Lindhe J and Wic´en PO: The effects on the gingivae of chewing fibrous foods, J Periodont Res 4:193, 1969.

Löe H: Reaction of marginal periodontal tissues to restorative procedures, Int Dent J 18:759, 1968.

Löe H, Theilade E, and Jensen SB: Experimental gingivitis in man, J Periodontol 36:177, 1965.

Löe H et al: The natural history of periodontal disease in man: the rate of periodontal destruction before 40 years of age, J Periodontol 49:607, 1978.

Mannerberg F: Gingival changes following porcelain crown therapy, Odontol Revy 22:156, 1971.

Masters D and Hoskins S: Projection of cervical enamel in molar furcations, J Periodontol 35:49, 1964.

McCombie F and Stothard D: Relationships between gingivitis and other dental conditions, J Can Dent Assoc 30:506, 1964.

Moermann W, Regolati B, and Renggli HH: Gingival reactions to well-fitted subgingival proximal gold inlays, J Clin Periodontol 1:120, 1974.

Morris ML: Artificial crown contour and gingival health, J Prosthet Dent 12:1146, 1962.

Newcomb GM: The relationship between the location of subgingival crown margins and gingival inflammation, J Periodontol 45:151, 1974.

Podshadley AG: Gingival response to pontics, J Prosthet Dent 19:51, 1968.

Polson AM and Reed BE: Long-term effect of orthodontic treatment on crestal alveolar bone levels, J Periodontol 55:28, 1984.

Rateitschak KH, Herzog-Specht F, and Hotz R: Reaktion und Regeneration des Parodonts auf Behandlung mit festsitzenden Apparaten und abnehmbaren Platten, Fortschr Kieferorthop 29:415, 1968.

Reichenbach E: Untersuchungen zur Frage einer zweckmässigen Gestaltung des Brückenkorpers, Vjschr Zahnheilk 47:125, 1931.

Renggli HH and Regolati B: Gingival inflammation and plaque accumulation by well-adapted supragingival and subgingival proximal restorations, Helv Odontol Acta 16:99, 1972.

Sadowsky C and Begole E: Long-term effects of orthodontic treatment on periodontal health, Am J Orthod 8:156, 1981.

Silness J: Periodontal conditions in patients treated with dental bridges. III. The relationship between the location of the crown margin and the periodontal condition, J Periodont Res 5:225, 1970.

Silness J: Periodontal conditions in patients treated with dental bridges. IV. The relationship between the pontic and the periodontal condition of the abutment teeth, J Periodont Res 9:50, 1974.

Silness J: Fixed prosthodontics and periodontal health, Dent Clin North Am, p 317, April 1980.

Silness J, Gustavsen F, and Maugersnes K: The relationship between pontic hygiene and mucosal inflammation in fixed-bridge recipients, J Periodont Res 17:434, 1982.

Silness J and Hegdahl T: Area of the exposed zinc phosphate cement surfaces in fixed restorations, Scand J Dent Res 78:163, 1970.

Silness J and Ohm E: Periodontal conditions in patients treated with dental bridges. V. Effects of splinting adjacent abutment teeth, J Periodont Res 9:121, 1974.

Silness J and Röynstrand T: Effects on dental health of spacing of teeth in anterior segments, J Clin Periodontol 11:387, 1984.

Silness J and Röynstrand T: Relationship between alignment conditions of teeth in anterior segments and dental health, J Clin Periodontol 12:312, 1985.

Simon JH, Glick DH, and Frank AL: Predictable failures as a result of radicular anomalies, Oral Surg 31:823, 1971.

Stein RS: Pontic-residual ridge relationship: a research report, J Prosthet Dent 16:251, 1966.

Stolk AH: Morphological changes of the interdental gingiva, Academic thesis, Hilversum, The Netherlands, 1977, Free University of Amsterdam.

Sutcliffe P: Chronic anterior gingivitis: an epidemiological study in school children, Br Dent J 125:47, 1968.

Trossello VR and Gianelly AA: Orthodontic treatment and periodontal status, J Periodontol 50:665, 1979.

Valderhaug J: Prepareringsgrensens beliggenhet- kronebrosynspunkter, Nord Tannlaegeforen Tidskr 82:386, 1972.

Valderhaug J and Birkeland JM: Periodontal conditions in patients 5 years following insertion of fixed prostheses, J Oral Rehabil 3:237, 1976.

Valderhaug J and Helöe LA: Oral hygiene in a group of supervised patients with fixed prosthesis, J Periodontol 48:221, 1977.

Wachsmann C: Gingivitis in relation to irregularities of the teeth, Dent Items Interest 73:634, 1951.

Waerhaug J: Effect of rough surfaces upon gingival tissues, J Dent Res 35:323, 1956.

Waerhaug J: Histologic considerations which govern where the margins of restorations should be located in relation to gingiva, Dent Clin North Am, p 161, 1960.

Waerhaug J: The interdental brush and its place in operative and crown and bridge dentistry, J Oral Rehabil 3:107, 1976.

Wheeler RC: Complete crown form and the periodontium, J Prosthet Dent 11:722, 1962.

Yuodelis RA, Weaver JD, and Sapkos S: Facial and lingual contours of artificial complete crown restorations and their effect on the periodontium, J Prosthet Dent 29:61, 1973.

Zachrisson BU: Cause and prevention of injuries to teeth and supporting structures during orthodontic treatment, Am J Orthod 69:285, 1976.

Zachrisson BU and Alnaes L: Periodontal condition in orthodontically treated and untreated individuals. I. Loss of attachment, gingival pocket depth and clinical crown height, Angle Orthod 43:402, 1973.

Zachrisson BU and Alnaes L: Periodontal condition in orthodontically treated and untreated individuals. II. Alveolar bone loss: radiographic findings, Angle Orthod 44:48, 1974.

Zachrisson S and Zachrisson BU: Gingival condition associated with orthodontic treatment, Angle Orthod 42:26, 1972.

Chapter 14

PATHOGENESIS AND HOST RESPONSES IN PERIODONTAL DISEASE

Robert J. Genco

The pathogenesis of periodontal disease is a sequence of processes from health to the formation of characteristic lesions, including periodontal pocket formation, loss of the gingival and periodontal connective tissue attachments, and loss of the tooth-supporting alveolar bone. The recognition that periodontal diseases are infections is important in understanding their pathogenesis. *Infection* is defined as the process by which pathogenic microorganisms penetrate or invade the tissues or organs of the body and cause injury followed by reactive phenomena. For most forms of periodontal infection, organisms are present in the periodontal pocket, and hence the pocket can be considered to be infected. Penetration of *Bacteroides gingivalis* into the pocket epithelium has been documented in adult periodontitis. Bacterial penetration of ulcerated gingival lesions occurs in acute necrotizing ulcerative gingivitis (ANUG) and in the deep gingival connective tissues in localized juvenile periodontitis (LJP). Periodontal diseases are therefore infections caused by organisms whose products penetrate into the gingival connective tissue; furthermore, in some forms of the disease bacteria appear to penetrate or invade the deep gingival connective tissue. Plaque bacteria grow at the orifice of the gingival crevice, which sets the stage for periodontal pathogens to colonize the subgingival area, leading to the development of periodontal pockets and subsequent loss of the connective tissue and bony attachment to the tooth.

Bacteria are the primary causative agents of gingivitis and the various forms of periodontitis. Bacteria in dental plaques that accumulate at the gingival margin cause the early forms of gingivitis and also possibly moderately progressing periodontitis. These plaque organisms, by and large, may be part of the indigenous microflora, which overgrow and induce inflammation by their presence at the margin of the gingiva, which normally has a sparse flora in health. On the other hand, unusual forms of gingivitis, such as ANUG, and rapid and severe forms of periodontal disease are associated with specific bacteria or combinations of specific bacteria in the subgingival flora adjacent to rapidly progressing lesions. For example, in most patients with adult periodontitis there are large numbers of *B. gingivalis,* whereas in LJP, *Actinobacillus actinomycetemcomitans* is a primary pathogen. *Bacteroides intermedius* and *Actinobacillus* are also found in some patients with adult periodontitis. Other oral organisms, including *Wolinella recta, Bacteroides forsythus, Eikenella corrodens, Fusobacterium nucleatum, Eubacterium* species, *Peptostreptococcus micros, Capnocytophaga,* and spirochetes, have also been implicated as periodontal pathogens. *B. gingivalis* and *A. actinomycetemcomitans* are generally not a significant part of the normal oral flora. They can be thought of as exogenous or foreign pathogens whose colonization of the subgingival area is indicative, and most likely causative, of periodontitis. Knowing which specific organisms are found in different forms of periodontal disease has been essential in understanding the host response to these organisms (Genco et al., 1988).

Many host responses are unique, since they involve antibodies or cellular immune reactions directed to specific bacterial antigens. It is recognized that many of the specific bacteria associated with periodontal disease are gram-negative anaerobes, which can cause periodontal destruction. Many of the periodontal bacteria are virulent when they enter the body and colonize tissues or surfaces. For example, *A. actinomycetemcomitans* is found in actinomycotic lesions of the jaws in association with *Actinomyces* species. *A. actinomycetemcomitans* can also cause brain abscesses and subacute bacterial endocarditis. *B. gingivalis* is a serious pathogen of humans that can cause brain and lung abscesses and dissecting infections of the head and neck, which may be fatal. It is clear, then, that the host response to periodontal pathogens plays a major role in localizing these organisms to the periodontium, preventing their spread to other areas of the body where they cause fulminating and often fatal infections. Serious systemic infections with periodontal bacteria are rare; hence the host's protective responses are effective. However, a common result of infections with the pathogenic periodontal microflora is localized destruction of the connective tissue and alveolar bone supporting the teeth, which we know as periodontal disease. Hence, the net effect of the host responses to the organisms causing periodontal infections is localization of tissue destruction to the periodontium and *protection* from extensive local or systemic infections with these pathogens.

HISTOPATHOLOGY OF PERIODONTAL DISEASES

Gingivitis affects over one half of the adult population in the United States. Gingivitis in many remains stable and does not proceed to periodontitis. However, in some individuals gingivitis does proceed to periodontitis. It is not yet predictable which patient or which site will progress from gingivitis to periodontitis; however, the progression is frequent, since some form of periodontitis is found in 70% of adults. All of the factors needed to initiate periodontitis are not known, but it is likely that colonization of the subgingival flora with sufficient levels of virulent pathogens, such as *B. gingivalis, A. actinomycetemcomitans,* some forms of *B. intermedius,* and other periodontal pathogens as yet to be described, is responsible. A summary of the histologic and ultrastructural changes in gingivitis and periodontitis is given in Table 14-1. An understanding of the histopathology of periodontal diseases in humans comes from four sources: (1) studies of normal periodontal tissues, (2) studies of histologic changes in experimentally induced gingivitis in humans, (3) studies of established or spontaneous gingivitis lesions, and (4) studies of established periodontitis lesions.

Normal periodontal tissues

When the dentogingival junction of humans and animals is kept relatively free of dental plaques, very few leukocytes are found in the gingival sulcus, the junctional epithelium, or the underlying gingival connective tissue (Attström et al., 1975; Payne et al., 1975; Schroeder et al., 1975). Under plaque-free conditions, the gingival sulcus may be very shallow (<1 mm), and very few round cells such as lymphocytes and plasma cells are found in the connective tissue (Attström et al., 1975; Payne et al., 1975). The junctional epithelium in health does not have rete pegs and is supported by highly oriented connective tissue bundles (Page et al., 1974; Attström et al., 1975). Histologically, normal gingiva is found only adjacent to plaque-free dentitions. This state of gingival health with few or no round cells in the connective tissue is probably rare. The usual condition in humans is characterized by varying levels of plaque accumulation, causing subclinical changes in the gingiva, such as round cell infiltrate of the connective tissue and rete peg formation of the junctional epithelium. This condition is what we designate as clinically healthy.

Experimental gingivitis

Starting from a clean tooth surface, plaque accumulation over a period of 2 to 3 weeks results in overt gingivitis in most subjects at most sites. The earliest changes detected microscopically and clinically are manifestations of vasculitis in the plexis of vessels lateral to the junctional epithelium. The junctional epithelium is infiltrated by large numbers of neutrophils that migrate from the gingival blood vessels subjacent to the junctional epithelium and the gingival sulcus. Macrophages and a few transforming lymphocytes also appear in the junctional epithelium and gingival connective tissue (Schroeder et al., 1975). At this early stage, large amounts of collagen are lost (Payne et al., 1975), and the gingival connective tissue subjacent to

Table 14-1. Histologic and ultrastructural findings in gingivitis and periodontitis

Diagnosis	Gingival crevice or pocket	Junctional or pocket epithelium	Gingival connective tissue attachment	Periodontal connective tissue attachment	Alveolar process
Normal	Few bacteria at orifice	Tight intercellular junctions, JE at CEJ	Supracrestal attachment intact	Intact	Intact
Early gingivitis	Complex flora fills gingival pocket	Widened intercellular spaces containing leukocytes; JE at CEJ	Loss of attachment; CT infiltrated by round cells, mainly lymphocytes	Intact	Intact
Chronic gingivitis	Complex flora fills gingival pocket; calculus may be present	Greater leukocytic infiltrate of JE, but JE still at CEJ	Loss of attachment; CT infiltrated by round cells, mainly plasma cells	Intact	Intact
Adult periodontitis	Subgingival flora contains specific pathogens; calculus to bottom of the pocket	JE apical to CEJ and converted to pocket epithelium	Loss of attachment; plasma cells predominant in CT	Loss of attachment of periodontal ligament; infiltrated with inflammatory cells; cemental resorption	Loss of crestal bone by osteoclastic resorption

the junctional epithelium is occupied by inflammatory cells. These changes begin after 2 to 4 days of accumulation of dental plaque, prior to overt manifestations of redness, bleeding, and gingival swelling, which would be termed *clinical gingivitis*. These early stages constitute subclinical gingivitis and may represent the common condition of the gingiva of humans resulting from the daily cycles of removal and accumulation of dental plaques at the gingival margin. Four to seven days after the initiation of experimental gingivitis, clinical signs of gingivitis, including redness, swelling, and bleeding on probing, are observed (Zachrisson, 1968). Histologically, the tissues are characterized by the accumulation of a dense lymphoid cell infiltrate in the gingival connective tissue subjacent to the junctional epithelium (Zachrisson, 1968; Payne et al., 1975). The junctional epithelial cells have widened intercellular spaces.

Lymphoid cells, mainly lymphocytes, constitute up to 75% of the total gingival connective tissue infiltrate in these early lesions. Most of the lymphocytes are T lymphocytes, with about 5% to 10% identified as B lymphocytes. Very few plasma cells are present, but when plasma cells are found, they are near the lateral and apical borders of the infiltrate. The infiltrated area may occupy from 5% to 15% of the connective tissue of the marginal gingival tissue (Schroeder et al., 1973), and collagen loss may reach 60% to 70% in this area, with a majority of fibroblasts manifesting histopathologic changes (Payne et al., 1975). Often the altered fibroblasts are associated with lymphoid cells and exhibit electron-lucent nuclei, swollen

mitochondria, and vacuolization of the endoplasmic reticulum with rupture of the cell membrane (Schroeder and Page, 1972; Newman et al., 1974; Simpson and Avery, 1974).

This early gingivitis is also characterized by increased gingival fluid flow with migration of crevicular leukocytes, mostly neutrophils, into the gingival fluid. The junctional epithelium develops widened intercellular spaces that are increasingly infiltrated by neutrophils and small numbers of mononuclear cells, especially monocytes (Lindhe et al., 1974).

Spontaneous, chronic gingivitis

The characteristic established lesion of chronic or spontaneous gingivitis differs markedly from the early stages of experimental gingivitis. The distinguishing feature of the chronic gingivitis lesion is the predominance of plasma cells (rather than lymphocytes) in the gingival connective tissue infiltrate, with inflammation limited to the soft tissues. There is no evidence of alveolar bone loss at this stage, or of apical migration of the junctional epithelium. This histologic picture is also seen after 14 to 21 days of cessation of oral hygiene in adults undergoing induction of experimental gingivitis (Zachrisson, 1968). Gingivitis at this point, and at all preceding stages, is reversible (Suomi et al., 1971). There is some evidence that established spontaneous gingivitis may become long-standing and not proceed to periodontitis in some patients at certain sites. However, it is also clear that periodontitis may occur at other sites in the same dentition, with destruction of alveolar bone and apical migration of the junctional epithelium. This has been documented in animals, where in time (6 to 18 months) destructive periodontitis appears if proper conditions of plaque accumulation are present (Saxe et al., 1967; Schroeder and Lindhe, 1975). It is likely that sensitive measurements of alveolar bone loss and attachment loss will show that this distinction may not be as clear as formerly thought. For example, in areas with gingival inflammation characterized as chronic gingivitis, low levels of marginal alveolar bone loss may be occurring, which is hard to detect clinically or radiographically and may even be reversible.

HISTOPATHOLOGY OF PERIODONTITIS LESIONS

By definition, periodontitis occurs when there is apical migration of the junctional epithelium from the cemento-enamel junction (CEJ) with loss of connective tissue attachment, and eventually loss of periodontal attachment and alveolar bone. This is easily determined histologically but very difficult to measure clinically, especially in its early stages. Loss of periodontal attachment can be detected clinically by probing from the CEJ. In later stages radiographically detectable loss of crestal alveolar bone occurs; however, often 50% to 60% of the alveolar crestal mass of bone has to be lost before it is clearly detectable on standard periapical or bitewing radiographs. The clinical and histologic hallmarks of adult periodontitis include apical migration of the epithelial attachment, the presence of gingival or periodontal pockets (often with suppuration and ulceration of the pocket epithelium), and associated alveolar bone loss. These changes may be present in areas where resolution of superficial gingivitis and fibrosis of the gingiva has taken place.

Periodontitis appears to be site specific and episodic, undergoing cycles of active destruction and remission. The long-term course of periodontitis, however, is often a net progressive destruction of the connective tissue attachment, periodontal ligament, and alveolar bone. The process progresses in an episodic manner over months or years, which varies markedly in rate among patients. In some patients it may lead to extensive periodontal attachment loss, tooth mobility, pathologic migration of teeth with spacing, and, eventually, tooth exfoliation. Periodontal abscesses are also seen in areas of severe periodontal pocket formation.

The inflammatory cell infiltrate of the gingival connective tissue adjacent to areas of periodontal attachment and alveolar bone loss contains mainly plasma cells and macrophages, with few lymphocytes. There are also variable, but low, numbers of neutrophils in the connective tissue. The neutrophils are found mainly in the pocket and between the epithelial cells lining the pocket, as well as around the blood vessels subjacent to the pocket. There is reduction in the collagen of the gingival connective tissue

subjacent to the pocket wall; however, fibrosis may be seen peripheral to this region. Bone resorption may be cyclic and variable (McHenry et al., 1981; Hausmann and McHenry, 1982), leading to net destruction of alveolar supporting bone. Clinically detectable root resorption is uncommon but may be seen, especially adjacent to deep pockets in severe lesions. However, microscopic evidence of resorption of the root surfaces adjacent to periodontal pockets is common.

Alterations of the connective tissue of the gingiva and the periodontal ligament are severe. There is a net reduction in soluble matrix collagen and an increase in the amounts of poorly cross-linked collagen, which is soluble. An inflammatory type collagen, the type I trimer, appears in inflamed gingiva. As a result of the loss of integrity of the gingival connective tissue matrix, the gingiva may detach from the tooth, forming a pocket that is almost always filled with dental plaque and calculus reaching to the bottom of the pocket.

Frank (1980) has proposed that microulceration of the pocket epithelium allows bacteria to directly invade periodontal tissues in severe adult periodontitis. There is invasion of the gingival connective tissue by *A. actinomycetemcomitans* in LJP patients (Christersson et al., 1987a, 1987b) and invasion of the pocket epithelium and connective tissue subjacent to the pocket epithelium by *B. gingivalis* in patients with adult periodontitis (Albini et al., 1988).

MECHANISM OF TISSUE DESTRUCTION

Several mechanisms may operate alone or cooperatively to produce the destruction of periodontal tissues. These tissue destructive mechanisms may be classified as direct or indirect. *Direct* mechanisms result from the actions of bacterial components that damage tissue directly. In contrast, *indirect* mechanisms are destructive host responses often triggered by the infecting organisms.

Direct effects

Factors elaborated by microorganisms that can damage tissue directly include histolytic enzymes, endotoxins, exotoxins, and factors that are not toxic but interfere with cell function. An example of histolytic enzymes are the proteases, including collagenase produced by *B. gingivalis*. This collagenase is capable of hydrolyzing native collagen to small fragments, contributing to destruction of the connective tissue attachment. *B. gingivalis* also produces potent proteases that can hydrolyze host components such as complement, immunoglobulins, fibrin, protease inhibitors, tissue procollagenases, and the clotting factors. Other bacterial enzymes such as hyaluronidase, which hydrolyzes tissue hyaluronic acid, and lipases and carbohydrates may also be operative in the pathogenesis of periodontal diseases. *A. actinomycetemcomitans* produces a toxin that kills human neutrophils, and to a lesser extent, monocytes

(Baehni et al., 1979). Other plaque substances that exhibit cytotoxicity or destructive effects on cells include mucopeptides, ammonia, hydrogen sulfide, indole, toxic amines, and formic and butyric acids. Bacterial components such as endotoxin, lipoteichoic acid, and other molecules are potent stimulators of bone resorption.

Indirect effects

It is clear that the candidate periodontal pathogens such as *B. gingivalis* and *A. actinomycetemcomitans* are virulent and can cause extensive tissue destruction directly. They are also capable of triggering host destructive mechanisms that amplify their local destructive effects. The indirect, or host-mediated, tissue destruction effects result from induction, stimulation, or activation of host cells or humoral factors, which then lead to local periodontal tissue destruction. Many of these are immunologic processes resulting in pathologic alterations of fibroblasts, activation of macrophages with release of collagenase and other hydrolytic enzymes, activation of lymphocytes, modulation of fibroblast growth and synthesis of collagen, and bone resorption stimulated by products of activated mononuclear cells, such as interleukin-1, prostaglandins, tumor necrosis factor (TNF), and other endogenous bone resorption factors.

BONE RESORPTION: LOCALIZED VERSUS SYSTEMIC

Bone resorption is a term given to the cellular removal of mineral and matrix components from bone. In healthy adult bone there is an overall equilibrium between bone resorption and the formation of new bone, and these two coupled processes constitute bone turnover. Disturbance of this equilibrium leads to either a net increase or a decrease of bone mass. Bone resorption is a necessary component of normal physiologic remodeling of the bone. It is more rapid in cancellous bone than in dense cortical bone. Bone remodeling in health is under the control of several hormones, including parathyroid hormone, vitamin D metabolites, calcitonin, sex steroids, glucocortoids, and growth hormones. Bone resorption is also influenced by local factors such as mechanical stress and prostaglandins.

Bone resorption as a pathologic process occurs when the balance between resorption and deposition is upset, with more resorption than deposition. When such an imbalance occurs systemically, it is called *osteoporosis*, which results in a generalized loss of bone mass. When the rate of loss exceeds the rate of deposition in a localized area, it is usually caused by local factors, including prostaglandins and the cytokines IL-1 and TNF. Localized, prostaglandin- or cytokin-mediated bone resorption occurs in periodontal disease where the loss of alveolar supporting bone appears to be largely independent of systemic bone turnover.

Several mechanisms are involved in bone resorption in periodontal disease, and the relative importance of each in various patients and at various periodontal sites is not very well understood. It first should be noted that the alveolar process in subjects with teeth is relatively independent from systemic calcium depletion in the body. Moderate systemic calcium depletion does not cause marked resorption of the alveolar process comparable to that seen for other bones, including the body of the mandible. Nutritional secondary hyperparathyroidism, for example, does not result in marked loss of alveolar bony support in experimental animals, and there is no evidence that systemic abnormalities in calcium metabolism, except in the extreme, are a major reason for loss of alveolar bone in humans. The implication of these findings is that calcium therapy is probably of little value in either the prevention or the treatment of periodontal disease in the otherwise healthy patient.

Most of the bony changes seen in periodontal disease are related to the release of factors that act locally to stimulate bone resorption, inhibit bone deposition, or both, with the net effect of loss of alveolar bone. These local factors are (1) factors associated with periodontopathic bacteria and other components in plaque, (2) factors derived from the arachidonic acid pathway, and (3) the biologic response modifiers, such as interleukin-1 and TNF, which are triggered during periodontal inflammation.

Bacterial factors that stimulate bone resorption

Considerable evidence has accumulated over the last 20 years for the participation of bacterial components such as endotoxin and lipoteichoic acid as potent stimulators of bone resorption. There are probably other components of bacteria, such as peptidoglycan components, that can also exert direct effects on bone (Table 14-2). The effects of these bacterial factors are most likely mediated through osteoclasts and result in localized bone resorption.

Table 14-2. Bone resorption in periodontal disease

Source	Factor	Reference
Bacteria	Lipopolysaccharide	Hausmann et al. (1970)
	Lipoteichoic acid	Hausmann et al. (1975)
	Amphipathic molecule from *A. viscosus*	Hausmann et al. (1982)
	Peptidoglycans (MDP)	Raisz et al. (1982)
Gingival	High molecular weight factor	Goldhaber et al. (1973)
	PGE_2	Goodson et al. (1974)
	6-keto-PGF_α	Wong et al. (1980)
	IL-1 (OAF)	Horton et al. (1972) Dinarello (1988)
	TNF (tumor necrosis factor)	Dinarello (1988)

Products of the arachidonic pathway

Many of the products of arachidonic acid metabolism can cause bone resorption or alter bone deposition. One of the best studied is prostaglandin E_2 (PGE_2). PGE_2 is a potent stimulator of bone resorption and functions as such at concentrations that have been found in periodontal lesions (Table 14-2). PGE_2 is sensitive to the effects of prostaglandin synthetase inhibitors such as nonsteroidal antiinflammatory drugs, and there are experimental treatment regimens directed to interfering with periodontal bone resorption by administering these drugs. The effects of low levels of PGE_2, possibly even in enhancing bone formation, need to be evaluated fully before prostaglandin synthetase inhibitors can be safely used for treatment.

Inflammatory mediators

Inflammatory mediators are the cytokines, which include lymphokines and products of mononuclear, epithelial, and other cells. The cytokines are protein or polypeptide hormone-like substances that have many effects, including bone resorption. Interleukin-1 and TNF are two of the most potent cytokines that may play a role in localized bone resorption. It is clear that interleukin-1 and TNF can stimulate other changes seen in periodontal disease, such as fibrosis (Table 14-3). The net effects of the cytokines is most likely dependent on their concentration, time of appearance in the lesion, and activity of inhibitors.

STAGES IN THE PATHOGENESIS OF HUMAN PERIODONTAL DISEASE

Recent advances in our understanding of the tissue changes and the host-bacterial interactions occurring in periodontal diseases led us to propose four stages in the pathogenesis of periodontal disease (Genco and Slots, 1984; Slots and Genco, 1984). This scheme helps to organize information about the pathogenesis of periodontal disease, as well as to expose areas of incomplete knowledge. The division of the pathogenesis of periodontal disease into these four operational stages may lead to approaches for intervention to prevent or treat the disease at a susceptible stage. The stages in the pathogenesis of human periodontal disease are (1) colonization, (2) invasion, (3) destruction, and (4) healing. They are shown graphically in Fig. 14-1.

Colonization

Initially a salivary pellicle is deposited onto the enamel or cementum surface. This pellicle soon becomes colonized by organisms such as *Streptococcus sanguis* and *Actinomyces* species, which bind both specifically and nonspecifically to the pellicle-coated surface. In turn, other organisms bind to these lightly colonized tooth surfaces. Once attached to the tooth surface, the organisms grow and the plaque mass increases. The plaque also progresses apically by bacterial growth and by migration of motile or-

Table 14-3. Biologic response modifiers of importance in periodontal diseases

Biological property	Interleukin-1	Tumor necrosis factor
Systemic effects		
Fever	+	+
Hepatic acute-phase proteins	+	+
Slow-wave sleep	+	+
In vitro effects		
Decreased lipoprotein lipase	+	+
Endothelial cell activation	+	+
Fibroblast proliferation	+	+
PGE_2 production*	+	+
Bone resorption*	+	+
Collagen synthesis	+	+
Induction of IL-2, other cytokines	+	+
Cytotoxicity*	+	+
Neutrophil superoxide stimulation	−	+
T-lymphocyte activation	+	±

From Dinarello CA: FASEB J 2:108, 1988.
*Effects where strong synergism between the two cytokines has been seen.

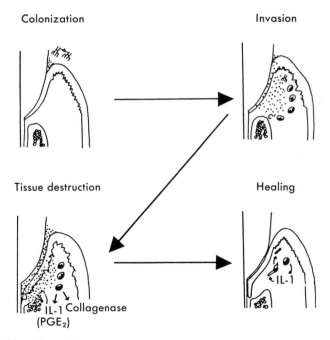

Fig. 14-1. Stages in pathogenesis of periodontal disease. Symbols include secretory IgA antibodies in colonization stage, and serum antibodies and complement (C′) in invasion stage.

ganisms. Gingival fluid, growth factors, and chemotactic factors draw spirochetes to migrate into the gingival crevice or the periodontal pocket. Similarly, the motility of other organisms allows them to migrate apically into the gingival crevice or periodontal pocket. Among the motile organisms found in the periodontal pocket are gliding organisms such as *Capnocytophaga* and flagellated anaerobic *Vibrios*. Organisms that colonize the subgingival area have mechanisms to attach to the tooth, the pocket epithelium, or other organisms, since they must resist the outward flow of gingival fluid.

Invasion

At this stage, whole organisms, components of organisms such as blebs, and/or their products penetrate or invade the gingiva through the sulcus or the pocket epithelium. These bacteria or their products penetrate the connective tissue to a variable extent, even to the surface of the alveolar bone. Bacterial penetration appears to be limited in most forms of periodontal disease; however, invasion of the deep gingival connective tissue by viable *A. actinomyectemcomitans* has been regularly observed in LJP (Christersson et al., 1987a, 1987b). In most gingival biopsy specimens taken from patients with LJP, *A. actinomycetemcomitans* can be demonstrated immunologically and ultrastructurally within the deep gingival connective tissue adjacent to infected periodontal pockets (Christersson et al., 1987a, 1987b). It is also well known that bacteria, particularly spirochetes, invade the tissue in ANUG. In adult periodontitis, *B. gingivalis* is found in the spaces between the pocket epithelial cells and in the connective tissues immediately below the epithelium, but not often in deep connective tissues, even in biopsy specimens taken from lesions undergoing active progressive breakdown in patients with adult periodontitis (Albini et al., 1988). Penetration of the tissue by bacterial antigens is suggested by the systemic immune responses seen that are specific to suspected periodontal pathogens in the subgingival flora. Bacterial antigens most likely penetrate or adhere to the tissues in order to induce an immune response. It is reasonable, then, that antigens, including molecules, such as collagenase, and macromolecular toxins, such as endotoxin, enter gingival tissues, where they trigger host responses and cause direct tissue destruction.

Destruction

Once the organism or the products of the organism have penetrated the tissue, destruction may ensue. There are two groups of mechanisms that account for tissue destruction: (1) *direct* effects of bacteria or their products and (2) *indirect*, or host-mediated, effects. Direct toxic effects, such as those exerted by exotoxins or histolytic enzymes such as bacterial collagenase, lead to periodontal tissue destruction. In addition, host-mediated toxic products and reactions are triggered by bacterial components, which then lead to tissue destruction. An example of this is the triggering of macrophages to produce collagenase by plaque bacterial endotoxins. Another example is bacterial triggering of cellular immune responses with local release of cytokines such as interleukin-1, and prostaglandin PGE_2, leading to bone resorption.

Healing

In the healing stage, resolution of inflammation and healing of the periodontal tissues occur. Very little is known about this stage; however, it is clear from histopathologic and clinical studies that periodontal disease is episodic, going through periods of exacerbation and remission. Periods of remission are characterized by reduction of inflammation, restoration of gingival collagenous tissues, and often gingival fibrosis. Changes in the alveolar bony contours, with remodeling and formation of radiographically apparent sclerotic linings of infrabony pockets, occurs during remission, suggesting that healing has occurred. Spontaneous healing in remission seldom restores lost alveolar crestal height or connective tissue attachment. These remain as evidence of previous periodontitis.

Although four distinct stages in the pathogenesis of periodontal disease can be described, the time sequence of these changes is complex. Colonization most likely precedes all other stages, but tissue invasion and tissue destruction may occur together. Tissue invasion may be transient, immediately preceding the tissue destructive phase, but tissue invasion may continue, resulting in progression of the periodontal lesion. Factors that affect tissue invasion, such as increased permeability of the gingiva, are likely to be important in initiating periodontitis. The healing stage is clearly distinct from both colonization and tissue invasion, and terminates tissue destruction.

COMPONENTS OF THE IMMUNE SYSTEM

Components of the immune system that have been shown to be operative in one or another of these stages in the pathogenesis of periodontal disease are listed in Table 14-4. They include the secretory immune system, the antibody-neutrophil-complement axis, and the lymphocyte-macrophage-lymphokine axis. Other systems such as IgE-mediated immediate hypersensitivity and immunoregulatory systems also may play a role in periodontal disease.

Secretory immune system

The secretory immune system consists of mucosa-associated lymphoid tissues such as Peyer's patches and local IgA-containing cells. IgA antibodies appear as the predominant antibodies in secretions such as saliva, which bathe mucosal surfaces.

Neutrophil-antibody-complement axis

The neutrophil-antibody-complement system comprises the phagocytic blood and tissue neutrophilic polymorpho-

Table 14-4. Principal components of immune systems affecting periodontal infections

System	Main functions in periodontal diseases	Cells	Humoral components	Mediators
Secretory immune	Reduce bacterial colonization of mucosal surfaces	Mucosa-associated lymphoid tissues (e.g., Peyer's patch), and local IgA-plasma cells	Secretory antibodies, mainly sIgA	—
Neutrophil, antibody, complement	Bactericidal; also secretory, producing extracellular enzymes and reactive oxygen species	Neutrophils, plasma cells	IgG antibodies; complement, especially C3	Bactericidal activity, reactive oxygen species, and granule components
Lymphocyte, macrophage, lymphokine	Tissue destruction	T- and B-effector cells, macrophages, and monocytes	—	Cytokines (TNF, Il-1, Il-2), macrophage enzymes (e.g., collagenase), and reactive oxygen species

nuclear granulocytes. These cells are highly mobile, and large numbers migrate from the gingival blood vessels through the gingival connective tissue and epithelium into the gingival crevice or periodontal pockets, and finally into the oral cavity. Ninety-five percent of the cells found in the gingival fluid are neutrophils. The neutrophils phagocytoses and kills organisms and hence to some extent regulates the subgingival flora. Neutrophils also probably limit the invasion of subgingival organisms into the tissue.

The neutrophil acts in concert with antibodies and complement in phagocytosis and killing of bacteria. IgG antibodies produced locally and derived from the blood coat the organisms, and the IgG-coated organism then binds to neutrophil surface receptors via the Fc portion of IgG. This enhances phagocytosis. Serum or locally derived IgM antibodies may also coat the organisms. When this occurs, the coated organisms bind components of the complement system, particularly the third component of complement, C3. There is a receptor for a fragment of C3 called C3b on the neutrophil, which binds the C3b opsonin on the bacteria and results in enhanced phagocytosis of the complement-coated organism. The antibody-complement-coated bacteria is phagocytosed very efficiently as compared with uncoated bacteria.

Once the bacteria are phagocytosed by the neutrophils, they can be killed intracellularly by oxidative or nonoxidative mechanisms. The neutrophil oxidative killing mechanisms involve the activity of reactive oxygen species such as hydrogen peroxide, the superoxide ion, and possibly hydroxyl radicals. The hydrogen peroxide effects may be inhibited by catalase, produced either by the organism or the neutrophil. On the other hand, neutrophil hydrogen peroxide–dependent killing is enhanced by myeloperoxidase, which in the presence of chloride forms the hypochlorous ions, which is highly antimicrobial. It is the

same ion that exerts antimicrobial effects in chlorinated water. Nonoxidative intracellular killing of organisms results from the action of neutrophil components such as lysozyme, lactoferrin, and the cathepsins, which kill directly in the absence of oxygen and would be expected to be important in anaerobic environments.

Lymphocyte-macrophage-lymphokine axis

The lymphocyte-macrophage-lymphokine axis consists mainly of effector T lymphocytes, which exert a variety of functions, including killing of target cells. T-helper and T-suppressor lymphocytes regulate both T-effector cell activity and the production of antibodies by B lymphocytes. Macrophages function as antigen-processing and antigen-presenting cells and can also act as effector cells by the production of substances such as collagenase. Macrophages are subject to control by the products of T lymphocytes. Lymphocytes, when stimulated either specifically by antigens or nonspecifically by mitogens such as lipopolysaccharide, produce highly active substances called lymphokines, such as interleukin-2. In addition, stimulated macrophages secrete a lymphokine, interleukin-1, as well as PGE_2. Activated macrophages can release enzymes and reactive-oxygen species that cause tissue destruction.

HOST RESPONSES

In Table 14-5 the stages of periodontal disease are depicted, and important host responses are summarized for each stage. In the *colonization* stage, antibody-mediated inhibition of adherence may play a decisive role in determining which organisms colonize the gingival margin and eventually become a part of the subgingival microflora. Antibodies of the secretory IgA class can be expected to exert effects on the early colonizing organisms. Later, in the presence of gingival inflammation, gingival fluid anti-

Table 14-5. Host responses operative in each stage in the pathogenesis of periodontal diseases

Stage of disease	Host factors
Colonization	Antibody-mediated inhibition of adherence; sIgA and gingival fluid antibodies limit colonization
Invasion	Neutrophil chemotaxis, phagocytosis, and bactericidal activity, with opsonic effects of antibody and C′ protect against periodontal infections; macrophage bactericidal activity and extracellular killing may also be protective
Destruction	Toxic effects on tissues of lymphocytes and macrophages exerted via cytokines and toxic phagocyte products such as collagenase and reactive oxygen species
	Direct toxic effects of bacteria controlled by antibodies, which neutralize toxins and enzymes
Healing	Bacteria and bacterial products removed by phagocytes
	Cytokines (Il-1), which may result in repair of connective tissue and epithelium

bodies, which are serum derived as well as locally produced, may further limit colonization of the subgingival area by periodontopathic organisms. Antibodies exert their effect on colonization by inhibiting adherence of organisms, leading to clearing into the gastrointestinal tract. In addition, plasma-derived or locally produced IgG and IgM antibodies in the gingival fluid can lead to antibody-complement–mediated bactericidal activity or to opsonization with removal by phagocytosis.

The neutrophil-antibody-complement axis is thought to exert a net protective role against the pathogenic periodontal bacteria, primarily through the ability of this system to limit tissue penetration by the organisms. There is considerable evidence that neutrophils are important in protecting against the periodontal microflora. For example, patients with compromised neutrophil numbers or neutrophil function, such as those with agranulocytosis, the Chediak-Higashi syndrome, or diabetes, are known to have severe periodontal disease (Van Dyke et al., 1985). Furthermore, in severe forms of periodontal disease in juveniles, such as LJP, neutrophil chemotaxis is depressed (Cianciola et al., 1977).

Periodontopathic organisms often have virulence factors that allow then to evade neutrophil protective mechanisms (Slots and Genco, 1984). It appears that in the absence of neutrophils, periodontal organisms or their products invade the tissue at a much greater rate. Hence under normal circumstances the neutrophils and their accessory factors, antibodies and complement, are likely to exert critical protective effects in preventing or limiting invasion of the tissue by periodontal pathogens.

The lymphocyte-macrophage-lymphokine axis, on the other hand, has a potential to exert marked pathologic effects and may contribute to the loss of periodontal tissues seen in the destructive phase. Lymphocytes activated by antigens or mitogens of the periodontal pathogens can stimulate the production of lymphokines (Genco and Slots, 1984). Stimulation of macrophages, either by bacterial products or by the lymphokine interleukin-2, results in the production of collagenase, which leads to dissolution of tissue collagen. Stimulation of macrophages by lymphokines or bacterial products can lead to production of reactive-oxygen species that are toxic to local cells. Furthermore, stimulated macrophages may produce interleukin-1 and PGE_2, which play a role in bone resorption. The potential, then, is clear for the lymphocyte-macrophage axis to exert pathogenic effects when stimulated by invading organisms or their products. Hyperreactive lymphocytes or macrophages, either genetically determined or locally activated, may result in accelerated peridontal destruction.

The role of host responses in the healing stage of periodontal disease is largely unknown; however, certain speculations can be made. It is reasonable that for remission and healing of a periodontal lesion to occur, the organisms and their products must largely by removed from the tissues. Tissue macrophages may play a role as scavengers in removing organisms, as well as in removing damaged tissue components. In addition, it is clear that there are cytokines, such as interleukin-1, that may stimulate the production of collagen and proliferation of fibroblasts, leading to regeneration of gingival and periodontal ligament collagen and eventually to gingival fibrosis, which often characterizes the healing stage. Interleukin-1 is produced by inflammatory cells such as macrophages and also by other cells, including the resident keratinocytes, and hence may play a role after the round cell infiltrate had been resolved.

SUMMARY

Great progress has been made in our understanding of the pathogenesis of periodontal disease, the primary role of bacterial etiologic agents, and the critical modifying role of host responses. In the absence of control of the virulence of periodontopathic organisms by the host, these organisms produce serious fulminating systemic infections. However, it is also clear that the periodontium is often destroyed in this fight to protect the host from systemic infections. Intervention at critical stages in the pathogenesis of periodontal disease will be possible when more information is available. For example, vaccines that prevent colonization or enhance phagocytosis, antiinflammatory agents that may block tissue-destroying mechanisms, and drugs that enhance protective functions all hold promise for future therapy and prevention.

Chapter 14 Pathogenesis and host responses in periodontal disease   **193**

REFERENCES

Albini B et al: Bacteria in periodontal tissues in adult periodontitis, J Dent Res 67(special issue), 1988 (abstract 794).

Attström R et al: Clinical and stereologic characteristics of normal gingiva, J Periodont Res 10:115, 1975.

Baehni P et al: Interaction of inflammatory cells and oral microorganisms. VIII. Detection of leukotoxic activity of a plaque derived Gram-negative organism, Infect Immun 24:233, 1979.

Christersson LA et al: Tissue localization of *Actinobacillus actinomycetemcomitans* in human periodontitis. I. Light, immunofluorescence and electron microscopic studies, J Periodontol 58:529, 1987a.

Christersson LA et al: Tissue localization of *Actinobacillus actinomycetemcomitans* in human periodontitis. II. Correlation between immunofluorescence and culture techniques, J Periodontol 58:540, 1987b.

Cianciola LJ et al: Defective polymorphonuclear leukocyte function in a human periodontal disease, Nature 265:445, 1977.

Dinarello CA: Biology of interleukin 1, FASEB J 2:108, 1988.

Frank RM: Bacterial penetration in the apical pocket wall of advanced human periodontitis, J Periodont Res 15:63, 1980.

Genco RJ: Pathogenesis of periodontal disease: new concepts, J Can Dent Assoc 5:391, 1984.

Genco RJ and Slots J: Host responses in periodontal diseases, J Dent Res 63:441, 1984.

Genco RJ, Zambon JJ, and Christersson LA: The origin of periodontol infections, Adv Dent Res 2(2):245, 1988.

Goldhaber P et al: Bone resorption in tissue culture and its relevance to periodontal disease, J Am Dent Assoc 87(special issue):1027, 1973.

Goodson JM, Dewhirst FE, and Brunetti A: Prostaglandin E_2 levels and human periodontal disease, Prostaglandins 6:81,1974.

Hausmann E et al: Structural requirements for bone resorption by endotoxin and lipoteichoic acid, J Dent Res 54(special issue B):94, 1975.

Hausmann E and McHenry KR: Alveolar bone mass measurements by ^{125}I absorptiometry in untreated periodontal patients: proceedings of international symposium on osteoporosis, Chichester, UK, 1982, John Wiley & Sons, Ltd.

Hausmann E, Raisz LG, and Miller WA: Endotoxin stimulation of bone resorption in tissue culture, Science 168:862, 1970.

Hausmann E et al: Partial purification and characterization of the bone resorption factor from *Actinomyces viscosus,* Calcif Tissue Int 34:53,1982.

Horton JE et al: Bone resorbing activity in supernatant fluid from cultured human peripheral blood leukocytes, Science 177:793, 1972.

Lindhe J et al: Clinical and stereologic analysis of the course of early gingivitis in dogs, J Periodont Res 9:314, 1974.

McHenry KR et al: [125]I absorptiometry: alveolar bone loss measurements in untreated periodontal patients, J Dent Res 60(special issue A), 1981, (abstract 306).

Newman MG, Socransky SS, and Listgarten MA: Relationship of microorganisms to the etiology of periodontosis, J Dent Res 53(special issue), 1974, (abstract 324).

Page RC, et al: Collagen fibre bundles of the normal marginal gingiva in the marmoset, Arch Oral Biol 19:1039, 1974.

Payne WA et al: Histopathologic features of the initial and early stages of experimental gingivitis in man, J Periodont Res 10:51, 1975.

Raisz LG et al: Effects of two bacterial products, muramyl dipeptide and endotoxin, on bone resorption in organ culture, Calcif Tissue Int 34:365, 1982.

Saxe SR, Greene JC, and Bohannan HM: Oral debris, calculus, and periodontal disease in the beagle dog, Periodontics 5:217, 1967.

Schroeder HE, Graf-de Beer M, and Attström R: Initial gingivitis in dogs, J Periodont Res 10:128, 1975.

Schroeder HE and Lindhe J: Conversion of established gingivitis in dog into destructive periodontitis, Arch Oral Biol 20:775, 1975.

Schroeder HE, Munzel-Pedrazzoli S, and Page R: Correlated morphometric and biochemical analysis of gingival tissue in early chronic gingivitis in man, Arch Oral Biol 18:899, 1973.

Schroeder HE and Page RC: Lymphocyte-fibroblast interaction in the pathogenesis of inflammatory gingival disease, Experientia 28:1228, 1972.

Simpson DM and Avery BE: Histopathologic and ultrastructural features of inflamed gingiva in the baboon, J Periodontol 45:500, 1974.

Slots J and Genco RJ: Black-pigmented *Bacteroides* species, *Capnocytophaga* species, and *Actinobacillus actinomycetemcomitans* in human periodontal disease: virulence factors in colonization, survival, and tissue destruction, J Dent Res 63:412, 1984.

Suomi JD, Smith LW, and McClendon BJ: Marginal gingivitis during a 16-week period, J Periodontol 42:268, 1971.

Van Dyke TE, Levine MJ, and Genco RJ: Neutrophil function and oral disease, J Oral Pathol 14:95, 1985.

Wong PYK, Ross JR, and Sticht FD: Metabolism of arachidonic acid in inflamed human gingivae. I. Formation of 6-keto-prostaglandin $F_{1\alpha}$, J Dent Res 59:670, 1980.

Zachrisson BU: A histological study of experimental gingivitis in man, J Periodont Res 3:293, 1968.

Chapter 15

ROLE OF OCCLUSION IN PERIODONTAL DISEASE

Leonard Abrams
Steven R. Potashnick

Occlusal analysis and therapy traditionally have been a part of periodontal treatment since the turn of the century when it was postulated that there was a relationship between occlusal stress and periodontitis. The relationship of occlusion to the pathogenesis of periodontal lesions and to periodontal therapy, however, was not clear until recently, and several theories were proposed to explain this relationship. For example, early workers (Stillman, 1917; Box, 1935) believed that excessive occlusal load on the dentition was a primary etiologic factor leading to pocket formation, gingival changes, and osseous and connective tissue destruction. These authors believed that occlusal trauma was therefore integral to periodontitis. Still others (Glickman, 1965) thought that occlusal stress led to angu-

lar defects or infrabony pockets by altering the pathway of spread of plaque-induced inflammation, and therefore that occlusal trauma was an aggravating factor in periodontal disease. A third concept, proposed by Waerhaug (1979), considered that excessive occlusal forces resulted in changes distinct from periodontitis and that there was little or no relationship between occlusal trauma and the changes associated with inflammatory or plaque-associated periodontitis. According to this school of thought there was no rationale for treating occlusion as part of the management of periodontal disease. Recent research has put much of this controversy to rest and we now have a clearer understanding of the effects that occlusal forces have on the periodontium and the relationship of these periodontal changes to inflammatory infectious periodontitis.

EVIDENCE OF OCCLUSAL TRAUMA

The periodontal attachment apparatus is the target for trauma from occlusion and manifests clinical, radiographic, and histologic changes when excessive occlusal loads are placed on the attachment apparatus (Goldman and Cohen, 1980). Tooth mobility is a clinical hallmark of occlusal traumatism. Widening of the periodontal ligament space, especially at the alveolar crest, which is often described as crestal funneling; alteration in furcation quality; and variations in the appearance of the lamina dura are noted radiographically with excessive occlusal loading. Clinical mobility per se depends on several factors. For example, it is affected by the height of the remaining alveolar bone around the tooth, the integrity of the surrounding tissues, and the level and repetitiveness of the force applied to the tooth. Root length, shape, and number and coronal form dictate crown-to-root ratios and therefore the mechanical resistance of the tooth to applied force.

When subjected to a force on the occlusal surface, the tooth moves about a fulcrum that is located within the clinical root length and is determined by the height of the remaining supporting alveolar bone. A tooth can move, however, only as far as the width of the ligament space allows, and then actual bone and possibly even tooth deformation occur. When occlusal forces become excessive because of their duration, magnitude, direction, distribution, or frequency, they may overwhelm the physical limitations of the periodontal ligament, which then becomes traumatized.

Histologically, a tooth subjected to occlusal trauma in the periodontal ligament space is seen to undergo a transient increase in vascularity, increase in vascular permeability, and osteoclastic resorption on the pressure side. Widening of the socket wall then occurs, as well as cemental resorption, resulting in a broader or wider periodontal ligament space. This often is an adaptive response, with widening of the socket allowing movement of the tooth out of trauma. When this occurs, there is no permanent vascular embarrassment to the ligament tissues. When traumatic forces continue, the tooth and the tissues of the attachment apparatus come to a level of accommodation that adapts to the chronic occlusal stress. Vasculitis resolves, and osteoclastic activity returns to within normal limits. Mobility of the tooth remains, and the ligament is widened; however, mobility does not grow progressively worse. The tooth may be displaced within its socket without additional damage to the tissues of the periodontal ligament at this point.

PRIMARY OCCLUSAL TRAUMA

A tooth subject to excessive occlusal forces but otherwise exhibiting health, with intact periodontal support, no loss of gingival connective tissue attachment, and no apical migration of junctional or sulcular epithelium is classically described as a tooth in pure, primary occlusal trauma. In Fig. 15-1 a tooth in primary occlusal traumatism can be seen during the trauma and after it has been removed. Teeth in primary occlusal traumatism may reach a state of stability in which mobility is no longer increasing and the clinical, radiographic, and histologic changes become no worse over time. Most likely, this rarely occurs in its pure form with a completely healthy periodontium.

Teeth that have adapted to occlusal stress and are mobile but do not experience increasing mobility with time may not necessarily require treatment. That is, mobility per se can be accepted as long as there are no symptoms, or as long as the tooth does not increase in mobility and the patient can function properly with the dentition. With a healthy periodontium (i.e., one showing no loss of gingival connective tissue or apical migration of the junctional epithelium) adaptive changes of the ligament and alveolar bone due to trauma from occlusion alone are reversible when the trauma is removed. These reversible changes are seen in Fig. 15-2. Under these circumstances, alveolar bone height and volume may be completely restored (Polson et al., 1976). In situations where an onlay has placed a tooth in occlusal trauma, the resulting widening of the periodontal ligament space and development of a periapical radiolucency are reversed by occlusal adjustment.

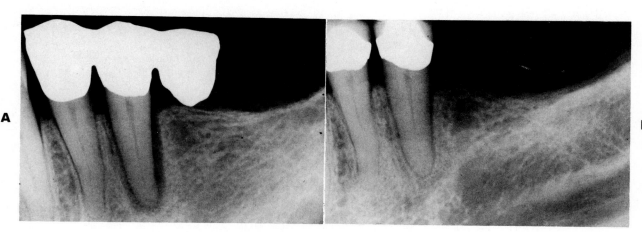

Fig. 15-1.   A, Radiograph of a patient presenting with discomfort and awareness of mobility around a three-unit cantilever splint. She was undergoing emotional stress and was aware of bruxing habit. **B,** Radiographic appearance 4 months after clinical presentation. Treatment consisted of immediate removal of cantilever unit followed by scaling and replacement of splint with two individual crowns. Note dramatic narrowing of periodontal ligament space. (Courtesy Dr. Richard Yamada, Chicago.) (From Potashnick S and Abrams L: Alpha Omegan 78:25, 1985.)

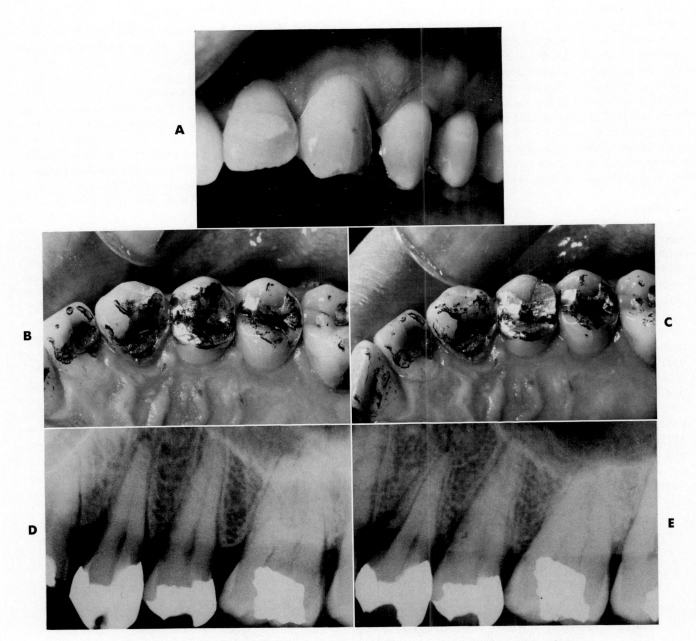

Fig. 15-2. **A,** Presenting appearance of a patient with a recently placed gold onlay on first premolar. Tooth was temperature sensitive, and patient was aware of parafunctional action on these teeth. Note wear facet on canine and length of buccal cusp of first premolar. **B,** Occlusal examination revealed working and balancing contacts. Onlay has "locked" tooth into position. **C,** Following occlusal adjustment by selective grinding of first premolar, working and balancing contacts have been removed and centric contacts are present in central fossa, marginal ridge, and on palatal cusp tip. Tooth is freed in lateral contacting movements while maintaining axially directed contact in maximum intercuspation. **D,** At initial presentation, depth of onlay on first premolar and widening at apex may easily be mistaken for changes of pulpal origin. Note widened ligament space and crestal funneling. What appears to be a mesial infrabony periodontal lesion probes within normal limits. **E,** View 8 months following occlusal adjustment. On first premolar note narrowing of ligament space, resolution of apical widening, and change in crestal morphology. (From Potashnick S and Abrams L: Alpha Omegan 78:25, 1985.)

SECONDARY OCCLUSAL TRAUMA

Secondary occlusal trauma is defined as occurring on a tooth having a major loss of support (e.g., with a reversed crown-to-root ratio), which is displaced in the remaining alveolus by any force applied to it, even the force of the tongue and cheek or of chewing soft foods. This often occurs where there has been loss of connective tissue attachment, as well as apical migration of the junctional epithelium, usually in association with infectious periodontitis. Secondary occlusal traumatism may occur with active periodontitis or may persist after the infectious periodontitis has been resolved. Again, the seriousness depends on whether or not the tooth is progressively, increasingly mobile; where a final judgment as to mobility cannot be reached, the tooth may have to be splinted.

OCCLUSAL TRAUMA AND PLAQUE-ASSOCIATED INFECTIOUS PERIODONTITIS

Trauma from occlusion may occur in the absence of, or concomitant with, infectious periodontitis. Infectious periodontitis can also occur in the absence or presence of occlusal trauma. The pathogenesis and lesions of various combinations of occlusal trauma and infectious periodontitis are discussed in this section.

Healthy periodontium

Trauma from occlusion on a healthy periodontium does not initiate gingival connective tissue attachment loss or create periodontal pocket formation. Trauma from occlusion as described above may result, however, in widening of the periodontal ligament space with loss of alveolar volume and possibly even loss of alveolar height if there is pressure on the alveolar crestal region. Since the maximum compressive stress occurs just apical to the alveolar crest as the tooth is intruded in the socket, there is often loss of alveolar crestal height. Since the tooth is a truncated cone, pressure would be greatest at the rim of the alveolar socket. This loss of both height and volume occurs in response to excessive occlusal loading and often leads to the development of an angular or vertical bony defect that is noted on the radiograph. This is not a pocket, since there is no loss of gingival connective tissue attachment or apical migration of the junctional or sulcular epithelium. It is simply loss of the alveolar crest. It is of considerable importance that widening of the periodontal ligament space and vertical alveolar crestal bone loss (funnel-shaped lesion) are completely reversible once the excessive occlusal stress has been removed. The lesion of the periodontal ligament associated with primary occlusal trauma in the absence of infectious periodontitis does not cause changes in the gingival connective tissue or the epithelium, probably because there is structural and functional independence of the periodontal and gingival blood circulation (Gaengler and Merte, 1983).

Is a tooth in occlusal trauma more susceptible to infectious periodontitis? It is clear that a tooth with a widened periodontal ligament and alveolar crestal bone loss due to occlusal stress that has occurred in the absence of periodontal infection is *not more susceptible* to plaque-induced inflammation and attachment loss. Connective tissue attachment loss around teeth with widened and normal periodontal ligament progresses at a rate that is independent of the mobility of the teeth and unrelated to periodontal ligament width (Ericsson and Lindhe, 1984). Another way of stating this is that the loss of connective tissue attachment is not related to the absence or presence of bony component of the periodontium (Nyman et al., 1984).

Furthermore, teeth with supporting tissues not infected by plaque that are markedly reduced because of previously treated periodontitis or apical resorption respond the same as those with intact periodontium. That is, there is no additional loss of attachment, adaptation will occur, and accommodation will be reached in the ligament tissues even though the reduction of alveolar bone height through previous periodontal disease may be marked (Lindhe and Ericsson, 1976). Indeed, it has been estimated that the reduction of alveolar bone height may have little effect on the degree of periodontal ligament stress until as much as 60% of the bone support has been lost (Reinhardt et al., 1984).

Plaque-induced inflammatory periodontitis

Periodontitis is an inflammatory disease caused by bacterial infection of the subgingival area. The tissue loss in inflammatory periodontitis is seen mainly in the supraalveolar soft connective tissue, with loss of gingival connective tissue attachment to the tooth and migration of the epithelium apical to the cementoenamel junction. Histologically, the supraalveolar connective tissue is infiltrated primarily by round cells; collagen has been resorbed; and the epithelium has migrated, proliferated, and may be ulcerated, forming a pocket wall. The region of inflammation subjacent to the subgingival plaque and calculus that results from periodontal infection is separate and distinct from the underlying lesion of trauma. The two lesions often are divided by a cell-poor, collagen-rich zone of connective tissue at or near the alveolar crest.

When trauma from occlusion is superimposed on plaque-induced inflammatory periodontitis, accommodation and adaption of the vascular and connective tissue attachment apparatus do not occur (Lindhe and Svanberg, 1974). However, vascularity and osteoclast activity remain elevated, and mobility of the tooth and the width of the ligament increase without approaching a stable plateau. There is an enhanced loss of alveolar bone height and volume as compared with inflammatory periodontitis alone. Plaque-associated inflammation in dog studies appears to prevent an accommodation of the attachment apparatus to jiggling-type occlusal forces. As a result, the mobility takes on an increasing character and does not reach a stable level (Lindhe and Svanberg, 1974; Lindhe and Nyman, 1977).

Control of trauma from occlusion may affect infrabony pocket formation in lesions in which trauma from occlusion is superimposed on plaque-induced periodontitis. It has been proposed that trauma from occlusion superimposed on plaque-induced periodontitis would lead to infrabony vertical pockets by altering the pathway of spread of plaque-induced inflammation (Macapanpan and Weinman, 1954; Glickman and Smulow, 1962) This proposed combined lesion with an altered pathway of spread of plaque-induced inflammation has been difficult to duplicate in animal models, and when shown to occur, it is in the presence of extremely high levels of force, in response to which the teeth may have actually been intruded in the jaw (Ericsson and Lindhe, 1982). Hence alteration of the pathway of spread of plaque-induced inflammation with diversion into the ligament space probably does not occur. The heavily infiltrated connective tissue associated with plaque-induced inflammation remains distinct from the changes occurring in the attachment apparatus in response to trauma from occlusion (Glickman and Smulow, 1962; Stahl, 1968).

Having shown that there is no alteration of the pathway of spread of plaque-induced inflammation with a coexisting lesion does not mean that there is no relationship between the two destructive processes. Indeed, vascular labeling is increased in the supraalveolar connective tissue when trauma is present and mobility is increasing in healthy or inflamed periodontal conditions. Changes in the extracellular matrix of the supraalveolar connective tissue can be measured with tritiated proline autoradiography (Svanberg and Lindhe, 1974; Simmons et al., 1979). The extent to which the vascular metabolic changes in the supraalveolar connective tissue in response to trauma from occlusion affect adaptation or periodontal ligament lesions is unclear. However, clinical experience suggests that a small number of patients are highly susceptible to the destructive capacity of plaque-induced infection combined with trauma from occlusion. Further research is needed to resolve this issue and to identify these susceptible patients.

Occlusal therapy and trauma control in periodontal inflammation

When trauma from occlusion is controlled in the presence of continued inflammation, a reduction in mobility is often noted. This occurs without restoration of marginal alveolar bone volume or accommodation of the periodontal ligament. Removal of occlusal interferences and the subsequent reduction in mobility without control of periodontal inflammation will not, however, improve the condition of the attachment apparatus (Polson et al., 1976). It is clear that the presence of gingival inflammation inhibits the po-tential for alveolar bone regeneration, although the lesions are histologically distinct. In experimental model systems, bone regeneration restoring volume and height of bone of the combined lesion (i.e., the lesion caused by bone loss and periodontitis) does not occur (Kantor et al., 1976).

Control of infective periodontitis without control of occlusal trauma. Vascular adaptation with incomplete bone regeneration occurs when inflammation is controlled but trauma from occlusion persists. Therefore bone regeneration may occur in the presence of continued active hypermobility if plaque-induced inflammation is resolved. The clinical implication is that if a healthy periodontium is maintained, a loose tooth will likely get no looser, and the periodontium will remain healthy unless reinfected.

Control of both marginal infection and occlusal trauma. Maximum repair of the periodontal ligament and alveolar regeneration often occur when both marginal infection and trauma from occlusion are controlled. This regeneration does not result in complete restoration of the original height of the tooth; however, the periodontal ligament space of the remaining periodontium may return to within normal limits. Therefore it is clear that maximum repair of the periodontal tissues is most likely to occur with the resolution of both infectious periodontitis and occlusal trauma.

EVALUATION OF THE ROLE OF OCCLUSION IN PERIODONTAL DISEASE

Clinical and radiographic parameters are measured to assess the role of occlusion in patients with periodontal disease. Mobility, fremitus, the presence of plaque-induced inflammation, the quality of the remaining support, and the radiographic signs of trauma from occlusion are assessed.

Mobility

Mobility is a measurement of horizontal and vertical tooth displacement created by the examiner's force. Blunt ends of two dental instruments are placed approximately at the buccal and lingual height of contour of the tooth, and forces are applied in the buccolingual direction. The horizontal mobility is assessed by comparing a fixed point on the tooth against a fixed point on the adjacent tooth. It is Class I, II, or III as follows:
Class I: Mobility less than 1 mm
Class II: Mobility within 1 to 2 mm
Class III: Mobility greater than 2 mm
Mobility can also be assessed in the axial direction. If a tooth is mobile in the axial direction, this is termed *depressible,* and most depressible teeth have a poor prognosis. Automated measurement of mobility can be carried out using a vibrating device (Periotest).*

*Siemans Corporation, Dental Division, 186 Wood Ave., S. Iselin, NJ 08830.

Fremitus

Fremitus is a measurement of the vibratory patterns of the teeth when the teeth are placed in contacting positions and movements. To measure fremitus, a dampened index finger is placed along the buccal and labial surfaces of the maxillary teeth. The patient is asked to tap the teeth together in the maximum intercuspal position and then grind systematically in the lateral, protrusive, and lateral protrusive contacting movements and positions. The teeth that are displaced by the patient in these jaw positions are then identified. Generally, this is limited to the maxillary teeth; however, in cases of edge-to-edge occlusion or when there is little overlap of the teeth, mandibular teeth can also be assessed. The following classification system is used:

Class I fremitus: Mild vibration or movement detected

Class II fremitus: Easily palpable vibration but no visible movement

Class III fremitus: Movement visible with the naked eye

Fremitus differs from mobility in that fremitus is tooth displacement created by the patient's own occlusal force. Therefore the amount of force varies greatly from patient to patient, unlike mobility, wherein the force with which it is measured tends to be the same for each examiner. Fremitus is a guide to the ability of the patient to displace and traumatize the teeth. If there is mobility but not fremitus, it is likely that there is sufficient movement of the tooth in the alveolus under occlusal loading to create the vascular embarrassment and other findings typical of occlusal traumatism.

Effects of antiinfective periodontal therapy on tooth mobility

Diagnosis of occlusal trauma, either primary or secondary, in a periodontal patient is not readily done in one appointment. It requires reevaluation after a sequence of initial therapeutic procedures. For example, loose teeth in a state of increased stable mobility or increasing and progressive mobility must be distinguished from one another. Teeth that are mobile in the presence of plaque-associated inflammation can tighten once this plaque-associated inflammation is resolved. The response of a patient to an appropriate sequence of therapy helps to distinguish between primary and secondary occlusal trauma and to determine the diagnosis and subsequent treatment needs. Unless there is overwhelming evidence of occlusal disease, such as a tooth that is in pain on occlusion with an obvious occlusal discrepancy, there is no need for aggressive occlusal management during the early stages of periodontal therapy. Also, it is not reasonable to establish a diagnosis of secondary occlusal trauma and subsequent need to splint by an assessment of the percentage of remaining alveolar bony support assigned to a tooth based on some hypothetical rule.

Active assessment of the role of occlusion and whether it threatens the dentition cannot be determined in the presence of plaque-induced inflammation. Control of infective periodontitis begins with patient personal plaque control instruction, scaling, root planing, and local systemic antibiotic medication where needed. After this course of therapy, with resolution of obvious inflammation and elimination of pathogenic microflora, reexamination of the occlusion is necessary.

There is often marked reduction in fremitus and mobility. Aggressive surgical curettage and surgical flap treatment should be avoided early in treatment if trauma from occlusion is suspected, since surgical therapy risks the removal of osteogenic connective tissue left at the expense of the widened periodontal ligament space. Loss of alveolar height and volume may occur by simple occlusal trauma in the absence of inflammatory disease. If, following initial resolution of inflammation, the teeth exhibit little decrease in previously recorded fremitus, or increase in fremitus or mobility in the absence of periodontal inflammation, there is reason to analyze the occlusion in greater detail. Now an evaluation of whether or not the mobility is not simply increased but stable, or increasing and progressive, can be made. Fig. 15-3 illustrates the effect of resolution of inflammation on mobility. In this patient scaling and root planing and the establishment of oral hygiene carried out prior to insertion of the provisional restoration resulted in reduction of mobility that ranged from I^+ to III before scaling to I^- to I after therapy. No occlusal therapy was needed, and the restorative work was completed to replace missing teeth and restore various teeth.

ANALYSIS OF OCCLUSAL FINDINGS

When fremitus and mobility patterns are correlated in both location and degree, this indicates that the existing occlusal arrangement is contributing a destructive role and that trauma from occlusion is present. If fremitus does not correlate, either by location or degree, with mobility or with occlusal discrepancies, trauma from occlusion is less likely. When fremitus and mobility correspond, but they are both less than expected, trauma from occlusion is still possible. Here, the percentage of remaining alveolar bone must be evaluated. Radiographic signs of trauma from occlusion may suggest an adverse response to occlusal activity.

If after resolution of the inflammation and reevaluation of the occlusion there is still doubt as to the role the occlusal forces may play, longitudinal monitoring is indicated. Fremitus, mobility, the degree of plaque-induced inflammation, and radiographic signs of trauma are recorded over a period of months, and possibly up to a year, to allow for full healing. This longitudinal record allows better evaluation of the role of trauma, if any, on the dentition.

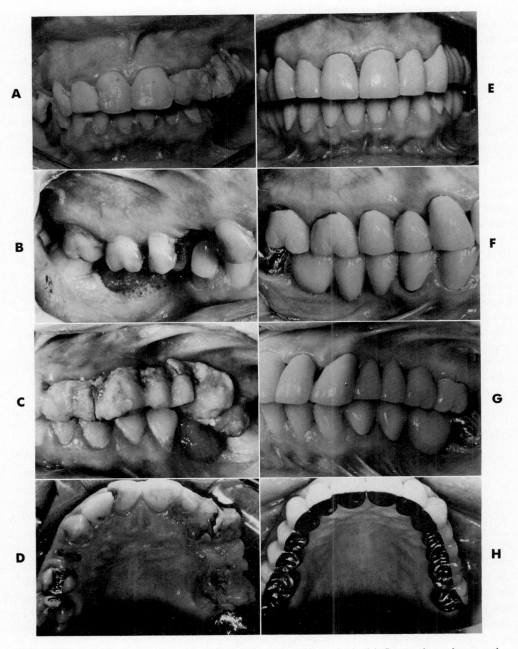

Fig. 15-3. A to **D,** Appearance on clinical presentation. Note gingival inflammation, plaque and calculus, extensive caries, and occlusal arrangement. **E** to **H,** View after final restoration. Note in occlusal view, **H,** that except for a three-unit bridge from Nos. 4 to 6, replacing No. 5, and a bridge from Nos. 10 to 15, replacing Nos. 12, 13, and 14, all crowns are individual units in maxillary arch. (From Potashnick S and Abrams L: Alpha Omegan 78:25, 1985.)

Physiologic and pathologic occlusions

Once the decision is made that occlusal trauma exists, an evaluation of the occlusal arrangement is made. Is it physiologic or pathologic? A *physiologic occlusion* is one that has demonstrated the ability to survive despite anatomic aberrations from the hypothetical normal or preconceived "ideal form" of occlusion and function. A physiologic occlusion may be an anatomic malocclusion, but it is a masticatory system functioning free of occlusally induced disease.

Pathologic occlusions, on the other hand, show evidence of disease attributable to occlusal activity. A pathologic occlusion is a dentition that often requires therapeutic alteration of the existing occlusion. This diagnosis is made only after careful documentation of the signs and symptoms of occlusal disease. If trauma from occlusion is documented, treatment of the intact dentition is directed to the elimination of occlusal interferences, creation of a stable interarch relationship, and actual loading of forces over a favorable distribution of teeth. Furthermore, the establishment of nonrestrictive mandibular movements with acceptable tooth guidance patterns that reduce and minimize fremitus is desirable. In a patient with previous periodontal disease, actual direction of force over a reasonable number of teeth is extremely important. The majority of the principal fibers of the periodontal ligament are oblique; therefore actual directed force will stimulate, as well as be resisted best, by the periodontal ligament fiber bundles.

After establishing a stable maxillomandibular relationship with axial loading and maximum distribution of force, excursive movements of the mandible must be evaluated and modified if necessary. Fremitus is an essential guide to the amount of correction necessary and to the distribution of force in contacting movements. The occlusal adjustment techniques used to modify guidance in contacting movements should reduce fremitus as much as allowed by the mechanical limitations of the dentition. It is not necessary to establish a predetermined occlusal pattern or cuspal anatomy. Anterior guidance in contacting movements with posterior disarticulation of the teeth is desirable; however,

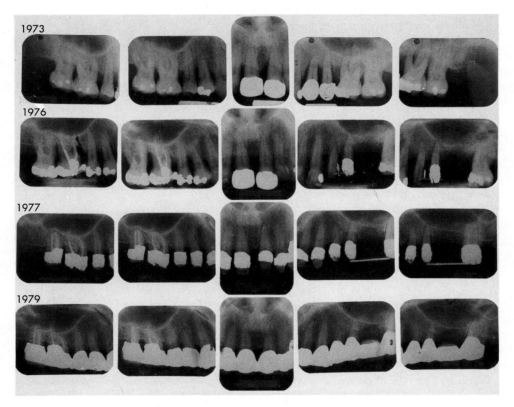

Fig. 15-4. Periodontal ligament spaces and crestal funneling remain widened in spite of control of marginal inflammation and antiinfective periodontal therapy from 1973 to 1976. Radiographic evidence corresponds to clinical documentation and supports diagnosis of secondary occlusal trauma. Tooth mobility and fremitus were increasing during this period. Full maxillary arch splinting was provided in 1977. Note positive radiographic changes following provisional split fabrication in 1977. There was continued narrowing of periodontal ligament spaces, character of lamina dura, and crestal morphology as case was taken to final restoration in 1979. (From Potashnick S and Abrams L: Alpha Omegan 78:25, 1985.)

orthodontic malocclusions, missing anterior teeth, severely weakened anterior teeth, or the need to reduce anterior crown-to-root ratios or generalized fremitus patterns may require that patterns of group function in lateral contacting movements on the working side be modified. Cross-tooth working contacts and cross-arch balancing contacts are often destructive and are to be avoided or eliminated. Furthermore, the goals of occlusal intervention must preserve a patient's negative occlusal sense and preserve or improve the esthetics, phonetics, and function. If successful, occlusal intervention will result in reduced mobility with a narrowing in the periodontal ligament space and in stability of the tooth.

If secondary occlusal trauma is the diagnosis, made after successful antiinfective treatment, then splinting may be necessary. *Secondary occlusal trauma* is characterized as mobility, fremitus, and the radiographic appearance of the supporting tissues remaining unchanged or progressively getting worse after antiinfective therapy. A case illustrating this is shown in Fig. 15-4. In this patient mobility ranged from I⁻ to III in 1973 and increased on many teeth in 1976 when it ranged from I to III with a shift to more II and III readings. This happened in spite of resolution of infectious periodontitis and occlusal adjustments; hence a diagnosis of secondary occlusal trauma was made, and splintings were undertaken. In 1979 resolution of the radiographic features of occlusal trauma was seen.

Constant evaluation and reevaluation is required throughout treatment, and adequate time must be allowed for the attachment apparatuses to respond before irreversible procedures are undertaken. Often, repair can be seen within the first several weeks; however, it is more resonable to evaluate the occlusion after several months to make sure the changes are stable, or that progression is truly worse and not transient. Before making major changes in occlusal arrangement based on perceived necessity for splinting, the clinician should be certain that trauma from occlusion is indeed present and that the patient will respond to the splinting in a desirable fashion.

• • •

Briefly, then, trauma from occlusion and infectious periodontitis often occur in the same patient. Control of both is often necessary for maximum resolution of the disease. A rational approach involving evaluation of antiinfective therapy and evaluation of occlusal therapy is necessary in determing if the occlusal trauma is leading to a deteriorating situation wherein the tooth must be splinted or extracted. This is defined as a tooth or segment of the dentition that is getting progressively worse or that does not allow the patient to function.

REFERENCES

Box HK: Experimental traumatogenic occlusion in sheep, Oral Health 25:9, 1935.

Ericsson I and Lindhe J: Effect of long-standing jiggling on experimental marginal periodontitis in the beagle dog, J Clin Periodontol 9:497, 1982.

Ericsson L and Lindhe J: Lack of significance of increased tooth mobility in experimental periodontitis, J Periodontol 55:447, 1984.

Gaengler P and Merte K: Effects of force application on periodontal blood circulation, J Periodont Res 18:86, 1983.

Glickman I: Clinical significance of trauma from occlusion, J Am Dent Assoc 70:607, 1965.

Glickman I and Smulow JB: Alterations in the pathway of gingival inflammation to the underlying tissues induced by excessive occlusal forces, J Periodontol 33:7, 1962.

Goldman HM, and Cohen DW: Periodontal therapy, ed 6, St Louis, 1980, The CV Mosby Co.

Kantor M, Polson AM, and Zander HA: Alveolar bone regeneration after removal of inflammatory and traumatic factors, J Periodontol 47:687, 1976.

Lindhe J and Ericsson I: The influence of trauma from occlusion on reduced but healthy periodontal tissues in dogs, J Clin Periodontol 3:110, 1976.

Lindhe J and Nyman S: The role of occlusion in periodontal disease and the biologic rationale for splinting in treatment of periodontitis, Oral Sci Rev 10:11, 1977.

Lindhe J and Svanberg GK: Influence of trauma from occlusion on progression of experimental periodontitis in the beagle dog, J Clin Periodontol 1:3, 1974.

Macapanpan IC and Weinman JP: The influence of injury to the periodontal membrane on the spread of gingival inflammation, J Dent Res 33:263, 1954.

Nyman S et al: The significance of alveolar bone in periodontal disease, J Periodont Res 19:520, 1984.

Polson AM, Meither S, and Zander HA: Trauma and progression of periodontitis in squirrel monkeys. IV. Reversibility of bone loss due to trauma alone and trauma superimposed upon periodontitis, J Periodont Res 11:290, 1976.

Reinhardt RA, Pao YC, and Krejci RF: Periodontal ligament stresses in the initiation of occlusal traumatism, J Periodont Res 19:238, 1984.

Simmons TA, Avery JK, and Svanberg GK: Periodontal collagen formation in juggling beagle dog teeth, J Dent Res 58(A):328, 1979.

Stahl SS: The responses of the periodontium to combined gingival inflammation and occluso-functional stresses in four human surgical specimens, Periodontics 6:14, 1968.

Stillman PR: The management of pyorrhea, Dent Cosmo 59:405, 1917.

Svanberg GK, and Lindhe J: Vascular reactions in the periodontal ligament incident to trauma from occlusion, J Clin Periodontol 1:58, 1974.

Waerhaug J: The angular bone defect and its relationship to trauma from occlusion and downgrowth of subgingival plaque, J Clin Periodontol 6:61, 1979.

Chapter 16

PERIODONTAL COMPLICATIONS AND NEUTROPHIL ABNORMALITIES

Robert J. Genco
Mark E. Wilson
Ernesto De Nardin

Neutrophil development
Neutrophil migration
Neutrophil function
Intracellular killing of microbes by neutrophils
Neutrophil secretory function and tissue destruction
Periodontal diseases associated with neutrophil abnormalities
    Congenital neutropenia
    Leukocyte adhesion deficiency
Periodontal disease as a complication of systemic diseases
   in which neutrophil function is compromised
    Chédiak-Higashi syndrome
    Diabetes
    Down's syndrome
    Phagocytic disorders

Neutrophils (also referred to as polymorphonuclear leukocytes, or PMNs) are the most abundant type of leukocytes present in the peripheral blood of humans, constituting approximately 40% to 70% of the total circulating leukocytes. As the primary circulating phagocytic cells, neutrophils play a key role in host defense against extracellular bacteria, especially pyogenic bacteria. They also play a role in the acute phase of inflammatory reactions. The importance of these cells in combating infectious disease is demonstrated through the increased susceptibility to recurrent bacterial infections observed in patients with defective neutrophil production or function.

Patients with neutrophil defects, which are either quantitative (neutropenia) or qualitative (adherence, chemotaxis, microbicidal activity), often suffer from oral mucosal ulcerations, gingivitis, and/or periodontitis. Severe oral disease occurs with both *primary* and *secondary* neutrophil abnormalities. The primary neutrophil disorders characterized by severe periodontal disease include neutropenia (chronic or cyclic), leukocyte adhesion deficiency (LAD), Chédiak-Higashi syndrome, and drug-induced agranulocytosis. Neutrophil abnormalities that occur secondary to underlying systemic disease and that are also associated with severe periodontal disease include insulin-dependent (type I) and non-insulin-dependent (type II) diabetes, Papillon-Lefèvre syndrome, Down's syndrome, hyperimmunoglobulinemia E–recurrent infection syndrome (HIE, or "Job's syndrome"), inflammatory bowel disease (Crohn's disease), preleukemic syndrome, acquired immunodeficiency syndrome (AIDS), and acute myeloid leukemia.

In contrast to the pattern of association between periodontal disease and neutrophil disorders, patients with mononuclear phagocyte defects do not exhibit an apparent predisposition to severe periodontitis. Thus patients with neoplastic disease or autoimmune disease such as Sjögren's syndrome, mixed cryoglobulinemia, dermatitis herpetiformis, or chronic, progressive multiple sclerosis do not have more severe periodontal disease than do normal individuals. It deserves mention, however, that a number of biochemical abnormalities affect both polymorphonuclear (neutrophils) and mononuclear phagocyte function, as in the case of LAD, Chédiak-Higashi syndrome, and Job's syndrome. In such instances the possible association between mononuclear phagocyte defects and severe periodontal disease is less clear.

It is instructive to note that individuals with immunodeficiencies in either T or B lymphocytes do not suffer from more severe periodontal disease than do immunocompetent persons. Patients with AIDS exhibit neutrophil abnormalities, as well as lymphocyte and mononuclear phagocyte defects, and they often have a severe form of ulcerative periodontal disease. In general, then, it appears that patients with systemic diseases associated with neutrophil abnormalities have more severe periodontal disease than do those with normal neutrophils. These observations have led to the concept of the neutrophil as a key protective cell against periodontal bacteria.

The importance of the neutrophil in the defense against periodontal infections has also been strongly supported by studies of localized juvenile periodontitis (LJP) (Van Dyke et al., 1985; Genco et al., 1986). Neutrophil abnormalities have been demonstrated in patients with LJP, as well as in those with rapidly progressing forms of periodontitis (Cianciola et al., 1977; Lavine et al., 1979). In addition, many of the periodontal pathogens have virulence factors such as antiphagocytic factors and leukotoxins, which subvert or abrogate neutrophil protective responses (Genco and Slots, 1984). Most patients with severe neutropenia or functional neutrophil impairment suffer from recurrent oral, as well as extraoral, infections. In contrast, patients with LJP or rapidly progressing periodontitis are characterized by severe periodontitis but do not appear to be predisposed to extraoral infections (Van Dyke, 1985; Genco et al., 1986; Gallin et al., 1988). These observations suggest that the periodontal tissues are one of the first organ systems to be compromised by reductions in neutrophil protective functions.

Evidence indicating that the neutrophil is a key protective cell against periodontal infection has engendered the concept that impaired neutrophil function is a *risk factor* for the development of periodontal disease. This certainly is the case with respect to primary and secondary neutrophil abnormalities. It may also be the case for other factors that are suspected of increasing the risk of periodontal disease (Wilton et al., 1988). These factors include smoking, drugs that depress neutrophils transiently (e.g., corticosteroids), nutritional deficiencies in which neutrophils are suppressed (especially in severe cases of protein-calorie malnutrition), and severe bacterial infections with endotoxemia. Stress-distress has also been implicated as a risk factor in certain forms of periodontal disease, such as acute necrotizing ulcerative gingivitis (ANUG). Stress-distress can function in two ways: (1) indirectly by changing behavior, which results in poor oral hygiene, and (2) directly by suppressing host resistance through immunomodulators such as adrenocorticosteroids, substance P, and bombastin, which are produced during stress.

Neutrophils function as a two-edged sword; although they are primarily protective, they also can act as proinflammatory cells capable of causing significant tissue destruction. Since the neutrophil is a critical cell in periodontal infections, a description of its development and function is necessary to gain appreciation for its role in disease.

NEUTROPHIL DEVELOPMENT

In normal adults neutrophils are found in the bone marrow, blood, and tissues (Fig. 16-1). In the bone marrow, neutrophils undergo development and proliferation from blast cells through promyelocytes to myelocytes. After the myelocyte stage, the cells become metamyelocytes, "band" cells (characterized by a single kidney-shaped nucleus), or segmented cells with characteristic multilobular nuclei that are no longer capable of mitosis. These cells are released from the marrow into the blood where they circulate for about 10 hours. They then migrate into the tissues where they survive for only 1 or 2 days. This migration is either random or in response to specific chemical signals called chemoattractants.

NEUTROPHIL MIGRATION

Egress from bone marrow, transit across vascular endothelial barriers (diapedesis), and migration to sites of infection or inflammation are critical steps in the expression of neutrophil function. Infection, inflammation, and stress can lead to elevation in circulating neutrophil levels (neutrophilia) as a result of mobilization of bone marrow reserves. Such factors can also enhance the kinetics of neutrophil maturation and consequently lead to the release of immature neutrophils into the general circulation, as manifested by increased numbers of "band forms." In healthy adults more than 100 billion neutrophils are in transit from the bone marrow daily; but this may increase almost tenfold in patients with a serious infection. The normal neutrophil count of 3000 to 5000 cells/mm^3 of peripheral blood may increase to 30,000 cells/mm^3 during infection; this results mainly from mobilization of the reserve pool in bone marrow. The final destination of neutrophils in the normal host has not been resolved; however, it appears that loss of neutrophils to sites of infection is important. For example, migration of neutrophils into the gingival crevice occurs in those who suffer from gingivitis and is increased in periodontitis. The neutrophils in the gingival crevice may represent an important and continuous form of host defense (Charon et al., 1985; Van Dyke et al., 1985).

Neutrophils produced in the bone marrow must cross two endothelial cell barriers in order to arrive at sites of tissue inflammation and/or infection (Fig. 16-1). Interaction between surface adhesins on the neutrophils and their corresponding ligands, the cell attachment molecules, on endothelial cells is a necessary first step in migration of the leukocyte across the endothelial borders. Modulation of neutrophil adhesins and endothelial cell attachment molecules by inflammatory mediators triggers neutrophil migration across blood vessel walls. The endothelial cell ligands

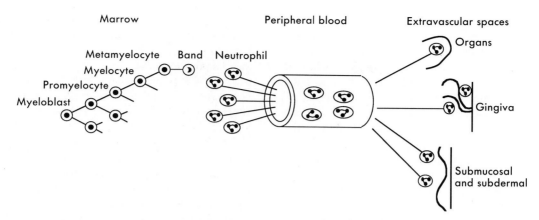

Fig. 16-1. Production and distribution of neutrophils. Neutrophils are produced and distributed into the following three compartments: marrow, peripheral blood, and tissue or extravascular spaces. In bone marrow, stem cells differentiate into myeloblasts, promyelocytes, and myelocytes under control of regulatory factors such as granulocyte-monocyte colony-stimulating factor (GMCSF), and granulocyte colony-stimulating factor (GCSF). When stem cells reach intermediate maturation stage known as metamyelocyte, they stop proliferating but continue differentiating to bands and eventually to segmented neutrophils. Segmented neutrophils and bands leave marrow when needed but generally spend about 5 days in marrow storage pool. Once neutrophils enter blood, about half the cells circulate, and these can be measured by a blood count. Other half of marginating neutrophils move out of main column of flowing blood and are closely associated with vascular endothelial cells. When needed, cells in peripheral circulation migrate to extravascular compartments of most organs, where they engage in phagocytosis of foreign particles. They then die in 1 or 2 days.

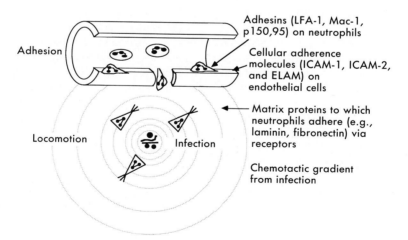

Fig. 16-2. Invasion of extravascular spaces by neutrophils. Neutrophils in venules undergo margination in response to humoral factors such as cytokines and chemotactic factors. These factors increase levels of cellular adherence molecules on endothelial cells (ICAM-1, ICAM-2, and ELAM), which act as ligands for surface adhesins of neutrophils. Leukocyte adhesins include LFA-1, Mac-1, and p150,95 (CR4). After adhering to endothelial cells, neutrophils leave vessel by migrating between endothelial cells, a process termed *diapedesis*. They then travel through extravascular spaces by adhering to matrix proteins such as laminin, fibronectin, and collagen, in response to a gradient of chemotactic factors that are found in highest concentrations at site of infection. Chemotactic factors include small peptides produced by microbes and cleavage fragments (notably C5a) generated during activation of complement cascade. Once at site of infection, neutrophils ingest microbial particles, which have been opsonized with antibody and complement.

are normally at low levels, and increases in their concentration by processes such as upregulation enhances neutrophil attachment to endothelial cells and facilitates transendothelial migration (Fig. 16-2). The process of neutrophil migration from the marrow to the blood and then into the tissues is extremely important. When this migration is altered, the number of neutrophils in the circulation or the tissues can be significantly affected, thereby influencing phagocyte protective effects. For example, maintenance of a constant number of neutrophils in the gingival crevice or periodontal pocket is critical for defense against periodontal pathogens. Sluggish neutrophil locomotion, resulting in a reduced rate of accumulation of these cells at the gingival sulcus, has been demonstrated in patients with LJP and refractory periodontitis (Genco et al., 1986).

The ability of phagocytes to migrate to sites of infection was recognized more than a century ago, and it was speculated even then that they did so in response to chemical mediators. This process is *chemotaxis,* defined as directed movement of leukocytes along a concentration gradient of substances called chemoattractants or chemotaxins. The chemotaxins may be derived from the tissue or from infecting organisms, and they stimulate leukocytes by binding to receptors on the neutrophil surface. Chemotaxins that are known to bind to neutrophil receptors include the N-formyl-methionyl peptides (e.g., FMLP), complement fragment C5a, and leukotriene B_4 (LTB_4). Hence the process by which neutrophils leave the blood vessels and then proceed to a site of infection has two stages. The first is leukocyte adhesion to the endothelium, and the second is directed migration toward areas of increased chemotaxin concentration (Fig. 16-2).

The molecular basis of leukocyte adhesion is just being unraveled. From Table 16-1 it can be seen that leukocyte adherence proteins are found not only on neutrophils, but also on monocytes and lymphocytes. The process of leukocyte homing is in general probably highly dependent on leukocyte surface adhesins and their corresponding endothelial cell ligands (Fig. 16-2). The adhesion molecules on the leukocyte surface are termed CR3, LFA-1, and p150,95 (CR4) and together constitute one subfamily of a larger family of adhesion molecules called integrins. Cell attachment molecules on endothelial cells include intercellular adhesion molecules 1 and 2 (ICAM-1 and ICAM-2) and endothelial leukocyte adhesion molecule 1 (ELAM-1). ICAM-1 is a 90-kilodalton endothelial cell surface glycoprotein that mediates PMN adherence by serving as a ligand for LFA-1 (Springer and Anderson, 1986; Anderson and Springer, 1987; Bevilacqua et al., 1989). As we learn more about the molecular basis of these surface glycoproteins that mediate the interaction between leukocytes and blood vessels, we will be better able to modulate this important process for the benefit of the patient.

NEUTROPHIL FUNCTION

Once neutrophils have entered the circulation and migrated into infected or inflamed tissues, they are ready to perform their phagocytic function. The initial step is target recognition. This involves coating (opsonizing) the infecting organism or host tissue component with plasma proteins. Opsonization facilitates adherence and subsequent phagocytosis of the infecting organism followed by intracellular killing. There are both heat-stable and heat-labile opsonins in human sera that dramatically enhance the ability of phagocytes to ingest bacteria (Fig. 16-3). The heat-stable opsonins include antibodies of the IgG and IgM classes. The labile factors include components of the complement system, of which the C3b and iC3b fragments of C3 are the most important. These C3 fragments are deposited on the bacterial surface during activation of the complement cascade. Phagocytes recognize the coated bacteria via specific receptors on the phagocyte surface for IgG,

Table 16-1. Leukocyte adherence-promoting receptors

Receptor	Structure	Cellular distribution	Function
CR3	α170 / β	Neutrophils, macrophages	Endothelial cell adherence, iC3b receptor, LPS receptor
LFA-1	α180 / β	Neutrophils, macrophages, lymphocytes	Endothelial cell adherence (possible ICAM-1 receptor), natural killer (NK) and T-cell target binding, tumorolytic macrophage binding, LPS receptor
p 150,95 (CR4)	α150 / β	Neutrophils, macrophages	iC3b receptor on tissue macrophages, LPS receptor

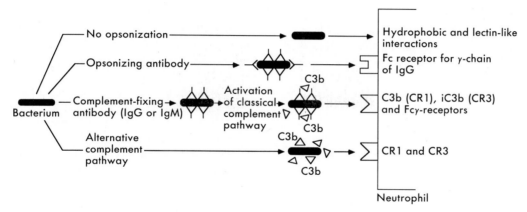

Fig. 16-3. Opsonization and phagocytosis. Process of coating particles with host proteins and thereby enhancing phagocyte recognition and ingestion is termed *opsonization*. Occasionally bacteria are phagocytosed in absence of such opsonins; however, majority of pathogenic bacteria require opsonization for efficient phagocytosis to occur. The two principal opsonins present in serum include antibodies (IgG and IgM) and fragments (C3b and iC3b) of third component of complement (C3). Antibodies of IgG class can effectively opsonize some bacteria for subsequent Fc receptor–mediated phagocytosis in absence of complement. However, for most pathogens, complement-fixing antibodies (IgG and IgM) bind to antigens on surface of bacterium, resulting in deposition of C3b on particle surface. These complement fragments can mediate recognition via neutrophil membrane receptors (CR1) for C3b. Fluid-phase regulatory proteins (C3b inactivator and s1H) can degrade membrane-bound C3b to its iC3b cleavage product, which remains bound to particle. These bacteria-bound iC3b fragments are recognized by a second class of complement receptors on neutrophil called CR3, which can also mediate phagocytosis. Finally, some bacteria may be effectively opsonized by complement alone in absence of antibody through alternative complement pathway, resulting in bacteria-bound C3b and, after degradation, iC3b, which bind to CR1 and CR3, respectively, on neutrophil surface.

C3b, and iC3b. The receptor for IgG is called the Fcγ-receptor, and the receptor for C3b is called CR1. C3b is converted to a cleavage fragment, iC3b, via the action of C3b inactivator in the presence of its cofactor β1H. This fragment is recognized by a second class of C3 receptors on phagocytic cells, termed CR3. As discussed earlier, CR3 is also a leukocyte adhesin. The principal role of opsonins is to facilitate the recognition and phagocytosis of infectious microorganisms, since most are otherwise poorly phagocytosed. Once the microorganism or particle is coated with opsonins such as immunoglobulin and/or complement components, binding to the neutrophil occurs and ingestion follows. The particle is taken into the cell in an "inside-out" cell membrane called the phagosome. The phagosome then fuses with neutrophil granules, forming a phagolysosome in which the bacteria are killed.

INTRACELLULAR KILLING OF MICROBES BY NEUTROPHILS

Neutrophils kill microorganisms by means of oxygen-dependent and oxygen-independent mechanisms. *Oxygen-independent* antimicrobial activity is carried out by a battery of substances, including cathepsin G, lactoferrin, lysozyme, defensins, proteases, and certain cationic proteins that increase bacterial permeability. Acidification of

the phagosome may result in either a bactericidal or a bacteriostatic effect on many ingested organisms. The *oxygen-dependent* killing mechanisms are linked to the production of toxic oxygen metabolites such as superoxide anion and hydrogen peroxide. Hydrogen peroxide, in addition to its direct antimicrobial properties, also serves as a cofactor in the myeloperoxidase-mediated antimicrobial system. The hydroxyl radical and singlet oxygen produced by this system are also thought to be toxic for many microorganisms.

The substances involved in microbial killing by neutrophils are contained in two major types of granules: primary, or azurophil, granules and secondary, or specific, granules. The azurophilic granules contain microbicidal enzymes such as myeloperoxidase and lysozyme; neutral proteinases, including elastase and cathepsin G; acid hydrolases, including beta-glucuronidase; and the cationic proteins. The specific granules contain the microbicidal enzyme lysozyme, a collagenase and lactoferrin.

NEUTROPHIL SECRETORY FUNCTION AND TISSUE DESTRUCTION

It is becoming increasingly clear that the neutrophil can lead to acute inflammatory tissue damage and is involved in inflammatory diseases such as rheumatoid arthritis, myocardial reperfusion, certain collagen vascular diseases, respiratory distress syndrome, blistering skin disorders, and ulcerative colitis (Weiss, 1989). Neutrophils usually sequester toxic products in the phagolysosomes. However, when large, nonphagocytosable particles are encountered or when the neutrophil is otherwise stimulated to secretion, these products may be released outside the cell, where they damage host tissues.

As discussed previously, the neutrophil contains a number of acid hydrolases and neutral proteinases capable of mediating injury not only to foreign microbes, but also, in certain instances, to host tissues. For example, the neutrophil plasma membrane contains an unusual enzyme, NADPH oxidase, which generates a family of reactive oxygen species through sequential univalent reduction of molecular oxygen. The powerful oxidants generated by this enzyme are by nature short-lived and nonspecific, and antioxidant enzymes such as superoxide dismutase and catalase often limit tissue damage produced by these substances. Neutrophil proteinases, on the other hand, are held in check by either their own latency or powerful antiproteinases.

It has recently been found that relatively small amounts of hypochlorous acid (HOCl), a major product of oxidative metabolism in neutrophils, can inhibit the tissue antiproteases such as alpha-2 macroglobulin, alpha-1 proteinase inhibitor, and a secretory leukoproteinase inhibitor. Hence HOCl from neutrophils can inactivate the tissues' own proteinase inhibitory shield, thereby allowing proteolytic enzymes such as elastase and collagenase to become active. Furthermore, collagenase and gelatinase are normally present in inactive precursor forms that are activated by HOCl. Hence in inflammatory sites with activated neutrophils, neutrophil elastase is protected from antiproteases by HOCl, and collagenase is activated by HOCl. This is a potent set of weapons that the neutrophils trigger to cause local tissue destruction.

During the normally acute inflammatory response, infiltrating neutrophils contain and eliminate the infectious or inflammatory agent, and damage to host tissue is localized and self-limited. Inability to eradicate the noxious agent may, however, lead to continued tissue infiltration by neutrophils and other phagocytic cells. Under such circumstances, subacute or chronic inflammation may result in significant phagocyte-mediated tissue injury. Fortunately, the net effect of normal neutrophil function in most infections, including periodontal disease, is protective, resulting in elimination of the inflammatory agent with variable levels of damage to surrounding host tissues.

PERIODONTAL DISEASES ASSOCIATED WITH NEUTROPHIL ABNORMALITIES
Congenital neutropenia

The total white blood cell count in the peripheral blood varies from 5000 to 10,000 cells/mm^3 in normal individuals. Since the circulating leukocytes consist of heterogeneous cell types, a differential blood cell count is necessary to determine the cell(s) responsible for alterations in the total white blood cell count. Neutropenia exists when the peripheral neutrophil count is less than 2000 cells/mm^3. However, neutrophil protective functions remain relatively intact if the neutrophil count is above 1000 cells/mm^3. When the neutrophil count drops below 500 cells/mm^3, the incidence of serious, recurrent, and recalcitrant infections rises markedly.

Neutropenias can be classified relative to the three compartments in which the neutrophils reside: the *marrow*, the *peripheral blood*, and the *tissue* (or extravascular) compartments. Abnormalities in any one of these compartments may result in neutropenia.

Abnormalities in the marrow, which account for the majority of neutropenias, can result from direct injury or from maturational defects of hematopoietic cells. Drug- or chemically induced injury is also common, resulting from cytotoxic agents or environmental hazards such as benzene, dichlorodiphenyltrichloroethane (DDT), or dinitrophenol. There are primary maturational abnormalities that manifest as congenital and hereditary neutropenias. Secondary maturational abnormalities associated with folic acid or vitamin B$_{12}$ deficiency may also cause neutropenia. Bone marrow replacement, which occurs in the rheumatoid disorders, infections, and infiltrative diseases such as malignancies, can also lead to neutropenia.

Abnormalities in the peripheral blood include hereditary or constitutional benign pseudoneutropenia in which there are fewer circulating and more marginating neutrophils (see Fig. 16-1). There are also acquired transient neutropenias in which severe infections and endotoxemia cause increased neutrophil margination. Acquired neutropenias may also be chronic, including those seen in patients with protein-calorie malnutrition or malaria. Intravascular sequestration of neutrophils as a result of complement-mediated leukagglutination in the lung or from hypersplenism may lead to neutropenia.

Abnormalities in the extravascular component associated with neutropenia include increased utilization of neutrophils in severe bacterial, fungal, viral, or rickettsial infections. Increased utilization or destruction of neutrophils is also observed in patients with hypersplenism and some forms of drug-induced leukopenia. Neutropenia is often observed in patients with certain autoimmune disorders. In some cases autoantibodies can lead to enhanced destruction of circulating neutrophils or can suppress myeloid development in the bone marrow. In other autoimmune disorders, such as systemic lupus erythematosus and Felty's syndrome, neutropenia may result from adsorption of destructive immune complexes to the leukocyte membrane rather than from the presence of cytolytic antibodies directed toward neutrophil-specific antigens.

Clinical manifestations. Neutropenias can be transient, cyclic, or persistent. Although the manifestations of neutropenia may be severe, many neutropenic patients may remain asymptomatic (e.g., when the neutrophil count is low but above 1000 cells/mm^3 of peripheral blood or when monocytes functionally compensate for the neutropenia). Asymptomatic patients may also exhibit cyclic neutropenia that is limited to 1 to 4 weeks, thereby modifying the risk.

The respiratory and genitourinary tracts and the oropharynx are the most frequent sites of infection in the neutropenic patient. In general, the infecting organisms are the usual pathogens for the given anatomic site. However, if antibiotics are given, unusual organisms may colonize the site and subsequently cause infection.

Diagnosis includes determining the temporal characteristics of neutropenia (cyclic or persistent) and identifying the underlying systemic disease that may be causative. Management of neutropenic patients follows the diagnosis and, if possible, involves *treatment* of the underlying cause, such as discontinuation of suspected toxins or drugs. In the neutropenic periodontal patient, treatment of the neutropenia should precede periodontal therapy or be carried out at the same time that periodontal treatment is initiated.

Oral manifestations. Drug-induced agranulocytosis (Bauer, 1946) and cyclic neutropenia (Cohen and Morris, 1961) are associated with severe periodontitis. Radiographic evidence of periodontal disease in a teenager and in a 4-year-old with cyclic neutropenia is provided in Figs. 16-4 and 16-5, respectively. Periodontal disease in children with infantile hereditary agranulocytosis (congenital neutropenia) has been recognized for 3 or 4 decades. Often the oral infections have been the first in a series of infections and have led to the parents' seeking health services for the child. In children and young adults with congenital neutropenia, the mucosa may present with black or gray necrotic ulcerations that are sharply demarcated from the uninvolved areas. There may be hemorrhage and necrosis of the gingival margin, and the patients may exhibit in-

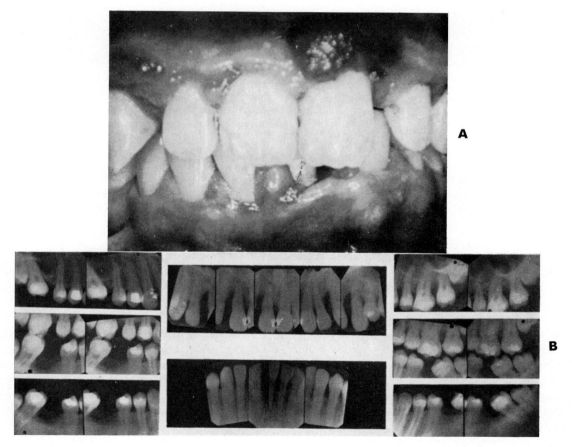

Fig. 16-4. A, Cyclic neutropenia in which red enlarged gingival tissues are observed about maxillary left central incisor and maxillary right canine in a 16-year-old girl. **B,** Teeth of patient seen in **A.** Note advanced resorptive lesion of alveolar process about permanent maxillary and mandibular left central incisors, maxillary right canine, and maxillary right posterior teeth. (From Cohen DW and Goldman HM: PDM, p 3, July 1962. © 1962 Year Book Medical Publishers, Inc. Reproduced with permission.)

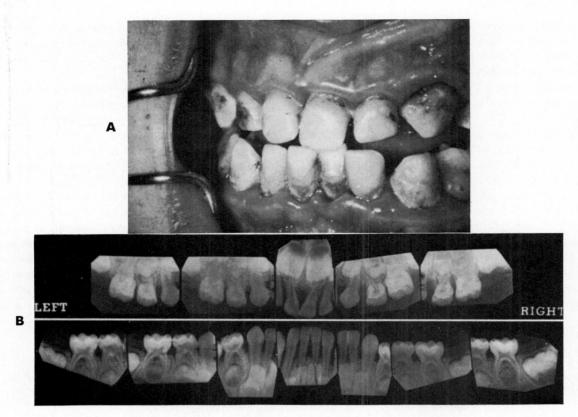

Fig. 16-5. A, Heavy stain, calculus formation, and gingival inflammation in a 4-year-old boy with cyclic neutropenia. **B,** Teeth of patient seen in **A.** Note horizontal resorption of alveolar and supporting bones around primary dentition throughout mouth. (From Cohen DW and Goldman HM: PDM, p 3, July 1962. © 1962 Year Book Medical Publishers, Inc. Reproduced with permission.)

creased salivation. In a histopathologic description of periodontal changes in neutropenia, Bauer (1946) described hemorrhage into the periodontal ligament with destruction of the principal fibers and osteoporosis of the cancellous bone with osteoclastic resorption. He also found small fragments of necrotic bone in the periodontal ligament and hemorrhage into the marrow.

The treatment of periodontal patients with cyclic neutropenia requires meticulous attention to debridement, plaque control, and the use of antibiotics. Treatment of periodontal disease in chronic neutropenia is less successful, often resulting in loss of teeth despite aggressive therapy. However, symptomatic relief can often be obtained with thorough subgingival scaling and root planing, along with adjunctive topical antimicrobial agents, systemic antibiotics, and long-term use of an antiplaque agent such as chlorhexidine.

Often the periodontal ulcerations in patients with neutropenia have a "punched-out" appearance and may proceed to a progressive periodontitis with sharply demarcated hyperemic zones along the marginal gingiva (Figs. 16-4 and 16-5). Such signs warrant a hematologic exami-

nation, including a differential count. Since the condition may be cyclic, repeated leukocyte counts at weekly intervals for at least 4 consecutive weeks are required to establish the diagnosis.

Leukocyte adhesion deficiency

Patients with a deficiency in expression of leukocyte adhesins suffer from recurrent infections with pyogenic bacteria, including severe periodontal disease. These patients, mostly children, have multiple defects in neutrophil and mononuclear phagocyte adhesion-dependent functions, including chemotaxis and CR3-mediated phagocytosis. They also have a persistent leukocytosis, delayed wound healing, and depressed leukocyte mobilization in vivo (Anderson et al., 1985; Anderson and Springer, 1987). Patients suffering from LAD lack CR3, the iC3b receptor, as well as two other cell membrane glycoproteins, LFA-1 and p150,95 (CR4), which are related to CR3 through a common subunit, the beta chain. As described previously (see Fig. 16-2 and Table 16-1), these adhesion glycoproteins are responsible for neutrophil binding to cell attachment molecules on the endothelial cell, a necessary first step in

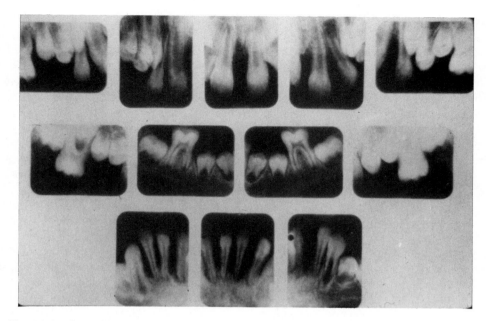

Fig. 16-6. Chédiak-Higashi syndrome in a 7-year-old boy. Note severe bone loss around incisors and bone loss in furcation of maxillary right first molar. (Courtesy Dr. Thomas Tempel.)

neutrophil migration through blood vessels.

There are two phenotypic variants of LAD described on the basis of the severity of the recurrent infections. These appear to be related to the reduced (90% to 95% deficient in the moderate phenotype) or absent (>99% deficient severe phenotype) expression of CR3. The biochemical basis of this autosomal recessive abnormality is the inability to synthesize the chromosome-21 encoded beta subunit common to CR3, LFA, and p150,95. This results in failure to insert these adhesins into the cell membrane (Anderson et al., 1985). Heterozygous family members, whose leukocytes express approximately half-normal amounts of these molecules, have apparently normal adhesion-dependent leukocyte function and are not susceptible to systemic infections. Although prepubescent heterozygotes appear periodontally healthy, a 31-year-old female heterozygote has been described who exhibited clinical and radiographic features characteristic of postjuvenile periodontitis (Waldrop et al., 1987).

Quantitative assessment of leukocyte CR3 expression can be made and is probably best performed by cytofluorography. Severe periodontal disease in children should raise suspicion of a neutrophil abnormality, with referral to a pediatric hematologist.

Oral and periodontal manifestations. Several children with LAD have been shown to have marked periodontal disease and severe gingivitis (Thompson et al., 1984). Periodontitis with attachment loss and severe alveolar bone loss is described in a series of children with LAD by Waldrop et al. (1987).

PERIODONTAL DISEASE AS A COMPLICATION OF SYSTEMIC DISEASES IN WHICH NEUTROPHIL FUNCTION IS COMPROMISED

In systemic diseases exhibiting neutrophil abnormalities, oral manifestations, including periodontitis, are common. This observation suggests that the common feature (i.e., neutrophil defects) in these patients accounts in part for their increased susceptibility to periodontal disease. It should be noted that there are many systemic diseases in which neutrophils are normal, and for these patients periodontitis is no more prevalent or severe than it is in systemically healthy individuals. Systemic diseases with neutrophil abnormalities and severe periodontal disease include Chédiak-Higashi syndrome, diabetes mellitus, Down's syndrome, Job's syndrome, Papillon-Lefèvre syndrome, Crohn's disease, acute monocytic leukemia, and AIDS. Crohn's disease and acute monocytic leukemia are discussed in Chapter 20, and AIDS is discussed in Chapter 23. The other conditions are discussed here.

Chédiak-Higashi syndrome

Chédiak-Higashi syndrome is a rare autosomal recessive disorder characterized by neutropenia, gingivitis, periodontal disease, and recurrent pyogenic infections (Tempel et al., 1973). This disease is also associated with partial oculocutaneous albinism, photophobia, nystagmus, and progressive peripheral neuropathy. Abnormal lysosomal granules are seen in many cells, resulting from the fusion of azurophil and specific granules. Severe periodontal disease and gingivitis at an early age have been reported in patients with Chédiak-Higashi syndrome. For example, Fig. 16-6 shows severe bone loss around a 7-year-old's permanent teeth with furcation involvement in the molars. A similar disease has been described in Aleutian mink, partial albino Hereford cattle, albino whales, and beige mice. Impaired neutrophil and monocyte migration and defective degranulation are thought to be linked to the increased susceptibility to infection, including periodontal disease, often observed in these animals (Wolff et al., 1972).

Diabetes

Approximately 6 million people in the United States have diagnosed diabetes, and an estimated additional 5 million have diabetes that is undiagnosed. The prevalence of diabetes increases with age, and estimates for the over-65 population are 25%. Infections create special problems in diabetic persons by further disturbing the control of glucose metabolism, and some of these infections are associated with significant morbidity and mortality. However, with the use of insulin to control glucose metabolism and the advent of antimicrobial agents, the high incidence of infection and resulting mortality among diabetic persons has diminished. Nevertheless, once infections are established, they may be difficult to control because of depressed host defense and repair mechanisms. Successful management of diabetes, therefore, requires daily attention to regimens (including oral hygiene) that minimize infection.

Diabetes mellitus comprises several diseases that have different causes and mechanisms of transmission but share glucose intolerance as the cardinal feature. Most cases of diabetes fall into two clinical types: type I diabetes, or insulin-dependent diabetes mellitus (IDDM), and type II diabetes, or non-insulin-dependent diabetes mellitus (NIDDM). Each type has a different prognosis, treatment, and cause, although periodontal disease can be a complication for patients with either type.

Insulin-dependent (type I) diabetes mellitus. The clinical symptoms of IDDM usually become manifest before age 40 but may appear at any age. The patient is prone to ketosis and is dependent on exogenous insulin to maintain life. The patient exhibits endogenous insulinopenia resulting from reduction of insulin production by the pancreas. IDDM is associated with certain genetically determined HLA haplotypes and abnormal autoimmune reactions, including production of antibodies reacting against insulin and pancreatic islet cells. The concordance of IDDM is only 50% in monozygotic twins over 40 years of age, suggesting that environmental factors also play a role in precipitating IDDM. One such factor, viral infection, has been shown to precede the development of IDDM. There is a strong relationship between viruses such as cox-

sackie group B virus, mumps, rubella, and cytomegalovirus infections and the development of IDDM. Concerning pathogenesis, there is general agreement that immunologic processes, both humoral and cell-mediated, are involved in destruction of the insulin-producing beta cells of the pancreas. Experimental modulation of IDDM has been successful with drugs such as cyclosporine, which interfere with these immunopathologic mechanisms.

Non-insulin-dependent (type II) diabetes mellitus. NIDDM usually occurs after the age of 40 but can occur at a younger age. Patients are usually not dependent on exogenous insulin to maintain life; however, for some patients, exogenous insulin may be needed for glucose control. Obesity is a common trait. Patients are ketosis resistant and may have a resistance to insulin, as evidenced by hyperinsulinemia and lack of the usual hypoglycemic response to insulin. There is a strong inherited tendency with concordance as the rule for diabetes in monozygotic twins. However, environmental factors also play a role in inducing glucose intolerance in NIDDM, since about 60% to 70% of patients with NIDDM form a subset characterized by obesity. In obese patients glucose tolerance is often improved with weight control.

Tests and diagnostic criteria. Accurate measurement of the plasma, serum, or blood glucose level is needed to identify patients with diabetes mellitus. Currently the National Diabetes Data Group recommends the following levels as defining normal: either a fasting plasma glucose of less than 140 mg/dl or a 2-hour plasma glucose of less than 200 mg/dl in the glucose tolerance test. The oral glucose tolerance test is indicated if (1) the fasting plasma or serum glucose is elevated on two occasions, (2) a high fasting plasma or serum glucose level is associated with glycosuria and/or ketonuria, or (3) there is a family history of diabetes.

Secondary diabetes mellitus. Secondary diabetes mellitus includes a variety of diseases that result in glucose intolerance severe enough to meet the diagnostic criteria for diabetes mellitus. Acute conditions such as cerebrovascular accident, myocardial infarction, and thyrotoxicosis may disturb glucose tolerance. Serial testing of blood glucose levels shows that most individuals with these diseases revert to normal; others show no significant change in the degree of intolerance, and a small percentage manifest clinical deterioration.

Gestational diabetes mellitus. Gestational diabetes mellitus (GDM) is a special problem in which glucose intolerance develops during pregnancy, and may be associated with an increased perinatal risk and fetal mortality. Hormonal interplay and insulin resistance are most likely responsible for the glucose intolerance. Retesting following pregnancy is necessary to determine if glucose intolerance persists.

Treatment. Diabetes is a chronic disease, and long-term control of blood glucose levels is necessary to minimize complications such as retinopathy, neuropathy, nephropathy, and microvascular and macrovascular changes. Control of blood glucose levels is important in preventing ketoacidosis in IDDM patients. Control of glucose levels is also important in controlling bacterial infection, as well as accelerating wound healing, and in promoting normal growth and development in the young diabetic patient. Diet remains a cornerstone of diabetic therapy in both IDDM and NIDDM. Oral hypoglycemic agents have been used for many years in NIDDM, although their use remains controversial. However, oral hypoglycemic agents are still used in the treatment of certain patients who have NIDDM with residual beta cell–secreting capacity.

Insulin therapy. The object of diabetic management is to keep the patient's glucose metabolism within reasonable limits and to prevent complications. Insulin is required for the IDDM patient and is also used for the insulin-resistant overweight patient who does not comply with the prescribed diet. Insulin may also be used in some patients with GDM, severe infection, and stress. Blood glucose levels are used for diabetes monitoring both in the office and at home. Much evidence has accumulated that suggests that good metabolic control can delay or prevent microvascular complications in diabetic patients. The level of glycosylated hemoglobin can also be used to monitor glucose control. The levels are normally 3% to 6% of the total hemoglobin value, but when blood glucose levels are elevated, the levels of glycosylated hemoglobin may increase to 15%. Since glycosylated hemoglobin is present during the life of the red blood cell, it can be used as a reflection of glucose control over a prolonged period of time.

Minor oral surgical procedures carried out with the patient under local anesthesia often require no change in the oral hypoglycemic or insulin regimen; however, major surgical procedures may involve a variety of methods, including intravenous glucose administration or low, continuous-dose infusion of insulin.

Complications. Complications of diabetes mellitus include atherosclerotic disease, often resulting in coronary artery, cerebrovascular, or peripheral vascular disease. Uncontrolled diabetes may be accompanied by reversible blurred vision. Cataracts and diabetic retinopathy may result from long-term uncontrolled diabetes. Diabetic nephropathy is a clinical syndrome of progressive renal dysfunction leading to hypertension, varying degrees of the nephrotic syndrome, and eventually renal failure. Typically, proteinuria is the first manifestation of renal complications. The nervous system is affected by diabetes mellitus in many ways. Diabetic neuropathy may also occur and results in functional abnormalities of the peripheral and cranial nerves. Motor and sensory dysfunction, resulting in numbness, loss of position or vibratory sensation, and

wasting and deformation of the foot, may occur. Susceptibility to infections, including chronic foot infections, is also a complication of diabetes, especially in those suffering from loss of sensation. Other infections, including severe, early-onset periodontal disease, are also a complication of diabetes.

Periodontal disease in insulin-dependent (type I) diabetes mellitus. During the preinsulin era of the 1930s and 1940s, severe periodontitis was commonly reported in patients with diabetes. More recent studies have also shown that children with IDDM are clearly less resistant to periodontal infection. For example, Gislen et al. (1980) showed that diabetic children who had poor metabolic control had more gingivitis than children who were not diabetic. A study of 263 IDDM patients compared with 208 control subjects was conducted by Cianciola et al. (1982) in the United States. Among subjects 11 to 18 years of age, periodontitis was found in 10% of the IDDM patients and in only 1.7% of the nondiabetic controls. A more recent update of this study on 437 IDDM patients (Fig. 16-7) shows an increased prevalence of periodontitis from 4% in 11- to 12-year-olds to 15% in 17- to 18-year-olds. Periodontitis in IDDM is illustrated in Fig. 16-8, in which oral radiographs of 9-year-old twin sisters with IDDM show generalized severe bone loss in the transitional dentition. In the 1982 study by Cianciola et al., there was little or no difference in supragingival plaque accumulation between the diabetic and control groups when comparisons were made at comparable levels of gingivitis or periodontitis. In a study of a Scandinavian population, there was a twofold greater prevalence of severe periodontitis in IDDM patients than in nondiabetic individuals (Hugoson et al., 1989). These researchers also found that the greater prevalence of periodontal disease in diabetic patients could not be explained by plaque or calculus levels, since these irritants were at similar levels in diabetic as compared with nondiabetic patients.

The subgingival microflora in IDDM patients with periodontitis was studied by Mashimo et al. (1983). It was found that the cultivable microflora was predominantly *Capnocytophaga* and anaerobic vibrios. In the majority of periodontitis patients, *Actinobacillus actinomycetemcomitans* was also found. However, few black-pigmented *Bacteroides*, such as *B. gingivalis* or *B. intermedius* species, were found. Serum antibody to *A. actinomycetemcomitans* was also seen, suggesting that these patients were infected with this organism. These studies have shown that the flora in IDDM patients with periodontitis resembles that seen in other juvenile forms of periodontal disease with *A. actinomycetemcomitans* as a major candidate pathogen. Thus, decreased host response most likely leads to an increased risk for periodontal disease in juvenile diabetics that is probably directly related to the lack of diabetic control. Most of the diabetic patients in the study by Cianciola

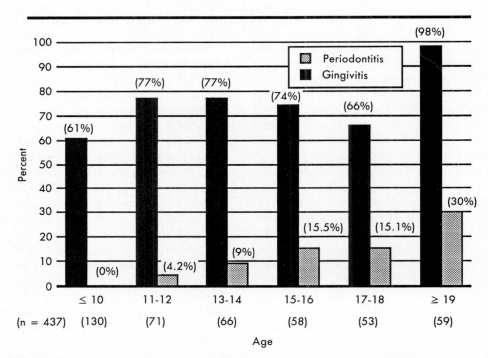

Fig. 16-7. Prevalence of gingivitis and periodontitis according to age in IDDM. (From Genco RJ: Unpublished continuation of study of Cianciola et al: J Am Dent Assoc 104:643, 1982.)

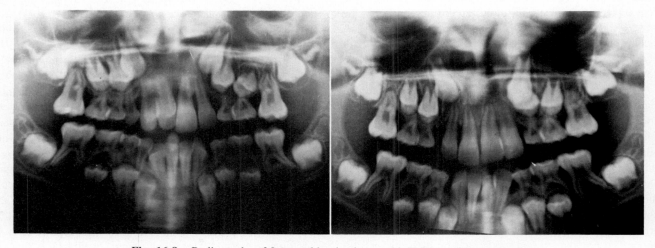

Fig. 16-8. Radiographs of 9-year-old twin sisters with IDDM and periodontitis.

et al. (1982) who suffered from periodontal disease had glycosylated hemoglobin levels of 12% to 15%, suggesting that their long-term control of diabetes was poor. Dentists seeing IDDM patients with severe periodontal disease should work with the patient and the primary physician to achieve control of the diabetes at the same time that they are treating the periodontal infection.

Periodontal findings in non-insulin-dependent (type II) diabetes mellitus. Early studies pointed to a greater rate of progression of periodontitis in NIDDM patients than in nondiabetic patients (Cohen et al., 1970). In a study by Glavind et al. (1968), it was found that periodontitis was most severe in NIDDM patients who had retinop-

athy as compared with nondiabetic or other diabetic patients. A large-scale epidemiologic study of the oral health of a population of Pima Indians has recently been completed and establishes the relationship between NIDDM and periodontal disease (Emrich et al., 1989; Shlossman et al., 1989). The Pimas are a tribe of native American Indians living in the southwestern United States who have the highest recorded incidence and prevalence of diabetes in the world (i.e., 50% of those over age 40 are diabetic). Diabetes mellitus among the Pima Indians is almost exclusively type II, or non-insulin-dependent.

The periodontal status of 3219 Pima subjects was evaluated using measurement of attachment loss and bone

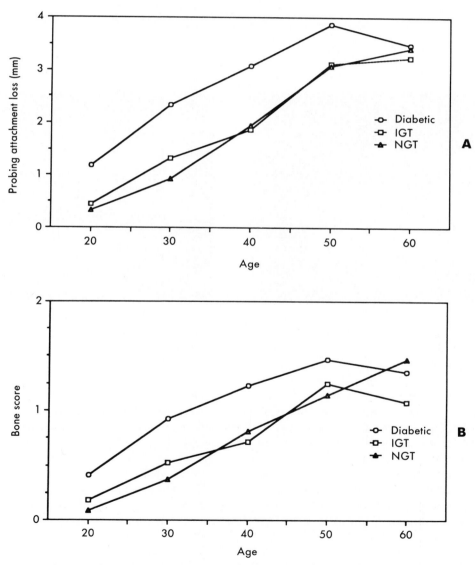

Fig. 16-9. Severity of periodontitis in Pima Indians with NIDDM (n = 1242). **A,** Attachment loss in diabetic patients as compared with loss in patients with impaired *(IGT)* or normal *(NGT)* glucose metabolism. **B,** Crestal alveolar bone loss in same groups.

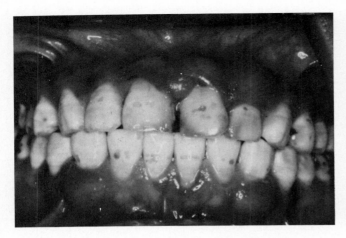

Fig. 16-10. Patient with NIDDM and multiple periodontal abscesses.

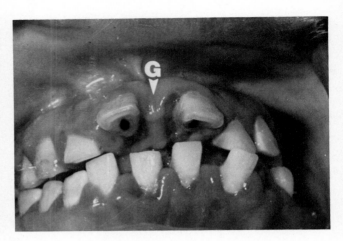

Fig. 16-11. Severe periodontitis with pathologic migration of teeth and abscesses in a 25-year-old woman with NIDDM. *G* points to interproximal gingiva, which is granulomatous near teeth. Three years previously, this woman did not have diabetes and had little or no periodontal disease.

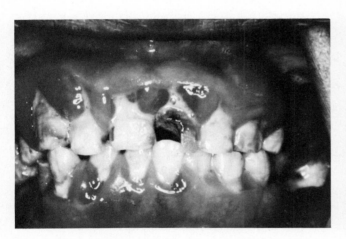

Fig. 16-12. Severe periodontal disease in a 45-year-old woman with NIDDM. Patient had poor metabolic control, as evidenced by a glycosylated hemoglobin level of 15.7%.

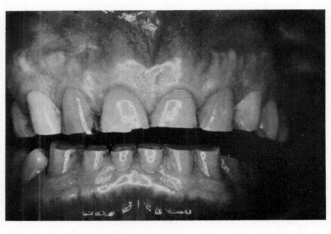

Fig. 16-13. Elderly NIDDM patient with retained dentition exhibiting healthy periodontal tissues.

score as independent but correlated measures of destructive periodontitis. The prevalence of periodontitis in NIDDM patients within this group is shown in Fig. 16-9. It can be seen that the prevalence of periodontal disease is greater in diabetic patients than in nondiabetic controls from ages 20 to 50. Clinical characteristics of periodontitis in diabetic patients often are not different from those of nondiabetic patients except for greater severity and earlier age of onset. Figs. 16-10 to 16-13 illustrate several cases of the periodontal condition of patients with NIDDM. Periodontal disease in diabetics is often characterized by multiple abscesses and granulation tissue (Fig. 16-10). Rapid onset and severe bone loss observed in young indi-

viduals with NIDDM is illustrated in Fig. 16-11.

Periodontal disease severity is often correlated with diabetic control as indicated by the level of glycosylated hemoglobin. As diabetic control deteriorates, the glycosylated hemoglobin level increases. This is illustrated in Fig. 16-12, which depicts a 45-year-old woman who has had NIDDM for 3 years and has an elevated glycosylated hemoglobin level of 15.7%, indicating poor glucose control. She suffers from severe periodontitis. However, not everyone with diabetes has periodontitis. Fig. 16-13 depicts an elderly diabetic patient who has retained the natural dentition and a healthy periodontium; this is most likely in large part a result of preventive maintenance.

It is clear, then, that diabetes is a major risk factor for periodontal disease. Patients with diabetes can be identified, and long-term metabolic control of the diabetes, along with intensive periodontal preventive regimens, offers hope for preventing periodontal diseases in diabetic patients.

Down's syndrome

Down's syndrome is one of the best-known and most frequently occurring autosomal trisomic disorders. It is trisomy-21 characterized by 47,XX,21+ or 47,XY,21+. The syndrome affects 1 in 700 live births. The phenotype of Down's syndrome is characterized by an atypical facial appearance with epicanthic folds, a broad bridge of the nose, a protruding tongue, an open mouth, square-shaped ears, and a flattened facial profile. There is variable mental retardation, muscular hypotonia, and, often, congenital heart disease. Patients with Down's syndrome are often susceptible to infections, and about one half suffer from neutrophil functional defects.

Periodontal disease has also been associated with Down's syndrome (Saxen et al., 1977). A comparison of the oral condition of Down's syndrome patients with that of age-matched and mentally retarded patients who did not have Down's syndrome revealed that the prevalence and severity of periodontal disease were much higher in patients with Down's syndrome than in similarly institutionalized mentally retarded patients not suffering from Down's syndrome. A prevalence of periodontal disease ranging from 60% to 100% of young adults under 30 years of age with Down's syndrome has been reported (Barnett et al., 1986; Izumi et al., 1989). The increased susceptibility of these patients to periodontitis has been associated with endogenous and exogenous factors (see review by Reuland-Bosma and Van Dijk, 1986). For example, abnormal neutrophil function has been described in many patients with Down's syndrome. Such defects include depressed bactericidal function, chemotaxis, and respiratory burst activity. Izumi et al. (1989) found that those individuals with the most severe periodontal disease among patients with Down's syndrome had a lower neutrophil chemotactic index than those with mild bone loss. These results suggest that neutrophil dysfunction is associated with a greater severity of periodontal disease in patients with Down's syndrome. An 18-year-old man with Down's syndrome suffering from severe periodontitis is shown in Fig. 16-14.

Phagocytic disorders

Job's syndrome (hyperimmunoglobulinemia E– recurrent infection syndrome). Job's syndrome is associated with otitis, sinusitis, staphylococcal pneumonia, furunculosis, and cellulitis. These patients exhibit characteristic coarse facies with hypertelorism, a prominent jaw,

cranial synostosis, and osteoporosis (Hill, 1982). They also suffer from cutaneous and sinopulmonary infection with *Staphylococcus aureus* and *Haemophilus influenzae*. Some become infected with *Aspergillus* species, and approximately 50% have mucocutaneous candidiasis. By definition, patients with Job's syndrome have extreme elevation of serum IgE levels, including IgE antibodies against *S. aureus* and *Candida albicans*. Patients with Job's syndrome have depressed acute inflammatory responses, as evidenced by cold abscesses. The basis for the depressed inflammation and the recurrent infections is unknown. However, abnormal neutrophil and monocyte chemotaxis has been documented. Abnormality of phagocyte chemotaxis may contribute to the recurrence of infections, but the chemotactic defect is variable and probably does not fully explain the tendency for recurrent infections. The presence of depressed T-suppressor activity and B-lymphocyte function in patients with Job's syndrome suggests a regulatory defect that has yet to be defined. There have been reports of more severe periodontal disease in patients with Job's syndrome; however, a systematic study of a large series of these patients has not been described that clearly establishes the association of Job's syndrome with oral infections.

Papillon-Lefèvre syndrome. Papillon-Lefèvre syndrome is a rare, autosomal recessive disorder characterized by hyperkeratotic palms and soles. Less common abnormalities include intracranial calcifications and mental retardation. Patients often exhibit increased infection, including furunculosis and pyoderma, and less frequently they exhibit liver abscesses and pneumonia.

Severe periodontal disease resulting in exfoliation of the primary and permanent dentition is one of the most constant features of Papillon-Lefèvre syndrome and therefore is important in its diagnosis. In most cases the keratotic changes of the palms and soles are noted within the first 3 years of life, and periodontal lesions begin shortly after eruption of both the primary and permanent dentitions. The periodontium is often affected in the order of tooth eruption; in addition, the teeth exhibit marked inflammation and suppuration, and there is bleeding of the gingiva, pocket formation, and loosening and spontaneous exfoliation, often without root resorption. After loss of the deciduous teeth, the tissues heal rapidly and without sequelae until the eruption of the permanent dentition, when the process begins anew. After loss of the permanent dentition, healing is uneventful and dentures are tolerated (Fig. 16-15).

The immunologic status of patients with Papillon-Lefèvre syndrome has been elucidated, and defects in cellular immunity (Djawari, 1978), neutrophil motility (Van Dyke et al., 1984), and reduced neutrophil bactericidal activity (Shams El Din et al., 1984) are found. The abnormality in neutrophil locomotion is associated with a de-

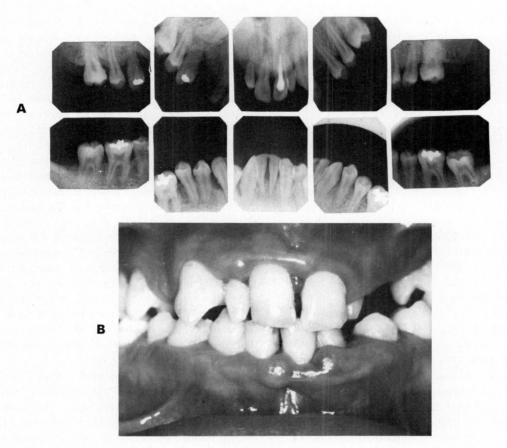

Fig. 16-14. Radiographs, **A,** and clinical photograph, **B,** of an 18-year-old man with Down's syndrome and periodontitis. (From Izumi Y et al: J Periodontal 60:238, 1989.)

crease in random migration, which manifests itself as a decrease in chemotaxis (Van Dyke et al., 1984).

The flora found in the periodontal lesions of patients with Papillon-Lefèvre syndrome is made up of *A. actinomycetemcomitans, B. intermedius,* and *Capnocytophaga,* which are typically found in periodontitis lesions of other juvenile patients.

• • •

In summary, it can be seen that neutrophil disorders that are either primary or secondary to systemic disease are often associated with severe periodontal disease. Hence neutrophil dysfunction is a risk factor for periodontitis, most likely lowering the host's resistance to periodontal infection by periodontal organisms.

REFERENCES

Anderson DC and Springer TA: Leukocyte adhesion deficiency: an inherited defect in the Mac-1, LFA-1, and P150-95 glycoproteins, Ann Rev Med 38:175, 1987.

Anderson DC et al: The severe and moderate phenotypes of heritable Mac-1, LFA deficiency: their quantitative definition in relationship to leukocyte dysfunction and clinical features, J Infect Dis 4:668, 1985.

Barnett ML et al: The prevalence of periodontitis and dental caries in a Down's syndrome population, J Periodontol 57:288, 1986.

Bauer WH: The supporting tissues of the tooth in acute secondary agranulocytosis (Arsphenanin neutropenia), J Dent Res 25:501, 1946.

Bevilacqua MP et al: Endothelial leukocyte adhesion molecule 1: an inducible receptor for neutrophils related to complement regulatory proteins and lectins, Science 243:1160, 1989.

Charon JA, Mergenhagen SE, and Gallin JI: Gingivitis and oral ulceration of patients with neutrophil dysfunction, J Oral Pathol 14:150, 1985.

Cianciola LJ et al: Defective polymorphonuclear leukocyte function in human periodontal disease, Nature 265:445, 1977.

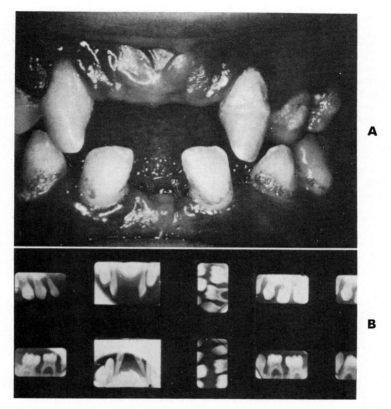

Fig. 16-15. A, Periodontosis as part of Papillon-Lefèvre syndrome in a 3-year-old girl. **B,** Teeth of patient seen in **A.** Note severe resorptive lesion affecting alveolar process. (Courtesy Manuel Album, Philadelphia.) (From Cohen DW and Goldman HM: PDM, p 3, July 1962. © 1962 Year Book Medical Publishers, Inc. Reproduced with permission.)

Cianciola LJ et al: Prevalence of periodontal disease in insulin-dependent diabetes mellitus (juvenile diabetes), J Am Dent Assoc 104:643, 1982.

Cohen DW and Morris AL: Periodontal manifestations of cyclic neutropenia, J Periodontol 32:159, 1961.

Cohen DW et al: Diabetes mellitus in periodontal disease: two year longitudinal observations, I, J Periodontol 41:709, 1970.

Djawari D: Deficient phagocytic function in Papillon-Lefèvre syndrome, Dermatologica 156:189, 1978.

Emrich LJ et al: Prevalence and severity of periodontal disease in non-insulin-dependent (type II) diabetes mellitus, J Periodontol, 1989 (in press).

Gallin JI, Goldstein IM, and Snyderman R: Inflammation: basic principles and clinical correlates, New York, Raven Press, 1988, p 505.

Genco RJ and Slots J: Host responses in periodontal diseases, J Dent Res 63:441, 1984.

Genco RJ et al: Molecular factors influencing neutrophil defects in periodontal disease, J Dent Res 65:1379, 1986.

Gislen G, Nilsson KO, and Matsson L: Gingival inflammation in diabetic children related to degree of metabolic control, Acta Odontol Scand 38:212, 1980.

Glavind L, Lund B, and Löe H: The relationship between periodontal state and diabetes duration, insulin dosage, and retinal changes, J Periodontol 39:341, 1968.

Hill HR: The syndrome of hyperimmunoglobulinema-E and recurrent infections, Am J Dis Child 136:767, 1982.

Hugoson A et al: Periodontal conditions in insulin-dependent diabetics, J Clin Periodontol 16:215, 1989.

Izumi Y et al: The effect of neutrophil chemotaxis in Down's syndrome patients and its relationship to periodontal destruction, J Periodontol 60:238, 1989.

Lavine WS et al: Impaired neutrophil chemotaxis in patients with juvenile and rapidly progressing periodontitis, J Periodont Res 14:10, 1979.

Mashimo PA et al: The periodontal microflora of juvenile diabetics: culture, immunofluorescence, and serum antibody studies, J Periodontol 54:420, 1983.

Reuland-Bosma W and Van Dijk LJ: Periodontal disease in Down's syndrome: a review, J Clin Periodontol 13:64, 1986.

Saxen L, Aula S, and Westermark T: Periodontal disease associated with Down's syndrome: an orthopantomographic evaluation, J Periodontol 48:337, 1977.

Shams El Din A et al: Hyperkeratosis, periodontosis, and chronic pyogenic infections in a 15 year old boy, Ann Allergy 53:11, 1984.

Shlossman M et al: Type II diabetes and periodontal disease, J Am Dent Assoc, 1989 (in press).

Springer TA and Anderson DC: The importance of Mac-1, LFA-1 glycoprotein family in monocyte and granulocyte adherence, chemotaxis and migration into inflammatory sites: insights from an experiment of nature. In Biochemistry of macrophages, Seppa Foundation Symposium 118, London, 1986, Pitman Publishing, Ltd.

Tempel TR et al: Host factors in periodontal disease: periodontal manifestations of the Chédiak Higashi syndrome, J Periodont Res 7(suppl 10):26, 1973.

Thompson RA, Candy DCA, and McNeish AS: Familial defect of polymorph neutrophil phagocytosis associated with absence of a surface glycoprotein antigen (OKM-1), Clin Exp Immunol 58:229, 1984.

Van Dyke TE: Role of the neutrophil in oral disease: receptor deficiency in leukocytes in patients with juvenile periodontitis, Rev Infect Dis 7:419, 1985.

Van Dyke TE, Levine MJ, and Genco RJ: Neutrophil function and oral disease, J Oral Pathol 14:95, 1985.

Van Dyke TE et al: The Papillon-Lefèvre syndrome: neutrophil dysfunction with severe periodontal disease, Clin Immunol Immunopathol 31:419, 1984.

Waldrop TC et al: Periodontal manifestations of the heritable Mac-1, LFA-1: deficiency syndrome, clinical histopathologic and molecular characteristics, J Periodontol 58:400, 1987.

Weiss SJ: Tissue destruction by neutrophils, N Engl J Med 32:365, 1989.

Wilton JM et al: Detection of high-risk groups and individuals for periodontal diseases: systemic predisposition and markers of general health, J Clin Periodontol 15:339, 1988.

Wolff SM et al: The Chédiak-Higashi syndrome: studies of host defenses, Ann Intern Med 76:293, 1972.

Chapter 17

SEX HORMONAL IMBALANCES, ORAL MANIFESTATIONS, AND DENTAL TREATMENT

Louis F. Rose

Pregnancy
    Oral manifestations
    Dental treatment
Oral contraceptive use
    Oral manifestations
    Dental treatment

It is believed that the gingival inflammation and hyperplasia frequently seen during puberty, pregnancy, and the menstrual cycle are induced by increased concentrations of female sex hormones in the circulation (Löe et al., 1965; Cohen et al., 1971; Arafat, 1974). This theory is supported by findings of gingival inflammation in women taking oral contraceptives, steroid hormones, and other medications containing estrogen and progesterone derivatives (Lindhe and Björn, 1967; Kalkwarf, 1978; Pankhurst et al., 1981), as well as by the findings of gingival hyperplasia in subjects treated with male sex hormones such as androgens (Ziskin, 1941; Michaelides, 1981). In addition, an induction of similar pathologic conditions was demonstrated in experimental animals treated systemically with male and female sex hormones (Lundren et al., 1973; Mohamed et al., 1974; Vittek et al., 1983).

Progesterone has been reported to have a significant impact on the gingival vascular system, causing increased exudation, as well as affecting the integrity of the capillary endothelial cells (Lindhe et al., 1968; Mohamed et al., 1974). Researchers have also demonstrated the influence of progesterone on the biosynthesis of prostaglandins in gingiva (El-Attar et al., 1973; Albers et al., 1979). Sex hormone–mediated alteration of the subgingival flora and a subsequent increase in periodontal inflammation have been noted by a number of investigators (Kornman and Loesche, 1980; Jensen et al., 1981).

PREGNANCY

Gingival changes during pregnancy were reported as early as 1877 (Pinard and Pinard, 1877). Observations differ on the incidence of "pregnancy gingivitis," its course during pregnancy, and the role that local and hormonal factors play in the etiology. Some investigators report a variable increase in the incidence of gingivitis during pregnancy (Hilming, 1950; Löe and Silness, 1963), whereas others believe such a phenomenon is lacking (Maier and Orban, 1949; Ringsdorf, 1962; Glickman, 1983).

It has been well established that the severity of gingival inflammation is significantly greater during pregnancy than in the postpartum period. The effects of pregnancy on the preexisting gingival inflammation is usually first seen in the second month of gestation and reaches a maximum in the eighth month. Furthermore, it has been found that the state of gingiva immediately after parturition is similar to that of the second month of pregnancy (Löe and Silness, 1963). The same investigators also found that the gingiva of the molar teeth demonstrated the highest scores throughout pregnancy, although the greatest relative increase was noted around the anterior teeth. Increased tooth mobility during the gestational period has also been reported, as has increased pocket depth (Rateitschak, 1967; Hugoson, 1970b).

The onset of increased gingival inflammation in the second month of gestation coincides with an increase in the circulating levels of estrogen and progesterone. Levels of the hormone rise in the eighth month, at which time the severity of gingival inflammation is at its greatest. In addition, a marked reduction in gingival inflammation following the eighth month correlates with an abrupt decrease in the excretion of these hormones. Thus there appears to be a definite relationship between the level of these hormones and the observed gingival response.

It has also been suggested that immune mechanisms play an important role in the initiation and development of chronic gingivitis and periodontitis (Lehner et al., 1970; Horton et al., 1974; Page and Schroeder, 1976; O'Neil, 1979a, 1979b). O'Neil confirmed that gingival inflammation increased between the fourteenth and thirtieth weeks of pregnancy despite a decrease in the amount of dento-gingival plaque. The presence of inflammation implicated a factor other than plaque accumulation. O'Neil was able to demonstrate that during pregnancy the cell-mediated response is depressed, which could contribute to the altered responsiveness of the gingival tissue to plaque.

Several studies have suggested that gingival inflammation during pregnancy results from an alteration in the subgingival flora to a more aerobic state. Kornman and Loesche (1980) found that the anaerobe-to-aerobe ratio increased significantly during the thirteenth through sixteenth weeks of pregnancy and remained high until the third trimester. The only organism whose proportions increased to a significant level during pregnancy was *Bacteroides intermedius*. At the peak of gingival bleeding, the plaque proportions of this organism were fivefold greater than initial levels. The authors concluded that the increase in *B. intermedius* appeared to be associated with increased systemic levels of estrogen and progesterone, based on the fact that steroid uptake by plaque samples paralleled increased plaque proportions of *B. intermedius*. Subsequent pure culture studies have shown that estrogen and progesterone can substitute menadione as an essential growth factor in *B. intermedius*. Also, at peak gingival bleeding, gram-negative anaerobic rods had increased fourfold over initial levels. Of note is the fact that shifts in endogenous steroid levels may have a significant influence on the subgingival flora.

The studies reported to date indicate that female sex hormones may be capable of altering the gingival vascular system, the immune system, and the normal subgingival flora.

Oral manifestations

Clinically, the gingiva of pregnant women is frequently characterized by inflammatory changes. The tissue appears edematous, hyperplastic, and dark red. The gingival surface is often shiny and tends to bleed when the individual brushes her teeth or chews food. These changes are noted on the marginal, gingival, and particularly the interdental papilla and may be generalized or localized (Fig. 17-1). During the second and third trimester the inflammation often becomes more severe (Goldman and Cohen, 1978; Lindhe, 1983).

During pregnancy a tumorlike mass may form interproximally (Brown et al., 1970). A classic lesion appears as an isolated, hyperplastic, protruding, bright red or magenta growth with a mulberry-like surface and often appears during the second trimester. This tissue mass frequently occurs in the interproximal area. It may bleed on the slightest provocation (Fig. 17-2). The tissue growth may cause migration and increased mobility of the adjacent teeth. Histologically, the pregnancy tumor is identical to a pyogenic granuloma (Kerr, 1961; Shafer et al., 1974), with the distinction based solely on occurrence during pregnancy. It has been suggested that some form of trauma or irritation, such as plaque, initiates the lesion and that the hormonal alterations occurring during pregnancy exaggerate the tissue response. Generally, the lesion will regress somewhat postpartum; however, surgical excision is often required for complete resolution. Whenever possible, surgery should be delayed until after pregnancy. Before parturition, scaling and root planing, as well as intensive oral hygiene instruction, should be initiated to reduce the plaque retention.

In addition to gingival changes, investigators have reported increased pocket depth, minimal loss of attachment apparatus, and increased tooth mobility (Rateitschak, 1967; Cohen et al., 1969; Hugoson and Lindhe, 1971). The gingival changes have decreased in severity postpartum (Cohen et al., 1971), possibly because of lowered hormonal levels, which allow the anaerobic bacterial flora to reestablish a normal state (Kornman and Loesche, 1980).

Dental treatment

Normal pregnancy does not necessarily contraindicate dental treatment if the stage of gestation and the extent of the dental procedures are taken into account. The first trimester is the period of organogenesis. In addition, approximately 75% to 80% of spontaneous abortions occur before the sixteenth week of gestation. The fetus is thus very sensitive to environmental influences at this time. In the last half of the third trimester, premature delivery becomes a hazard. Prolonged chair time should be avoided, since supine hypotensive syndrome may occur. Whether the pregnant woman is in a semireclining or a supine position, the great vessels, particularly the inferior venicava, are compressed by the uterus. By interfering with venus return, this compression causes hypotension, decreased cardiac output, and eventual loss of consciousness. Supine hypotension syndrome can usually be reversed by turning the patient on her left side and thereby relieving the pressure on the vena cava and allowing blood to return to the lower

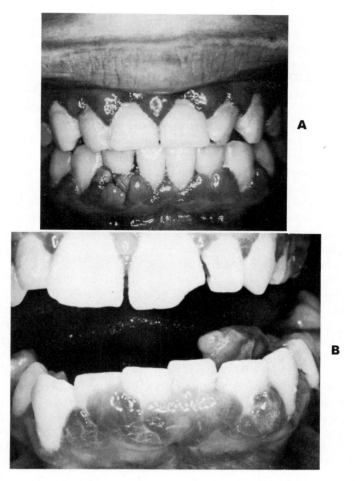

Fig. 17-1. Appearance and severity of gingival changes during pregnancy may vary. **A,** Generalized gingival inflammation. Tissue is edematous, dark red, smooth, and shiny. **B,** Inflammation of gingival tissues is most severe interdentally, producing lobulated hyperplastic tissue.

extremities and pelvic area. However, because of these hazards, no elective procedures, such as definitive periodontal surgery, should be performed during the first and third trimesters.

The second semester is the safest period during which routine dental care can be provided. Even so, it is advisable to limit care to minimal treatment. Based on numerous studies that emphasize the role of local irritants in the initiation of periodontal disease during pregnancy, it is prudent to educate the pregnant woman in good plaque control techniques early in pregnancy (Cohen et al., 1969, 1971; Löe and Silness, 1963). All local irritants should be removed as soon as possible, before the effects of pregnancy are manifested in the gingival tissues.

If emergency treatment is indicated, it should be performed any time during gestation to eliminate any associated physical or emotional stress. The pain and anxiety precipitated by a dental emergency may be more detrimental to the fetus than the treatment itself.

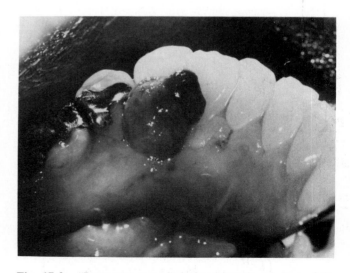

Fig. 17-2. "Pregnancy tumor": isolated interdental mass of tissue frequently occurring in interproximal areas.

One controversial area in the treatment of the pregnant patient involves taking dental radiographs. Only serious dental emergencies require a radiographic evaluation, especially during the first trimester when the developing fetus is particularly susceptible to the effects of radiation. Routine radiographs should be avoided and taken only when necessary. If radiographs are taken, the patient should wear a protective lead apron to reduce the amount of radiation to which the abdominal area is exposed.

Another area of concern involves drug therapy, since any drug given to the pregnant patient can affect the fetus by diffusion across the placental barrier. The dentist must carefully evaluate the indications and contraindications of drug usage. Before any drugs, whether anesthetics, analgesics, or antibiotics, are given, consultation with the patient's physician is recommended. Most pharmaceutical companies caution against the use of many of their products during pregnancy because little well-controlled research has been done to determine the effects on the developing fetus. Fortunately, most of the drugs commonly used in dental practice can be given with relative safety.

In most cases it is safe practice to use a local anesthetic with a vasoconstrictor (1:1000,000). Analgesics, including acetaminophen and aspirin (except during the third trimester, when bleeding problems can occur during or after delivery), are also safe. Both mother and fetus are similarly protected against antibiotics, such as penicillin, cephalosporins, and erythromycin.

Certain drugs occasionally prescribed by dentists are known to cause complications during pregnancy and therefore should be avoided. These include diazepam (Valium), chlordiazepoxide (Librium), flurazepam (Dalmane), meprobamate (Miltown), streptomycin, and tetracycline. Nitrous oxide should not be administered during organogenesis (first trimester), and neither general anesthesia nor intravenous sedation should be used at all during pregnancy.

If a "pregnancy tumor" develops that is uncomfortable for the patient, disturbs the alignment of teeth, and bleeds easily on mastication, it should be excised. "Pregnancy tumors" excised before term may recur; therefore the patient should be advised that revision of the surgical procedure may have to be performed postpartum. It is misleading to tell the pregnant patient that the gingival disease is a transitory condition and will disappear after delivery. The severity of gingival disease is reduced after childbirth, but the gingiva does not necessarily return to a state of health. Patients with untreated gingival disease during pregnancy will most likely have gingival disease after pregnancy, although it may decrease in severity (Lyon and Wishan, 1965).

In summary, the exaggerated inflammatory response seen during pregnancy can be eliminated or prevented by efficient oral hygiene procedures. Bacterial plaque appears to be responsible for the initiation and maintenance of gingival inflammation during pregnancy, and the accentuated response is due to altered tissue metabolism, vascular permeability, and changed anaerobic bacterial flora (Silness and Löe, 1964; Kornman and Loesche, 1980).

ORAL CONTRACEPTIVE USE

The number of women taking oral contraceptives has reached an estimated 8 to 10 million in the United States and 50 million worldwide. As a result of such widespread use, many systemic and oral side effects have been detected. Among the undesirable systemic effects associated with the use of oral contraceptives are an increased incidence of thromboembolic events, increased risk of myocardial infarction, and, in certain circumstances, significant elevation in blood pressure.

Oral manifestations

Gestational hormones, used as oral contraceptives, produce hormonal situations similar to pregnancy (Kalkwarf, 1978). Various investigators have reported women taking oral contraceptives as having an increased prevalence of gingivitis accompanied by higher levels of gingival crevicular fluid flow (Lindhe and Björn, 1967; Lindhe et al., 1969; El-Ashiry et al., 1970) (Fig. 17-3). Also, Hugoson (1970a) has demonstrated that pregnancy and the use of oral contraceptives elevate the serum levels of female sex hormones. These hormones have been positively associated with increased gingival crevicular fluid. Similarly, Lindhe and Attström (1967), Lindhe and Brånemark (1968), and Samant et al. (1976) found that regular administration of gestational hormones used in oral contraceptives resulted in increased gingival crevicular fluid.

Although most, if not all, reports reveal an increased prevalence of gingivitis with the use of oral contraceptives, not all women respond in this manner. In fact, many do not have a clinically altered gingival condition. It has been well established that the incidence or prevalence of gingivitis is very closely correlated with increased dental plaque (Greene, 1963; Löe et al., 1965; Lang et al., 1973; Loesche and Syed, 1978). More recent studies have noted the relationship of increased gingivitis with increased supragingival *Actinomyces* species and increased gram-negative microorganisms in subgingival human plaque (Palenstein–van Helderman, 1975; Slots, 1979). Jensen et al. (1981) monitored the crevicular microbial flora (i.e, *Bacteroides* and *Fusobacterium* species) in women taking oral contraceptives. Clinical measurements of gingivitis, gingival crevicular flow, and periodontal pocket depth were all evaluated. The most dramatic change noted was the increased proportion of *Bacteroides* species in the women taking oral contraceptives. In fact, the increased proportion of *Bacteroides* proved to be a more sensitive indicator of altered systemic hormonal conditions than the usual clinical parameters. Jensen suggested that substitution of

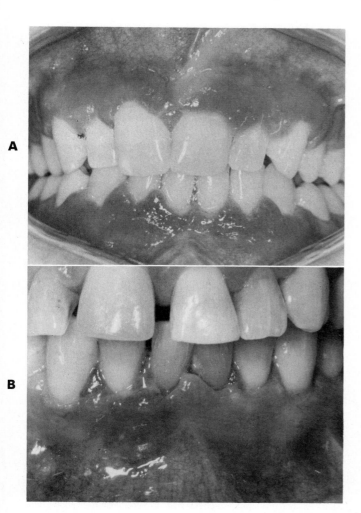

Fig. 17-3. Increased prevalence of gingivitis due to gestational hormones (oral contraceptives). Clinical manifestations are similar to those found during pregnancy. **A,** Diffuse gingival inflammation in a woman taking oral contraceptives. **B,** Localized response of gingiva to female hormones.

the increased female sex hormones for the naphthoquinone requirement of certain *Bacteroides* species was most likely responsible for this increase.

Other investigators have shown that the addition of sex hormones to gingival tissue can cause a significant increase in the synthesis of prostaglandin E_2. Since E-type prostaglandins are potent mediators of inflammation, this may be another mechanism whereby sex hormones increase the inflammatory response (El-Attar et al., 1973). Another factor under consideration is the disruption of gingival mass cells, liberating stores of histamine and proteolytic enzymes and thus aggravating the inflammation produced by local irritants (El-Ashiry et al., 1970).

Several studies have addressed the effects of oral contraceptives on the periodontal attachment. Knight and

Wade (1974) found no significant difference in the plaque and gingival indices or in loss of attachment between subjects taking oral contraceptives and control subjects. However, subjects who had taken the hormonal drug for more than 1½ years showed a trend toward a higher gingival index score and more loss of periodontal attachment than those who had taken drugs for less time or who were not taking hormones. Pankhurst et al. (1981) compared the responses of the periodontal tissue to plaque in subjects who were taking oral contraceptives at various periods of time and in control subjects. They found a significant increase in gingival inflammation in correlation with the duration of drug therapy, although there was no significant difference in the level of attachment between the groups of subjects.

There appears to be no correlation between the severity of inflammation and the particular type of progesterone and estrogen in the oral contraceptives, but there may be a direct relationship between severity of inflammation and duration of hormone therapy. This suggests that oral contraceptives may have cumulative effects in altering host resistance.

Measurable changes have been observed in the saliva of women taking sex hormones. Specifically, the concentrations of protein, sialic acid, hexosamine, fructose, hydrogenione, and total electrolytes have decreased (Magnusson et al., 1975).

Since another side effect of oral contraceptives is spotty malanoic pigmentation of the skin, the relationship between the use of oral contraceptives and the occurrence of gingival melanosis in individuals with light complexions has also been suggested (Hertz et al., 1980).

The dental literature reports that women taking oral contraceptives have a two- to threefold increase in the incidence of localized osteitis following extraction of mandibular third molars (Sweet and Butler, 1977). The higher incidence of osteitis in these patients may be attributed to the effects of oral contraceptives and estrogen on blood-clotting factors. Since a patient's coagulation and fibrinolytic factors are cyclic when oral contraceptives are being taken, there may be a temporary shift when fibrolytic components are increased in relation to clotting factors. If this shift occurs while a patient is recovering from a third molar extraction, the loss of surgical clot may result. Another mechanism to be considered is the presence of tissue activators after teeth are removed, which may allow high fibrinolytic activity and consequently clots.

In summary, oral contraceptive therapy apparently has a bearing on the health of periodontal tissues of patients. The majority of studies to date indicate that the ingestion of hormones affects one or more of the clinical signs of inflammation, ranging from measurable increases in gingival exudate to pregnancy-like gingivitis and pregnancy tumors. Although in most instances the changes noted with alterations in female sex hormones are reversible, there is some indication that long-term, irreversible changes can occur. Many case reports have noted that when the oral contraceptive is stopped or the dosage is reduced, the inflammation tends to subside (Kaufman, 1969; Lynn, 1967). The divergence of opinion is most likely due to differences in drug composition, dosage, duration of treatment, and species.

Dental treatment

The dental management of patients taking oral contraceptives should include the establishment of a plaque control program and the elimination of all local predisposing factors. Ideally, the oral contraceptives should be discontinued or at least reduced in dosage to truly control the periodontal health of the patient.

REFERENCES

Albers Von HK, Koning T, and Lisboa BP: Biochemische und morphologische Untersuchungen über die Prostaglandine E und F in der normalen und entzündlich veränderten Gingiva, Dtsch Zahnaerztl Z 34:440, 1979.

Arafat A: The prevalence of pyogenic granuloma in pregnant women, J Baltimore Coll Dent Surg 29(2):64, 1974.

Brown GM et al: Pituitary-adrenal function in the squirrel monkey, Endocrinology 86:519, 1970.

Cohen DW et al: A longitudinal investigation of the periodontal changes during pregnancy, J Periodontol 40:563, 1969.

Cohen DW et al: A longitudinal investigation of the periodontal changes during pregnancy and 15 months post partum, part II, J Periodontol 42:653, 1971.

El-Ashiry GM et al: Comparative study of the influence of pregnancy and oral contraceptives on the gingivae, Oral Surg 30:472, 1970.

El-Attar TMA, Roth GD, and Hugoson A: Comparative metabolism of 4-C progesterone in normal and chronically inflamed human gingival tissue, J Periodont Res 8:79, 1973.

Glickman I: Clinical periodontology, ed 6, Philadelphia, 1983, WB Saunders Co.

Goldman HM and Cohen DW: Periodontal therapy, ed 6, St Louis, 1978, The CV Mosby Co.

Greene JC: Oral hygiene and periodontal disease, Am J Public Health 53:913, 1963.

Hertz RS, Beckstead PC, and Brown WJ: Epithelial melanosis of the gingiva possibly resulting from the use of oral contraceptives, J Am Dent Assoc 100(5):713, 1980.

Hilming F: Gingivitis gravidarum, dissertation, Copenhagen, 1950, Royal Dental College.

Horton JE, Oppenheim JJ, and Mergenhagen SE: A role for cell-mediated immunity in the pathogensis of periodontal disease, J Periodontol 45:351, 1974.

Hugoson A: Gingival inflammation and female sex hormones—clinical investigation of pregnant women and experimental studies in dogs, J Periodont Res 5(suppl):1, 1970a.

Hugoson A: Gingivitis in pregnant women, Odontol Revy 21:1, 1970b.

Hugoson A and Lindhe J: Gingival tissue regeneration in non pregnant female dogs treated with sex hormones: clinical observations, Odontol Revy 22:237, 1971.

Jensen J, Liljemark W, and Bloomquist C: The effect of female sex hormones on subgingival plaque, J Periodontol 52:588, 1981.

Kalkwarf KL: Effect of oral contraceptive therapy on gingival inflammation in humans, J Periodontol 49:560, 1978.

Kaufman A: An oral contraceptive as an etiologic factor in producing hyperplastic gingivitis and a neoplasm of the pregnancy tumor type, Oral Surg 28:666, 1969.

Kerr DA: Granuloma pyogenicum, Oral Surg 4:158, 1961.

Knight GM and Wade AB: The effects of hormonal contraceptives on the human periodontium, J Periodont Res 9:18, 1974.

Kornman KS and Loesche WJ: The subgingival microbial flora during pregnancy, J Periodont Res 15:111, 1980.

Lang NP, Cumming BR, and Löe H: Toothbrushing frequency as it is related to plaque development and gingivitis, J Periodontol 44:396, 1973.

Lehner T, Wilton JA, and Ward RG: Serum antibodies in dental caries in man, Arch Oral Biol 15:481, 1970.

Lindhe J: Textbook on clinical periodontology, Philadelphia, 1983, WB Saunders Co.

Lindhe J and Attström R: Gingival exudation during the menstrual cycle, J Periodont Res 2:194, 1967.

Lindhe J, Attström R, and Björn AL: The influence of progestogen on gingival exudation during menstrual cycles, J Periodont Res 4:97, 1969.

Lindhe J and Björn AL: Influence of hormonal contraceptives on the gingiva of women, J Periodont Res. 2:1, 1967.

Lindhe J and Brånemark PI: The effects of sex hormones on vascularization of granulation tissue, J Periodont Res 3:6, 1968.

Lindhe J, Brånemark PI, and Birch J: Microvascular changes in cheekpouch wounds of oophorectomized hamsters following intramuscular injections of female sex hormones, J Periodont Res 3:180, 1968.

Löe H and Silness J: Periodontal disease in pregnancy. I. Prevalence and severity, Acta Odontol Scand 21:533, 1963.

Löe H, Theilade E, and Jensen SB: Experimental gingivitis in man, J Periodontol 36:177, 1965.

Loesche WJ and Syed SA: Bacteriology of human experimental gingivitis. II. Effect of plaque and gingivitis score, Infect Immun 21:830, 1978.

Lundren D, Magnusson B, and Lindhe J: Connective tissue alterations in gingivae of rats treated with estrogen and progesterone, Odontol Revy 24:49, 1973.

Lynn B: "The pill" as an etiologic agent in hypertrophic gingivitis, Oral Surg 24:333, 1967.

Lyon LZ and Wishan MS: Mangement of pregnant dental patients, Dent Clin North Am, p 623, Nov 1965.

Magnusson T, Ericson T, and Hugoson A: The effect of oral contraceptives on some salivary substances in women, Arch Oral Biol 20:119, 1975.

Maier AW and Orban B: Gingivitis in pregnancy, Oral Surg 2:334, 1949.

Michaelides PL: Treatment of periodontal disease in a patient with Turner's syndrome, J Periodontol 52:386, 1981.

Mohamed AH, Waterhouse JP, and Frederici HH: The microvasculature of the rabbit gingiva as affected by progesterone: an untrastructural study, J Periodontol 45:50, 1974.

O'Neil TCA: Maternal t-lymphocyte response and gingivitis in pregnancy, J Periodontol 50(4):178, April 1979a.

O'Neil TCA: Plasma female sex hormone levels and gingivitis in pregnancy, J Periodontol 50(6):279, June 1979b.

Page RC and Schroeder HE: Pathogenesis of inflammatory periodontal disease, Lab Invest 33:235, 1976.

Palenstein–van Helderman WH: Total viable count and differential counts of *Vibrio (Campylobacter) sputorum*, *Fusobacterium nucleatum*, *Selenomonas sputigena*, *Bacteroides ochraceus* and *Veillonella* in the inflamed and noninflamed human gingival crevice, J Periodont Res 10: 294, 1975.

Pankhurst CL et al: The influence of oral contraceptive therapy on the periodontium—duration of drug therapy, J Periodontol 52(10):617, 1981.

Pinard A and Pinard D: Treatment of the gingivitis of puerperal women, Dent Cosmos 19:327, 1877.

Rateitschak KH: Tooth mobility changes in pregnancy, J Periodont Res 2:199, 1967.

Ringsdorf WM et al: Periodontal status and pregnancy, Am J Obstet Gynecol 83:258, 1962.

Samant A: Gingivitis and periodontal disease in pregnancy, J Periodontol 47:415, 1976.

Shafer WG, Hine MK, and Levy BM: A textbook of oral pathology, ed 3, Philadelphia, 1974, WB Saunders Co.

Silness J and Löe H: Periodontal disease in pregnancy. II. Correlation between oral hygiene and periodontal condition, Acta Odontol Scand 22:121, 1964.

Slots J: Subgingival microflora and periodontal disease, J Periodontol 6:351, 1979.

Sweet JB and Butler DP: Increased incidence of postoperative localized osteitis in mandibular third molar surgery associated with patients using oral contraceptives, Am J Obstet Gynecol 127:518, 1977.

Vittek J et al: Phenytoin effect on the proliferation of rat oral epithelium is mediated by a hormonal mechanism, Cell Differ 12:335, 1983.

Ziskin D: Effect of the male sex hormones on the gingival and oral mucous membranes of rhesus monkeys and humans, J Dent Res 20:419, 1941.

Chapter 18

DISEASES OF THE SKIN AND MUCOUS MEMBRANES WITH ORAL MANIFESTATIONS

Russell Nisengard
Mirdza Neiders

Diagnosis
Pemphigus
Cicatricial pemphigoid (benign mucous membrane pemphigoid)
Bullous pemphigoid
Lichen planus
Psoriasis
Desquamative gingivitis
Lupus erythematosus
   Systemic lupus erythematosus
   Discoid lupus erythematosus
Erythema multiforme (Stevens-Johnson syndrome)
Idiopathic gingival fibromatosis
Recurrent aphthous stomatitis
Systemic sclerosis (scleroderma)

Several diseases may involve the oral mucosa, as well as the skin and other organs. The lesions may be localized exclusively to the oral cavity, be localized to the skin and other organs, or involve both intraoral and extraoral sites. When the lesions are only intraoral, identification may be difficult because many of them have erythematous and ulcerative areas. This chapter considers several conditions that may involve the gingiva and manifest as erythema, ulcerations, or combinations of both. The etiologies or triggering mechanisms for many of these entities are unknown, making specific treatment difficult.

DIAGNOSIS

This group of diverse diseases is diagnosed on the basis of one or more criteria: clinical, histologic, and immunologic. Conditions such as aphthous ulcers, with characteristic, easily recognizable lesions, can be diagnosed solely by a careful clinical examination. A diagnosis of fibromatosis requires not only a clinical examination, but also histologic evaluation of a biopsy specimen. For a third group, including pemphigus, pemphigoid, lichen planus, psoriasis, desquamative gingivitis, and lupus erythematosus, diagnosis requires clinical, histologic, and often immunologic evaluation.

Direct immunofluorescent examination of biopsy specimens and/or of sera frequently allows identification of the underlying etiology when routine histology does not. Direct immunofluorescence can identify immune deposits in lesional specimens and often in perilesional and normal specimens. This is particularly important in oral vesicular-bullous disease wherein lesions quickly ulcerate and in connective tissue diseases, which often present as erythematous vesicles.

For collection and handling of biopsy and serum specimens, it is important to follow the laboratory protocols.

PEMPHIGUS

Pemphigus is an autoimmune disease with chronic bullous lesions involving the skin and mucous membranes. Its forms include pemphigus vulgaris, pemphigus vegetans, pemphigus foliaceus, and pemphigus erythematosus (Lever and Schaumberg-Lever, 1975).

Pemphigus vulgaris, the most common form, characteristically occurs in elderly patients, with a predilection for patients of Jewish and Mediterranean origin (Pesanti et al., 1974). In over 50% of patients the initial lesions are intraoral with subsequent extraoral involvement (Ryan, 1971; Meyer et al., 1977). Eventually, oral lesions develop in over 90% of patients.

The oral lesions initially occur as crops of fluid-filled

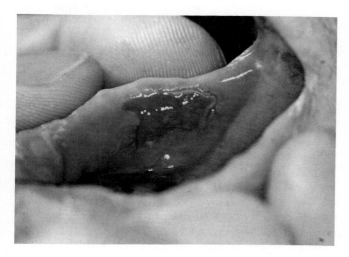

Fig. 18-1.   Oral pemphigus. A large area of ulceration is observed.

bullae, which rapidly rupture, leading to denuded areas covered with necrotic debris (Fig. 18-1). The gingiva is not a major intraoral site; however, when gingival lesions occur, they are desquamative. Skin lesions may be flaccid bullae or ulcerated. Patients with bullae frequently exhibit a positive Nikolsky's sign, whereby lateral pressure on normal skin or mucosa results in dislodgment of the epithelium similar to that seen with a ruptured blister. While a positive Nikolsky's sign is useful in the diagnosis of pemphigus, it can also be elicited in pemphigoid and other vesiculobullous diseases.

Histologically, pemphigus is characterized by acantholysis, or loss of coherence between epithelial cells. This results from the degeneration of intercellular substance with the resultant development of intraepithelial blisters (Lever and Schaumberg-Lever, 1975) (Table 18-1). The epithelium superficial to the acantholytic process usually is hyalinized and degenerated. Acantholytic or rounded squamous cells (Tzanck cells) occur freely within the blister cavity. The base of the blister is lined with partially separated basal epithelial cells attached to an intact basement membrane (Fig. 18-2). The underlying lamina propria is usually intact with an inflammatory cell infiltrate.

Immunologically, direct immunofluorescence on biopsy specimens reveals diagnostic findings of intercellular deposits of IgG in the epithelium (Fig. 18-3). Indirect immunofluorescence on serum demonstrates diagnostic findings of IgG antibodies reactive with the intercellular substance of squamous epithelium in almost all patients (Beutner et al., 1987a). Both the biopsy and serum antibody findings

Table 18-1. Histopathology and immunopathology in dermatoses associated with desquamative gingival lesions, generalized red conditions, and multiple ulcerations

Disease	Immunopathology	Histopathology
Cicatricial pemphigoid (benign mucous membrane pemphigoid)	Basement membrane deposits of IgG and C3*	Subepithelial bullae (blisters) with epithelium separated from lamina propria; inflammatory infiltrate in lamina propria
Bullous pemphigoid	Similar to cicatricial pemphigoid	Similar to cicatricial pemphigoid
Lichen planus	Globular deposits or cytoid bodies of IgG, IgM, and C3 in dermis and epidermis†; fibrin deposits along dermoepidermal junction	Bandlike inflammatory infiltrate in lamina propria; degeneration of basal epithelium with sawtooth interdigitation of epithelium and lamina propria
Pemphigus, all forms	Intercellular IgG in gingival epithelium*	Epithelial acantholysis; intraepithelial bullae (blisters); inflammatory infiltrate in lamina propria
Psoriasis	Stratum corneum deposits of IgG and C3†	Epithelial hyperplasia with thickened stratum corneum and parakeratosis; epithelial microabscesses; inflammatory infiltrate in lamina propria
Erythema multiforme	IgM and C3 in blood vessel walls*	Subepithelial clefts with mononuclear infiltrate and necrosis of keratinocytes

*Findings are diagnostic.
†Findings are suggestive but not diagnostic.

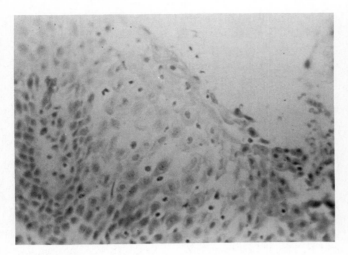

Fig. 18-2. Histopathology of pemphigus characterized by intercellular bullae.

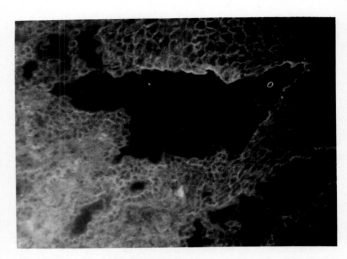

Fig. 18-3. Direct immunofluorescence for IgG in oral biopsy specimen from a patient with pemphigus demonstrating intercellular deposits of IgG.

are diagnostic for pemphigus. Serum intercellular antibody titers also reflect the severity of disease. Titers usually decrease during remission and increase during clinical relapse. At times, an elevation in titers precedes a clinical exacerbation, providing prognostic information. With this in mind, indirect immunofluorescence tests on serum are often performed at intervals, and changes in antibody titers of two doubling dilutions or more indicate when to modulate therapy.

Treatment.   According to Nisengard and Rogers (1987a, 1987b), the treatment of pemphigus may be outlined as follows:

1. Oral hygiene reinforcement (where there is gingival involvement)
2. Frequent scaling and root planing (also where there is gingival involvement)
3. Systemic corticosteroids—40 mg of prednisone every other day with or without adjunctive immunosuppressant agent every day (usually 100 mg of azathioprine per day)

These measures are effective in mild, relatively stable disease.

Corticosteroids are the drugs of choice for treatment of pemphigus (Lever and Schaumberg-Lever, 1977, 1984). While early cases of oral pemphigus may partially respond to topical steroids alone, systemic treatment is necessary because skin lesions develop. In the early stages prompt remission may be induced by systemic corticosteroids, often in conjunction with immunosuppressants. Because of systemic manifestations of the disease and systemic complications of therapy, pemphigus patients are usually referred to dermatologists for treatment.

Treatment of mild cases with only intraoral lesions usually includes 20 to 40 mg of prednisone every other day,

sometimes with an immunosuppressant drug such as azathioprine, 100 mg/day (Nisengard and Rogers, 1987a, 1987b). If control is not achieved, or the condition worsens, the dosage of prednisone can be increased. Prednisone at a dosage of 40 mg every other day combined with an immunosuppressant is relatively safe and can be given for a year or longer when lesions persist. With extensive intraoral and cutaneous involvement or progressive disease, higher doses of corticosteroids may be prescribed initially.

In the past, approximately 10% of patients with pemphigus died of complications of prednisone treatment. This appears to have resulted from prolonged intermediate dosages of prednisone (over 40 and up to 200 mg/day). Short-term doses of 200 to 400 mg for up to 10 weeks (provided patients have not previously received intermediate doses of prednisone) are not associated with such fatalities.

Where there is gingival involvement, establishment of plaque control and frequent scaling and root planing are also recommended.

CICATRICIAL PEMPHIGOID (BENIGN MUCOUS MEMBRANE PEMPHIGOID)

Cicatricial pemphigoid, frequently called benign mucous membrane pemphigoid, is a chronic bullous disease affecting mucous membranes of the mouth, conjunctiva, nose, pharynx, penis, vagina, and anus, but rarely the skin (Hardy et al., 1971; Nisengard and Drinnan, 1982). In contrast, bullous pemphigoid, which is clinically, histologically, and immunologically similar, mainly involves the skin and affects the oral mucosa only about 30% of the time. Cicatricial pemphigoid occurs most often after 40 years of age, and women are more commonly affected than men.

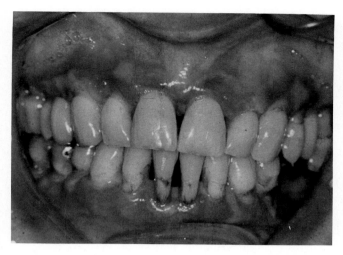

Fig. 18-4. Desquamative gingivitis in a 70-year-old woman. Erythematous and erosive lesions were present for at least 1 year and localized to buccal and lingual aspects of free and attached gingiva. (Courtesy Dr. S.L. Fischman, SUNY at Buffalo.)

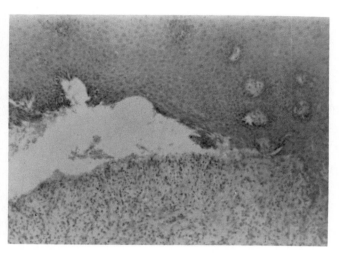

Fig. 18-5. Section from perilesional gingival biopsy specimen revealing a subepithelial bulla consistent with cicatricial pemphigoid. (Hematoxylin and eosin; ×400.) (Courtesy Dr. S.L. Fischman, SUNY at Buffalo.)

Cicatricial pemphigoid is a vesiculobullous disease characterized by erythema, bullae, and ulcerated areas lasting for months to years. Lesions may heal spontaneously, and then periodic breakouts may occur in new sites. In oral lesions, termed *desquamative gingival lesions* (Fig. 18-4), the epithelium overlying the bullae usually sloughs, leaving ulcerated, denuded areas. When the conjunctiva is affected, blindness may ensue. Conjunctival lesions have been reported in 50% to 70% of patients seeing dermatologists for cicatricial pemphigoid and in only 10% of patients seeing dentists for desquamative gingivitis. One explanation for the lower incidence of eye involvement in patients with desquamative gingival lesions may be that they seek professional care earlier because of their sore mouths. Alternatively, they may represent a subset of patients with cicatricial pemphigoid who do not manifest eye lesions as frequently.

Histologically, cicatricial pemphigoid and bullous pemphigoid are identical (see Table 18-1). Both are characterized by subepithelial bullae. Typically, intact epithelium is separated along the basement membrane from the underlying lamina propria (Fig. 18-5). The rete ridges are shortened, with minimal interdigitation of epithelium and lamina propria. Both an acute and a chronic infiltrate may be seen in the lamina propria, depending on the age of the lesion. Lymphocytes and plasma cells dominate the infiltrate of established lesions.

Immunologically, useful diagnostic immunofluorescence findings are made with biopsy specimens from potential lesions and adjacent tissue (Beutner et al., 1987a) (see Table 18-1). Almost all biopsy specimens have unique basement membrane zone deposits of IgG and C3

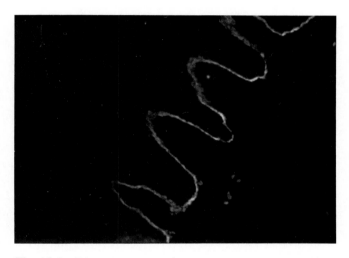

Fig. 18-6. Direct immunofluorescence for C3 on section from a clinically normal biopsy specimen. C3 deposits along basement membrane are consistent with cicatricial pemphigoid.

(Fig. 18-6). Approximately 10% of patients with desquamative gingival lesions associated with cicatricial pemphigoid have serum antibodies reactive with the basement membrane zone (Rogers et al., 1976; Person et al., 1977; Fine and Weathers, 1980; Laskaris et al., 1981; Nisengard and Neiders, 1981).

In comparing the relative merits of light microscopy and immunofluorescence in the diagnosis of cicatricial pemphigoid, it can be noted that direct immunofluorescence identifies more cases. This slight but consistent advantage probably reflects the fact that oral lesion specimens are frequently ulcerated, making complete interpreta-

Treatment of cicatricial pemphigoid

Asymptomatic disease with gingival involvement

1. Oral hygiene reinforcement
2. Frequent scaling and root planing

Symptomatic mild disease

1. Oral hygiene reinforcement (with gingival involvement)
2. Frequent scaling and root planing (with gingival involvement)
3. Topical application of fluorinated corticosteroids two to three times daily until sufficient control is achieved (e.g., 0.05% Lidex cream or 0.01% Synalar cream)

Symptomatic moderate to severe disease involving other mucosal surfaces

1. Oral hygiene reinforcement (with gingival involvement)
2. Frequent scaling and root planing (with gingival involvement)
3. Systemic dapsone therapy, increasing the dose stepwise to 150 mg, adjusting the dose until sufficient control is achieved, and then stepwise decreasing the dose:
    - 25 mg daily for 3 days
    - 25 mg twice a day for 3 days
    - 25 mg three times a day for 3 days
    - 50 mg twice a day for 1 week
    - 75 mg in the morning plus 25 mg in the evening for 1 week
    - 75 mg in the morning plus 75 mg in the evening until symptoms subside
4. Topical application of fluorinated corticosteroids two to three times daily as possible supplement to dapsone

Modified from Nisengard RJ and Rogers RS III: J Periodontol 58:167, 1987.

tion possible. However, even clinically normal gingival biopsy specimens from patients can be examined immunologically and demonstrate diagnostic basement membrane zone immune deposits. Histologically, such clinically normal biopsy specimens would usually demonstrate only chronic inflammation, which is not diagnostic.

Treatment. Treatment of localized oral cicatricial pemphigoid is determined by the degree of involvement (Rogers et al., 1982a, 1982b; Nisengard and Rogers, 1987a, 1987b) (see box above). In asymptomatic patients no specific treatment is necessary. Oral hygiene should be maintained, and patients should receive periodic scaling and root planing. In symptomatic patients with localized lesions, topical application of fluorinated corticosteroids two to three times each day, usually for long periods of time extending to several months, may be sufficient to control the process. Lidex cream (0.05%) and Synalar cream (0.01%) have proved to be effective. Wray and McCord (1987) have recently suggested that acrylic labial ve-

neers may act as a vehicle to maintain topical steroids in contact with the lesions for longer periods of time and may be used in symptomatic mild disease.

In patients with moderate, progressive disease, systemic therapy is indicated. While most inflammatory diseases usually respond to systemic corticosteroids, cicatricial pemphigoid is an exception. Even high doses of prednisone may have minimal effect. A better response has been reported to dapsone (DeGowin, 1967).

Dapsone (4-4' diaminodiphenylsulfone) has been widely used for the treatment of dermatitis herpetiformis and leprosy. More recently it has proved to be highly effective in the treatment of cicatricial pemphigoid and other bullous diseases with predominantly neutrophilic and eosinophilic infiltrates (Rogers et al., 1982a, 1982b). Its antiinflammatory effect results partially from inhibition of lysosomal enzyme activity and interference with the myeloperoxidase-mediated cytotoxic system in polymorphonuclear leukocytes.

Side effects of dapsone therapy include hemolysis and methemoglobinemia, particularly in patients with glucose-6-phosphate dehydrogenase deficiency. Therefore, before beginning dapsone therapy, patients should be tested for this deficiency and have a complete blood count (CBC). CBC examinations should then be obtained weekly or every other week during the first 3 months and every other month thereafter.

Eighty-five percent of patients will respond to dapsone and do so within 6 to 12 weeks. Once control has been established and maintained for an additional 6 to 12 weeks, the dapsone may be tapered by 25 mg every week until the lowest effective dose for control is achieved. At times, the dapsone can eventually be discontinued without exacerbation.

For those patients not responding to 150 mg of dapsone per day, sulfapyridine in a dose of 500 mg/day for 7 days, then twice a day for 7 days, then three times a day thereafter, may be used as primary therapy or added to the dapsone therapy (Katz, 1982).

BULLOUS PEMPHIGOID

In bullous pempigoid, skin lesions usually precede the infrequent oral lesions. The skin lesions are characterized by large tense bullae, denuded areas where the bullae have broken, and erythematous areas.

Immunologically, bullous pemphigoid demonstrates basement membrane immune deposits as seen in cicatricial pemphigoid (Beutner et al., 1987a). It differs from cicatricial pemphigoid in that over 70% of patients have circulating antibodies, generally in high titers, to the epithelial basement membrane (see Table 18-1). As discussed above, patients with cicatricial pemphigoid infrequently have such antibodies, and when they are present, titers are low. The basement zone serum antibodies in bullous pemphigoid do not correlate with disease activity, as do the intercellular antibodies of pemphigus.

Treatment. Because bullous pemphigoid has primarily cutaneous involvement, treatment should be provided by a dermatologist. Patients with symptomatic cases are usually treated with systemic steroids. Once lesions are asymptomatic or in remission, treatment is discontinued because of the untoward responses to steroids.

LICHEN PLANUS

Lichen planus affects the skin and mucous membranes. The majority of patients are 30 to 65 years of age; both sexes are affected equally. While the etiology is unknown, many cases are associated with psychic or emotional trauma. At times, there is a spontaneous remission of the disease following resolution of emotional problems. The lesions vary considerably and range from keratotic lesions, which appear linear, reticulate, annular, or plaquelike, to ulcerative or erosive lesions. The erosive form may appear as desquamative gingival lesions (Nisengard and Neiders, 1981). Usually the keratotic forms are asymptomatic, whereas the erosive and ulcerative forms are chronically irritated.

Histologically, lichen planus is characterized by a band-like infiltrate below the basement membrane zone; a damaged basal cell layer, including degeneration of the basal cells with Civatte bodies (possibly the "cytoid" bodies observed by immunofluorescence) above and below the basement membrane zone; hyperkeratosis; hypergranulosis; and a "sawtooth" interdigitation of the epithelium and lamina propria (Lever and Schaumberg-Lever, 1975) (see Table 18-1). The lamina propria is infiltrated by lymphocytes and occasionally leukocytes that abut the basement membrane zone and extend into the epithelium.

Immunologically, biopsy specimens of lichen planus have characteristic but not diagnostic findings, including (1) cytoid bodies in the epidermis and dermis and (2) fibrin (fibrinogen) deposits along the basement membrane (Nisengard and Neiders, 1981; Bergfeld et al., 1987) (see Table 18-1 and Fig. 18-7).

Treatment. The treatment regimen for lichen planus is similar to that for asymptomatic and mild, symptomatic cicatricial pemphigoid (Nisengard and Rogers, 1987a, 1987b) (see box on opposite page). Asymptomatic cases require no treatment unless there is gingival involvement. With gingival lesions, plaque-associated inflammation should be controlled by oral hygiene reinforcement and frequent scaling and root planing. Symptomatic lichen planus is treated by topical application of fluorinated corticosteroids two to three times a day until sufficient control is achieved. This usually requires treatment lasting from several weeks to months.

PSORIASIS

Psoriasis of the skin commonly appears as well-circumscribed papules covered by scales, but in some cases there may be pustules. Oral lesions of psoriasis are uncommon; however, lesions of the gingiva, buccal mucosa, tongue,

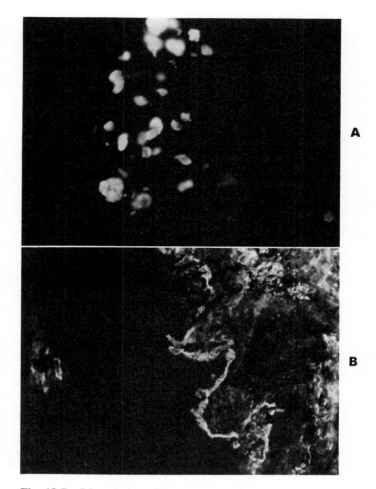

Fig. 18-7. Direct immunofluorescence on biopsy specimen from a patient with lichen planus. **A,** Cytoid bodies containing IgG in dermis. **B,** Fibrin deposits along dermoepidermal junction.

and lips can occur. Gingival lesions may appear desquamative (Brayshaw and Orban, 1953; DeGregori et al., 1971; Jones and Dolby, 1972; Beutner, et al. 1977; Nisengard and Neiders, 1981).

Histologically, psoriasis is characterized by hyperkeratosis and hyperplasia of the malpighian stratum, with thinning of the epithelium over the connective tissue papillae. Also, increased mitotic figures within the nuclei of the basal cells and epidermal microabscesses are seen (Lever and Schaumberg-Lever, 1975) (see Table 18-1). The lamina propria contains a chronic inflammatory cell infiltrate that is scattered and diffuse. In acute lesions, a polymorphonuclear leukocyte infiltrate may be noted in the lamina propria and epithelium.

Immunologically, gingival and skin biopsy specimens show features similar to those of psoriasis of the skin: antibodies and complement bound in vivo to the stratum corneum antigen (see Table 18-1) (Beutner et al., 1987c). No unique serologic findings are associated with psoriasis.

Most, if not all, sera, whether from healthy subjects or from patients with psoriasis, have naturally occurring antibodies to the stratum corneum. These antibodies may play a physiologic role in epidermal repair (Beutner et al., 1987d).

Treatment. Treatment of psoriasis is similar to the regimen used for asymptomatic or symptomatic but mild oral cicatricial pemphigoid and for lichen planus (Nisengard and Rogers, 1987a, 1987b). This includes plaque control as well as scaling and root planing where there is gingival involvement. In addition, fluorinated corticosteroids are given topically two to three times daily until control is achieved.

DESQUAMATIVE GINGIVITIS

Desquamative gingivitis is a chronic gingival disease characterized by erythematous, erosive, vesiculobullous, and/or desquamative involvement of the free and attached gingivae (see Fig. 18-4). The majority of patients are female (80%) and in the fourth through sixth decade of life. However, lesions have been reported in individuals from 7 to 78 years of age. In half of the cases lesions are localized solely to the gingivae, and in the remainder they concurrently involve other intraoral and extraoral sites, including the buccal mucosa, palate, tongue, lips, skin, and conjunctiva of the eye. With time, lesions localized exclusively to the gingivae sometimes extend to other sites (Zeskin and Zegarelli, 1945; Engel et al., 1950; McCarthy et al., 1960; Glickman and Smulow, 1964; Rogers et al., 1976; Forman and Nally, 1977; Chaiken, 1980; Barnett et al., 1981; Laskaris et al., 1981; Nisengard and Neiders, 1981).

The disease entity was described by Tomes more than 100 years ago, and the name "chronic diffuse desquamative gingivitis" was coined by Prinz in 1932. While early reports suggested that desquamative gingivitis was a specific disease entity, Glickman, as early as 1953, speculated that it may represent a manifestation of several disease processes. Since then, histologic and immunologic findings have supported that speculation. McCarthy et al. (1960) and more recently Shklar (1984) proposed a provisional classification based on etiologic considerations. This has been expanded by observations of others (Rogers et al., 1976; Forman and Nally, 1977) and is summarized in the box at right.

While many diseases and conditions have been associated with desquamative gingivitis, the majority (75%) are dermatologic. The most common dermatologic diseases are cicatricial pemphigoid and lichen planus, which constitute over 95% of desquamative gingivitis with a dermatologic etiology. Other, nondermatologic diseases associated with desquamative gingival lesions, such as hormonal imbalances, chronic infections, and idiopathic disorders, occur less frequently.

The diagnosis of the underlying etiology is important for appropriate treatment and subsequent long-term management. This requires evaluation of clinical, histologic,

---

Diseases associated with desquamative gingival lesions

Dermatoses
  Cicatricial pemphigoid
  Lichen planus
  Pemphigus
  Psoriasis
  Bullous pemphigoid
  Epidermolysis bullosa acquisita
  Contact stomatitis
Endocrine imbalance
  Estrogen deficiencies following oophorectomy and in postmenopausal women
  Testosterone imbalance
  Hypothyroidism
Aging
Abnormal response to bacterial plaque
Idiopathic
Chronic infections
  Tuberculosis
  Chronic candidiasis
  Histoplasmosis

From Nisengard RJ and Rogers RS III: J Periodontol 58:167, 1987.

---

and immunologic criteria (Nisengard et al., 1978; Laskaris et al., 1981; Rogers et al., 1982a, 1982b; Nisengard and Rogers, 1987a, 1987b). Specimens for the laboratory diagnosis of desquamative gingival lesions should include (1) a perilesional specimen to be divided and one half placed in formalin for histologic study and the other in Michele's buffer for immunofluorescence study, and (2) a normal specimen placed in Michele's buffer for immunofluorescence (Nisengard and Neiders, 1981). The examination of sera from patients with desquamative gingivitis by indirect immunofluorescence usually yields negative results except in cases of pemphigus and in less than one third of the cases of cicatricial pemphigoid. Except for pemphigus, serum tests are not usually informative. The characteristic histologic and immunologic findings associated with desquamative gingival lesions are summarized in Table 18-1.

The direct immunofluorescence biopsy findings in 174 cases of desquamative gingivitis are summarized in Table 18-2 (Forman and Nally, 1977; Barnett et al., 1981; Laskaris et al., 1981; Nisengard and Neiders, 1981; Rogers et al., 1982a, 1982b). In almost one half of the cases (48.9%) diagnostic findings for cicatricial pemphigoid were found. Pemphigus was uncommon and occurred in 2.3% of the cases. Findings suggestive, but not diagnostic, of lichen planus and psoriasis occurred in 23.6% and 0.6%, respectively. Negative findings suggesting a nondermatologic etiology were observed in 24.6% of the cases. Thus, on the basis of direct immunofluorescence of oral lesion biopsy specimens, approximately one half of the desquamative lesions are cicatricial pemphigoid, one fourth are lichen planus, and one fourth have no significant immunopathology. In addition, a small number are pemphigus and psoriasis. Serum studies by indirect immunofluorescence indicate that approximately 10% of patients with cicatricial pemphigoid have basement membrane zone antibodies and 100% of patients with pemphigus have intercellular antibodies.

The early diagnosis of cicatricial pemphigoid and pemphigus in patients whose presenting signs and symptoms indicate "desquamative gingivitis" is of the utmost importance. Cicatricial pemphigoid can cause blindness, and pemphigus is a life-threatening disease. In cases of cicatricial pemphigoid, an ophthalmologist and a dermatologist should be consulted. With pemphigus, a dermatologist should be consulted.

Treatment. A variety of drugs and clinical therapeutic modalities have been suggested for the treatment of desquamative gingival lesions (Glickman and Smulow, 1964; Chaiken, 1980; Lozada and Silverman, 1980; Rogers et al., 1982a, 1982b; Shklar, 1984; Nisengard and Rogers, 1987a, 1987b). Drug therapy has included (1) topical corticosteroids: triamcinolone (e.g., Kenalog in Orabase, Aristocort) and fluocinolone (e.g., Synalar), (2) systemic corticosteroids (e.g., prednisone), (3) antibiotics (e.g., penicillin and tetracycline), (4) methotrexate, (5) dapsone, (6) estrogens, (7) androgens, and (8) vitamins. Periodontal clinical treatment has included (1) oral hygiene, (2) scaling and root planing, (3) curettage, (4) gingivectomy, and (5) free gingival grafts. This extensive list has evolved because desquamative lesions heal slowly or not at all in response to therapy. This is partially a result of failure to diagnose the underlying disease, leading to selection of inappropriate therapy. In addition, success of a particular therapy has been claimed when there was actually spontaneous remission, which sometimes occurs with desquamative gingival lesions. The experiences of Nisengard and Rogers (1987b) with 62 cases are summarized in Table 18-3.

Recommended treatments for desquamative gingivitis caused by pemphigoid, pemphigus, lichen planus, and psoriasis are outlined with the discussions of these specific diseases. As already stated, selection of a treatment modality first requires diagnosis of the underlying etiology. In some cases histologic and immunologic examination does not allow identification of the etiology. Either these lesions are idiopathic or the biopsy specimens do not have characteristic histopathologic or immunopathologic findings. In these cases another biopsy specimen taken several months later may prove diagnostic. If none of the clearly defined disease entities is identified, symptomatic, idiopathic desquamative gingival lesions may be treated with topical steroids in a manner similar to their use in mild localized cicatricial pemphigoid.

LUPUS ERYTHEMATOSUS

Lupus erythematosus, a connective tissue disease with autoimmune manifestation, is divided into two groups: systemic lupus erythematosus (SLE), with systemic in-

Table 18-2. Summary of direct immunofluorescence findings in desquamative gingivitis

Immunologic diagnosis*	No. of patients	% of total
Cicatricial pemphigoid†	85	48.9
Pemphigus†	4	2.3
Lichen planus‡	41	23.6
Psoriasis‡	1	0.6
Negative§	43	24.6
TOTAL	174	

From Nisengard RJ and Rogers RS III: J Peridontol 58:167, 1987.
*Based on direct immunofluorescence findings in gingival biopsy specimens.
†Immunologic findings are diagnostic: immune deposits along the basement membrane zone in cicatricial pemphigoid and intercellular in pemphigus.
‡Immunologic findings are suggestive but not diagnostic: large numbers of cytoid bodies and/or fibrin deposits along the basement membrane zone in lichen planus and immune deposits in the stratum corneum in the psoriasis form of psoriasis.
§No significant immune findings.

Table 18-3. Treatment of desquamative gingivitis

Underlying disease	Therapy	No. of cases	Response NR*	Response PR	Response R
Cicatricial pemphigoid	No treatment	8	7	-	1
	Topical corticosteroid	17	2	6	9
	Systemic corticosteroid	3	3	-	-
	Systemic dapsone or sulfapyridine	16	1	3	12
	SUBTOTAL	44			
Lichen planus	No treatment	5	4	1	
	Topical corticosteroid	7	2	1	4
	Systemic corticosteroid	1		1	
	SUBTOTAL	13			
Pemphigus	Systemic corticosteroid	2			2
	SUBTOTAL	2			
Etiology unknown	Topical corticosteroid	3	1	1	1
	SUBTOTAL	3			
	TOTAL	62			

From Nisengard RJ and Rogers RS III: J Periodontal 58:167, 1987.
*NR, No resolution; PR, partial resolution; R, resolution during time of treatment.

volvement, and discoid lupus erythematosus (DLE), with primarily localized skin involvement.

Systemic lupus erythematosus

SLE clinically offers a wide range of clinical manifestations depending on the organs involved (Nisengard and Drinnan, 1982). These may include the skin, kidneys, central nervous system, vascular system, bone marrow, heart, and mucous membranes. Skin lesions often include the characteristic "butterfly" erythematous rash over the malar areas and the bridge of the nose. Oral lesions occur in approximately 45% of SLE patients, mainly as erythematous areas often accompanied by edema and petechiae (Jonsson et al., 1984). Other findings may include arthritis, arthralgia, nephritis, seizures, psychosis, pericarditis, endocarditis, and pleurisy.

Histologic findings depend on the organ(s) involved. Skin and mucous membrane changes include hydropic degeneration of the basal epithelial cells, hyperkeratosis, parakeratosis, pseudoepitheliomatous hyperplasia interspersed with atrophy, and edema in the upper dermis (Lever and Schaumberg-Lever, 1975) (see Table 18-1).

Immunologically, SLE is characterized by a polyclonal B-cell activation to tissue, particularly the nuclear antigens. Direct immunofluorescent examination of normal as well as lesional biopsy specimens reveals in vivo bandlike deposits of IgG and sometimes IgM, IgA, and complement along the dermoepidermal junction (see Table 18-1) (Beutner et al., 1987b). This "lupus band finding" in normal biopsy specimens is diagnostic for SLE. The disease occurs more frequently in sun-exposed areas than in sun-protected sites, so skin biopsies are usually preferred over oral biopsies. Serum tests reveal antibodies to a variety of nuclear and cytoplasmic components, including antinuclear antibodies (ANA) and antibodies to DNA and other cellular antigens: RNP, Sm, Ro, and La. High titers to ANA (usually ≥160) occur in SLE but are not diagnostic for SLE, since they are associated with other connective tissue diseases as well. DNA antibodies are highly specific for SLE, and antibodies to RNP, Sm, Ro, and La occur principally in SLE and in a limited number of other connective tissue diseases.

Treatment. Treatment of SLE depends to some degree on the organs involved but generally includes systemic steroids. Endothelial damage to heart valves occurs in 50% of patients with SLE (Zysset et al., 1987), leading to an increased incidence of endocarditis similar to that seen in rheumatic heart disease. As a consequence, prophylactic antibiotics should be considered before dental procedures causing transient bacteremias are undertaken.

Discoid lupus erythematosus

DLE is usually confined to the skin and oral mucous membranes. Skin involvement appears as well-defined, erythematous, scaly lesions that mainly appear on the face, neck, arms, and scalp (Nisengard and Drinnan, 1982). Oral manifestations of DLE occur in approximately 20% of patients with skin involvement and may even occur in the absence of skin lesions (Schiodt et al., 1978). Early oral lesions are characterized by erythema. Well-developed oral lesions often have central erythema with white spots and a border of radiating striae similar to striae in lichen planus.

Histologically, DLE lesions are characterized by hyperkeratosis with keratotic plugging, epithelial atrophy, hydropic degeneration of the basal cells, a patchy lymphocytic infiltration, and edema with vasodilation (Lever and Schaumberg-Lever, 1975) (see Table 18-1).

Immunologically, lesional DLE biopsy specimens have immunofluorescence findings similar to those found in both lesional and normal SLE biopsy specimens (Beutner et al., 1987a). In contrast to normal biopsy specimens from SLE patients, DLE specimens, however, have no significant immunopathologic findings. As a result, immunofluorescent examination of normal biopsy specimens often aids in differentiating SLE from DLE. DLE usually has no associated serum antibodies to nuclear antigens, as is seen in SLE.

Treatment. Treatment of DLE is similar to but less intense than that of SLE. Although treatment commonly includes systemic steroids, topical steroids are sometimes applied to intraoral lesions.

ERYTHEMA MULTIFORME (STEVENS-JOHNSON SYNDROME)

Erythema multiforme is an acute, self-limiting vesiculobullous inflammatory disease with distinctive skin lesions and sometimes mucosal involvement (Huff et al., 1983; Fischman et al., 1985). Recurrences are frequent (Leigh et al., 1985). Most cases occur in young adults 20 to 40 years of age, but children and adolescents may also be affected.

The clinical appearance of erythema multiforme is quite variable, and the disease is classified as being minor or major. Erythema multiforme minor is the less severe cutaneous form, usually lasting less than 4 weeks (Fig. 18-8). Erythema multiforme major (also called Stevens-Johnson syndrome) is the more severe mucocutaneous form, lasting considerably longer than a month, depending on systemic

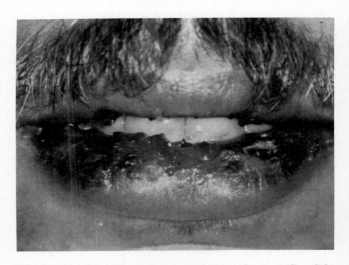

Fig. 18-8. Erythema multiforme of lips. (Courtesy Dr. S.L. Fischman, SUNY at Buffalo.)

complications (Edmond et al., 1983; Huff et al., 1983; Nethercott and Choi, 1985). Typical skin lesions have concentric zones of erythema called "iris" or "target" lesions, depending on the number of color zones (Fig. 18-9), and these are more common in erythema multiforme minor.

Mucosal involvement in erythema multiforme occurs in 25% to 60% of cases (Huff et al., 1983). In erythema multiforme major, mucosal involvement is severe and usually affects the eyes and mouth. Genital, upper respiratory tract, and pharyngeal lesions also may occur. Lozada and Silverman (1978) described cases having mucosal involvement alone; however, dermatologists often are reluctant to consider cases without skin lesions as representing erythema multiforme (Huff et al., 1983). The dentist should be aware of patients who have mucosal lesions in the absence of skin lesions, in addition to clinical findings, natural history, and histopathologic findings indistinguishable from erythema multiforme.

Erythema multiforme has a tendency to recur, and these recurrences are often associated with infectious agents or drugs. Herpes simplex infections have been implicated in up to 65% of erythema multiforme cases (Leigh et al., 1985). Erythema multiforme minor usually occurs approximately 10 days following recurrent herpes infections. *Mycoplasma pneumoniae* infections with systemic manifestations of fever and prostration have been reported to precede erythema multiforme major. Sulfonamides are also associated with erythema multiforme major (Huff et al., 1983).

Histologically, erythema multiforme is characterized by a subepithelial cleft, accumulation of mononuclear cells within blood vessel walls in the upper dermis, and necrosis of keratinocytes. These findings may be obscured in ulcerated lesions. Immunologically, IgM and C3 deposits are identified in the walls of superficial blood vessels within

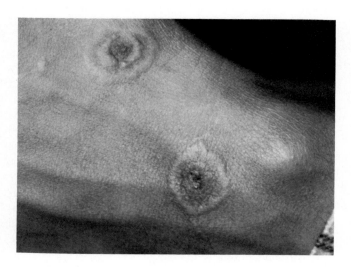

Fig. 18-9. Erythema multiforme of wrist demonstrating typical target lesions. (Courtesy Dr. S.L. Fischman, SUNY at Buffalo.)

the lesions. Accompanying this are immune complexes in the sera of up to half of the cases (Leigh et al., 1985; Beutner et al., 1987a).

Diagnosis of erythema multiforme is made on history, clinical, and histologic criteria. In addition to a biopsy for light microscopic examination, an additional biopsy for immunofluorescence is important in ruling out a diagnosis of pemphigoid, pemphigus, and dermatitis herpetiformis (Beutner et al., 1987a).

Treatment. Since erythema multiforme is a self-limiting disease, treatment is supportive and directed toward reduction of pain and prevention of infection. For erythema multiforme major, hospitalization is recommended to manage the frequent serious complications (Edmond et al., 1983). While steroid therapy is common for serious cases of erythema multiforme major, its use actually increases time in the hospital without definite efficacy (Rasmussen, 1976).

Recently, postherpetic erythema multiforme has been managed with acyclovir (Zovirax). This approach focuses on controlling the precipitating disease (Green et al., 1985; Lemak et al., 1986). Thus patients prone to developing erythema multiforme after recurrent herpes simplex infections are placed on a maintenance dose of acyclovir to prevent recurrent herpetic infections. Acyclovir has also been recommended after herpes lesions appear (Goldberg and Sperber, 1986). If the herpes lesions are controlled by the acyclovir, development of postherpetic erythema multiforme is also controlled. Acyclovir is not effective in managing erythema multiforme once the lesions of erythema multiforme appear.

IDIOPATHIC GINGIVAL FIBROMATOSIS

Idiopathic gingival fibromatosis is characterized by gingival enlargement associated with increased mature collagen. It is usually painless and can be generalized or localized. These cases can be divided into two subgroups: those associated with drugs and those that appear to be idiopathic. The drug-induced forms are discussed in Chapter 21. The idiopathic cases with a genetic basis are termed *hereditary gingival fibromatosis*. This is generally an autosomal dominant trait, although some recessive cases have been described.

Clinically, the degree of overgrowth is variable, with the gingiva covering significant portions of the crowns of teeth in severe cases (Fig. 18-10). The lobulated masses of tissue may produce an unsightly appearance and make it difficult to bring the lips together. In half of the cases patients have only gingival enlargement, whereas in the remainder of cases the fibromatosis is associated with a variety of conditions and syndromes (Witkop, 1971; Sciubba and Niebloom, 1985; Pina-Neto, 1986). The most common disease associated with fibromatosis is hypertrichosis; oligophrenia and epilepsy are generally also present (Horning et al., 1985).

Gingival fibromatosis also occurs in Murray-

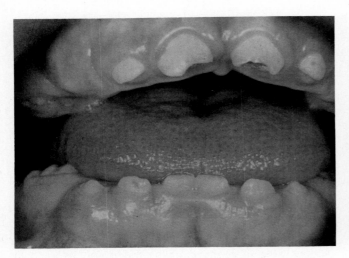

Fig. 18-10. Gingival fibromatosis. (Courtesy Dr. A. Uthman, SUNY at Buffalo.)

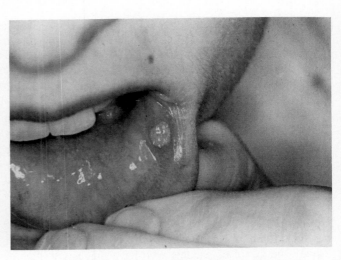

Fig. 18-11. Aphthous ulcer of labial mucosa.

Puretic-Drescher syndrome, or juvenile hyaline fibromatosis (Sciubba and Niebloom, 1985; Aldred and Crawford, 1987; Fayad et al., 1987). This autosomal recessive disease is characterized by multiple, subcutaneous, fibrous tumors on the scalp, back, and legs. Flexural contractures and osteolytic bone lesions also occur. Other rare entities occurring with gingival fibromatosis include Zimmerman-Laband syndrome, with anomalies of the digits, ear, nose, and nails, as well as hepatosplenomegaly; Cross syndrome, with micro-ophthalmia, hypopigmentation oligophrenia, and athetosis; Rutherford's syndrome, with corneal dystrophy and disturbed tooth eruption; and Cowden syndrome, with hypertrichosis and fibroadenomas of the breasts (Sciubba and Niebloom, 1985; Chodirker et al., 1986).

Treatment. The clinical management of hereditary fibromatosis consists of gingivectomy (Horning et al., 1985; Sciubba and Niebloom, 1985; Aldred and Crawford, 1987). Recurrences of the gingival overgrowth appear common. While recurrences of hyperplasia associated with dilantin therapy are controlled in part by rigid oral hygiene, it is unknown whether such plaque control is effective in hereditary gingival fibromatosis. Regardless, it appears to be good clinical practice to maintain plaque control in patients with hereditary fibromatosis following gingivectomy procedures.

RECURRENT APHTHOUS STOMATITIS

Recurrent aphthous stomatitis (RAS) is characterized by single or multiple, painful, oral ulcers that recur after variable periods of time (Fig. 18-11). Aphthous ulcers commonly occur in 10% to 60% of the population (Axell and Henricsson, 1985). Cooke (1969) divided the disease into three forms: (1) minor aphthous ulcers, (2) major aphthous

ulcers (sometimes called periadenitis mucosa necrotica recurrens), and (3) herpetiform aphthous ulcers. This classification is accepted in both the dental and dermatologic fields (Rogers, 1977; Rennie et al., 1985).

The most common form of RAS is the minor aphthous ulcer, which appears as groups of 2 to 4 mm round or oval painful, yellow ulcers with erythematous margins (Rennie et al., 1985). The lesions are normally located in the lining mucosa, with the masticatory mucosa of the palate and attached gingiva infrequently involved. The ulcers heal in 5 to 14 days without scarring. The lesions often recur, and in some patients recurrence may be as often as weeks between episodes, whereas in others it is years between episodes. Recurrence is often preceded by a premonitory stage lasting up to 24 hours that is characterized by a tingling and burning sensation. This is followed by painful, preulcerative lesions consisting of erythematous macules and papules that last from 18 hours to 3 days prior to ulceration (Rogers, 1977).

Approximately 10% of patients with RAS suffer from major aphthous ulcers. These are larger, deeper, usually solitary lesions that last longer, destroy deep tissue, and heal with scarring. Another 10% develop herpetiform aphthous ulcers occurring as multiple, small, pinpoint lesions that may involve the entire oral mucosa, occur in large numbers, and resemble herpes simplex stomatitis. This variant occurs more commonly in women and develops during the third decade (Rennie et al., 1985).

While a number of etiologic factors have been suggested for RAS, no single factor has been identified. Immune mechanisms, local trauma, deficiency disorders, and psychologic factors have all been implicated (Rogers, 1977; Rennie et al., 1985).

The diagnosis of RAS is primarily based on past history and clinical findings. Precipitating factors such as foods, stress, and other diseases may be considered. Other local and systemic causes of recurrent ulcerations must be excluded, including trauma, lichen planus, cyclic neutropenia, erythema multiforme, celiac disease, and foliate deficiency (Rennie et al., 1985).

Treatment. Treatment of mild cases of RAS is generally palliative to reduce pain. Tetracycline therapy alters to some degree the ulcer duration, size, and associated pain (Graykowski and Kingman, 1978). In severe, generalized cases, topical corticosteroids are commonly used to reduce symptoms and the duration of lesions (Glass et al., 1986). It is usually best to start the corticosteroids during the premonitory stage (Pimlott and Walker, 1983; Rennie et al., 1985). Kenalog in Orabase and 0.05% fluocinonide in Orabase have both been recommended (Pimlott and Walker, 1983; Glass et al., 1986). In severe cases systemic corticosteroids may be required and should be administered in consultation with the patient's physician.

If ulcers do not heal within the normal 2- to 4-week period, reassessment of the lesion has to be made, and other diagnoses, including malignancies and other ulcerative lesions, must be considered. The most important step to be taken for nonhealing ulcers is a biopsy to rule out malignancies.

SYSTEMIC SCLEROSIS (SCLERODERMA)

Systemic sclerosis and systemic scleroderma are synonomous terms applied to a disease of unknown etiology characterized by excessive deposition of collagen and other connective tissue components in skin and multiple internal organs. The disease is associated with prominent and often severe alterations in the microvasculature and the autonomic nervous system. Because of the frequent presence of immunologic abnormalities, systemic sclerosis has been included in a group of autoimmune diseases.

Systemic sclerosis affects women two to four times more frequently than men, and there is no racial predilection. The initial symptoms appear usually within the third to fifth decade of life, although the disease has been described in children and the elderly. Systemic sclerosis is a complex and clinically heterogeneous disease with clinical forms ranging from localized skin involvement with minimal systemic alterations to forms with severe internal organ disease and a fulminate course.

The pathologic changes in systemic sclerosis represent variable stages of progression and the development of at least three major processes occurring in the affected tissues:

1. Connective tissue alteration, with fibroblast proliferation, fibrosis, and increased ground substance
2. Inflammation, occurring predominantly in the early stages of disease and characterized by infiltration with large numbers of mononuclear cells, predominantly lymphocytes
3. Vascular disease, characterized by intimal proliferation, deposition of collagen and mucinous material, and narrowing of the vessel lumen and thrombosis

Progression of the vascular and fibrotic reaction and decrease in the inflammatory component lead to the final stage of atrophic changes in the affected organs.

Clinical manifestations. The most impressive and most common clinical features of systemic sclerosis are related to the generalized thickening and infiltration of the skin, but some degree of multiple organ involvement is almost always present. The skin is affected in almost all cases, but, rarely, classic visceral involvement can be demonstrated without clinical evidence of skin disease.

Raynaud's phenomenon is the second most common manifestation of systemic sclerosis and is present in more than 85% of patients. It usually appears simultaneously with other manifestations but may precede them by several years. Raynaud's phenomenon is usually triggered by exposure to cold and occasionally by stressful circumstances. Episodes are often painful and are characterized by involvement of the fingers, toes, and occasionally the face. Initial vasoconstriction and blanching are followed by a dusky cyanosis. With return of blood flow there is reactive erythema. Other systems that are involved include the musculoskeletal, gastrointestinal, respiratory, cardiac, renal, hepatic, and neurologic systems.

Dental considerations. The most common dental finding in systemic sclerosis is rigidity and thinness of the lips. In addition to contributing to the masklike comic expressionless appearance of patients with the disease, the circumoral fibrosis causes puckering and pallor when an attempt is made to open the mouth wide (Fig. 18-12). The collagination may progress to produce a microstomia. This inability of the patient to open his mouth may hinder oral hygiene, mastication, speech, and placement of a prosthesis.

The diffuse hyperpigmentation of the skin commonly seen in systemic sclerosis occasionally involves the oral mucous membrane. The mucous membrane may become ulcerated by the teeth as pressure and rigidity of the collagenated skin intensifies. Inhibition of the wound-healing process following trauma to the oral mucosa may also be a complication.

Telangiectasias, a common manifestation of several forms of systemic sclerosis, are often found on the lips and in the mouth. They are histologically identical to the lesions of hereditary hemorrhagic telangiectasia. A distinction can usually be made by the additional presence of Raynaud's phenomenon and a lack of family history.

A classic radiographic finding that has been associated with systemic sclerosis is widening of the periodontal ligament spaces. This is usually seen in posterior teeth (Fig.

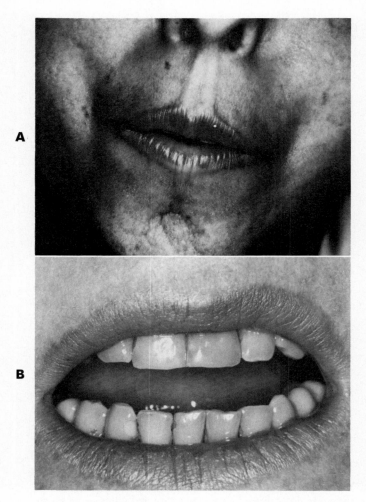

Fig. 18-12. Patient with systemic sclerosis demonstrating, **A,** circumoral puckering of lips and, **B,** limited ability to open mouth.

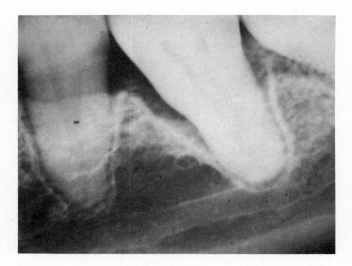

Fig. 18-13. Radiographic manifestation of systemic sclerosis revealing widened periodontal ligament spaces and prominent lamina dura.

18-13). This finding, however, appears to be highly variable. One report noted thickening of the periodontal ligament in only 7% of 127 cases, whereas another found it in 37% of 35 patients studied (Stafne and Austin, 1944; White et al., 1977). Additional radiographic changes that have been reported include resorption of the angle of the mandible, the condyle, and the coronoid process (Seifert et al., 1975). Pathologic fractures of the mandible may result from progression of the osseous resorption. These osseous changes apparently are related to pressure atrophy or ischemia and are associated with the advanced stages of systemic sclerosis.

Treatment. The most common complication encountered in attempting to perform routine dentistry on patients with systemic sclerosis is lack of access to the oral cavity because of microstomia. An attempt should therefore be made to improve the plaque control of the patient to prevent dental problems from occurring. Inability to open the mouth, however, may limit even basic oral hygiene. If there is sufficient crippling of the hands, toothbrushing and other means of plaque control may require specially designed instruments and techniques, as well as more frequent professional assistance. The periodontist should attempt to provide supportive therapy, including scaling, root planing, and prophylaxis, to assist the patient in maintaining good periodontal health.

A bilateral commissurotomy may be considered when the overall disease process appears controlled and the limitation of opening sufficiently interferes with mastication, speech, or insertion of dental prostheses.

Practitioners performing surgical procedures should be cognizant of the serious bleeding problem that can occur when oral telangiectasias are inadvertently involved.

REFERENCES

Aldred MJ and Crawford JM: Juvenile hyaline fibromatosis, Oral Surg 63:71, 1987.

Axell T and Henricsson V: The occurrence of recurrent aphthous ulcers in an adult Swedish population, Acta Odontol Scand 43:121, 1985.

Barnett ML, Wittwer JW, and Miller RL: Desquamative gingivitis in a 13-year-old male case report, J Periodontol 52:270, 1981.

Bergfeld WF, Valenzuela R, and Beutner EH: Lichen planus. In Beutner EH, Chorzelski TP, and Kumar V, editors: Immunopathology of the skin, ed 3, New York, 1987, John Wiley & Sons, Inc.

Beutner EH, Chorzelski TP, and Joblonska S: Clinical significance of immunofluorescence tests of sera and skin in bullous diseases: a cooperative study. In Beutner EH, Chorzelski TP, and Kumar V, editors: Immunopathology of the skin, ed 3, New York, 1987a, John Wiley & Sons, Inc.

Beutner EH, Chorzelski TP, and Kumar V: Comments on clinical significance of immunological findings in connective tissue diseases. In Beutner EH, Chorzelski TP, and Kumar V, editors: Immunopathology of the skin, ed 3, New York, 1987b, John Wiley & Sons, Inc.

Beutner EH, Nisengard RJ, and Binder WL: Differentiation of autoantibodies to hidden and accessible antigens in oral mucosa, J Dent Res 56(special issue B):B92, 1977.

Beutner EH et al: Autoimmunity in psoriasis. In Beutner EH, Chorzelski TP, and Kumar V, editors: Immunopathology of the skin, ed 3, New York, 1987c, John Wiley & Sons, Inc.

Beutner EH et al: Nature and function of stratum corneum/keratinocyte cytoplasm autoantibodies and their antigens. In Beutner EH, Chorzelski TP, and Kumar V, editors: Immunopathology of the skin, ed 3, New York, 1987d, John Wiley & Sons, Inc.

Brayshaw HA and Orban B: Psoriasis gingivae, J Periodontol 24:156, 1953.

Chaiken BS: A treatment of desquamative gingivitis by the use of free gingival grafts, Quintessence 9:105, 1980.

Chodirker BN et al: Brief clinical report: Zimmerman-Laband syndrome and profound mental retardation, Am J Med Genet 25:543, 1986.

Cooke BE: Recurrent oral ulceration, Br J Dermatol 81:159, 1969.

DeGowin RL: A review of therapeutic and hemolytic effects of dapsone, Arch Intern Med 120:242, 1967.

DeGregori G, Pippen R, and Davies E: Psoriasis of the gingiva and the tongue: report of a case, J Periodontol 42:97, 1971.

Edmond BJ, Huff JC, and Weston WL: Erythema multiforme, Pediatr Clin North Am 30:631, 1983.

Engel MD, Ray HG, and Orban B: The pathogenesis of desquamative gingivitis: a disturbance of the connective tissue ground substance, J Dent Res 29:410, 1950.

Fayad MN et al: Juvenile hyaline fibromatosis: two new patients and review of the literature, Am J Med Genet 26:123, 1987.

Fine RM and Weathers DR: Desquamative gingivitis: a form of cicatricial pemphigoid? Br J Dermatol 102:393, 1980.

Fischman SL, Nisengard RJ, and Blozis GG: Generalized red conditions and multiple ulcerations. In Wood NK and Goaz PW, editors: Differential diagnosis of oral lesions, St Louis, 1985, The CV Mosby Co.

Forman L and Nally FF: Oral non-dystrophic bullous eruption mainly limited to the gingivae: a mechano-bullous response, Br J Dermatol 96:111, 1977.

Glass BJ, Kuhel RF, and Lanlois RP: Treatment of common orofacial conditions, Dent Clin North Am 30:421, 1986.

Glickman I and Smulow JB: Chronic desquamative gingivitis: its nature and treatment, J Periodontol 35:397, 1964.

Goldberg LH and Sperber J: Erythema multiforme due to herpes simplex: treatment with oral acyclovir, South Med J 79:757. 1986.

Graykowski EA and Kingman A: Double-blind trial of tetracycline in recurrent aphthous ulceration, J Oral Pathol 7:376, 1978.

Green JA et al: Post-herpetic erythema multiforme prevented with prophylactic oral acyclovir, Ann Intern Med 102:632, 1985.

Hardy KM et al: Benign mucous membrane pemphigoid, Arch Dermatol 104:467, 1971.

Horning GM et al: Gingival fibromatosis with hypertrichosis, J Periodontol 56:344, 1985.

Huff JC, Weston WL, and Tonnesen MG: Erythema multiforme: a critical review of characteristics, diagnostic criteria and causes, J Am Acad Dermatol 8:763, 1983.

Jones LE and Dolby AE: Desquamative gingivitis associated with psoriasis, J Periodontol 43:35, 1972.

Jonsson R et al: Oral mucosal lesions in systemic lupus erythematosus: a clinical, histopathological and immunopathological study, J Rheumatol 11:38, 1984.

Katz SE: Commentary: sulfoxone (diasone) in the treatment of dermatitis herpetiformis, Arch Dermatol 118:809, 1982.

Lamak MA, Duvie M, and Bean SF: Oral acyclovir for the prevention of herpes-associated erythema multiforme, J Am Acad Dermatol 15:50, 1986.

Laskaris G, Demetriou N, and Angelopoulos A: Immunofluorescent studies in desquamative gingivitis, J Oral Pathol 10:398, 1981.

Leigh IM et al: Recurrent and continuous erythema multiforme: a clinical and immunological study, Clin Exp Dermatol 10:58, 1985.

Lever WF and Schaumburg-Lever G: Histopathology of the skin, ed 5, Philadelphia, 1975, JB Lippincott Co.

Lever WF and Schaumberg-Lever G: Immunosuppressants and prednisone in pemphigus vulgaris: therapeutic results obtained in 63 patients between 1961 and 1975, Arch Dermatol 113:1236, 1977.

Lever WF and Schaumberg-Lever G: Treatment of pemphigus vulgaris: results obtained in 84 patients between 1961 and 1982, Arch Dermatol 120:44, 1984.

Lozada F and Silverman S Jr: Erythema multiforme: clinical and natural history in fifty patients, Oral Surg 46:628, 1978.

Lozada F and Silverman S Jr: Topically applied fluocinonide in an adhesive base in the treatment of oral vesiculoerosive diseases, Arch Dermatol 116:898, 1980.

McCarthy FP, McCarthy PL, and Shklar G: Chronic desquamative gingivitis: a reconsideration, Oral Surg 13:1300. 1960.

Meyer M et al: Oral pemphigus vulgaris: a report of ten cases, Arch Dermatol 113:1520, 1977.

Nethercott JR and Choi BCK: Erythema multiforme (Stevens-Johnson snydrome): chart review of 123 hospitalized patients, Dermatologica 171:383, 1985.

Nisengard RJ, Alpert AM, and Krestow V: Desquamative gingivitis: immunologic findings, J Periodontol 49:27, 1978.

Nisengard RJ and Drinnan A: Oral mucosal diseases of unknown etiology. In Hooks JJ and Jordan GW, editors: Viral infections in oral medicine, New York, 1982, Elsevier/North Holland.

Nisengard RJ and Neiders M: Desquamative lesions of the gingiva, J Periodontol 52:500, 1981.

Nisengard RJ and Rogers RS III: Desquamative gingivitis. In Beutner EH, Chorzelski TP, and Kumar V, editors: Immunopathology of the skin, ed 3, New York, 1987a, John Wiley & Sons, Inc.

Nisengard RJ and Rogers RS III: The treatment of desquamative gingivitis, J Periodontol 58:167, 1987b.

Person JR, Rogers RS III, and Jordon RE: Cicatricial pemphigoid with circulating antibasement membrane antibodies, Dermatologica 154:90, 1977.

Pesanti S et al: Pemphigus vulgaris: incidence in Jews of different ethnic groups according to age, sex and initial lesion, Oral Surg 38:382, 1974.

Pimlott SJ and Walker DN: A controlled clinical trial of the efficacy of topically applied fluocinonide in the treatment of recurrent aphthous ulceration, Br Dent J 195:174, 1983.

Pina-Neto JM et al: Cherubism, gingival fibromatosis, epilepsy and mental deficiency (Ramon syndrome) with juvenile rheumatoid arthritis, Am J Med Genet 25:433, 1986.

Prinz H: Chronic diffuse desquamative gingivitis, Dent Cosmos 74:331, 1932.

Rasmussen JE: Erythema multiforme in children: response to treatment with corticosteroids, Br J Dermatol 95:181, 1976.

Rennie JS, Reade PC, and Scully C: Recurrent aphthous stomatitis, Br Dent J 159:361, 1985.

Rogers RS III: Recurrent aphthous stomatitis: clinical characteristics and evidence for an immunopathogenesis, J Invest Dermatol 69:499, 1977.

Rogers RS III, Sheridan PJ, and Jordon RE: Desquamative gingivitis, Oral Surg 42:316, 1976.

Rogers RS III, Seehafer JR, and Perry HO: Treatment of cicatricial (benign mucous membrane) pemphigoid with dapsone, J Am Acad Dermatol 6:215, 1982a.

Rogers RS III, Sheridan PJ, and Nightingale SH: Desquamative gingivitis: clinical, histopathologic, immunopathologic and therapeutic observations, J Am Acad Dermatol 7:729, 1982b.

Ryan JG: Pemphigus, Arch Dermatol 104:14, 1971.

Schiodt M, Halberg P, and Hentzer B: A clinical study of 32 patients with oral discoid lupus erythematosus, Int J Oral Surg 7:85, 1978.

Sciubba JJ and Niebloom T: Juvenile hyaline fibromatosis (Murray-Puretic-Drescher syndrome): oral and systemic findings in siblings, Oral Surg 62:397, 1985.

Seifert MH, Stergerwald JC, and Cliff MM: Bone resorption of the mandible in progressive systemic sclerosis, Arthritis Rheum 18:507, 1975.

Shklar G: Desquamative gingivitis and oral mucous membrane diseases. In Carranza F Jr, editor: Glickman's clinical periodontology, Philadelphia, 1984, WB Saunders Co.

Stafne EC and Austin LT: A characteristic dental finding in athero-sclerosis and diffuse scleroderma, Am J Orthod 30:25, 1944.

White SC et al: Oral radiographic changes in patients with progressive systemic sclerosis, J Am Dent Assoc 94:1178, 1977.

Witkop CJ: Heterogeneity in gingival fibromatosis, Birth Defects 7:210, 1971.

Wray D and McCord JF: Labial veneers in the management of desquamative gingivitis, Oral Surg 64:41, 1987.

Zeskin DE and Zegarelli EF: Chronic desquamative gingivitis: a report of twelve cases, Am J Orthod Oral Surg 31:1, 1945.

Zysset MK et al: Systemic lupus erythematosus: a consideration for antimicrobial prophylaxis, Oral Surg 64:30, 1987.

Chapter 19

INFECTIVE FORMS OF GINGIVOSTOMATITIS

Louis F. Rose

Herpetic gingivostomatitis
Herpes zoster
Herpangina
Syphilis
Candidiasis
Actinomycosis
Histoplasmosis

HERPETIC GINGIVOSTOMATITIS

The two strains of herpes simplex virus (HSV) differ in their antigenicity and anatomic distribution. HSV-1 is more frequently associated with oral lesions, and HSV-2 is usually isolated from the genital area. Most strains are found throughout the world. Large-scale epidemics do not occur, but small outbreaks are seen.

The initial infection with HSV is asymptomatic in 80% to 90% of patients. In children the majority of infections are caused by HSV-1, which is transmitted nonvenereally. HSV-2 is increasingly common after puberty, primarily as a result of spread by the genital route.

Acute herpetic gingivostomatitis is commonly caused by HSV-1, but occasionally HSV-2 may be found. The renewed interest in this disease arises from the recognition that it attacks not only infants and young children, but also adults in their second and third decades.

Pathogenesis. After inoculation at the primary site on the skin or mucosa, HSV replicates locally. In the intact host, viremia has been infrequently observed; however, despite an immune response, the virus spreads to local ganglion cells via ascension along the neuron. Various lo-

cal and systemic insults, such as trauma or fever, as well as stress, can produce reactivation of the latent virus.

In light of the pathogenesis of HSV infection, it has been suggested that multiplication of the herpes virus in a site that has access to the oral tissues can account for the occurrence of the virus in oral secretions and for the high frequency of recurrence in the oral cavity. It has been hypothesized that the occurrence may also be present in extraneural tissues and that the gingiva may act as an additional reservoir site for the HSV (Zakay-Rones et al., 1982, 1986). The crevicular environment provides the virus with a central location from which relapse can commence during trauma, stress, etc. The virus is often induced following routine dental treatment in association with patient stress and injury to the sulcular tissue during procedures such as scaling, root planing, or tooth preparation. The spread of the infection in the oral cavity may be due to the turnover of the sulcular epithelial cells (Löe et al., 1969) or to the transfer by leukocytes, whose main port of entry into the oral cavity is provided by the gingival sulcus (Cimasoni, 1974).

The hypothesis of an extraparametral reservoir for HSV is corroborated by several experimental data (Zakay-Rones et al., 1973, 1982, 1986; Ehrlich et al., 1983). The presence of viral antigens and antibodies, as well as the sensitivity of gingival sulcus tissues to infection with HSV in vitro (Rones et al., 1983), emphasizes the potential of the sulcus to serve as a site for viral primary replication and infection, and later as a reservoir site for occult virus.

Dental considerations. The incubation period ranges from 2 to 20 days, with the average being 1 week. Primary infections produce clinically apparent lesions on the skin and/or oral mucosa in 10% to 20% of cases. Acute gingi-

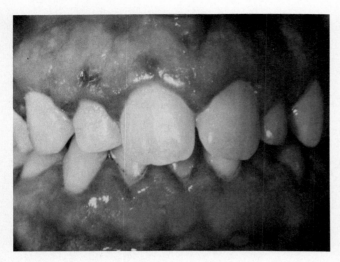

Fig. 19-1. Acute gingivostomatitis: ruptured vesicular lesions of gingiva with formation of shallow ulcers.

vostomatitis is the most common manifestation in childhood and is increasingly seen among young adults. The illness begins with fever and inflammation of the oral mucosa. Over the next 1 to 2 days painful, vesicular lesions appear in the oral tissues. These vesicles rupture easily and lead to the formation of shallow ulcers with smooth margins surrounded by a red halo. The lesions occur on all areas of the mouth, with the most dramatic signs appearing on the labial mucosa and gingiva (Fig. 19-1).

The gingiva shows signs of acute inflammation resulting from the viral infection, which is further aggravated by the accumulation of dental plaque due to poor oral hygiene and the interruption of masticatory function. Superinfection by the normal oral flora may further complicate the picture. Ulcers develop on the gingival tissues, and bleeding from the marginal gingiva is not uncommon. Severe pain and marked difficulty in chewing, talking, and swallowing are the chief complaints of patients with primary herpetic gingivostomatitis. Drooling of saliva is apparent. In infants lack of food and fluid ingestion may result in dehydration, requiring hospitalizaiton and parenteral fluid administration. Swollen, tender regional lymph nodes are frequently observed. The ulcerations heal in approximately 14 days, although the gingival inflammation may take longer to resolve.

Histologic evidence of intranuclear intrusions and multinucleated giant cells at the base of a vesicle or in tissue suggests an HSV infection. Immunofluorescent staining may prove useful clinically. A definitive diagnosis is made by isolation of the virus. Inoculation of tissue cultures produces cytopathic changes rapidly, often in 48 hours. Acute and convalescent sera can be tested for antibodies using a complement fixation, immunofluorescent,

or neutralization assay. A fourfold rise in titer points to a recent lesion.

The differential diagnosis of gingivostomatitis includes herpangina as a result of group A coxsackieviruses and thrush caused by *Candida* species. The lesions in herpes simplex are located predominantly in the anterior portion of the mouth, whereas those resulting from coxsackieviruses are seen in the posterior oral pharynx. Also, the duration of illness is longer with herpes simplex virus.

When primary herpetic gingivostomatitis occurs during the first trimester of pregnancy, as a result of a viremia, the herpes virus may cross the placental barrier and infect the fetus, resulting in severe congenital malformations. If the oral infection is diagnosed close to delivery, a pelvic examination is indicated, and if a vaginal or cervical involvement coexists, a caesarian section must be considered. Both primary and reactivation herpetic oral lesions in immunocompromised patients are characterized by their severity and intensity of local complications.

Treatment. Treatment of acute herpetic gingivostomatitis is mainly supportive and aimed at alleviating pain and reducing the chance of secondary infection. Mouth rinses with a 2% lidocaine viscous solution are beneficial and facilitate drinking, eating of soft foods, and oral hygiene. A milder anesthetic action may be obtained by the use of a 5% aqueous diphenhydramine (Benadryl) solution. Abundant bicarbonate or saline solution mouthwashes provide mechanical cleansing. Antibiotics are of no benefit. In severe cases secondary monilial infection occurs and is treated with antimycotic agents, such as nystatin suspension (100,000 units/ml) or amphotericin B lozenges (four to six times a day).

A recently introduced agent, acyclovir, selectively inhibits the replication of the virus without affecting noninfected cells. It inhibits herpes simplex virus types 1 and 2, varicella zoster viruses, and cytomegalovirus in vitro. Acyclovir blocks the replication of the virus by inhibiting viral DNA polymerase activity.

HERPES ZOSTER

Herpesvirus varicellae, the cause of both zoster and varicella (chickenpox), has a worldwide distribution. Herpes zoster occurs predominantly in older adults. More than 60% of episodes are in individuals over 45 years of age, although the disease is seen occasionally in childhood. There is an increased incidence of zoster in the immunocompromised host. In one study of patients with Hodgkin's disease, herpes zoster developed in 22%.

Since a reactivation of latent virus is the antecedent of the eruption in zoster, an individual does not acquire this disease from an exogenous source. Viral shedding occurs until all lesions are crusted, usually after 7 to 10 days in the normal host.

Pathogenesis. Entry of the virus, probably through the

oropharynx, is followed in the susceptible host first by local replication and then by dissemination via the blood or the lymphatics. Presumably, viremia occurs after exposure to the virus and before the onset of the exanthema, but this has not been demonstrated. However, investigators have recovered virus from the blood of immunocompromised patients with progressive disease. Specific humoral and cellular immune responses terminate the viremic stage, but enlargement of cutaneous lesions continues for several days. The interdermal vesicles become pustular after invasion of polymorphonuclear leukocytes. Multinucleated giant cells are located at the base of the vesicles.

It has been postulated that during episodes of varicella, virus invades sensory nerve endings and ascends along the nerve fibers to the dorsal route ganglion, where it becomes latent. Zoster represents reactivation of this latent virus, which then migrates along the nerve to the skin. Occasional vesicle formation outside a single dermatone occurs in 25% of healthy individuals with zoster, probably as a result of viremia. In some immunosuppressed patients extensive disease can occur outside a dermatone, and virus can be isolated from the blood. In essence, the primary infection causes varicella (chickenpox), chiefly in children, and reactivation of the virus results in herpes zoster (shingles), mainly in adults.

Among cranial nerves the trigeminal nerve (especially its ophthalmic division), is most commonly involved (approximately 10% of all cases of herpes zoster) (Fig. 19-2). In recent years herpes zoster infection of the mandibular and maxillary divisions of the trigeminal nerve has been reported as causing aseptic alveolar bone necrosis and spontaneous exfoliation of teeth (Schwartz and Kvorning, 1982; Wright et al., 1983).

Dental considerations. Oral lesions occur in herpes zoster only when the trigeminal nerve is involved. Symptoms include severe pain, described as stabbing, burning, or aching. The pain may appear during the prodromal stage and persist during healing or even after the mucocutaneous lesions disappear. Persistent neuralgia is one of the severe sequelae of the disease. It has been proposed that a severe insult to the localized vascular supply directly affected by herpes zoster infection can result in necrosis of the alveolar bone, periodontal ligament, nerve supply, and adjacent gingival tissues (Wright et al., 1983). The evidence of local vasculitis in herpes zoster infection is limited but has been well described in cases with central nervous system involvement (Cravioto and Feigin, 1959; Linnemann, 1980; Ferguson, 1981). The evidence of virally affected vascular and nerve pathosis is of interest when one is considering the etiology of herpes zoster infection and alveolar bone complications, since virus-infected fifth cranial nerve branches traverse close to the blood vessels that supply the necrosing oral tissues.

A rising prevalence of trigeminal herpes zoster has been

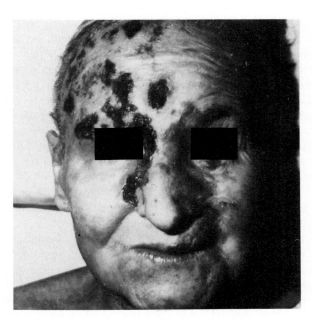

Fig. 19-2. Herpes zoster: crusted lesions of herpes zoster noted along divisions of trigeminal nerve.

accompanied by alveolar bone necrosis and tooth loss. Until 1973 there were three cases; from 1974 to 1979 there were eight; and from 1980 to 1986 there were four reported cases.

Treatment. Treatment of oral lesions is usually symptomatic and is similar to that of herpes simplex virus infection.

HERPANGINA

Herpangina, unlike herpes virus oral infection, involves the posterior half of the mouth, pharynx, and tonsils. The gingiva, buccal mucosa, floor of the mouth, and lips are involved less frequently. The lesions consist of small vesicles surrounded by an erythematous area. As many as 20 vesicles may be present. The vesicles erupt shortly after they are formed, leaving small ulcerated areas. The oral symptoms of herpangina tend to be milder than those of herpes virus infection; however, throat involvement is twice as severe. Lesions of herpangina in the pharynx and tongue make drinking, chewing, and talking difficult. Herpangina may occasionally be associated with bilateral parotitis.

Bacterial pharyngitis, acute herpetic gingivostomatitis, and aphthous stomatitis must be considered in the differential diagnosis.

Treatment. There is no specific therapy for herpangina; however, symptomatic relief with anesthetic mouthwashes and/or analgesic medication is often helpful to reduce the pain, allowing the patient to eat.

SYPHILIS

Syphilis is a specific infection associated with the spirochete *Treponema pallidum*. The disease is chronic with subacute symptomatic periods and asymptomatic intervals during which the diagnosis can be made only serologically. Because of its ability to involve all organ systems and the variability of its clinical presentation, syphilis has been called "the great imitator." The infection is acquired almost entirely by sexual contact, although it must be recognized that the term *sexual contact* encompasses far more than coitus.

Pathogenesis.   *T. pallidum* can penetrate intact mucous membranes or infect via tiny cuts or abrasions in cornified epithelium. The minimal infecting dose in experimental syphilis is two spirochetes injected intradermally. Organisms divide every 30 to 33 hours, and lesions appear when the organisms have attained the concentration of approximately $10^7/g$ of tissue. Very early in infection, well before the first lesion appears or the blood test becomes reactive, spirochetes enter the blood and lymphatic system and disseminate widely.

Clinical manifestations.   There are three stages of syphilis: primary, secondary, and tertiary. The incubation period for syphilis ranges from 10 to 90 days but generally lasts approximately 3 weeks. At that time a lesion, the chancre, develops at the point of initial inoculation of the spirochete. The chancre typically begins as a papule that subsequently erodes to form a gradually enlarging ulcer with a clean base and indurated edge. Although most chancres appear on the genitalia, the clinician must always bear in mind the possible syphilitic origin of sores on other parts of the body. Chancres of the gingiva, throat and tonsils, lip, nipple, hand, and a variety of other anatomic sites are well described. The patient with an oral, gingival, tonsillar, or pharyngeal chancre often manifests anterior cervical adenopathy.

In secondary syphilis all lesions are protean in nature, including the characteristic intraoral mucous patches that resemble the macular and maculopapular skin lesions. The mucous patches are raised on the mucosal surface and appear inflamed, with an area of central erosion covered by a white membrane (Fig. 19-3). On removal of the membrane, a clear flat, erythematous base is seen. Patches are found on the tongue, buccal mucosa, oropharynx, palate, the inner aspect of the lips, and occasionally on the gingival surface. Maculopapular lesions when present on the corners of the mouth are called "split" papules. They form a painless fissure between the upper and lower lip. These lesions must be differentiated from angular chelosis caused by riboflavin deficiency. Syphilitic, mucous patches are highly contagious, and during this phase infected saliva droplets can easily transmit the disease.

Gummatous infiltration of oral tissue and diffuse glossitis are manifestations of tertiary syphilis. Gummas are painless granulomas that become necrotic. They develop on the lips, oral mucosa, salivary glands, palate, and jawbone. Involvement of the palate will eventually be followed by its perforation. Gummas on the tongue will produce lingual lobulations, and ulcerations and fibrosis will induce surface irregularities.

CANDIDIASIS

Oral candidiasis (moniliasis) is a well-recognized common fungal infection, mainly associated with extremes of age, debilitation, immunodeficiency, and prolonged antimicrobial therapy. Specifically, the principal defects in the immune system that predispose an individual to oral candidiasis are granulocytopenia and cell-mediated immunity.

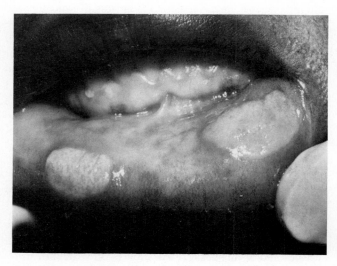

Fig. 19-3. Secondary syphilis: mucous patches on labial mucosa covered by a grayish white membrane.

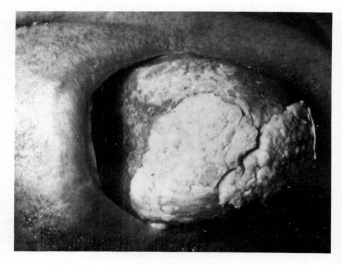

Fig. 19-4. Candidiasis of dorsal surface of tongue.

Dental considerations. The typical oral candidal lesion is pearly/bluish white and covers any part or all of the oral mucosa. The patches of candidiasis resembling "milk curds" and extending to the mouth corners are called *perleche*. The white plaques are attached to the underlying mucosa and, when scraped, leave erythematous mucosa with bleeding spots. The creamy whitish material is almost pure *Candida albicans* culture. In the absence of white lesions, erythematous atrophy (acute or chronic form) is also seen, particularly on dental-bearing mucosa.

Pain is the most common symptom encountered, although it is not invariably present and tends to be most severe in the acute atrophic form of candidiasis. Other frequent complaints include a burning sensation of the oral mucosa, especially the tongue, a loss of taste, and the onset of a metallic taste in the mouth (Fig. 19-4). Painful dysphasia develops dramatically when candidal lesions involve the throat and extend to cause candidal esophagitis (Fig. 19-5). In spite of the considerable suffering, patients remains afebrile.

Oral candidiasis is considered an opportunistic infection. Furthermore, in severely immunocompromised patients the dangers of oral candidiasis are not limited to the local disease manifestations; candidemia and systemic metastatic dissemination of fungi occur, resulting in life-threatening sequelae, including candidal endophthalmitis, meningitis osteomyelitis, and renal abscesses. Today, candidiasis is a common infection of patients infected with the human immunodeficiency virus (Figs. 19-6 and 19-7).

Chronic mucocutaneous candidiasis. This is a rare congenital syndrome characterized by chronic and relapsing candidal infection of the oral mucosa, lips, perioral skin, and nails. In vitro studies have identified specific defects in cell-mediated immunity in relation to candidal antigen, whereas T-cell function in response to other antigens is normal. The clinical manifestations are often severe, unrelenting, and hypertrophic or atropic in nature, yet systemic manifestations and visceral spread are extremely rare.

Another clinical syndrome characterized by chronic oral candidal infection has been noted to be associated with familial hypoparathyroidism, mental retardation, and often additional hypoadrenalism. The finding of chronic or recurrent oral candidal infection in otherwise healthy patients should alert the dental practitioner of the possibility of undiagnosed endocrinopathy or defective immunity

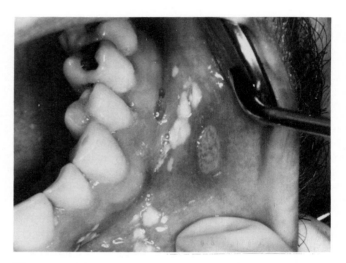

Fig. 19-6. Patches of candidiasis: labial mucosa and large aphthous ulcer in a patient infected with human immunodeficiency virus.

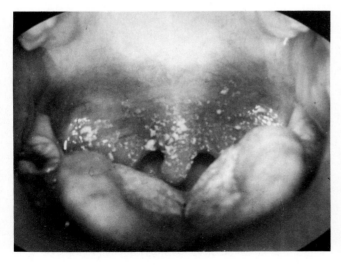

Fig. 19-5. Candidiasis involving soft palate and throat, and extending into esophagus.

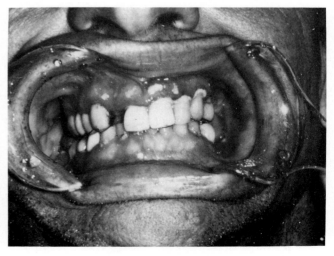

Fig. 19-7. Candidiasis of gingiva.

(e.g., acquired immunodeficiency syndrome [AIDS]), justifying further investigation.

Treatment. Where possible, the eradication of predisposing factors should be attempted and sometimes may be sufficient to control and cure the oral candidiasis. In the acute symptomatic phase, however, treatment is justified.

One milliliter of nystatin in suspension (100,000 to 200,000 units/ml) is held in the mouth for approximately 5 minutes and then swallowed. This treatment should be repeated four times a day while the disease is still active and for several days after the signs and symptoms have improved. Nystatin is not well absorbed through the mucous membrane, and when taken orally, almost all of the drug is excreted in the feces.

The direct contact needed between the drug and the fungus is better achieved when nystatin ointment is used. A plastic tray is custom fabricated to fit the upper jaw of the patient. On its inner surface nystatin (100,000 units/ml) is applied, and the tray is worn for about 2 hours. This treatment is repeated four times a day. This ensures the prolonged presence of a high concentration of the agent in the oral cavity.

Regular nystatin tablets are not effective for treatment of oral moniliasis, because their dissolving time is slow and the bitter taste is not tolerated by patients. Vaginal nystastin tablets, however, can be used for treatment of oral moniliasis. These are taken four times a day and allowed to dissolve in the mouth. There is no known resistance of *C. albicans* to this drug, even after prolonged use. Recently ketoconazole (200 to 440 mg daily) has become available as oral systemic therapy for oral and pharyngeal candidal infections and has had excellent results even in immunocompromised hosts.

In general, the use of these drugs for prevention of oral candidiasis is not very effective. However, antifungal medications can be used on a continuous basis in immunocompromised or leukemic patients prone to developing oral candidiasis.

ACTINOMYCOSIS

Actinomyces israelii, a normal inhabitant of the oral cavity, has been isolated from dental plaque, calculus, necrotic dental pulps, and tonsils. In spite of its prevalence, clinical infection from *Actinomyces* is relatively rare.

Poor oral hygiene is one of the contributing factors in oral actinomycosis. The infection extends from the necrotic tooth pulp to the periapical area and alveolar bone and penetrates through the periosteum into the muscles. The infection becomes apparent as sinus tracts on the skin. Cases have been described in which the infection ascended along the mandibular ramus and penetrated the middle cranial fossa, causing intracranial infection.

In typical cases the mandibular area is involved, a condition known as "lumpy jaw" (Fig. 19-8). Involvement of

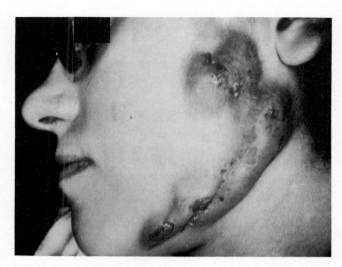

Fig. 19-8. Actinomysis infection in mandibular area (lumpy jaw).

the gingiva, oral mucosa, floor of the mouth, and palate may follow localized infection. *Actinomyces* species are part of the normal flora of the oral cavity in at least 70% of adults. In periodontal disease the numbers of *Actinomyces* and other bacteria increase in dental plaque and calculus. Aspiration of dental plaque and calculus into the lungs must be considered during periodontal therapy. Seating of tooth-associated materials containing *Actinomyces* into the pulmonary field could cause pulmonary actinomycosis (Suzuki and Delisle, 1984).

Ascending infection of salivary glands is possible through their ducts. Further spread of the disease may involve the muscles of mastication, resulting in severe trismus.

Actinomycosis of the tongue is rare. It involves the anterior third of the tongue as an indurated nodule that is deep seated, painful to palpation, and adherent to the musculature. The absence of regional lymphadnopathy is a striking feature.

The tongue or buccal mucosa is occasionally the primary site of the disease. It starts with a deep-seated painless nodule that grows slowly and eventually breaks through the mucosa, discharging a yellowish purulent material. On the gingiva the picture is somewhat similar. It takes about 4 to 6 weeks for an actinomycotic nodule to soften and discharge its contents.

The exudate from the lesion is collected from the draining sinuses. It is examined grossly for yellow sulfur granules in order to make the diagnosis. Microscopic and cultural examination of such actinomycotic lesion exudates show that there are often two organisms present: *Actinomyces* and *Actinobacillus actinomycetemcomitans*. *A. actinomycetemcomitans* has been implicated as a periodontal pathogen (see Chapter 11) and is virulent and tissue invasive. Its role in the pathogenesis of actinomycotic lesions is not known; however it probably contributes significantly to these lesions.

Treatment. The prognosis of cervicofacial actinonmycosis is relatively good, except in the presence of chronic osteomyelitis. Present therapy consists of prolonged parenteral penicillin administration. Because *A. actinomycetemcomitans* is found in these lesions and is often penicillin resistant, it is reasonable to obtain antibiotic sensitivities of the cultivable organisms in the lesions and select an antibiotic regimen accordingly.

HISTOPLASMOSIS

Histoplasmosis is caused by *Histoplasma capsulatum,* a fungus encountered in many parts of the world. It is highly endemic in areas of the central and mid-Atlantic United States. Up to 80% of adults are positive on skin testing. The fungus grows as a mold in nature, and its spores reach the lung by inhalation. In the lung the fungus changes to a small budding yeast that results in pneumonia, which is usually self-limited and causes only a few days of fever, dry cough, and chest ache.

Dissemination beyond the lung and hylar nodes can occur in self-limited primary pulmonary infection. Progressive extrapulmonary dissemination is a rare but highly lethal form of the disease. Most patients are either young children or immunosuppressed adults, but previously normal adults can also acquire the disease. The clinical manifestations are extremely variable, depending on which organs are involved.

Dental considerations. About one third of patients with progressive disseminated histoplasmosis develop oral lesions. Ulcers and granulomas are the dominant manifestations noted. Cases have been described in which primary lesions were diagnosed in the mouth. Extreme destruction of the palate, pharynx, and nasal septum is known to follow the infection of these respective areas. Histoplasmosis of the jawbone will induce mobility in the area and possibly oroantral fistulas. Radiographs show diffuse osteolysis of the alveolus without subperiosteal new bone formation. These oral lesions may occur anywhere in the oral cavity, including the gingiva, but the tongue is the most frequent site. The most common form is an indurated ulcer, although nodular lesions as well as verrucous or granular masses have been reported (Bennett, 1967). Purpuric, macular areas may accompany the ulcerations.

The diagnostic process requires a biopsy and culture. Microscopic examination reveals a granuloma with enlarged histiocytes containing spores of histoplasma.

Treatment. As in the case of systemic histoplasmosis, the treatment of choice for oral involvement is amphotericin B. Miconazole has been used with varying success.

REFERENCES

Bennett DE: Histoplasmosis of the oral cavity and larynx, Arch Intern Med 120:417, 1967.

Cimasoni G: The crevicular fluid, Monogr Oral Sci 3:1, 1974.

Cravioto H and Feigin I: Noninfectious granulomatous angiitis with predilection for the nervous system, Neurology 9:599, 1959.

Ehrlich J, Cohen GH, and Hochman N: Specific herpes simplex virus antigen in human gingiva, J Periodontol 54:357, 1983.

Ferguson RH: Vasculitis associated with herpes zoster, Mayo Clin Proc 56:524, 1981.

Linnemann CC Jr and Alvira MM: Pathogenesis of varicella zoster angeitis in the CNS, Arch Neurol 37:239, 1980

Löe H and Karring T: A quantitative analysis of the epithelium connective tissue interface in relation to assessments of the mitotic index, J Dent Res 48:634, 1969.

Rones Y et al: Sensitivity of oral tissues to herpes simplex virus in vitro, J Periodontol 54(2):91, 1983.

Schwartz O and Kvorning SA: Tooth exfoliation, osteonecrosis of the jaw and neuralgia following herpes zoster of the trigeminal nerve, Int J Oral Surg 11:364, 1982.

Suzuki JB and Delisle AL: Pulmonary actinomycosis of periodontal origin, J Periodontol 55(10):581, Oct 1984.

Wright WE et al: Alveolar bone necrosis and tooth loss: a rare complication associated with herpes zoster infection of the fifth cranial nerve, Oral Surg 56(1):39, 1983.

Zakay-Rones Z, Hochman N, and Rones Y: Immunological response to herpes simplex virus in gingival fluid, J Periodontol 53:42, 1982.

Zakay-Rones Z et al: The sulcular epithelium as a reservoir for herpes simplex virus in man, J Periodontol 44:779, 1973.

Zakay-Rones Z et al: Hypothesis: the gingival tissue as a reservoir for herpes simplex virus, Microbiologica 9:367, 1986.

SUGGESTED READINGS

Arondor TM and Walker DM: The prevalence and intraoral distribution of *Candida albicans* in man, Arch Oral Biol 25:1, 1980.

Babajews A, Poswillo DE, and Griffin GE: Acquired immune deficiency syndrome presenting as recalcitrant *Candida,* Br Dent J 159:106, 1985.

Cawson RA and Lehner T: Chronic hyperplastic candidiasis—candidal leukoplakia, Br J Dermatol 80:9, 1968.

Chow AW: Infectious syndromes of the head and neck, Infect Dis Clin North Am 2(1), 1988.

Daramola JO et al: Maxillary African histoplasmosis mimicking malignant jaw tumour, Br J Oral Surg 16(3):241, 1979.

Davies RM et al: Disseminated histoplasmosis: a case report, Br Dent J 142:372, 1977.

Fiumara NJ et al: Papular secondary syphilis of the tongue, report of a case, Oral Surg 45(4):540, 1978.

Gorlin RJ and Goldman HM, editors: Thoma's oral pathology, ed 6, St Louis, 1970, The CV Mosby Co.

Kirkpatrick CH and Smith TK: Chronic mucocutaneous candidiasis: immunologic and antibiotic therapy, Ann Intern Med 80:310, 1974.

Krolls SO, Westbrook SD, and Hess DS: Actinomycosis as periapical pathology case report, J Oral Med 32(2):41, 1977.

Krolls SO et al: Oral manifestations of syphilis, Hosp Med 8:14, 1972.

Kuepper RS and Harrigan WT: Actinomycosis of the tongue: report of a case, J Oral Surg 37(2):123, 1979.

Mace MC: Oral African histoplasmosis resembling Burkitt's lymphoma, Oral Surg 46(3):407, 1978.

Manz HJ, Canter HG, and Melton J: Trigeminal herpes zoster causing mandibular osteonecrosis and spontaneous tooth exfoliation, South Med J 79(8):1026, 1986.

Miller RL et al: Localized oral histoplasmosis, Oral Surg 53(4):367, 1982.

Nahmias AJ and Roizman B: Infection with herpes simplex viruses 1 and 2 (in three parts), N Engl J Med 289:667, 719, 781, 1983.

Neisel P and Taylor DS: Chronic mucocutaneous candidiasis: treatment of the oral lesion with miconazole, Br J Oral Surg 18:51, 1980.

Nicholls M, Robertson TI, and Jennis F: Oral histoplasmosis treated with miconazole, Aust NZ J Med 10:563, 1980.

Rose LJ and Kaye D: Internal medicine for dentistry, St Louis, 1983, The CV Mosby Co.

Smith JW and Utz JP: Progressive disseminated histoplasmosis, Ann Intern Med 76:557, 1972.

Sparling PF: Diagnosis and treatment of syphilis, N Engl J Med 284:642, 1977.

Syphilis: a synopsis, Washington, DC, 1968 USPHS recommendation, J Am Vener Dis Assoc 3:98, 1976.

Weese EC and Smith IM: A study of 57 cases of actinomycosis over a 36 year period, Arch Intern Med 135:1562, 1975.

Yusef H et al: Disseminated histoplasmosis presenting with oral lesions: report of a case, Br J Oral Surg 16(3):234, 1979.

Chapter 20

DISEASES OF OTHER ORGAN OR TISSUE SYSTEMS WITH PERIODONTAL MANIFESTATIONS

Louis F. Rose

Acute leukemias
Thrombocytopenia
Hemophilia
Sturge-Weber syndrome
Wegener's granulomatosis
Ehlers-Danlos syndromes
Crohn's disease
Hypoadrenocorticism
Hypophosphatasia
Paget's disease (osteitis deformans)
Osteoporosis
Stress
Nutritional deficits
    Vitamin D (calcium and phosphorus)
    Vitamin C
    Proteins

ACUTE LEUKEMIAS

Acute leukemias are cancers of the blood-forming organs causing marrow failure and infiltration of various organs and tissues by blast cells. If the disease is untreated, death ensues in a few weeks to several months.

The cause of human acute leukemia remains uncertain, but of the many possible causes that have been suggested, ionizing radiation, certain chemicals, and viruses have received the most attention. Radiation exposure from atomic bomb blasts, radiation therapy, and inadequate shielding of radiologists have been associated with an increased incidence.

Pathogenesis. Once the leukemic process has been initiated, there is a progressive expansion of the leukemic population. In particular, there is an increase in the population of leukemic stem cells. These cells retain their ability to multiply in the future. This process is associated with a maturation defect, thereby preventing the cells from maturing more than minimally beyond the blast stage, so that mature functional cells capable of fighting infection are not produced. In addition, the presence of leukemic cells in the marrow inhibits production of normal blood cells; this seems to be caused not only by the space-occupying effect of the leukemic infiltrate but also by the inhibitory effect on normal cell growth.

Clinical manifestations. The signs and symptoms of acute leukemia are caused by marrow failure and by infiltration of the blood and other organs and tissues by leukemic cells. Easy fatigability, dyspnea, palpitations, and other symptoms of anemia may be present. Fever with or without demonstrable infection is very common. Bleeding or easy bruising, or both, are occasionally noted. Bone or joint pain may be permanent, especially in children.

The physical examination can be negative or demonstrate fever, pallor, petechiae or purpura, enlargement of cervical and other peripheral lymph nodes, splenomegaly, and sometimes hepatomegaly. Signs of an infection may be muted in patients with severe granulocytopenia. A variety of neurologic signs and symptoms may occur during the course of the disease, especially meningeal leukemia, but these are not usually overt at the time of initial diagnosis.

Dental considerations.   Intraoral signs and symptoms of leukemia are related to the severity of the deficiency of the mature normal white blood cells, red blood cells, and platelets. Other oral signs are caused by infiltration of leukemic cells into the oral tissues and side effects of chemotherapeutic drugs used to treat the disease.

It has been reported that there are oral lesions in over 80% of patients with acute monocytic leukemia, in 40% of patients with acute myeloid leukemia, and in over 20% of those with lymphoid leukemia.

Acute leukemia frequently causes a massive infiltration of leukemic cells into the gingival tissues. The gingiva appears to have lost its normal contour and texture. It is hyperplastic, edematous, and bluish red, with blunting of the interdental papillae. Varying degrees of gingival inflammation, ulceration, and necrosis have been described (Burket, 1944; Wentz et al., 1949; Lindhe, 1983) (Fig. 20-1).

The clinical and histologic appearances of the gingiva are indicative of the degenerative changes that have occurred. This tissue is therefore more susceptible to bacterial infection, and the severity of such an infection may exacerbate the leukemic state. Such intraoral manifestations are probably secondary to the presence of dental plaque, since good plaque control can lead to a reduction of gingival inflammation in leukemias.

Also, oral mucosal ulcers are a common finding in patients with leukemia. These lesions may result from bacterial invasion due to severe leukopenia or mucosal atrophy caused by the direct effect of the chemotherapeutic drugs on the epithelial cells. Trauma from a dental prosthesis or teeth may result in large secondarily infected ulcers progressing to facial cellulitis and septicemia.

Candidiasis is almost universally seen in hospitalized leukemic patients undergoing chemotherapy. It is important to remember that infections with unusual organisms

(e.g., *Pseudomonas* and *Klebsiella*) are common in this group of patients.

Treatment.   The oral complications that occur during leukemia may cause considerable difficulty for the patient. Toxemia, septicemia, gingival hemorrhage, marked discomfort and pain, and loss of appetite are a few of the complications that may arise. During the acute phase of the disease only those procedures that are necessary to alleviate the discomfort and hemorrhaging should be performed. On the other hand, during a period of remission every attempt should be made to achieve a state of periodontal health. The treatment should be conservative, consisting of the removal of all local irritants and instruction in good plaque control techniques. Treatment procedures involving long periods of time should be avoided.

Severe gingival bleeding resulting from thrombocytopenia can often be managed successfully with localized treatment. The use of an absorbable gelatin sponge with topical thrombin or placement of microfibrillar collagen is often sufficient. Some authors have reported successful management of gingival bleeding with oral rinses of antifibrinolytic agents. If these measures are not successful in stopping blood flow from an oral site, platelet transfusions may be necessary.

Management of oral ulcers in leukemic patients should be directed toward preventing the spread of localized infection and bacteremia, promoting healing of the lesion, and decreasing pain. Oral ulcers serve as the source of septicemia in patients with leukemia. Topical antibacterial and antifungal medication should be used on these patients. Chlorhexidine, which is used extensively in Europe but which to date has had limited use in the United States, is a very successful topical antibacterial agent. Also, povidone-iodine solution is a typical drug that can be placed directly on the lesion. Severe ulcers showing clinical signs of infection should be treated with a combination of topical medication and systemic antibiotics.

Candidiasis may be treated with topical nystatin, as a solution or in the form of troches. In severe cases of infiltrating lesions of candidiasis or when the oral lesions are associated with esophogeal lesions, systemic use of amphotericin is recommended.

THROMBOCYTOPENIA

Thrombocytopenia purpura is a blood dyscrasia associated with a decrease in circulating platelets. Thrombocytopenia of clinical significance exists when the whole blood platelet count is below $150,000/mm^3$, although the precise limits for normal vary slightly among laboratories.

The most common manifestation of thrombocytopenia purpura is spontaneous hemorrhage into the skin and mucous membranes. The disease is also characterized by prolonged bleeding.

Two major forms of thrombocytopenic purpura have been described. *Primary (idiopathic) thrombocytopenic*

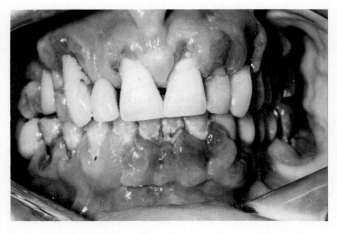

Fig. 20-1.   Acute leukemia in a 19-year-old woman. Note dramatic changes in gingival contour and texture.

purpura (ITP) is of unknown etiology. This is a relatively common form of the disease and is seen at any age. *Secondary thrombocytopenia* is due to a known etiologic factor such as chemicals or drugs.

Two forms of ITP are recognized: acute and chronic. Acute ITP is a self-limited disease that generally remits permanently without sequelae. The onset is usually sudden, with thrombocytopenia manifested by bruising, bleeding, and petechiae a few days to several weeks after an otherwise uneventful viral illness. On the other hand, chronic ITP is usually a disease of adults and can be sudden or insidious in onset. It is three times more frequent in women than in men, and the course is characterized by remissions and exacerbations. In both acute and chronic ITP, thrombocytopenia and its manifestation are the only physical or laboratory abnormalities.

Oral manifestations. The oral manifestations of thrombocytopenia may represent the initial signs of the disease. Purpura, the most common oral sign, is defined as any escape of blood into subcutaneous tissues and includes

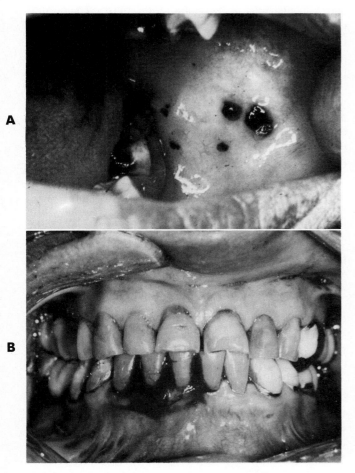

Fig. 20-2. A, Purpura on buccal mucosal surface due to idiopathic thrombocytopenia. **B,** Spontaneous gingival hemorrhage of a thrombocytopenic patient.

petechiae, ecchymoses, hemorrhagic vesicles, and hematomas. These may appear on any mucosal surface and are often seen on the tongue, lips, and occlusal line of the buccal mucosa secondary to minor trauma (Fig. 20-2, *A*). Purpura may be differentiated from vascular lesions by applying pressure directly to the area. These lesions will not blanch and may be induced on the palate from the suction created by a full denture. Other oral signs include spontaneous gingival hemorrhage and prolonged bleeding following trauma, toothbrushing, extractions, or periodontal therapy (Fig. 20- 2, *B*). Similar purpuric findings are seen on the skin. The patient may have a positive history of epistaxis, hematuria, melena, and increased menstrual bleeding.

Gingival biopsy is helpful in the diagnosis of thrombotic thrombocytopenic purpura, since the gingiva is readily accessible, highly vascular, and amenable to hemostasis.

Treatment. Spontaneous gingival bleeding can usually be managed by oxidizing mouthwashes, but platelet transfusions may be required to stop the bleeding. Good oral hygiene and conservative periodontal therapy will help to remove plaque and calculus, which potentiate the bleeding. Accidental trauma can be avoided by replacing ill-fitting prostheses and removing all orthodontic appliances. These patients should be cautioned not to sleep with any removable prosthesis in place.

Emergency care during severe thrombocytopenic episodes consists of endodontic therapy, antibiotics, and nonsalicylate analgesics. A stab incision and drainage may be performed, but blunt dissection of an abscessed area is to be avoided. Definitive dental treatment should be delayed until normal platelet function returns. Platelet levels greater than 50,000/mm^3 are desired before dental treatment, and further transfusions are given as needed postoperatively to maintain hemostasis.

Block injections are to be avoided if the platelet count is below 30,000/mm^3, because of the possibility of hematoma formation and airway obstruction. Infiltration anesthesia is used instead. Aspirin-containing analgesics are contraindicated, since they may potentiate bleeding. Any drug that has previously induced a thrombocytopenic episode should not be used. Frequently these patients are treated with steroids, which may further complicate dental treatment.

HEMOPHILIA

Classic hemophilia (hemophilia A) is an inherited deficiency of functional factor VIII with an associated bleeding tendency proportional to the severity of the deficiency. It is the most common inherited disorder of coagulation. Severe hemophilia (factor VIII levels less than 1% of the normal value) is associated with serious and often apparently spontaneous bleeding. Individuals with mild hemophilia (5% to 25% of normal levels of factor VIII) may have little or no increase in bleeding and escape detection for years, whereas those with hemophilia of intermediate severity (factor VIII levels 1% to 4% of normal) usually have no spontaneous bleeding but may have bleeding with surgery or trauma (Fig. 20-3).

Hemophilia A is caused by the presence of a functionally deficient factor VIII molecule rather than by the absence of production of factor VIII. Nearly all cases of hemophilia are inherited, and carrier detection or family history reveals the presence of the trait.

Hemophilia is carried on the X-chromosome of the female carrier. Although her factor VIII antigen-to-activity ratio is abnormal, she is unlikely to manifest any bleeding tendency because of the production of normal factor VIII via her own X-chromosome. However, 50% of her offspring will inherit the abnormal chromosome, with the daughters being carriers and the sons having the clinical disease. Conceivably, the daughter of a hemophiliac male and a carrier female could be severely affected with two abnormal chromosomes, but this is obviously a rare occurrence.

Clinical manifestations. The clinical manifestations of hemophilia A are directly related to the factor VIII level. Although mild hemophilia is not detected until later in life, severe hemophilia can usually be diagnosed in infancy or early childhood. Because of the limited activity of infants, spontaneous bleeding is frequently not a problem during the first year. With increased activity, one notes hematomas, oral bleeding, and hemarthroses.

Hemarthroses are common clinical problems. In decreasing order of frequency, they involve the knee, ankle, hip, elbow, wrist, and shoulder. There is often a history of preceding trauma or stress, but this may be relatively minor. With repeated hemarthroses, extensive destructive changes within the joint may occur, leading eventually to loss of cartilage, osteoporosis, contractures, and functionally useless joints.

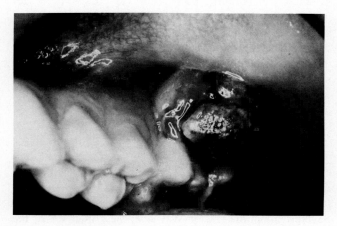

Fig. 20-3. Hemophilia: hematoma in a hemophiliac patient secondary to a local anesthetic injection.

Hematomas and other soft tissue bleeding may occur into subcutaneous tissues or muscles, most commonly in calves, thighs, buttocks, or forearms. Bleeding may occur in critical areas such as the tongue, floor of the mouth, or pharynx and may compromise the airway.

Although clinical manifestations may be suggestive, the specific diagnosis of hemophilia A is made in the laboratory. Whole-blood clotting time is usually abnormal in severe hemophilia but can be normal in mild cases. The partial thromboplastin time (PTT), which assesses the intrinsic coagulation pathway, is prolonged, and the prothrombin time (PT) and bleeding time are normal. Specific diagnosis requires a functional assay for factor VIII activity demonstrating decreased or absent activity. Antigenic assays for factor VIII reveal normal or elevated values, demonstrating the presence of a functionally deficient factor VIII molecule.

Classic hemophilia is treated by intravenous infusion of normal human factor VIII in the form of cryoprecipitate or lyophilized concentrate. A plasma factor VIII level above 30% must be achieved to halt bleeding.

Oral manifestations. Episodic, prolonged bleeding, either spontaneous or traumatic, is the most common oral presentation. Bleeding from the nose, mouth, and lips may be severe. Hemarthroses, which may lead to ankylosis and erosion of the temporomandibular joint surface, are incapacitating and painful.

The high incidence of dental problems among hemophiliacs is the result of neglect and the fear of bleeding during treatment. These patients will benefit from a good comprehensive multidisciplinary treatment plan. The dentist should be aware of a factoring period so that required dental treatment can be accomplished at that time.

Treatment. Dental management should be directed toward prevention. Good oral hygiene will aid in the reduction of gingival bleeding. Oral prophylaxis can generally be accomplished without factor replacement. Bleeding caused by supragingival ultrasonic scaling or rubber cup prophylaxis is controlled by the platelets. However, deep scaling can cause serious hemorrhage in patients who have not had factor replacement.

Hematomas can be prevented by taking care during x-ray film placement, when using high-speed vacuum and saliva ejectors, and in all oral tissue management. Foam rubber–tipped or gauze-padded instruments can minimize this hematoma formation.

The administration of local anesthesia is a major concern in dental treatment. Dissecting hematomas, airway obstruction, and death are known complications of block anesthesia in hemophiliac patients. Injections should not be given unless the patient has a plasma factor level of 50% or greater. Additional plasma factors are required if blood is aspirated, a hematoma develops, or other symptoms of bleeding such as pain in the area of injection occur. In severe hemophilia, replacement therapy should precede any anesthetic technique. Local anesthesia may be accomplished by infiltration or pericemental injections with an interligamentary injection syringe.

Most restorative treatment can be performed without factor replacement. A rubber dam should be used to protect the oral tissues against accidental lacerations. Wedges should be placed before any interproximal preparations to both protect and retract the papilla.

Endodontics is preferable to extraction. Pulpal bleeding is readily controlled in any conventional manner. Overinstrumentation and overfilling are to be avoided.

Orthodontic treatment can be performed in the well-motivated patient. Care should be exercised in the placement of bands. Minor intraoral bleeding caused by orthodontics will respond to pressure within 5 minutes. Meticulous plaque control is absolutely necessary in these patients.

Primary teeth are to be removed soon after they become loose. When radiographs reveal only soft tissue attachment, a vigorous oral hygiene program is initiated for at least 2 days, followed by tooth extraction. Initial bleeding can be controlled by pressure or local hemostatic measures such as thrombin or microfibrillar collagen (Avitene). Antihemophiliac factor (AHF) as a topical agent to prevent postextraction bleeding has been reported to stop the bleeding within 12 hours. The extraction site need not be covered or protected. No replacement therapy is needed when using this technique.

Periodontal surgery should be performed only if the anticipated therapeutic benefits outweigh the possibility of severe postoperative complications. No factor replacement is needed for probing and careful supragingival scaling. Replacement is necessary preceding deep scaling, curettage, and surgery.

The objective of periodontal therapy in hemophiliac patients is to control gingival inflammation to an extent that allows the patient to perform oral hygiene and allows the therapist to perform maintenance and instrumentation with minimal fear of bleeding problems.

Surgical treatment has often been avoided because of the potential for continued bleeding. Before any surgery, complete coagulation studies, factor levels, and red cell types should be obtained. The patient should be tested for inhibitors, and replacement therapy should be available.

Chemical cautery or electrosurgery should be avoided because of the possibility of tissue necrosis and secondary bleeding. Aspirin-containing analgesics should not be prescribed. All hemophiliacs should be tested for hepatitis and acquired immunodeficiency syndrome (AIDS) because of the quantity of blood products and transfusions they have received. Dental treatment is maximized while the patient is receiving replacement therapy. The number of visits to achieve the desired results are minimized.

STURGE-WEBER SYNDROME

Sturge-Weber syndrome consists of craniofacial angiomatosis and cerebral calcification. The cutaneous vascular nevus ("port wine stain") varies in size and shape and is present at birth. It is usually located along the course of the superior and middle branches of the trigeminal nerve. There is an associated meningeal hemangioma on the same side, with calcification and cortical atrophy of adjacent brain tissue, often resulting in contralateral Jacksonian convulsions, paralysis, sensory deficit, and mental retardation. Although the nevus is usually unilateral with a sharp border, it may be bilateral or midline. The oral mucous membranes may be affected on the same side, and glaucoma may be present in the ipsilateral eye. This is not an inherited disorder, although occasionally more than one member of the family may be affected. The etiology of the Sturge-Weber syndrome is unknown.

Characteristic calcification in the outer layer of the cerebral cortex may be seen in radiographs of the skull as sinuous, double-contoured lines ("tram lines") that follow the convolutions of the cerebral cortex on the affected side. It is demonstrated quite well with computed tomography (CT) scanning. Treatment is directed at the neurologic manifestations. Since the occurrence is sporadic and cannot be determined before birth, there are no preventive measures available.

The diagnosis of Sturge-Weber syndrome should be suspected in all children with a typical facial nevus and neurologic symptoms.

Dental considerations. Angiomas of the face and mucosa are readily seen. Generally, a cutaneous vascular nevus will occur over an area of the trigeminal nerve. Oral involvement, seen in about 40% of patients, consists of a bluish red lesion that blanches on pressure and is found most commonly on the buccal mucosa and lips. Occasionally seen are lesions involving the gingiva and palate. The floor of the mouth and tongue are rarely involved (Fig. 20-4).

Gingival changes range from slight vascular hyperplasia to extremely large masses that make closure of the mouth impossible (Royle et al., 1966; El-Mostehy and Stallard, 1969; Tarsitano et al., 1970; Gorlin et al., 1976; Lynch, 1984). This complication of gingival enlargement may be due to the increased vascular component and/or the phenytoin (Dilantin) therapy usually employed to manage the epileptic seizures common to the syndrome (Gorlin and Goldman, 1970; Wannenmacher and Forck, 1970).

Only two descriptions of alveolar bone changes have been reported. Royle et al. (1966) found bone loss in the ipsilateral body of the mandible, with rarification apical to the first molar on a panoramic radiograph in one case, and El-Mostehy and Stallard (1969) reported a case in which intraoral radiographs showed bizarre bone resorption, widening of trabeculations, and total loss of lamina dura

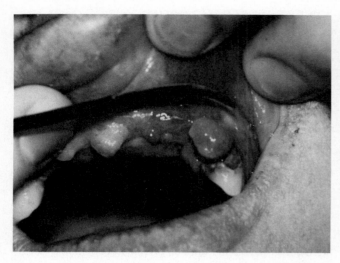

Fig. 20-4. Sturge-Weber syndrome: vascular hyperplasia of gingiva in a patient with Sturge-Weber syndrome.

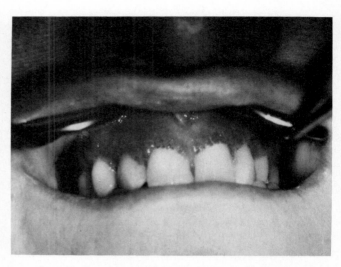

Fig. 20-5. Generalized granular gingival tissue with significant amount of petechiae in a patient with Wegener's granulomatosis.

around the first and second molars on the affected side. Other intraoral changes cited have included excessive tooth mobility to the point of depressibility and extensive angiomatous tissue in the dental pulp.

Treatment. Since periodontal and oral surgical procedures in the involved area may be associated with severe and at times fatal hemorrhage, there is a need for hemostatic precautions such as splints, dressings, and hospitalization. Treatment has ranged from total extraction to selective extraction to splinting of involved teeth, coupled with management of the hyperplastic gingival enlargment by means of complete surgical excision, injection of sclerosing solutions, radiation therapy, carbon dioxide snow, and electrodissection (Thoma, 1952; Royle et al., 1966; El-Mostehy and Stallard, 1969; Tarsitano et al., 1970).

WEGENER'S GRANULOMATOSIS

Wegener's granulomatosis (WG) is a disseminated granulomatous necrotizing vasculitis of the small vessels of the upper and lower respiratory tract. In the generalized form, glomerulonephritis is an important component of the disease process. Although a localized, limited form confined to the airways has been described, this probably represents an early stage of generalized disease before the development of detectable renal disease. The histologic features characteristic of WG include necrotizing vasculitis of small arteries and veins with coexistent granuloma formation.

Clinical manifestations. The mean age at onset of WG is 40 years, and the male-to-female ratio is 3:2. Early in the disease the clinical picture is dominated by upper respiratory tract signs, including rhinorrhea, paranasal discharge, septal perforations, saddle nose deformity, and osteitis media. However, virtually any manifestation of the

disease may be seen at the time of presentation. Nonspecific pulmonary complaints may include cough, hemoptysis, chest discomfort, and shortness of breath. It is not uncommon for asymptomatic pulmonary infiltrates to be seen on radiographs of the chest.

Bone lesions are usually present radiographically as multiple, bilateral nodular infiltrates with a tendency to cavitate. Renal disease in WG is characterized by focal and segmental glomerulonephritis with accompanying crescent formation.

Virtually any organ system may be involved in WG, but these manifestations are usually less dramatic in comparison with the respiratory tract and renal disease. Skin disease results from vasculitis with or without granuloma formation and is manifested in up to 50% of patients as petechiae, palpable purpura, papules, vesicles, ulcerations, or subcutaneous nodules. Oral and other mucosal membrane ulcerations can also occur.

Dental manifestations. A variety of oral lesions have been described in association with WG. The most common oral lesion is a distinctive hyperplastic gingivitis originating in the interdental papilla areas. The gingiva is generally described as granular and red to purple in color with many petechiae (Fig. 20-5). The lesion extends to the labial and buccal aspects, eventually involving the entire gingiva and periodontium, resulting in tooth mobility and loss of teeth. Once the teeth are lost, extraction sites fail to heal.

There have also been reports of extensive ulcerative stomatitis. In many cases the lesions are the initial manifestation of the disease (Edwards and Buckerfield, 1978; Karmody, 1978; Cohen and Meltzer, 1981; Israelson et al., 1981). The distinct histologic feature of the gingival lesion is the unusual combination of well-formed multinucleated

Table 20-1. Ehlers-Danlos syndromes

Classification	Type	Inheritance*	Clinical features	Basic defect
I	Gravis	AD	Generalized severe joint hypermobility, skin hyperextensibility, easy bruisability, molluscoid pseudotumors, subcutaneous spheroids, poor wound healing, premature rupture of fetal membranes	Unknown
II	Mitis	AD	Similar to ED I but milder, joint laxity limited to hands and feet, little cutaneous involvement and tissue friability	Unknown
III	Benign hypermobility	AD	Severe hypermobility of all joints	Unknown
IV	Arterial, ecchymotic, Sack's	AD/AR	Spontaneous rupture of large arteries, perforation of bowel, thin skin with prominent underlying veins	Reduced synthesis of type III collagen
V	X linked	XL	Marked hyperextensibility of skin, minimal joint hypermobility	Deficiency of lysyl oxidase
VI	Ocular	AR	Severe scoliosis, moderate joint involvement, ocular fragility with scleral rupture or retinal detachment, or both	Deficiency of lysyl hydroxylase
VII	Arthrochalasis multiplex congenita	AR	Short stature, generalized joint hypermobility with multiple subluxations, abnormal facies	Deficiency of procollagen peptidase
VIII	Periodontal	AD	Mild to moderate skin hyperextensibility and joint hypermobility, marked skin friability, generalized periodontitis	Unknown

From Rose LF and Kaye DK: Internal medicine for dentistry, St Louis, 1983, The CV Mosby Co.
*AD, Autosomal dominant; *AR,* autosomal recessive; *XL,* X linked.

giant cells in the midst of an acute inflammatory infiltrate in the absence of a demonstrable pathogen.

Treatment. The prognosis before chemotherapy was hopeless. There is no doubt that early diagnosis and institution of treatment are important factors in determining survival. The gingival involvement diminishes following cytotoxic therapy in responsive patients.

The dentist may play an important role in the early detection of WG by associating the oral manifestations with the systemic changes of mild anemia, leukocytosis, thrombocytosis, and an elevated erythrocyte sedimentation rate.

EHLERS-DANLOS SYNDROMES

The Ehlers-Danlos (ED) syndromes are a group of conditions characterized by hypermobility of joints, hyperextensibility of skin, and increased tissue friability. It was originally described in 1682 by the Dutch surgeon Job van Meekeran. For many years the disorder was thought to be a single entity, but it has since been shown to exhibit extensive heterogenicity with at least eight entities, each distinguishable by clinical and genetic criteria (Table 20-1).

Dental considerations. Dental abnormalities could serve as important diagnostic clues when associated with other features of ED syndrome. Both hard and soft oral tissues appear to be affected in this disorder. Excessive fragility of the mucous membranes of the gingival tissues is apparent. Dental hard tissue findings include hypoplastic enamel and structural changes associated with the den-

tinoenamel and cementodentinal junction, irregular dentin formation, and increased tendency to develop pulp stones. Several of these developmental pulpal aberrations result in calcification of pulp tissue and/or malformed, stunted roots. There may be a direct developmental relationship to the degree of calcification of the dental papilla and deformation of the roots. In addition, reports in the literature have indicated that the hypermobility of the temporomandibular joint can result in repeated joint dislocation in some individuals.

The recognition of ED syndrome is especially important in treating oral problems associated with wound healing. It is possible to perform intraoral surgical procedures on patients with ED syndrome without any untoward effects, although it has been suggested that all surgical procedures, including exodontia, be conducted in a hospital dental environment and that special precaution be taken to prevent postoperative hemorrhage. In addition, great care should be exercised in placing sutures to minimize tissue tearing.

Cases have been reported of ED syndrome in association with severe destructive periodontitis (Baer and Sheldon, 1974; Stewart et al., 1977). These associated findings must be considered as possibly emanating from other disorders with similar intraoral features, such as degenerative periodontal disease, neutropenia, hypophosphatasia, Papillon-LeFèvre syndrome, and juvenile periodontitis (Linch and Acton, 1979). It is important to recognize severe destructive periodontitis associated with ED syndrome, so that postoperative bleeding and poor wound healing may be anticipated.

CROHN'S DISEASE

Crohn's disease is an inflammatory disease of the small or large intestine. The inflammation involves all layers of the gut; thus the term *transmural colitis* has been used to describe this disease in the colon. Although ulcerative colitis is usually contiguous, beginning in the rectum and extending retrograde to involve various portions of the colon, Crohn's disease is usually segmental, and there is normal intestine between areas of inflammation. Most commonly, the terminal ileum and right colon are involved. Lesions also have been reported in the esophagus, stomach, and duodenum. Gross examination may reveal mucosal ulceration, aphthous ulcers within mucosa that appears normal, deep ulcers within areas of swollen mucosa, and long linear ulcers; serpiginous areas of mucosal hemorrhage may alternate with areas of gross hemorrhage.

Clinical manifestations.   Although bleeding is a prominent feature of ulcerative colitis, it is present in only 50% of patients with transmural colitis. Bleeding is rare in cases of small bowel Crohn's disease. Diarrhea is the most common feature in both large and small bowel disease. Patients with disease limited to the terminal ileum may have a tender right lower quadrant mass and obstructive symptoms of pain, nausea, vomiting, and distension. Weakness, fatigue, anorexia, and fever are common symptoms of active disease. An intraabdominal abscess or enterocutaneous fistula may be the initial manifestation of the disease or may develop during its course. Other manifestations depend on the location of the disease. Inflammation of the small intestine may impair its absorption of vital nutrients. Extraintestinal manifestations also develop in Crohn's disease, usually in association with colonic involvement. Arthritis, pyoderma gangrenosum, erythema nodosum, uveitis, and liver disease have all been reported.

Crohn's disease is a protean illness characterized by exacerbations and remissions. It is estimated that 5% to 10% of infected patients die of the illness. The initial location of the disease may provide some clue as to its probable course. The incidence of carcinomas of the small bowel is increased in patients with Crohn's disease. Life tables indicate that up to 80% of patients require surgery within 20 years.

Dental considerations.   Oral lesions have been found in approximately 6% to 20% of patients with Crohn's disease. It can occur at any time during the course of the disease and may be present before intestinal involvement is demonstrable. These lesions may recur in various forms in different locations in the same patient and may or may not be correlated with the exacerbation and remission of intestinal symptoms.

Oral lesions occur more commonly in patients with colonic disease than in those with disease confined to the small bowel. Patients with extraintestinal manifestations of Crohn's disease, such as skin and joint lesions, have a greater chance of developing oral manifestations.

The oral lesions seen in patients with Crohn's disease are either "specific" or "nonspecific," as differentiated by clinical and histologic features. "Specific" oral lesions are histologically similar to the intestinal lesions of the disease. They most commonly occur in the mucobuccal fold or buccal mucosa, where they are described as having a lobulated, hypertrophic fissured appearance, with or without linear ulcerations. The diffuse buccal lesions have a "cobblestone" appearance that is characteristic of Crohn's disease. Lesions on vestibular and retromolar mucosa are indurated and polypoid, often resembling denture granulomas (epulis fisuratom). Specific lesions of the gingiva, alveolar mucosa, and lips appear as areas of diffuse red swelling, sometimes accompanied by angular cheilitis (Fig. 20-6).

"Nonspecific" lesions are recurrent aphthous ulcers and

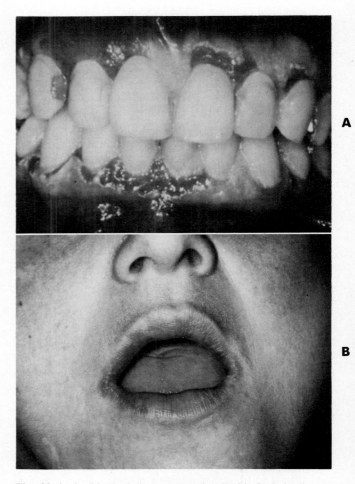

A

B

Fig. 20-6. A, Gingival changes associated with Crohn's disease. Tissue is red, edematous, and somewhat granular at dentogingival junction. **B,** Angular cheilitis in a patient suffering from Crohn's disease.

are probably the most common oral sign of Crohn's disease. The onset of these ulcers, which are generally widespread and severe, may be concurrent with bowel symptoms. The cause is not certain, but it is suspected that since measurably lower IgA secretion rates have been found in patients with active Crohn's disease, the oral mucous membrane may be more likely to undergo an immunologic reaction to exogenous oral antigens, resulting in these lesions.

Oral lesions generally regress when intestinal symptoms are brought under control. Local steroids may reduce inflammation in some patients, and 2% viscous lidocaine rinses are prescribed to reduce pain.

A possible association between Crohn's disease and periodontal disease has been reported (Lamster et al., 1978; Van Dyke et al., 1986). The manifestations are similar to those of a rapidly progressing form of periodontal disease.

HYPOADRENOCORTICISM

The clinical syndrome of glucocorticoid deficiency in humans is due to inadequate production of a single hormone, cortisol. When this results from lesions directly involving the adrenal cortex, the disorder is termed *primary adrenal failure,* hypoadrenocorticism, or Addison's disease. If, however, the deficiency is due to failure of adrenocorticotrophic hormone (ACTH) to stimulate cortisol production, the resulting syndrome is termed *secondary adrenal failure.*

Two important distinctions between primary and secondary adrenal failure are noteworthy:

1. Addison's disease is commonly associated with loss of adrenal steroids other than cortisol, particularly aldosterone; by contrast, secondary adrenal failure is not associated with aldosterone deficiency.
2. Primary adrenal failure is accompanied by marked elevated levels of plasma ACTH as a physiologic feedback consequence of cortisol deficiency; by definition, plasma ACTH is low or undetectable in secondary adrenal failure.

Clinical manifestations.   Adrenal failure occurs as either an acute or a chronic syndrome. The predominant feature of acute adrenal failure is hypotension. Sudden, unexpected shock may be the only finding that raises suspicion of the diagnosis. This commonly occurs during the course of a serious illness.

Chronic adrenal failure develops progressively over several years, the course being variable in duration and severity, depending on the destructive process. Weakness is a universal complaint, noted initially as easy fatigue, but increasing in time to profound exhaustion that limits normal activity. Weight loss is also a regular occurrence, usually accompanied by a poor appetite and sometimes by episodes of nausea and vomiting. Hypotension, particularly with upright posture, is frequently noted. Occasionally this is symptomatic, with episodes of dizziness occurring after standing.

Hyperpigmentation is the single most characteristic physical finding of primary adrenal failure; it represents melanocyte stimulation induced by high levels of ACTH and thus is absent in secondary adrenal failure. The skin darkening is generalized but most intense over sunexposed areas, sometimes described as a summer tan that never fades. Other involved areas, particularly in whites, reveal bluish black mottling of the lips, gingiva, buccal mucosa, palate, and under the tongue. On the skin freckles and moles become more intense, the nipple areolae darken, recent scars are heavily pigmented, the palmar and finger creases of the hand acquire pigmentation, linear pigmented lines appear on the fingernails, and the exterior (pressure) surface of the extremities, such as the elbows and knees, acquires a dirty brown color.

Dental considerations.   The oral pigmentations appear as irregular spots that may vary in color and intensity, ranging from pale brown to gray or even black. They occur most frequently on the buccal mucosa but may be found on the gingiva, palate, tongue, or lips.

Administration of corticosteroids is the usual treatment for Addison's disease and often leads to suppression of the individual's immune response. Consequently, patients receiving steroid therapy are more prone to developing periodontal disease, chronic mucocutaneous candidiasis, and oral infections that may be difficult to treat with conventional therapy.

Treatment.   Dental management is the same for patients with primary or secondary adrenal insufficiency. Patients who have been taking steroids within the past year present two potential problems: an increased susceptibility to infection and the possibility of adrenal crisis.

Dental patients taking corticosteroids are at increased risk of developing severe dental infection, since corticosteroids alter the host's normal inflammatory response. The chance of infection can be minimized by employing atraumatic and aseptic technique and by adequate antimicrobial therapy.

Stress induced by infection, trauma, surgery, and anesthesia may lead to adrenal crisis in any patient with adrenal insufficiency. In these patients there is atrophy of the adrenal glands with inhibition of the production of cortisol by suppression of the pituitary-adrenal feedback system. During physical or emotional stress there is an increased metabolic demand for corticoids. Since this demand cannot be met by the adrenal cortex, the dosage of exogenous corticoids must be increased. It is generally accepted that significant adrenal suppression will occur within 2 to 4 weeks of the daily administration of any corticosteroids (equivalent to hydrocortisone, 30 mg). The patient continues to be at risk of experiencing adrenal crisis even if steroids were taken within 1 year, since this length of time is required for complete restoration of adrenal function. Consultation and close cooperation with the patient's physician are absolutely essential before dental treatment is initiated, in order to adjust the dosage of corticosteroids.

Despite all precautions, an acute adrenal crisis may occur, and the dentist should be able to recognize and initially manage the condition. Signs and symptoms of crisis include hypotension, weakness, nausea, vomiting, headache, and fever. Immediate treatment consists of 100 mg of hydrocortisone administered intravenously or intramuscularly. The patient should be transferred to a hospital facility as soon as possible.

HYPOPHOSPHATASIA

Hypophosphatasia is a familial disease in which the skeletal deformities of rickets and osteomalacia develop in the presence of normal metabolism of vitamin D, parathyroid hormone, and bone mineral. It is inherited as an autosomal recessive trait. The disease may appear in infancy, childhood, or adulthood.

Cardinal features of the disease are rickets and/or osteomalacia of variable severity with a low serum and bone alkaline phosphatase level and the excretion of excessive amounts of phosphoethanolamine in the urine. The primary defect is thought to be a lack of the normal amount of alkaline phosphatase in bone matrix vesicles, leading to delay or inhibition of the nucleation of bone mineral crystals. There is no definitive treatment, but continuous high phosphate intake has been reported to lead to an improvement in some cases.

Dental considerations. Dental abnormalities have been described only in the juvenile type of hypophosphatasia, the first clinical symptom of which is often the premature loss of primary teeth. The teeth most frequently involved are the primary mandibular central and lateral incisors, followed by the maxillary incisors and, less commonly, the posterior teeth. Additional signs of juvenile hypophosphatasia are loss of alveolar bone, lack of periodontal ligament integrity, and reduced or complete absence of cementum (Fig. 20-7).

Radiographic evidence of the disorder consists of enlarged pulp chambers and root canals, sometimes giving the tooth a "shell" appearance; reduction in the thickness of the dentin and irregular dentin formation with large dentinal tubules and many areas of interglobular dentin; enamel hypoplasia; and irregular calcifications and lesions in the alveolar bone. The histologic features of the jawbone are similar to those of rickets and osteomalacia (Jedrychowski and Duperon, 1979; Rose and Kaye, 1983).

PAGET'S DISEASE (OSTEITIS DEFORMANS)

Paget's disease of bone is a chronic disease characterized by excessive osteoblastic and osteoclastic activity that results in poorly mineralized, distorted bones. Most cases

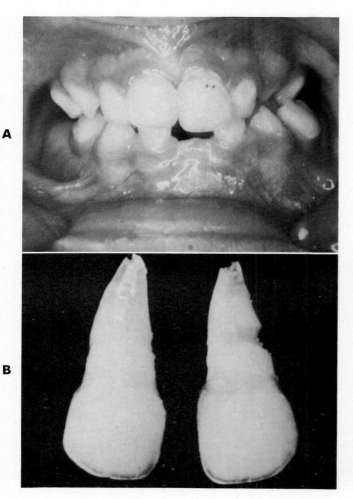

Fig. 20-7. A, Patient afflicted with hypophosphatasia. **B,** Maxillary central incisors demonstrate loss of significant amount of cementum in a patient with hypophosphatasia.

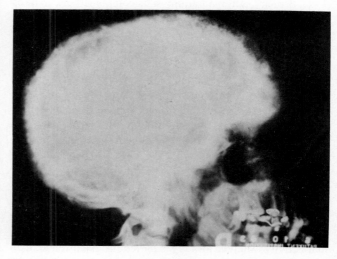

Fig. 20-8. Paget's disease of skull characterized by osteoblastic and osteoclastic activity resulting in poorly mineralized bones (cotton wool appearance).

are not clinically apparent. Pagetic bones usually produce typical radiographic changes, and the diagnosis is often made when radiographs are taken during the evaluation of another problem (Fig. 20-8). The incidence of disease rises with age, and men have a slight predominance. There are some reports of familial clustering.

Pain is the most common complaint in symptomatic Paget's disease. It may be present before radiographic changes, and the diagnosis at that time is often missed. The pain is aggravated by weight bearing if the lower extremity or spine is involved.

Headache, dizziness, and reduced hearing result from disease in the skull. Cranial enlargement develops over many years. With marked involvement of the skull, patients may have cranial nerve compression. Other skeletal deformities can include distortion of the clavicles, multiple compression fractures, pagetic vertebrae resulting in severe kyphosis, and unsuspected pathologic fractures. Patients who have one third or more of the skeleton involved can have increased cardiac output, only to increase vascularity of the bone lesions. This can ultimately lead to congestive heart failure.

Dental considerations. Jaw involvement in Paget's disease is common; most commonly, the maxilla is targeted. Jaw involvement is usually symmetric, although unilateral lesions have been reported (Tillman, 1962; Akin et al., 1975).

The characteristic osteolytic, osteoblastic, and combined phases are evident in Paget's disease of the jaw. The initial demineralization is reflected by an increased trabeculation and ground glass appearance of bone. Radiolucent, ill-defined demineralized areas may also be apparent. The osteoblastic and combined phases produce the well-known cotton wool appearance associated with the disease. Bone during the final "burnout" stage is extremely dense and radiopaque.

A gradual encroachment by Paget's bone on the teeth is occasionally observed. Radiographic changes include a gradual loss of lamina dura, hypercementosis, and occasional calcification of pulp chambers. Increased periapical radiolucencies have been associated with involved teeth, with little or no differentiation between tooth and bone (Stafne and Austin, 1938; McGowan, 1975). A case of Paget's disease of the mandible has been reported, in which three teeth required extraction because of progressive resorption of the roots by the disease process (Ripp, 1972).

The primary oral manifestation of Paget's disease is a gradual enlargement of the maxilla and the mandible. This osseous enlargement in the edentulous patient often causes an inability to wear existing dentures. In patients with teeth, the expansion of the jaws results in spreading, flaring, and mobility of the dentition and the production of an abnormal occlusal pattern.

Bleeding is the most important complication encoun-

tered in performing periodontal surgery during the early stages of Paget's disease. Nonunion extraction sites, bone exposure, and osteomyelitis commonly occur during the late stages of the disease. The use of antibiotics before, during, and after surgical procedures has been advocated to minimize the risk of osteomyelitis. Excision has been recommended if sequestration should occur (McGowan, 1975).

OSTEOPOROSIS

Osteoporosis is a metabolic bone disorder and the most common cause of osteopenia in the elderly. It represents a disease state of skeletal metabolism in which the rate of bone matrix formation is depressed and unable to compensate for the excessive resorption. Ossification is normal, but there is inadequate matrix to ossify. It is known that loss of bone mass accompanies normal physiologic aging, but in osteoporosis the rate of atrophy is accelerated well beyond the usual 1% per year.

Clinical osteoporosis, characterized by bone pain and pathologic fractures, develops when 30% or greater of the bone mass is lost. The rate of loss determines the age at which the disease is clinically apparent.

Dental considerations. The mandible, in addition to the long bones and vertebrae, may exhibit changes related to generalized osteoporosis. Although most patients with osteoporosis do not suffer from an underlying systemic disease, certain disease states cause a decrease in mineral density that may become apparent in the mandible and alveolar bone. For this reason, changes in the mandible and alveolar bone can be an important means of recognizing systemic diseases.

Most of the systemic disorders causing secondary osteoporosis produce in the mandible, as in other bones, a decrease in trabeculation. The demineralization associated with secondary osteoporosis due to hyperparathyroidism may cause a ground glass appearance of bone and a loss of lamina dura (Dreizen et al., 1971; Warren, 1977).

The effect of osteoporosis on alveolar bone has been investigated. Ward and Manson (1973) noted no correlation between the amount of alveolar bone loss and the extent of osteoporosis as measured by the metacarpal index. Dreizen et al. (1971) found that steroid-induced osteoporosis involved alveolar bone, as well as the vertebral and appendicular skeleton. Carranza et al. (1969) observed marked osteoporosis with decreased trabeculation of interradicular bone in animals fed a protein-deficient diet.

Osteoporosis of the mandible is usually manifested by a decrease in trabeculation. However, a decrease in mineral content of 30% to 50% is required before diminished bone density becomes apparent on dental radiographs. It has been shown that the densities of the mandible and radius are similarly affected by age; both show a comparable decrease in mineral density with increasing age (Carranza et al., 1969; Hemikson and Wallenius, 1974). Periodic, routine dental radiographs provide a means to compare density changes in the mandible over a period of time.

STRESS

There are many forms of stress, such as trauma, drug intoxication, and muscular fatigue, that may compromise the health of an individual. The systemic reactions that affect the body generally or produce an interrelated nonspecific tissue change resulting from continued exposure to stress have been termed the *general adaptation syndrome (GAS)* by Selye (1946). Selye considered GAS to be the basis for the pathogenesis of numerous diseases. This syndrome is thought to be a group of psychologic mechanisms that represent an attempt by the body to resist the damaging effects of stress. Three stages of the syndrome have been identified:

1. The initial response (the alarm reaction)
2. The adaptation to stress (the resistant stage)
3. The final stage, marked by inability to maintain adaptation to stress (the exhaustion stage)

The inferior lobe of the pituitary gland and the adrenal cortex are extremely active during periods of stress. They produce the morphologic functional changes that compromise the GAS. The adrenal glands are enlarged, with increased secretion of adrenocortocoid hormones; involution of lymphatic organs; hyalinization and inflammatory changes in blood vessels; gastrointestinal ulceration; and malignant nephrosclerosis. Thus the adaptive mechanisms of the body in response to stress may produce disease.

Relationship to periodontal disease. Osteoporosis of alveolar bone (Gupta et al., 1960), epithelial sloughing, degeneration of the periodontal ligament, reduced osteoblastic activity (Ratcliff, 1956), and the formation of periodontal pockets (Shklar, 1966), as well as delayed wound healing of connective tissue and bone (Stahl, 1961), have all been associated with stress.

Acute necrotizing ulcerative gingivitis (ANUG) is the periodontal disease having a significant relationship to stress (Schluger, 1943, 1949; Goldhaber and Giddon, 1964) (Fig. 20-9). Many authors have found a positive correlation between ANUG and psychologic stress (Manson and Rand, 1961; Shields, 1977; Pollman and Dietrich, 1979). Moulton et al. (1952) pointed out that emotional stress may affect the gingiva directly or indirectly. The direct route involves overt habits partially or incompletely under voluntary control, which may include such problems as poor oral hygiene, poor dietary habits, and smoking. The indirect route may alter the resistance of the periodontium to infection by acting on the autonomic nervous system and the endocrine system to affect such factors as circulating antibodies (reduced resistance) and gingival circulation. Manhold (1956) hypothesized that the constriction of blood vessels that results from continual severe emotional upset may be a complicating or causative factor in the pathogenesis of periodontal disease. Constant

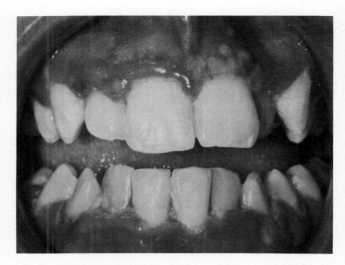

Fig. 20-9. Acute necrotizing ulcerative gingivitis (ANUG) commonly noted in patients experiencing stress.

vasoconstriction could result in a lack of oxygen and nutrients to the periodontal tissues (Gupta, 1966). A variety of stress stimuli have been used in experimental animals to alter emotional stability. Both histologic and clinical observations demonstrated that stress is capable of altering the psychologic state of the periodontium (Manhold, 1956; Manhold et al., 1971) (Fig. 20-10).

Loesche et al. (1982) shed light on the interrelationship of stress and the bacterial flora associated with periodontal disease. They identified specific bacteria that were considered to be pathogenic for ANUG and implicated *Bacteroides intermedius* as a significant bacterial entity in ANUG. These authors have noted that increased clinical steroid levels associated with stress may be a precipitating factor in ANUG that enhances bacterial invasion of the interdental region by weakening host inflammatory response or by inducing relative ischemia in the gingival papillary regions. Also, they have proposed that corticosteroid may be an important nutritional factor for *B. intermedius,* thus providing the organism with a selective nutrient advantage, with subsequent overgrowth and increased inflammatory response.

Cogen et al. (1983) have suggested that elevated levels of cortisol may produce alterations in the immune system. These alterations may account for the decreased chemotactic and phagocytic response of polymorphonuclear leukocytes (PMNS). Other authors have reported on the relationship of stress and its impact on the immune system, indicating that hydrocortisone and epinephrine reduce host resistance, rendering the host more susceptible to bacterial infection (Goldhaber and Giddon 1964; Shields, 1977).

Treatment. In severely stressed patients periodontal therapy is frequently dictated by the dentist's ability to communicate and motivate the patient. The dentist should

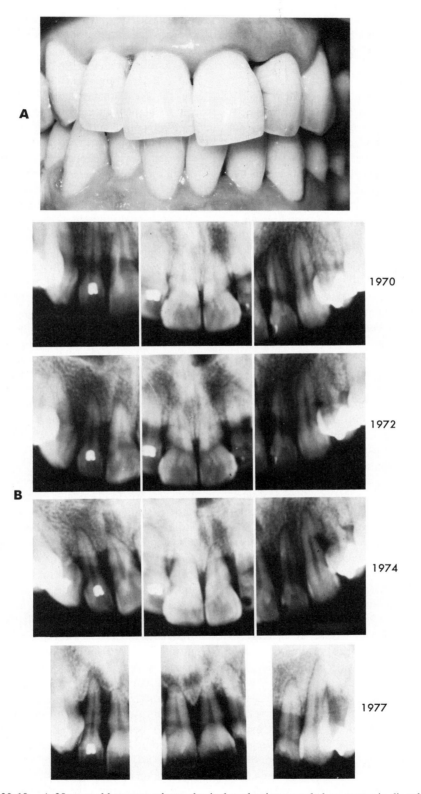

Fig. 20-10.   A 29-year-old woman whose physical evaluation revealed no systemic disorders, although she had been experiencing severe emotional instability since 1969, had had several episodes of ANUG and had noted increased mobility and migration of her teeth. **A,** Acute symptoms of ANUG have been eliminated, and interproximal cratering is evident, especially about maxillary anterior teeth. **B,** Radiographs demonstrate rapid destruction of alveolar process.

consider referral of the patient to a psychiatrist or clinical psychologist for additional therapy if necessary. This may significantly enhance the result of periodontal treatment.

NUTRITIONAL DEFICITS

Nutritional disorders are not only the result of inadequate dietary intake, but also may be due to disturbances in absorption and utilization, economic and educational limitations, self-imposed dietary restrictions, and geographic isolation from an adequate food supply.

Dental considerations. The relationship between nutritional factors and maintenance of periodontal health, or the role of nutritional factors in the pathogenesis of periodontal disease, is controversial. Although dental plaque is recognized as the major etiologic factor of periodontal disease, inadequate nutrition may render the host susceptible to periodontal disease or accelerate the progress of an existing condition.

The components of host defense that are of particular significance in the maintenance of oral health and that may be adversely affected by inadequate nutrition include (1) optimal, inflammatory immune response, (2) functional capacity of salivary glands and composition of saliva, (3) gingival fluid production, (4) responsiveness of the repair process, and (5) integrity of the oral mucosa.

The oral epithelial tissues are able to play a protective role by virtue of their capacity to replace cells rapidly and to act as a functional barrier. The epithelial lining of the gingival sulcus has one of the fastest turnover rates and requires a continuous and adequate supply of nutrients. Dietary studies in experimental animals demonstrate that 70% to 80% caloric restriction or protein calorie malnutrition reduces microtic activity in epithelial tissues, including that of the oral cavity (Alvares et al., 1976).

The barrier function of the oral epithelium and its permeability depend on the cumulative integrity of an intraepithelial barrier: the basement membrane and the plasma membrane of the epithelial cells. Such a barrier serves to limit the passage of antigenic material, such as bacterial endotoxins and other metabolic by-products, from the surface into the underlying connective tissue. An increase in mucosal permeability has been shown to occur with ascorbic acid–, folate-, and zinc-deficient experimental animals (Alfano et al., 1975, 1978; Joseph et al., 1982).

PMNs play a vital role in the protection of periodontal tissues. It has been demonstrated that nonhuman primates are vulnerable to periodontitis as a result of chronic ascorbic acid deficiency (Alvares et al., 1981). This suggests that the susceptibility may be related to impaired PMN chemotactic and phagocytic activities. Therefore subclinical nutritional deficiencies may influence periodontal health.

The properties of the salivary defense include adequate flow rate, buffering capacity, and antimicrobial activity. The antimicrobial activity stems from salivary immunologic and nonimmunologic constituents. These proteins perform the vital task of inhibiting bacterial adherence, growth, and colonization.

Gingival crevicular fluid contains many of the humoral and cellular components found in blood. Several of the constituents, notably immunoglobulins (IgG, IgA, and IgM), complement factors, and neutrophils, are capable of exerting a protective influence in the gingival sulcus. Studies in humans have shown that gingival fluid flow decreases following supplementation of otherwise healthy individuals with vitamin C and folic acid (Vogel and Deasy, 1978; Vogel et al., 1978). This decrease in flow may be due to a decrease in permeability of the gingival sulcular and junctional epithelium.

The process of tissue repair, including repair of periodontal tissues, is influenced by several factors, notably integrity of the inflammatory immune response, hormones, and an adequate supply of nutrients, particularly immunoacids, ascorbate, riboflavin, folic acid, vitamin A, and zinc.

The local nutrient requirement of human tissues may be considerably elevated. The gingival sulcus, owing to the ever-present toxic and antigenic challenge, is probably in a state of continuous repair. It is conceivable that inadequate nutrient levels in this tissue may result in "end organ" deficiency, causing impairment of the repair process, and facilitate the progression of periodontal disease (Mallek, 1978; Vogel and Deasy, 1978; Vogel et al., 1978).

Vitamin D (calcium and phosophorus)

Vitamin D is a fat-soluble vitamin that is essential for the absorption of calcium from the gastrointestinal track for the maintenance of the calcium/phosphorus balance and for the formation of teeth and bones. The metabolism of calcium and phosphorus and vitamin D are interrelated. A deficiency in vitamin D and/or imbalance in the calcium/phosphorus intake results in rickets in the very young and osteomalacia in adults.

Vitamin D deficiency with normal dietary calcium and phosphorus in young dogs is characterized by osteoporosis of alveolar bone (Becks et al., 1946); osteoid forming at a normal rate but remaining uncalcified; failure of osteoid to resorb, leading to its excessive accumulation; reduction in the width of the periodontal space; and a normal rate of cementum formation but defective calcification and some cementum resorption (Weinmann and Schour, 1945). Oliver (1969) reported in rats that the periodontium is unaltered in vitamin D deficiency, provided that the diet is adequate in minerals.

In animals that demonstrate osteomalacia, there is a rapid, generalized severe osteoclastic resorption of alveolar bone, proliferation of fibroblasts replacing bone and marrow, and new bone formation around remnants of unresorbed bone trabeculae (Dreizen et al., 1967). Radiographically, there is generalized partial to complete disappearance of the lamina dura and reduced density of the supporting bone, loss of trabeculae, increased radiolucence of the trabecular pattern, and increased prominence of the remaining trabeculae.

In vitamin D and calcium deficiency with normal dietary phosphorus, there is generalized bone resorption in the jaws, fibro-osteoid hemorrhage in the marrow spaces, and destruction of the periodontal ligament (Becks and Weber, 1931). The pattern is suggestive of changes in hyperparathyroidism. Vitamin D and phosphorus deficiency with normal dietary calcium presents rachitic changes characterized by marked osteoid deposition (MacCollum et al., 1921).

In phosphorus deficiency with normal dietary vitamin D and calcium, jaw growth is disturbed and tooth eruption and condylar growth are retarded (Burrill, 1943; Weinmann 1946).

Vitamin C

The effect of ascorbic acid on the periodontium has been evaluated more than any other nutrient. Attempts to correlate the ascorbic acid level of the blood with the incidence and severity of gingival and periodontal disease have produced conflicting results. Weisberger et al. (1938), Blockley and Baenzinger (1942), and Keller et al. (1963) were able to demonstrate a relationship between ascorbic acid levels in the blood and periodontal disease. However, other investigators did not agree with these results (Grandon et al., 1940; Spies, 1955; Perlitsh et al., 1961).

Ever since the discovery that vitamin C affects the gingiva, many dentists have advocated large doses of such vitamins to treat bleeding, inflamed gingiva, and mobile teeth (Parfitt and Speris, 1970) (Fig. 20-11).

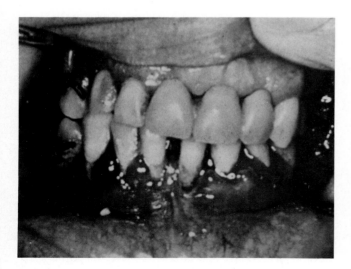

Fig. 20-11. Ascorbic acid deficiency causing severe gingival inflammation and tooth mobility.

The value of vitamin C supplementation on the periodontal status has been studied by many investigators. Grandon et al. (1940) consumed a vitamin-deficient diet for 5 months without incurring gingival changes. However, after 6 months the authors observed some slight changes at the gingival margin. El-Ashiry et al. (1964) stated that significant reduction in gingivitis was noted in individuals in whom both local periodontal treatment and systemic administration of vitamin C was given. Similar results were also reported by the same group of investigators in relation to sulcus depth before and after both local periodontal therapy and additional vitamin C supplementation were given.

Coven (1965) reported on a double-blind study in which 267 healthy children were treated with prophylaxis plus a placebo versus vitamin C and multivitamin supplementation for a 28-day period. Coven concluded that vitamin supplementation resulted in a trend toward improvement over the placebo. In addition, Dachi et al. (1966) attempted to study the effects of vitamin C and multivitamin supplementation on gingival sulcus depth over a period of 4 days. They found no significant changes in the sulcus depth values in either the group taking multivitamins or the group taking a placebo.

Many researchers have studied the effects of vitamin C supplementation on tooth mobility. Cheraskin et al. (1968b) noted a positive correlation between the lingual vitamin C test and tooth mobility. A reduction in tooth mobility following orthodontic movement was reported by Karlson et al. (1959) with the use of massive doses of vitamin C supplementation over a 14-day period. Also, O'Leary et al. (1969) reported on the results of a study to determine the effects of ascorbic acid supplementation (300 mg/day) on tooth mobility. They concluded that under the conditions of their study, in which the subjects did not have overt symptoms of ascorbic acid deficiency, ascorbic acid supplementation did not decrease tooth mobility.

In brief, it has been suggested that human gingivitis and alveolar bone loss results from ascorbic acid deficiency. However, clinical, epidemiologic, and histologic studies have failed to link vitamin C with the prevalence or severity of periodontal disease or tooth mobility (Ferguson, 1969; Grant et al., 1973). One should not ignore the fact that vitamin C plays an important role in the formation of the amino acids hydroxyproline and hydroxylysine, which are almost unique to collagen, the major protein of the periodontium (Drummond, 1971). Experimental data may suggest that periodontal tissues respond to vitamin C deficiencies in a manner similar to that of connective tissue in general. However, while gingival repair following injury may be disturbed in scorbutic animals, no experimental evidence exists that vitamin C deficiency initiates inflammatory periodontal disease (Ferguson, 1969; Grant et al., 1973).

Proteins

Protein deficiency has been reported to cause osteoporosis of alveolar bone and a narrowing of the periodontal ligament fibers. It does not appear to affect the epithelial attachment, nor does it initiate any local inflammatory reaction (Chawla and Glickman, 1951; Person et al., 1958). In addition, protein deprivation has been known to retard the healing of wounds, as well as the repair of local tissue irritation (Levenson et al., 1950; Dunphy, 1960; Stahl, 1965; Stahl et al., 1965). South Indian children with severe protein deficiencies (kwashiorkor) were examined for oral mucosal lesions and periodontal disease. The children with kwashiorkor had a greater incidence of ANUG and higher periodontal disease index scores than were observed in the healthy children (Pindborg et al., 1967). Cheraskin et al. (1967, 1968a) evaluated the effects of prophylaxis and protein supplementation on gingival tissues and tooth mobility. They concluded that local therapy alone, or protein supplementation alone, was not as effective as combined therapy (protein and prophylaxis). This combined approach to therapy is thought to increase host resistance and decrease local irritants.

Protein deprivation in the presence of periodontal tissue injury will decrease the rate of connective tissue and bone repair and frequently cause a breakdown of the healing wound (Stahl, 1962, 1966, 1965). When Stahl et al. (1970) evaluated the effects of low-protein feeding in young adult rats using audioradiographic analysis of the gingival response to injury, they noted that animals fed a low-protein diet demonstrated less proliferative activity in noninjured periodontal sites than animals on an adequate dietary regimen, although the healing response to injury over 30 days was similar irrespective of diet. It is believed that the stimulus created by inflicting a wound in the animals fed a low-protein diet resulted in tissue compensation for the reduction in proliferative activity.

Published data related to the systemic influence of nutrition on the periodontium in health and disease have led to the following conclusions:

1. Animal studies have demonstrated inconclusively that when a large number of nutrients are either withheld from the diet or ingested in excessive amounts, a deleterious effect may be seen. Animal experiments give us a clue as to what to study in humans, but we cannot make conclusions about the pathogenesis of human periodontal disease solely from results obtained from animal experiments.

2. Nutitional imbalance in humans does not cause periodontal disease without the presence of local irritating factors. Deficiencies in nutrition appear to modify the severity and extent of periodontal disease by altering the host resistance and the potential for repair of the affected tissues. To date, evidence is lacking to support nutritional disorders as a factor in the initiation of periodontal disease.

3. Well-controlled nutritional studies in human subjects with severe periodontal disease will be essential and very helpful for definitive and valid assessment of the systemic role of nutrition in periodontal health and disease.

It is clear that periodontal disease is primarily an infectious process involving an inflammatory response to local tissue irritants (e.g., bacterial plaque). Current knowledge suggests that the response can be conditioned by nutritional factors. However, prevention or reversal of this disease by short-term nutritional therapy has not been demonstrated. Thus the fundamental basis for patient counseling relative to diet, nutrition, and periodontal disease rests with instructing the patient to ingest a nutritionally adequate diet in the long term. If periodontitis responds positively to plaque control and conventional modes of treatment, nutritional supplementation is usually unwarranted.

REFERENCES

Akin RK, Barton K, and Walters PJ: Paget's disease of bone: a case report, Oral Surg 39(5):707, 1975.

Alfano MC: Effect of acute ascorbic acid deficiency on the DNA content and permeability of guinea-pig oral mucosal epithelium, Arch Oral Biol 23:929, 1978.

Alfano MC, Miller SA, and Drummond JF: Effects of ascorbic acid deficiency on the permeability and collagen biosynthesis of oral mucosa epithelium, Ann NY Acad Sci 258:253, 1975.

Alvares 0, Altman LC, and Springmeyer S: The effect of subclinical ascorbate deficiency on periodontal health in non-human primates, J Periodont Res 16:628, 1981.

Alvares 0, Worthington B, and Enwonwu CO: Regional differences in the effects of protein calorie malnutrition on oral epithelium, J Dent Res 55(B):173, 1976.

Baer P and Sheldon B: Periodontal disease in children and adolescents, Philadelphia, 1974, JP Lippincott Co.

Becks H, Collins DA, and Freytog RM: Changes in oral structures of the dog persisting after chronic overdoses of vitamin D, Am J Orthod 32:463, 1946.

Becks H and Weber M: Influence of diet in bone system with special reference to alveolar process and labyrinthine capsule, J Am Dent Assoc 18:197, 1931.

Blockley CH and Baenziger PE: An investigation into the connection between the vitamin C content of the blood and periodontal disturbances, Br Dent J 73:57, 1942.

Burket LW: Histopathologic explanation for the oral lesion in the acute leukemias, Am J Orthod Oral Surg 30:516, 1944.

Burrill DY: The effect of low phosphorus intake on the growth of the jaws in dogs, J Am Dent Assoc 30: 513, 1943.

Carranza FA et al: Histometric analysis of interradicular bone in protein deficient animals, J Periodont Res 4:292, 1969.

Chawla TN and Glickman I: Protein deprivation and the periodontal structures of the albino rat, Oral Surg 4:578, 1951.

Cheraskin E et al: An ecologic analysis of gingiva state: effect of prophylaxis and protein supplementation, J Periodontol 39:316, 1968a.

Cheraskin E et al: A lingual vitamin C test. X. Relationship to tooth mobility, Int J Vitam Nutr Res 38:434, 1968B.

Cheraskin WM, Steyaadmadja ATSH, and Ray DW: An ecologic analysis of tooth mobility: effect of prophylaxis and protein supplementation, J Periodontol 38: 227, 1967.

Cogen RB et al: Leukocyte function in the etiology of ANUG, J Periodontol 54:402, 1983.

Cohen PS and Meltzer JA: Strawberry gums: a sign of Wegener's granulomatosis, JAMA 246:2610, 1981.

Coven EM: Effect of prophylaxis and vitamin supplementation upon periodontal index in children, J Periodontol 36:494, 1965.

Dachi SF, Saxe SR, and Bohannan HM: The failure of short-term vitamin supplementation to reduce sulcus depth, J Periodontol 37:221, 1966.

Dreizen S, Levy B, and Bernick S: Studies on the biology of the periodontium of marmosets: cortisone induced periodontal and skeletal changes in adult cottontop marmosets, J Periodontol 42:217, 1971.

Dreizen S et al: Studies on the biology of the periodontium of marmosets. III. Periodontal bone changes in marmosets with osteomalacia and hyperparathyroidism, Isr J Med Sci 3:731, 1967.

Drummond JF: Note and comments, Dent Abstr 16:73, 1971.

Dunphy JE: On the nature and care of wounds, Ann R Coll Surg Engl 26:69, 1960.

Edwards MB and Buckerfield JP: Wegener's granulomatosis—a case with primary mucocutaneous lesions, Oral Surg 46:53, 1978.

El-Ashiry GM, Ringsdorf WM, and Cheraskin E: Local and systemic influences in periodontal disease. II. Effect of prophylaxis and natural versus synthetic vitamin C upon gingivitis, J Periodontol 35:250, 1964.

El-Mostehy MR and Stallard RE: The Sturge-Weber syndrome: its periodontal significance, J Periodontol 40:243, 1969.

Ferguson HW: Effect of nutrition on the periodontium. In Melcher AH and Bower WH, editors: Biology of the periodontium, New York, 1969, Academic Press, Inc.

Goldhaber P and Giddon DB: Present concepts concerning etiology and treatment of acute necrotizing ulcerative gingivitis, Int Dent J 14:468, 1964.

Gorlin RJ and Goldman HM: Thoma's oral pathology, ed 6, St Louis, 1970, The CV Mosby Co.

Gorlin RJ, Pindborg JJ, and Cohen MM Jr: Syndromes of the head and neck, ed 2, New York, 1976, McGraw Hill Book Co.

Grandon JH, Lund CC, and Dill DB: Experimental human survey, N Engl J Med 223:353, 1940.

Grant DA, Stern IB, and Everett FG: Orban's periodontics, ed 4, St Louis, 1973, The CV Mosby Co.

Gupta OP: Psychosomatic factors in periodontal disease, Dent Clin North Am, p 11, March 1966.

Gupta OP, Bleechman H, and Stahl SS: The effects of stress on the periodontal tissues of young adult male rats and hamsters, J Periodontol 32:413, 1960.

Hemikson P and Wallenius K: The mandible and osteoporosis, J Oral Rehabil 1:67, 1974.

Israelson H, Binnie WH, and Hurt WC: The hyperplastic gingivitis of Wegener's granulomatosis, J Periodontol 52:8 1981.

Jedrychowski JR and Duperon D: Childhood hypophosphatsia with oral manifestations, J Oral Med 35:18, 1979.

Joseph CE et al: Zinc deficiency changes in the permeability of rabbit periodontium to 14C-phenytoin and 14-C albumin, J Periodontol 54:251, 1982.

Karlson FA, Cheraskin E, and Dunbar JB: Subclinical scurvy and subclinical tooth mobility, Periodontol Abstr 7:6, 1959.

Karmody C: Wegener's granulomatosis: presentation as an otologic problem, Otolaryngology 86:573, 1978.

Keller SE, Ringsdorf WM, and Cheraskin E: Interplay of local and systemic influences in the periodontal diseases, J Periodontol 34:259, 1963.

Lamster I et al: An association between Crohn's disease, periodontal disease and enhanced neutrophil function, J Periodontol 475, 1978.

Levenson SM, Burkhill FR, and Waterman DF: The healing of soft tissue wounds, the effects of nutrition, anemia and age, Surgery 28:905, 1950.

Linch DC and Acton CHC: Ehlers-Danlos syndrome presenting with juvenile destructive periodontitis, Br Dent J 147:95, 1979.

Lindhe J: Textbook on clinical periodontology, Philadelphia, 1983, WB Saunders Co.

Loesche WJ et al: The bacteriology of ANUG, J Periodontol 53:223, 1982.

Lynch MA, editor: Burket's oral medicine, ed 8, Philadelphia, 1984, JP Lippincott Co.

MacCollum EV et al: The production of rickets by diets low in phosphorus and fat soluble, Am J Biol Chem 47:507 1921.

Manhold JH: Introductory psychosomatic dentistry, New York, 1956, Appleton-Century Crofts, Inc.

Manhold JH, Doyle JL, and Weisinger EH: Effects of social stress on oral and other bodily tissues, J Periodontol 42:109, 1971.

Manson MJ and Rand D: Recurrent Vincent's disease—a survey of 61 cases, Br Dent J 110:386, 1961.

McGowan DA: Clinical problems in Paget's disease affecting the jaws, Br J Oral Surg 11:230, 1975.

Moulton R, Ewen S, and Theiman W: Emotional factors in periodontal disease, Oral Surg 5:883, 1952.

O'Leary TJ et al: The effect of ascorbic acid supplementation on tooth mobility, J Periodontol 40:284, 1969.

Oliver WM: The effect of deficiencies of calcium, vitamin D or calcium and vitamin D and of variations in the source of dietary protein on the supporting tissues of the rat molar, J Periodont Res 4:56, 1969.

Parfitt GJ and Speris DM: Role of nutrition in the prevention and treatment of periodontal disease, J Can Dent Assoc 36:224, 1970.

Perlitsh M, Nielsen AG, and Stanmeyer WR: Ascorbic acid and plasma levels and gingival health in personnel wintering over in Antarctica, J Dent Res 40:789, 1961.

Person P, Wannamacher R, and Fine A: The response of adult rat oral tissues to protein depletion: histologic, observations and nitrogen analysis, J Dent Res 37:292, 1958.

Pindborg JJ, Bhat M, and Roed-Petersen B: Oral changes in South Indian children with severe protein deficiency, J Periodontol 38:218, 1967.

Pollman L and Dietrich A: ANUG in young men, Dtsch Zahnartl 34:222, 1979 (English abstract).

Ratcliff PA: The relationship of the general adaptation syndrome to the periodontal tissues in the rat, J Periodontol 27:40, 1956.

Ripp GA: A complication after extraction in a patient with advanced Paget's disease, Oral Surg 33:35, 1972.

Rose LF and Kaye DK, editors: Internal medicine for dentistry, St Louis, 1983, The CV Mosby Co.

Royle HE, Lapp R, and Ferrara ED: The Sturge-Weber syndrome: its periodontal significance, J Periodontol 22:490, 1966.

Schluger S: The etiology and treatment of Vincent's infection, J Am Dent Assoc 39:524, 1943.

Schluger S: Necrotizing ulcerative gingivitis in the Army: incidence, communicability and treatment, J Am Dent Assoc 38:174, 1949.

Selye H: The general adaptation syndrome and diseases of adaptation, J Clin Endocrinol 6:117, 1946.

Shields WD: ANUG—a study of some of the contributing factors and their validity in an Army population, J Periodontol 48:346, 1977.

Shklar G: Periodontal disease in experimental animals subjected to chronic cold stress, J Periodontol 37:377, 1966.

Spies TD: Nutrition and disease, Postgrad Med 17:2, 1955.

Stafne EC and Austin LT: A study of dental roentgenograms in cases of Paget's disease (osteitis deformans), osteitis fibrosa, cystica, and osteoma, J Am Dent Assoc 25:1202, 1938.

Stahl SS: Healing gingival injury in normal and systemically stressed young adult male rats, J Periodontol 32:63, 1961.

Stahl SS: The effect of a protein-free diet on the healing of gingival wound in rats, Arch Oral Biol 7:551, 1962.

Stahl SS: The healing of experimentally induced gingival wounds in rats on prolonged nutritional deprivations, J Periodontol 36:283, 1965.

Stahl SS: Influence of prolonged low-protein feedings on epithelized gingival wounds in adult rats, J Dent Res 45:1448, 1966.

Stahl SS, Sandler HC, and Cahn LR: The effects upon the oral tissues of the rat and particularly upon periodontal structures under irritation, Oral Surg 8:760, 1965.

Stahl SS, Tonna EA, and Weiss R: Autoradiographic evaluation of gingival response to injury. IV. Surgical trauma in low-protein fed young adult rats, J Dent Res 49:531, 1970.

Stewart RE, Hollister DW, and Rimoin DL: A new variant of Ehlers-Danlos syndrome: an autosomal dominant disorder of fragile skin, abnormal scarring and generalized periodontitis, Birth Defects 13(3B):85, 1977.

Tarsitano JJ, Wooten NW, and Munford AG: Sturge Weber syndrome: a possible dental complication, Ill Dent J 39:236, 1970.

Thoma KH: Sturge-Kalischer-Weber syndrome with pregnancy tumors, Oral Surg 5:1125, 1952.

Tillman HH: Paget's disease of bone: a clinical, radiographic and histopathologic study of 24 cases involving the jaws, Oral Surg 15:1225, 1962.

Van Dyke TE et al: Potential role of microorganisms isolated from periodontal lesions in the pathogenesis of inflammatory bowel disease, Infect Immun 53(3):671, 1986.

Vogel RI and Deasy MJ: The effect of folic acid on experimentally produced gingivitis, J Prev Dent 5:30, 1978.

Vogel RI et al: The effect of topical application of folic acid on gingival health, J Oral Med 33:20, 1978.

Wannenmacher VMF and Forck G: Mundschleimhautveranderungen Beim Sturge-Weber Syndrome, Dtsch Zahnarztl Z 25:1030, 1970.

Ward VJ and Manson JD: Alveolar bone loss in peridontal disease and the metacarpal index, J Periodontol 44:763, 1973.

Warren R: Osteoporosis, J Oral Med 32(4):113, 1977.

Weinmann JP and Schour I: Experimental studies in calcification, Am J Pathol 21:821, 1945.

Weinmann JP: Rachitic changes of the mandibular condyle of the rat, J Dent Res 25:509, 1946.

Weisberger D, Young AP, and Mouse FW: Study of ascorbic acid blood levels in dental patients, J Dent Res 17:101, 1938.

Wentz FM, Anday G, and Orban B: Histopathologic changes in the gingiva in leukemia, J Periodontol 20:119, 1949.

Chapter 21

LOCAL AND SYSTEMIC ACTIONS OF DRUGS AND OTHER CHEMICAL AGENTS ON PERIODONTAL TISSUES

Thomas M. Hassell

Systemic medications
    Phenytoin
    Sodium valproate
    Cyclosporine
    Dihydropyridines: nifedipine and nitrendipine
Compounds with local effects
Heavy metals

Some therapeutic agents and medicaments may lead to pathologic changes in the periodontal tissues, especially the gingiva. Such agents are classified as (1) systemic medications with periodontal side effects, (2) topically applied compounds with direct local adverse effects on periodontal tissues, or (3) heavy metals (for reviews see Hassell and Jacoway, 1980a, 1980b; Jones and Mason, 1980; Roth and Calmes, 1981; Rye, 1984; and Wright, 1984).

SYSTEMIC MEDICATIONS
Phenytoin

Phenytoin (sodium 5,5-diphenylhydantoin) has been the drug of choice in grand mal epilepsy for over 50 years and was first described by Putnam and Merritt (1937). Marketed under numerous trade names, including Dilantin Sodium, Dilantin, and Phenytoin, it is among the 20 most-prescribed drugs in the world, used not only in epilepsy but in other neurologic disorders, including depression.

Overgrowth of the gingiva is one of the most common and troublesome side effects of phenytoin (Fig. 21-1, *A*). Since 1939, when Kimball first reported gingival lesions, over 1500 related articles have appeared in the scientific literature (for review see Hassell, 1981). Gingival overgrowth occurs in about half of all individuals who ingest phenytoin on a chronic regimen as their sole antiepileptic medication (Nacimento et al., 1985). However, the prevalence of gingival overgrowth is much higher when phenytoin is taken in combination with other antiepileptic agents (Table 21-1).

Both sexes and all races are susceptible to phenytoin-induced gingival overgrowth. Teenagers and young adults to about 30 years of age are affected more frequently than middle-aged or elderly persons. Neither prevalence nor severity of the gingival lesions is positively correlated with drug dosage or with blood or saliva concentrations of phenytoin. The earliest clinical signs of gingival change are soreness and tenderness and may occur 2 to 3 weeks after initiation of phenytoin therapy. Gingival overgrowth often becomes clinically apparent during the first 6 to 9 months of therapy as interdental papillae overgrow and extrude, forming firm, mobile, triangular tissue masses. These increase in magnitude during the ensuing 1 to 2 years and may fuse mesially and distally and form a continuous curtain of overgrown marginal gingiva, with maximum size usually achieved within that time (Hassell et al., 1978). The attached gingiva often exhibits firm nodules, with a

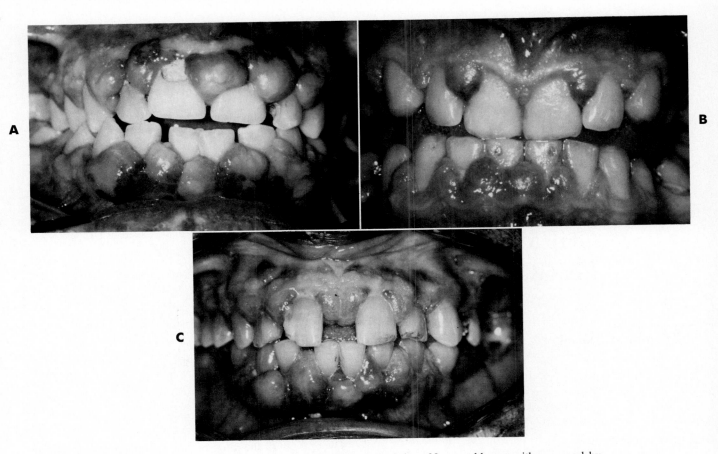

Fig. 21-1. A, Phenytoin-induced gingival overgrowth in a 29-year-old man with poor oral hygiene and gingival inflammation. Note also Class V and Class III carious lesions, anterior diastemata (possibly caused by expanding interdental connective tissue), anterior and posterior segment malocclusion, and fusion of adjacent overgrown papillae. This patient had been taking phenytoin on a chronic daily regimen for 4 years. **B,** Gingival overgrowth elicted by long-term treatment with cyclosporine following kidney transplantation in a 41-year-old woman. Interdental papillae balloon from proximal areas, and secondary inflammation is observed as a result of heavy plaque accumulation. There is fusion of tissue lobules in mandibular anterior segment. **C,** Firm, fibrous gingival overgrowth in a 56-year-old woman who had been taking nifedipine for 18 months following a heart attack. Diastema between central incisors had doubled in size since drug regimen was instituted. In addition to pseudopockets caused by redundant tissue, patient had alveolar bone loss and true periodontal pockets to 10 mm, with hemorrhage and suppuration on probing. (**B** courtesy Dr. Edith Rateitschak-Plüss.)

granular appearance on the labial surface. In the absence of papillary enlargement, gingival overgrowth may develop as a distinct marginal festoon or crescent that gradually reduces the apparent clinical crown length. There is rarely apical migration of the junctional epithelium; thus deep pseudopockets are created as the accumulation of redundant tissue continues. Oral hygiene may be extremely difficult, resulting in plaque accumulation with gingival inflammation and often enamel as well as cervical caries. Halitosis is also common.

The histopathology of excised gingiva is characterized at the light microscopic level by moderate epithelial acanthosis with rete ridge elongation. The gross increase in gingival size is due to a dramatic expansion of the connective tissue compartment, which exhibits abundant tortuous and nonoriented collagenous fiber bundles (Fig. 21-2). The collagen is biochemically distinct from that in normal gingiva, with twice as much type III and less type I collagen (Narayanan and Hassell, 1985). Electron microscopic studies have demonstrated that the excessive connective tissue also has a significantly greater volume density of noncollagenous matrix and ground substance (Bernstein and Hassell, 1987). These morphologic findings are supported by the finding of increased proteoglycans and glycosaminoglycans in excised gingiva and cultured cells from phenytoin-related overgrown gingiva (Kantor and

Table 21-1. Prevalence of gingival overgrowth associated with various antiepileptic drug regimens in a nonretarded outpatient population

Antiepileptic drug regimen	Prevalence of gingival overgrowth (%)
Phenytoin alone	52
Phenytoin + sodium valproate	56
Phenytoin + carbamazepine	71
Phenytoin + carbamazepine + phenobarbital	83
Phenytoin + polypharmacy	88
Carbamazepine alone*	0

From Maguire et al: Phenytoin-induced gingival overgrowth incidence is dependent upon co-medication, J Dent Res 65:249, 1986.
*Data from Eeg-Olofsson et al: The influence of antiepileptic medication on oral cavity structures, Eleventh International Epilepsy Symposium, Florence, Italy, 1979.

Hassell, 1983; Dahllöf et al., 1986). Hence, the excess gingival tissue that results from phenytoin ingestion represents neither hypertrophy nor hyperplasia, nor is it a true fibrosis; it is best described as *gingival overgrowth.*

Phenytoin causes gingival overgrowth in genetically susceptible individuals (Cockey et al., 1987) by enhancing the proliferation of a discrete and phenotypically stable subpopulation of highly active fibroblasts that produce elevated quantities of collagen and ground substance macromolecules (Hassell et al., 1976). These fibroblasts also secrete a collagenolytic enzyme that is largely inactive (Hassell, 1982). The drug is known to be mitogenic for some strains of cells (Hassell and Stanek, 1983), which may in part explain the predominance of these active fibroblasts.

An hypothesis currently being tested is that it is the phenytoin metabolites that may be responsible for the gingival overgrowth. Phenytoin is metabolized by hepatic cytochromes P450 to a series of well-characterized compounds (Fig. 21-3). In humans the major metabolite is 5-para-hydroxyphenyl-5-phenylhydantoin (*p*-HPPH), which is present in blood, saliva, and gingival tissue (Conard et al., 1972). *p*-HPPH causes gingival overgrowth in the cat model when administered orally on a chronic regimen (Hassell and Cooper, 1980). In addition, *p*-HPPH and the minor phenytoin metabolites (dihydrodiol, catechol and 3-0-methyl-catechol; see Fig. 21-3) have direct effects on in vitro proliferation and protein production by fibroblasts.

Treatment. Treatment of gingival enlargement is often necessary if there is gingival inflammation, dental caries, or a problem with esthetics, speech, function, or comfort. Esthetically objectionable gingival overgrowth may be effectively treated by any one or a combination of three strategies (for review see Hutchens, 1981):

1. Replacing phenytoin with an alternate drug (e.g.,

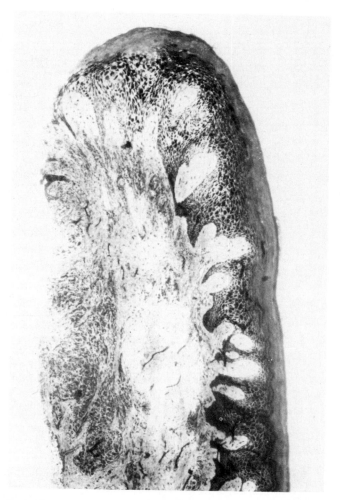

Fig. 21-2. Light microscopic photomicrograph of faciolingual section through interdental papilla excised from a 29-year-old woman who had taken phenytoin for over 6 years and who manifested gross clinical gingival enlargment with moderate inflammation. Note thickening of oral epithelium and accumulation of redundant connective tissue matrix, which contains an inflammatory cell infiltrate. (×70.) (Courtesy Dr. Aaron Bernstein.)

carbamazepine or sodium valproate) in counsel with the patient's neurologist. After such replacement, spontaneous regression of excess tissue may occur within 12 months if the patient's oral hygiene is good (Brunsvold et al., 1985).

2. Conservative periodontal therapy, including frequent professional prophylaxis and a rigorous home care regimen. This will reduce the inflammatory component of the enlargement (redness and edema) and may reduce the need for surgical resection (Fig. 21-4). Effective oral hygiene will also delay or prevent lesion recurrence after resection (Donnenfeld et al., 1974; King et al., 1976). Daily rinsing with chlorhexidine is indicated (O'Neil and Figures, 1982).

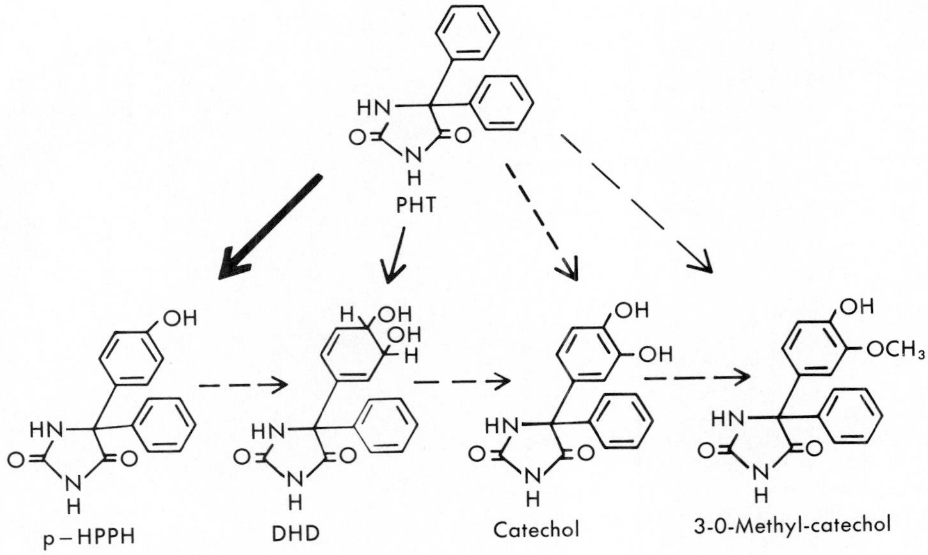

Fig. 21-3. Metabolic pathways for phenytoin in humans. Major metabolite (*p*-HPPH, *heavy arrow*), accounting for about 65% of daily dose, is hydroxylated at *para*-position on one of the aromatic rings. Dihydrodiol (DHD), a minor metabolite, can be formed by direct enzymatic action on parent compound by way of an arene oxide intermediate (which is believed to be highly teratogenic). DHD also can be further metabolized to catechol and 3-0-methyl-catechol compounds, which are likewise minor metabolites of phenytoin. It remains speculative whether the two catechol metabolites can be formed directly from parent molecule in vivo. All of the metabolites have direct effects on gingival fibroblasts in vitro; *p*-HPPH elicits gingival overgrowth when administered to experimental animals. Therefore it is likely that drug metabolism plays a pathogenetic role in etiology of gingival enlargement.

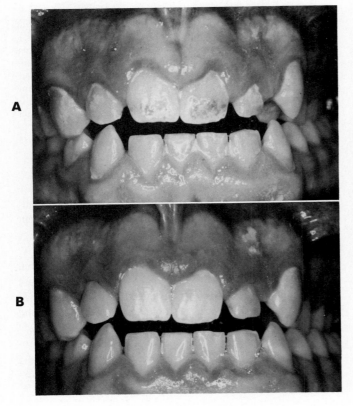

Fig. 21-4. A, Gingival inflammation in a 22-year-old male epileptic patient treated with phenytoin for 4 years. Extremely poor oral hygiene led to inflammatory response, with edema and erythema, in addition to enlargement caused by antiepileptic medication. This patient, who had never seen a dentist before, came for treatment to have his "gums cut back." **B,** Same patient, 1 month after periodontal therapy including plaque and calculus removal plus patient motivation and repeated oral hygiene instruction. In this patient sufficient esthetic improvement was achieved by plaque control and debridement, and surgical removal of tissue was not required. (Courtesy Dr. James Cady.)

3. Surgical elimination of redundant tissue by means of a scalpel (Rateitschak et al., 1985) or electrosurgery (Sherman, 1982). This is a relatively straightforward gingivectomy procedure and can be performed in the dental office with local anesthesia. Healing is routinely uneventful. Recurrence of overgrowth should be expected within 1 to 2 years, particularly in individuals under the age of 25, if the phenytoin regimen is continued. If oral hygiene is inadequate, regrowth may occur extremely quickly.

Sodium valproate

Sodium valproate (valproic acid; di-*n*-propylacetic acid; Depakene) has been used as an antiepileptic in the United States since 1978. Its mechanism of anticonvulsant action involves elevating the brain content of gamma-aminobutyric acid (Godin et al., 1969), a mechanism probably similar to that of phenytoin and several other antiepileptic agents (Halpern and Julian, 1972). "Hyperplastic gingivitis" was reported in a 15-month-old boy in Finland who was given valproate for a severe seizure disorder (Syrjanen and Syrjanen, 1979). Biopsy examination revealed an increased expanse of the connective tissue compartment with marked inflammation and dilation of capillaries, and the generalized overgrowth regressed when the drug dose was reduced. Sodium valproate can cause platelet dysfunction, which has been reported to elicit spontaneous gingival hemorrhage in the absence of inflammatory symptoms (Hassell et al., 1979). It is possible that this latter effect of valproate could account for the edematous overgrowth described by Syrjanen and Syrjanen (1979).

Public health and economic realities virtually ensure that phenytoin will maintain its rank as the drug of choice in epilepsy, since Dilantin capsules are presently one half to one fourth the cost of carbamazepine or sodium valproate. Hence, the dental community will continue to be confronted with phenytoin-induced gingival overgrowth in the forseeable future.

Cyclosporine

Cyclosporine (Sandimmune; see Fig. 21-1, *B*) has been used in the United States since 1984 for prevention of rejection phenomena following solid organ and bone marrow transplantation. It is dramatically effective, having increased the success rate in, for example, heterologous kidney transplants from 50% to 96%. In Europe and the Far East, cyclosporine is also employed in the treatment of type II diabetes mellitus, rheumatoid arthritis, psoriasis, multiple sclerosis, malaria, sarcoidosis, and some other diseases with an immunologic basis. Clinical trials currently ongoing in the United States may lead to Food and Drug Administration approval for greatly expanded use of cyclosporine in the near future. Because of its effectiveness in so many disorders, it has been estimated that over

a billion persons worldwide will be taking cyclosporine in the next decade. Cyclosporine exerts its effects by selective suppression of specific subpopulations of T lymphocytes, interfering with production of lymphokines and interleukins 1 and 2 (Bunjes et al., 1981; Koponen et al., 1985).

Accumulation of excess connective tissue is a major adverse effect of long-term cyclosporine therapy; pulmonary, pericardial, and renal fibrosis have been reported (Janin-Mercier et al., 1985). Cyclosporine-induced gingival overgrowth has also been observed (Rateitschak-Plüss et al., 1983; Adams and Davies, 1984; Bennett and Christian, 1985; Rostock et al., 1986). The gingival lesions are often clinically indistinguishable from those elicited by phenytoin (see Fig. 21-1, *A*). The clinical course is likewise similar in that the lesions generally originate in the interdental area; all segments of the dental arch may be affected.

The histopathologic picture of cyclosporine-induced gingival overgrowth is also reminiscent of the phenytoin lesion in that apparent fibroplasia, redundant collagenous elements, epithelial thickening, and secondary manifestations of inflammation are exhibited. Recent experiments show that cyclosporine can exert direct effects on human gingival fibroblasts, causing enhanced production of matrix macromolecules (Coley et al., 1986).

Dihydropyridines: nifedipine and nitrendipine

Nifedipine (Procardia; see Fig. 21-1, *C*) is a substituted dihydropyridine used widely since 1978 in the treatment of angina pectoris and postmyocardial syndrome. It blocks the influx of calcium ions into myocardial cells, thus reducing oxygen consumption (Stern and Levy, 1981). *Nitrendipine* (Bayotensin) is a structurally related dihydropyridine calcium antagonist that is used for treatment of hypertension. It has been reported that nifedipine induces gingival overgrowth in patients with heart disease (Lucas et al., 1985). The gingival lesions elicited by nifedipine in humans are clinically similar to those elicited by phenytoin or by cyclosporine. In an animal model (beagle), nitrendipine elicited dramatic gingival overgrowth after a 20-month regimen of oral administration (Heijl and Sundin, 1987) (Fig. 21-5).

All segments of the dentition are susceptible to dihydropyridine-induced overgrowth, but the anterior facial aspects are most frequently and severely affected. Secondary inflammatory manifestations are common because oral hygiene is compromised by the excess tissue. The histopathologic picture is one of thickened epithelium exhibiting elongation of epithelial rete, with the preponderance of redundant tissue composed of connective tissue with abundant fibroblasts (Ramon et al., 1984). Extracellular ground substance also appears to be in excess, as depicted by electron photomicrographs (Lucas et al., 1985). Clinical experience suggests that establishment of excellent plaque con-

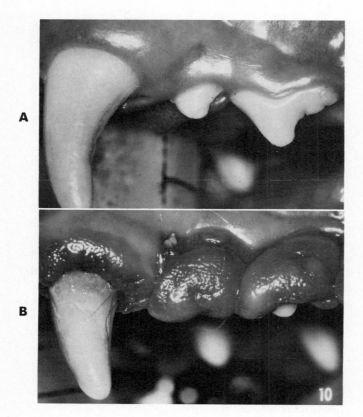

Fig. 21-5. A, Maxillary left canine and premolars of a young beagle after 6 weeks of professionally administered daily oral hygiene. Note healthy-appearing gingival contour and absence of plaque or inflammatory symptoms. **B,** Same animal as in **A** after a 20-week regimen of daily oral administration of a dihydropyridine (in this case, nitrendipine) and no tooth-cleaning procedures. Note massive accumulation of redundant gingival tissue, completely obscuring premolars and causing apparent "shortening" of canine. Gross plaque accumulation and hair impaction have occasioned secondary inflammation in overgrown gingivae, which are primarily composed of dense fibrous connective tissue. It was subsequently possible to almost entirely eliminate excess gingiva by rigorous oral hygiene and withdrawal of dihydropyridine medication. (Courtesy Dr. Lars Heijl.)

trol and regular scaling and root planing will aid in preventing and moderating dihydropyridine-induced gingival overgrowth.

Another commonly prescribed calcium antagonist used in cardiology is verapamil hydrochloride (Calan). Although structurally similar to the dihydropyridines (see Fig. 21-1, *C*), verapamil hydrochloride has *not* been associated with gingival enlargement or with fibrosis elsewhere in the body.

COMPOUNDS WITH LOCAL EFFECTS

Aspirin (acetylsalicylic acid) is one of mankind's most useful drugs. It alleviates pain by inhibiting the enzyme prostaglandin synthetase; the prostaglandins are now ac-

knowledged as a biologic source of pain. Unfortunately, many individuals attempt to use aspirin for the relief of oral pain of various types (pulpitis, operculitis, periostitis, abscess) by applying whole or crushed tablets locally, generally by placement in the vestibulum near the perceived site of the pain (Glick et al., 1974). Not only is this practice ineffective, but the consistent adverse effect is the creation of a whitish, raw, bleeding, cauterized, and painful lesion on cheek mucosa and gingiva. Such an aspirin-elicited lesion is like other chemical burns (e.g., one caused by accidental exposure to one of many agents commonly used in the dental operatory, including eugenol, trichloroacetic acid, phenol, alcohol, hydrogen peroxide, and beechwood creosote). If the offending agent is removed and the area flushed generously with water, healing will ensue within days if the sloughed area does not become secondarily infected by opportunistic microorganisms.

HEAVY METALS

Pigmentation of the gingivae or other oral mucosa results when heavy metals, primarily heavy metal sulfides, are present in the body. The oral manifestations of mercury (Hg), lead (Pb), and bismuth (Bi) intoxication are well described; however, the prevalence of such manifestations has decreased significantly in the United States in recent years as exposure to the heavy metals by way of occupational hazards and metal-containing products has declined. Bismuth pigmentation, for example, was common when bismuth salts were prescribed for the treatment of syphilis. Bismuth today may be found in the occasional over-the-counter remedy for gastrointestinal distress and is used rarely in dermatology. In the oral cavity the "bismuth line" is a blue-black, easily discernible and diffuse pigmentation on the marginal gingiva. The patient may complain of a metallic taste in the mouth and a general burning sensation (bismuth stomatitis). If the gingivae are severely inflamed, bismuth sulfides may be more readily deposited as a result of increased capillary permeability. Treatment and prevention therefore are limited to the institution of a scrupulous oral hygiene regimen.

Lead poisoning is exceedingly rare today in the United States, in major part as a result of environmental awareness and technologic advances in the automotive, paint, smelting, printing, and other industries. However, lead intake may occur by ingestion or by aspiration of vapors created during, for example, removal of old, lead-containing paint. A possible result is the "lead line," a grayish pigmentation typically located a few millimeters apical to the gingival margin. On close inspection, the lead line is seen to be composed of clusters of discrete granules, in contrast to the diffuse bismuth line. Gingival manifestations of lead intoxication are insignificant, however, compared with systemic problems, which may include anemia, pallor, anorexia, peripheral neuritis, and more severe neurologic disorders. Treatment of the oral manifestation is limited to improving oral hygiene; the prognosis is good if the source of lead intake is discovered and eliminated.

Mercury poisoning is similarly rare in the United States today, despite the current revitalized furor over mercury in dental restorations and in the dental office atmosphere. Inorganic mercurial salts, mainly mercuric sulfide, may be deposited in the gingivae, resulting in a "mercury line" identical in pathogenesis to the bismuth and lead lines described above. Recent reports from Western Europe describe potentially serious consequences in children treated topically with antiseptics that contain organic mercurials. Such antiseptics (e.g., Mercurochrome and Glyceromerfen) are frequently used for omphalocele (Stanley-Brown and Frank, 1971), and some are used intraorally as well (Schaad and Kehrer, 1983). Acrodynia (Feer's disease) has been reported in such patients (Hertl et al., 1982), as well as true mercury poisoning (Rützler, 1973; Clark et al., 1982). Mercury and other heavy metals such as cadmium, lead, and even plutonium adsorb to and traverse the oral mucosa when these elements are present in, for example, drinking water, medicaments in liquid form, or the atmosphere (Bhattacharyya et al., 1985). Cases of true allergy to the mercury present in silver amalgam dental restorations are rare (Finne et al., 1982; Fuchsjager et al., 1983; Simeone et al., 1985).

REFERENCES

Adams D and Davies G: Gingival hyperplasia induced by cyclosporin-A, Br Dent J 157:89, 1984.

Bennett J and Christian J: Cyclosporine-induced gingival hyperplasia: case report and literature review, J Am Dent Assoc 111:272, 1985.

Bernstein A and Hassell T: Morphometric analysis of phenytoin-enlarged human gingiva at the level of ultrastructure, J Dent Res 66:235, 1987.

Bhattacharyya M et al: Adsorption of Pu, Pb and Cd to mouth surfaces during oral administration to mice, Health Phys 48:207, 1985.

Brunsvold M, Tomasovic J, and Ruemping D: The measured effect of phenytoin withdrawal on gingival hyperplasia in children, J Dent Child 52:417, 1985.

Bunjes D et al: Cyclosporin-A mediates immunosuppression of primary cytotoxic T cell response by impairing the release of interleukin 1 and interleukin 2, Eur J Immunol 11:657, 1981.

Clark J et al: Mercury poisoning from merbromin (Mercurochrome) therapy of omphalocele, Clin Pediatr 21:445, 1982.

Cockey G et al: Effects of the methyl-catechol metabolite of phenytoin on human gingival fibroblasts, J Dent Res 65:353, 1986.

Coley C, Jarvis K, and Hassell T: Effect of cyclosporin-A on human gingival fibroblasts in vitro, J Dent Res 65:353, 1986.

Conard G et al: Levels of 5,5-diphenylhydantoin and its major metabolite in human serum, saliva and hyperplastic gingiva, J Dent Res 53:1323, 1972.

Dahllöf G et al: Proteoglycans and glycosaminoglycans in phenytoin-induced gingival overgrowth, J Periodont Res 21:13, 1986.

Donnenfeld O, Stanley H, and Bagdonoff L: A nine month clinical and histological study of patients on diphenylhydantoin following gingivectomy, J Periodontol 45:547, 1974.

Finne K, Goransson K, and Winckler L: Oral lichen planus and contact allergy to mercury, Int J Oral Surg 11:236, 1982.

Fuchsjager E et al: Regional heavy metal deposits in presence of amalgam restorations, Osterr Z Stomatol 80:228, 1983.

Glick G et al: Oral mucosal chemical lesions associated with acetyl-salicylic acid: two case reports, NY State Dent J 40:475, 1974.

Godin Y et al: Effects of di-n-propylacetate, an anticonvulsant compound, on GABA metabolism, J Neurochem 16:869, 1969.

Halpern L and Julian R: Augmentation of cerebellar Purkinje cell discharge rate after diphenylhydantoin, Epilepsia 13:377, 1972.

Hassell T: Epilepsy and the oral manifestations of phenytoin therapy, Basel, Switzerland, 1981, S Karger.

Hassell T: Evidence for production of an inactive collagenase by fibroblasts from phenytoin-enlarged human gingivae, J Oral Pathol 11:310, 1982.

Hassell T and Cooper C: Phenytoin-induced gingival overgrowth in a mongrel cat model. In Hassell T, Johnston M, and Dudley K: Phenytoin-induced teratology and gingival pathology, New York, 1980, Raven Press.

Hassell T and Jacoway J: Clinical and scientific approaches to gingival enlargement, I, Quintessence 11:53, 1980a.

Hassell T and Jacoway J: Clinical and scientific approaches to gingival enlargment, II, Quintessence 11:51, 1980b.

Hassell T, Page R, and Lindhe J: Histologic evidence for impaired growth control in diphenylhydantoin gingival overgrowth in man, Arch Oral Biol 23:381, 1978.

Hassell T and Sobhani S: Effects of dihydropyridines on connective tissue cells in vitro, J Dent Res 66:282, 1987.

Hassell T and Stanek E: Evidence that healthy human gingiva contains functionally heterogeneous fibroblast subpopulations, Arch Oral Biol 28:617, 1983.

Hassell T et al: Diphenylhydantoin (Dilantin) gingival hyperplasia: drug-induced abnormality of connective tissue, Proc Natl Acad Sci USA 73:2909, 1976.

Hassell T et al: Valproic acid: a new antiepileptic drug with potential side effects of dental concern, J Am Dent Assoc 99:983, 1979.

Hassell T et al: Quantitative histopathologic assessment of developing phenytoin-induced gingival overgrowth in the cat, J Clin Periodontol 9:365, 1982.

Heijl L and Sundin Y: Nitrendipine-induced gingival overgrowth in dogs, J Dent Res 66:282, 1987.

Hertl M et al: Akrodynie (Feer-Krankheit)—wieder aktuell durch ein quecksilberhaltiges Stomatologicum, Kinderarzt Prax 13:677, 1982.

Hutchens LH Jr: Phenytoin gingival overgrowth: treatment. In Hassell T: Epilepsy and the oral manifestations of phenytoin therapy, Basel, Switzerland, 1981, S Karger.

Janin-Mercier A et al: Lesions pulmonaires à pres grette de moelle osseus: etude de 35 cas, Ann Pathol 5:183, 1985.

Jones J and Mason D: Oral manifestations of systemic disease, Philadelphia, 1980, WB Saunders Co.

Kantor M and Hassell T: Increased accumulation of sulfated glycosaminoglycans in cultures of human fibroblasts from phenytoin-induced gingival overgrowth, J Dent Res 62:383, 1983.

Kimball 0: The treatment of epilepsy with sodium diphenylhydantoinate, JAMA 112:1244, 1939.

King D, Hawes R, and Bibby B: The effect of oral physiotherapy on Dilantin gingival hyperplasia, J Oral Pathol 5:1, 1976.

Koponen M et al: Interference of cyclosporin with lymphocyte proliferation: effects on mitochondria and lysosomes of cyclosporin-sensitive or -resistant cell clones, Cell Immunol 93:486, 1985.

Lucas R, Howell L, and Wall B: Nifedipine-induced gingival hyperplasia: a histochemical and ultrastructural study, J Periodontol 56:211, 1985.

Nacimento A et al: Interaction of phenytoin and inflammation induces gingival overgrowth in rats, J Periodont Res 20:386, 1985.

Narayanan A and Hassell T: Characterization of collagens in phenytoin-enlarged human gingiva, Coll Rel Res 5:513, 1985.

O'Neil T and Figures K: The effects of chlorhexidine and mechanical methods of plaque control on the recurrence of gingival hyperplasia in young patients taking phenytoin, Br Dent J 152:130, 1982.

Putnam T and Merritt H: Experimental determination of the anticonvulsant properties of some phenyl derivatives, Science 85:525, 1937.

Ramon Y et al: Gingival hyperplasia caused by nifedipine: a preliminary report, Int J Cardiol 5:195, 1984.

Rateitschak K et al: Color atlas of periodontology, New York, 1985, Theime Medical Publishers, Inc.

Rateitschak-Plüss E et al: Initial observation that cyclosporin-A induces gingival enlargement in man, J Clin Periodontol 10:237, 1983.

Rostock M, Fry R, and Turner J: Severe gingival overgrowth associated with cyclosporine therapy, J Periodontol 57:294, 1986.

Roth G and Calmes R: Oral biology, St Louis, 1981, The CV Mosby Co.

Rützler L: Passageres tubulares Syndrom durch Vergiftung mit einer organischen Quecksilberverbindung (Glyceromerfen) bei einem 1½-jährigen Mädchen, Schweiz Med Wochenschr 103:678, 1973.

Rye L: Drug interactions: facts you should know about what physicians are prescribing, Dent Management, p 54, Oct 1984.

Schaad U and Kehrer B: Phenymercuriborat in Glycerin (Glycero-Merfen) im Kleinkindesalter: unerwünschte Quecksilberresorption auch bei intakter Mundschleimhaut, Schweiz Med Wochenschr 113:148, 1983.

Sherman J: The effective removal and treatment of Dilantin hyperplasia, Dent Clin North Am 26:825, 1982.

Simeone M et al: Allergy to mercury in dental amalgam: clinical report, Arch Stomatol 26:311, 1985.

Stanley-Brown E and Frank J: Mercury poisoning from application to omphalocele, JAMA 216:2144, 1971.

Stern Z and Levy N: Nifedipine—a new antianginal agent, Harefuah (J Isreal Med Assoc) 10:494, 1981.

Syrjanen S and Syrjanen K: Hyperplastic gingivitis in a child receiving sodium valproate treatment, Proc Finn Dent Soc 75:95, 1979.

Wright J: Oral manifestations of drug reactions, Dent Clin North Am 28:529, 1984.

Chapter 22

TUMORS OCCURRING IN THE PERIODONTIUM

Steven D. Vincent
Murray W. Hill

DIFFERENTIAL DIAGNOSIS

Acquired enlargements or tumors of the periodontal soft tissues can result from inflammatory or neoplastic processes. Acute inflammatory enlargements of soft tissues are characterized by rapid growth, pain, and occasionally spontaneous regression. They may be diffuse or localized, fluctuant or hard on palpation, and associated with regional tender lymphadenopathy. In contrast, benign and malignant neoplasms of soft tissue are characterized by progressive growth without remarkable symptoms. They may be diffuse or localized, but seldom show regional lymphadenopathy until late in their clinical course.

The growth of benign neoplasms is measured in terms of months or years, and they are often found incidentally on routine examination. Benign neoplasms usually move teeth rather than resorb them, although occasionally unidirectional resorption may be evident.

Malignant neoplasms in soft tissue show rapid clinical growth but are usually asymptomatic unless secondarily ulcerated. Their growth may loosen rather than move teeth. Oral malignant neoplasms are seldom associated with regional lymphadenopathy until late in their development.

Fixation is a valuable clinical characteristic in determining the nature of some soft tissue tumors. However, fixation is of little value in evaluating soft tissue lesions of the periodontium because normal gingiva or tissues of the dorsal tongue and hard palate are bound to the underlying structures. Hence most enlargements of these tissues, whether benign or malignant, exhibit clinical fixation.

Because the periodontal tissues are intimately associated with bone, radiographic features may be of value in establishing a differential diagnosis.

Differential diagnosis by exclusion also makes use of site-specific features to further narrow the possibilities. For example, salivary gland tissue and therefore tumors of the salivary glands are not usually found on the dorsal tongue, anterior hard palate (except at the incisal foramen), gingiva, and attached alveolar mucosa. While salivary choristomas or tumors in the body of the mandible (Browand

and Waldron, 1975) or gingiva (Brannon et al., 1986) are reported occasionally, these are rare. In contrast, peripheral odontogenic fibromas and peripheral giant cell granulomas are lesions that occur exclusively in the gingiva or attached alveolar mucosa.

Finally, individual lesions may be included or excluded from consideration based on their individual features, such as color, pain on palpation, and consistency. Tumors showing increased vascularity such as hemangioma, pyogenic granuloma, and peripheral giant cell granuloma are usually purple or blue in color and bleed easily when traumatized. Neuromas are painful when palpated, even without secondary inflammation. Myxomas, lipomas, hemangiomas, and lymphangiomas are usually soft and compressible when palpated, whereas most benign tumors of fibrous connective tissue, nerve, or muscle origin are usually firm to palpation.

LESIONS OF SURFACE MUCOSA

Lesions of the gingival surface epithelium can be divided into four categories, each with distinct features: (1) vesicular and ulcerated lesions, (2) pigmented lesions, (3) benign tumors, and (4) surface thickening with cellular abnormality or dysplasia. Vesicular and ulcerative lesions are discussed in Chapters 18 and 19.

Localized pigmentation of the oral cavity

Pigmentations in the oral mucosa can be generalized or localized. Generalized pigmentations are often associated with systemic or genetic diseases and are not discussed here.

Pigmented lesions that blanch when compressed have a high degree of vascularity, such as hemangiomas, varices, and newly formed hematomas, ecchymoses, or petechiae. These lesions can usually be distinguished by clinical and historical features. A hematoma, ecchymosis, or petechia is usually of traumatic origin unless the patient has a bleeding diathesis such as von Willebrand's disease. Hemangiomas may become more characteristic as they enlarge, and most are congenital lesions and usually have a long history.

Ephelides (freckles) and *lentigines* (simplex and senile) do not blanch and therefore can be readily distinguished from the blood-containing pigmentations. They are brown to black in color because of the presence of melanin in the basal and parabasal cells of the epithelium. These lesions can be distinguished microscopically, but since they generally do not develop into more serious lesions, they are seldom removed.

Tattoos are localized pigmentations resulting from the implantation of foreign material in the submucosa and are by far the most commonly acquired intraoral pigmentation in adults. Many inert foreign materials may cause tattoos, but the most common intraoral tattoo results from implan-

tation of silver amalgam particles. Clinically, these lesions do not blanch and are usually blue-gray.

Blue-gray pigmentations may also be evaluated using intraoral radiographs. If sufficient metallic foreign material is present, they appear on an intraoral radiograph. However, some clinically obvious tattoos do not contain enough metallic foreign material to be visualized on a radiograph. Therefore the finding of metallic radiopaque particles may help confirm the diagnosis of a tattoo, but the lesion cannot be excluded if not visualized on a film. Tattoos may increase in diameter over months or years as a result of phagocytosis and redistribution of the foreign material.

Cellular nevi.   Intraoral *nevocellular nevi* and their malignant relatives, the *melanomas,* can usually be distinguished from vascular pigmentations because they do not blanch, from most tattoos by their brown-black color associated with melanin, and from ephelides and lentigines because of their palpation characteristics. Both nevi and melanomas result from cellular proliferation, which usually produces a clinically palpable lesion.

The common nevocellular nevus undergoes progressive evolution over many years or decades (Greene et al., 1985). Initially they appear as small (1 to 2 mm in diameter) brown or black macules, which progressively enlarge to about 4 to 6 mm. These early developmental nevocellular nevi are histologically classified as junctional nevi, having theques of nevus cells in the epithelium near the basal cell layer. With continued maturation these theques penetrate into the superficial connective tissue and form a compound nevus that is a clinically palpable, slightly raised papule. Eventually the nevus cells completely separate from the epithelium to produce an "intradermal nevus" or, if located in oral mucosa, an "intramucosal nevus," which varies in degree of pigmentation from black to a normal mucosal hue. The intramucosal nevus is the most common variety, with junctional and compound types quite rare in the oral mucosa (Buchner and Hansen, 1987). Oral nevocellular nevi are slightly more common in females and are located most frequently on the hard palate, buccal mucosa, vermilion of the lip, and gingival mucosa (Fig. 22-1).

The nevus cells may further differentiate along the lines of other neural crest cells into neural or schwannian morphology. The papule may then become pedunculated and slough, or simply return to a normal configuration. Most adults have from 10 to 40 nevocellular nevi (Greene et al., 1985). Any nevus, mucosal or dermal, may suddenly stop evolving and remain stable at any point along its developmental pathway.

Most dermal melanomas develop from preexisting nevocellular nevi, with the junctional stage of nevus development carrying the greatest risk of becoming malignant (Goldsmith, 1979). While the potential for oral nevi to be-

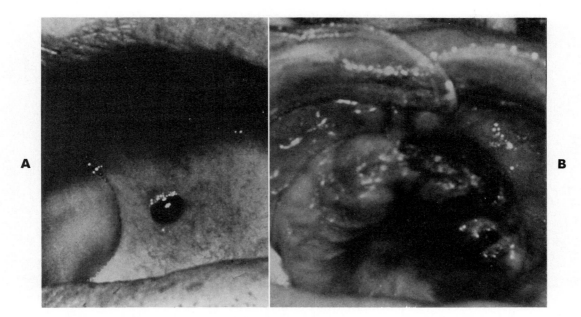

Fig. 22-1. **A,** Raised, black, smooth-surfaced, well-demarcated, asymptomatic, nonblanchable nodule (7 × 4 mm in diameter) of unknown duration on buccal mucosa. Excision revealed an intramucosal nevocellular nevus. **B,** Diffuse, poorly demarcated, slightly raised, variably pigmented, nonblanchable lesion of unknown duration of alveolar and palatal mucosa. Incisional biopsy revealed malignant melanoma. (Courtesy G.E. Lilly.)

come melanomas may be similar to that of skin nevi, only a small number have been documented. However, in a retrospective review, Rapini et al. (1985) found that about one third of oral melanomas were preceded by a clinically evident mucosal pigmentation.

Malignant melanomas. Melanomas of oral mucosa are rare, accounting for less than 8% of all melanomas in a study by Rapini et al. (1985). Eighty percent of the patients in their study were over 40 years old, and 37% were over 60. Fifty-eight percent were men. Most lesions occurred on the palate or the maxillary gingival mucosa.

Mucosal melanomas appear clinically the same as melanomas of skin, with irregular borders, patchy pigmentation, and rapid growth (Fig. 22-1). The rapid growth may result in secondary ulceration of the mucosa and irregular resorption of underlying bone, features common to most malignant diseases.

The prognosis for cutaneous melanoma depends on the depth of invasion of the lesion, with patients having a 10-year survival rate of 99.5% if their melanoma shows invasion of less that 0.76 mm when completely excised. Conversely, patients having cutaneous melanomas with invasion of 3 mm or greater have a 10-year survival rate of only 48% (Friedman et al., 1985).

Unfortunately, the depth of invasion has not always been considered in the documentation of cases of oral melanoma, and therefore it is not known whether these figures

are appropriate for oral melanomas. However, the prognosis for primary oral melanoma appears to be worse than the prognosis for its cutaneous counterpart, with only 13% of patients surviving 5 years (Rapini et al., 1985). This poor outcome may be due to a failure to detect oral melanomas early in their development, the difficulty in achieving a complete surgical excision for lesions arising near the maxilla, or a combination of both. Therefore all localized oral pigmentations that show clinical features suggesting cellular proliferation should be removed.

Benign lesions of surface epithelium

Benign (self-limiting) surface lesions of oral mucosa are clinically pale relative to the surrounding normal mucosa. They are well demarcated, rough and firm when palpated, asymptomatic, and exhibit no fixation to underlying submucosa. Lesions in this category may be reactive in origin or possibly viral related.

Papillomas. Papillomas are benign proliferations of surface epithelium found occasionally on the gingiva and attached alveolar mucosa. They are usually characterized by a pedunculated base, which can be of value in differentiating them from verrucae (warts). Immunologic laboratory techniques have revealed viral DNA and sometimes viral particles within papillary lesions of oral mucosa, but it remains unclear whether all papillomas may be caused by one or more viruses of the Papovaviridae family.

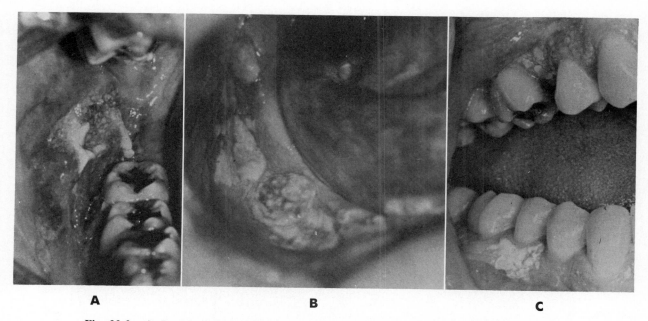

Fig. 22-2.   A, Rough, indurated, asymptomatic, hyperkeratotic, and erythematous lesion (2.5 × 3 cm in diameter) of right posterior buccal mucosa, fixed to underlying alveolus and masseter muscle. Incisional biopsy revealed a well-differentiated squamous cell carcinoma. **B,** Diffuse white plaques noted on alveolar and vestibular mucosa. Centrally, a 1 × 1 cm, slightly raised, indurated, hyperkeratotic, and erythematous nodule was noted. Excision revealed a well-differentiated squamous cell carcinoma. **C,** Foci of hyperkeratosis on buccal gingiva, asymptomatic and of unknown duration. A change in toothbrushes from hard to soft and a change in oral hygiene technique resulted in resolution in 2 weeks.

Histopathology. Microscopic examination of papillomas reveals irregular acanthosis of the stratified squamous epithelium forming exophytic, fingerlike projections. There may or may not be evidence of hyperkeratosis at the surface. The epithelial cells show an apparently normal maturation pattern with virtually no cellular dysplasia. Each fingerlike projection shows a central fibrovascular connective tissue core.

Surface-thickening lesions

Lesions in which the surface epithelium is thickened are clinically asymptomatic, rough to palpation, opaque compared with the surrounding mucosa, and usually white, erythematous, or a combination of both. White lesions include hyperkeratosis, in which the surface mucosa exhibits increased thickness of the stratum corneum.

Hyperkeratosis. Simple hyperkeratosis occurring in the so-called high-risk areas (the floor of the mouth, lateral and ventral tongue, and retromolar trigone) is associated with the development of carcinomas in about 10% of lesions. This is not true of gingival hyperkeratosis, since gingival hyperkeratosis is often a response to chronic mechanical or chemical trauma such as improper tooth brushing (Fig. 22-2). However, should a causal factor such as toothbrush irritation be identified and eliminated, lesions that then persist after 3 weeks should be considered for biopsy.

Epithelial dysplasia. Epithelial dysplasia, carcinoma-in-situ, and squamous cell carcinoma can all appear white as a result of hyperkeratosis or epithelial thickening, or red as a result of decreased maturation of the squamous cells, or both red and white (Fig. 22-2). Ulceration not due to secondary trauma is rare in either dysplastic lesions or superficially invasive squamous cell carcinoma. Therefore the characterization of oral cancer as "an ulcer that does not heal" is seldom accurate until late in the development of the disease. The cause of preneoplastic epithelial dysplasia is unknown, although both combustible and smokeless tobacco, and alcohol consumption are causally related (Mashberg et al., 1981).

Histopathology. Microscopically, dysplastic epithelium shows characteristic cellular abnormalities such as pleomorphism, increased and abnormal mitosis (which may also be present in the suprabasal layer), nuclear hyperchromasia, dyskeratosis, and acantholysis (Fig. 22-3). When the epithelial cells, which normally replicate near the basal cell layer, migrate to the surface and undergo keratinization, the microscopic and clinical appearance of the lesion is one of hyperkeratosis.

Conversely, if the cells fail to mature, the lesion may be red. This explains why the erythroplastic lesions are more likely to develop into squamous cell carcinoma.

Carcinoma-in-situ. Carcinoma-in-situ differs from epithelial dysplasia only in the degree of abnormality. Car-

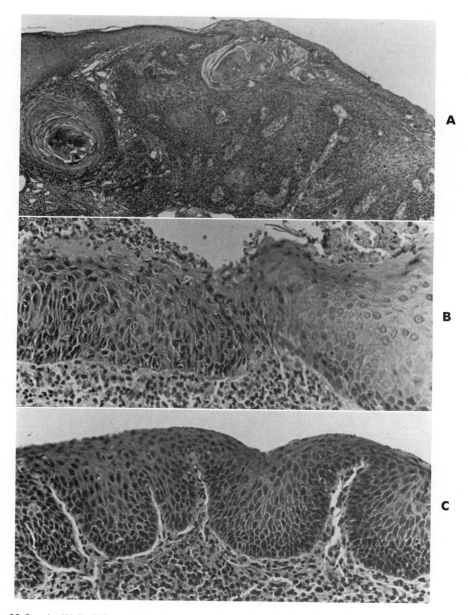

Fig. 22-3. **A,** Well-differentiated squamous cell carcinoma of gingiva. (Hematoxylin and eosin; original magnification ×25.) **B,** Junctional area showing relatively normal parakeratinized stratified squamous epithelium on right side and moderate epithelial dysplasia on left. (Hematoxylin and eosin; original magnification ×63.) **C,** Carcinoma-in-situ showing little evidence of cellular maturation with nuclear hyperchromasia, cellular pleomorphism, and increased mitotic activity. (Hematoxylin and eosin; original magnification ×63.)

cinoma-in-situ clinically is usually a velvety erythematous or combined red and white lesion that is rough when palpated and asymptomatic unless secondarily ulcerated. As the name suggests, it is considered a true malignancy even though it does not metastasize. Unlike epithelial dysplasia, which may or may not be a reversible process, carcinoma-in-situ is an irreversible, anaplastic lesion that if left untreated will presumably develop into frank squamous cell carcinoma.

Histopathology. Microscopically, carcinoma-in-situ differs from epithelial dysplasia in that it is an anaplastic lesion with no evidence of epithelial maturation from the basal cell layer to the surface (Fig. 22-3). However, the epithelial cells have not penetrated the basement membrane or invaded the subjacent connective tissue.

Squamous cell carcinoma. Squamous cell carcinoma is the most common primary oral malignant disease. All oral primary malignancies account for 4% of new cancers identified each year in males, 2% of all cancer-related deaths in males, and 1% of cancer-related deaths in fe-

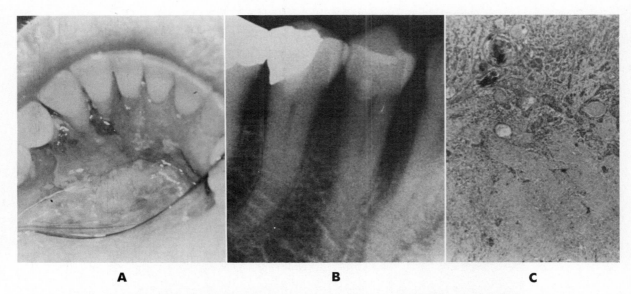

A   **B**   **C**

Fig. 22-4. A, Focal gingival erythema, asymptomatic and associated with hyperkeratosis of floor of mouth in a 57-year-old woman. **B,** Radiographs showed focal crestal alveolar bone loss. Area did not respond favorably to root planing and scaling. Incisional biopsy, **C,** revealed moderately differentiated squamous cell carcinoma. (Hematoxylin and eosin; original magnification ×25.)

males. The male-to-female ratio has changed remarkably from a predominantly male disease to a male-to-female ratio of 2:1 (Silverberg and Lubera, 1987).

Squamous cell carcinoma is rarely a primary lesion of the gingiva or the attached alveolar mucosa. When it occurs, it is usually seen in men over the age of 40. Clinically, it may be indistinguishable from simple hyperkeratosis, epithelial dysplasia, or carcinoma-in-situ (see Fig. 22-2). It may also exhibit induration. Although fixation to underlying structures cannot be assessed on gingiva or alveolar mucosa, radiographic evaluation of the underlying bone is often valuable in evaluating the extent of the neoplasm and formulating a therapeutic protocol (Fig. 22-4).

The use of both combustible and smokeless tobacco products has been linked to an increased risk of developing squamous cell carcinoma. An early study by Wynder et al. (1957) showed that only 3% of 659 patients with oral cancer had never smoked. The risk is greatest in heavy smokers (more than 40 cigarettes per day) (Rothman and Keller, 1972). In India 48% of primary carcinomas are found in the oral cavity, and between one half to three quarters of the population use some form of smokeless tobacco (Jayant et al., 1977). Smokeless tobacco use as a high-risk factor has been confirmed by data from the southeastern United States (Winn et al., 1981).

For nonsmokers, the use of 1.6 ounces or more of alcohol per day increases the risk of oral cancer 2.3-fold (Mashberg et al., 1981). Of particular significance is Mashberg's finding that alcohol and tobacco have a synergistic effect in increasing the risk of developing oral cancer. The combined effect of heavy cigarette smoking (more than 40 cigarettes per day) and the consumption of more than 1.6 ounces of alcohol per day increased the long-term relative risk of oral cancer 15.5-fold.

Of significance to the clinician is the concept of field cancerization, implying that oral and pharyngeal mucosa will show an increased incidence of second primary lesions in persons previously treated for oral squamous cell carcinoma. Patients followed after treatment for cancer of the oral cavity developed second primary carcinomas of the pharynx and larynx in 8% to 19% of cases studied (Wynder et al., 1969; Fu et al., 1976).

Grading and staging. Once an oral squamous cell carcinoma has been identified, therapeutic management is based on the location of the lesion, the patient's age and state of health, and the grade and stage of the lesion.

The stage of the tumor is especially important in establishing a patient management protocol and a prognosis (Baker, 1983). Most oncology centers rely on the TNM system: *T* for primary tumor size in centimeters, *N* for regional lymph node involvement, and *M* for distant metastasis. It is important for the clinician to remember that regional lymph node evaluation should be performed in detail prior to an incisional or excisional biopsy. The biopsy may evoke an inflammatory reaction sufficient to cause enlargement of regional nodes, making postbiopsy assessment difficult for several days.

Prognosis. The 5-year survival rate recorded for oral cancers increased from 45% in whites during the years 1960 to 1963, to 53% during the years 1977 to 1983 (Silverberg and Lubera, 1987). The vast majority of these oral cancers are squamous cell carcinomas that develop in oral mucosa from clinically recognizable lesions as described above. It is clear that most oral cancers are preventable by early detection and intervention.

Initial therapy for surface lesions

The therapeutic management of surface lesions varies from no treatment for some forms of simple hyperkeratosis to radical excision, radiation, and chemotherapy for squamous cell carcinoma. The clinical appearance of simple hyperkeratosis, epithelial dysplasia, and squamous cell carcinoma may be identical; hence it is essential to establish a definitive diagnosis with a biopsy. The biopsy may be excisional, with orientation for microscopic evaluation of clinically small lesions, or incisional for diffuse superficial or large, deeply invasive lesions.

Toluidine blue, a vital nuclear stain, has been advocated as a screening tool for evaluating "leukoplakias" and "erythroplakias" of the oral cavity. Unlike normal oral mucosa, some severely dysplastic or carcinomatous lesions exhibit hypercellularity at their external surfaces and therefore show relative retention of the dye. However, the rate of false negative and false positive findings is too high for this clinical tool as presently configured to be used as a screen to determine if a biopsy is indicated (Silverman, 1981). Toluidine blue should be used only on diffuse surface lesions to determine where an incisional biopsy would be most likely to reveal the most significant disease.

Exfoliative cytology has also been advocated as a preliminary diagnostic tool when evaluating surface-thickening lesions. However, the high rate of false negative and false positive findings (Dabelsteen et al., 1971) and the inability to grade the invasive lesion accurately make this procedure of questionable value.

BENIGN LESIONS OF PERIODONTAL SUBMUCOSA

Benign submucosal lesions of the periodontium may be categorized as being derived from nonodontogenic or odontogenic mesenchyme, or odontogenic epithelium. They present clinically as slow-growing lesions, asymptomatic and usually without alteration of the overlying mucosal epithelium. Large benign lesions may resorb the underlying alveolar bone. Peripheral odontogenic fibromas and peripheral ossifying fibromas, congenital epulides, and giant cell granulomas are site-specific lesions occurring only in periodontal soft tissues. While no further discussion of peripheral odontogenic tumors of epithelial origin is given here, it is important to recognize that their reported behavior suggests they are less aggressive than their central bony counterparts, with conservative excision the treatment of choice even for ameloblastoma. An excellent review is provided by Buchner and Scuibba (1987).

Pyogenic granulomas

Pyogenic granulomas are hyperplastic lesions of mesenchymal tissue that may develop in response to a nonspecific low-grade irritation. They may be sessile or pedunculated and frequently are reddish purple as a result of their high vascularity (Fig. 22-5). Although the surface of a pyogenic granuloma may be ulcerated, it is not usually purulent, as the name suggests. The lesion commonly involves the interdental papilla. The "pregnancy tumor" in females is a pyogenic granuloma.

Histopathology. Pyogenic granulomas are composed of highly vascular granulation tissue that has a delicate fibrous stroma with numerous proliferating fibroblasts and endothelial cells. The overlying epithelium is usually thin and may be ulcerated. Frequently there is an inflammatory infiltrate composed predominantly of polymorphonuclear leukocytes, but the extent of the inflammatory response depends on the degree of ulceration of the lesion. Long-standing lesions have a greater proportion of mature collagen fibers with fewer capillary spaces than younger lesions.

Hemangiomas

Hemangiomas consist of a mass of vascular channels that are probably hamartomatous (developmental) rather than neoplastic in origin. Although the vascular channels themselves have a normal structure, they lack proper organization. Usually lesions of the oral mucosa are present at birth or are identified in early childhood. The lesions can be variable in shape, may be flat or raised, and are usually dark red or purple.

Peripheral giant cell granulomas

Peripheral giant cell granulomas occur only on the gingiva or alveolar mucosa and are more common in women than in men (Andersen et al., 1973). The lesions are vascular and red or purple, and they are most frequent anterior to the molar teeth in the interdental region.

Histopathology. Since the majority of peripheral giant cell granulomas occur in areas in which primary teeth were present, it has been suggested that the lesion represents hyperplasia of the tissues involved in root resorption. A number of reports indicate that minor trauma often precedes the development of the lesions, and several authors have suggested that peripheral giant cell granuloma represents aberrant osteogenic granulation tissue (Bhaskar et al., 1971). This view is supported by the ultrastructural similarity of the giant cells and osteoclasts (Sapp, 1972).

Microscopically, these lesions show loose, nonencapsulated cellular fibrous connective tissue with numerous thin-walled vascular channels, hemorrhage, and usually hemosiderin pigment. Important to the diagnosis is the finding of numerous multinucleated osteoclast-like giant cells distributed throughout the lesion.

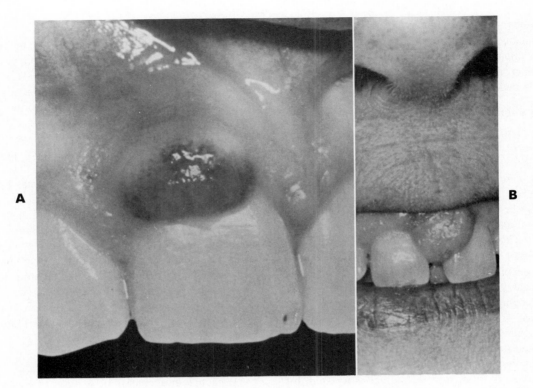

Fig. 22-5. **A,** Smooth-surfaced, raised, erythematous, easily bleeding lesion (1.5 × 1 cm in diameter) of marginal gingiva labial to maxillary right central incisor. Excisional biopsy revealed a pyogenic granuloma. **B,** Smooth-surfaced, raised, firm nodule (1.8 × 1.3 cm in diameter) causing separation of central incisors. Excisional biopsy revealed an ossifying fibroma.

Peripheral ossifying fibromas

Peripheral ossifying fibromas are relatively common lesions, occurring only on the gingiva or alveolar mucosa as a sessile or pedunculated mass covered with normal surface epithelium (Fig. 22-5). They can occur at any age but are most common in children and young adults (Shafer et al., 1983) and may be derived from the periodontal ligament.

Histopathology. Histologically, peripheral ossifying fibromas show numerous fibroblasts supported by a collagenous stroma. The surface of the lesion is covered by a normal stratified squamous epithelium that may be ulcerated as a result of trauma. Throughout the lesion there is a variable amount of mineralization, which may resemble bone, osteoid, acellular cementum, or dystrophic calcification. Occasional rests of odontogenic epithelium may also be present.

Treatment

The management of these four lesions, as well as of other benign submucosal neoplasms, is complete surgical excision. While the creation of wide surgical margins or the removal of underlying bone is usually not indicated, the margins should be clear of tumor cells in order to decrease the risk of recurrence.

DISEASES OF THE JAW BONES

Diseases of the jaw bones can be classified into one of eight categories: (1) cysts, (2) benign odontogenic neoplasms, (3) benign nonodontogenic neoplasms, (4) malignant neoplasms, (5) inflammatory diseases, (6) dysplastic diseases, (7) primary or systemic diseases, or (8) idiopathic diseases. Each of these categories has distinct, often unique features, which usually allow a clinician to include or exclude an entire category when establishing a differential diagnosis.

The growth rate of intrabony lesions is valuable in determining the nature of the disease. Slow-growing lesions within bone are usually surrounded by a thin (1 to 2 mm) rim of reactive, hyperostotic bone, which is apparent on conventional radiographs. It is characteristic of cysts, benign odontogenic tumors, and benign nonodontogenic tumors (Fig. 22-6). Static lesions, such as surgical defects or the well-documented mandibular salivary gland defect, appear to be surrounded by smooth, dense bone, 3 to 4 mm in diameter and sometimes similar to normal cortical plate (Fig. 22-7). In contrast, rapidly growing lesions, whether of inflammatory or malignant origin, are poorly delineated and lack a uniform peripheral hyperostotic border (Fig. 22-8).

Although any central bony lesion may cause pain, this

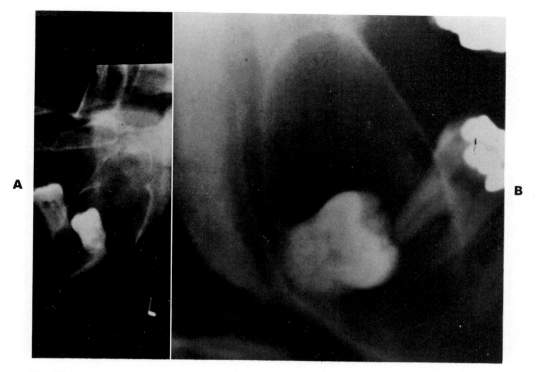

Fig. 22-6. A, Asymptomatic buccal expansion, multiloculated radiolucency with a hyperostotic border having displaced mandibular left third molar inferiorly and eroded inferior cortical plate. Enucleation revealed a dentigerous cyst. **B,** Asymptomatic, buccal expansion radiolucency with a hyperostotic border having displaced third molar and mandibular canal inferiorly. Enucleation revealed a parakeratinized odontogenic keratocyst.

symptom is most often associated with malignant and inflammatory lesions and seldom with the slow-growing lesions. Paresthesia is also characteristic of rapidly growing, malignant, or inflammatory diseases.

Perforation of the overlying bone cortex by a central lesion is a characteristic of rapid growth and therefore is usually indicative of malignant or inflammatory disease. However, the posterior maxilla-tuberosity region, where the cortical bone is normally thin, can be perforated readily, even by a relatively slow-growing cyst or benign neoplasm.

Teeth will often be moved by slow-growing lesions, but if pressure resorption does occur, it is characteristically unidirectional. By contrast, malignant or inflammatory diseases seldom move teeth and may cause multidirectional resorption. Rapidly expanding tumors resorb bone at a faster rate than healthy tooth structure, and once the periodontal membrane is involved, malignant or inflammatory cells quickly involve this entire soft tissue space. The tumor cells will therefore surround a tooth root prior to causing resorption of a significant amount of root structure. This is the reason for the radiographic phenomenon of widened periodontal ligament spaces, often reported in association with an intrabony malignancy (Fig. 22-9).

Palpation of a bony expansion is also a useful clinical

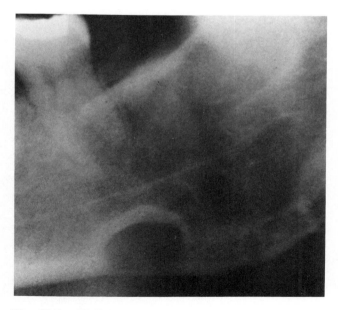

Fig. 22-7. Well-demarcated radiolucency found incidentally with a 3 to 4 mm thick corticated margin without clinical expansion or symptoms. Radiographic diagnosis: static lesion, consistent with lingual salivary defect.

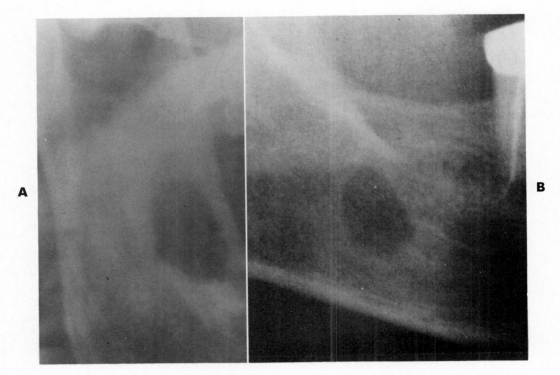

Fig. 22-8. A, Poorly demarcated radiolucency without a hyperostotic border associated with buccal expansion and pain of 1 month's duration. Biopsy revealed a metastatic adenocarcinoma. Primary lesion was of prostate. **B,** Poorly demarcated radiolucency without a hyperostotic border, imposed over mandibular canal. Patient had right mandibular region pain and paresthesia of chin at right of midline. Biopsy revealed metastatic adenocarcinoma. Primary lesion was of lung.

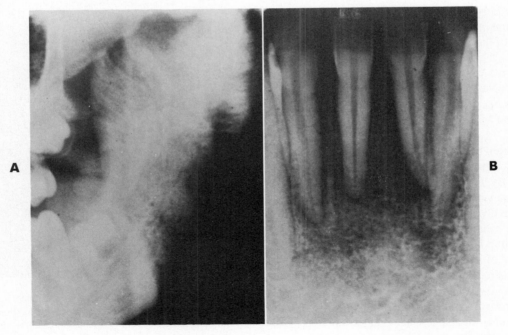

Fig. 22-9. Osteosarcoma of mandible showing a sun ray pattern, **A,** and radiolucent appearance, **B,** with widening of periodontal ligament space of left lateral incisor. (**B** courtesy Axel Ruprecht.)

tool. The feature of crepitus, often described as incomplete or spongy bone, suggests rapid growth. The palpation of a thrill or bruit would suggest a central osseous arteriovenous fistula. Regional lymphadenopathy suggests an inflammatory process, since patients with central bony malignancies rarely exhibit regional lymphadenopathy until late in the course of the disease. Other systemic manifestations or laboratory tests may be necessary to further refine the clinical differential diagnosis.

Cysts

Development of odontogenic cysts. In contrast to other bones of the skeleton, the maxilla and mandible are uniquely involved with epithelium-lined cysts that can be categorized as either developmental or inflammatory in origin. The frequent occurrence of jaw cysts is due to the presence of numerous remnants of epithelium, which may be of odontogenic origin, the remnants of the vestigial nasopalatine ducts, or the ectoderm that covers the developing embryonic facial processes.

The cysts most commonly associated with the periodontium are derived from odontogenic epithelium: (1) the dental lamina or its remnants (the rests of Serres), (2) the enamel organ, (3) the reduced enamel epithelium, or (4) the epithelial cell rests of Malassez. The type of cyst that develops is determined by the putative origin of the epithelium and the mechanism of its reactivation. Thus cysts developing from the less-differentiated epithelium, such as the dental lamina, may have a more aggressive behavior than those developing from epithelium that has completed its normal function, such as the epithelial rests of Malassez. Although any of the odontogenic cysts may develop in association with the periodontium and must be considered as part of any differential diagnosis of cystic jaw lesions, the present discussion is limited to the odontogenic keratocyst, the keratinizing and calcifying odontogenic cyst, the lateral periodontal cyst, the gingival cyst, and the radicular (apical periodontal) cyst. A detailed discussion of the entire range of jaw cysts can be found in Shafer et al. (1983), Shear (1983), and Hoffman et al. (1987).

Radiologic features. The radiologic features of all odontogenic and nonodontogenic cysts are quite similar to those of benign tumors. Since they are slow growing, they are characterized by a thin hyperostotic peripheral border of reactive bone. They generally move teeth rather than resorb them, but if tooth resorption occurs, it is unidirectional rather than multidirectional. All cysts are radiolucent with the possible exception of the calcifying epithelial odontogenic cyst, which varies, depending on matrix mineralization, from completely radiolucent to mostly radiopaque. Although the odontogenic keratocyst and calcifying epithelial odontogenic cyst are diagnosed on the basis of their histopathologic features, the remaining odontogenic and nonodontogenic cysts are diagnosed on the basis of their location and relation (if any) to surrounding tooth structures.

Odontogenic keratocysts. Odontogenic keratocysts have a characteristic histopathology and, unlike the majority of jaw cysts, may behave in a relatively aggressive manner. Although the World Health Organization uses the term *keratocyst* synonymously with *primordial cyst,* it is generally accepted that only some primordial cysts are keratocysts; keratocysts may also develop from other epithelial remnants of odontogenic origin (Soskolne and Shear, 1967). Keratocysts can occur at any age, with about 60% of lesions diagnosed in patients between 10 and 40 years of age, and are more frequent in males than in females (Shear, 1983). These lesions occur most often in the mandibular third molar area but may be located anywhere in the alveolar bone, including the apex of tooth roots or between the tooth roots.

Multiple odontogenic keratocysts may be associated with the nevoid basal cell carcinoma syndrome (Gorlin and Goltz, 1960). This is a hereditary condition, transmitted as an autosomal dominant trait, which may include numerous basal cell carcinomas, skeletal abnormalities such as bifid ribs and kyphoscoliosis, frontal and temperoparietal bossing, and mild hypertelorism.

Histopathology. The lining of the odontogenic keratocysts consists of a thin connective tissue capsule lined with a stratified squamous epithelium, 5 to 10 cells thick, which is devoid of rete ridges. The basal cell layer consists of uniform cuboidal or columnar cells with polarized nuclei. The luminal surface usually has a characteristic corrugated appearance with either orthokeratinization or parakeratinization.

Odontogenic keratocysts may appear clinically and radiographically as any other jaw cyst—dentigerous, lateral periodontal, or radicular—and may also mimic the appearance of benign odontogenic and benign nonodontogenic tumors. The diagnosis of odontogenic keratocyst is based entirely on the histopathologic features. Unlike other jaw cysts, the keratocyst tends to recur even after apparent total removal. The parakeratinized variant has a recurrence rate of 26% (Browne, 1971), and the orthokeratinized variant has a much lower recurrence rate (Wright, 1981). Occasionally both patterns of keratinization occur in the same lesion (Wright, 1981).

Calcifying odontogenic cysts. Calcifying odontogenic cysts have recently been described as being composed of two distinct entities: a cyst and a neoplasm (Praetorius et al., 1981). Clinically, the lesion usually presents as a slowly enlarging, painless swelling that is most frequently located anterior to the molar teeth. It can occur within either the bone or the soft tissues of the gingiva. The importance of correctly identifying this lesion lies in the propensity of this lesion to recur following treatment.

Histopathology. Microscopically, the cystic component of the calcifying odontogenic cyst is classified into three subtypes. The first subtype (1A) is a unilocular lesion lined with cuboidal or squamous epithelium. In some areas the epithelial cells resemble stellate reticulum, and large ghost cells, which are a characteristic feature of this lesion, may occur. These ghost cells are believed to represent an aberrant form of keratinization and are histologically indistinguishable from ghost cells in other lesions. Occasionally deposits of a dentinoid material may be present. In the second subtype (1B) the lesion is histologically similar, but it also contains components similar to odontomas, whereas in the third subtype (1C) there is proliferation of the epithelium to produce ameloblastomatous foci. The neoplastic component (type II) is a solid mass of tissue containing infiltrative strands of ameloblastomatous odontogenic epithelium, which is associated with both ghost cells and dentinoid material (Praetorius et al., 1981).

Lateral periodontal cysts. Lateral periodontal cysts are rare developmental lesions occurring predominantly in the premolar region of the mandible of adults (Wysocki et al., 1980). Frequently the lesion is symptomless, but it may present as a gingival swelling. The lateral periodontal cyst develops from odontogenic epithelium. The lesion may develop from the reduced enamel epithelium of a dentigerous cyst, which does not impede the eruption of the tooth but becomes laterally displaced by the existing tooth. Alternatively, the lateral periodontal cyst may represent a nonkeratinizing primordial cyst that develops from a supernumerary tooth, which occurs commonly within this region. Finally, based on the epithelial morphology of the cyst lining, this cyst may be derived from the clear cells of the postfunctional dental lamina (Wysocki et al., 1980). If this latter view is correct, it has been suggested that the lateral periodontal cyst and the gingival cyst (see below) are essentially the same lesion, differing only in anatomic location. The botryoid odontogenic cyst (Weathers and Waldron, 1973) is essentially a multiloculated variant of the lateral periodontal cyst.

Histopathology. The lining of the lateral periodontal cyst is a stratified squamous epithelium, usually one to five cell layers thick with no evidence of keratinization. Focal epithelial thickenings may be present, and the cells in these plaques may be large with pyknotic nuclei and clear cytoplasm. Inflammatory cells are uncommon and when present most likely result from secondary infection.

Gingival cysts of adults. Gingival cysts are uncommon developmental soft tissue lesions occurring most often in the free or attached gingiva of the premolar area of the mandible. They are usually seen in patients over 40 (Buchner and Hansen, 1979) and present as a small (<1 cm), circumscribed and slowly enlarging, painless mass. The lesion is fluctuant, and the overlying mucosa is clinically normal. It has been suggested that gingival cysts are derived from traumatically implanted epithelial cells from the gingiva. The most widely held view is that this lesion arises by cystic degeneration of postfunctional epithelial rests derived from the dental lamina (Wysocki et al., 1980) and thus represents an extraosseous variant of the

lateral periodontal cyst. This latter view is supported by the similar behavior, morphologic appearance, and anatomic distribution of these lesions (Shafer et al., 1983).

Histopathology. Gingival cysts are located in the lamina propria of the gingiva and are usually lined with a flattened stratified squamous epithelium that, like the lateral periodontal cyst, may display localized epithelial thickenings. The lumen is filled with fluid but may also contain keratin squames (Hoffman et al., 1987).

Radicular cysts. Radicular or apical periodontal cysts, the most common cystic lesions of the jaws, account for 55% to 70% of jaw cysts (e.g., Shear, 1983). They can occur at any age but are seen predominantly in persons between 20 and 60 years of age. These cysts are always associated with the root of a nonvital tooth, usually at the apex, but they may also appear on the lateral aspect of the root in association with a lateral canal.

Pathogenesis. Radicular cysts develop within a periapical granuloma in two stages: (1) initiation and (2) growth. Initially there is proliferation of the epithelial cell rests of Malassez within the periapical granuloma to form arcades of epithelium surrounding islands of connective tissue. It is not known how the proliferating epithelium comes to line a cavity, but it is generally considered that as the mass of epithelial cells increases in size, there is necrosis of the central cells (Shear, 1983). It has also been suggested that a cyst could be formed by proliferating epithelium lining the connective tissue of a chronic periapical abscess arising from degeneration of the central portion of a granuloma (Summers, 1974).

The subsequent growth in size of a radicular cyst is due to the accumulation of fluid within the cyst lumen. Opening the cyst cavity into the mouth leads to a progressive reduction in the size of the lesion, an observation that forms the basis of the surgical procedure of marsupialization.

Histopathology. The cyst is lined by a stratified squamous epithelium that is of irregular thickness, with epithelial cords often penetrating into the underlying connective tissue of the cyst wall. The epithelial lining, which may be incomplete, shows a variable pattern of differentiation. Mucous cells are relatively frequent (Browne, 1972) in the lining epithelium, occurring as isolated groups of cells. Occasionally they may form a large portion of the lining epithelium. Since mucous cells occur in radicular cysts of the maxilla or mandible, it seems likely that these cells arise by metaplasia rather than being derived from respiratory epithelium. Carcinomatous change in the cyst epithelium is rare.

The epithelial lining of the cyst may contain amorphous structures known as Rushton's hyaline bodies, which are composed of a core of granular material surrounded by a clear eosinophilic outer layer and are of unknown origin. These structures occur in other lesions with an inflammatory origin.

Lesions of cementum

Hypercementosis, manifested as an increase in the amount of cementum uniformly deposited on a tooth root, can occur simply as a response to a chronic periapical inflammatory process or occlusal trauma, or in association with Paget's disease. Based on clinical, radiographic, and histologic features, central bony lesions of cementum may be classified as periapical cemental dysplasia, benign cementoblastoma, cementifying fibroma, or the rare gigantiform cementoma (Pindborg et al., 1971).

Periapical cemental dysplasia. Periapical cemental dysplasia is a self-limiting bone abnormality and is therefore not a true neoplasm. The term *cementoma,* which is usually ascribed to these lesions, is discouraged, since it implies a benign neoplastic nature. These lesions are site specific, forming at the apices of teeth. They are not the result of pulpal degeneration and do not cause devitalization of a tooth. Therefore associated teeth should be vital unless involved by a secondary process. The lesions, which are usually multiple, are more frequent in women than in men and are usually seen between the fourth and fifth decades of life. The cause of periapical cemental dysplasia is not known, but it appears to progress through three distinct stages. In the first (osteolytic) phase, periapical bone is replaced by a fibrous connective tissue. In the second (cementoblastic) stage, islands and spicules of cementum-like matrix form within the connective tissue until, in the third (mature) stage, the lesion is predominantly composed of irregular cementum-like material. Lesions displaying different stages of development may be seen concurrently in the same patient. Since this lesion is innocuous and self-limiting, its significance is in distinguishing it, especially during the radiolucent phase, from inflammatory periapical lesions such as a periapical granuloma or cyst.

Radiologic features. Periapical cemental dysplasia is usually first detected during routine radiographic examination when the lesion is identified as a well-circumscribed radiolucency at the apex of a tooth. As these lesions mature, mineralized cementum-like material accumulates to produce irregular radiopacities within the radiolucent area. In later stages it may appear as a well-circumscribed radiopacity with a distinct radiolucent margin.

Benign cementoblastomas. Benign cementoblastomas are slow-growing neoplasms of cementoblasts that form a mass of hard tissue at the apex of a tooth. The lesion eventually forms a bulbous mass that is firmly attached to the tooth root. It occurs most commonly on the mandibular first molar, affects men and women equally (Farman et al., 1979), and is seen most commonly in patients in their early 20s. The associated tooth is usually vital. Although the tumor has a margin of soft connective tissue between the lesion and alveolar bone, enucleation of the lesion may be incomplete, and the lesion recurs in up to 50% of cases (Hoffman et al., 1987).

Radiologic features. The tumor appears as a large (1 to 8 cm) periapical radiopaque lesion, often with a fine radiolucent margin, and is confluent with the roots of a tooth. The apex of the tooth may be obscured by the tumor mass, and occasionally there may be root resorption (Abrams, et al., 1974).

Histopathology. Histologically, the tumor mass consists of sheets of cementum-like tissue, which may contain a very large number of reversal lines and be unmineralized at the periphery of the mass or in the more active growth areas. It is attached to the involved tooth, which may show partial root resorption. Cementoblasts are present throughout the tissue but tend to be more numerous at the periphery.

Odontogenic tumors

Ameloblastomas. Ameloblastomas are benign epithelial neoplasms that develop from odontogenic epithelium. They occur equally in both sexes and at all ages but are most common between 20 and 40 years of age (Small and Waldron, 1955). The majority of cases occur in the region of the third molars, with 80% of the lesions occurring in the mandible. Frequently they are associated with an unerupted tooth. The lesions are slow growing, which causes expansion of the cortical bone rather than perforation. Large lesions may be associated with mobile or displaced teeth, thinning of the inferior border of the mandible, and extension into the ramus. Occasionally ameloblastomas develop in association with dentigerous cysts, but the relationship of the two lesions is not clear. Rarely, an ameloblastoma may develop as a submucosal mass in the mucosa overlying the alveolar process.

Radiologic features. The radiologic features of ameloblastomas vary. Most frequently they appear as a unilocular or multilocular lesion with scalloped margins. When associated with an unerupted tooth, the lesion may appear as a pericoronal radiolucency that is indistinguishable from a dentigerous cyst. If associated with the root of a tooth, it is indistinguishable from a radicular cyst (Fig. 22-10).

Histopathology. Ameloblastomas consist of masses of cuboidal or columnar epithelial cells with polarized nuclei that resemble ameloblasts. These cells may surround a mass of stellate cells that resemble the stellate reticulum, squamous epithelium with keratinization, or polygonal cells with a granular or clear cytoplasm. Based on the histologic appearance of ameloblastomas, a number of variants have been described. There is no correlation between the histologic pattern and the lesion's clinical behavior. The exception is the granular cell ameloblastoma, an unusual variant in which the stellate reticulum-like cells are replaced by large cells with a granular cytoplasm. This variant appears to have a greater rate of recurrence than the other types of ameloblastoma (Hartman, 1974).

Calcifying epithelial odontogenic tumors. Calcifying epithelial odontogenic tumors are epithelial neoplasms that

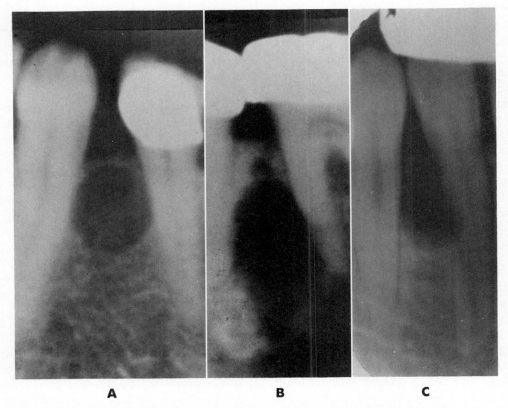

A   **B**   **C**

Fig. 22-10. Three interproximal radiolucencies with hyperostotic borders. **A** and **C** have moved roots of adjacent teeth. **B** lies adjacent to chronic focal sclerosing osteitis subjacent to premolar. Differential diagnosis included cysts, benign odontogenic neoplasms, and benign nonodontogenic neoplasms. Biopsies revealed parakeratinized odontogenic keratocyst, **A,** lateral periodontal cyst, **B,** and ameloblastoma, **C.**

usually occur within bone at any age with no significant difference between the sexes (Franklin and Pindborg, 1976). The lesions are more common in the mandible than in the maxilla and usually occur in the molar or premolar areas, frequently in association with the crown of an unerupted tooth. They may arise peripherally as a painless, firm swelling of the periodontal submucosa.

Histopathology. Histologically, the tumor consists of sheets of closely packed polyhedral epithelial cells within a connective tissue stroma. The epithelial cell nuclei, which are pleomorphic and contain distinct nucleoli, are hyperchromatic. Cells may be multinucleate, and mitotic figures are rare. Areas of hyaline material that are dispersed within the epithelium react positively for amyloid. It has been suggested that some matrix material may represent unmineralized enamel (Chaudhry et al., 1972), keratin, or glycoprotein. Also distributed within the epithelium are characteristic ovoid lamellar mineralizations, which apparently form within the amorphous hyaline material.

Adenomatoid odontogenic tumors. Adenomatoid odontogenic tumors are infrequent benign epithelial tumors

occurring within the bone, primarily in the incisor and canine regions of the maxilla. They occur most commonly in young women and are frequently associated with an unerupted tooth.

Histopathology. In contrast to ameloblastomas, adenomatoid odontogenic tumors are encapsulated lesions consisting of a scanty stroma and masses of epithelial cells that occur either as (1) polyhedral and spindle-shaped cells arranged in swirls or clusters or as (2) ordered cuboidal or columnar cells that resemble ameloblasts organized into tubular structures. The lumena often contain an eosinophilic material that has been described as preenamel matrix (Gorlin and Chaudhry, 1958), predentin matrix (Shear, 1962), or amyloid-like material (Smith et al., 1979).

Ameloblastic fibromas. Ameloblastic fibromas are relatively uncommon odontogenic neoplasms that involve proliferation of both the epithelial and mesenchymal elements. They are benign, slow-growing lesions that occur most commonly in the mandibular molar region of persons under 20 years of age (Slootweg, 1981). The lesions are usually asymptomatic and may be associated with an unerupted tooth.

Histopathology. Histologically, the tumor consists of a highly cellular fibromyxoid mesenchymal component resembling the primitive dental papilla. Strands and islands of cuboidal or columnar odontogenic epithelium are distributed throughout the lesion. Occasionally an eosinophilic hyalinized material may separate the epithelial cells from the mesenchymal component, and it has been suggested that this results from an inductive stimulus from the epithelial cells.

Odontomas. Odontomas are a group of relatively common lesions in which both the epithelium and the mesenchymal elements undergo normal patterns of histodifferentiation but in which there is aberrant morphodifferentiation. Hence these lesions are considered to be hamartomas rather than true neoplasms. Two major types are commonly identified depending on the organization of the component tissues: (1) the compound odontoma and (2) the complex odontoma. In both types the normal hard and soft tissues of the tooth (i.e., enamel, dentin, cementum, pulp) are present. In the compound variety small toothlike denticles are formed, whereas in the complex variety the various tissues are disorganized. It is not known how these lesions develop, but both trauma and genetic factors have been suggested as etiologic agents. These lesions, which are usually seen in adolescents, may occur at any location in the alveolar process of the maxilla and mandible. However, whereas the compound type occurs primarily in the anterior segment, the complex type is more frequent in the molar region. They may be associated with an unerupted tooth or seen in place of a missing tooth.

Radiologic features. The radiologic features of the lesion are characteristic, consisting of an irregular central radiopacity of varying density surrounded by a radiolucent margin. The compound odontoma consists of a variable number of small lobular, radiopaque toothlike structures, whereas the complex odontoma appears as an irregular homogeneous, radiopaque mass.

Ameloblastic fibro-odontomas. Ameloblastic fibro-odontomas are benign lesions with features of both ameloblastic fibromas and complex odontomas, with foci of calcified dental tissues. Since these lesions are seen in the molar region in children, it is likely that they represent an immature form of the complex odontoma.

Histopathology. Histologically, these lesions differ from complex odontomas in that they have a greater proportion of cellular myxoid fibrous tissue and numerous strands of odontogenic epithelium.

Malignant tumors of bone

Although malignant diseases of bone constitute a very small portion of periodontal lesions, they require a great deal of insight to ensure the earliest possible definitive diagnosis, thereby giving the patient the greatest chance of survival.

Malignant bone disease most closely mimics inflammatory disease of bone. Radiographically, both usually show poorly defined radiopacities or radiolucencies, along with features of rapid growth. Both are usually characterized by pain. Therefore, if a suspected inflammatory disease does not respond to therapeutic management, two possibilities should be considered: (1) the therapeutic management is inadequate or improper, or (2) the diagnosis may be wrong, in which case a malignancy should be considered.

Primary malignancies of the maxilla and mandible may be derived from undifferentiated mesenchyme, hematopoietic or other mesenchymal soft tissues, odontogenic or enclaved epithelium, or the bone matrix producing cells, primarily osteoblasts and chondroblasts. The two most common primary bone sarcomas are *osteosarcomas* and *myelomas*.

Osteosarcomas. Osteosarcomas are second only to multiple myelomas as the most common primary malignant bone disease (Dahlin, 1978). Malignant neoplasms of osteoblastic origin are aggressive sarcomas occurring principally in young persons between 10 and 30 years of age. They may originate in any bone and many soft tissues but are most common in the long bones of the leg. They are characteristically painful and rapidly growing.

Persons who have received therapeutic radiation have an increased risk of developing osteogenic sarcoma (Huvos et al., 1985). This risk is particularly evident in patients in whom fibrous dysplasia has been inappropriately treated by irradiation (Mock and Rosen, 1986).

Radiologic features. Radiographically, osteosarcoma presents as a poorly delineated, diffuse lesion, varying from radiopaque to radiolucent or any combination thereof. The variable radiographic appearance depends on the degree of differentiation of the neoplasm. Poorly differentiated osteosarcomas are very cellular, with little mineralized tissue, and thus present a radiolucent appearance. Tumors showing greater degrees of differentiation are less cellular, with more mineralized matrix and hence a more radiodense appearance. The so-called sun ray appearance, often associated with osteosarcoma, is produced by radiating poorly formed spicules and trabeculae of neoplastic bone (see Fig. 22-9). This pattern is often reported, though relatively seldom seen, with malignant bone disease. In the jaws osteosarcoma may cause perforation of the cortical bone, widened periodontal ligament spaces (see Fig. 22-9), local loss of the normal anatomic features of bone, and multidirectional resorption of teeth, similar to other malignant, rapidly growing diseases of bone.

Several classifications for the various subtypes of osteosarcoma exist; these are based on radiographic, clinical, or histopathologic features. Most authors prefer the clinical, or location-based classification, even though individual case reports may emphasize specific histopathologic variants (Martin et al., 1982, Chan et al., 1986).

Periosteal osteosarcoma is a less aggressive variant, arising from periosteum and having a radiating outward growth pattern (Unni et al., 1976; Zarbo et al., 1984).

Juxtacortical osteosarcoma also arises in close association with the bone cortex but may involve the medullary cavity (Spjut et al., 1971). This variant also has a much better prognosis as compared with medullary osteosarcoma. True osteogenic sarcomas arising in soft tissue are rare and rapidly fatal (Sordillo et al., 1983).

Osteosarcoma of the jaws. Osteosarcoma of the jaws accounts for about 6% of all osteosarcomas (Dahlin, 1978) and occurs equally in the maxilla and mandible (Clark et al., 1983). The most frequent histopathologic subtype that occurs in the jaws is the chondroblastic variant. The 5-year survival rate for these patients was found to be only 39.7%, even after radical surgery. This prognosis, although bleak, is much better than that for non-jaw-related osteosarcoma, which has a 5-year survival as low as 12% (Uribe-Botero et al., 1977).

Metastatic disease of the periodontium. Metastatic disease is uncommon in the jaws and represents about 1% of all oral malignancies (Stypulkowska et al., 1979). However, the identification of a metastatic lesion in the jaws may be the first evidence of distant malignant disease. The mandible is more frequently involved than the maxilla, and the surrounding soft tissues are involved with even less frequency (Clausen and Poulsen, 1963). Although metastatic tumors may originate in any tissue or organ, the most common sites of origin are breast, lung, kidney, thyroid, prostate, and colon (Clausen and Poulsen, 1963).

In general terms, a metastatic lesion in the periodontal tissues appears and behaves like a primary malignant lesion. A metastatic lesion affecting the gingival or alveolar mucosa clinically appears as a painless, smooth, relatively rapid growing, submucosal nodule that is firm to palpation (Finkelstein et al., 1983) (Fig. 22-11). Destruction of underlying bone and tooth, as well as overlying epithelium, with resultant ulceration and secondary inflammation, occurs at a later stage.

Radiologic features. Metastases to the maxilla or mandible are poorly demarcated, diffuse lesions, usually associated with pain and sometimes paresthesia as a result of impingement of the rapidly growing mass on peripheral nerve bundles. The diffuse soft tissue lesions may be completely radiolucent or predominantly radiopaque, depending on the reactivity of surrounding normal bone to the neoplasm. Metastatic tumors most commonly showing a radiopaque appearance originate from prostate, breast, kidney, and lung.

Treatment. The initial management of tumors thought to be possibly metastatic in origin is the same as for primary malignancies (i.e., the establishment of a definitive diagnosis), which usually requires an incisional biopsy. Grading and staging of the lesion are then accomplished prior to definitive therapeutic management.

LYMPHOMAS OF THE PERIODONTIUM

Diseases of the reticuloendothelial system may arise within any oral soft or hard tissue either as a solitary lesion or as part of a generalized disease. These diseases are classified as reactive, neoplastic, and Hodgkin's diseases. Hodgkin's disease, although well-defined and extensively studied, remains an enigma, showing features of both a reactive and a neoplastic process. Hodgkin's disease is divided into four distinct subtypes, all of which contain the Reed-Sternberg cell with varying involvement of other cells. These four subtypes—lymphocyte predominant, nodular sclerosing, mixed cellular, and lymphocyte depleted—have distinctly different histopathologic and prognostic features (Ioachim, 1982).

Non-Hodgkin's lymphomas are somewhat unique in that there are no recognized benign neoplastic counterparts. Numerous classification schemes, based on cellular morphology, architecture, and immunologic features, have been proposed. The first, widely accepted classification was that of Rappaport et al. (1956), which was based on architectural features, such as the presence or absence of neoplastic germinal centers, as well as specific cytologic features. Recent advances in immunology have facilitated the classification of lymphocytes into those of T, B, histiocytic, or null cell origin. Using this tool, most neoplasms originally characterized as histiocytic by the Rappaport system have been subsequently identified as lymphocytes in various stages of transformation. Accordingly, the Lukes-Collins classification of non-Hodgkin's lymphomas, which is based on anatomic and immunologic features,

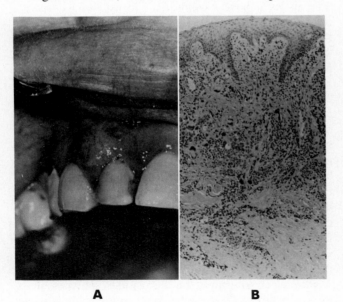

A   **B**

Fig. 22-11. A, Enlargement of 1 × 1 cm submucosal lesion asymptomatic and of 3 weeks' duration with a noticeable increase in size since first noticed. **B,** Biopsy revealed metastatic adenocarcinoma. Primary lesion was of breast. (Hematoxylin and eosin; original magnification ×75.) (From Finkelstein M, Hammond H, and Van Heuklom J: Int Dent J 69:53, 1983. By permission of the publishers, Butterworth & Co (Publishers) Ltd © 1983.)

was proposed (Lukes and Collins, 1974). On the basis of these immunologic cell surface markers, about 70% of lymphomas are found to be of B cell origin, 20% of T cell origin, and 10% unknown. Less than 1% of lymphomas are of true histiocytic origin.

While slow to gain acceptance, a new scheme incorporating components of previously used classifications without specification as to immunologic cell type has been proposed by the National Institutes of Health. This classification, the International Working Formulation, attempts to identify the more aggressive variants of non-Hodgkin's lymphoma (Non-Hodgkin's lymphoma pathologic classification project, 1982; Hart et al., 1985).

Clinical features. Lymphomas in the oral soft tissues are clinically indistinguishable from other rapidly growing submucosal neoplasms. They are usually painless and therefore may go unnoticed by the patient until they have reached a significant clinical size. They are most often localized and unilateral, and occasional involvement of regional lymph nodes may occur early in the course of the disease. As the tumor progresses in size, it may cause ulceration of the overlying epithelium or erode the underlying bone in a manner similar to that of other malignant diseases.

A lymphoid entity unique to the oral cavity was described by Tomich and Shafer (1975) as lymphoproliferative disease of the hard palate. These lesions presented as soft, fluctuant enlargements of the palate of elderly patients. Based on morphologic and cytologic features, these cases were eventually diagnosed as lymphomas. These observations are significant for two reasons: (1) because of the lack of normal lymphoid tissue on the hard palate, these lymphomas would be described as extranodal or soft tissue in origin; and (2) no examples of benign lymphoid proliferations originating on the hard palate were found in a review of over 45,000 surgical specimens. Therefore a palatal biopsy showing signs of a lymphoproliferative disease should be considered either malignant or premalignant.

Non-Hodgkin's lymphoma arising within bone shows clinical and radiographic features that are similar to those of other rapidly growing malignant lesions. Radiographically, lymphomas appear as radiolucencies without distinct borders and without hyperostotic peripheries. They often cause pain or paresthesia even in the absence of secondary inflammation.

Handlers et al. (1986) reported 34 cases of extranodal oral lymphoma, 97% identified as being of B-cell origin. The so-called T-cell lymphoma (mycosis fungoides) is rare in the oral cavity (Wright et al., 1981). Burkitt's lymphoma (a B-cell lesion), so named because of its undifferentiated nature, defies cytologic or immunologic classification. It was originally recognized as a lymphoma involving the jaw in about 60% of presentations. This tumor was frequently seen in Equatorial Africa (Burkett and O'Connor,

1961). Subsequently, a histologically identical "American" Burkitt's lymphoma has been identified, having jaw involvement in only about 18% of cases reported (Saraban et al., 1984).

DISEASES OF THE JAWS THAT MAY RESEMBLE PERIODONTAL DISEASE

Numerous systemic or metabolic diseases may contribute to accelerated, focal, or diffuse alveolar crestal bone loss. Two diseases of bone that can mimic periodontal disease without displaying any other clinically evident features are *multiple myeloma* and *idiopathic histiocytosis*. Both of these diseases cause bone loss from a central or peripheral location and radiographically lack a hyperostotic border surrounding the radiolucent lesions. Neither of these diseases produces a "tumor" until late in development, so that the true nature of the disease is masked. Hence the clinical and radiographic pictures of these two diseases may be identical to those of periodontal disease (Figs. 22-12 and 22-13).

Multiple myelomas

Multiple myelomas are primary malignant lesions of bone occurring most commonly in persons over 40 years of age. The lesions are reported in men much more often than in women. Because of its insidious nature and predilection to involve bone, the initial manifestation of myeloma may be pain, the result of pathologic fractures, often localized to the spinal column. Although myeloma may involve any bone, there appears to be greater involvement in bones in which there is hematopoiesis. Cataldo and Meyer (1966) studied the maxilla and mandible in 44 cases of myeloma and found that 70% demonstrated lesions.

Radiographically, the classic presentation of multiple myeloma is one of numerous, well-circumscribed "punched out" radiolucencies with no hyperostotic peripheral borders. However, this disease may present initially as a localized or diffuse lesion with loss of either crestal alveolar or central bone (see Fig. 22-12).

Histopathology. The cells of some cases of multiple myeloma bear a distinct resemblance to plasma cells, whereas in other, less-differentiated neoplasms the cell of origin is difficult to determine. Although many reactive inflammatory cell infiltrates may be composed predominantly of plasma cells, central bony myeloma lesions lack the mixed cellular infiltrate with neutrophils, lymphocytes, histiocytes, and other inflammatory cells. Myeloma lesions are composed of sheets of relatively uniform plasmacytoid cells.

Immunopathology. Laboratory studies often reveal an increased sedimentation rate, hypergammaglobulinemia, a reversed serum albumin-to-globulin ratio, and a Bence-Jones proteinuria. However, these features may be absent in some cases of myeloma and therefore should not be re-

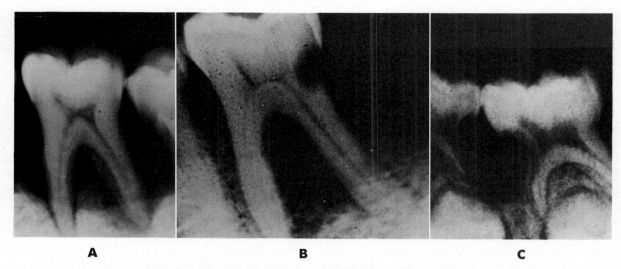

Fig. 22-12.   Three poorly demarcated foci of crestal alveolar bone loss. All were asymptomatic and had no evidence of clinical expansion. Biopsy revealed chronic inflammation consistent with periodontitis, **A,** plasmacytoma consistent with multiple myeloma, **B,** and idiopathic histiocytosis, **C.**

lied on to exclude the disease from a differential diagnosis.

Immunologic methods to identify long- and short-chain immunoglobulin proteins are usually helpful in establishing a diagnosis. In contrast to inflammatory infiltrates, myelomas exhibit monoclonal immunoglobulin production, usually of the IgG class (Bataille and Sany, 1981). It has also been suggested that solitary myeloma lesions may be clinically different from actual multiple myeloma; however, most patients with a solitary plasmacytoid lesion of bone will eventually develop multiple myeloma.

Patients with diagnosed or occult myeloma occasionally present with secondary amyloidosis involving visceral organs, skin, or submucosa. In the oral cavity primary or secondary amyloidosis most often involves the tongue (Babajews, 1985).

Idiopathic histiocytosis

Idiopathic histiocytosis, or histiocytosis X, is a disease or group of diseases involving a reticuloendothelial disturbance of unknown cause. While some forms of histiocytosis X may behave in a neoplastic manner, these diseases remain classified under the idiopathic inflammatory disease category. These diseases were previously categorized as one of three entities: eosinophilic granuloma, Hand-Schüller-Christian, or Letterer-Siwe disease; however, most investigators now refer to the disease as being localized, chronic disseminated, or acute disseminated.

The diagnosis of localized idiopathic histiocytosis (eosinophilic granuloma) is based on the detection of a single lytic lesion of bone or, rarely, a single soft tissue infiltration. The prognosis for this form of the disease is excel-

lent, and curettage is considered curative.

In contrast, chronic disseminated histiocytosis involves widespread involvement of bone and sometimes soft tissue. It usually occurs in children under the age of 10, in boys more often than in girls, and is characterized by chronic progression. The classic triad of chronic disseminated histiocytosis (Hand-Schüller-Christian disease) presents with multiple "punched out" radiolucencies of the skull, exophthalmos, and diabetes insipidus as a result of involvement of the pituitary gland. The prognosis for chronic disseminated histiocytosis is very good, with excellent patient response to local curettage, chemotherapy, and radiation.

Acute disseminated histiocytosis (Letterer-Siwe disease) is an acute, rapidly progressive form of idiopathic histiocytosis found most often in children under the age of 5. Visceral soft tissue, as well as multiple bone involvement, is often seen early in the disease. Despite chemotherapy and radiation, the prognosis is very poor, with the majority of cases resulting in death in a short period of time.

Soft tissue involvement may result in a submucosal enlargement, but lesions in bone seldom result in loss of alveolar bone with no enlargement, and these bony lesions may resemble changes seen in periodontitis. Most lesions of bone are clinically asymptomatic. The oral features of histiocytosis X have been reviewed by Jones et al. (1970).

Central lesions of bone present with well-defined borders but with no evidence of hyperostotic margins. Involvement of the periodontium may produce localized or diffuse crestal alveolar bone loss, thereby mimicking primary periodontal disease (Fig. 22-12).

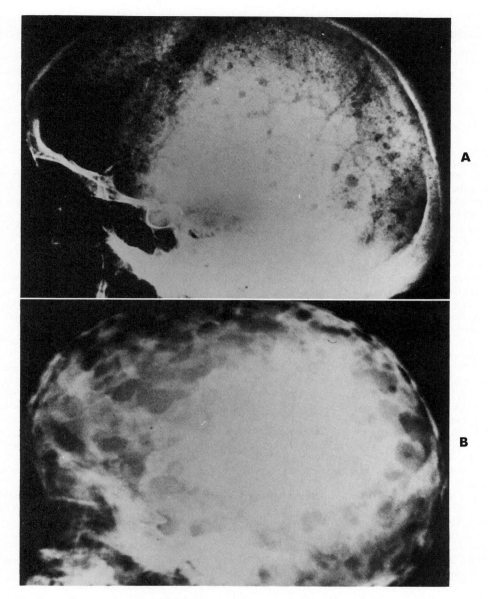

Fig. 22-13. Further evaluation of patients in Fig. 22-12, *B* and *C*, revealed multiple bone involvement. **A,** Multiple myeloma. **B,** Acute disseminated idiopathic histiocytosis.

Histopathology. The microscopic features of the clinical variants of idiopathic histiocytosis are similiar. There are sheets of histiocytic-type cells with a variable degree of cellular dysplasia and pleomorphism. Eosinophils are present in most, but not all, lesions. Chronic lesions may show xanthomatous cellular changes and fibrosis. In general, the more aggressive lesions of idiopathic histiocytosis show fewer eosinophils and more dysplasia of the histiocytic cells, becoming microscopically difficult to distinguish from a large-cell lymphoma.

Immunologic and electron microscopic studies suggest that the histiocytic cells are related to the dendritic Langerhans' cells of skin and mucosa (Favara et al., 1983), leading some authors to rename the disease Langerhans' cell disease (Lieberman, 1982).

Since both multiple myeloma and idiopathic histiocytosis may present clinical, historical, and radiographic features similiar to those of periodontitis, the astute clinician should consider biopsy to exclude these diseases in patients with periodontal disease that is not responsive to conventional therapy.

ACKNOWLEDGMENTS

We wish to thank Dr. Gilbert E. Lilly, Professor and Head, Department of Oral Pathology and Diagnosis, The University of Iowa, for his guidance in the differential diagnostic schemes presented herein.

REFERENCES

Abrams AM, Kirby JW, and Melrose RJ: Cementoblastoma, Oral Surg 38:394, 1974.

Andersen L, Fejerskov O, and Philipsen HP: Oral giant cell granulomas: a clinical and histological study of 129 new cases, Acta Pathol Microbiol Scand A81:606, 1973

Babajews A: Occult multiple myeloma associated with amyloid of the tongue, Br Assoc Oral Maxillofac Surg 23:298, 1985.

Baker H: Staging of cancer of the head and neck: oral cavity, pharynx, larynx, and paranasal sinuses, CA 33:130, 1983.

Bataille R and Sany J: Solitary myeloma, Cancer 48:845, 1981.

Bhaskar SN et al: Giant cell reparative granuloma (peripheral): report of 50 cases, J Oral Surg 29:110, 1971.

Brannon RB, Houston GD, and Wampler HW: Gingival salivary gland choristoma, Oral Surg Oral Med Oral Pathol 61:185, 1986.

Browand BC and Waldron CA: Central mucoepidermoid tumors of the jaws, Oral Surg Oral Med Oral Pathol 40:631, 1975.

Browne RM: The odontogenic keratocyst: clinical aspects, Br Dent J 128:225, 1970.

Browne RM: The origin of cholesterol in odontogenic cysts in man, Arch Oral Biol 16:107, 1971.

Browne RM: Metaplasia and degeneration in odontogenic cysts in man, J Oral Pathol 1:145, 1972.

Buchner A and Hansen LS: The histomorphologic spectrum of the gingival cyst in the adult, Oral Surg 48:532, 1979.

Buchner A and Hansen LS: Pigmented nevi of the oral mucosa: a clinicopathologic study of 36 new cases and review of 155 cases from the literature, Oral Surg Oral Med Oral Pathol 63:676, 1987.

Buchner A and Scuibba J: Peripheral epithelial odontogenic tumors: a review, Oral Surg Oral Med Oral Pathol 63:688, 1987.

Burkett D and O'Connor G: Malignant lymphoma in African children, Cancer 14:258, 1961.

Cataldo E and Meyer I: Solitary and multiple plasma cell tumors of the jaws and oral cavity, Oral Surg Oral Med Oral Pathol 22:628, 1966.

Chan C, Kung T, and Lily M: Telangiectatic osteosarcoma of the mandible, Cancer 58:2110, 1986.

Chaudhry AP et al: Calcifying epithelial odontogenic tumor: a histochemical and ultrastructural study, Cancer 30:519, 1972.

Clark J et al: Osteosarcoma of the jaws, Cancer 51:2311, 1983.

Clausen F and Poulsen H: Metastatic carcinoma to the jaws, Acta Pathol Microbiol Scand 57:361, 1963.

Dabelsteen E et al: The limitations of exfoliative cytology for the detection of epithelial atypia in oral leukoplakias, Br J Cancer 25:21, 1971.

Dahlin D: Bone tumors: general aspects and data on 6,221 cases, ed 3, Springfield, Ill, 1978, Charles C Thomas, Publisher.

Farman AG et al: Cementoblastoma: report of a case, J Oral Surg 37:198, 1979.

Favara B, McCarthy R, and Mierau G: Histiocytosis X, Hum Pathol 14:663, 1983.

Finkelstein M, Hammond H, and Van Heuklom J: Localized soft tissue enlargement of the gingiva, Int Dent J 69:53, 1983.

Franklin CD and Pindborg JJ: The calcifying epithelial odontogenic tumor, Oral Surg 42:753, 1976.

Friedman R, Rigel D, and Kopf A: Early detection of malignant melanoma: the role of physician examination and self-examination of the skin, CA 35:131, 1985.

Fu KK et al: External and interstitial radiation therapy of carcinoma of the oral tongues, Am J Roentgenol 126:107, 1976.

Goldsmith H: Melanoma, an overview, CA 29:194, 1979.

Gorlin RJ and Chaudhry AP: Adenomeloblastoma, Oral Surg 11:762, 1958.

Gorlin RJ and Goltz RW: Multiple nevoid basal cell epithelioma, jaw cysts and bifid rib: a syndrome, N Engl J Med 262:908, 1960.

Greene M et al: Acquired precursors of cutaneous malignant melanoma, N Engl J Med 312:97, 1985.

Handlers J et al: Extramodal oral lymphoma. I. A morphologic and immunoperoxidase study of 34 cases, Oral Surg Oral Med Oral Pathol 61:362, 1986.

Hart W, Farber L, and Codman E: Non-Hodgkin's lymphoma for the non-oncologist, JAMA 253:1431, 1985.

Hartman KS: Granular cell ameloblastoma: a survey of twenty cases from the Armed Forces Institute of Pathology, Oral Surg 38:241, 1974.

Hoffman S, Jacoway JR, and Krolls SO: Intraosseous and periosteal tumors of the jaws. In Hartman WH, editor: Atlas of tumor pathology, series 2, Fascicle 24, Washington, DC, 1987, Armed Forces Institute of Pathology.

Huvos A et al: Postradiation osteogenic sarcoma of bone and soft tissues, Cancer 55:1244, 1985.

Ioachim H: Hodgkins lymphoma. In Lymph node biopsy, Philadelphia, 1982, JB Lippincott Co.

Jayant K et al: Qualification of the role of smoking and chewing tobacco in oral, pharyngeal and oesophogeal cancers, Br J Cancer 35:232, 1977.

Jones J, Lilly G, and Marlette R: Histiocytosis X, J Oral Surg 28:461, 1970.

Lieberman P: Langerhans cell (eosinophilic) granulomatosis and related syndromes. In Wyngaarden J and Smith L, editors: Cecil's textbook of medicine, Philadelphia, 1982, WB Saunders Co.

Lukes R and Collins R: Immunologic characterization of human malignant lymphomas, Cancer 34:1488, 1974.

Martin S et al: Small cell osteosarcoma, Cancer 50:990, 1982.

Mashberg A, Garfindel L, and Harris S: Alcohol as a primary risk factor in oral squamous cell carcinoma, CA 31(3):146, 1981.

Mock D and Rosen I: Osteosarcoma in irradiated tibious dysplasia, J Oral Pathol 15:1, 1986.

Morgan PR and Johnson NW: Histological, histochemical and ultrastructural studies on the nature of hyalin bodies in odontogenic cysts, J Oral Pathol 3:127, 1974.

Non-Hodgkin's lymphoma pathologic classification project: National Cancer Institute study of classifications of non-Hodgkin's lymphomas: summary and description of a working formulation for clinical usage, Cancer 49:2112, 1982.

Pindborg J, Kramer I, and Torloni H: Histological typing of odontogenic tumors, jaw cysts and allied lesions, International Histological Classification of Tumors, No 5, Geneva, 1972, World Health Organization.

Praetorius F et al: Calcifying odontogenic cyst, Acta Odontol Scand 39:227, 1981.

Radden BG and Reade PC: Odontogenic keratocysts: a review and clinicopathological study of 368 odontogenic cysts, Aust Dent J 18:218, 1973.

Rapini R et al: Primary malignant melanoma of the oral cavity: a review of 177 cases, Cancer 55:1543, 1985.

Rappaport H, Winter W, and Hicks E: Follicular lymphoma: a reevaluation of its position in the scheme of malignant lymphoma based on a survey of 253 cases, Cancer 9:792, 1956.

Rothman K and Keller A: The effect of joint exposure to alcohol and tobacco on the risk of cancer of the mouth and pharynx, J Chronic Dis 25:711, 1972.

Sapp JP: Ultrastructure and histogenesis of peripheral reparative giant cell granuloma of the jaws, Cancer 30:1119, 1972.

Saraban E, Donahue A, and Magrath I: Jaw involvement in American Burkitt's lymphoma, Cancer 53:1777, 1984.

Sedano HO and Gorlin RJ: Hyaline bodies of Rushton: some histochemical considerations concerning their etiology, Oral Surg 26:198, 1968.

Shafer WG, Hine MK, and Levy BM: A textbook of oral pathology, ed 4, Philadelphia, 1983, WB Saunders Co.

Shear M: Cysts of the oral regions, ed 2, Littleton, Mass, 1983, Wright-PSG.

Shear M: The histogenesis of the turnover of enamel organ epithelium, Br Dent J 112:494, 1962.

Sigurdson A: Toluidine blue staining as a malignancy test, Acta Otolaryngol 75:308, 1973.

Silverberg E and Lubera J: Cancer statistics, CA 37(1):2, 1987.

Silverman S: Diagnosis. In Silverman S, editor: Oral cancer, New York, 1981, American Cancer Society.

Slootweg PJ: An analysis of the interrelationship of the mixed odontogenic tumors—ameloblastic fibroma, ameloblastic fibro-odontoma, and the odontomas, Oral Surg 51:266, 1981.

Small IA and Waldron CA: Ameloblastomas of the jaws, Oral Surg 8:281, 1955.

Smith RRL et al: Adenomatoid odontogenic tumor: ultrastructural demonstration of two cell types and amyloid, Cancer 43:505, 1979.

Sordillo P et al: Extraosseous osteogenic sarcoma, Cancer 51:727, 1983.

Soskolne WA and Shear M: Observations on the pathogenesis of primordial cysts, Br Dent J 123:321, 1967.

Spjut H et al: Tumors of bone and cartilage. In Firminger HI, editor: Atlas of tumor pathology, Fascicle 5, Bethesda, Md, 1971, Armed Forces Institute of Pathology.

Stypulkowska J et al: Metastatic tumors to the jaws and oral cavity, J Oral Surg 37:805, 1979.

Summers L: The incidence of epithelium in periapical granulomas and the mechanism of cavitation in apical dental cysts in man, Arch Oral Biol 19:1177, 1974.

Tomich C and Shafer W: Lymphoproliferative disease of the hard palate: a clinicopathologic entity, Oral Surg Oral Med Oral Pathol 39:754, 1975.

Unni K, Dahlin D, and Beabout J: Periosteal osteogenic sarcoma, Cancer 37:2476, 1976.

Uribe-Botero G et al: Primary osteosarcoma of bone: a clinicopathologic investigation of 243 cases with necropsy studies in 54, Am J Clin Pathol 67:427, 1977.

Weathers DR and Waldron CA: Unusual multilocular cysts of the jaws (botryoid odontogenic cysts), Oral Surg 36:235, 1973.

Winn DM et al: Snuff dipping and oral cancer among women in the southern United States, N Engl J Med 304:745, 1981.

Wright JM: The odontogenic keratocyst: orthokeratinized variant, Oral Surg 51:609, 1981.

Wright JM, Balcuinas B, and Muus J: Mycosis fungoides with oral manifestations, Oral Surg Oral Med Oral Pathol 51:24, 1981.

Wynder EL, Bross IJ, and Feldman RM: A study of etiologic factors in cancer of the mouth, Cancer 10:1300, 1957.

Wynder EL et al: Epidemiologic investigation of multiple primary cancers of the upper alimentary and respiratory tracts. I. A retrospective study, Cancer 24:730, 1969.

Wysocki GP et al: Histogenesis of the lateral periodontal cyst and the gingival cyst of the adult, Oral Surg 50:609, 1980.

Zarbo R, Regezi J, and Baker S: Periosteal osteogenic sarcoma of the mandible, Oral Surg Oral Med Oral Pathol 57:643, 1984.

Chapter 23

ACQUIRED IMMUNODEFICIENCY SYNDROME

Oral and periodontal changes

John S. Greenspan
Deborah Greenspan
James R. Winkler
Patricia A. Murray

Essentials of the disease
    The virus
    Pathogenesis
    HIV testing
    Clinical features
    Epidemiology
    Treatment and prevention
Oral manifestations
    Fungal and bacterial lesions
    Virus-associated lesions
    Neoplastic lesions
    Other lesions
HIV-associated gingivitis and periodontitis
    Etiology
    HIV-associated gingivitis
    HIV-associated periodontitis
    Differential diagnosis
    Treatment

In the ninth year of the epidemic of the acquired immunodeficiency syndrome (AIDS), with well over 200,000 cases known or suspected worldwide and several million individuals thought to be infected with the causative agent, it is now clear that we are dealing with an epidemic or

□Parts of this chapter are slightly modified from Greenspan JS: The problem: etiology, pathogenesis and epidemiology of HIV infection, CDA J 15(1):15, 1987.

pandemic of enormous significance. In this chapter some of the current knowledge concerning AIDS and its etiologic agent, the human immunodeficiency virus (HIV), is presented. The pathogenesis and nature of the group of diseases due to HIV are discussed, as well as the status of the epidemic and some of the oral manifestations. Finally, a more detailed description of the gingival and periodontal lesions seen in HIV-infected persons is given, including preliminary information on the microbiology of and therapy for these newly described conditions.

ESSENTIALS OF THE DISEASE
The virus

The causative agent of AIDS is a human retrovirus of the lentivirus group. Originally described by the group at the Pasteur Institute in Paris and named lymphadenopathy-associated virus (LAV) (Barre-Sinoussi et al., 1983), this virus was subsequently studied in more detail by researchers at the National Institutes of Health, who named it the human T-lymphotropic virus III (HTLV-lll) (Popovic et al., 1984), and by investigators at the University of California, San Francisco, who characterized it as the AIDS-associated retrovirus (ARV) (Levy et al., 1984). In 1986 an international committee chose the name *human immunodeficiency virus* (International Committee, 1986).

HIV is an RNA virus. The genome contains at least seven known genes. These include *gag,* which encodes the inner core protein, and *env,* which encodes the envelope glycoprotein. The *pol* gene is related to viral reverse transcriptase. The virus attaches to and enters target cells where the RNA, through the action of the enzyme reverse transcriptase, causes the cell to produce a DNA copy of itself. The proviral DNA becomes incorporated in the genome of the host cell and, through the agency of the cell's DNA and RNA mechanisms, causes the production of viral proteins. These assemble at the cell surface along with the viral RNA to produce budding particles of new virus, which are then available to infect other cells. In the course of this process of infection and replication, the target cell may or may not become damaged and die. HIV can also be transmitted by cell-to-cell contact, evading a cell-free tissue fluid or plasma phase. This is of significance when one is considering the routes and efficacy of antiviral drugs, as well as the significance of antibody and antigen testing for the presence of the virus in serum.

The virus binds predominantly, but not exclusively, to lymphocytes of the helper series, which carry a unique cell surface antigen and are known as T-4 lymphocytes. This binding involves the unique T-4 molecule itself (McDougal et al., 1986), but it is not clear whether other proteins are also required for binding and penetration. In addition to its cytopathic effects on infected target cells, the virus may become latent, causing little untoward effect but being available for subsequent, often explosive, replication under the influence of its own *tat* (transactivating gene) or other cofactors (Fisher et al., 1986), which may include gene products or proteins of herpes simplex virus (Mosca et al., 1987) or Ebstein-Barr (EB) virus (Purtilo, 1986).

Different isolates of HIV show genetic variability, especially in *env*, the gene coding for the envelope glycoprotein (Montagnier et al., 1985). This is, of course, the very molecule that would be used for the production of vaccines, and its variability is a cause for great concern. However, well-conserved regions of the envelope gene do exist, some of which are highly antigenic, and it is on this factor that hopes for vaccine production currently rest (Starcich et al., 1986).

Simian retroviruses have been isolated that have some cross-reactivity with isolates of HIV and are thought to belong to the same group of primate retroviruses (Barin et al., 1985). Furthermore, other human isolates from West Africa (LAV-2 and HTLV-IV [now known as HIV-2]), isolated from asymptomatic or AIDS patients, show similar biologic properties to the HIV-1 studied in Paris, Bethesda, and San Francisco but have dissimilar envelope proteins and do not produce significant amounts of cross-reacting antibodies (Kanki et al., 1986; Guyader et al., 1987; Kornfeld et al., 1987). It thus seems that the retroviruses, of which HIV is an example, have been evolving for some time in Africa. It also seems possible that newer forms of these retroviruses, some of which may be at least as pathogenic as HIV and may even have different ranges of host and tissue specificity, may become apparent as time goes by. Thus the current epidemic of AIDS and HIV infection may unfortunately be the first of a series of such epidemics caused by human retroviruses.

Pathogenesis

The pathogenesis of AIDS is now quite well understood. The virus can be transmitted from person to person by three main routes (Sande, 1986). The predominant mechanism is through sexual contact. Any individual engaging in unprotected sexual intercourse with an HIV carrier is now known to be at risk. This includes heterosexual intercourse, the source of a growing number of cases of AIDS (Clumeck, 1986; Fischl et al., 1987). The second route is through the agency of blood and blood products. Recipients of transfused HIV-infected blood, hemophiliacs receiving HIV-contaminated blood-clotting products, and individuals who share contaminated needles (e.g., intravenous drug abusers) are the prime examples of this route of transmission (Chaisson et al., 1987; Moss, 1987).

Finally, HIV-infected pregnant women can pass the virus on to their babies (Pahwa et al., 1986), probably at birth or by transplacental transmission (Cowan et al., 1984; La Pointe et al., 1985). In the Western world the main risk groups are thus homosexual and bisexual men, recipients of blood transfusions and blood products, intravenous drug abusers, the heterosexual partners of HIV carriers, and the children of HIV-infected mothers. In Africa AIDS and HIV infection show a more or less equal predilection for both sexes, and it is believed that heterosexual transmission is the major route there (Biggar, 1986). Additional risk factors in Africa include preexisting venereal disease and genital ulcers (Katzenstein et al. 1987; Plummer et al., 1987).

In infected individuals the virus can be isolated from certain blood cells, from serum and plasma, and from semen, vaginal secretions, and cerebrospinal fluid (Levy et al., 1985). Much lower levels of the virus are present in tears, saliva (Ho et al., 1985a), feces, and breast milk, and the virus is also present in infected tissues, notably lymph node and brain, although other tissues have yet to be fully explored.

While the predominant target cell of HIV is the helper T cell, other lymphocytes, monocytes and macrophages, dendritic reticular cells of lymph nodes, Langerhans' cells, cells in the brain (probably oligodendrocytes but possibly brain neurons), and other target cells can be infected to some extent (Ho et al., 1985b, 1986; Asjo et al., 1987).

HIV testing

Antibodies to HIV become detectable approximately 1 to 3 months after infection. These antibodies can be detected by indirect immunofluorescence, enzyme-linked immunosorbent assay (ELISA), and Western blot, as well as radioimmunoassay. In general, ELISA is used as the screening assay, and Western blot is used for confirmation and for studies of antibodies to individual HIV proteins. Culture for HIV is laborious, time consuming, and expensive, and is confined to limited research applications. However, newer antigen assays are becoming more widespread, and their use may solve problems presented by individuals who are viremic but antibody negative (Chaisson et al., 1986; Lange et al., 1986).

Clinical features

Initial infection by HIV can probably be asymptomatic but sometimes produces an acute illness resembling infectious mononucleosis, with malaise, fever, lymphadenopathy, pharyngitis, and a skin rash (Cooper et al., 1985). The initial infection is accompanied or followed shortly by seroconversion, with the appearance of antibodies to HIV. HIV can be cultured from the blood, in some cases before antibody seroconversion has occurred.

The acute mononucleosis-like episode may be followed by an asymptomatic period of unknown length. Alternatively, the individual may enter a chronic phase of overt HIV infection. This may take the form of persistent diffuse lymphadenopathy or of more widespread constitutional disease, with loss of weight, night sweats, and malaise. Or the disease may present as the more notable effects of HIV infection (CDC, 1986). These include the classic surveillance criteria for AIDS, consisting mainly of fatal opportunistic infections and neoplasia, such as Kaposi's sarcoma and non-Hodgkin's lymphoma (Gottlieb et al., 1983; Klein et al., 1984). A much wider range of less fatal but equally significant opportunistic infections and other diseases is also found. Among these are nonfatal secondary infectious complications such as oral candidiasis and oral hairy leukoplakia (Greenspan et al., 1984, 1985b). These oral complications are notable for their predictive significance for the development of full-blown AIDS, as defined by the Centers for Disease Control (CDC). Another of these secondary infectious complications is multidermatomal herpes zoster, which can affect the face and mouth.

In addition to these opportunistic infections and neoplasms that take advantage of the suppressed immune system, other features of HIV infection include autoimmunity and neurologic manifestations. Autoimmunity is expressed as overactivity of the B-cell system, resulting in hypergammaglobulinemia and sometimes the production of specific autoantibodies. The latter include lymphocytotoxic antibodies (Pollack et al., 1983; Kloster, et al., 1984), which may further aggravate the immunodeficiency, and antibodies to platelets, which can cause immune thrombocytopenic purpura (Stricker et al., 1985; Abrams et al., 1986). The neurologic effects are probably the result of the direct infection of brain elements—oligodendrocytes, endothelial cells, or neurons—by the HIV. The effects are widespread and potentially devastating, and include dementia and specific, histologically characteristic neuroencephalopathy (Sharer et al., 1986). The ultimate consequences of the neurologic effects of HIV infection are as yet unknown but could be enormously significant, both in terms of seriousness and in terms of the widespread nature and long-term chronicity that they threaten.

Thus it is clear that the original clinical features of HIV infection, notably *Pneumocystis carinii* pneumonia (PCP) and Kaposi's sarcoma, seen in male homosexuals in New York, San Francisco, and Los Angeles in 1981, have given way to a very wide range of clinical manifestations. Although the majority of these have as their final common pathway the well-known and now quite well understood immunodeficiency due to HIV ablation of helper T-4 cells, other and potentially equally serious manifestations due to direct effects or as yet unknown effects of the AIDS virus are becoming apparent.

Epidemiology

On February 22, 1988, there were in the United States 54,233 diagnosed cases of CDC-defined AIDS, with 30,355 deaths having been reported. In California 11,994 cases of AIDS and 6647 AIDS-related deaths had been reported. In San Francisco the figures were 4514 cases of AIDS and 2707 deaths at that time. In the month of February 1988 in San Francisco alone, 143 new cases of AIDS were diagnosed and 78 deaths were reported. These figures for the United States, California, and San Francisco must be considered in the light of some additional statistics. First, it is probable that the rate of development of AIDS in seropositive individuals ranges from 3% to 10% per year and is increasingly likely with the passage of time since seroconversion (Moss, 1985). There are thus as many as 30 times more people with HIV infection as there are individuals with AIDS. Second, significant underreporting, probably 50%, is thought to occur. Third, it has been estimated that over 1.5 million individuals in the United States are infected with the AIDS virus. Very rough estimates indicate that at least a similar number of individuals are involved worldwide. This would give a world total as of June 1987 of over 100,000 cases of AIDS and approximately 3 million infected individuals worldwide.

The risk groups for HIV infection and for AIDS remain very much the same as they have been since the beginning of the epidemic. People of Haitian origin were among the original risk groups; for a while it was thought that they were no longer particularly susceptible, but more recently it has become clear that, as in Africa, the prevalence of AIDS among such individuals is significant (Pape et al., 1986) and is equally distributed between the sexes, presumably because of heterosexual transmission (Collaborative Study Group of AIDS in Haitian-Americans, 1987). Changes in sexual practices among homosexual men are leading to a slight slowing of the epidemic in the gay community (McKusick et al., 1985). Conversely, the heterosexual partners of HIV carriers continue to show a steady increase in figures and an increase in the proportion of cases that they represent (Redfield et al., 1985; Clumeck,

1986). Similarly, AIDS and HIV infection among intravenous drug abusers (Pape et al., 1986; Moss, 1987) is an increasing problem, as it is among children (New York City Department of Health AIDS Surveillance, 1986; Fischl et al., 1987).

The potential extent of the epidemic of HIV infection and AIDS is best illustrated by some predictions for the coming year 1991 (Curran and Morgan, 1987), just 10 years since the first description of AIDS in 1981. By 1991 the Centers for Disease Control estimate that there will be in the United States 270,000 cases of AIDS and 170,000 deaths due to AIDS. In that year it is estimated that worldwide there will be 300,000 new cases of AIDS. It is also estimated that in 1991 the costs of AIDS in the United States alone (i.e., for AIDS education, health care, and research) will be $8 billion.

Treatment and prevention

No specific effective treatment is available for HIV infection or AIDS. Several antiviral agents are being tested, of which one, azidothymidine (AZT) has been licensed (Yarchoan et al., 1986). Prospects for an HIV vaccine are still remote (Francis, 1985), and evidence of autoantibodies induced by the HIV-1 and reactive with the major histocompatibility II antigen may further delay vaccine development (Golding et al., 1988). Therapy for the myriad infectious and neoplastic complications of HIV infection is complex and requires the expertise of many medical specialties. Meanwhile, the only real hope for prevention lies in widespread educational programs directed at the risk groups and at those who can inform them. It is also essential to inform the general public about risk behaviors and modes of transmission, not only to reduce the spread of the virus, but also to decrease the ignorance and false assumptions that lead to inappropriate discrimination against those infected with HIV (Black, 1986; Price, 1986).

ORAL MANIFESTATIONS

As knowledgeable and conscientious health care professionals, dentists are aware of the need to understand the essential nature of the diseases that may appear in their patient population, and especially to know about the causes, features, and treatment of those general diseases that affect the mouth or have implications for dental practice. Failure to understand these general diseases may prejudice the health of patients and even of the practitioner and his or her colleagues, staff, and family. Examples include several important infectious diseases, such as tuberculosis, syphilis, hepatitis, and herpesvirus infections (Greenspan, 1983).

The group of diseases caused directly or indirectly by HIV, including AIDS, is particularly notable for several reasons (Greenspan et al., 1986a). First, it is now clear that oral lesions, detectable on careful examination by the well-trained practitioner (Reichart et al., 1985, 1987; Greenspan and Greenspan, 1987; Greenspan and Silver-

man, 1987), are often the first clinical expression of HIV infection. Second, the immunosuppression and susceptibility to opportunistic infection that are caused by HIV may alter the responses of the oral soft tissues, gingiva, and periodontium, as well as the oral flora, and thus modify both treatment plans and the probable outcome of therapy. Third, the dentist has a responsibility to know and understand the current state of knowledge about AIDS in order to advise and educate patients (Gerbert, 1987). The dental profession has an ethical and moral obligation to help in the education process. We must also recognize the impact that a rational understanding of AIDS has on the safety and effectiveness of the dental office environment.

The tragedy of AIDS and the challenge it poses for biomedicine, including dentistry, also offer some unique opportunities for research and discovery. The epidemic has opened new avenues in the exploration of RNA viruses and viral transmission, the human immune system, and neoplasia, among other areas. Two notable examples that concern the mouth are the pathogenesis of periodontal disease and the effects of viruses on epithelial cells.

Finally, the AIDS epidemic has stimulated much-needed efforts to improve infection-control measures in dental practice. These have long been appropriate on the basis of knowledge concerning hepatitis B virus and other infectious agents, but the fatal nature of full-blown AIDS and the mystery surrounding the disease in its first few years have certainly caught our attention and made us devote energy and efforts to this problem.

Fungal and bacterial lesions

The fungal disease most commonly seen in the oral cavity is candidiasis, and the *Candida* species most often involved is *C. albicans,* although *C. stellatoides* and *C. tropicalis* are occasionally seen. *C. albicans* may occur as a commensal organism in the mouth (Epstein et al., 1984). Candidiasis of the esophagus is one of the opportunistic infections seen in AIDS, and, indeed, its presence along with HIV infection is diagnostic of AIDS according to the CDC surveillance definition (Tavitian et al., 1986). Oral candidiasis is a very prevalent feature, occurring in about three fourths of patients with AIDS-related complex (ARC) or AIDS (Pindborg et al., 1986). Furthermore, oral candidiasis among risk group individuals may be predictive of the subsequent development of full-blown AIDS (Chandrasekar and Molinari, 1985; Murray et al., 1985). In one study as many as 59% of individuals with oral candidiasis in the high-risk groups developed AIDS (Klein et al., 1984).

Oral candidiasis associated with HIV infection may present as clinically distinct forms. These forms include pseudomembranous candidiasis, atrophic candidiasis, and angular cheilitis. Pseudomembranous candidiasis (thrush) is characterized by the presence of creamy plaques on the oral mucosa, which may appear bright red where visible (Fig. 23-1). These white plaques can be removed, reveal-

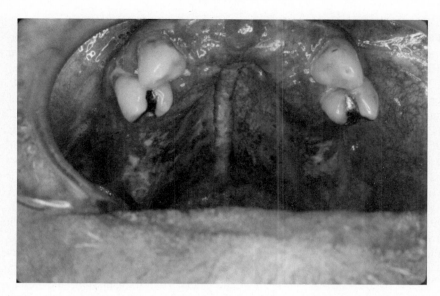

Fig. 23-1.   Pseudomembranous candidiasis in a 27-year-old seropositive man with AIDS-related complex.

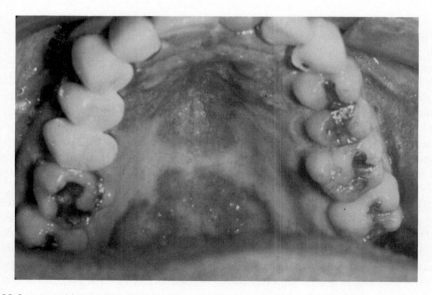

Fig. 23-2.   Atrophic candidiasis on palate of a 32-year-old seropositive man who was otherwise asymptomatic.

ing a bleeding surface. The atrophic form of candidiasis appears clinically as a red lesion, and the most common locations are the palate and the dorsum of the tongue (Fig. 23-2). When candidiasis affects the dorsal surface of the tongue, patchy depapillated areas appear. Angular cheilitis may occur alone or in conjunction with either of the other forms.

Diagnosis of oral candidiasis is made from cultures and examination of potassium hydroxide suspensions of smears, showing hyphae and blastospores. Little is known of the pathogenesis of HIV-associated oral candidiasis. In other populations the development of oral candidiasis can be associated with a number of predisposing factors, including antibiotic therapy, diabetes, xerostomia, and defects in cell-mediated immunity. The destruction of helper T cells by the cytopathic effects of HIV and the subsequent profound immunodeficiency are presumably steps in the pathway that leads to oral candidiasis. However, the

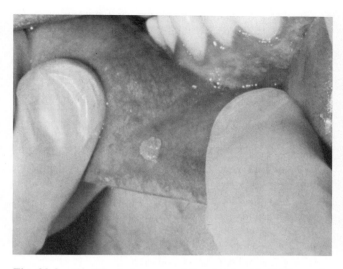

Fig. 23-3. Wartlike lesions resembling focal epithelial hyperplasia in a 28-year-old asymptomatic seropositive man.

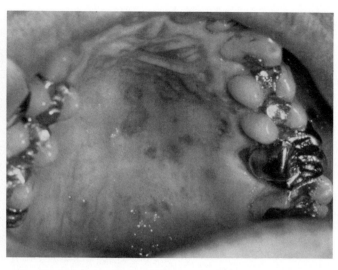

Fig. 23-4. Herpes simplex of palate. Ulcers and vesicles have been present for 2 weeks in a 21-year-old man who developed AIDS 1 month later.

exact mechanisms whereby these systemic abnormalities are expressed as local mucosal changes that permit colonization and even invasion by candidal hyphae are unknown. Treatment involves the use of systemic or topical antifungal drugs. In association with HIV infection, oral candidiasis may persist for months if untreated.

As the epidemic grows, it is likely that other opportunistic organisms will be found causing oral lesions in HIV-infected individuals (Volpe et al., 1985; Greenspan et al., 1986b).

Virus-associated lesions

In the same way that potentially pathogenic fungi are able to take advantage of the immune changes induced by HIV infection, several viruses become able to colonize or become reactivated in the mouth, producing lesions. These include herpes group viruses and papillomaviruses.

Human papilloma viruses cause warts, including oral papillomas, condylomas, and focal epithelial hyperplasia (Scully et al., 1985). Immunosuppressed individuals show an increased tendency to develop skin warts, and anogenital warts occur as a sexually transmitted disease in male homosexuals (Owen, 1980) and in promiscuous heterosexual individuals of both sexes. We have seen many cases of oral warts of all three kinds in HIV-infected individuals (Fig. 23-3).

Herpes simplex virus can produce recurrent painful episodes of ulceration on the lips and intraorally, most commonly on the palate (Fig. 23-4) (Quinnan et al., 1984). The patient may report small vesicles that erupt to form ulcers. The disease can be diagnosed from culture or from cytologic smears showing characteristic viral giant cells.

Recently more accurate confirmation by monoclonal antibodies has become available (Fung et al., 1985).

Herpes zoster caused by the varicella-zoster virus, another member of the herpes group, can also produce oral ulcerations and lesions of the facial skin. The lesions can be seen in young people with HIV infection, whereas zoster is otherwise seen in older people. Herpes zoster, when seen in HIV seropositives or those in the risk groups for AIDS, is highly predictive of the development of the full-blown syndrome.

Oral hairy leukoplakia is a white lesion that does not rub off and is found predominantly on the lateral margins of the tongue. The lesion was discovered in San Francisco in 1981 (Greenspan et al., 1984). Virtually all patients with hairy leukoplakia are antibody-positive to the AIDS virus (Greenspan et al., 1987b). Patients with hairy leukoplakia have a similar clinical and laboratory profile to those with asymptomatic HIV infection or ARC (Greenspan et al., 1984; Eversole et al., 1986). The lesion was originally seen in homosexual men and has been reported in the other risk groups for AIDS, except children (Greenspan et al., 1986b). It is found on the tongue and occasionally also on the buccal or labial mucosa. The surface may be smooth, corrugated, or markedly folded and hairy (Figs. 23-5 and 23-6). The folds tend to run vertically, along the lateral surface of the tongue. The surface may become so thick that hairlike projections appear (Fig. 23-7). Microscopically, there are characteristic changes, with folds or "hairs," hyperparakeratosis, acanthosis, vacuolation of bands or clumps of prickle cells, and little if any subepithelial inflammation (Fig. 23-8).

Hairy leukoplakia is probably a virally induced lesion.

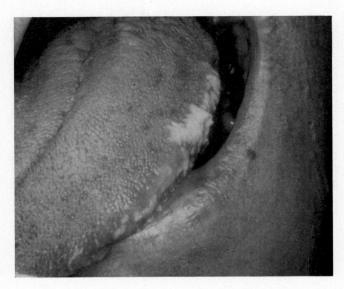

Fig. 23-5. Innocuous lesion of hairy leukoplakia on tongue of an asymptomatic seropositive 39-year-old man.

Studies have revealed the presence of EB virus in hairy leukoplakic tissue as EB viral capsid antigen on immunofluorescence, as typical particles on electron microscopy, and as the complete linear form of EB viral DNA in very high copy number in Southern blot hybridization (Fig. 23-9) (Greenspan et al., 1985b). This is the first lesion in which EB virus has been found in this prolific and fully replicating form. As to the relationship of hairy leukoplakia with the development of AIDS, data on 143 homosexual patients who had hairy leukoplakia but not AIDS have been analyzed. The data indicate that more than one half of the patients with hairy leukoplakia will develop AIDS, and that more patients with hairy leukoplakia develop *P. carinii* pneumonia as their first manifestation of AIDS than is seen in the general San Francisco AIDS population (Greenspan et al., 1987b).

Hairy leukoplakia is a remarkable lesion. It serves as a model of virally induced oral epithelial hyperplasia, presents new opportunities to study the biology of EBV infection, and is a significant clinical marker or early warning sign of HIV infection. Recent studies have suggested that very high doses of acyclovir or moderate doses of a prodrug of acyclovir, desciclovir, are effective in the short term in eliminating the lesion of hairy leukoplakia and the EB virus that infects the epithelial cells of the lesion (Greenspan et al., 1987a).

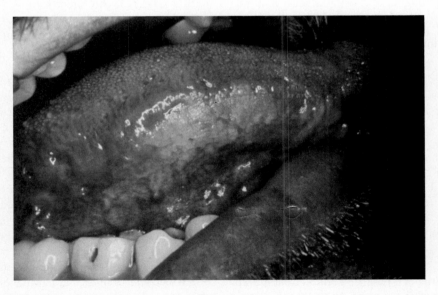

Fig. 23-6. This 31-year-old patient with AIDS-related complex had typical lesions of hairy leukoplakia on both sides of tongue.

Neoplastic lesions

The neoplastic diseases associated with AIDS may be analogous to the opportunistic infections seen in the same group of individuals. Carcinogens and oncogenic viruses are probably rendered more effective by failure of some part of the immune system, such as the tumor surveillance mechanism. These neoplastic diseases include Kaposi's sarcoma and non-Hodgkin's lymphoma.

Kaposi's sarcoma is a multicentric vascular-like neoplasm found primarily in the skin. However, Kaposi's sarcoma may occur intraorally, either alone or in association with skin, visceral, and lymph node lesions. In one study oral lesions were found in 53% of AIDS patients with Kaposi's sarcoma, and in almost 10% of cases the mouth was the only site of Kaposi's sarcoma (Lozada-Nur et al., 1984). Oral Kaposi's sarcoma can appear as red, blue, or purple lesions that may be flat or raised, solitary or multiple (Lozada-Nur et al., 1984). The most common oral site reported is the palatal mucosa, although lesions may be found on any part of the oral mucosa, including the gingiva, soft palate, and buccal mucosa (Figs. 23-10 to 23-13).

The lesion is thought to arise from either lymphatic or blood vessel endothelium. Histologic examination of early lesions shows atypical vascular channels and chronic inflammatory cells, and examination of more advanced le-

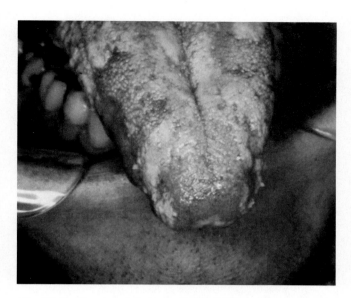

Fig. 23-7. Very extensive hairy leukoplakia covering entire dorsal surface of tongue in a 41-year-old homosexual man with AIDS-related complex.

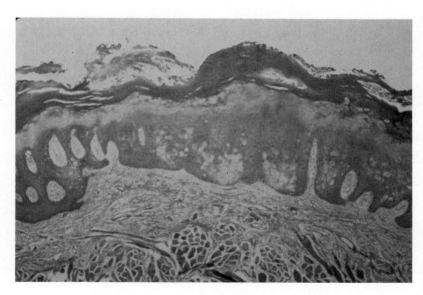

Fig. 23-8. Histologic section of hairy leukoplakic lesion showing epithelial thickening, surface projection, and ballooning cells (koilocytes).

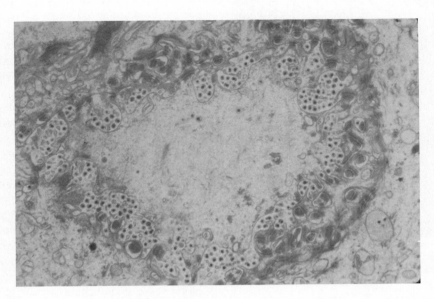

Fig. 23-9.   Electron micrograph showing typical appearance of Epstein-Barr virus in an epithelial cell in hairy leukoplakia.

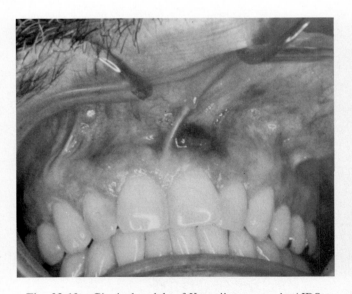

Fig. 23-10.   Gingival nodule of Kaposi's sarcoma in AIDS.

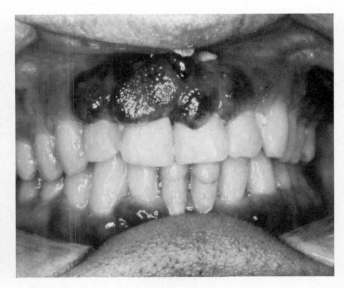

Fig. 23-11.   Extensive gingival masses of late-stage Kaposi's sarcoma.

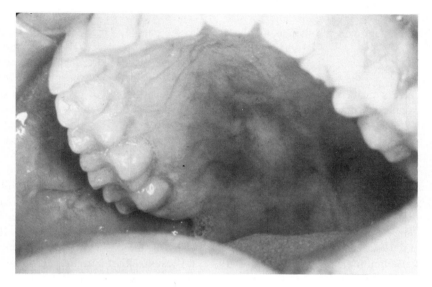

Fig. 23-12.   Purple flat lesion of Kaposi's sarcoma of hard palate in a 28-year-old male homosexual.

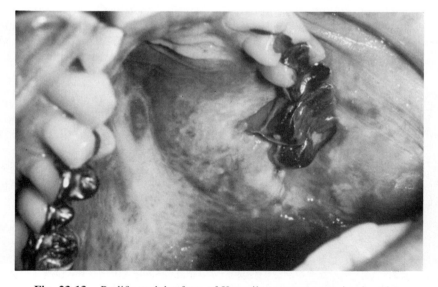

Fig. 23-13.   Prolific nodular form of Kaposi's sarcoma occurring in palate.

sions shows a prominent spindle-cell component and mitotic figures, as well as red blood cells and eosinophilic bodies (Green et al., 1984). The nature of the cofactors that cause Kaposi's sarcoma in the presence of HIV immunodeficiency is unknown, although both cytomegalovirus and angiogenic factors are being investigated. Treatment for aggressive or extensive lesions involves localized radiation therapy and chemotherapeutic agents such as vinblastine.

Other lesions

Recurrent aphthous ulcers are common oral lesions. The cause of recurrent aphthous ulcers is unknown, but hormonal factors, food allergy, stress, and viral factors have been implicated. A role for cellular immune mechanisms in the pathogenesis has been suggested (Greenspan et al., 1985a). It is our impression that there may be a recurrence of aphthous ulcers in HIV-positive patients who have not experienced any bouts for many years. Perhaps the local and systemic host defects in HIV infection are the cause of recurrent aphthous ulcers in this group of patients. The lesions have the typical appearance of aphthous ulcers, appearing as well-circumscribed ulcers with an erythematous margin (Fig. 23-14).

Salivary gland swelling and xerostomia have been reported in children (Ammann, 1985), and xerostomia alone has been reported in adults (Greenspan and Silverman, 1987).

The varied nature and important implications of the oral lesions associated with HIV infection are among the factors that make an understanding of oral soft tissue diseases increasingly important in dental practice. The dentist is in a unique position to recognize some of the earliest signs of

immunosuppression and to refer the patient for appropriate investigation and treatment.

HIV-ASSOCIATED GINGIVITIS AND PERIODONTITIS

Periodontal diseases generally progress over an extended period of time with little or no pain or discomfort to the patient. This lack of signs and symptoms frequently masks the presence of periodontal disease until severe damage has occurred. In fact, its progression normally goes undetected by the patient. On the other hand, periodontal lesions that result in pain or other marked rapidly appearing signs and symptoms usually represent more acute conditions and require immediate attention. A variety of periodontal lesions that cause generalized pain have been described previously and include acute necrotizing ulcerative gingivitis (ANUG) and the recently described periodontal lesions associated with HIV infection. Clinically, these lesions can appear to be similar.

In this section the clinical features of HIV-associated periodontal disease (HIV-P) and HIV-associated gingivitis (HIV-G) are described and compared with other periodontal lesions. Furthermore, the diagnosis, management, and treatment of HIV-P and HIV-G are discussed. Patients not clearly identified as belonging to HIV risk groups present a challenging differential diagnosis. However, it is important that the correct diagnosis be made to determine appropriate therapy. Whereas most acute periodontal lesions are self-limiting and respond to conventional therapy, those lesions associated with HIV infection often do not effectively respond and can rapidly cause extensive periodontal disease and potentially life-threatening nomalike lesions (Grassi, 1987a, 1987b; Murray et al., 1987a; Winkler and Murray, 1987; Winker et al., 1987).

Etiology

The oral cavity represents a unique microenvironment where the host is continuously defending against microbial infection (Genco and Slots, 1984; Listgarten, 1987). Microbial organisms are always present in the mouth as a heterogeneous population, although the numbers and relative proportions are constantly changing and are influenced by a wide variety of factors (Gibbons and van Houte, 1975; Slots, 1979; Socransky, 1977; Kornman and Loesche, 1980; Loesche et al., 1982; Newman, 1985). However, soft tissues of the mouth rarely become infected by microbial organisms in healthy individuals (Gibbons, 1980). Evidence suggests that the host's immune system plays a critical role in preventing microbial colonization of these tissues (Genco and Slots, 1984; Taubman et al., 1984; Listgarten, 1987).

It is well recognized that the development of periodontal disease depends on the interaction between the resident oral microbiota found in the dentogingival plaque and the host response (Listgarten, 1987). The bacteria attempt to

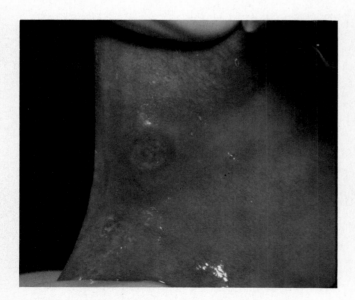

Fig. 23-14. This 31-year-old seropositive man experienced his first bout of aphthous ulcers in 15 years.

colonize and invade the periodontal tissue while the host uses a variety of defense mechanisms to maintain a dynamic equilibrium with the resident oral microbial flora (Gibbons, 1980). In fact, in the attempt to inhibit bacterial colonization, the sequence of host immune mechanisms may be activated even at the expense of damaging the periodontium in the process (Oshrain et al., 1979; Robertson et al., 1980; Genco and Slots, 1984; Taubman et al., 1984).

The etiology of the HIV-associated periodontitis (HIV-P) and gingivitis (HIV-G) remains unclear. It is likely that the compromised immune system contributes to the pathogenesis of the lesions. However, the consequences of changes in the resident flora and altered host response in the oral cavity remain unknown. We hypothesize that the periodontitis observed in HIV-infected patients, by analogy with ANUG (Loesche et al., 1982), represents an infection resulting from a shift in the oral microbiota in virulence potential or by pathogens overgrowing during periods when the tissue defense mechanisms have been compromised (Murray, 1987b).

HIV-associated gingivitis

Gingivitis is an inflammation of the free gingival margin that is associated with the presence of bacterial plaque. Typically, gingivitis has been shown to be reversible (i.e., removal of plaque and maintenance of good oral hygiene results in the return of gingival health) (Löe et al., 1965; Theilade and Theilade, 1976). On the other hand, HIV-G is characterized as not responding to plaque removal therapy. As with typical gingivitis, HIV-G is a subtle periodontal change and may easily go unnoticed by the un-

trained eye. Our data demonstrate that individuals with HIV-associated gingivitis frequently show no other intraoral or extraoral signs or symptoms of HIV infection (Figs. 23-15 and 23-16) and frequently are unaware of their HIV-sero status.

In evaluating the clinical features of HIV-G, it is necessary to be systematic. A systematic clinical approach requires an orderly examination of the gingiva for the following features: color, ease of bleeding, pain, involvement of the attached gingiva, and involvement of the alveolar mucosa. HIV-G is characterized by a red linear band on the free gingival margin, red patellae, and/or diffuse red lesions on the attached gingiva and a fiery red appearance to the mucosa (Fig. 23-17). In addition, spontaneous bleeding is frequently observed in the interproximal regions.

Color. A distinct linear red band can be noted on the free gingival margin (Fig. 23-17). On close inspection, the red margin usually has a translucent appearance with distinct capillary loops. In some cases this linear band is very subtle but definitely apparent to the trained eye (Fig. 23-18).

Bleeding. Interproximal spontaneous bleeding is characteristic of HIV-G even after treatment (see Fig. 23-17). This presence of gingival bleeding is frequently the chief complaint of patients seeking treatment.

Pain. Pain is not characteristically a feature of the early HIV-G lesion but may be present immediately prior to progression to HIV-P.

Lesions of the attached gingiva. A unique feature of HIV-G is the distinctive red petechiae often seen on the attached gingiva. These petechiae are distinct from the small

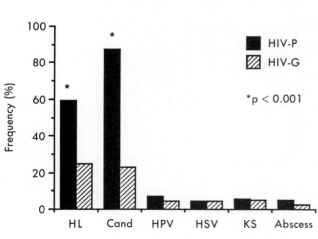

Fig. 23-15. Relationship of other HIV-associated intraoral lesions to HIV-P and HIV-G. *HL,* Hairy leukoplakia; *Cand,* candidiasis; *HPV,* human papilloma virus; *HSV,* herpes simplex virus; *KS,* Kaposi's sarcoma.

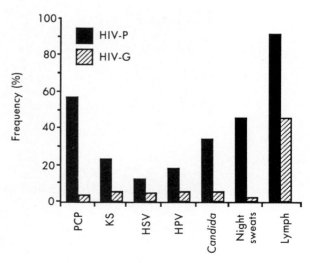

Fig. 23-16. Relationship of selected HIV-associated extraoral features to HIV-P and HIV-G. *PCP, Pneumocystis carinii* pneumonia; *KS,* Kaposi's sarcoma; *HSV,* herpes simplex virus; *HPV,* human papilloma virus.

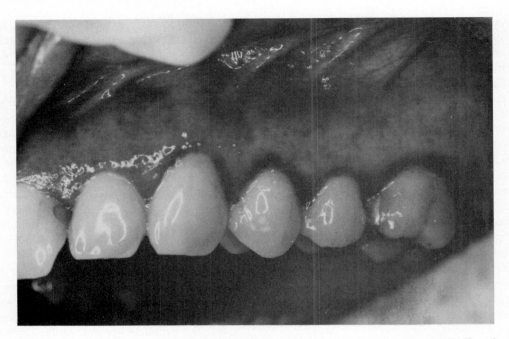

Fig. 23-17.   Close-up view of HIV-G. This photograph shows clinical features of HIV-G and lack of response to therapy after 2 weeks of extensive scaling and root planing and excellent oral hygiene.

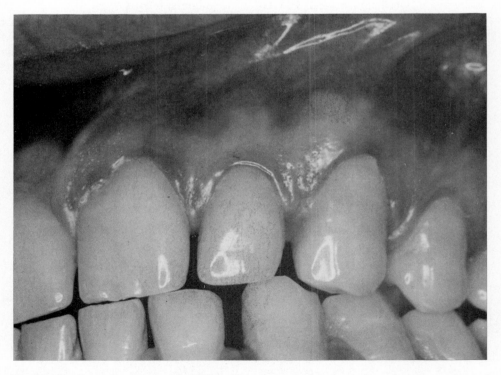

Fig. 23-18.   Example of very early HIV-G. Note changes occurring in free gingival margins and attached gingiva of central incisor.

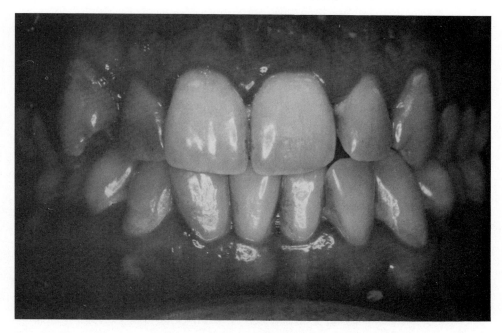

Fig. 23-19. Colonization of attached gingiva and vestibular mucosa by *Candida*. Removal of these white lesions by wiping will leave red, bleeding ulcerations. These lesions are easily confused with petechiae seen in HIV-G.

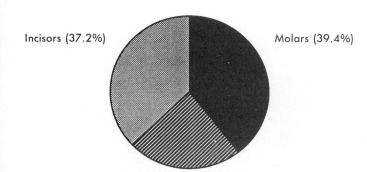

Incisors (37.2%) Molars (39.4%)

Premolars (23.4%)

Fig. 23-20. Distribution of HIV-G.

areas of bleeding ulceration that result from the removal of *Candida* colonies from the mucosa by wiping with a gauze (Fig. 23-19). The petechiae are most frequently seen as isolated lesions and are uniformly spread over the attached gingiva (see Fig. 23-17). Occasionally they appear to coalesce into a diffuse red band involving the entire attached gingiva.

Lesions of the alveolar mucosa. An additional distinctive feature of HIV-G is the presence of a bright red vestibular mucosa. The mucosa is typically a diffuse red but may show isolated petechiae. In cases of generalized HIV-G the vestibular changes are seen throughout the mouth.

Location. HIV-G most frequently involves the entire mouth and is usually distributed equally to all quadrants (Fig. 23-20). In some mouths, however, it is found in limited regions involving one or two teeth.

Lack of response to therapy. The most distinguishing feature of HIV-G is its lack of response to conventional therapy. Repetitive scaling and root planing, prophylaxis, and good oral hygiene do not appear to substantially improve the clinical appearance (see Fig. 23-17). Unlike conventional gingivitis, the distinct red band seen on the free gingival margin of these patients is not specifically associated with the accumulation of plaque. In fact, plaque scores are frequently quite low in these patients (Fig. 23-21).

Differential diagnosis. Many systemic diseases may cause color changes in the oral mucosa including the gingiva (Dummett, 1979). In general, these abnormal color changes are nonspecific in nature and should stimulate further diagnostic efforts or referral to the proper specialist. The importance of diagnosing HIV-G is twofold. First, this lesion may represent one of the first signs of HIV infection and consequently aid in the identification of HIV-positive individuals (Winkler and Murray, 1987). Second, available clinical data suggest that HIV-G may be the ini-

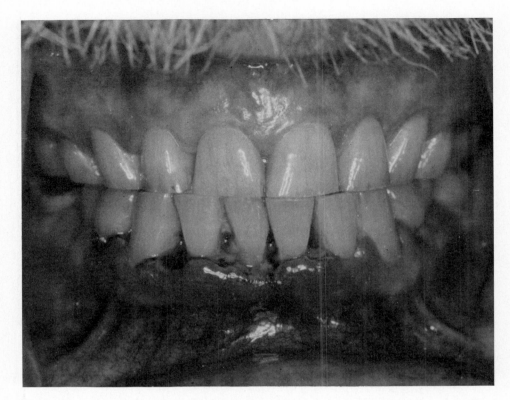

Fig. 23-21. HIV-seropositive patient with low plaque scores. Note lack of disease on maxillary arch but definite signs of HIV-P on mandibular arch.

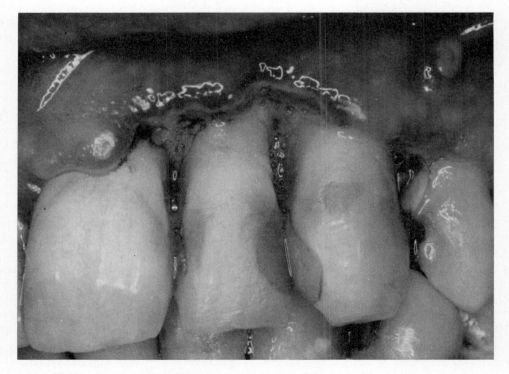

Fig. 23-22. Close-up view of HIV-P in a 30-year-old HIV-seropositive homosexual patient.

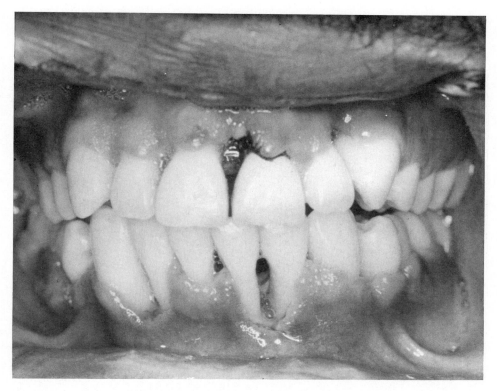

Fig. 23-23.   Generalized HIV-P in a 28-year-old HIV-seropositive man. Note spontaneous interproximal bleeding.

tial stage of HIV-P (Winkler et al., 1987). Consequently, efforts to control HIV-G may prevent the unnecessary breakdown of periodontal tissues.

HIV-associated periodontitis

On first inspection it is difficult to differentiate HIV-P from ANUG (Johnson and Engel, 1986; Sabiston, 1986). HIV-P resembles ANUG superimposed on a rapidly progressive severe periodontitis (Figs. 23-21 to 23-23; see also Fig. 23-25, *A*). In fact, further studies may show that HIV-P is a form of ANUG (Pindborg et al., 1967). However, it seems to us that the rapidly progressive nature of HIV-P clearly distinguishes this lesion clinically from ANUG (Williams et al., 1988).

Individuals with HIV-P, in contrast to those with HIV-G, are frequently aware of their seropositive status and/or have other manifestations of HIV infection such as candidiasis, hairy leukoplakia, Kaposi's sarcoma, or PCP (see Fig. 23-16). Consequently, early identification of these lesions is a particularly important role for the dental professional.

The major clinical features of HIV-P are intense erythema of attached and marginal gingiva; interproximal necrosis, ulceration, and cratering; extremely rapid bone loss; pain, including severe "deep" pain; and spontaneous

gingival bleeding. As with HIV-G, HIV-P appears to respond poorly to conventional therapy. Patients show little response to scaling and root planing and improved oral hygiene (Figs. 23-24 and 23-25). Available clinical data clearly suggest that the atypical gingivitis may indeed be the initial stage of HIV-associated periodontitis (Winkler and Murray, 1987; Winkler et al., 1988).

Color.   The free gingiva is bright, fiery red. In most cases the free gingival margin has a red linear border similar to that seen in HIV-G. In severe cases of HIV-P, there is no distinct border or separation between the free and attached gingiva.

Interproximal necrosis, ulceration, and cratering. The HIV-P lesion typically starts with changes in gingival contour such as interproximal necrosis, ulceration, and cratering. Unlike ANUG, the soft tissue involvement is not limited to the papillary region and free gingival margin. Soft tissue destruction can extend on to the attached gingiva and alveolar mucosa as well (Fig. 23-26).

Odor.   Fetor oris may or may not be present, but does not appear to be of diagnostic significance for HIV-P. In most cases of HIV-P, fetor oris is apparent. However, in contrast to ANUG, there is no detectable correlation between severity of disease and fetor oris.

Spontaneous bleeding/nocturnal bleeding.   Sponta-

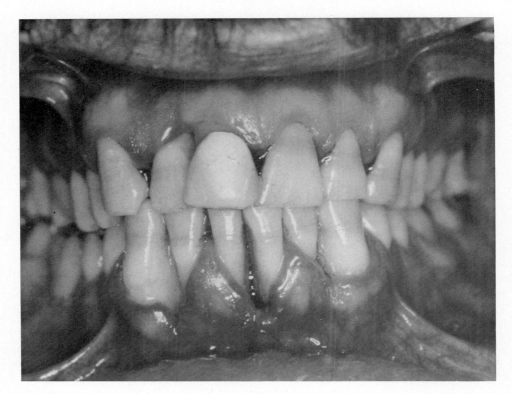

Fig. 23-24.   Generalized HIV-P in a 32-year-old HIV-seropositive man after treatment. Note extensive destruction. Interestingly, spontaneous interproximal bleeding still exists after 1 month of extensive treatment.

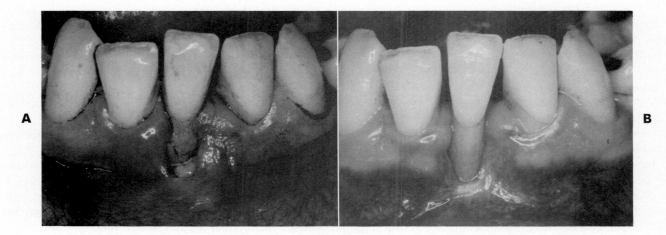

Fig. 23-25.   **A,** HIV-P localized to a mandibular incisor. **B,** HIV-P lesion seen in **A** 1 month after treatment.

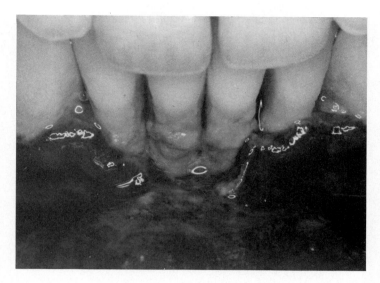

Fig. 23-26.   Necrotic involvement of vestibular mucosa in direct relationship to HIV-P.

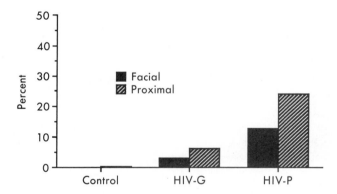

Fig. 23-27.   Percentage of sites in control, HIV-G, and HIV-P individuals showing spontaneous bleeding at initial visit.

neous and/or nocturnal bleeding is frequently reported. Patients report waking up with a blood clot in their mouth, blood on their pillow, and excessive bleeding on brushing and flossing. On initial clinical examination as many as 25% of the interproximal sites show spontaneous bleeding (Fig. 23-27).

Severe pain.   Severe pain is a distinguishing feature of HIV-P. In fact, this is the chief complaint of many patients and the reason that causes them to seek dental treatment. Unlike the ANUG patient, in whom pain is located in the "gums" (Johnson and Engel, 1986), the pain of HIV-P is described as being localized to the jaw bones, or as being a deep, aching pain. Frequently patients report that it feels as if their teeth are hitting the jaw bone when chewing. Often this deep pain precedes the development of the clin-

ically obvious HIV-P lesion. The cause of this pain is not clear but is probably the result of rapid bone destruction.

Lesions of the attached gingiva and alveolar mucosa. It appears that the inflammatory response of HIV-P also involves the attached gingiva, as well as the vestibular mucosa. HIV-P lesions have similar soft tissue clinical features to those seen in HIV-G. For example, the free marginal gingiva has the distinct red band, the attached mucosa appears to have the petechiae lesions, and the vestibular mucosa also is a diffuse fiery red. Frequently the necrosis of gingival tissue extends onto the alveolar mucosa (see Fig. 23-26).

Rapid bone loss.   The most distinguishing feature of HIV-P is its rapid destruction of the periodontal attachment and bone (Murray et al., 1987; Winkler and Murray, 1987; Winkler et al., 1987). In HIV-P lesions the loss of >90% attachment loss has been seen in some teeth in as little as 3 to 6 months (Fig. 23-28) and in many cases has resulted in exodontia. Soft tissue cratering, interproximal necrosis, and ulceration are seen in direct relationship to the regions of bone loss. In HIV-P it appears that tissue destruction is not limited to the soft tissues and rapidly spreads to the next naturally occurring anatomic structures. Consequently, the periodontal and alveolar bone may be rapidly destroyed. In contrast, the lesions of ANUG are normally self-limiting to the soft tissue of the periodontium (Pindborg et al., 1967; Johnson and Engel, 1986). Although bone loss can be seen in some cases of recurrent severe ANUG, this is usually the result of multiple attacks over many years. Individuals with HIV-P, on the other hand, typically report no previous long-term ANUG history.

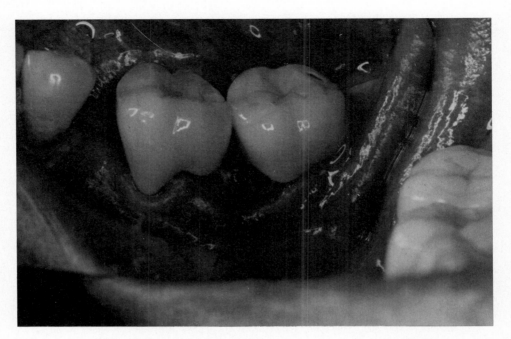

Fig. 23-28. Interproximal bone loss between two molars in less than 3 months in a 40-year-old HIV-seropositive male homosexual patient.

In some cases we have noted that necrosis of the connective tissue progresses at a greater rate than the subjacent bone. This results in denudation and eventual sequestration of bone (Fig 23-29). Osseous involvement does not appear to be limited to the periodontal bone (Fig. 23-30). Sequestration of bone has been seen in combination with aggressive soft tissue lesions suggestive of noma.

Location of lesions.   Severe cases of HIV-P can affect all of the teeth and surrounding periodontium. More frequently HIV-P affects several localized areas independently, resulting in islands of severely involved periodontium surrounded by relatively normal tissue. In fact, it is frequently observed that only one surface of the tooth, (e.g., the distal) is severely involved with HIV-P while the remaining surfaces are only slightly involved. The reason for such discrete localization is unclear. On the other hand, all regions of the mouth appear to have similar chances of being affected (Fig. 23-31). An important observation is that the HIV-P lesions are always associated with areas of preexisting or coexisting HIV-G. This observation, along with longitudinal clinical data, suggests that HIV-G is the precursor lesion to HIV-P.

Pocket depth.   Pocket depth is not a distinguishing factor between HIV-G and HIV-P. In HIV-P, the loss of periodontal soft tissue occurs at such a rapid rate that little or no pocket formation occurs. This is in definite contrast to chronic inflammatory periodontal disease wherein the loss of attachment precedes the loss of overlying periodontal tissues and results in the formation of pockets.

Differential diagnosis

Proper diagnosis is essential for rational treatment. First, an overall appraisal of the patient should be made. This includes a thorough medical history. The systemic history aids in (1) the diagnosis of oral manifestations of systemic disease, (2) the detection of systemic conditions that may affect the periodontal tissues, and (3) the detection of systemic conditions that require careful modification of treatment procedures. This is of particular importance in the treatment of HIV-infected individuals because of their propensity for a variety of opportunistic infections (Gottlieb et al., 1983). As seen above, HIV-P can quickly progress to rapid periodontal destruction and exodontia. In fact, this rapid progression can involve tissues other than the periodontium. Besides the unnecessary loss of hard and soft tissues, misdiagnosis can further endanger the HIV-infected individual by the inappropriate use of antibiotics. Unfortunately, many of the clinical features are easily confused with a variety of other periodontal diseases.

Treatment

In most periodontal diseases, the removal of the primary etiologic agent, bacterial plaque, is generally sufficient to reverse the inflammation (Löe et al., 1965). In contrast, conventional treatment by scaling and root planing alone has not proved to be sufficient therapy to obtain substantial resolution of HIV-P and HIV-G lesions. The intriguing question of why HIV-G and HIV-P do not respond in the typical manner is not clear at this point and is

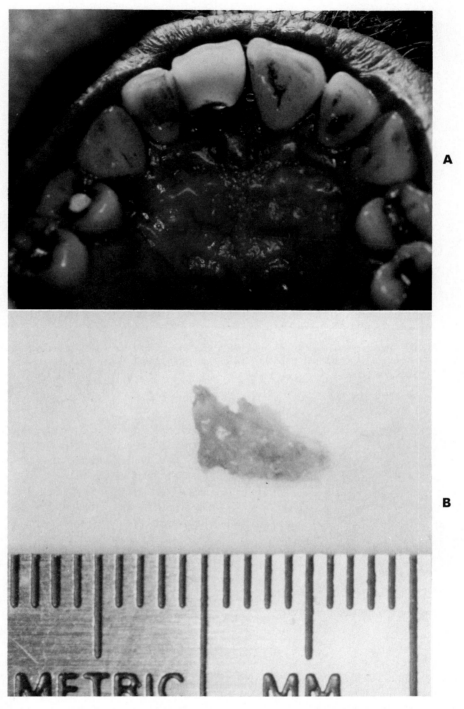

Fig. 23-29.   A, Bone sequestrum between central incisors as a result of HIV-P. This sequestrum was noticed approximately 1 month after treatment had begun. **B,** Bone sequestrum removed from patient seen in Fig. 23-28 during scaling and root planing. Multiple sequestra were removed from other sites.

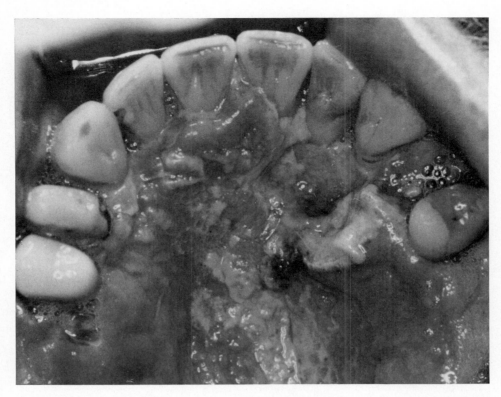

Fig. 23-30. Aggressive HIV-P involving palate of a 30-year-old male homosexual who tested HIV seropositive 1 week earlier. Four days before this photograph was taken, only a redness of palatal tissues was seen.

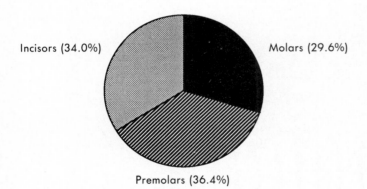

Fig. 23-31. Site frequency distribution of HIV-P.

undergoing active investigation. The answer may lie in either the flora involved or the alterations that have occurred in the immune system of HIV-infected individuals.

In general, antibiotics are contraindicated for the treatment of HIV-G and HIV-P because of their potential for increasing candidal superinfection. The use of broad-spectrum antibiotics such as penicillins and tetracycline is associated with increased superinfection of *Candida* even in in-dividuals with intact immune systems. As mentioned above, *Candida* is a frequent opportunistic infection of HIV-infected individuals and can cause life-threatening systemic manifestations. In cases where it is deemed necessary to use antibiotic therapy, the use of antifungal therapy is a necessity and should be done in consultation with the patient's primary physician.

At present, our treatment for HIV-P involves the use of scaling and root planing, in conjunction with povidone-iodine (Betadine) and Peridex (Grassi et al., 1989). Povidone-iodine is most familiar as a surgical scrub. The active agent, iodine, is one of the oldest antimicrobials known. Iodine is a contact antimcrobial and is effective against bacteria, fungus, and some viruses (Molinari 1983).

Treatment is usually divided into two phases: the acute phase and the maintenance phase. The primary problem in the acute phase of treatment of the HIV-P lesion is pain control. Povidone-iodine, interestingly, has a topical anesthetic effect immediately after application that is usually profound enough to allow for adequate initial debridement. This is particularly important when the entire mouth is involved. In addition to the problem of pain control, bleeding can be quite severe, compounding the difficulty in achieving adequate debridement. Since povidone-iodine tends to cause an increased coagulation of blood during the debridement procedure, the use of this agent allows for timely and efficient initial debridement to occur. This combination of properties—topical antimicrobial, topical anesthetic, and aid in blood coagulation—has made it our current agent of choice for the acute treatment of HIV-P and HIV-G.

Povidone-iodine is used in both office treatment and home treatment of patients. In the office, povidone-iodine is placed into the pockets and/or onto the necrotic tissues using a syringe equipped with a blunt needle. After a few minutes the tissues can usually be curettaged without undue discomfort. It is necessary to apply povidone-iodine frequently during the procedure for maximum effect. The patient is then given the irrigation syringe to take home and instructed to "squirt" some povidone-iodine interproximally, a minimum of five times a day, and told not to rinse for at least one half hour. Approximately 3 to 5 ml of povidone-iodine is used for each application.

With this treatment most patients return the next day with significant reduction of pain and are able to brush, floss, and/or use interproximal brushes for oral hygiene. Patient compliance has been excellent, presumably because of the pain relief that the agent provides. Before povidone-iodine is recommended for a patient, however, the practitioner should ascertain that no history of sensitivity to iodine exists.

Frequently, the povidone-iodine regimen is continued for several weeks until healing is well under way. Unfortunately, it appears that long-term use of povidone-iodine for maintenance may not be the answer. First of all, it stains both hard and soft tissues and is difficult to remove even with a professional prophylaxis. More important, we have observed that those of our patients who have used povidone-iodine for longer than 1 month show a tendency to relapse clinically.

For long-term maintenance we are using chlorhexidine-containing preparations such as Peridex. Peridex, besides being an effective antimicrobial, has the advantage of substantivity (i.e., binding to hard and soft tissues) and need not be applied as frequently (Löe et al., 1976; Lang and Brecx, 1986). In addition, the staining seen with Peridex occurs at a slower rate and is more easily removed. At present, Peridex is not recommended for the acute treatment of HIV-P lesions, because the alcohol vehicle found in Peridex is extremely irritating to the necrotic soft tissue and exposed bone. Furthermore, Peridex does not provide the topical anesthetic effect seen with povidone-iodine. However, once epithelialization has successfully occurred, Peridex is well tolerated. Many of our patients who have been maintained on a regimen of Peridex have not had relapses for as long as 6 months.

Metronidazole has been used for some time in the treatment of ANUG and other related anaerobic infections (Loesche et al., 1981, 1987). In severe infections we have used this antibiotic in conjunction with scaling and root planing and the topical antimicrobial agents mentioned above. This combination of treatment has proved to be very successful and has not resulted in candidal superinfection. However, the use of this antibiotic should probably be limited to aggressive lesions involving large areas of denuded bone. One advantage of metronidazole, when compared with other antibiotics, is that it can be administered effectively for a very short course of 3 to 5 days. Furthermore, it is fairly specific for anaerobes, which are probably the primary flora involved in HIV-G and HIV-P (Grassi et al., 1987a, 1987b). It does not appear to substantially affect the aerobic flora. Consequently, the niches for candidal colonization are not made available, as is the case with other antibiotics. Both properties reduce the risk of candidal superinfection.

In summary, it appears that scaling and root planing alone are insufficient to handle the periodontal lesions associated with HIV-infection, particularly HIV-P. The indiscriminate use of antibiotics for treatment of this local infection is contraindicated because of the risk of fungal overgrowth that can be life-threatening in this patient population. In some severe cases, metronidazole has been used, but with great caution. Treatment by frequent application of povidone-iodine in conjunction with debridement and scaling and root planing seems to be an effective therapy during the acute phases of HIV-P. Long-term maintenance with povidone-iodine does not seem adequate, and the condition may require the use of chlorhexidine-containing agents.

REFERENCES

Abrams DI et al: Antibodies to human T-lymphotropic virus type III and development of the acquired immunodeficiency syndrome in homosexual men presenting with immune thrombocytopenia, Ann Intern Med 104:47, 1986.

Ammann AJ: The acquired immunodeficiency syndrome in infants and children, Ann Intern Med 103:734, 1985.

Asjo B et al: Susceptibility to infection by the human immunodeficiency virus (HIV) correlates with T4 expression in a parental monocytoid cell line and its subclones, Virology 157:359, 1987.

Barin F et al: Serological evidence for virus related to simian T-lymphotropic retrovirus III in residents of west Africa, Lancet 2:1387, 1985.

Barre-Sinoussi F et al: Isolation of a T-lymphotropic retrovirus from a patient at risk for acquired immune deficiency syndrome (AIDS), Science 220:868, 1983.

Biggar RJ: The AIDS problem in Africa, Lancet 1:79, 1986.

Black JL: AIDS: preschool and school issues, J Sch Health 56:93, 1986.

Centers for Disease Control (CDC): Oral viral lesion (hairy leukoplakia) associated with acquired immunodeficiency syndrome, MMWR 34:549, 1985.

Centers for Disease Control (CDC): Current trends: Classification system for human T-lymphotropic virus type lll/lymphadenopathy-associated virus infections, MMWR 35:334, 1986.

Chaisson RE et al: Significant changes in HIV antigen level in the serum of patients treated with azidothymidine, N Engl J Med 315:1610, 1986.

Chaisson RE et al: Human immunodeficiency virus infection in heterosexual intravenous drug users in San Francisco, Am J Public Health 77:169, 1987.

Chandrasekar PH and Molinari JA: Oral candidiasis: forerunner of acquired immunodeficiency syndrome (AIDS), Oral Surg 60:532, 1985.

Clumeck N: Heterosexual transmission of AIDS: no time for complacency, Eur J Clin Microbiol 5:609, 1986.

Collaborative Study Group of AIDS in Haitian-Americans: Risk factors for AIDS among Haitians residing in the United States: evidence of heterosexual transmission, JAMA 257:635, 1987.

Cooper DA et al: Acute AIDS retrovirus infection: definition of a clinical illness associated with seroconversion, Lancet 1:537, 1985.

Cowan MJ et al: Maternal transmission of acquired immunodeficiency syndrome, Pediatrics 73:382, 1984.

Curran JW and Morgan WM: AIDS in the United States: future trends. In Gluckman JC and Vilmer E, editors: Acquired immunodeficiency syndrome (international conference on AIDS, Paris 1986), Paris, 1987, Elsevier.

Dummett CO: Oral tissue color changes, Ala J Med Sci 16:274, 1979.

Epstein JB, Truelove EL, and Izutzu KT: Oral candidiasis: pathogenesis and host defense, Rev Infect Dis 6:96, 1984.

Eversole LR et al: Oral condyloma planus (hairy leukoplakia) among homosexual men: a clinicopathologic study of thirty-six cases, Oral Surg 61:249, 1986.

Fischl MA et al: Evaluation of heterosexual partners, children, and household contacts of adults with AIDS, JAMA 257:640, 1987.

Fisher AG et al: The trans-activator gene of HTLV-lll is essential for virus replication, Nature 320:367, 1986.

Francis DP: The prospects for and pathways toward a vaccine for AIDS, N Engl J Med 313:1586, 1985.

Fung JC, Shanley J, and Tilton RC: Comparison of herpes simplex virus-specific DNA probes and monoclonal antibodies, J Clin Microbiol 22:748, 1985.

Genco RJ and Slots J: Host responses in periodontal diseases, J Dent Res 63:441, 1984.

Gerbert B: AIDS and infection control in dental practice: dentists' attitudes, knowledge, and behavior, J Am Dent Assoc 114:311, 1987.

Gibbons RJ: Adhesion of bacteria to surfaces in the mouth. In Berkley RCW et al., editors: Microbial adhesion to surfaces, Chichester, England, 1980, Ellis Howard, Ltd.

Gibbons RJ and van Houte J: Bacterial adherence in oral microbial ecology, Ann Rev Microbiol 29:19, 1975.

Golding H et al: Identification of homologous regions in HIV 1 gp41 human MHC Class II beta 1 domain. I. Antibodies against the gp41 derived peptide react with native HLA Class II antigens suggesting a role for autoimmunity in the pathogenesis of AIDS, J Exp Med 167:914, 1988.

Gottlieb MS et al: The acquired immunodeficiency syndrome, Ann Intern Med 99:28, 1983.

Grassi M, Murray PA, and Winkler JR: Microbiologic evaluation of AIDS virus associated periodontitis, Third International Conference on AIDS, Washington, DC, 1987a (abstract).

Grassi M et al: Zahnartz und HIV-Infektionen, Schweiz Monatsschr Zahnmed, 1987b.

Grassi M et al: Local treatment of HIV-associated periodontal disease, Manuscript submitted for publication, 1989.

Green TL et al: Histopathologic spectrum of oral Kaposi's sarcoma, Oral Surg 58:306, 1984.

Greenspan D and Greenspan JS: Oral mucosal manifestations of AIDS. In Disorders of mucous membranes, Dermatol Clin 5:733, 1987.

Greenspan D and Silverman S, Jr: Oral lesions of HIV infection, CDA J 15(1):28, 1987.

Greenspan D et al: Oral "hairy" leucoplakia in male homosexuals: evidence of association with papillomavirusus and a herpes-group virus, Lancet 2:831, 1984.

Greenspan D et al: AIDS and the dental team, Copenhagen, 1986a, Munksgaard.

Greenspan D et al: Oral hairy leukoplakia in two women, a hemophiliac, and a transfusion recipient, Lancet 2:978, 1986b (letter).

Greenspan D et al: Efficacy of BWA515U in treatment of EBV infection in hairy leukoplakia, Third International Conference on AIDS, Washington, DC, 1987a (abstract).

Greenspan D et al: Relation of oral hairy leukoplakia to infection with the human immunodeficiency virus and the risk of developing AIDS, J Infect Dis 155:475, 1987b.

Greenspan JS: Infections and non-neoplastic diseases of the oral mucosa, J Oral Pathol 12:139, 1983.

Greenspan JS et al: Lymphocyte function in recurrent aphthous ulceration, J Oral Pathol 8:592, 1985a.

Greenspan JS et al: Replication of Epstein-Barr virus within the epithelial cells of oral "hairy" leukoplakia, an AIDS-associated lesion, N Engl J Med 313:1564, 1985b.

Guyader M et al: Genome organization and transactivation of the human immunodeficiency virus type 2, Nature 326:662, 1987.

Ho DD, Rota TR, and Hirsch MS: Infection of monocyte/macrophages by human T lymphotropic virus type III, J Clin Invest 77:1712, 1986.

Ho DD et al: Infrequency of isolation of HTLV-lll virus from saliva in AIDS, N Engl J Med 313:1606, 1985a (letter).

Ho DD et al: Isolation of HTLV-lll from cerebrospinal fluid and neural tissues of patients with neurologic syndromes related to the acquired immunodeficiency syndrome, N Engl J Med 313:1493, 1985b.

International Committee for the Taxonomy of Viruses, AIDS Subcommittee: Human immunodeficiency viruses, Science 232:697, 1986.

Johnson BD and Engel D: Acute necrotizing ulcerative gingivitis, J Periodontol 57:141, 1986.

Kanki PJ et al: New human T-lymphotropic retrovirus related to simian T-lymphotropic virus type III (STLV-lll$_{AGM}$), Science 232:238, 1986.

Katzenstein DA et al: Risks for heterosexual transmission of HIV in Zimbabwe, Third International Conference on AIDS, Washington, DC, 1987 (abstract).

Klein RS et al: Oral candidiasis in high-risk patients as the initial manifestation of the acquired immunodeficiency syndrome, N Engl J Med 311:354, 1984.

Kloster BE, Tomar RH, and Spira TJ: Lymphocytotoxic antibodies in the acquired immune deficiency syndrome (AIDS), Clin Immunol Immunopathol 30:330, 1984.

Kornfeld H et al: Cloning of HTLV-4 and its relation to simian and human immunodeficiency viruses, Nature 326:610, 1987.

Kornman KS and Loesche WJ: The sub-gingival microbial flora during pregnancy, J Periodont Res 15:111, 1980.

La Pointe N et al: Transplacental transmission of HTLV-lll virus, N Engl J Med 312:1325, 1985.

Lang NP and Brecx MC: Chlorhexidine digluconate—an agent for chemical plaque control and prevention of gingival inflammation, J Periodont Res (suppl 16):74, 1986.

Lange JM et al: Persistent HIV antigenaemia and decline of HIV core antibodies associated with transition to AIDS, Br Med J 293:1459, 1986.

Levy JA et al: Isolation of lymphocytopathic retroviruses from San Francisco patients with AIDS, Science 225:840, 1984.

Levy JA et al: Isolation of AIDS-associated retroviruses from cerebrospinal fluid and brain of patients with neurological symptoms, Lancet 2:586, 1985.

Listgarten MA: Nature of periodontal disease: pathogenic mechanisms, J Periodont Res 22:172, 1987.

Löe H, Theilade E, and Jensen B: Experimental gingivitis in man, J Periodontol 36:177, 1965.

Löe H et al: Two years' oral use of chlorhexidine in man. I. General design and clinical effects, J Periodont Res 11:135, 1976.

Loesche WJ et al: Treatment of periodontal infections due to anaerobic bacteria with short-term treatment with metronidazole, J Clin Periodontol 8:29, 1981.

Loesche WJ et al: The bacteriology of acute necrotizing ulcerative gingivitis, J Periodontol 53:223, 1982.

Loesche WJ et al: Metronidazole therapy for periodontitis, J Periodont Res 2:224, 1987.

Lozada-Nur F et al: The diagnosis of AIDS and AIDS related complex in the dental office: findings in 171 homosexual males, CDA J, p 21, June, 1984.

McDougal JS et al: Binding of HTLV-III/LAV to T4+ T cells by a complex of the 110K viral protein and the T4 molecule, Science 231:382, 1986.

McKusick L et al: Reported changes in the sexual behavior of men at risk for AIDS, San Francisco, 1982-1984—the AIDS Behavioral Research Project, Public Health Rep 100:622, 1985.

Molinari JA: Sterilization and disinfection. In Schuster GS, editor: Oral microbiology and infectious disease, ed 2, Baltimore, 1983, Williams & Wilkins.

Montagnier L et al: Identification and antigenicity of the major envelope glycoprotein of lymphadenopathy-associated virus, Virology 144:283, 1985.

Mosca JD et al: Herpes simplex virus type-1 can reactivate transcription of latent human immunodeficiency virus, Nature 325:67, 1987.

Moss AR: What proportion of HTLV-III antibody positives will proceed to AIDS? Lancet 2:223, 1985 (letter).

Moss AR: AIDS and intravenous drug use: the real heterosexual eipdemic (editorial), Br Med J 294:389, 1987.

Murray HW et al: Patients at risk for AIDS-related opportunistic infections, N Engl J Med 313:1504, 1985.

Murray PA, Grieve WG, and Winkler JR: The humoral immune response in HIV-associated periodontitis, Third International Conference on AIDS, Washington, DC, 1987a (abstract).

Murray PA et al: The bacteriology of the HIV-associated perio lesions, Manuscript submitted for publication, 1987b.

New York City Department of Health AIDS Surveillance: The AIDS epidemic in New York City, 1981-1984, Am J Epidemiol 123:1013, 1986.

Newman MG: Current concepts of the pathogenesis of periodontal disease: microbiology emphasis, J Periodontol 56:734, 1985.

Oshrain HI, Mender S, and Mandel ID: Periodontal status of patients with reduced immunocapacity, J Periodontol 50:185, 1979.

Owen WF: Sexually transmitted disease and traumatic problems in homosexual men, Ann Intern Med 92:805, 1980.

Pahwa S et al: Spectrum of human T-cell lymphotropic virus type III infection in children: recognition of symptomatic, asymptomatic, and seronegative patients, JAMA 255:2299, 1986.

Pape JW et al: Risk factors associated with AIDS in Haiti, Am J Med Sci 291:4, 1986.

Pindborg JJ, Bhat M, and Roed-Petersen B: Oral changes in South Indian children with severe protein deficiency, J Periodontol 38:218, 1967.

Pindborg JJ et al: Suggestion for a classification of oral candidiasis in patients with AIDS, ARC, and serum antibodies for LAV/HTLV-III, J Dent Res 65:765, 1986.

Plummer FA et al: Incidence of human immunodeficiency virus (HIV) infection and related disease in a cohort of Nairobi prostitutes, Third International Conference on AIDS, Washington, DC, 1987 (abstract).

Pollack MS et al: Lymphocytotoxic antibodies to non-HLA antigens in the sera of patients with acquired immunodeficiency syndrome (AIDS), Prog Clin Biol Res 133:209, 1983.

Popovic M et al: Detection, isolation, and continuous production of cytopathic retroviruses (HTLV-III) from patients with AIDS and pre-AIDS, Science 224:497, 1984.

Price JH: AIDS, the schools, and policy issues, J Sch Health 56:137, 1986.

Purtilo DT: Lymphotropic viruses, Epstein-Barr virus (EBV), and human T-cell lymphotropic virus-I (HTLV-I), adult T-cell leukemia virus (ATLV), and HTLVIII/human immune deficiency virus (HIV) as etiological agents of malignant lymphoma and immune deficiency, AIDS Res 1(suppl):S1, 1986.

Quinnan GV et al: Herpes virus infections in the acquired immunodeficiency syndrome, JAMA 252:72, 1984.

Redfield RR et al: Heterosexually acquired HTLV-III/LAV disease (AIDS-related complex and AIDS): epidemiologic evidence for female-to-male transmission, JAMA 254:2094, 1985.

Reichart PA, Pohle HD, and Gelderblom H: Oral manifestations of AIDS, Dtsch Z Mund Kiefer Gesichts Chir 9:167, 1985.

Reichart PA et al: AIDS and the oral cavity, The HIV-infection: virology, etiology, origin, immunology, precautions and clinical observations in 110 patients, Int J Oral Maxillofac Surg 16:129, 1987.

Robertson PB et al: Periodontal status of patients with abnormalities of the immune system. II. Observations over a 2-year period, J Periodontol 51:70, 1980.

Sabiston CB: A review and proposal for the etiology of acute necrotizing gingivitis, J Clin Periodontol 13:727, 1986.

Sande MA: Transmission of AIDS: the case against casual contagion, N Engl J Med 314:380, 1986 (editorial).

Scully C et al: Papillomaviruses: their possible role in oral disease, Oral Surg 60:166, 1985.

Sharer LR et al: Pathologic features of AIDS encephalopathy in children: evidence for LAV/HTLV-III infection of brain, Hum Pathol 17:271, 1986.

Slots J: Subgingival microflora and periodontal disease, J Clin Periodontol 6:351, 1979.

Socransky SS: Microbiology of periodontal disease—present status and future considerations, J Periodontol 48:497, 1977.

Starcich BR et al: Identification and characterization of conserved and variable regions in the envelope gene of HTLV-III/LAV, the retrovirus of AIDS, Cell 45:637, 1986.

Stricker RB et al: Target platelet antigen in homosexual men with immune thrombocytopenia, N Engl J Med 313:1375, 1985.

Taubman MA et al: Host response in experimental periodontal disease, J Dent Res 63:455, 1984.

Tavitian A, Raufman JP, and Rosenthal LE: Oral candidiasis as a marker for esophageal candidiasis in the acquired immunodeficiency syndrome, Ann Intern Med 104:54, 1986.

Theilade E and Theilade J: Role of plaque in the etiology of periodontal disease and caries, Oral Sci Rev 9:23, 1976.

Volpe F, Schimmer A, and Barr C: Oral manifestation of disseminated *Mycobacterium avium intracellulare* in a patient with AIDS, Oral Surg 5:567, 1985

Williams CA, Winkler JR, and Grassi M: Necrotizing stomatitis associated with AIDS, Fourth International Conference on AIDS, Stockholm, 1988 (abstract).

Winkler JR, Grassi M, and Murray PA: Periodontal disease in HIV-infected male homosexuals, Third International Conference on AIDS, Washington, DC, 1987 (abstract).

Winkler JR and Murray PA: Periodontal disease: a potential intraoral expression of AIDS may be rapidly progressive periodontitis, CDA J 13:20, 1987.

Winkler JR et al: Periodontal indices of HIV-seropositive individuals, Manuscript submitted for publication, 1988.

Yarchoan R et al: Administration of 3'-azido-3'-deoxythymidine, an inhibitor of HTLV-III/LAV replication, to patients with AIDS or AIDS-related complex, Lancet 1:575, 1986.

Antiinfective and Adjunctive Management of Periodontal Diseases

Antiinfective and Adjunctive Management of Periodontal Diseases

Part II

Chapter 24

MEDICAL AND DENTAL HISTORY AND SYSTEMIC LABORATORY TESTS

Louis F. Rose
Barbara J. Steinberg

Patient evaluation
Medical history
Interpretation of clinical laboratory studies
    Complete blood count
    Blood glucose
    Blood urea nitrogen
    Serology
    Screening tests for hemorrhagic disorders
Medical risk assessment
Dental history

PATIENT EVALUATION

Medical emergencies can occur in any patient; however, they are most prevalent in geriatric or medically compromised patients. There is a rapidly growing segment of the population whose physical or psychosocial problems may complicate dental treatment. The elderly or medically compromised patient, who is frequently taking one or more medications, such as steroids, anticoagulants, cardiac drugs, or immunosuppressive agents, may require special consideration before undergoing dental treatment. As ever-increasing numbers of such individuals seek dental care, it becomes the responsibility of the dentist to avoid adverse therapeutic interactions and to deal with medical emergencies when they occur.

Careful study has shown that the compromised patient is actually in the majority, with more than 50% of 4365 patients recently surveyed giving a history of more than one significant medical problem. Sophisticated surgical manipulation and medical intervention have made possible the ambulatory treatment of patients with cardiovascular, endocrine, and degenerative diseases—disorders that just a few years ago would have meant confinement or death. These medical advances, along with the increasing public awareness of dental health, probably explain the increased numbers of elderly and chronically ill patients seeking dental treatment.

With an increasing likelihood of medical emergencies in this population, the practicing dentist and auxiliary staff is responsible for identifying patients with a potential for medical risk by obtaining a comprehensive pretreatment physical evaluation. This evaluation is performed to determine patients' physical and emotional status and how well they will tolerate a specific dental procedure.

Little and King (1971) have presented the reasons for an evaluation of general health in the dental office, and these are summarized as follows:

1. To identify patients with undetected systemic disease that could be a serious threat to the life of the patient or whose condition could be complicated by dental treatment
2. To identify patients who are taking drugs or medications that could adversely interact with drugs prescribed, that would complicate dental therapy, or that may serve as a clue to an underlying systemic disease the patient has failed to mention

3. To provide information for the dentist to modify the treatment plan for the patient in light of any systemic disease or potential drug interactions
4. To enable the dentist to select and communicate with a medical consultant concerning the patient's possible systemic problems
5. To help establish a good patient-doctor relationship by showing patients the clinician's interest in them as individuals and concern for their overall well-being

The information obtained from a comprehensive health evaluation may prevent a medical emergency. A well-conceived evaluation of the patient includes the following: (1) recording a complete medical history; (2) recording appropriate findings on physical examination; (3) when indicated, ordering and interpreting necessary laboratory studies; and (4) initiating medical consultation or referral as needed.

In addition, the medical evaluation must be updated every time the patient is seen during maintenance therapy (e.g., every 3 to 6 months) and at appropriate intervals during protracted active therapy to detect changes in general health that may affect dental treatment.

MEDICAL HISTORY

History taking is a technique for eliciting subjective information. These data are organized logically to convey the patient's physical and emotional status. Diagnosis of a specific medical disorder may require consultation. The medical history puts the physical examination into perspective by supplying information that should alert the examiner to suspected abnormalities. Even in a life-threatening situation, once the immediate threat has been contained, a history should be obtained from the patient if possible, or from a relative or friend if the patient is unable to respond.

Two basic methods for obtaining a medical history are the questionnaire and the personal interview. At first, it might seem that a great deal of time and trouble could be saved if we were to have each patient complete a printed questionnaire and then have the answers coded. There are, however, several problems with this approach. For instance, a "no" answer may mean the patient never had the symptoms or the disease, or that the question is not understood or is thought to be irrelevant, since the patient only wants to have a tooth restored or extracted. On the other hand, a personal history elicited by dialogue allows for observation of the patient and reactions to questions. This is often more important than the answer itself. The personal dialogue interview allows the practitioner to evaluate the patient's mental status in a nonthreatening atmosphere. The patient who is afraid or uninterested will respond quite differently from the one who is self-confident and truly concerned about oral health.

A questionnaire can be used in conjunction with the di-

alogue history to obtain a more complete medical history. The questionnaire may help a patient recall frequently used medications and various symptoms that indicate disease. It can also assist the dentist in determining which areas to emphasize and further explore when conducting the dialogue. The questionnaire completed by the patient in privacy can also alleviate embarrassment in answering questions concerning habits or addictions, sexual preferences, or venereal diseases, all of which are important components of a complete medical history.

A comprehensive medical history helps the dentist evaluate present health status, past medical history, allergies, medications, and pertinent familial and social history, as well as conduct a body systems review. The following information may be elicited under each area of the medical history.

Present health status. The patient should be asked the date and results of his last complete physical examination. If the patient states, for example, that he has diabetes, it is important to determine the date of the initial diagnosis, the degree of success in controlling the disease, and the therapeutic regimen, as well as the date, type, and results of the last blood glucose study. If the patient has not had a recent physical examination, it may be advisable to make a recommendation for an examination, especially if the patient is in a high-risk group. The patient's perception of his present health status may be an important indication of his psychologic makeup and potential compliance with treatment.

Past medical history. The date, diagnosis, and treatment rendered at significant hospitalizations and illnesses during childhood and adult life will help evaluate the patient's past medical history and clearly indicate whether his average state of health has been one of normal vigor or chronic illness.

Allergies. The patient should be asked if he is allergic or has reactions to any foods, medications, or environmental factors. Specifically, aspirin, local anesthetics, antibiotics, and any other allergens that may be used in dental therapy should be mentioned.

Medications. In questioning about medications, it is imperative to determine the brand and/or generic name of the drug, why and by whom it was prescribed, the dosage, and the length of time the medication has been taken. Patients may not include medications used for allaying anxiety or for inducing sleep, such as tranquilizers and sedative-hypnotic drugs. An effective way of obtaining this information is by asking patients if they ever have to take anything to help them rest, relax, or sleep. Also, some women will not include oral contraceptives or supplemental hormones, either of which may affect the oral tissues.

Review of systems. The review of body systems (see box on opposite page) is the main component of the interview approach to history taking. It provides additional data about each system and reveals signs and symptoms not al-

Review of systems

1. *Skin:* Itching, rash, ulcers, excessive dryness, pigmentary change, changes in hair or nails, hair loss
2. *Eyes:* Vision, inflammation, diplopia, blurring
3. *Ears, nose, throat:* Hearing, earache, epistasis, sore throat, hoarseness, sinus pain
4. *Respiratory:* Cough, sputum (describe quantity, color, odor, blood), wheezing, infections, exposure to tuberculosis, prior chest x-ray examination
5. *Cardiac:* Chest pain on exertion, palpitation, dyspnea, orthopnea, swelling of ankles, history of rheumatic fever, rheumatic heart disease, "heart attack," high blood pressure, murmur
6. *Gastrointestinal:* Appetite, nausea, vomiting, dysphagia, heartburn, indigestion, food intolerance, abdominal pain, jaundice, hepatitis
7. *Genitourinary:* Dysuria, nocturia, polyuria, hematuria, frequency, difficulty starting stream, sexually transmitted diseases, kidney infection
   For women:
   a. Menstrual history—last menstrual period and previous menstrual periods; dysmenorrhea
   b. Menopause—age of occurrence, hot flushes
   c. Obstetric history—pregnancies, miscarriages, living children
8. *Extremities*
   a. Vascular—varicose veins, phlebitis.
   b. Joints—pain, stiffness, swelling of joints
   c. Muscles—weariness, pain, tenderness, cramps
9. *Nervous system:* Syncope, convulsions, headache, vertigo, tremor, paralysis, paresthesias, anesthesias
10. *Hematopoietic:* Bleeding tendency, excessive bruising, anemia, known exposure to radiation or toxic agents
11. *Psychiatric:* "Nervousness," irritability, depressions, history of previous "nervous breakdown," family history of mental illness

ready elicited that may indicate a previously treated or undiagnosed disorder. The review of systems helps to refresh the patient's memory, hopefully preventing inadvertent forgetfulness.

Family history. The family history is taken to determine if there is a familial predisposition to diseases or if there are diseases in which inheritance is an important factor, such as diabetes. For example, a patient with a strong family history of diabetes mellitus, with no apparent signs or symptoms of the disease, should be evaluated periodically, since clinical manifestations may appear later in life. Also, those with a history of diabetes may have a greater risk for developing infections such as periodontal disease. The dentist should inquire specifically about a family history of diabetes, cancer, heart disease, high blood pressure, seizure disorders, mental disorders, and other diseases that may be familial.

Social history. The social history may assist in determining the patient's response to the demands and conflicts of modern society. In addition, it may help to explain the untoward reactions of a patient to his health problems and to the therapeutic recommendations. For example, the alcoholic patient may be unwilling to follow recommendations about diet and oral hygiene. Also, the alcoholic patient is an anesthetic risk and may develop prolonged and profound hypotensive episodes secondary to certain anxiety and pain-control drugs. The social history should include the patient's occupation and any associated health hazards, marital status, diet, and use of alcohol, tobacco, or other drugs. Possible exposure to various infectious diseases—hepatitis B, herpes, or acquired immunodeficiency syndrome (AIDS)—should also be determined. The social history is therefore important in assessing whether a patient is in a high-risk group for conditions such as alcoholism, drug addiction, or contagious infections such as herpes, hepatitis, or AIDS. Direct confirmation of these conditions often requires testing and consultation.

Medical summary and recommendations. Positive findings should be summarized and recommendations recorded. This will enable the dentist and the dental staff to quickly review a patient's medical status at each visit and facilitate the diagnosis and treatment of any medical emergency that may arise.

Initially, the medical history form described here represents one of the most accurate methods for determining the physical and emotional status of the patient, the patient's tolerance for specific procedures, and the presence of any medical risk factors. In essence, this form aids in decisions to proceed with dental treatment with relative safety or to seek medical consultation before beginning therapy.

In conclusion, the comprehensive medical history is an important procedure for dentists to adopt and routinely use to ensure that their patients are receiving the optimum benefit from all available health resources. A form for recording the medical history as suggested by the American Dental Association is given in the box on pp. 328 and 329.

INTERPRETATION OF CLINICAL LABORATORY STUDIES

On occasion the patient's medical history and physical examination warrant laboratory tests to confirm a diagnosis or to uncover incidental findings separate from the chief complaint. Depending on the dentist's background and experience in interpreting such tests, he will refer directly to either a clinical laboratory or a physician for appropriate examination, tests, and opinion. With the first alternative the dentist assumes responsibility for the interpretation and then the referral to a physician for confirmation and treatment if indicated. With the second alternative the physician assumes all responsibility for preparing the patient and evaluating the findings.

Table 24-1 lists some commonly used clinical laboratory tests.

Medical history

Date _____

Name _____   Address _____
    Last   First   Middle   Number and Street

City _____ State _____ Zip code _____ Home phone _____ Business phone _____

Date of birth _____ Sex _____ Height _____ Weight _____ Occupation _____

Social Security No. _____ Single ____ Married ____ Name of spouse _____

Closest relative _____   Phone _____

If you are completing this form for another person, what is your relationship to that person? _____

Referred by: _____

In the following questions, circle yes or no, whichever applies. Your answers are for our records only and will be considered confidential.

1. Are you in good health? . . . . **Yes** **No**
2. Has there been any change in your general health within the past year? . . . . **Yes** **No**
3. My last physical examination was on _____
4. Are you now under the care of a physician? . . . . **Yes** **No**
   a. If so, what is the condition being treated? _____
5. The name and address of my physician is _____
   _____
   _____

6. Have you had any serious illness or operation? . . . . **Yes** **No**
   a. If so, what was the illness or operation? _____
7. Have you been hospitalized or had a serious illness within the past 5 years? . . . . **Yes** **No**
   a. If so, what was the problem? _____
8. Do you have or have you had any of the following diseases or problems?
   a. Damaged heart valves or artificial heart valves . . . . **Yes** **No**
   b. Congenital heart lesions . . . . **Yes** **No**
   c. Cardiovascular disease (heart trouble, heart attack, coronary insufficiency, coronary occlusion, high blood pressure, arteriosclerosis, stroke) . . . . **Yes** **No**
      (1) Do you have pain in your chest on exertion? . . . . **Yes** **No**
      (2) Are you ever short of breath after mild exercise? . . . . **Yes** **No**
      (3) Do your ankles swell? . . . . **Yes** **No**
      (4) Do you get short of breath when you lie down, or do you require extra pillows when you sleep? . . . . **Yes** **No**
      (5) Do you have a cardiac pacemaker? . . . . **Yes** **No**
   d. Allergy . . . . **Yes** **No**
   e. Sinus trouble . . . . **Yes** **No**
   f. Asthma or hay fever . . . . **Yes** **No**
   g. Hives or a skin rash . . . . **Yes** **No**
   h. Fainting spells or seizures . . . . **Yes** **No**
   i. Diabetes . . . . **Yes** **No**
      (1) Do you have to urinate (pass water) more than six times a day? . . . . **Yes** **No**
      (2) Are you thirsty much of the time? . . . . **Yes** **No**
      (3) Does your mouth frequently become dry? . . . . **Yes** **No**
   j. Hepatitis, jaundice, or liver disease . . . . **Yes** **No**
   k. Arthritis . . . . **Yes** **No**
   l. Inflammatory rheumatism (painful swollen joints) . . . . **Yes** **No**
   m. Stomach ulcers . . . . **Yes** **No**
   n. Kidney trouble . . . . **Yes** **No**

o. Tuberculosis . . . . **Yes** No

p. Do you have a persistent cough or cough up blood? . . . . **Yes** No

q. Low blood pressure . . . . **Yes** No

r. Venereal disease . . . . **Yes** No

s. Other _____

9. Have you had abnormal bleeding associated with previous extractions, surgery, or trauma? . . . . **Yes** No

a. Do you bruise easily? . . . . **Yes** No

b. Have you ever required a blood transfusion? . . . . **Yes** No

If so, explain the circumstances _____

_____

10. Do you have any blood disorder such as anemia? . . . . **Yes** No

11. Have you had surgery or x-ray treatment for a tumor, growth, or other condition of your head or neck? . . . . . **Yes** No

12. Are you taking any drug or medicine? . . . . **Yes** No

If so, what? _____

13. Are you taking any of the following:

a. Antibiotics or sulfa drugs . . . . **Yes** No

b. Anticoagulants (blood thinners) . . . . **Yes** No

c. Medicine for high blood pressure . . . . **Yes** No

d. Cortisone (steroids) . . . . **Yes** No

e. Tranquilizers . . . . **Yes** No

f. Antihistamines . . . . **Yes** No

g. Aspirin . . . . **Yes** No

h. Insulin, tolbutamide (Orinase), or similar drug . . . . **Yes** No

i. Digitalis or drugs for heart trouble . . . . **Yes** No

j. Nitroglycerin . . . . **Yes** No

k. Oral contraceptive or other hormonal therapy . . . . **Yes** No

l. Other _____

14. Are you allergic or have you reacted adversely to:

a. Local anesthetics . . . . **Yes** No

b. Penicillin or other antibiotics . . . . **Yes** No

c. Sulfa drugs . . . . **Yes** No

d. Barbiturates, sedatives, or sleeping pills . . . . **Yes** No

e. Aspirin . . . . **Yes** No

f. Iodine . . . . **Yes** No

g. Codeine or other narcotics . . . . **Yes** No

h. Other _____

15. Have you had any serious trouble associated with any previous dental treatment? . . . . **Yes** No

If so, explain _____

_____

16. Do you have any disease, condition, or problem not listed above that you think I should know about? . . . . . . **Yes** No

If so, explain _____

_____

17. Are you employed in any situation that exposes you regularly to x-rays or other ionizing radiation? . . . . **Yes** No

18. Are you wearing contact lenses? . . . . **Yes** No

WOMEN

19. Are you pregnant? . . . . **Yes** No

20. Do you have any problems associated with your menstrual period? . . . . **Yes** No

21. Are you nursing? . . . . **Yes** No

CHIEF DENTAL COMPLAINT:

_____

Signature of patient

_____

Signature of dentist

Courtesy American Dental Association

Table 24-1. Normal values

Test	Normal values*
Blood chemistry	
Albumin	3.8-5.0 g/dl
Bilirubin	
Direct	<0.3 mg/dl
Indirect	0.1-1.0 mg/dl
TOTAL	0.1-1.2 mg/dl
Calcium	9.2-11.0 mg/dl
	4.6-5.5 mEq/l
Creatinine	0.6-1.2 mg/dl
Glucose	70-110 mg/dl
Lactate dehydrogenase	25-100 IU/l
Phosphatase, alkaline	
Child	20-150 IU/l at 30° C
Adult	20-90 IU/1 at 30° C
Transferases	
Aspartate amino (SGOT)	16-60 U/ml at 30° C
Alanine amino (SGPT)	8-50 U/ml at 30° C
Urea nitrogen	8-23 mg/dl
Hematology	
Leukocyte count (WBC)	5000-10,000/mm^3
	$5\text{-}10 \times 10^3/\mu l$
Neutrophils	
Segmented	50%-70%
Band	0%-5%
Lymphocytes	25%-40%
Monocytes	4%-8%
Eosinophils	1%-4%
Basophils	0%-1%
Erythrocyte count (RBC)	
Male	4.6-6.2 million/mm^3
	$4.6\text{-}6.2 \times 10^5/\mu l$
Female	4.2-5.4 million/mm^3
	$4.2\text{-}5.4 \times 10^6/\mu l$
Hemoglobin	
Male	13.5-18.0 g/dl
Female	12.0-16.0 g/dl
Hematocrit	
Male	40%-54%
Female	37%-47%
RBC indices	
Mean corpuscular hemoglobin	27-31 pg
Mean corpuscular volume	80-96 μm^3
Mean corpuscular hemoglobin concentration	32%-36%
Platelet count	150,000-400,000/mm^3
	$150\text{-}400 \times 10^3/\mu l$
Bleeding time (Ivy)	1-7 min
Partial thromboplastin time	60-70 sec
Prothrombin time	12-14 sec

*These values vary with the laboratory used.

Complete blood count

The complete blood count (CBC) will routinely include the hemoglobin (HgB), hematocrit (Hct), red blood cell (RBC) count, and white blood cell (WBC) count, with a differential WBC count and a statement on the adequacy of platelets.

Hemoglobin. HgB is the oxygen carrier of the blood. The HgB is decreased in hemorrhage and anemias and increased in hemoconcentration and polycythemia. The normal range is 14 to 18 g/dl of blood in men and 12 to 16 g/dl of blood in women.

Hematocrit. The Hct reflects the relative volume of cells and plasma in the blood. In anemias and after blood loss, the Hct is lowered. In polycythemia and dehydration, it is raised. The normal Hct range is 40% to 54% for men and 37% to 47% for women, or roughly three times the HgB value.

RBC count. The RBCs contain HgB. An increase in RBCs may indicate hemoconcentration or polycythemia. A decrease in the number of RBCs may be indicative of blood loss or one of the anemias.

WBC count. WBCs are important in the bodily defense against invading microorganisms. An increase in the WBC count is seen in the leukemias, bacterial infections, infectious mononucleosis, and certain parasitic infections, as well as after exercise and emotional stress. A decrease in the WBC count is seen in aplastic anemia, lupus erythematosus, acute viral infections, and drug and chemical toxicity. A normal WBC count is 5000 to 10,000/mm^3.

There are several kinds of WBCs that can be identified microscopically; such identification is called the differential. It is important to know whether the proportions of these cells have changed, since they may be indicative of a particular type of ailment.

1. Neutrophils (50% to 70%) are increased in most bacterial infections. An increase in the number of immature neutrophils is frequently found in acute infections. This is the so-called shift to the left.
2. Eosinophils (1% to 4%) are increased in allergic conditions and parasitic infections.
3. Basophils (0% to 1%) may be increased in some blood dyscrasias.
4. Lymphocytes (25% to 40%) are noted to be increased in measles and in several bacterial or chronic infections.
5. Monocytes (4% to 8%) may be increased during recovery from severe infections and Hodgkin's disease.

Blood glucose

Blood glucose tests are performed to evaluate glucose metabolism. Basic tests for disorders of blood glucose are the fasting blood sugar (FBS), the 2-hour postprandial blood sugar test, the glucose tolerance test, and the random blood sugar test. The normal range for blood glucose is 70 to 110 mg/dl of serum.

Blood urea nitrogen

Blood urea nitrogen (BUN) is used as a screening test for kidney function; however, it is not entirely specific. An increased value may be seen in extensive kidney disease, congestive heart failure, and dehydration. Protein intake may also directly affect the BUN value. If renal disease is suspected, a more reliable assessment is the serum creatinine test. The ratio of BUN to creatinine is 10:1. The normal range for BUN is 8 to 23 mg/dl of blood.

Serology

There are a variety of serologic tests for the screening of syphilis. All are nonspecific tests for syphilis and may give both false positive and false negative results. Interpretation of these serologic tests requires correlation with the patient's history and clinical findings. Normally, results of these tests are negative; if results are positive, confirmation with the fluorescent treponemal antibody-absorption test (FTA-abs) or the microhemagglutination treponemal pallidum test (MHA-tp) is indicated.

Screening tests for hemorrhagic disorders

Bleeding time.   Bleeding time is the time required for hemostasis to occur in a standard wound of the capillary bed. Bleeding time varies with vascular and platelet abnormalities. The normal range is 1 to 7 minutes.

Platelet count.   Platelets are decreased in thrombocytopenia purpura. In myeloproliferative diseases, platelets are increased. A normal platelet count is 150,000 to 400,000/mm^3.

Prothrombin.   The prothrombin (PT) test is an indirect test of the clotting ability of the blood. It is used to establish and control the anticoagulant effect of coumadin (Dicumarol) and similar drugs. This test gives an indication of prothrombin deficiency arising from liver disease, fibrinogen deficiency, and lack of or inability of the body to utilize vitamin K. The normal range is 12 to 14 seconds, depending on the type of thromboplastin used. In treatment with coumadin, the physician will attempt to keep the prothrombin time at 2 to 2½ times the normal value.

Partial thromboplastin time.   The partial thromboplastin time (PTT) test is designed to help the clinician recognize mild to moderate deficiencies of the intrinsic clotting factors. This test is necessary because the PT entirely bypasses the intrinsic clotting system. Another use for the PTT is to demonstrate a circulating anticoagulant in plasma. The normal PTT is 45 seconds or less; however, because variations in technique are widespread, the normal range for the PTT varies somewhat between laboratories.

Table 24-2. Medical risk categories (adopted in 1962 by the American Society of Anesthesiologists, ASA)

ASA classification	Dental consideration
Physical status 1 A patient without systemic disease; a normal healthy patient	Routine dental therapy without modification
Physical status 2 A patient with mild systemic disease	Routine dental therapy with possible treatment limitations or special considerations (e.g., duration of therapy, stress of therapy, prophylactic consideration, possible sedation and medical consultation)
Physical status 3 A patient with severe systemic disease that limits activity but is not incapacitating	Dental therapy with possible strict limitations or special considerations
Physical status 4 A patient with incapacitating systemic disease that is a constant threat to life	Emergency dental therapy only with severe limitations or special considerations

MEDICAL RISK ASSESSMENT

Having completed all of the components of the physical evaluation and a thorough oral examination, the dentist must gather all of the information and determine if the patient is capable, physiologically and psychologically, of tolerating in relative safety the stresses involved in the proposed dental treatment. Is there a greater risk (of morbidity or mortality) than normal during dental therapy? If the patient is determined to be medically compromised, then appropriate modifications in the planned dental treatment must be considered to minimize the risk.

To assist the dentist in categorizing dental patients from the standpoint of medical status, each patient should be assigned an appropriate medical risk category as adopted by the American Society of Anesthesiologists. This is commonly referred to as the ASA physical status classification system and is summarized in Table 24-2.

DENTAL HISTORY

Significant items of the past dental history that should be recorded at this visit include previous restorative, periodontic, endodontic, or oral surgical treatment; reasons for loss of teeth; untoward complications of dental treatment; attitudes toward previous dental treatment; experience with orthodontic appliances and dental prostheses; and radiation or other treatment for oral or facial lesions. General features of past treatment, rather than specific, detailed, tooth-by-tooth descriptions, are needed at this time. In the case of radiation or other treatment for oral or facial lesions, exact information regarding the date and nature of the diagnosis, the type and anatomic location of treatment, and the name, address, and telephone number of the physicians and/or dentists involved, as well as the facility (hospital, clinic) where the treatment was given, must be recorded. Likewise, clear details of any previous untoward complications of dental treatment must be recorded.

REFERENCE

Little JW and King OR: The significance of physical diagnosis, patient history, data and medical screening in the dental office, Ann Dentistry 3:31, 1971.

SUGGESTED READINGS

Bates B: A guide to physical examination, Philadelphia, 1974, JB Lippincott Co.

Brasher WJ and Rees TD: The medical consultation: its role in dentistry, J Am Dent Assoc 95:961, 1977.

Coltone JA and Kafrawy AH: Medications and health histories: a survey of 4,365 dental patients, J Am Dent Assoc 98:713, 1979.

DeGowin EL and DeGowin RL: Bedside diagnostic examination, ed 2, London, 1969, Macmillan, Ltd.

Halstead CL et al: Physical evaluation of the dental patient, St Louis, 1982, The CV Mosby Co.

Hendler BH and Rose JF: Common medical emergencies: a dilemma in dental education, J Am Dent Assoc 91:575, 1975.

Hooley JR: Hospital dentistry, Philadelphia, 1970, Lea & Febiger.

Kerr DA, Ash MM, and Millard DH: Oral diagnosis, ed 6, St Louis, 1983, The CV Mosby Co.

Little JW and King OR: The significance of physical diagnosis, patient history, data and medical screening in the dental office, Ann Dent 3:31, 1972.

Malamed SF: Handbook of medical emergencies in the dental office, St Louis, 1982, The CV Mosby Co.

McCarthy FM: Emergencies in dental practice, ed 2, Philadelphia, 1972, WB Saunders Co.

Redding SW and Rose LF: The consultation: a means of communication between dentists and physicians, Gen Dent, p 54, Sept/Oct 1979.

Rose LF: Hospital dental practice, Dent Clin North Am 19(4), 1975.

Rose LF: Diagnosis and management of medical emergencies in the dental office, U Pa School Dent Med 1(3), 1977.

Rose LF: Medical history as a dental procedure, Dent Dimens, p 13, Jan-March 1977.

Rose LF and Hendler BH: Medical emergencies in dental practice, Chicago, 1981, Quintessence Publishing Co, Inc.

Rose LF, Steinberg BJ, and Hendler BH: Physical evaluation, Alpha Omegan 77(4):17, 1984.

Sonis ST and Jandinski JJ: Physical and laboratory diagnosis, Dent Clin North Am 18(1), 1974.

Vazuka FA: Essentials of the neurological examination, Philadelphia, 1968, Smith, Kline & French Laboratories.

Wasserman BS: Teaching physical evaluation in a hospital setting, J Am Dent Assoc 95:103, 1977.

Zambito RF: Hospital dental practice: a manual, New York, 1978, Medical Examination Publishing.

Chapter 25

RADIOGRAPHIC EXAMINATION

Ernest Hausmann

A radiographic image of the periodontium, alveolar bone, and adjacent tooth root is formed by x-rays penetrating these structures to varying degrees and impinging on an x-ray detector such as film. Therefore, in order to interpret a radiograph properly, one must have an understanding of mineralized and unmineralized structures in the periodontium and how x-rays are attenuated by these structures.

A radiograph represents a two-dimensional image of a complex three-dimensional object. In relation to forming such an image of the periodontal tissues, the following is discussed in this chapter: (1) how different periodontal tissue components attenuate the x-ray beam, (2) how angulation of the x-ray beam influences the radiographic image and its fidelity to the radiographed structures, and (3) the significance of the lamina dura and radiographic appearance of trabeculation to the diagnosis of periodontal and systemic diseases.

ROLE OF THE X-RAY BEAM IN APPEARANCE OF THE RADIOGRAPHIC IMAGE

When 1 g of bone is exposed to x-rays, it attenuates the x-rays about 20 times more than if they were exposed to 1 g of soft tissue. As a consequence, fewer x-rays will sensitize the film passing through the bone than will sensitize the film passing through the soft tissue, this difference being responsible for the radiographic image produced. The gray level of the exposed x-ray film at any one point (range of black to white) is a function of the amount of bone or other calcified structure and, to a lesser extent, soft tissue in the path of the x-ray beam.

HEIGHT OF THE ALVEOLAR CREST

The level of the alveolar crest, especially the interproximal alveolar crest, is of great significance in the diagnosis of destructive periodontal diseases. The position of the image of the crest on a radiographic film of alveolar bone is influenced by the direction of the x-ray beam relative to the bone. The level of the radiographic crest and its position relative to the cementoenamel junction (CEJ) will correspond to the anatomic crest when (1) the x-ray beam is directed perpendicular to the bone and (2) the film is positioned parallel to the long axis of the tooth. When the parallel technique is being used for periapical radiographs, anatomic constraints frequently require compromise in the positioning of the film and consequently the x-ray beam. The crest then can give the radiographic appearance of being closer to the CEJ than it is in situ (Fig. 25-1). When bitewing radiographs are being taken, most frequently it is possible to position the film correctly, parallel to the long axis of the tooth and the x-ray beam perpendicular. Therefore bitewing radiographs, especially vertical bitewings, are recommended for obtaining an anatomically correct image of the position of the alveolar crest.

If there is no alveolar bone loss, the level of the crest will be from 1 to 2 mm apical to the CEJ of the immediately adjacent teeth (Fig. 25-2, *A*). In health, a line connecting the CEJ of adjacent teeth will parallel the alveolar

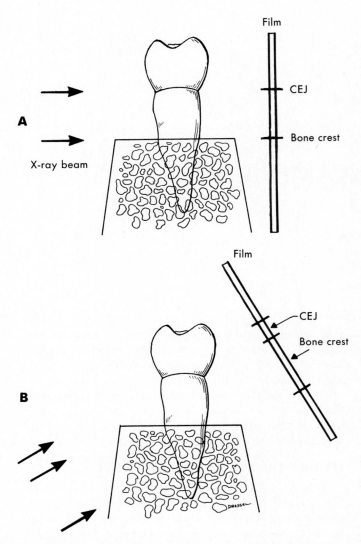

Fig. 25-1. Schematic illustration of projection of cemento-enamel junction *(CEJ)* and alveolar bone crest onto film as a function of angle of x-ray beam to tooth and bone, and of position of film. **A,** X-ray beam is perpendicular to tooth, and film is positioned parallel to long axis of tooth. **B,** Film is maintained perpendicular to x-ray beam, but relationships between x-ray and tooth and between film and tooth have been compromised.

crest. Crestal bone loss at an interdental site may be *horizontal* (Fig. 25-2, *B*), parallel to an imaginary line between the CEJs, but more apical than the 1 to 2 mm seen in health. Crestal bone loss may also be *vertical,* at an angle to the imaginary line connecting adjacent CEJs. Furthermore, it must be remembered that the crest has three dimensions, projected onto a two-dimensional radiograph. Bone loss, for example, may occur at a given interdental site to a different extent at the buccal and lingual cortical plate or may occur in the center of the interdental core of

bone, in which case no change in crestal height may be seen. Fig. 25-2, *C*, demonstrates a radiograph interpreted to represent different degrees of horizontal bone loss at the same site. Similarly, crestal loss may involve a combination of horizontal loss on one side and vertical loss on the other (Fig. 25-2, *D*). It is not possible to determine from the radiograph the number of walls of such an infrabony defect.

Under the most ideal circumstances, when two radiographs of the same location are taken with the identical geometric relation of x-ray collimator to bone and film, a difference in alveolar crest level of about 0.6 mm can be detected (Hausmann et al., 1985).

It must be recognized that identification of a decreased alveolar crestal height on a radiograph reflects only a historical record of bone loss and tells one nothing about whether bone loss continues to progress at that site at the time the radiograph was taken. Using subtraction radiography of serial standardized radiographs of patients with periodontitis, it has been demonstrated that about 9% of alveolar crestal sites with loss in radiographic bone height proceed to lose further bone in a 6-month period without any treatment (Hausmann et al., 1986; McHenry et al., 1987).

BONE CHEMISTRY AND STRUCTURE AS RELATED TO RADIOGRAPHY

Bone is composed of mineral consisting of hydroxyapatite, $Ca_{10}(PO_4)_6(OH)_2$, embedded within an organic matrix made up predominantly of collagen fibers. From a combination of analyses of autoradiographs and micrographs of histologic sections of undemineralized bone, it has been inferred that mineralization of organic matrix during bone formation takes place in essentially two steps: (1) rapid precipitation of mineral in a newly formed unit volume of matrix to about 70% of the maximum and (2) slow mineralization of the remaining matrix occurring over a span of about a month (Neuman and Neuman, 1958). Bone resorption, no matter if the inciting stimulus is systemic, such as parathyroid hormone, or local, such as interleukin-1, involves removal of both the mineral and matrix in the resorbing unit volume of bone (Meikle et al., 1986). Analyses of microradiographs of undecalcified sections from bone undergoing resorption indicates that mineral in any unit volume of bone is removed very rapidly, not slowly leached out over time.

On histologic grounds, bone can be divided into *cortical bone,* made up of haversian systems, and *trabecular bone,* made up of a network of spicules with soft tissue, marrow, or fat filling in the spaces within the network. The buccal and lingual aspects of the alveolar bone consist of cortical bone. The bone immediately adjacent to the root surfaces of teeth is also primarily cortical bone. Trabecular bone is found between the cortical buccal and lin-

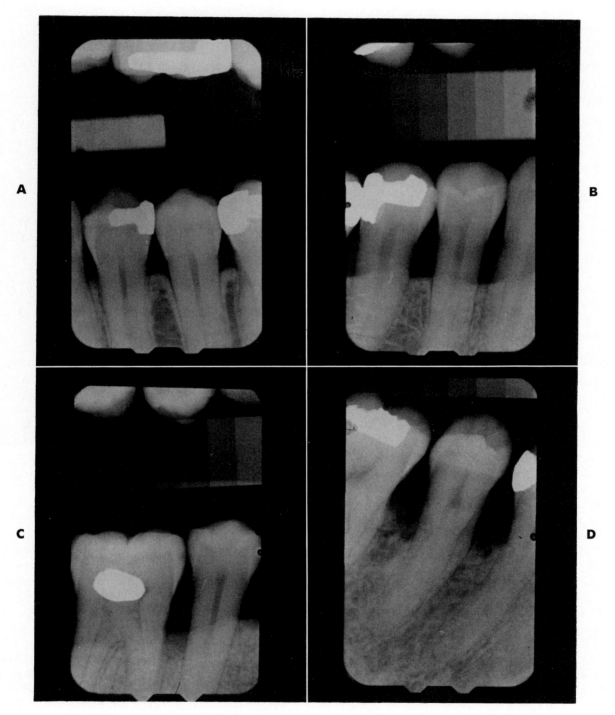

Fig. 25-2. Position and configuration of alveolar crest as seen in periapical radiographs without bone destruction and as a consequence of destructive periodontal disease. **A,** Level of alveolar crest without history of disease. **B,** Horizontal bone loss. **C,** Horizontal bone loss to a different extent in the two cortical plates at same anatomic location. **D,** Vertical bone loss.

gual plates and the lining adjacent to the tooth socket. The amount of mineral per unit mass (1 g) of cortical bone is the same as the amount of mineral per unit mass (1 g) of the spicules of trabecular bone freed of soft tissue in their interstices.

RELATING BONE STRUCTURE AND COMPOSITION TO THE RADIOGRAPHIC IMAGE

We can use physiologic facts about bone in general, specific anatomic facts about alveolar bone in particular, and the passage of x-rays through bone and their effects on film to interpret an oral radiographic image. It is important to keep in mind that an oral radiograph is a two-dimensional representation of a three-dimensional anatomic structure. For example, the gray level produced at a particular location of a film by an x-ray beam will be the same whether the beam passes through 1 g of cortical bone or 1 g of trabecular bone. However, it must be recognized that 1 g of trabecular bone is contained in a considerably larger volume than is 1 g of cortical bone. A significant consequence of this difference in relation to radiographic interpretation is the inability to predict the size of a crestal bone lesion from the size of a radiographic rarefaction.

Lamina dura

The radiographic image of the bone lining the tooth socket and the alveolar crest often appears as a dense continuous white line called the lamina dura. There exists considerable confusion in the dental literature concerning the anatomic basis of the lamina dura and alterations in the lamina dura that occur in periodontal disease and various systemic diseases. The appearance of this line is determined as much by the shape and position of the tooth root in relation to the x-ray beam as by the integrity of the bone lining the tooth socket and alveolar crest. The importance of the position of the x-ray beam to the bone is evidenced by the lack of correlation between lamina dura images on periapical and bitewing radiographs of the same location (Greenstein et al., 1981). Microradiographic evidence of undecalcified histologic sections indicate that the bone of the tooth socket wall has the same mineral content as the neighboring bone. This dense white line more likely is the result of this bone being more densely packed, with fewer and/or smaller marrow spaces than in the neighboring bone (Manson et al., 1963).

Although many clinicians believe that the absence of a continuous lamina dura is pathognomonic of active periodontal disease, crestal lamina dura when studied systematically did not appear to be related to the presence or absence of clinical inflammation, bleeding on probing, periodontal pockets, or loss of attachment (Greenstein et al., 1981). In any case, loss of lamina dura associated with periodontal disease has been associated by some with discontinuities along the alveolar crest around specific teeth.

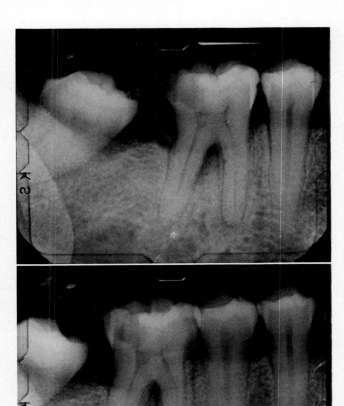

Fig. 25-3. Alveolar bone loss in a furcation as seen in two periapical radiographs taken of same site but with x-ray beam differing in horizontal angulation.

On the other hand, in systemic diseases, including hyperparathyroidism (Strock, 1941), Gaucher's disease, scleroderma, and Paget's disease, there is often complete loss of lamina dura around tooth sockets, along with alveolar crestal loss throughout the mouth (Kaffee et al., 1982).

Trabecular pattern

Attempts have been made to relate the image of the trabecular pattern, thickness of trabeculi, and their number per unit area with periodontal and systemic health status. Parfitt (1962) systematically divided the trabecular patterns seen on radiographs into coarse, medium, and fine. The predominant trabecular pattern in over 1000 individuals assessed by Parfitt fell into the medium category. The pattern observed appeared to be independent of age, sex, or tooth loss. van der Stelt et al. (1986) have suggested that the trabecular pattern in the jaw bone is characteristic of the individual and that computerized analysis of the trabe-

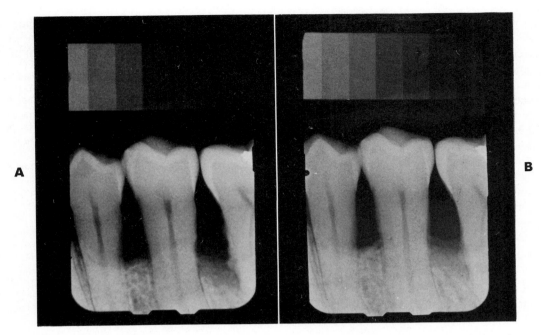

Fig. 25-4. Two radiographs of same anatomic area before and after scaling and root planing. **A,** Pretreatment radiograph showing mineralized deposits (calculus) along root surface of a molar tooth. **B,** Posttreatment radiograph; calculus has been removed.

cular pattern seen in periapical radiographs may be of forensic value for purposes of identification. No trabecular pattern has been observed, which is characteristic of periodontal disease.

The medical literature is replete with evidence of the influence of enhanced marrow activity on bone, such as in anemias due to the increased rate of red blood cell destruction and in cancer such as leukemia proliferating within the marrow spaces (Ascenzi, 1976). These influences are reflected in radiographs as thinning of trabeculi, increased size of trabecular spaces, and thinning of cortical plates resulting in rarefaction on x-rays. These radiographic changes have also been described on intraoral radiographs of most patients with sickle cell anemia (Prowler et al., 1955).

Furcations

Besides the crest, another area of alveolar bone for which change may be reflected in radiographs is in furcal regions, particularly in mandibular first molars. An area of reduced gray level, or rarefaction between the roots, may be seen as indicative of destructive periodontal disease extending into the furca. It is difficult to determine the anatomic form of a furcation defect on the basis of a radiograph. This is illustrated in the two radiographs of the same furcation lesion shown here (Fig. 25-3), which differ only in the horizontal angle of the x-ray beam to the lesion when the radiographs were made. The two radiographs

give the appearance of a difference in the anatomy of the lesion when none really exists.

Even though a rarefied area on a radiograph in a furca is indicative of bone loss in the area, a lack of rarefaction does not necessarily imply no bone loss. For example, if the x-ray beam is directed so that it penetrates a significant amount of tooth substance, loss of furcal bone may be masked.

Subgingival calculus

Radiographs may also be useful in the diagnosis of subgingival calculus (Fig. 25-4). The ability to radiographically diagnose calculus will depend on its degree of mineralization and on angulation factors of the x-ray beam. However, the radiographic appearance of calculus plates, or more often spicules, is useful in the diagnosis and monitoring of periodontal disease.

SUMMARY

The aim of this chapter on periodontal radiographic diagnosis has been to provide the reader with basic principles to use as a guide in radiographic decision making. One such principle is that the radiographic image is influenced by the angulation of the x-ray beam to the object being radiographed. The radiographic image as it is affected by x-ray beam angulation is illustrated (1) by shifts in the relationship of the alveolar bone crest to the CEJ, (2) by the inconsistency of the presence of a lamina dura in a periapical and bitewing radiograph of the same site, and (3) by apparent change of the anatomy of a furcal defect. A second principle is that a radiograph represents a two-dimensional image of a complex three-dimensional anatomic structure, making it difficult, for example, to determine the number of walls of an infrabony pocket from the radiograph. A third principle is that estimation of periodontal disease activity by assessment of bony changes presently requires comparison of radiographs of the same site taken at different times.

It is clear, then, that radiographs are invaluable aids in the diagnosis of periodontal diseases: however, their interpretation must be carried out with caution and with assessment of changes occurring in the periodontal tissues by other means such as probing, bleeding assessment, and microbiologic monitoring.

REFERENCES

Ascenzi A: Physiological relationship and pathological interferences between bone tissue and marrow. In Bourne GH, editor: The biochemistry and physiology of bone, vol 4, New York, 1976, Academic Press, Inc.

Greenstein G et al: Associations between crestal lamina dura and periodontal status, J Periodontol 52:362, 1981.

Hausmann E et al: Usefulness of subtraction radiography in the evaluation of periodontal therapy, J Periodontol 57(suppl):4, 1985.

Hausmann E et al: Progression of untreated periodontitis as assessed by subtraction radiography, J Periodont Res 21:716, 1986.

Kaffee I et al: Changes in the lamina dura as a manifestation of systemic diseases: report of a case and review of the literature, J Endod 8:467, 1982.

Manson JD: The lamina dura, Oral Surg Oral Med Oral Pathol 16:432, 1963.

McHenry K et al: Methodological aspects and quantitative adjuncts to computerized subtraction radiography, J Periodont Res 22:25, 1987.

Meikle MC et al: Advances in understanding cell interactions in tissue resorption: relevance to the pathogenesis of periodontal diseases and a new hypothesis, J Oral Pathol 15:239, 1986.

Neuman WF and Neuman MW: The chemical dynamics of bone mineral, Chicago, 1958, The University of Chicago Press,

Parfitt GJ: An investigation of the normal variations in alveolar bone trabeculation, Oral Surg Oral Med Oral Pathol 15:1453, 1962.

Prowler JR and Smith EW: Dental bone changes occurring in sickle-cell diseases and abnormal hemoglobin traits, Radiology 65:762, 1955.

Strock MS: The mouth in hyperparathyroidism, N Engl J Med 224:1019, 1941.

van der Stelt P et al: Forensic identification of trabecular patterns from dental radiographs, J Dent Res 65:176, 1986 (abstract 56).

Chapter 26

CLINICAL PERIODONTAL EXAMINATION

Gary C. Armitage

Assessment of potential etiologic factors
Recognition of gingival inflammation
Clinical assessment of damage to periodontal structures
Factors that may affect success of therapeutic intervention
    Reliability and reproducibility of periodontal probing
    Assessment of furcation involvement
    Potential mucogingival problems
    Assessment of tooth mobility
    Basics of periodontal charting

An oral examination should not be considered complete unless it includes an assessment of the patient's periodontal status. Information collected during a clinical periodontal examination is essential for determining the diagnosis and prognosis of a patient's dentition and for formulating a treatment plan. A thorough periodontal examination includes assessment of potential etiologic factors, the extent of gingival inflammation, and the amount of damage to periodontal structures, as well as an appraisal of factors that may affect the success of therapeutic intervention. To be considered clinically competent, all dentists must master the skills necessary to perform a complete periodontal examination.

ASSESSMENT OF POTENTIAL ETIOLOGIC FACTORS

In the past decade it has been well established that periodontal diseases are mixed infections associated with relatively specific groups of bacteria (Tanner et al., 1979; Moore et al., 1982, 1983; Zambon et al., 1983; Loesche et al., 1985; Slots et al., 1986). Consequently, during a peri-odontal examination it is necessary to assess the patient's current level of plaque control and to identify local conditions that might promote the colonization of teeth by periodontopathic bacteria. For example, notation should be made of dental restorations with overhanging subgingival margins, since they are difficult to clean and can enhance the proliferation of putative pathogens such as black-pigmented *Bacteroides* (Lang et al., 1983). Similarly, any situation that makes daily plaque removal difficult, such as crowded or malaligned teeth, furcation involvements, and poorly contoured restorations, should be recorded.

Even the clinical absence of heavy plaque deposits can be of significance and should be noted. For example, in some periodontal infections, such as localized juvenile periodontitis and refractory periodontitis, massive periodontal damage and considerable infection can exist with only slight amounts of clinically visible plaque. Indeed, a characteristic of sites harboring high percentages of *Actinobacillus actinomycetemcomitans*, *Bacteroides gingivalis*, or certain other gram-negative bacteria is *not* to exhibit thick deposits of plaque or calculus.

RECOGNITION OF GINGIVAL INFLAMMATION

Recognition of gingival inflammation is a basic skill required to detect infected periodontal tissues. When periodontal pathogens colonize subgingival sites in sufficient numbers, the host mounts an inflammatory response that can be observed clinically. In general, infected sites exhibit one or more of the four signs of gingival inflammation: color change, edema (swelling), bleeding on gentle probing, and gingival crevicular fluid or exudate (Figs. 26-1 and 26-2).

Inflamed gingival tissues can exhibit a wide range of

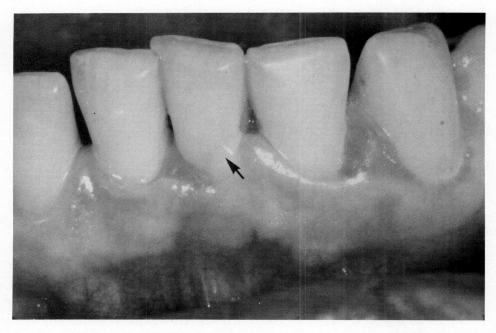

Fig. 26-1. Clinical signs of gingival inflammation in a 55- year-old woman with periodontitis. Gingival swelling and color change are particularly noticeable in interproximal areas. Purulent exudate *(arrow)* can be seen on distal half of left central incisor.

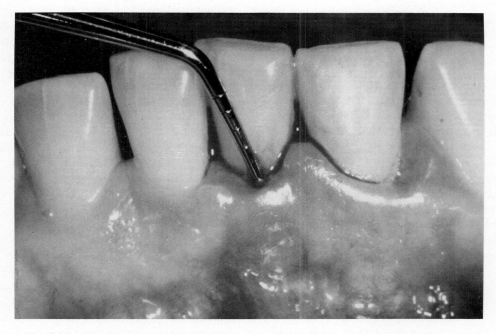

Fig. 26-2. Bleeding on gentle probing in same patient and location as shown in Fig. 26-1.

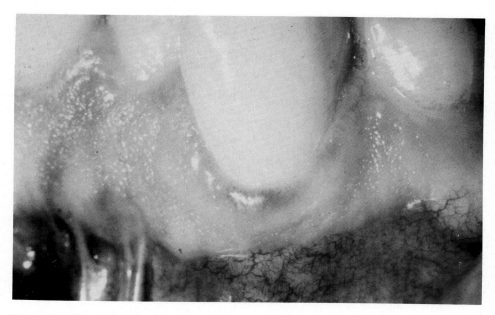

Fig. 26-3. Gingival color change (redness) of marginal gingiva of a lower right canine. Inflammatory change can be detected by comparing color of gingival margin with that of adjacent attached gingiva. (From Parr et al: Recognizing periodontal disease, San Francisco, 1978, Praxis Publishing Co.)

color changes. Most of the changes, however, are various hues of red. The redness is primarily due to an increased blood supply to the inflamed site. The best way to detect inflammatory color change is to compare the color of the gingival margin with the color of the adjacent attached gingiva (Fig. 26-3). In other words, one compares the area that is nearest the subgingival flora (and thereby inflamed) with the area least likely to be inflamed (Parr et al., 1978).

Gingival swelling or edema is a common feature of inflamed gingival tissues. Edematous gingival enlargement is due to accumulation of fluids in the inflamed gingival connective tissue. The fluid is primarily serum that has emerged from blood vessels with increased permeability due to local inflammation. Recognition of gingival edema is easy when it is marked. However, it is valuable to be able to recognize this sign of inflammation before it becomes strikingly obvious (Parr et al., 1978). In its earliest stages, gingival edema is usually confined to the first few millimeters of the gingival margin and involves changes in contour, form, texture, and consistency. Healthy sites generally have knife-edged gingival margins, and the surrounding tissues are firm and resilient. The gingiva fits snugly against the tooth. Edematous sites, on the other hand, usually have rounded gingival margins, and the adjacent tissues are somewhat enlarged and puffy. The gingiva does not fit tightly against the tooth. Detection of small amounts of gingival edema takes practice and re-

quires that the clinician have a very clear mental picture of what healthy gingiva looks like. Fortunately, gingival edema is frequently found in association with one or more of the other signs of inflammation, thereby making its recognition easier.

In clinical practice, bleeding on gentle probing is a relatively objective sign of gingival inflammation. Subjective decisions similar to those necessary for the detection of gingival redness or edema are not required, since bleeding is either present or absent. Inflamed gingival tissues bleed when probed because the epithelial lining of an infected pocket is either quite thin or has microulcerations (Fig. 26-4). Manipulation of an intact epithelial lining of a healthy gingival sulcus with a blunt instrument, such as a probe, does not elicit bleeding. Hence bleeding on probing is a simple, painless, and rapid way to identify inflamed sites.

There are many clinical situations wherein an underlying infection in deep pockets can be "hidden" by deceptively healthy-looking gingiva. Bleeding on probing can be particularly useful in identifying such sites, since it can detect inflammation at the base of periodontal pockets that would otherwise be masked from view.

The last major sign of gingival inflammation is the presence of gingival crevicular fluid that oozes from the pocket orifice. The fluid is produced by the inflamed soft tissue wall of the pocket and may range from a clear serous liquid to highly viscous pus (i.e., purulent exudate). Gingival

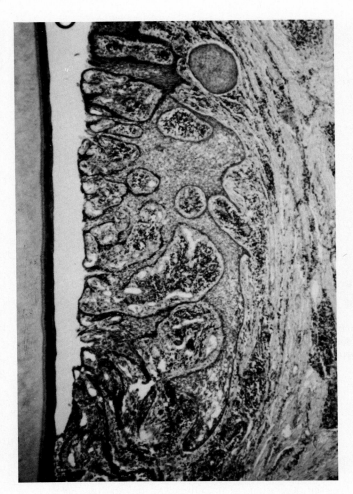

Fig. 26-4. Photomicrograph of thin, microulcerated epithelial lining of soft tissue wall of an infected pocket. Such sites readily bleed when gently probed. (×16.)

crevicular fluid is primarily composed of inflammatory cells (mostly polymorphonuclear neutrophilic leukocytes) and serum proteins. In addition, the fluid contains bacteria, tissue breakdown products, enzymes, antibodies, complement, and a wide variety of inflammatory mediators (Cimasoni, 1983). The amount and rate of fluid production at a given site are highly variable and are, in a very general way, related to the severity of inflammation.

Three basic methods can be employed for the detection of gingival crevicular fluid. The first involves isolating a site, gently drying it with an air syringe, and inserting a small filter paper strip into the crevice or pocket for 3 to 5 seconds. The strip is then removed from the site and placed in an electronic device (i.e., Periotron) that indirectly measures the volume of fluid absorbed by the strip (Golub and Kleinberg, 1976; Suppipat and Suppipat, 1977; Tsuchida and Hara, 1981). This method is particularly valuable as a research tool, since small amounts of

gingival fluid can be detected and measured objectively. Unfortunately, it has limited value in clinical practice, since the amount of gingival fluid provides no diagnostic or prognostic information. It does not distinguish between sites with gingivitis or periodontitis and cannot identify progressing or nonprogressing lesions. However, in the future it may be possible to use qualitative analyses of gingival crevicular fluid to detect, or even predict, important clinical events such as the progression of periodontitis (Armitage, 1987). Indeed, in preliminary experiments, Offenbacher et al. (1986) showed that the levels of prostaglandin E_2 in gingival crevicular fluid had some predictive value in determining if patients were in a state of remission or were about to undergo an episode of attachment loss.

The second way to detect crevicular fluid simply involves isolating and drying a site and waiting for visible amounts of fluid to collect at the pocket orifice. This method is not particularly useful in clinical situations, since sites that produce visible quantities of crevicular fluid also usually exhibit one or more of the other signs of inflammation.

In the third method, digital pressure is applied to the gingiva overlying the approximate base of the pocket and moved coronally. This is the best way to determine if purulent exudate (a form of crevicular fluid) is being produced at a given site.

CLINICAL ASSESSMENT OF DAMAGE TO PERIODONTAL STRUCTURES

Two of the main purposes of a periodontal examination are to systematically record (1) probing pocket depths and (2) probing attachment loss around each tooth. Periodontal pockets are pathologically deepened gingival sulci that develop at infected sites and are conceptually important because they represent the potential subgingival habitats for periodontopathic bacteria. The probing pocket depth is the distance from the gingival margin to the base of the probeable crevice. Probing attachment loss is the distance from the cementoenamel junction (CEJ) to the base of the probeable crevice. Attachment loss readings are important because they are the best assessment of how much damage has occurred to the periodontal apparatus.

Because a pocket can develop at any point around a tooth, its entire circumference must be probed. Probing involves "stepping" a calibrated periodontal probe around the tooth and recording the deepest point at each of six tooth surfaces: distofacial, facial, mesiofacial, distolingual, lingual, and mesiolingual (Fig. 26-5). As a general rule, a probe reading that falls between two calibrated marks on the probe should be *rounded upward* to the next highest millimeter. Thus, if the probe penetrates far enough to cover the 3 mm mark, it should be recorded as 4 mm (Parr et al., 1978).

Periodontal probing should be done gently. Ordinarily,

Facial view

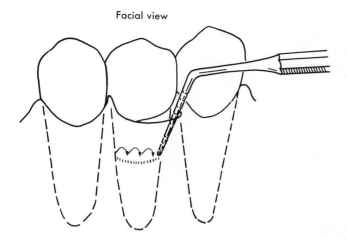

Fig. 26-5. Periodontal probing involves "stepping" a calibrated probe around tooth. (From Parr et al: Recognizing periodontal disease, San Francisco, 1978, Praxis Publishing Co.)

Proximal view

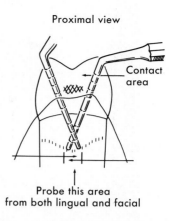

Contact area

Probe this area
from both lingual and facial

Fig. 26-6. Area under contact point should be probed from both facial and lingual aspects, since deep pockets frequently develop in this location. (From Parr et al: Recognizing periodontal disease, San Francisco, 1978, Praxis Publishing Co.)

patients should not experience discomfort from the procedure. As the probe is inserted into the pocket and moved apically along the root surface, a piece of subgingival calculus may be encountered. In such cases the probe is gently teased past the calculus and moved apically until "soft" resistance from tissues at the base of the probeable pocket is encountered. With a little practice, most examiners can readily determine when the soft tissue at the base of the lesion is reached.

In most locations an attempt should be made to probe parallel to the long axis of the tooth. Exaggerated probe angulations can lead to spuriously high pocket readings. A notable exception to this rule is when one is probing interproximal areas where it is necessary to angle the probe slightly so that the site directly under the contact point can be reached. Care should be taken to probe the area under the contact from both facial and lingual aspects, since deep pockets frequently develop in this location (Fig. 26-6).

Most practitioners do not record probing attachment loss readings at the initial examination but wait until the patient is ready to enter the maintenance phase of therapy. The two main reasons behind this approach are that many changes occur in probing attachment loss readings as a result of therapy, and the readings are easier to obtain once plaque and calculus have been removed and the inflammation has been controlled.

Probing attachment loss measurements taken at two different times are the best way to determine longitudinally if progression has occurred (Goodson, 1986). Collection of these readings can be difficult and time consuming, since it requires that one locate the CEJ as the landmark from which measurements are taken. This can be particularly difficult if there has been minimal gingival recession and

the gingival margin is located coronal to the CEJ. In such cases the position of the CEJ must be estimated by feeling for it with the probe tip. If there has been enough recession, the gingival margin will be located somewhere on the root and the CEJ will be in full view, thereby making attachment loss measurements easier to obtain. In any event, the time and trouble required to collect attachment loss measurements are worth the effort, since these readings serve as a baseline for future comparisons during the maintenance phase of therapy. (See Chapter 27 for charting.)

FACTORS THAT MAY AFFECT SUCCESS OF THERAPEUTIC INTERVENTION
Reliability and reproducibility of periodontal probing

Without question, properly used periodontal probes are the best current way to measure pocket depth and attachment loss under clinical conditions. However, periodontal probing has several drawbacks when it is used to monitor periodontal status longitudinally. From one visit to the next, it is difficult to duplicate precisely the insertion force and reproduce the site and angulation of probe insertion. Because of these technical problems, when consecutive readings of probing pocket depth are taken at a given site, it is generally expected that the probing depth may vary by up to 1 mm as a function of the limited sensitivity of this system of measurement (Glavind and Löe, 1967).

In addition, it has been established that the extent of probe penetration is influenced by the inflammatory status of the tissues (Armitage et al., 1977; Listgarten, 1980; Fowler et al., 1982; Van der Velden, 1982). In most instances when healthy tissues are examined, the probe tip stops coronal to the apical termination of the junctional ep-

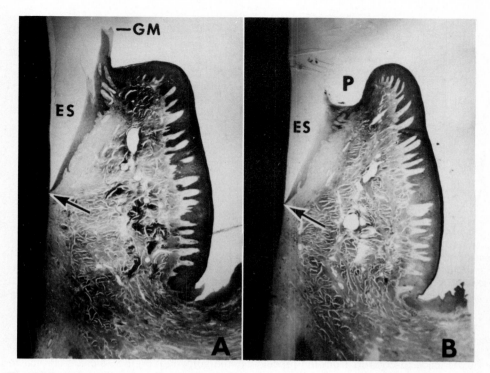

Fig. 26-7. Photomicrographs of clinically healthy facial gingiva of a lower incisor from a beagle. **A,** Site without periodontal probe. **B,** Adjacent site with probe. End of transparent plastic probe *(P)* is located coronal to apical termination of junctional epithelium *(arrows)*. *GM,* Gingival margin; *ES,* enamel space. (×30.) (From Armitage GC: J Clin Periodontol 4:173, 1977. © 1977 Munksgaard International Publishers, Ltd., Copenhagen, Denmark.)

ithelium (Fig. 26-7), whereas at inflamed sites the probe tip frequently passes apical to this point (Fig. 26-8). The depth of probe penetration partially depends on the extent to which the gingival connective tissue has been lysed or infiltrated by inflammatory cells. Stated differently, intact connective tissue underlying the crevicular epithelium is an important factor resisting probe penetration.

This has important implications as to how measurements taken with periodontal probes are interpreted. Since probes rarely stop at the exact location of the most apical cells of the junctional epithelium, probing measurements are clearly not precise assessments of the level of the connective tissue attachment. Probing overestimates connective tissue attachment loss at inflamed sites and underestimates it at noninflamed sites. Consequently, gains in probing attachment level as a result of treatment are not necessarily due to the formation of a new connective tissue attachment (Fowler et al., 1982).

In spite of these problems, properly used periodontal probes provide critically important information regarding the periodontal status of patients. Measurements obtained with periodontal probes are the best way to assess damage caused by periodontal infections and are essential for longitudinally monitoring the response to treatment. In the near future, electronic periodontal probes will become available that will allow insertion with a constant force and electronic measurement of probing pocket depths (Fuller et al., 1987; Gibbs et al., 1987; Magnusson et al., 1987). Furthermore, computer programs are being developed to provide for the automatic recording of probe readings or allow voice-activated data entry (Williams et al., 1987; Baumgarten, 1988).

Assessment of furcation involvement

When periodontal infections occur around multirooted teeth, destruction of the soft tissue and bone in the furcation area is frequently observed. Infection in these areas presents a considerable therapeutic problem, since furcations are difficult for both the patient and the therapist to clean. The type of treatment for furcation involvement is highly dependent on the extent to which the periodontal infection has destroyed tissues in the area. Therefore, for treatment planning purposes, it is important during a periodontal examination to assess the extent of furcation involvement. One of the best ways to detect furcation openings is with a curved instrument such as an explorer. A simple and useful classification system for assessing the severity of furcation involvements is as follows (Ramfjord and Ash, 1979):

Class I: Beginning involvement. The tissue destruction should not extend more than 2 mm (or not more than one third of the tooth width) into the furcation.

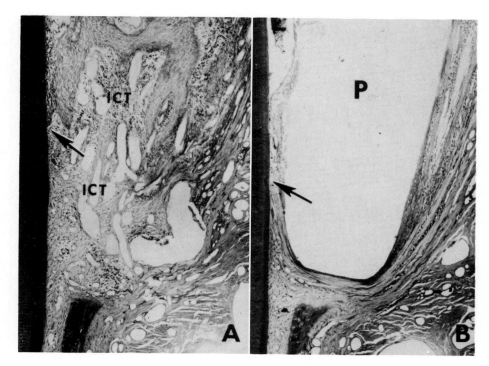

Fig. 26-8. Photomicrographs of facial gingiva of a lower premolar in a beagle with periodontitis. **A,** Site without periodontal probe. Note extensive inflamed connective tissue *(ICT)* and epithelial proliferation. **B,** Adjacent site with probe. Transparent plastic probe *(P)* has gone past apical termination of junctional epithelium *(arrows)*. Probe tip is in contact with connective tissue near alveolar crest. (×75.) (From Armitage GC: J Clin Periodontol 4:173, 1977. © 1977 Munksgaard International Publishers, Ltd., Copenhagen, Denmark.)

Class II: Cul-de-sac involvement. The tissue destruction extends deeper than 2 mm (or more than one third of the tooth width) into the furcation but does not completely pass from one furcation opening to the next.

Class III: Through-and-through involvement. The tissue destruction extends throughout the entire length of the furcation, so that an instrument can be passed between the roots and emerge on the other side of the tooth.

Potential mucogingival problems

During a periodontal examination notation is usually made of sites that have a narrow zone of attached gingiva. The boundary between keratinized attached gingiva and nonkeratinized alveolar mucosa is readily visible in most patients. It is called the mucogingival junction (Fig. 26-9). In general, sites with less than 1 mm of keratinized gingiva are usually noted, because some patients have difficulty in comfortably cleaning these areas. A toothbrush can usually be passed over keratinized gingiva without discomfort, whereas brushing of nonkeratinized alveolar mucosa can be painful. As a result, some patients avoid cleaning sites with little or no attached gingiva, and plaque-induced disease develops. It should be emphasized, however, that many patients with a "narrow" zone of at-

tached gingiva can maintain these areas quite well and require no therapeutic intervention other than routine professionally administered cleaning (Kennedy et al., 1985). In any event, it is advisable to record sites with potential mucogingival problems for treatment planning and monitoring purposes.

Assessment of tooth mobility

Since one of the major causes of increased tooth mobility is the loss of alveolar support secondary to periodontal infections, it is important that abnormal tooth mobility be recorded as part of a complete periodontal examination. Although longitudinal assessment of probing attachment loss is a superior method of determining the progression of periodontal disease, increasing tooth mobility over time suggests that some deterioration may be occurring. In addition, tooth hypermobility may have some prognostic significance (Fleszar et al., 1980). A simple classification system for recording tooth mobility is as follows:

Class I: The tooth can be moved less than 1 mm in a buccolingual direction.

Class II: The tooth can be moved 1 mm or more in a buccolingual direction but does not exhibit abnormal mobility in an occlusoapical direction.

Class III: The tooth can be moved buccolingually *and* occlusoapically.

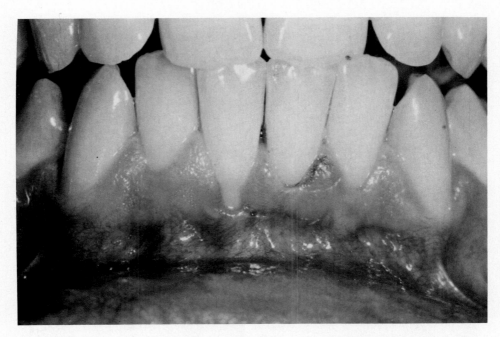

Fig. 26-9. Gingival recession on a lower right central incisor extending slightly past mucogingival junction into alveolar mucosa in a 26-year-old man. All other incisors have a relatively wide band of keratinized gingiva. Both canines have a very narrow zone of keratinized gingiva.

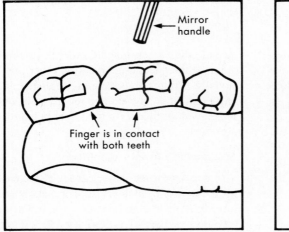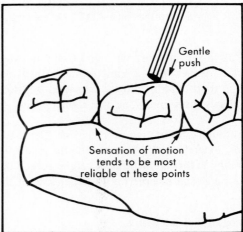

Fig. 26-10. Method for testing tooth mobility. (From Parr et al: Recognizing periodontal disease, San Francisco, 1978, Praxis Publishing Co.)

It should be emphasized that increased tooth mobility can have a variety of causes unrelated to periodontal infections. For example, hypermobility is commonly observed when teeth are under extremely heavy functional loads, for a time after orthodontic movement, and when teeth have extensive periapical disease (i.e., endodontic lesions).

It is important to remember that all teeth are mobile to some extent. However, with practice it is relatively easy to determine abnormal tooth mobility. To test for tooth mobility, it is best to place a finger on the lingual surface and gently push on the facial surface with the handle of an instrument such as a probe or mouth mirror. Usually, using an adjacent nonmoving tooth as a reference point, one can feel and see movement (Fig. 26-10).

Basics of periodontal charting

A periodontal chart should be uncomplicated, easy to read, and contain all of the basic information required for determining the patient's periodontal diagnosis, prognosis, and treatment plan. In addition, it should provide a permanent record that can be used to evaluate longitudinally the response to therapy.

Prior to therapy, essential information to be recorded on a periodontal chart should include probing pocket depths for each tooth, the amount of gingival recession on a site-by-site basis, furcation involvement, mobility, potential mucogingival problems, malalignment or crowding of teeth, defective restorations, and any other observations that may influence decisions relating to the diagnosis, prognosis, and treatment plan. An overall appraisal of the severity of inflammation, level of plaque control, and amount of supragingival and subgingival calculus is desirable. Conceptually, the periodontal chart represents a database from which one can assess the extent of damage and identify probable etiologic factors. (See Chapter 27 for charting.)

On completion of the periodontal therapy, before placing the patient on a maintenance/recall program, the periodontal examination should be repeated. The primary purposes of this examination are (1) to determine how successful the treatment was in controlling the etiologic factors and arresting the disease and (2) to provide a basis for future comparisons as the patient proceeds through the maintenance program. It is very important that probing attachment loss readings be taken during this examination, because such measurements are the most reliable way to determine if progression of disease is occurring over time.

REFERENCES

Armitage GC: Diagnosing periodontal diseases and monitoring the response to periodontal therapy. In Perspectives on oral antimicrobial therapeutics: proceedings of the symposium, Dec. 1986, Dallas, Tex., Littleton, Mass, 1987, PSG Publishing Co, Inc.

Armitage GC et al: Microscopic evaluation of clinical measurements of connective tissue attachment levels, J Clin Periodontol 4:173, 1977.

Baumgarten H: A voice input computerized dental examination system using high resolution graphics, Compend Contin Educ Dent 9(6):446, 1988.

Cimasoni G: Crevicular fluid updated, Monogr Oral Sci 12, 1983.

Fleszar TJ et al: Tooth mobility and periodontal therapy, J Clin Periodontol 7:495, 1980.

Fowler C et al: Histologic probe position in treated and untreated human periodontal tissues, J Clin Periodontol 9:373, 1982.

Fuller W et al: Reproducibility of probing pocket depth with a new constant force probe, J Dent Res 66:229, 1987 (abstract 978).

Gibbs CH et al: Florida's periodontal probe, J Dent Res 66:228, 1987 (abstract 975).

Glavind L and Löe H: Errors in the clinical assessment of periodontal destruction, J Periodont Res 2:180, 1967.

Golub LM and Kleinberg I: Gingival crevicular fluid: a new diagnostic aid in managing the periodontal patient, Oral Sci Rev 8:49, 1976.

Goodson JM: Clinical measurements of periodontitis, J Clin Periodontol 13:446, 1986.

Lang NP et al: Clinical and microbiological effects of subgingival restorations with overhanging or clinically perfect margins, J Clin Periodontol 10:563, 1983.

Listgarten MA: Periodontal probing: what does it mean? J Clin Periodontol 7:165, 1980.

Loesche WJ et al: Bacterial profiles of subgingival plaques in periodontitis, J Periodontol 56:447, 1985.

Kennedy JE et al: A longitudinal evaluation of varying widths of attached gingiva, J Clin Periodontol 12:667, 1985.

Magnusson I et al: Attachment level measurements with a constant-force probe, J Dent Res 66:228, 1987 (abstract 976).

Moore WEC et al: Bacteriology of severe periodontitis in young adult humans, Infect Immun 38:1137, 1982.

Moore WEC et al: Bacteriology of moderate (chronic) periodontitis in mature adult humans, Infect Immun 42:510, 1983.

Offenbacher S et al: The use of crevicular fluid prostaglandin E_2 levels as a predictor of periodontal attachment loss, J Periodont Res 21:101, 1986.

Parr RW et al: Recognizing periodontal disease, San Francisco, 1978, Praxis Publishing Co.

Ramfjord SP and Ash MM Jr: Periodontology and periodontics, Philadelphia, 1979, WB Saunders Co.

Slots J et al: The occurrence of *Actinobacillus actinomycetemcomitans, Bacteroides gingivalis* and *Bacteroides intermedius* in destructive periodontal disease in adults, J Clin Periodontol 13:570, 1986.

Suppipat N and Suppipat N: Evaluation of an electronic device for gingival fluid quantitation, J Periodontol 48:388, 1977.

Tanner ACR et al: A study of the bacteria associated with advancing periodontitis in man, J Clin Periodontol 6:278, 1979.

Tsuchida K and Hara K: Clinical significance of gingival fluid measurement by "Periotron," J Periodontol 52:697, 1981.

Van der Velden U: Location of probe tip in bleeding and non-bleeding pockets with minimal gingival inflammation, J Clin Periodontol 9:421, 1982.

Williams DD et al: Computer-assisted direct entry of clinical periodontal data, J Dent Res 66:229, 1987 (abstract 980).

Zambon JJ et al: *Actinobacillus actinomycetemcomitans* in human periodontal disease: prevalence in patient groups and distribution of biotypes and serotypes within families, J Periodontol 54:707, 1983.

Chapter 27

PERIODONTAL DIAGNOSIS, PROGNOSIS, AND TREATMENT PLANNING

Robert J. Genco

The oral examination of all patients in a dental practice should have a periodontal component that includes periodontal probing, tooth mobility measurements, and a radiographic survey of alveolar bone levels. The primary objective of the periodontal examination is to facilitate diagnosis and treatment planning. Another important objective of this examination is to establish baseline data so that periodontal disease changes can be detected early on subsequent examinations. Other goals of a periodontal examination are (1) to establish effective patient communication about periodontal disease and its prevention and treatment, (2) to create an awareness of periodontal disease among the dental office staff and to establish staff guidelines for early diagnosis and prevention, and (3) to obtain information on which a decision to treat or to refer the patient to a periodontal specialist can be made.

A recent survey of periodontal information in 2500 dental records from general dental practitioners showed that the status of diagnostic information describing periodontal conditions was, in general, inadequate (McFall et al., 1988). For example, conditions such as alterations in gingival color, probing pocket depths, furcation involvement, mobility, occlusal relationships, plaque, calculus, and mucogingival relationships were not described for most patients. Furthermore, a periodontal diagnosis was entered in only 16%, and gingival bleeding in only 13% of the records. Radiographs taken were mostly bitewing films of the horizontal type, which often fail to display adequately the alveolar process for a periodontal evaluation. In general, McFall et al. (1988) believed that the majority of patient records lacked sufficient diagnostic information to describe the patients' present periodontal status, and they also were inadequate to permit the practitioner to evaluate changes in the patients' periodontal status over time. This study and observations of the general inadequacy of periodontal documentation are the main impetus for providing a summary and a protocol for periodontal examination of patients in this chapter. Guidelines are provided for a *standard screening examination* for all patients and a *complete periodontal examination* for those patients who are either at high risk or in whom some signs or symptoms of periodontal disease are detected on the screening examination.

EXAMINATION

Periodontal diseases can occur in all patients regardless of age, although they are more prevalent in adults and the elderly. It was recently reported that only 15% of the U.S. population 18 years of age and older were free of any signs of periodontal disease; 50% had gingivitis, 33% moderate periodontitis, 8% advanced periodontitis, and in 4% periodontal disease was so severe that extraction of teeth was required (Brown et al., 1989). Hence since 85% of adults show some sign of periodontal disease, the standard screening periodontal examination should be carried out on all adults. Periodontal disease is less common in children and juveniles; however, when it does occur, it is often severe. Therefore it is also necessary to examine these patients for periodontal changes.

A flow chart for the standard screening periodontal examination is given in the box below and includes a gingival examination, periodontal probing for pockets, assessment of plaque control, tooth mobility measurements, and a radiographic survey of alveolar bone. This screening examination should be carried out along with an examination for caries and other oral problems, and all in-formation recorded on appropriate charts for future use and as a routine procedure for risk management. Fig. 27-1 is an example of an oral mucous membrane examination form, and examples of forms used for periodontal charting and recording are given in Fig. 27-2. Radiographic survey results, dietary analysis, medical consultation, and laboratory tests can be noted on the periodontics record (Fig. 27-2, *B*).

Changes detected at the screening examination that suggest periodontal disease include (1) probing pocket depths greater than 3 mm, (2) gingival bleeding on deep probing, (3) gingival redness or edema, (4) gingival suppuration, (5) excessive plaque and calculus deposits, (6) mobile teeth, (7) radiographic evidence of bone loss, and (8) probing attachment loss. If one or more of these abnormalities are detected in the standard screening examination, a further, more complete periodontal examination should be carried out, possibly at another visit. The elements of the complete periodontal examination are listed in the box on p. 350 and include full periodontal probing, including pocket depths, furcation probing, and probing attachment level measurements. It is important to reiterate the necessity for the minimum standard examination for *all* patients coming to the dental office. This not only aids in detecting periodontal disease, especially in its early stages, but also provides baseline gingival crevice depths and radiographic measurements against which future changes can be compared. The screening periodontal examination should be repeated at 2-year intervals.

Periodontal measurements are under intense evaluation and development. For example, developments are rapidly occurring in the automation of probes, with the potential for rapid and accurate pocket depth and attachment level measurements. There are currently available probes that make both measurements at a constant force, record the data, and give a computer printout of the results. These instruments are presently research instruments, but with further development these automated probes may be useful for the standard examination of a periodontal patient. Tooth mobility can be assessed with an instrument that provides an automated longitudinal assessment (Periotest*). Recent developments in computer-assisted radiographic technology have also taken place and are resulting in greater ease in obtaining quantitative assessment of bone density changes by computer subtraction radiography. Measurements of alveolar crest–to–cementoenamel junction (CEJ) levels using computer-aided techniques, and computer-assisted image enhancement to show subtle changes in the alveolar process are also on the horizon.

Reference laboratories are available for microbiologic analysis of the subgingival flora with identification of important periodontal bacteria. If periodontal disease is de-

---

Screening periodontal examination for all patients

1. Screening and medical history to evaluate risk for subacute bacterial endocarditis, allergies, or pregnancy, which would alter radiographic surveys
2. Chief dental complaint
3. Complete medical history
4. Complete dental history
5. General examination of the head, neck, mouth, and pharynx
6. Standard screening periodontal examination
   a. *Gingival examination* assessing color, swelling, texture, suppuration, bleeding, ulceration, recession, clefts, mucogingival abnormalities, loss of attached gingiva, furcations, high frenal attachments, and vestibular depth
   b. *Periodontal probing* at six points on each tooth and probing furcations to determine classification
   c. Assessment for *plaque retention areas,* abnormal root formations, retained grooves, mottled or decalcified enamel, or defective restorations, including open margins, overhanging margins, and overcontoured or undercontoured restorations
   d. *Oral hygiene evaluation,* assessment of supragingival plaque, subgingival and supragingival calculus, and tooth stains
   e. Assessment for tooth mobility
   f. Assessment of occlusal relationship; Angle classification
   g. *Radiographic examination,* periapical radiographs as necessary

---

*Siemans Corp., S. Iselin, N.J.

Complete periodontal examination procedures

1. Medical consultations with a physician in cases where diabetes or other systemic diseases that influence periodontal disease severity or healing response are suspected
2. Full-mouth periapical radiographs
3. Full periodontal probing, recording probing pocket depths at six points per tooth, furcation probing, and attachment level measured from the cementoenamel junction or another fixed point (e.g., a stent or the crown tip using an automated probe)
4. Microbial sampling of the subgingival flora of the deepest pocket in each sextant for identification and estimation of the periodontal bacterial level
5. Major occlusal analysis (intraoral)
6. Major temporomandibular dysfunction analysis
7. Major occlusal analysis on anatomic articulated casts if prostheses are contemplated
8. Pulp testing if endodontic or pulpal-periodontal problems are suspected
9. Clinical photographs to record surface topography such as recession for further reference
10. Bone sounding with the patient under local anesthesia for assessing infrabony pockets and unusual furcation defects
11. Tissue biopsy if unusual lesions are detected
12. Further radiographs, as necessary, for evaluation of temporomandibular dysfunction syndrome or to evaluate the alveolar process for implant patients (panoramic radiographs or maxillary and/or mandibular computed tomography scans)
13. Assessment for mucogingival abnormalities, including high frena, lack of attached gingiva, altered passive eruption, and other functional or cosmetic abnormalities

---

tected from the screening examination, it is important to test for periodontal pathogens, since the treatment plan may depend on whether or not there is *Actinobacillus actinomycetemcomitans* or other organisms present in the lesions. For example, a recent survey of periodontitis patients by Rodenburg et al. (1989) showed that among 138 untreated patients with periodontitis, 97% were infected with one or more of three prominent periodontal pathogens: *Bacteroides gingivalis, Bacteroides intermedius,* and *A. actinomycetemcomitans. A. actinomycetemcomitans* was found singly or in combination in over half of these patients, and there is evidence that intensive systemic antimicrobial treatment is often necessary to eliminate this periodontal bacteria.

A complete periodontal examination can often be accomplished in one or two visits by a clinician with some experience and is best incorporated in the total workup of the patient before an overall diagnosis, treatment plan, or prognosis is determined.

Comments on periodontal probing

The probing pocket depth, which is the distance from the gingival margin to the bottom of the gingival pocket, is measured by means of a probe with various gradations. The probe should be "walked along" each surface of the tooth and the greatest depth at each surface recorded. This will give three recordings from the buccal aspect and three recordings from the palatal or lingual aspect of each tooth, or a total of six recordings per tooth. The interproximal recordings should be made to the depths of the pocket; often the probe will have to be angled to reach the depths of the pocket, especially if the contact point is wide. All other probing measurements (except the horizontal measurements made to classify furcation lesions) should be made in the long axis of the tooth. The *probing pocket depth* is most often not the same as the *probing attachment level*, since the probing pocket depth measurement is made from the gingival margin to the bottom of the probeable pocket or sulcus. The gingival margin is subject to change in position; for example, with inflammation or recession the gingival margin may be several millimeters away from the CEJ (Fig. 27-3). Hence a fixed measurement —the probing attachment level—is desirable for monitoring patients over long periods of time. When the gingival margin is coincident with the CEJ, the probing pocket depth and probing attachment measurements are the same. Most often, however, the gingival margin is either coronal to the CEJ because of gingival swelling or apical to the CEJ because of gingival recession. In these instances the probing pocket depth will be either an overestimate (in the case of gingival swelling) or an underestimate (because of gingival recession). Hence separate measurements made from the CEJ or some other fixed point are necessary to record periodontal attachment levels. It is suggested that the full mouth be probed for pocket depth first and then another sweep made of the same sites for probing attachment levels. The gingival margin–to–CEJ measurement is recorded as a positive value if the margin is coronal to the CEJ or as a negative value if the gingival margin is apical to the CEJ. By subtracting (Fig. 27-3, *B*) or adding (Fig. 27-3, *C*) the gingival margin–to–CEJ measurements from the pocket depths, the probing attachment levels can be obtained. Several computer charting programs are available to facilitate these calculations and recordings; some even plot changes in attachment levels over time.

Errors inherent in periodontal probing are discussed in Chapter 26. Various factors influence the measurements made with the periodontal probe, including the thickness of the probe used, malposition of the probe because of anatomic features such as the contour of the tooth surface, the pressure applied during probing, and, probably most important, the degree of inflammatory cell infiltration in the soft tissue. Hence the apparent gain or loss of attachment often reflects changes in inflammation. Despite these difficulties, probing attachment levels give a reasonably

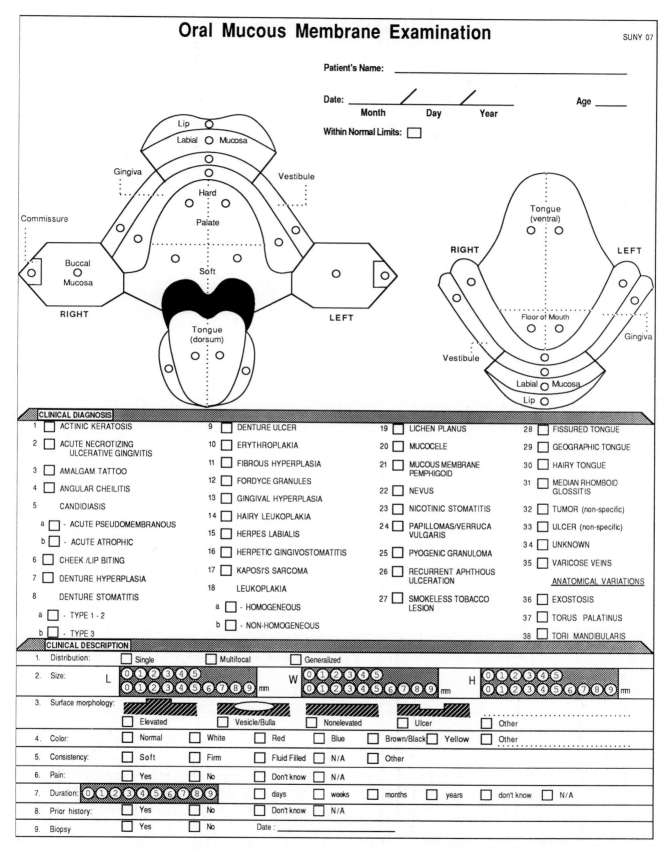

Fig. 27-1. Oral mucous membrane examination form. (Courtesy Department of Oral Biology, School of Dental Medicine, State University of New York at Buffalo, Buffalo, NY.)

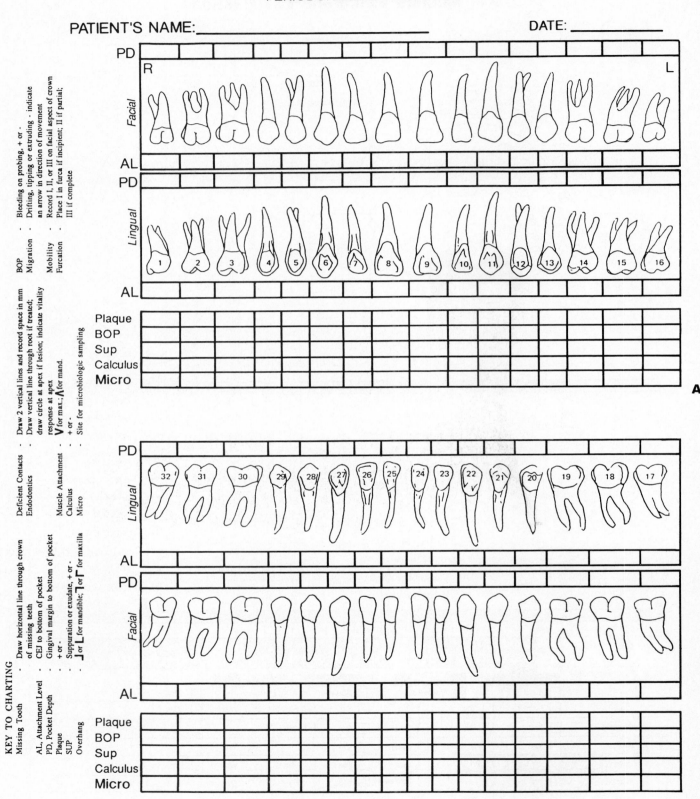

Fig. 27-2. A, Chart for periodontal examination.

PERIODONTICS RECORD

FILE NO.

NAME		BIRTHDATE	CLINICIAN	EXAM DATE

CHIEF PERIODONTAL COMPLAINT

ORAL HYGIENE METHODS
  Current:

  Rx:

HISTORY OF PERIODONTAL ILLNESS

PLAQUE INDEX (P.I.)

Date							
P.I.							

PREVIOUS PERIO (prophylaxis, other perio, inc. dates)

HABIT HISTORY

OCCLUSAL OBSERVATIONS

  Arch Rel. (angle):   Overbite: Overjet:

  Teeth in fremitus:

  C.R. ⟶ C.O.:

  C.O. ⟶ P.:

  P.:

  R.L. working:

    non-working:

  L.L. working:

    non-working:

  TMD:

RADIOGRAPHIC FINDINGS

B

SOFT TISSUE EXAM

ETIOLOGY

  Local Factors:

  Microbiological Findings:

  Occlusal Factors:

  Systemic Factors:

GINGIVAL EXAM (color, form, density, bleeding on probing, etc.)

DIAGNOSIS

TREATMENT PLAN

PRE-TREATMENT PROGNOSIS

SYSTEMIC FACTORS OF IMPORTANCE IN TREATMENT

Fig. 27-2, cont'd. B, Periodontics record. (Courtesy Department of Oral Biology, School of Dental Medicine, State University of New York at Buffalo, Buffalo, NY.)

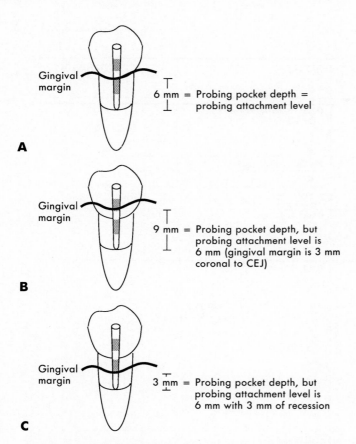

Fig. 27-3. Probing pocket depth and probing attachment level. **A,** Gingival margin is at CEJ. **B,** Gingival margin is coronal to CEJ (gingival swelling). **C,** Gingival margin is apical to CEJ (gingival recession). (Courtesy Department of Oral Biology, School of Dental Medicine, State University of New York at Buffalo, Buffalo, NY.)

accurate estimate of the degree of periodontal tissue destruction and indirectly reflect levels of the alveolar bony crest. With careful probing, a measured loss or gain of 2 mm or more in probing attachment is clinically meaningful.

Assessment of furcations

The precise identification of the presence and extent of periodontal tissue destruction around multirooted teeth is extremely important because these teeth often have the worst prognosis if the furcations are infected. In health the entire furcation is encased in the alveolar bone; however, the openings to furcations on most teeth are 2 to 5 mm from the CEJ. Hence often very little loss of periodontal attachment need occur before the furcation is infected. The classifications of furcation involvement are given in Chapter 26 but can be briefly stated as:

Class I: Horizontal loss of the supporting tissue not exceeding one third of the width of the tooth

Class II: Horizontal loss of the supporting tissue exceeding one third of the width of the tooth but not through the furcation from the buccal or lingual aspect, or the mesial or distal aspect

Class III: Horizontal through-and-through destruction of the supporting tissues of the furcation

This classification deals with the horizontal loss. Vertical loss is of critical importance in healing. Hence periodontal charting of the furcation vertical loss (measured as probing attachment loss on root surfaces involved in the furcation), as well as classification based on horizontal loss in furcations, is necessary. The maxillary molars have three furcations, and often the maxillary first premolar has two roots and a furcation that may become infected.

Assessment of tooth mobility

Progressive loss of the periodontal attachment apparatus may lead to tooth mobility. However, inflammatory changes in the periodontal ligament with minimal loss of attachment can also lead to tooth mobility. Increased tooth mobility (see Chapter 26) is as follows:

Degree I: The horizontal mobility of the crown is from detectable to 1 mm.

Degree II: The mobility of the crown ranges from 1 to 2 mm horizontally.

Degree III: The mobility of the crown is also observed in a vertical or apical direction (i.e., it is depressible).

It is extremely important to accurately establish criteria for identifying degrees I, II, and III and then to use these consistently. It has been shown that a single examiner grades tooth mobility consistently. Hence measurements taken years apart by the same dentist that show changes in these gradations of mobility are likely to be clinically meaningful. Progressively increasing mobility indicates a poor prognosis for the tooth, whereas tooth mobility that is stable or decreases with time is a favorable prognostic factor. Also, teeth that have migrated out of their original position (pathologic migration) because of loss of periodontal support often have a poor prognosis.

Evaluation of the alveolar bone

Radiographic analysis of the alveolar bone with evaluation of the relationship of the alveolar crest to the CEJ, assessment of the quality of the crestal bone, and determination of the width and quantity of the bone surrounding the root is extremely important in evaluating periodontal disease. However, the x-ray image has severe limitations in that it is two dimensional, so that the image of the teeth and bony structures of the jaws often overlay important landmarks, making diagnosis of the bony crypt of the attachment apparatus difficult. Hence radiographic changes must be closely correlated with clinical measurements to accurately assess the existence or extent of periodontal destruction. Reproducibility of radiographs is also important, since a series of radiographs before and after treatment often show changes, especially at the alveolar crest, which indicate successful therapy or persistent infection. However, these changes are masked or not seen if the techniques are not standardized.

Panoramic radiographs and computed tomography (CT) scans of the maxilla or mandible are valuable in assessing bony dimensions and contours when implants are to be considered. It is important to obtain these and other radiographs before treatment planning, especially in partially edentulous cases, since inadequate bone may preclude the use of implants and change the treatment plan to one emphasizing preservation of periodontally involved teeth. If implants can be used, preservation of periodontally involved teeth is often less important.

Bone sounding

Occasionally, with complex periodontal lesions a detailed analysis of the pocket morphology is needed in order to select therapy. For example, determination of the number of infrabony walls and the extent of vertical or horizontal furcation involvements may not be possible with periodontal probing alone. It may be painful, or the probe may be too thick or not shaped properly to negotiate the contours of the lesion. In these instances the area should be anesthetized with a local anesthetic, and then the presence of angular bony defects or interdental osseous craters, the number of bony walls, and the confirmation of furcation defects can be determined by inserting the tip of a fine periodontal probe, furcation probe, curette, anesthesia needle, or other instrument through the connective tissue to make contact with the bone.

Reliability of laboratory or clinical diagnostic methods

The usefulness of a diagnostic test depends on its *veracity,* or its ability to correctly assess the feature in question. For example, the probing attachment level measurement is a noninvasive method used to estimate the true periodontal attachment. The actual periodontal attachment level can definitively be measured only on histologic sections and is the distance from the apical border of the junctional epithelium to the CEJ. Hence the veracity of a method must be judged according to how it truly reflects the definitive measure, or "gold standard," for that parameter.

Two other features of a diagnostic method are its rate of false negative results, or *sensitivity,* and its rate of false positive results, or *specificity.* Both sensitivity and specificity are also compared with a "gold standard" for that parameter. For example, in monitoring subgingival periodontal bacteria, the clinical microbiologic test (e.g., antibody-based assay or DNA probe) is compared with the culture of the organism from the subgingival flora, which is the "gold standard." To follow this example, sensitivity, or the ability to detect patients infected with one or another of the periodontal bacteria, is calculated as the number of

true positive results divided by the total number of results (true positive plus false negative). Specificity, or the ability to detect subjects who do not have the organism, is calculated as the number of true negative results divided by the total number of results (true positive plus false positive). A good clinical microbiologic test has high sensitivity and specificity (i.e., a low proportion of false negative and false positive results).

In a test such as that for periodontal organisms or probing attachment loss, the outcome is a continuous scale of values, and some cutoff point has to be determined that is clinically meaningful. In choosing a useful cutoff point, a comparison is made of the true positive and false positive or the true negative and false negative results. This is called the receiver operating characteristic curve. From this curve a cutoff point is chosen that has high sensitivity (few false negative results) and good specificity (few false positive results).

We presently have no single diagnostic test for early or recurrent periodontitis and have to rely on a series of measurements such as probing attachment loss, pocket depth, radiographic alveolar bone loss, periodontal inflammation, and the presence of periodontal pathogens in the subgingival flora. Each of these measurements has a clinical cutoff and a certain level of false positive and false negative results. However, when all or several of these measurements are positive, we can be reasonably assured of a diagnosis of periodontitis. Future refinement of our diagnostic methods, with strict measurement of *veracity, sensitivity,* and *specificity* and the establishment of meaningful *cutoff points,* will give us even better tools for early and more definitive diagnosis of periodontal diseases.

DIAGNOSIS

Once the clinical examination, laboratory analysis, medical history and examination, and all other necessary data are obtained, a diagnosis can be determined. The most common diagnoses include a periodontally healthy state, gingivitis, early periodontitis, moderate periodontitis, and advanced periodontitis. Less common conditions include pericoronitis, acute necrotizing ulcerative gingivitis (ANUG), and juvenile periodontitis. Table 27-1 offers a synopsis of common diagnoses and clinical, radiographic, and microbiologic features of the various periodontal diseases. Combinations of these can occur, and any one of these conditions may include complicating factors such as systemic disease or occlusal trauma. The common diagnoses and associated clinical features, along with codes useful for case reporting, are discussed here.

Periodontally healthy individuals

Periodontally healthy individuals have no probeable gingival crevice depths greater than 3 mm, no attachment loss ≥ 2 mm, and no signs of alveolar bone loss on radiographs. Often there are no signs of gingival inflammation;

Table 27-1. Clinical, radiographic, and microbiologic diagnosis of periodontal diseases

Periodontal diagnosis	Sign or feature					
	Gingival inflammation (bleeding on probing)	Periodontal pockets	Attachment loss	Radiographic bone loss	Subgingival A.a., B.g., B.i., others	Tooth mobility
Normal	No	No	No	No	No	No
Gingivitis (case type I)	Yes	May be pseudopockets	No	No	No B.g.; may be A.a. or B.i.	No, except during pregnancy
Periodontitis (case type II, III, or IV)	Yes	Yes	Yes	Yes	Yes	Yes, especially in advanced disease
Localized juvenile periodontitis	Yes	Yes	Yes	Yes, may be localized to first molars and incisors	Yes A.a.; may be B.i.; rarely B.g.	Yes, affected teeth

A.a., Actinobacillus actinomycetemcomitans; B.g., Bacteroides gingivalis; B.i., Bacteroides intermedius.

however, even in a clinically healthy individual 1 out of 10 or 20 gingival sites may bleed on probing. Since gingivitis is very transient and reversible, this low level of inflammation is probably insignificant. Little plaque is present, although 1 out of 5 or 10 tooth surfaces may have flecks of plaque at the gingival margin, a level of supragingival plaque often consistent with health. No calculus is detected, with the possible exception of small amounts of supragingival calculus on the lingual aspects of the mandibular incisors or the buccal surfaces of the maxillary molars. There is no detectable mobility of the teeth, with the possible exception of Class I mobility on the lower incisors, and no radiographic changes associated with loss of periodontal attachment. It is important to note that a patient with periodontitis who has been successfully treated exhibits a healthy periodontium but may have residual attachment loss and radiographically apparent bone loss.

Gingivitis

Gingivitis is detected when there is evidence of gingival inflammation, such as swelling, redness, and bleeding on probing. Often the probing pocket depths are ≥4 mm, but by definition there is no measurable loss of probing periodontal attachment associated with periodontal infection. Gingival recession may be associated with gingival abrasion or prominent radicular surfaces. Plaque is usually present but may be absent at the time of examination, since patients often brush vigorously just before coming to the dentist. Calculus may or may not be present. Tooth mobility is rarely present, and radiographic changes do not suggest bone loss. Gingivitis may be simple and uncomplicated (AAP Classification I, ADA Code No. 04500), or it may be complicated by systemic factors, such as drug therapy or hormonal imbalance, in which case the diagnosis is AAP Classification IA. Gingivitis may also occur in patients who were successfully treated for periodontitis previously. In these cases the patient must be followed carefully to determine if active periodontitis is also present or if the patient is suffering from gingivitis only. Careful serial radiographs and serial probing attachment measurements, as well as evaluation of the subgingival flora, may establish if active periodontitis is occurring or if the patient has gingivitis only.

Periodontitis

Periodontitis in adults is classified as early (AAP Classification II, ADA Code No. 04600), moderate (AAP Classification III, ADA Code No. 04700), or advanced (AAP Classification IV, ADA Code No. 04800). According to the AAP definition, in early periodontitis there are shallow pockets, minor to moderate bone loss, satisfactory topography, and generally no tooth mobility. Moderate periodontitis is characterized by moderate to deep pockets, moderate to severe bone loss, unsatisfactory topography, and slight tooth mobility. In advanced periodontitis there are deep pockets, many areas of severe bone loss, advanced tooth mobility patterns, and often a need for prostheses to replace missing teeth or to splint mobile teeth.

Periodontitis is by definition diagnosed when there is measurable attachment loss (e.g., >2 mm). Probing attachment loss may be generalized or localized and is often associated with pocket depths ≥4 mm. Plaque and calculus are usually present, and in over 90% of untreated cases one or more of the predominant periodontal bacteria, such as *B. gingivalis*, *B. intermedius*, and *A. actinomycetemcomitans*, are found in the deepest periodontal pockets. Tooth mobility may also occur, and gingivitis is often present. Radiographic changes seen in periodontitis include alveolar crestal resorption of varying degrees and, in advanced cases, loss of alveolar bone in furcations. If attachment loss and radiographic evidence of bone loss are localized to the first molars and incisors of an individual under age 20, this is clinical evidence of localized juvenile periodontitis (LJP). The deepest periodontal pockets in LJP are almost always heavily infected with *A. actinomycetemcomitans* and rarely with *B. gingivalis*. Most often, adults with periodontitis have localized areas of severe bone loss and pocketing along with generalized horizontal loss affecting most of the other teeth.

Early, moderate, or advanced periodontitis may occur with complicating factors, in which case the case type is designated IIA, IIIA, or IVA, respectively. These complications include systemic diseases such as diabetes, acquired immunodeficiency syndrome (AIDS), and Down's syndrome and affect the severity of the periodontitis.

Occlusal trauma may also be a complicating factor and may be of the primary or secondary type, depending on the amount of attachment remaining. Secondary trauma is associated with inadequate remaining periodontal attachment, so that even normal forces are not resisted. Mobility and radiographic signs of secondary occlusal trauma often persist after complete resolution of periodontal infection. Primary occlusal trauma is associated with excessive occlusal function, such as occlusal stress in bruxers. It should be noted that tooth mobility is also often associated with periodontal inflammation. Mobility associated with primary occlusal trauma is often reversed by relieving the excessive occlusal stress. Tooth mobility associated with periodontal inflammation can be reversed by antiinfective therapy.

Various combinations of periodontal diseases and occlusal trauma are commonly seen. For example, gingivitis may occur with primary occlusal trauma. Periodontitis most often is seen with gingivitis, and periodontitis is often associated with primary or secondary occlusal trauma. Advanced periodontitis is most often found in patients who also suffer from gingivitis and secondary occlusal trauma. However, some patients with longstanding periodontitis may have few superficial signs of gingival inflammation, and indeed their gingiva may appear pink and often fibrotic.

Pericoronitis

Pericoronitis is a dental abscess associated with the crown of an incompletely erupted tooth (Kay, 1960, 1966; McGowan et al., 1977; Leone et al., 1986). Mandibular third molars are the teeth most frequently associated with pericoronitis; however, maxillary third molars or the distal molars on either arch may also be affected. In pericoronitis the occlusal surface of the affected tooth is often covered with a flap of gingival tissue, termed the *operculum*. The operculum partially covers the crown of the tooth during eruption and may persist after full or partial eruption of the tooth, particularly if there is too little space for full passive eruption of the gingiva after the tooth is erupted. With the

accumulation of bacteria, the flap over the occlusal surface may become acutely inflamed, swell, and be extremely painful. The flap may also be so swollen that it is in occlusion with the opposing tooth and becomes traumatized during mastication. With increased inflammation the condition becomes more severe, swelling increases, and trismus and an elevated temperature may occur. There may also be an accumulation of inflammatory exudate in the adjacent tissues.

Treatment often resolves the inflammation. Successful treatment using antibiotics, as well as lavage and curettage to establish drainage, is important. An ANUG type of lesion may also occur, in which case the patient is handled as for ANUG. Prevention of pericoronitis often is achieved by removal of impacted or partially erupted third molars, with care being taken not to damage the distal aspect of the second molar in the process. Complications of pericoronitis include cyst formation (Craig, 1976), Ludwig's angina, and fascial space abscesses, which are rare but serious.

PROGNOSIS

The prognosis is essentially a clinical prediction of outcomes under various circumstances. For example, there is a *prognosis* for the tooth or the dentition *without therapy* and a *prognosis with periodontal therapy alone*. The *prognosis* may also differ if the *periodontal therapy* is *coupled with prosthetic therapy*. The patient should be informed of the prognosis under all of these circumstances, as well as others (e.g., with or without orthodontic therapy, with or without endodontic therapy, and with or without implant therapy), as appropriate. The prognosis is also affected by systemic diseases that affect the severity of periodontal disease and/or healing after therapy. Hence the prognosis is affected by the diagnosis and is intimately associated with the treatment plan. The prognosis is usually expressed as excellent, good, fair, guarded, poor, or hopeless.

Determining a prognosis for a patient before any therapy is often difficult. Where the prognosis is not clear-cut, it is prudent to inform the patient that the initial prognosis is provisional and that a reevaluation of the prognosis will be made after various stages of therapy. For example, the prognosis is often markedly different after successful antiinfective therapy. The prognosis for the entire dentition depends on a careful evaluation of the prognosis for individual teeth, particularly for those that may function as abutments for prostheses.

The prognosis for the patient is affected by general and local factors. General factors include the patient's desire and motivation to maintain an infection-free dentition. General factors, often outside the control of the patient, such as general systemic health, are extremely important in the overall prognosis. For example, diabetes, particularly uncontrolled diabetes, is a risk factor for periodontal disease and affects healing. Hence a poor prognosis is usually made for a patient with periodontal disease and poorly controlled diabetes. This may, however, be revised to a good or even an excellent prognosis after successful antiinfective therapy coupled with successful control of the diabetes. The effect of stress and the patient's ability to cope with it on the prognosis of periodontal disease is suggested to be significant but is poorly understood.

Previously accepted concepts of advanced age as compromising the success of therapy are being revised, with age becoming a less important prognostic factor. For individuals in their 70s, 80s, and even 90s, the prognosis for periodontal therapy may not be so much affected by age per se as by other factors, such as general health status. For example, if other factors such as motivation and systemic health are favorable, then the prognosis for periodontal therapy in an aged individual may be the same as that for a much younger patient who is otherwise comparable.

Individual tooth prognostic factors, including whether or not one or more sites are undergoing an episode of active periodontal disease, are important. The concept of periodontal destruction not occurring at a constant rate but rather being episodic has been shown experimentally but is difficult to document clinically. However, some patients may be undergoing active disease at multiple sites, and other patients may be in remission. Careful, standardized serial probing, attachment measurements, and radiographic measurements may help distinguish the patient who is in remission from one who is experiencing sites of active periodontal destruction. Another factor affecting the prognosis, which is probably related to disease activity, is the virulence of the periodontal microflora. There are slowly progressive forms of periodontal disease associated with common plaque organisms such as *Actinomyces,* and these are probably the easiest to treat; hence their prognosis is best. Other forms of periodontal disease associated with bacteria such as *A. actinomycetemcomitans* are more difficult to treat, since these organisms are more virulent, are often associated with rapid periodontal destruction, and are more difficult to suppress. The prognosis appears to be poor for patients infected with subgingival *A. actinomycetemcomitans,* either singly or in combination with *B. gingivalis* or *B. intermedius.* For example, Rodenburg et al. (1989) and Bragd et al. (1985) found these organisms persisting in periodontitis patients refractory to treatment (i.e., those for whom the prognosis was evidently poor or guarded as evidenced by the fact that therapy was not successful).

The presence or absence of infections in furcations is another factor affecting the prognosis. For example, Hirschfeld and Wasserman (1978) showed that furcations may be a hazard, especially in patients who are not "well maintained." However, in their evaluation of over 500 patients who were well maintained (had good oral hygiene and faithfully visited their dentist), only 15% of mandibular first and second molars with furcation involvements were extracted over a period of 22 years. It appears that furcation involvement per se does not dictate a poor prognosis. However, if teeth with furcation involvements are not well treated and well maintained, a less than favorable prognosis results. Several studies have also shown that teeth with furcation involvements can be treated by tunneling, root amputation, or guided tissue regeneration; this may substantially improve the prognosis of molar teeth with furcation infections. However, when severe vertical loss of attachment has occurred, the prognosis is less favorable, especially if the furcation defects are narrow and deep as compared with wide and shallow defects (Pontoriero et al., 1989).

Increasing tooth mobility over time, particularly if the tooth is symptomatic, also indicates a poor prognosis. Teeth that are depressible (exhibiting degree III mobility) generally have a poor prognosis if they do not respond to initial antiinfective, endodontic, or occlusal therapy.

In summary, patients have a good prognosis if an initial course of therapy, including all required antiinfective therapy, occlusal therapy, and establishment of plaque control, results in resolution of periodontal inflammation and reduction or stabilization of tooth mobility. Once these endpoints are obtained, a definitive periodontal and prosthetic treatment plan and definitive prognosis can be developed. The prognosis is guarded if plaque or calculus control is poor or if resolution of inflammation is inadequate, with persistent bleeding on probing, continuing suppuration, persistent pocket depths, or persistent periodontal pathogens. If increasing attachment loss, radiographic evidence of increasing bone loss, increasing mobility, or persistent third-degree mobility are found 1 to 3 months after antiinfective and initial occlusal therapy, the prognosis may be guarded to poor. These signs of persistent periodontal disease dictate use of aggressive antiinfective therapy and, as appropriate, occlusal therapy and evaluation of the response to treatment again before a definitive prognosis is made. If signs of persistent periodontal infection or occlusal trauma persist after repeated antiinfective therapeutic attempts, the prognosis for periodontal therapy and for prosthetic therapy is then fair to poor. Little or no prosthetic therapy should be attempted until there is a good or excellent overall periodontal prognosis. It should be noted, however, that individual teeth may not respond to even repeated antiinfective therapy because of intractable endodontic/periodontal lesions, or the tooth may have hard-to-detect root fractures or other abnormalities that preclude resolution of the infection and adequate healing. These "refractory" teeth often can be extracted or offending roots amputated, and the prognosis for the rest of the dentition may be good to excellent.

TREATMENT PLAN

The prognosis of untreated patients is often very different from the prognosis after treatment. Hence the dentist must develop a treatment plan before assessing the overall prognosis. The treatment plan depends on the following major factors:

1. The patient's degree of interest and cooperation, as well as ability to participate in therapy
2. The findings of the examination and the nature and extent of disease diagnosed
3. The prognosis of individual teeth, segments, and arches

The general treatment plan for various forms of periodontal disease fits into the following major categories:

1. *Emergency therapy*
   a. Alleviate pain.
   b. Treat acute infections.
   c. Treat traumatic lesions.
   d. Repair defective prostheses.
2. *Antiinfective therapy*
   a. Oral hygiene instructions are begun.
   b. Supragingival calculus and plaque are removed.
   c. Plaque retention areas are removed, and iatrogenic habits modified.
   d. Subgingival plaque and calculus are completely removed.
   e. Root planing is carried out.
   f. Strategic extraction is done for hopeless teeth.
   g. Occlusal therapy is begun.

Adjunctive procedures that may be necessary during the antiinfective phase of therapy include topical antimicrobial or systemic antibiotic medication for treatment of refractory periodontal infections, surgical access procedures for complete removal of subgingival plaque and calculus as necessary, occlusal therapy to relieve gross occlusal discrepancies, endodontic and orthodontic therapy, temporary splinting, and temporary restorations as required.

3. *Reevaluation.* Reduction of infection, resolution of inflammation, and reduced tooth mobility are sought. After this, a more accurate prognosis can be made and a further, more definitive treatment plan formulated.
4. *Reconstructive or surgical therapy*
   a. Mucogingival and periodontal surgery, including tooth- or root-lengthening procedures, gingivoplasty, osseous recontouring, ostectomy, and treatment of furcation involvements by tunneling or root amputation, and cosmetic procedures such as ridge augmentation, subepithelial connective tissue or gingival grafts, and lateral or pedicle grafts
   b. Regenerative therapy, including osseous grafting and guided tissue regenerative procedures
   c. Endodontic therapy
   d. Extraction of teeth refractory to therapy (e.g., suspected fractured root or recalcitrant periodontal-endodontic lesion)
   e. Surgery for first-phase insertion of osseointegrated dental implants

Adjunctive procedures during this phase may include temporary or provisional restorations, completion of orthodontic procedures, and, after healing, second-phase surgery for implants.

5. *Prosthetic phase.* Prostheses are fabricated as needed.
6. *Long-term maintenance therapy.* During this time there are periodic recall appointments at 3- to 6-month intervals, during which gingival bleeding and suppuration, oral hygiene, probing pocket depths, and probing attachment levels are measured. Also, serial radiographs are taken if further breakdown is suspected. At these appointments plaque and calculus removal and polishing of the teeth are performed. Treatment of recurrent periodontal disease or caries, and repair or replacement of defective restorations are carried out as necessary.

REFERENCES

Bragd L, Wikström M, and Slots J: Clinical and microbiological study of "refractory" adult periodontitis, J Dent Res 64:234, 1985.

Brown LJ et al: Periodontal diseases in the U.S. in 1981: prevalence, severity, extent, and role in tooth mortality, J Periodontol 60(7), 1989.

Craig GT: The paradental cyst: a specific inflammatory odontogenic cyst, Br Dent J 41:9, 1976.

Hirschfeld L and Wasserman B: A long-term survey of tooth loss in 600 treated periodontal patients, J Periodontol 49:225, 1978.

Kaye HLW: The management of pericoronitis, Dent Pract 11:80, 1960.

Kaye HLW: Investigation into the nature of pericoronitis, Br J Oral Surg 4:52, 1966.

Leone S et al: Correlation of acute pericoronitis in a position of the mandibular third molar, Oral Surg 6:245, 1986.

McFall WT et al: Presence of periodontal data in patient records of dental practitioners, J Periodontol 59:445, 1988.

McGowan DA, Murphy KJ, and Sheiham A: Metronidazole in the treatment of a severe acute pericoronitis: a clinical trial, Br Dent J 142:221, 1977.

Pontoriero R et al: Guided tissue regeneration in the treatment of furcation defects in mandibular molars: a clinical study of Class III involvements, J Clin Periodontol 16:170, 1989.

Rodenburg JP et al: Occurrence of *Bacteroides gingivalis, Bacteroides intermedius* and *Actinobacillus actinomycetemcomitans* in progressive periodontal disease in relation to age, J Clin Periodontol, 1989 (in press).

Chapter 28

PREVENTING PERIODONTAL DISEASE

Irene R. Woodall

Maintaining a clean oral environment
    Evaluation of plaque
    Periodontal evaluation
    Effects of brushing
    Effects of flossing
    Other mechanical aids
    Chemical agents for controlling plaque and gingivitis
Maintaining good general physical and mental health

There have been many advances in the treatment of periodontal disease as research has developed a more scientific understanding of its etiology and its response to treatment modalities. Despite this emphasis on treatment, an important objective in periodontal care is preventing the initiation or recurrence of the disease. Patients seeking dental care should learn how to care for their oral health so that periodontal disease does not occur.

Preventing the initiation and recurrence of periodontal disease focuses on minimizing or eliminating the etiologic factors that are currently believed to contribute to it. Those measures fall into two major categories: (1) maintaining a clean oral environment so that pathogenic bacteria are not able to proliferate and contribute to the breakdown of supporting tissue (Löe et al., 1965) and (2) maintaining overall host defense capabilities through good physical and mental health. The patient ultimately has more control over health-related life-style changes than does the clinician. However, a well-planned educational program can affect the patient's attitudes and behavior and ultimately help that person stay healthy.

The task of developing such a program has two major components: determining what specific procedures the patient needs to perform in order to improve health and presenting those suggestions in such a way that the patient is likely to adopt the changes.

MAINTAINING A CLEAN ORAL ENVIRONMENT

Research currently suggests that certain bacteria in plaque are associated with periodontal disease and that others may play an ameliorative role or be associated with an absence of inflammation (Socransky et al., 1986; Genco et al., 1988). It may be possible someday to cultivate or encourage "healthy plaque," but until that time the accepted procedure for preventing periodontal disease is keeping the teeth and other oral tissues relatively plaque free. Fastidious daily supragingival plaque control can help control subgingival bacterial populations (Smulow et al., 1983), although this effect is difficult to obtain by personal oral hygiene only and may require professional maintenance at regular intervals.

Evaluation of plaque

The degree of plaque control can be determined through the use of plaque disclosants (Squillaro et al., 1975). Several commercial products stain plaque so that it is visible. Some colored dyes stain plaque red and stain plaque and calculus differentially. Typically, colored dyes are less acceptable to patients than the relatively colorless fluorescein dye, which is visible when blue-filtered light is shown on the plaque (O'Brien and Fanian, 1984). Colored dyes often stain the lips and gingiva and will be obvious hours after use. The fluorescein dye is less obvious and thus may be used more routinely at home or with fewer objections being raised when it is used to disclose plaque in the dental office.

At the start of oral hygiene instructions, disclosants can show the clinician and the patient how much plaque is on the teeth and where it is located; this serves as a baseline. The patient can then use a disclosant weekly after brushing and flossing to evaluate the effectiveness of the efforts. At subsequent appointments the plaque can be evaluated against the baseline to measure improvement.

Periodontal evaluation

It is possible to have minimal supragingival plaque but substantial evidence of periodontal breakdown (van der Velden et al., 1986b). The pathogenic plaque is often present in the subgingival pocket despite supragingival plaque control or other factors. Bleeding on probing can clinically detect the presence of inflammation in the tissues, and the extent of inflammation can be determined through the number of areas that bleed following periodontal probing and the amount of bleeding at each site. When bleeding affects more than 10% to 15% of sites, procedures that specifically aim at removing subgingival plaque are indicated. The effectiveness of those efforts is evaluated by observing reduction in bleeding tendency.

Patients can watch for bleeding following flossing or the use of interdental toothpicks. Again, bleeding sites should be charted initially for comparison with results obtained at subsequent appointments.

Effects of brushing

Brushing remains the most universally recommended procedure for removing supragingival plaque from the broad surfaces of the teeth and from the occlusal surfaces. However, the proximal surfaces and subgingival areas are difficult for the brush to reach (Lang et al., 1973), and for these areas other aids such as dental floss and rubber tips are needed.

Numerous styles of brushes are available, with different head sizes and shapes, angled handles, and filament dimensions. Standard recommendations in selecting a brush are (1) soft bristles, (2) a multitufted head, (3) flat bristles with rounded-end filaments, and (4) the head of the brush in the same plane with the handle. Double-headed brushes work as well as single-headed brushes, with some superiority on lingual surfaces (Bastiaan, 1984, 1986).

Soft nylon, multitufted bristles remove more plaque with less pressure than hard bristles (Burgett and Ash, 1974). Bristles that are rounded rather than cut straight across create less gingival abrasion (Breitenmoser et al., 1979). Brushes with a prominent "toe" of bristles can cause tissue damage when pressure is applied to force the shorter bristles to contact the teeth. Many believe that the brush is easier to manipulate if it is in the same plane as the handle. These criteria can be varied to meet individual needs in reaching particularly difficult areas of the denti-

tion or to compensate for physical limitations (Fig. 28-1). A clinician may recommend a brush whose head is at an acute angle to the plane of the handle, or one with small head size or a tapered head.

Patients with periodontal problems often have exposed dentin, with abrasion at the cementoenamel junction. Dentin abrasion is affected by brush hardness and the concentration of the abrasive in the dentifrice (Harte and Manly, 1975). Less abrasion is caused by soft bristles and smaller toothpaste particle sizes (DeBoer et al., 1985), and the soft-bristled toothbrushes and relatively nonabrasive toothpastes now available in developed countries result in little abrasion.

Brushing techniques. An important step in addressing good oral hygiene is to assess the brush the patient is currently using. The patient should be requested to bring it to

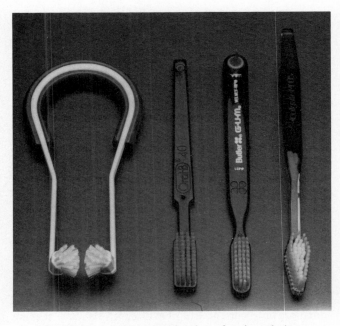

Fig. 28-1. Available toothbrushes of various designs.

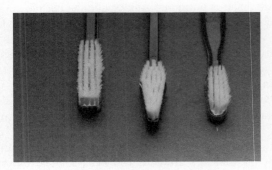

Fig. 28-2. Splayed bristles on used toothbrushes signifying need for replacement.

the first appointment. Its design and apparent age are then discussed with the patient. If the bristles are splaying out (Fig. 28-2), a new brush is needed. Individual differences in use will determine how long a brush will last, but a new one is indicated approximately every 2 to 4 weeks.

The Bass technique is generally the method of choice in removing plaque, particularly from the area adjacent to the margins of the gingivae. The bristles are placed at the gingival margin and angled toward the soft tissue (Fig. 28-3). They are vibrated in place, the bristles being worked between the soft tissue and tooth, so that the bristles move slightly subgingivally. The angulation and vibratory motion help the bristles clean the area most critical to the initiation of gingivitis and aid in keratinizing the most coronal aspect of the lining of the sulcus (Fry and App, 1978). The modified Bass method includes an additional step.

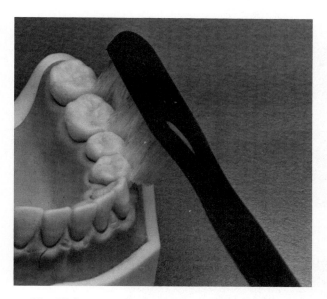

Fig. 28-3. Placement of bristles for Bass technique.

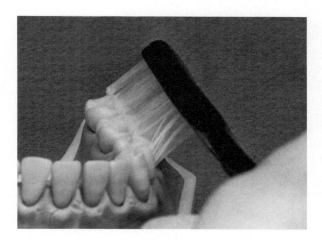

Fig. 28-4. Bass technique in operation demonstrating interproximal bristle placement with a rotary motion.

Following the vibratory motion, the bristles are swept toward the occlusal surface of the tooth (Fig. 28-4), cleaning the remaining facial or lingual surface. Occlusal surfaces are brushed with simple back-and-forth horizontal strokes.

When giving instructions in brushing, it is helpful to ask patients to demonstrate their techniques. In many cases the patient is using a horizontal stroke. It is easier to replace a horizontal stroke with the Bass method if the stroke is described as "very short horizontal strokes that cover only one or two teeth." Once the patient has shortened the stroke, the concept of angling the bristles into the sulcus area can be introduced.

If the patient faithfully uses the "roll technique," advocated by the American Dental Association during the 1950s and 1960s, which tends to skip over the area adjacent to the soft tissue (Hansen and Gjermo, 1971), a slight alteration to the modified Bass technique can be made by asking the patient to angle the bristles and vibrate them into the sulcus area prior to rolling the bristles up over the teeth.

Typically, people being observed in their brushing habits will take from 33 seconds to 2 minutes to brush their teeth (MacGregor et al., 1986). Unobserved brushers probably spend less time, and most remove less than half of all plaque present on their teeth with those efforts (De la Rosa et al., 1979). Missed areas occur at the gingival margin, particularly on the lingual areas and on the proximal surfaces of the teeth (Lang et al., 1973). Following a routine sequence of brushing each time reduces the risk of missing an entire area. To maximize the effectiveness of toothbrushing, a number of vibratory or elliptic strokes should be used for every two teeth (for instance, five vibratory circles). The patient should then move to the next two teeth, overlapping slightly with the area just cleansed.

Brushing thoroughly twice daily or at least every 12 hours keeps reachable plaque under control. Plaque left undisturbed for 48 or more hours becomes thick and covers much of the tooth surface (Lang et al., 1973).

Electric toothbrushes can be recommended to patients who show little dexterity with a hand brush or who are unwilling to abandon a cursory scrubbing. The stroke employed seems not to matter. The stroke size is sufficiently small with most brands that they function in a manner similar to that of hand brushing with a small elliptic or vibratory motion. Two brands of electric brushes stand out from most others. The Rotodent brush (Fig. 28-5) has a single brush head that rotates. It fits well interdentally and can be applied at the gingival margin to remove plaque. The Interplak (Fig. 28-6) uses several tufts that rotate individually a turn and a half in one direction and back again. Electric toothbrushes are not significantly more abrasive to the teeth and gingivae than are regular toothbrushes (Padbury and Ash, 1974; Stookey et al., 1985). Most studies have failed to show that electric toothbrushes are superior to hand toothbrushes when good oral hygiene instructions

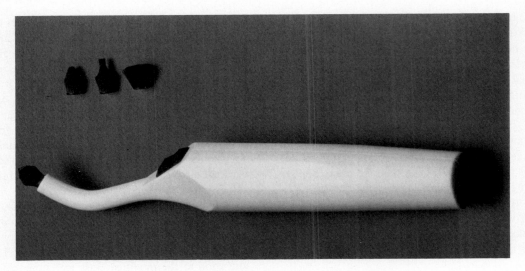

Fig. 28-5. Electric rotary brush with single tip.

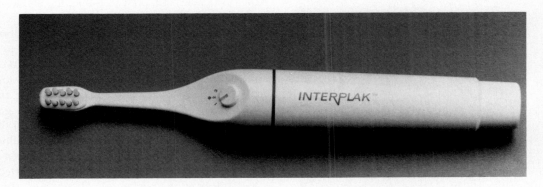

Fig. 28-6. Electric brush with multiple tufts that rotate individually.

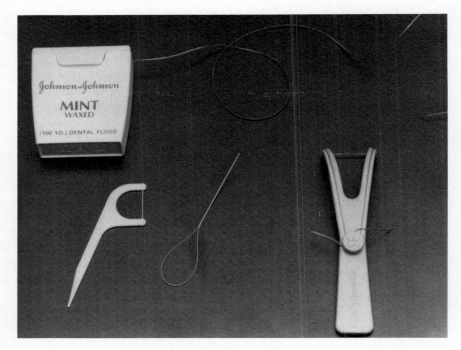

Fig. 28-7. Dental floss and floss holders.

are given. However, for some patients electric toothbrushes may help remove more plaque in the amount of time spent brushing by virtue of their continuous motion.

On completion of brushing the teeth and adjacent soft tissue, the brush should be drawn along the tongue with several overlapping strokes to cleanse it of plaque and debris. The stroke should start at the back of the tongue and move firmly forward toward the tip. Keeping the tongue clean helps reduce the the bacterial population in the mouth and may influence the amount of plaque that grows on the teeth (van der Velden et al., 1986a).

Effects of flossing

Flossing and other mechanical aids are necessary to remove plaque from the interproximal and gingival crevice areas, which are often not effectively reached by the toothbrush. Flossing is often recommended to remove plaque from the proximal surfaces, where the brush is not effective. In a study by Walsh and Heckman (1985), subjects who brushed and flossed experienced significant improvement in gingival health (Walsh and Heckman, 1985).

Clinicians develop personal preferences for waxed or unwaxed floss or wider tape. While many recommend unwaxed floss because it is believed to trap plaque more efficiently, no measurable difference exists between them (Hill et al, 1973). Ultimately the patient is the best judge of which floss or tape is easiest to manipulate or to move between tooth contact points (Fig. 28-7).

Floss is available in flavors and colors and in precut lengths. One style has a stiffened end for threading the

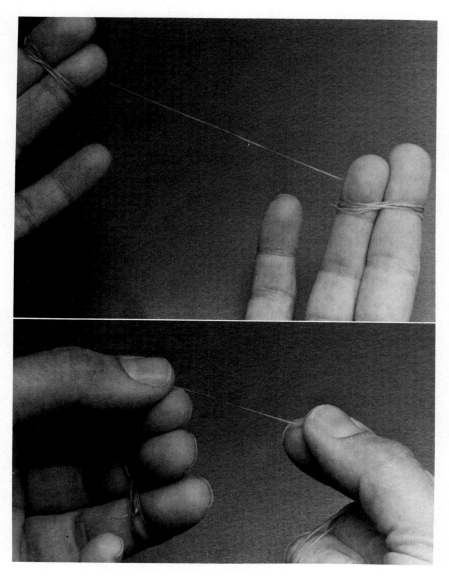

Fig. 28-8. Techniques for holding floss with fingers.

floss between the teeth, apical to the contact point. One type of floss is a bushy, flexible filament, which functions in a manner similar to that of a brush on a string. This type is particularly useful in large embrasures. A study comparing this "super floss" with waxed dental floss showed that the bushy filament was more effective in removing plaque, but that neither type of floss completely removed interproximal deposits. The super floss missed 49.9%, and waxed floss missed 54.7% (Wong and Wade, 1985).

Flossing methods. Holding the floss firmly is a challenge. Most methods call for winding the floss around one or two fingers on each hand and then grasping the floss between the thumbs and forefingers with just enough slack between the hands to allow for manipulating the floss between the teeth (Fig. 28-8).

The standard flossing method (Fig. 28-9) calls for moving the floss between the contacts of the teeth in a gentle sawing motion until it is past the contact point. The floss is then pressed against the mesial or distal surface of the teeth so that the floss contacts the tooth from one line angle across the proximal surface to the other line angle. The thumbs are used to control the floss as it moves past the contact points on the maxillary teeth. The forefingers are used to press the floss past the contact points on the man-

dibular teeth. The floss is then moved up and down the tooth, scraping away the plaque. The floss is moved up over the papilla to the adjacent proximal surface and pressed against it, covering the entire surface from line angle to line angle, and scraped over the surface. The floss is removed by gently drawing it out past the contact.

For particularly tight contacts, the patient may need to use floss threaders (Fig. 28-10). These are flexible plastic devices with a large loop, through which the floss can be threaded. The end of the device is pushed below the contact, between the teeth from the buccal to the lingual aspect, and pulled through, drawing the floss with it. The threader is then removed, and the floss is applied to the proximal surfaces as described above.

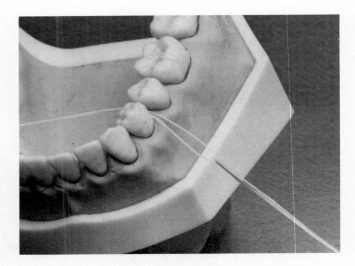

Fig. 28-10. Floss threading under a tight contact.

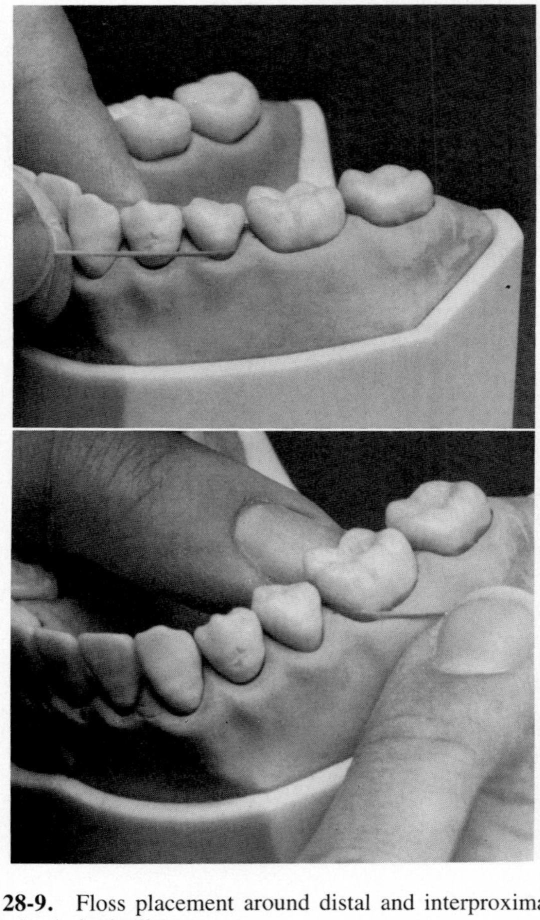

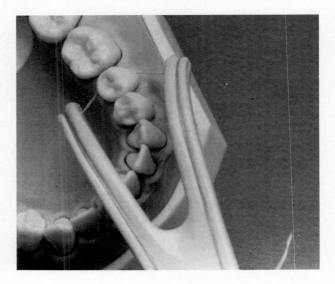

Fig. 28-11. Floss placement with an instrument.

Fig. 28-9. Floss placement around distal and interproximal areas and subgingivally.

Patients who cannot manipulate the floss or whose hands do not fit easily in the mouth may elect to use a floss holder (Fig. 28-11). The floss can be stretched between the two pronged "fingers" of the holder and worked past the contact points, scraped against the proximal surfaces, and then withdrawn from between the teeth. Patients should be advised to take care that gingival abrasion or clefting does not occur from overzealous flossing.

Other mechanical aids

Interdental brushes and rubber tips (Fig. 28-12) can be used to clean between teeth and in exposed furcation areas. *Toothpicks* can be used to clean between the teeth as well. Wedge-shaped Stim-u-dents (Fig. 28-13) can be ap-plied with the flat surface against the papilla, cleaning away plaque from the proximal surfaces coronal to the soft tissue. Standard, round toothpicks (Fig. 28-14) can be applied at the margin of the gingiva and even subgingivally. Careful instruction can prevent tissue damage and the lodging of a broken piece in a pocket. Round toothpicks can be fitted into a Perio-Aid handle for easier manipulation.

Pulsating irrigation has recently received increased attention as an important adjunct in oral health. The research of the late 1960s and early 1970s following its introduction demonstrated its effectiveness against gingivitis but not against plaque. The nonspecific plaque hypothesis was popular at that time; thus it was difficult to reconcile those

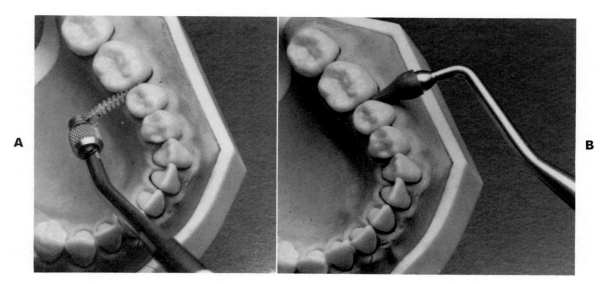

Fig. 28-12. **A,** Use of an interproximal brush. **B,** Use of an interproximal rubber tip.

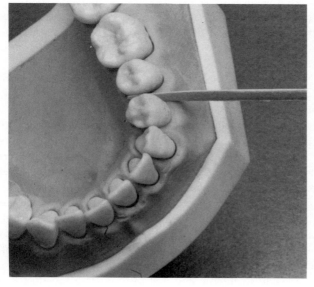

Fig. 28-13. Application of supragingival irrigation with a standard tip.

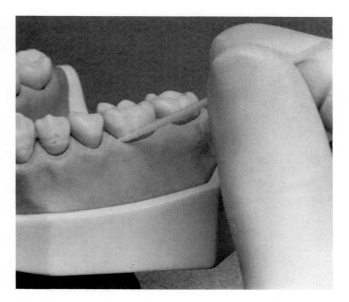

Fig. 28-14. Interproximal cleansing toothpick used subgingivally.

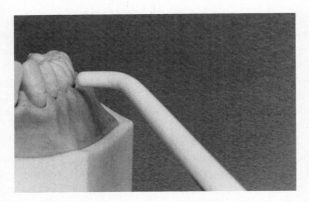

Fig. 28-15. Application of supragingival irrigation with a standard tip.

findings. It was believed that one had to reduce plaque quantity in order to effect tissue health. Since the concepts of plaque quality and of loosely adherent plaque (Fine et al., 1978) are now generally accepted in periodontal research, the research on irrigation is being reconsidered. Irrigation reduces gingivitis; adding an antimicrobial or antiplaque agent reduces plaque (Parsons et al., 1986). The pulsating action of the irrigant may influence the quality of the plaque, flushing away the more toxic, loosely adherent plaque in addition to stimulating circulation in the soft tissue. The addition of an active agent in the fluid may help reduce or inhibit adherent plaque and reduce the specific pathogen level in the plaque.

The application of supragingival irrigation at 70 psi with a standard tip (Fig. 28-15) will deliver fluid approximately one half to two thirds of the distance to the base of the attachment in periodontal pockets, depending on their depth (Eakle et al., 1986). Thus at-home irrigation with water or with an antimicrobial agent can reach the subgingival area; however, penetration of the irrigant to the base of the pocket is not achieved. Hence local supragingival irrigation cannot be considered to remove or detoxify all subgingival plaque. Professional scaling and root planing are required to remove subgingival plaque from moderate to deep periodontal pockets.

Chemical agents for controlling plaque and gingivitis

Even the most meticulous patients will not always completely remove plaque. Patients with a lesser commitment will leave larger amounts. As a result, clinicians have investigated the use of antimicrobial or antiplaque agents to boost mechanical removal efforts.

Chlorhexidine (0.2%) has been studied and used successfully in Europe for two decades as an antiplaque, antigingivitis topical rinse or gel. Research has been unequivocal in establishing the agent's effectiveness. A 0.12% rinse was introduced in the United States in 1986 as a prescription agent. Side effects of reversible tooth staining and altered taste sensation are reduced with the lower concentration but still occur. The agent can be used to help control plaque and gingivitis particularly during initial therapy when patients are mastering mechanical removal techniques and when healing is critical. Labeling information for the prescription agent does not limit the duration of its use. However, patients should be monitored for staining (Ellingsen et al., 1982), tissue response, and patient compliance during continued use.

An additional antimicrobial prescription agent is stannous fluoride. It is active against bacteria because the stannous ion is taken into the cells and retained, affecting the ability of the cells to grow and metabolize (Camosci and Tinanoff, 1984). Gel preparations of 0.4% can be used on a twice-daily basis to help control plaque (Leggott et al., 1986). The gel is brushed onto the teeth and then swished and expectorated. A 0.02% stannous fluoride can be self-administered with daily irrigation, improving health (Boyd et al., 1985). As with any prescription agent, stannous fluoride should be monitored for adverse effects and patient compliance. Long-term evaluation of the 0.4% stannous fluoride gel did not confirm earlier results (Wolff et al., 1988).

Other nonprescription agents are available for extended patient use between appointments. Listerine, with its "essential oils" has demonstrated efficacy against plaque when used as a rinse for 30 seconds twice daily. The studies used 20 ml of the product (Fine et al., 1985; Gordon et al., 1985). The alcohol content in Listerine is 26.8%. Baking soda (either used straight or in recently introduced toothpaste and powder form as Dental Care) has an effect on bacteria as well, disrupting the cell membranes. Salts need to be applied in high concentration and reapplied frequently to have an antibacterial effect (Newbrun et al., 1984).

The antimicrobial effect of the agent is potentiated when mixed with small amounts of hydrogen peroxide (Miyasaki et al., 1986). An 8-week study comparing fluoride toothpaste with a mixture of hydrogen peroxide and sodium bicarbonate showed no differences between the regimens (Lyne et al., 1986).

Iodine- and chlorine-based preparations are often used by clinicians as irrigants. They are active antimicrobially and can reduce subgingival plaque.

Cepacol and Glister concentrate contain cetylpyridinium chloride (CPC) as an antiplaque ingredient. A study using 0.1% CPC over a 48-hour period during which no other oral hygiene was allowed showed improved results over previous studies using 0.05% CPC, where only mild antiplaque effects were noted (Ashley et al., 1984). Scope contains CPC and domiphen bromide, which was significantly better than CPC alone in mouth rinses in one study using 21 subjects in three groups (Sturzenberger and Leonard, 1969).

Viadent toothpaste and oral rinse contain sanguinarine,

an alkaloid extract from the bloodroot plant. The cationic sanguinarine molecule chemically combines with dental plaque and remains detectable in the plaque for up to 4 hours after use. It is antimicrobial (Dzink and Socransky, 1985), and it appears to alter the receptor sites in freshly formed pellicle, reducing the ability of bacteria to adhere to it (Babu et al., 1986). Short-term studies (1 month or less) have indicated effectiveness for both the toothpaste and the oral rinse (Klewansky and Vernier, 1984; Wennstrom and Lindhe, 1985). Two clinical studies have shown the efficacy of the toothpaste and oral rinse in controlling plaque and gingivitis in orthodontic patients. Miller et al. (1988) reported efficacy from a 9-week study, and Hannah et al. (1989) documented efficacy over 6 months' use. When used after scaling and root planing in another study, the oral rinse reduced gingival inflammation as well as 0.2% chlorhexidine (Wennstrom and Lindhe, 1986).

Plax is described as a prebrushing rinse that enables the mechanical action of the brush and floss to more easily remove plaque. Short-term studies have shown activity (Emling and Yankell, 1985). However, several studies have shown moderate or no observable efficacy (Beiswanger et al., 1989; Grossman, 1988; Kazmierczak, 1989; Sharma, 1989). The active ingredient is not specified; the concentrations of sodium laurel sulfate and sodium borax (soaping agents) suggest that it may have a surfactant action on plaque.

This area of plaque control is relatively new in dentistry. New products and reports of clinical studies will undoubtedly emerge in the coming years.

MAINTAINING GOOD GENERAL PHYSICAL AND MENTAL HEALTH

For some patients, periodontal disease will progress in spite of careful therapy and meticulous daily oral hygiene, and the reasons for this are not understood. They may relate to failure to eliminate specific periodontal pathogens that are active at low levels or to depressed host resistance to low levels of plaque.

While the connection between specific dietary patterns and periodontal disease has not been established (Lee et al., 1985), nutrition undoubtedly plays a role in the ability of the tissue to regenerate, produce specific enzymes, and ward off bacterial invasion. A diet high in sucrose promotes rapid, heavy supragingival plaque formation (Lim et al., 1986) but has not been tied directly to periodontitis. A comprehensive assessment of a periodontal patient should include an assessment of the dietary habits of the patient to determine if there are any extreme dietary abnormalities that may possibly affect host resistance.

An assessment of the patient's overall general health should be performed with particular attention given to any systemic disease that may render the patient more susceptible to periodontal disease, that may slow healing, or that may hamper the patient's ability to follow oral hygiene instructions. Stress levels should also be considered as a factor that may influence the ability of the patient to maintain a sound defense system against disease.

Research on the etiology of periodontal disease continues, with increased emphasis being placed on natural immunity and host defense mechanisms. General health will be more closely related to the occurrence of or susceptibility to periodontal disease in the future. There are a few clear-cut systemic conditions that increase susceptibility to periodontal disease: diabetes mellitus, Down's syndrome, and neutrophil disorders such as congenital neutropenia. Patients with these conditions require more rigorous plaque control for prevention of initiation, as well as recurrence, of periodontal disease.

Good oral hygiene is an integral part of overall health practices, such as regular exercise, stress management, diet and weight control, smoking cessation, and moderation in alcohol consumption. If the clinician assesses general health levels and can establish the link between oral health and general health for the patient, the patient may be more willing to establish oral hygiene as an integral part of good prevention practices for overall health. Changing one's oral hygiene practices by taking more time to brush, floss, and irrigate with special antiplaque agents is a life-style change. Patients who are already in the midst of changing a life-style pattern to include good general health practices may be more willing to change oral health practices as well.

The whole notion of changing one's life-style is the more difficult part of designing a program for patients to begin practicing good oral hygiene. The principles of brushing and flossing are easy to learn. Integrating them into one's daily routine is far more difficult (Chen and Rubinson, 1982) and a source of frustration for clinicians who believe that because they have taught the skills, patients will change their behaviors.

REFERENCES

Ashley F et al: Effect of a 0.1% cetylpyridinium chloride mouthrinse on the accumulation and biochemical composition of dental plaque in young adults, Caries Res 18:465, 1984.

Babu J et al: Antiplaque activity of a sanguinaria-containing oral rinse: an in vitro study, Compend Contin Educ Dent 7(suppl):S209, 1986.

Bastiaan R: Comparison of the clinical effectiveness of a single and a double headed toothbrush, J Clin Periodontol 11:331, 1984.

Bastiaan R: The cleaning efficiency of different toothbrushes in children, J Clin Periodontol 13:837, 1986.

Beiswanger BB et al: Plaque removal by a pre-brushing rinse, J Dent Res 68(special issue), 1989 (abstract 1472).

Boyd R et al: Effect of self-administered daily irrigation with 0.02% SnF$_2$ on periodontal disease activity, J Clin Periodontol 12:420, 1985.

Breitenmoser J, Mormann W, and Muhlemann H: Damaging effects of bristle end form on gingiva, J Periodontol 50:212, 1979.

Burgett F and Ash M: Comparative study of the pressure of brushing with three types of toothbrushes, J Periodontol 45:410, 1974.

Camosci D and Tinanoff N: Anti-bacterial determinants of stannous fluoride, J Dent Res 63:1121, 1984.

Chen M and Rubinson L: Preventive dental behavior of white American families: a national dental health survey, J Am Dent Assoc 105:43, 1982.

De la Rosa M et al: Plaque growth and removal with daily toothbrushing, J Periodontol 50:661, 1979.

DeBoer P, Duinkerke A, and Arends J: Influence of tooth paste particle size and tooth brush stiffness on dentine abrasion in vitro, Caries Res 19:232, 1985.

Dzink J and Socransky S: Comparative in vitro activity of sanguinarine against oral microbial isolates, Antimicrob Agents Chemother 27:663, 1985.

Eakle WS, Ford C, and Boyd RL: Depth of penetration in periodontal pockets with oral irrigation, J Clin Periodontol 13(1):39, 1986.

Ellingsen J, Rolla G, and Eriksen H: Extrinsic dental stain caused by chlorhexidine and other denaturing agents, J Clin Periodontol 9:317, 1982.

Emling R and Yankell S: First studies of a new prebrushing mouthrinse, Compend Contin Educ Dent 6:637, 1985.

Fine D, Letizia J, and Mandel I: The effect of rinsing with Listerine antiseptic on the properties of developing dental plaque, J Clin Periodontol 12:660, 1985.

Fine D et al: Studies in plaque pathogenicity. I. Plaque collection and limulus lysate screening of adherent and loosely adherent plaque, J Periodont Res 13:17, 1978.

Fry H and App G: Histologic evaluation of the effects of intrasulcular toothbrushing on human sulcular epithelium, J Periodontol 49:163, 1978.

Genco RJ, Zambon JJ, and Christersson LA: The origin of periodontal infections, Adv Dent Res 2(2):245, 1988.

Gordon J, Lamster I, and Seiger M: Efficacy of Listerine antiseptic in inhibiting the development of plaque and gingivitis, J Clin Periodontol 12:697, 1985.

Grossman E: Effectiveness of a prebrushing mouthrinse under single-trial and home-use conditions, Clin Prev Dent 10(6):4, 1988.

Hannah JJ et al: Long-term clinical evaluation of toothpaste and oral rinse containing sanguinaria extract in controlling plaque, gingival inflammation, and sulcular bleeding during orthodontic treatment, Am J Orthod, 1989 (in press).

Hansen F and Gjermo P: The plaque-removing effect of toothbrushing methods, Scand J Dent Res 79:502, 1971.

Harte D and Manly R: Effect of toothbrush variables on wear of dentin produced by four abrasives, J Dent Res 54:993, 1975.

Hill H, Levi P, and Glickman I: The effects of waxed and unwaxed dental floss on interdental plaque accumulation and interdental gingival health, J Periodontol 44:441, 1973.

Kazmierczak M: Clinical evaluation of Plax as a prebrushing rinse, J Dent Res 68(special issue), 1989 (abstract 1474).

Klewansky P and Vernier D: Sanguinarine and the control of plaque in dental practice, Compend Contin Educ Dent 5(suppl):S94, 1984.

Lang N, Cumming B, and Löe H: Toothbrushing frequency as it relates to plaque development and gingival health, J Periodontol 44:396, 1973.

Lee M, Jewson L, and Jaynes S: Diet and the prevention of periodontitis, Clin Prev Dent 7(1):11, 1985.

Leggott P, Boyd R, and Quinn R: Gingival disease during fixed orthodontic therapy, J Dent Res 65, 1986 (abstract 1465).

Lim L et al: A comparison of 4 techniques for clinical detection of early plaque formed during different dietary regimes, J Clin Periodontol 13:658, 1986.

Lobene R, Soparkar P, and Newman M: The effects of a sanguinaria dentifrice on plaque and gingivitis, Compend Contin Educ Dent 7(suppl):S185, 1986.

Löe H, Theilade E, and Jensen S: Experimental gingivitis in man, J Periodontol 36:177, 1965.

Lyne S, Glasscock N, and Allen D: Clinical effectiveness of hydrogen peroxide-sodium bicarbonate paste on periodontitis treated with and without scaling and root planing, Dent Hyg 60:450, 1986.

MacGregor I, Rugg-Gunn A, and Gordon P: Plaque levels in relation to the number of toothbrushing strokes in uninstructed English schoolchildren, J Periodont Res 21:577, 1986.

Miller RA et al: Effects of sanquinaria extract on plaque retention in orthodontic patients, J Clin Orthod 22:304, 1988.

Miyasaki K, Genco R, and Wilson M: Antimicrobial properties of hydrogen peroxide and sodium bicarbonate individually and in combination against selected oral, gram-negative, facultative bacteria, J Dent Res 65:1142, 1986.

Newbrun E, Hoover C, and Ryder M: Bactericidal action of bicarbonate ion on selected periodontal pathogenic microorganisms, J Periodontol 55:658, 1984.

O'Brien W and Fanian F: Use of a dual filter-mirror device with a fluorescent plaque disclosant, Clin Prev Dent 6(3):13, 1984.

Padbury A and Ash M: Abrasion caused by three methods of toothbrushing, J Periodontol 45:434, 1974.

Palcanis K et al: Longitudinal evaluation of sanguinaria: clinical and microbiological studies, Compend Contin Educ Dent 7(suppl):S179, 1986.

Parsons L et al: Effect of 0.03% sanguinaria rinse on plaque and gingivitis when delivered as a manual rinse and under pressure in an oral irrigator, Compend Contin Educ Dent 7(suppl):S205, 1986.

Sharma N: Efficacy of Plax prebrushing rinse in reducing dental plaque, J Dent Res(special issue), 1989 (abstract 1473).

Smulow J, Turesky S, and Hill R: The effect of supragingival plaque removal on anaerobic bacteria in deep periodontal pockets, J Am Dent Assoc 107:737, 1983.

Socransky S et al: Microbiota of destructive periodontal diseases. II. Probable beneficial species, J Dent Res 65, 1986 (abstract 669).

Squillaro R, Cohen D, and Laster L: A comparison of microbial plaque disclosants after personal oral hygiene instruction and prophylaxis, J Prev Dent 2(2):3, 1975.

Stookey G, Schemehorn B, and Choi K: In vitro studies of the hard-tissue abrasivity of a new home plaque-removal instrument, Compend Contin Educ Dent 6(suppl):152, 1985.

Sturzenberger O and Leonard G: The effect of a mouthwash as adjunct in tooth cleaning, J Periodontol 40:299, 1969.

van der Velden U, Abbas F, and Winkel E: Probing considerations in relation to susceptibility to periodontal breakdown, J Clin Periodontol 13:894, 1986a.

van der Velden U et al: Habitat of periodontopathic microorganisms, J Clin Periodontol 13:243, 1986b.

Walsh M and Heckman B: Interproximal subgingival cleaning by dental floss and the toothpick, Dent Hyg 59:464, 1985.

Wennstrom J and Lindhe J: Some effects of a sanquinarine-containing mouthrinse on developing plaque and gingivitis, J Clin Periodontol 12:867, 1985.

Wennstrom J and Lindhe J: The effect of mouthrinses on parameters characterizing human periodontal disease, J Clin Periodontol 13:86, 1986.

Wolff LF et al: Effect on gingivitis of toothbrushing with SnF_2 or NaF gel, J Dent Res 67(special issue), 1988 (abstract 768).

Wong C and Wade A: A comparative study of effectiveness in plaque removal by Super Floss and waxed dental floss, J Clin Periodontol 12:788, 1985.

Chapter 29

INFECTION CONTROL

Joseph J. Zambon

Hepatitis
Herpes
Acquired immunodeficiency syndrome
Protective measures

Control of transmission of infections among patients and therapists in dental offices has reached a high level of effectiveness in this century. The well-publicized concern over the acquired immunodeficiency syndrome (AIDS) epidemic has further focused attention on infection control in general and on infection control in the dental office in particular. Concerns have been further spurred by reports of health workers becoming infected with the virus that causes AIDS, the human immunodeficiency virus (HIV).

Infection control should always be a prime consideration in the dental office. Most dentists are aware, at least to some degree, of the potential risks posed by the transmission of infectious diseases. However, studies have shown that despite this knowledge, the practice of infection-control procedures is often erratic. Several infectious diseases, notably hepatitis, are of great concern in the dental office because of their prevalence in the general population. To prevent the transmission of these diseases, each office must establish an infection-control system that can deal with both the known risks, as in the case of diagnosed AIDS patients, and with unknown cases of transmissible disease. These latter patients not only are much more numerous, but they also pose much greater risks for the dental team by virtue of their anonymity. Hence infection-control procedures should be based on the assumption that any patient can be a source of infection.

Dentists and dental auxiliary personnel are exposed to various infectious microorganisms, including bacteria such as staphylococci, Streptococci, and *Mycobacterium tuberculosis,* which causes tuberculosis, and viruses such as the HIV, hepatitis virus, cytomegalovirus, and herpes simplex virus. Each of these agents may be transmitted directly from patient to dentist or dental auxiliary, or from dentist to patient. Transmission may occur by direct contact, by droplet infection (coughing), or by the formation of infectious aerosols generated by high-speed handpieces.

Indirect spread of infection can occur via contaminated instruments or dental charts, or via water used for rinsing or cooling. Indirect spread with water sprays or coolants occurs when microorganisms make contact with water from the handpiece, air syringe, or ultrasonic scaler and this water is sucked back into the water lines when the instrument is turned off, a process called *water retraction.* When the next patient is treated using this same dental unit, even if the instrument is autoclaved, the infectious agent can be sprayed when the water is turned back on, since the microorganisms were in the water lines, not the instrument. Check valves installed into the dental unit can avoid water retraction. Also, running the instrument for several minutes at the beginning of the clinic day and between patients can minimize contamination.

HEPATITIS

Hepatitis, while not receiving as much recent attention as AIDS, is a significant health risk to dentists and dental auxiliaries. There are three types of hepatitis: type A, formerly known as infectious hepatitis; type B, formerly known as serum hepatitis; and non-A, non-B hepatitis. Hepatitis A, which comprises only a small proportion of the total number of cases of hepatitis, is spread by an oral-fecal route and is associated with contaminated water and food. Hepatitis B is spread by contact with blood or saliva, as well as by urine, feces, sweat, and semen; this may involve direct or indirect inoculation by needlestick or absorption through mucosal surfaces. Approximately 500,000 to 1 million people carry hepatitis B virus, and approximately 200,000 cases occur each year.

Not surprisingly, dentists have a higher rate of infection by hepatitis B than does the general population because they are in daily contact with these potentially infectious materials. They exhibit a carrier rate of 0.9% to 12.3%. Recent estimates suggest that as many as 28% of all dentists have serologic evidence of prior hepatitis B infection, and 3% to 5% of dentists are thought to develop hepatitis each year. The risk for contracting hepatitis B is 3 to 5 times greater for general dentists than for the population at large; it is 5 to 10 times greater for dental specialists who perform large numbers of surgical procedures, which includes periodontists and oral surgeons. Dentists are thought to contract hepatitis B mainly by means of needlesticks or cuts.

Other people at higher risk for hepatitis B include hemophiliacs, patients receiving kidney dialysis, immunosuppressed patients, intravenous drug abusers, and prisoners.

In addition to barrier techniques and proper sterilization technique, the most effective means of preventing hepatitis B is through vaccination with a safe, effective vaccine: Heptavax. However, of a group of dentists surveyed, only half had been inoculated; among their office staff only 20% had had the vaccine. When the vaccine was introduced, there were concerns over its safety, since it was prepared from blood pools rich in blood from homosexual men. These concerns have been allayed by the rigorous processing procedure that inactivates hepatitis B virus, HIV, and all other viruses known to be present in human serum. Furthermore, a recombinant hepatitis B vaccine is in use and has also been proved to be safe and effective. Hepatitis vaccines are immunogenic and highly effective in preventing hepatitis B. However, a significant number of individuals over 40 years of age do not make antibodies to the hepatitis vaccine; hence serum testing is recommended to confirm the effectiveness of the vaccination in older individuals.

HERPES

Herpes affects the skin, mucous membranes, eyes, and central nervous system. There are two major types of herpesvirus: herpes simplex type 1 (HSV-1), which causes perioral lesions, and herpes simplex type 2 (HSV-2), which is associated with genital infections. With changing sexual practices, both types of virus can be found in either location.

Children are generally infected with the herpesvirus, so that by the time of adulthood, most people have antibodies to the virus. Approximately 30% to 80% of patients have antibodies to herpes simplex. However, some adults, especially those from higher socioeconomic groups, have not been exposed and may therefore develop primary herpetic gingivostomatitis as a result of contact with infected patients. After the primary exposure, recurrent lesions can occur, generally on the lips (herpes labialis). Recurrences are caused by reactivation of the latent herpesvirus, which is often associated with psychologic stress, sun exposure, trauma, and fatigue.

The virus is shed from active lesions and may be a prime threat to health professionals, in whom it causes infection and swelling of the fingers following oral examination. Herpetic whitlow is a specific form of herpetic infection that can cause blistering and swelling on the hands and fingers. It may be disabling to dentists and dental auxiliaries. The virus may also be spread to the eye and cause ocular herpes.

ACQUIRED IMMUNODEFICIENCY SYNDROME

It was estimated that approximately 1 to 1.5 million people in the United States were infected with HIV as of 1988. Between 1981 and 1986 there were over 20,000 deaths attributed to AIDS; 71% of those diagnosed with AIDS have died of the disease. By the end of 1991, it is projected that there will be 270,000 cases of AIDS, with 129,000 deaths. Studies have projected that most if not all individuals who are infected with HIV will develop fatal AIDS.

The potential risk to the dental profession from AIDS as a consequence of treating infected patients is great. However, the actual occurrence of transmission through exposure in a dental office is apparently low. The American Dental Association has reported 24 cases of dental personnel having AIDS. None of these were likely to have been infected as a result of occupational exposure, since they were all in high-risk groups. In a Centers for Disease Control (CDC) study of 1758 health care workers who experienced needlestick injuries, only 26 were seropositive for HIV. Of this number, 23 were in high-risk groups such as male homosexuals or intravenous drug users, two were apparently infected as a result of their needlestick injury, and the status of one subject was unknown. The preliminary data accumulated to date, therefore, suggest that dentists and health care workers are at a significant but low risk of developing AIDS as a result of occupational exposure.

PROTECTIVE MEASURES

In 1986 the CDC published its "Recommended Infection-Control Practices for Dentistry" (see box on opposite page), which are intended to minimize the risk of cross-infection in the dental setting. While these guidelines are not yet law, dental practitioners who do not follow them may be at risk for the transmission of infectious disease to themselves, their staffs, and their patients. Furthermore, failure to follow these guidelines could conceivably result in legal actions in which the dentist would be required to

---

Centers for Disease Control recommended infection-control practices for dentistry

1. Medical history
2. Use of protective attire and barrier techniques
   a. Gloves must be worn when handling blood, saliva, or mucous membranes; when touching items or surfaces contaminated by these substances; and when examining oral lesions.
   b. Change gloves between patients or more frequently when gloves are torn, cut, or punctured.
   c. Surgical masks and protective eyewear or face shields must be worn when splattering with body fluids is likely.
   d. Reusable or disposable gowns must be worn when clothing is likely to be splattered with body fluids. Gowns must be changed daily or when visibly soiled (white is a preferable color).
   e. Environmental surfaces that are difficult to disinfect may be covered with impervious material (aluminum foil, plastic wrap) and then discarded between patients.
   f. Dental procedures should be performed to minimize splatters and aerosol formation.
3. Handwashing and care of hands
   a. Hands must be washed between patients.
   b. Members of the dental team who have exudative lesions or weeping dermatitis should refrain from all patient care and from handling patient care equipment.
4. Use and care of sharp instruments
   a. Disposable sharp instruments (needles, scalpel blades, etc.) should be placed in puncture-resistant containers located as close to the work area as possible.
   b. To avoid needlestick injury, needles should not be recapped, bent, or broken before disposal. For procedures where multiple injections are required, the unsheathed needles should not be recapped, but placed in a "sterile field."
5. Indications for high-level disinfection or sterilization of instruments
   a. Instruments that penetrate soft tissue or bone should be sterilized after each use (forceps, bone chisels, scalers, surgical burs).
   b. Instruments that do not penetrate, but come in contact with, oral tissues should also be sterilized or, if that is not possible, should receive high-level disinfection.
6. Methods for high-level disinfection or sterilization
   a. Instruments should be cleaned to remove debris by scrubbing in soap and water or by ultrasonics. Personnel involved in cleaning should wear heavy-duty rubber gloves.
   b. Metal and other heat-stable instruments should be sterilized by steam under pressure, dry heat, or chemical vapor, and the pack should be marked with an appropriate indicator.
   c. The adequacy of sterilization should be verified by periodic spore testing.
   d. Heat-sensitive instruments may require 10 hours of exposure in an EPA-approved disinfectant/sterilant. This should be followed by rinsing with sterile water.
7. Decontamination of environmental surfaces
   a. Surfaces should be cleaned and then disinfected with a suitable chemical germicide.
   b. Sodium hypochlorite (household bleach) at a concentration of 1:10 to 1:100 prepared fresh daily is an effective germicide.
8. Decontamination of laboratory supplies and materials
   a. Laboratory supplies and materials that have been in the mouth (impressions) should be cleaned of blood and saliva and disinfected prior to shipment to a laboratory, as should material returned from the laboratory.
9. Use and care of ultrasonic scalers, handpieces, and dental units
   a. Routine sterilization of handpieces is desirable.
   b. Those handpieces, ultrasonic scalers, and air syringes that cannot be sterilized should be scrubbed with a detergent and water, and then thoroughly wiped with absorbent material saturated with a chemical germicide (EPA-approved and mycobactericidal at working concentration) so that the agent remains in contact with the handpiece for a period of time specified by the manufacturer. Chemical residue should be removed by rinsing with sterile water.
   c. Check-valves should be installed on dental units to prevent water retraction of potentially infective materials. Water-cooled handpieces should be run for 20 to 30 seconds after each patient and for several minutes at the beginning of each day. Sterile saline should be used as a coolant/irrigant when performing surgery.
10. Handling of tissue specimens
    a. These should be put in a sturdy container with a secure lid.
    b. If the outside of the container is visibly contaminated, it should be placed in an impervious bag.
11. Disposal of materials
    a. Blood, suctioned fluids, or other liquid waste may be poured into a drain connected to a sanitary sewer system.
    b. Contaminated solid waste should be placed in sealed, sturdy impervious bags and disposed of according to state and local requirements.

explain why these recommendations were not followed.

Dental offices, like hospital operating rooms, cannot be made sterile (i.e., cannot be made free of all microbial forms). Instruments, handpieces, and other materials that come into direct contact with the patient can be made sterile. Other things in this environment can only be disinfected. That is, agents can be used that kill surface vegetative pathogenic organisms, but not necessarily spore forms or viruses.

The first step is cleaning. This must be accomplished prior to disinfection or sterilization. Proteins and carbohydrates from blood and saliva can accumulate on instruments or surfaces. There they can cover pathogenic microorganisms and render sterilization or disinfection ineffective. For instruments, cleaning can be accomplished using a brush, soap or detergent, and water. Soaps have limited antibacterial activity and are effective mainly at basic pH. Detergents are bactericidal against gram-positive microorganisms and are effective in neutral and acidic solutions. Ultrasonic cleaners provide an alternative to manual cleaning. The cavitation bubbles produced by ultrasonic cleaners can effectively aid in debris removal prior to disinfection or sterilization.

Several agents can effectively disinfect surfaces, as follows:

1. Alcohols such as ethanol and isopropyl alcohols act by denaturing proteins and require at least 10 minutes of contact. The fact that they evaporate quickly makes them inappropriate for surfaces, since the time of contact will be less than optimal. Alcohols are most effective at concentrations of 70%. Their effectiveness is greatest against some gram-positive microorganisms and *M. tuberculosis;* they do leave spores and viruses unaffected.

2. Quaternary ammonium compounds such as benzalkonium chloride kill bacteria by increasing the permeability of the bacterial cell wall. They are effective against some gram-positive and gram-negative microorganisms, but not against spores, viruses, or *M. tuberculosis.*

3. Phenols can be used to disinfect surfaces and are active against viruses, fungi, and bacteria.

4. Aldehyde compounds such as formalin and glutaraldehyde will kill bacterial spores, fungi, and viruses, but only after extended periods of incubation. From 18 to 30 hours of contact are needed for formalin to exert bactericidal activity, although glutaraldehyde works after 10 hours of contact. Instruments treated with either of these agents must be rinsed with sterile water or alcohol to remove the agent before use.

5. Povidone-iodine is effective as a topical agent against HIV.

Effective methods of sterilization include (1) steam autoclaving, which will sterilize at 121° C, 15 psi pressure, after 15 to 30 minutes; (2) dry heat applied at 170° C for 1 hour; and (3) ethylene oxide in a 10% concentration in CO_2 at 55° to 69° C for 8 to 10 hours. It is important that the effectiveness of these sterilization techniques be assessed periodically, and biologic indicators are available commercially for this purpose. These indicators are included with instruments during sterilization, and the indicators are then cultured. A positive test (i.e., microbial growth) indicates ineffective sterilization.

In addition to sterilization and disinfection, the use of disposable supplies can reduce the risk of cross-contamination. Also, the use of a rubber dam where appropriate to reduce aerosol contamination in the operatory can reduce the risk of transmission of infectious agents.

SUGGESTED READINGS

CDC: Hepatitis B among dental patients—Indiana, Morbid Mortal Weekly Rep 34:73, 1985.

CDC: Recommended infection-control practices for dentistry, Morbid Mortal Weekly Rep 35:237, 1986.

Cottone JA: Hepatitis B virus infection in the dental profession, J Am Dent Assoc 110:617, 1985.

Gerbert B: AIDS and infection control in dental practice: dentists' attitudes, knowledge, and behavior, J Am Dent Assoc 114:311, 1987.

Hadler SC et al: An outbreak of hepatitis B in a dental practice, Ann Intern Med 95:133, 1981.

Infectious waste disposal in the dental office, American Dental Association publication S211, Chicago, 1989.

Kaplan JC et al: Inactivation of human immunodeficiency virus by Betadine, Infect Control 8:412, 1987.

Klapes NA et al: Effect of long-term storage on sterile status of devices in surgical packs, Infect Control 8:289, 1987.

Logan MK: Legal implications of infectious disease in the dental office, J Am Dent Assoc 115:850, 1987.

McClean AA: Hepatitis B vaccine: a review of the clinical data to date, J Am Dent Assoc 110:624, 1985.

Thomas LE et al: Survival of herpes simples virus and other selected microorganisms on patient charts: potential source of infection, J Am Dent Assoc 111:461, 1985.

Chapter 30

MEDICATIONS USED FOR PAIN AND ANXIETY CONTROL AND TOOTH SENSITIVITY, AND PROPHYLACTIC ANTIBIOTICS

Sebastian G. Ciancio

Many medications are available for the treatment and management of patients with periodontal disease. Patients seeking periodontal therapy are often older adults who may suffer from diseases for which medications are prescribed, and the effects of these medications on the management of periodontal disease must be considered. A thorough knowledge of the specifics of medications used for the treatment of periodontal disease, including antibiotics, and of medications used for pain and anxiety control, as well as prophylactic antibiotics used to prevent subacute bacterial endocarditis and bacterial implantation prostheses, is also necessary. In addition, interactions among the various medications prescribed by the physician and dentist must be taken into account in the management of patients undergoing periodontal therapy.

In this chapter medications used for pain and anxiety control, dental hypersensitivity, and prophylactic antibiotics are discussed. Drug interactions are also discussed; however, for detailed discussion of drug interactions the reader is referred to appropriate pharmacology texts.

ANALGESICS

Pain is a problem that is common to all areas of dentistry. The patient may be in pain because of abscessed teeth, caries, periodontal disease, orthodontic appliances, poorly fitting dentures, or other disease of the hard or soft oral structures. A patient's early experiences of dentally related pain may affect his approach to dental care, with fear of dental treatment and pain often leading to dental neglect. It is therefore important to understand pain, as well as to minimize or prevent it. The same noxious stimulus can produce varying degrees of pain in different individuals. It is interesting, however, that despite this wide variation in response, the pain threshold (the intensity of stimulus that is noticeable) is essentially the same for everyone (Nelson and Bourgault, 1978), suggesting that the difference in pain experienced by individuals is mainly based on differences in psychologic response to the painful stimulus.

At the present time the major drugs used to decrease or prevent pain can be divided into the following categories:

1. *General anesthetics:* Drugs that produce unconsciousness and as a result prevent pain; all sensory and motor function can be affected. These are rarely used in the management of periodontal disease in otherwise healthy individuals; however, they are useful in severely traumatized patients and in pa-

tients with handicaps or systemic diseases that preclude periodontal therapy carried out with local anesthesia alone.

2. *Local anesthetics:* Drugs that prevent activity in neurons when injected locally; they will prevent activity in all neurons when they are present in adequate quantity. All sensations, including pain, as well as motor function can be abolished; however, they are commonly used at levels that block pain but not touch or motor reactivity. These are the most commonly used drugs in periodontal therapy.

3. Drugs that have analgesic effects but are used primarily for treating other conditions (e.g., diazepam [Valium] for treatment of anxiety; carisoprodol [Soma], a central muscle relaxant; and nitrous oxide for sedation). These are sometimes used for patient management during periodontal therapy.

4. Drugs that are effective in specific painful conditions (e.g., antidepressants and antipsychotics in pain related to depression and psychosis, and antiepileptics in the treatment of trigeminal and other neuralgias).

5. *Analgesics:* Drugs that decrease pain in concentrations that have little or no effect on other sensations. There are two types of analgesics: aspirin-like drugs that inhibit prostaglandin synthesis and act primarily at the site of pain, and opiate drugs, such as morphine, which produce their effects in the central nervous system (CNS) in a manner similar to that of the endorphins. Analgesics that inhibit prostaglandins are those most commonly used in periodontal therapy.

Classification

It is apparent from the discussion above that the term *analgesic* is appropriate for drugs that decrease or abolish pain without significantly affecting other sensations such as touch, temperature, or pressure. The division in this chapter into mild, moderate, and strong analgesics represents common usage, as well as therapeutic effects. These classifications are obviously arbitrary, since pain cannot be strictly classified and is difficult to study (Ciancio and Bourgault, 1984).

The drugs classified as mild analgesics are used to treat pain that ranges from mild to moderate. They include the salicylates, such as aspirin, the aniline derivatives, such as acetaminophen (Tylenol), and propoxyphene (Darvon), a weak member of the opioid family (Rondeau et al., 1980).

Moderate analgesics treat pain that ranges from moderate to moderately severe. This group includes the nonsteroidal antiinflammatory drugs (NSAIDs) that are related to the salicylates in function, the weaker members of the opioids, such as codeine, as well as varying combinations of these weak opioids with salicylates, aniline derivatives, and NSAIDs (Watkins and Mayer, 1982).

All strong analgesics are drugs that are functionally similar to morphine, an active ingredient of opium. Mild to moderate analgesics are usually effective against pain of dental origin. However, a strong analgesic may be necessary if severe pain is present.

Analgesics are most effective when given prior to the onset of pain. If postoperative pain is expected from a periodontal procedure, analgesics are often effective when given while the patient is still "protected from pain" by a

Table 30-1. Analgesics used in dental treatment of mild to moderate pain

Drug	Dose (mg)*	Adminstration
Acetaminophen (Tylenol)	325-650	po every 4 hr
	Children:150-300 (6-12 yr)	Daily limit for adult: 2.4 g; daily limit
	60-120 (1-6 yr)	for child: 1.2 g
	60 (under 1 yr)	
Aspirin	325-650	po every 3-4 hr
	Children: 65/kg	
Choline salicylate (Arthropan)	870 (over 12 yr)	po every 3-4 hr; daily limit of 6 doses
Diflunisal (Dolobid)	250-500 (initial dose 500-1000)	po every 8-12 hr
Magnesium salicylate (Durasil)	600	po 3-4 times daily
Propoxyphene hydrochloride (Darvon)	65	po every 3-4 hr
Propoxyphene napsylate (Darvon-N)	100	po every 4 hr
Salicylamide	325-650	po 3-4 times daily
Salsalate (Disalcid)	325-1000	po 2-3 times daily
Sodium salicylate	325-650	po 3 times daily

Various mixtures of salicylates, acetaminophen, phenacetin, and caffeine are also available.

Reprinted from *Clinical Pharmacology for Dental Professionals, second edition,* by Sebastian G. Ciancio and Priscilla C. Bourgault, copyright 1984 by PSG Publishing Company, Littleton, Mass. Used with permission.
*Adult dose unless specified.

local anesthetic. The rationale for giving analgesics to patients immediately after periodontal surgery is based on the findings of Linden et al. (1986) that pain scores of patients peak 4 to 6 hours after surgery and then return to presurgical levels by 24 hours.

The analgesics of interest in dentistry are outlined in Tables 30-1, 30-2, and 30-3.

AGENTS FOR CONTROL OF ANXIETY

Anticipation of dental treatment can produce anxiety, excitement, and fear in a patient. Frequently this can be alleviated if the dentist and dental staff appear confident and carefully explain the procedure and the degree of discomfort that can be expected (Whall, 1986). When this approach fails, various groups of drugs can be administered to relax the patient.

Production of moderate sedation is achieved with oral administration of drugs classified as sedative-hypnotics, antianxiety drugs (minor tranquilizers), and sedative-antihistamines, as well as with inhalation of nitrous oxide.

Many of these same drugs, plus narcotics and the major tranquilizers, are given intravenously alone or in combination to produce deep sedation when severe anxiety exists or when prolonged or traumatic procedures are required (Foreman, 1974). Intravenous sedation should be administered by personnel qualified to give general anesthesia, since there is a danger that the patient may become unconscious.

Drug interactions

All drugs that depress the CNS have an additive effect when used together. Serious CNS depression can occur if this is not taken into consideration. The drugs in this category include general anesthetics, sedative-hypnotics, alcohol, tranquilizers, antihistamines, antidepressants, and narcotic analgesics.

Table 30-2. Analgesics used in dental treatment of moderate to moderately severe pain

Drug	Dose (mg)*	Administration
Codeine	30-60	po every 4 hr
Fenoprofen (Nalfon)	200	po every 4-6 hr
Ibuprofen (Motrin)	400	po every 4-6 hr
Naproxen (Naprosyn)	250 (initial dose, 500)	po every 6-8 hr
Oxycodone (mixture)	1 tablet of Percodan Children: 1 tablet of Percodan-Demi	1 hr preoperatively, then every 6 hr
Pentazocine with Naloxone (Talwin-Nx)	50-100 0.5-1	po every 3-4 hr; daily limit 600 mg
Pentazocine hydrochloride (Talwin)	50-100	po every 3-4 hr
Pentazocine lactate (Talwin)	30	IM every 3-4 hr
Various mixtures of opioids with salicylates, phenacetin, and acetaminophen.		

Reprinted from *Clinical Pharmacology for Dental Professionals, second edition,* by Sebastian G. Ciancio and Priscilla C. Bourgault, copyright 1984 by PSG Publishing Company, Littleton, Mass. Used with permission.
*Adult dose unless specified.

Table 30-3. Analgesics used in dental treatment of moderately severe to severe pain

Drug	Dose (mg)*	Administration
Anileridine (Leritine)	25-50	po or IM every 4-6 hr
Butorphanol (Stadol)	1-4 0.5-2	IM every 3-4 hr as needed IV every 3-4 hr as needed
Fentanyl citrate (Sublimaze)	0.05-0.1	IM; same dose IV every 2-3 min for preoperative and postoperative pain
Hydromorphone (Dilaudid)	2	po or parenterally every 4-5 hr
Meperidine (Demerol)	50-100; children: 25 (under 16 years)	po or parenterally every 4 hr
Methadone (Dolophine)	2.5-10	po, SC, IM every 4 hr
Morphine	5-20; Children: 0.1-0.2 mg/kg	SC or IM every 3 hr
Nalbuphine (Nubain)	10	IV, IM, SC, every 3-4 hr as needed

Reprinted from *Clinical Pharmacology for Dental Professionals, second edition,* by Sebastian G. Ciancio and Priscilla C. Bourgault, copyright 1984 by PSG Publishing Company, Littleton, Mass. Used with permission.
*Adult dose unless specified.

Antianxiety drugs (minor tranquilizers)

Considerable overlap occurs in the classification of antianxiety drugs and sedative-hypnotics. There is even greater difficulty in trying to differentiate between the effects of the two groups. In this section the two major groups of antianxiety drugs, the benzodiazepines and the propanediols, are frequently compared with the barbiturates in order to point out their advantages and disadvantages. Both antianxiety drugs and sedative-hypnotics can be used for treatment of overexcitement and anxiety caused by either a stressful situation or fear.

Although the use of antianxiety agents for premedication currently receives primary attention, these medications may be beneficial in the treatment of patients with symptoms of mild neurosis manifesting in the oral cavity. The administration of these agents should never be substituted for an explanation of the patient's problem. When symptoms are severe and border on psychosis, the patient should be referred to a psychiatrist.

Antianxiety drugs, especially the benzodiazepine derivatives, have distinct advantages over the barbiturates (Greenblatt and Shader, 1981). Reduction of anxiety with antianxiety drugs occurs at doses that produce fewer undesirable CNS side effects, such as drowsiness and ataxia and loss of coordination, than are seen with the barbiturates. Less mental and physical impairment also occurs when antianxiety drugs are used for oral preoperative sedation. In addition, the safety range between therapeutic doses and toxic doses is much greater with antianxiety drugs as compared with the barbiturates. Because of this, suicide attempts with drugs such as chlordiazepoxide rarely result in death. This is in contrast to the barbiturates, where death is a common sequela of overdosing.

Antianxiety drugs also produce skeletal muscle relaxation by action on the CNS. This central muscle relaxant effect is prominent when these drugs are administered parenterally. However, this relaxant effect has not been demonstrated to be greater than that produced with barbiturates administered orally. Most antianxiety drugs will produce some degree of muscle relaxation in relation to their sedative effects. Some of the more common antianxiety drugs are summarized in Table 30-4.

Major tranquilizers (antipsychotic drugs)

The primary use of the major tranquilizers is in the treatment of psychoses, which are disorders of mental functioning serious enough to impair severely the ability of an individual to cope with the normal demands of life. Such disorders are characterized by a distortion of reality frequently accompanied by hallucinations and delusions.

Table 30-4. Useful antianxiety drugs

Drug	Dose	Oral administraton route unless otherwise stated
Alprazolam (Xanax)	Adults: 0.25-1 mg	For sedation: 3-4 times daily
Diazepam (Valium)	Adults: 2-10 mg; children: 1-2.5 mg; elderly and debilitated: 2-5 mg	For sedation: 3-4 times daily
	5-10 mg	IM or IV preoperatively; inject IV 5 mg (1 ml) per min
Chlordiazepoxide (Librium)	Adults: 15-40 mg; elderly and debilitated: 10-20 mg; children over 6 years: 10-20 mg	For sedation: once daily
	Adults: 50-100 mg	IM preoperatively
Flurazepam (Dalmane)	15-30 mg	For hypnosis
Lorazepam (Ativan)	Adults: 1-3 mg	For sedation: 2-3 times daily
	2-4 mg	For hypnosis: as a single dose
	Debilitated: 0.5-1 mg	For sedation: twice daily
Hydroxyzine (Vistaril)	Adults: 25-100 mg	For sedation: 3-4 times daily
	Children under 6 years: 50 mg	For sedation: daily in divided doses
	Children over 6 years: 50-100 mg	For sedation: daily in divided doses
	Adults: 25-100 mg	IM preoperatively
	Children: 0.5 mg/kg body weight	
Chloral hydrate	Adults: 250 mg; children: 25 mg/kg body weight (capsule or syrup)	3 times daily after meals for sedation
		15-30 min preoperatively or before sleep
	Adults: 500 mg to 1 g	30-45 min preoperatively or before sleep
	Children: 50 mg/kg body weight (maximum 1 g)	
Promethazine (Phenergan)	Adults: 25-50 mg; children: 12.5-25 mg	1-1½ hr preoperatively or before sleep
Ethchlorvynol (Placidyl)	500-1000 mg 15 min preoperatively or before sleep	For hypnosis
Ethinamate (Valmid)	500-1000 mg 20 min preoperatively or before sleep	For hypnosis

Under the influence of these drugs, psychotic behavior tends to decrease and the ability to function improves. The major tranquilizers produce mental and physical slowing, an indifference to incoming stimuli, and an emotional quieting. This triad of actions is referred to as the neuroleptic syndrome, and these drugs are also called neuroleptics.

Rarely used in general dental practice, the major tranquilizers are administered intravenously along with other drugs to produce deep sedation. Like antianxiety drugs and sedative-hypnotics, the major tranquilizers produce sedation and drowsiness, but increasing the dose does not produce general anesthesia. Usually, a patient can be easily aroused even when drowsy from having received large doses. Tolerance to the sedative effects develops after chronic administration over a period of 2 weeks.

AGENTS FOR DENTAL HYPERSENSITIVITY

Agents that are effective against dentinal hypersensitivity can be categorized according to their mode of delivery and their clinical significance. Those agents that have been applied professionally are as follows:

Calcium acid phosphate
Calcium hydroxide
Corticosteroids
Formaldehyde
Periodontal dressings
Sodium fluoride
Silver nitrate
Zinc chloride
Dental adhesives

Reports of success or failure with these agents have varied. One product that has been reported to be successful is a mixture of 33⅓% sodium fluoride, kaoline, and glycerin (Hoyt and Bibby, 1943). Calcium hydroxide application has also resulted in some success (Green et al., 1977). These agents have been effective after one or two treatments for periods of up to 3 months, with efficacy criteria improved by about 50% for periods of up to 3 months.

When chemical methods have not been successful, periodontal dressings have been placed over sensitive tooth surfaces for periods of up to 6 weeks. The rationale is that the removal of irritants allows the pulpal tissues to become less irritable and the dentinal sensitivity is then reduced (Carranza, 1979).

Fluoride iontophoresis has also been used for desensitization; since iontophoresis assists the penetration of ions into tissues, there is a rational basis for using an electrical current to carry fluoride into the tooth. Many clinical observations indicate the effectiveness of fluoride iontophoresis, but only one study reported effectiveness and was adequately controlled and properly conducted (Murthy et al., 1973). Two groups that did not demonstrate the effectiveness of fluoride iontophoresis used the wrong polarity on the tooth electrode: one claimed the current alone was effective (Schaeffer et al., 1971) and the other (Minkov et al., 1975) claimed that the fluoride was effective with or without current. Studies on the iontophoretic toothbrush (Jensen, 1964) are generally supportive of fluoride iontophoresis. Nevertheless, iontophoretic toothbrushing has not gained acceptance over the years among dentists or patients for various reasons. One problem involves the present design of the electrode placement, which favors current flow through saliva rather than into the tooth. Another is that in some cases the application of a positive current cannot deliver fluoride to the tooth surface.

The problems with fluoride iontophoretic technology have involved (1) an inadequate power supply, (2) no provision for site insulation, and (3) poor adaptation of electrodes to the teeth. Relative to pulpal effects of iontophoresis, safety has been established.

The effect of 2% sodium fluoride applied iontophoretically to 73 teeth in 28 subjects using the method of Gangarosa was evaluated (Carlo et al., 1982). This study included only those patients in whom all other agents tried by the dentist had been applied without success. It was found that over 80% of the sites responded to one treatment, which persisted to the end of the study (i.e., 4 weeks). Other studies have found that the desensitization is long lasting (Gangarosa, 1983).

Agents that have been evaluated most often when applied by the patient as either a toothpaste or gel include:

Strontium chloride
Stannous fluoride
Potassium nitrate
Formaldehyde
Calcium hydroxide
Monofluorophosphate
Sodium citrate

In evaluating these agents, the best effects have been reported with strontium chloride, potassium nitrate, and sodium citrate. Assuming a peak effect to be a reduction in dentinal sensitivity by 50%, potassium nitrate peaks in 4 to 6 weeks and the other agents in 6 to 8 weeks. The duration of this effect is not known. Since these agents are effective by 8 weeks, for those products not containing fluoride, the effect of the absence of fluoride on the risk of caries must be considered. It is likely that if a nonfluoride desensitizing toothpaste is used for 8 weeks or less, the effect on caries risk is minimal. However, when nonfluoride agents are used for longer time periods, the caries risk probably increases, although there are no studies to support this concept. Root caries is a concern in these patients, since they usually have exposed root surfaces.

One approach to the treatment of dentinal hypersensitivity consists of first recommending one type of dentifrice. If no effect is seen in 4 weeks, a different type is recommended. If, after an additional 4 weeks, the patient is still not comfortable, iontophoresis or professionally applied topical desensitizers are used.

PREVENTION OF BACTERIAL ENDOCARDITIS

Dental treatment or surgical procedures or instrumentation involving mucosal surfaces or contaminated tissue may cause transient bacteremia. Blood-borne bacteria may lodge on damaged or abnormal heart valves or on endocardium near congenital anatomic defects and result in bacterial endocarditis or endarteritis. However, it is impossible to predict which patients will develop this infection or which procedures will be responsible. Certain patients, especially those with prosthetic heart valves and surgically constructed systemic-pulmonary shunts, are at higher risk of endocarditis than others. Likewise, certain dental (e.g., extractions) and surgical (e.g. genitourinary tract) procedures are much more likely to initiate significant bacteremia than are others. Although the importance of such factors is difficult to quantitate, they have been considered in developing these recommendations. Prophylactic antibiotics are recommended for patients at risk who are undergoing those procedures most likely to cause bacteremia.

Because there are no controlled clinical trials, the choice of antibiotic regimens for prevention of endocarditis in humans must be based on indirect information. The present recommendations are based on a review of all available data, including in vitro studies, anecdotal clinical experience, experimental animal model data, and assessment of both the bacteria most likely to produce bacteremia from a given site and those most likely to result in endocarditis. The substantial morbidity and mortality in infective endocarditis and the paucity of controlled clinical studies emphasize the need for continuing research into the epidemiology, pathogenesis, prevention, and treatment of endocarditis.

Antibiotic regimens used to prevent recurrences of acute rheumatic fever are inadequate for the prevention of bacterial endocarditis. Appropriate additional antibiotics should be prescribed at times of procedures associated with the risk of development of endocarditis.

A minority of cardiologists are recommending the use of a cephalosporin for patients who are allergic to both penicillin and erythromycin. The dosage regimen is 1 g 1 to 1½ hours before the appointment and 500 mg 6 hours later. A danger with this usage is that patients allergic to penicillin may also be allergic to the cephalosporins, although the incidence of cross allergy is low (about 5%). Also, this dosage regimen has not been approved by the American Dental Association or the American Heart Association.

Since the antibiotic recommendations for prevention of bacterial endocarditis are periodically changed, the practitioner must maintain an awareness of these changes. The American Dental Association and the American Dental Hygienist Association usually inform their members of changes.

Patients who have a history of rheumatic fever but have no associated cardiac problems do not require antibiotic prophylaxis. However, these patients should be evaluated by a cardiologist before being included in one's dental practice.

Table 30-5. Recommended antibiotic regimens for prevention of bacterial endocarditis*

Dental and upper respiratory procedures†	Dosage for adults	Dosage for children
Oral‡ penicillin V	2 g 1 hr before procedure and 1 g 6 hr later	>60 lb: adult dosage <60 lb: half the adult dose 1 hr before procedure and 6 hr later
Penicillin allergy: Erythromycin	1 g 1 hr before procedure and 500 mg 6 hr later	20 mg/kg 1 hr before procedure and 10 mg/kg 6 hr later
Parenteral‡ Ampicillin	1-2 g IM or IV 30 min to 1 hr before procedure plus gentamicin, 1.50 mg/kg IM or IV 30 min to 1 hr before procedure, followed by oral penicillin V, 1 g 6 hr later. Alternatively, the parenteral regimen may be repeated once 8 hr later.	50 mg/kg IM or IV 30 min to 1 hr before procedure plus gentamicin, 2 mg/kg IM or IV 30 min to 1 hr before procedure, followed by oral penicillin V, 500 mg 6 hr later. Alternatively, the parenteral regimen may be repeated once 8 hr later.
Penicillin allergy: Vancomycin	1 g IV infused over 1 hr beginning 1 hr before procedure	20 mg/kg IV infused over 1 hr beginning 1 hr before procedure

Reprinted from *Clinical Pharmacology for Dental Professionals, second edition,* by Sebastian G. Ciancio and Priscilla C. Bourgault, copyright 1984 by PSG Publishing Company, Littleton, Mass. Used with permission.

*For patients with valvular heart disease, prosthetic heart valves, most forms of cogenital heart disease (but not uncomplicated secundum atrial septal defect), idiopathic hypertrophic subaortic stenosis, and mitral valve prolapse.

†Data are limited on the risk of endocarditis with a particular procedure. For a review of the risk of bacteremia with various procedures, see ED Everett and JV Hirschmann, Medicine 56:61, 1977.

‡An oral regimen is safer and is preferred for most patients. Parenteral regimens are more likely to be effective; they are recommended especially for patients with prosthetic valves, those who have had endocarditis previously, or those taking continuous oral penicillin for rheumatic fever prophylaxis. An oral regimen can be substituted for the parenteral route when the procedure is considered to be of low risk in producing bactermia (i.e., prophylaxis in a patient with good oral hygiene).

Endothelial damage to heart valves occurs in 50% of patients with systemic lupus erythematosus (Zysset et al., 1987), leading to an increased incidence of endocarditis similar to that seen in rheumatic heart disease. As a consequence, prophylactic antibiotics should be considered before dental procedures causing transient bacteremias are undertaken.

Patients in whom joints have been replaced with prosthetic appliances are susceptible to subsequent infections in that area, which can be protracted, difficult to treat, and crippling. The association of prior dental therapy with the onset of prosthetic joint infection suggests that dental infections may serve as a source of infection of the tissue supporting the prosthesis. Although a cause-effect relationship has not been definitely established, the practitioner should consider prophylactic antibiotic coverage of the patient in conjunction with the recommendations of the patient's orthopedist (Ciancio and Bourgault, 1984). Many orthopedists suggest the same antibiotic coverage as discussed for the prevention of subacute bacterial endocarditis, including the use of cephalosporins.

The recommendations of the American Dental Association and the American Heart Association are summarized in Table 30-5 (Council on Dental Therapeutics, 1985).

REFERENCES

Carlo GT et al: An evaluation of iontophoretic application of fluoride for tooth desensitization, J Am Dent Assoc 105:452, 1982.

Carranza FA Jr: Glickman's clinical periodontology, ed 5, Philadelphia, 1979, WB Saunders Co.

Ciancio SG and Bourgault P: Clinical pharmacology for dental professionals, ed 2, Littleton, Mass, 1984, PSG Publishing Co, Inc.

Council on Dental Therapeutics: Prevention of bacterial endocarditis: a committee report of the American Heart Association, J Am Dent Assoc 110:98, 1985.

Foreman PA: Control of anxiety/pain complex in dentistry: intravenous psychosedation with techniques using diazepam, Oral Surg 36:337, 1974.

Gangarosa LP Sr: Iontophoresis in dental practice, Chicago, 1983, Quintessence Publishing Co, Inc.

Green BL et al: Calcium hydroxide and potassium nitrate as desensitizing agents for hypersensitive root surfaces, J Periodontol 48:667, 1977.

Greenblatt DJ and Shader RI: Clinical use of benzodiazepines, Ration Drug Ther 15:1, 1981.

Hoyt WH and Bibby BG: Use of sodium fluoride for desensitization, J Dent Res 22:208, 1943.

Jensen AL: Hypersensitivity controlled by iontophoresis: double-blind clinical investigation, J Am Dent Assoc 86:216, 1964.

Linden ET et al: A comparison of postoperative pain experience following periodontal surgery using two local anesthetic agents, J Periodontol 57:637, 1986.

Minkov B et al: The effectiveness of sodium fluoride treatment with and without iontophoresis on the reduction of hypersensitive dentin, J Periodontol 46:246, 1975.

Murthy KS et al: A comparative evaluation of topical application and iontophoresis of sodium fluoride for desensitization of hypersensitive dentin, Oral Surg 36:448, 1973.

Nelson JE and Bourgault PC: Current concepts of analgesic action, The Fourth Symposium of the Pharmacology, Therapeutics and Toxicology Group of the International Association of Dental Research, 1978.

Rondeau PL, Yeung E, and Nelso P: Dental surgery—pain—analgesics, J Can Dent Assoc 7:433, 1980.

Schaeffer ML et al: The effectiveness of iontophoresis in reducing crevical hypersensitivity, J Periodontol 42:695, 1971.

Watkins LR and Mayer DJ: Organization of endogenous opiate and nonopiate pain control, Syst Sci 216:1185, 1982.

Whall CW: ADA activities on nonpharmacologic pain and anxiety control, J Am Dent Assoc 113:734, 1986.

Zysset MK et al: Systemic lupus erythematosus: a consideration for antimicrobial prophylaxis, Oral Surg Oral Med Oral Pathol 64:30, 1987.

Chapter 31

WOUND HEALING AFTER PERIODONTAL THERAPY

Paul B. Robertson
Sally A. Buchanan

The response of the periodontium to injury, be it surgical incision or microbial insult, has many features in common with wound healing in other organ systems. After any wound, survival dictates that the host must invoke mechanisms to stop bleeding, protect against invasion by microorganisms, provide a temporary dressing, facilitate movement of phagocytic and reparative cells to the wound site, and initiate controlled replacement of the damaged tissue. Many of these mechanisms, including inflammatory events; migration of epithelium; angiogenesis; fibroblastic, cementoblastic, and osteoblastic elaboration of connective tissue; and remodeling, are detailed in earlier chapters on the response of the periodontium to microorganisms. Indeed, many investigators have characterized the various forms of periodontal disease as the host's response to microbially induced wounds. Thus descriptions of wound healing after periodontal therapy reflect the fact that surgical insult is often added to microbial injury.

The healing process is orchestrated by highly ordered cellular cascades that are regulated by a variety of chemoattractants, growth factors, and other chemical regulators, as well as by changing environmental conditions in the wound site. Healing events occur in highly predictable sequences, such that any particular event is dependent on others preceding it. Injury to the periodontium is always followed by inflammation. The wound debridement that occurs during inflammation is protective for the host and necessary to restore the area, but may result in a net loss of periodontal connective tissues. A number of factors, particularly microbial contamination of the wound, may extend and change the nature of the inflammatory process. Epithelial migration from the wound margins begins within 24 hours of injury and establishes surface continuity well before the connective tissue is repaired. Wound remodeling may continue for months.

Within these general biologic principles, healing of periodontal tissues has a number of unique aspects. These include the complex structural and functional interrelationships of cementum, periodontal ligament, and bone; the junction of epithelium with the tooth surface; and the microbial environment to which this organ system is constantly exposed. This chapter will examine the biology of wound healing with particular attention to clinical and histologic patterns of tissue restoration after periodontal therapy, factors that modify the healing process, and complications associated with periodontal treatment.

BIOLOGY OF PERIODONTAL WOUND HEALING: REGENERATION, NEW ATTACHMENT, AND REPAIR

Most forms of periodontal therapy cause injury to both epithelium and connective tissue. These tissues can be restored by two processes: regeneration and repair. In many biologic systems the term *regeneration* is limited to the regrowth of complex tissues or limbs that are identical to those lost. In general, mammals do not have the capacity for spontaneous regeneration of organ systems, although induction of regenerative processes is a rapidly advancing area of research. *Regeneration* is often used in the periodontal literature to describe instances where the structural and functional relationships of damaged periodontal tissues appear to be renewed. The most common use of the term *regeneration* describes new attachment, or the formation of new cementum, new alveolar bone, and new intervening periodontal ligament, in sites where all these structures were lost to periodontitis. Another example of periodontal regeneration is the formation of a junctional epithelial attachment to the tooth surface and reestablishment of functionally oriented gingival fibers in the lamina propria after wounding. Evidence to date suggests that the new junctional epithelium formed after gingival resection is essentially identical to that lost (Takata et al., 1986). Unlike other wounded connective tissues, which respond to injury by scar formation and poorly oriented connective tissue fibers, the lamina propria regenerates rapidly, and the gingival fiber system is restored.

However, complete regeneration of a periodontium severely damaged by periodontitis is rare, and most healing after periodontal therapy appears to occur by "repair," wherein damaged tissues are replaced by tissues that do not duplicate the function of the original tissues. For example, decreased probing depths after treatment of severe periodontal suprabony defects are frequently the result of connective tissue repair and the formation of a long junctional epithelial attachment rather than the regeneration of new alveolar bone and cementum (Caton et al., 1980). The connective tissue repair is termed *reattachment*.

Epithelial healing

Periodontal epithelial healing has been studied in two general wound conditions. The first is separation of the dentogingival junction from the tooth surface, as might occur after scaling or subgingival placement of a matrix band. Two days after introducing a steel blade into the sulcus of marmosets, investigators observed initial cellular reattachment by poorly differentiated hemidesmosomes in the apical third of the junctional epithelium (Taylor and Campbell, 1972). Three days after injury the junctional epithelial attachment extended to within one third of the distance from the gingival margin, and by 5 days it was totally restored. In cats an intact junctional epithelium with hemidesmosomes and a basal lamina was reestablished 1 week after scaling (Thilander and Hugoson, 1970). When the junctional epithelium has been disrupted but not removed, final healing is probably similar to normal turnover, whereby new cells originating at the apical end of the junctional epithelium displace older cells coronally, a process that requires approximately 5 days (Listgarten, 1967).

The second wound condition is the essentially complete removal of the junctional epithelium by extensive root planing/curettage or surgical resection. Studies in dogs, monkeys, and rats have shown that after removal of the epithelial attachment, new junctional epithelium originates from the cut edge of oral epithelium (Takata et al., 1986). The sequence of epithelial repair has been consistent in all studies. Migrating sheets of epithelium originating from the basal layer of oral epithelium at the wound edge were visible 1 to 2 days after surgery. The connective tissue bed was rapidly covered with regenerated junctional epithelium within 5 to 12 days. The ultrastructural appearance of the regenerated junctional epithelium was identical to its appearance before surgery. Moreover, the junction could occur on enamel, cementum, or dentin and, in one report (Listgarten and Ellegaard, 1973), on calculus that remained on the root surface. The environmental signals that influence cells from stratified squamous, keratinizing oral epithelium to become precursors of nonkeratinized junctional epithelium have not been determined.

Connective tissue healing

Therapeutic injury to periodontal connective tissues is always followed by inflammation. The features of this inflammation differ little from those of the periodontal response to bacteria and bacterial products, which is detailed in earlier chapters. Injury causes the release of acute biologic mediators, including histamine, serotonin, arachidonic acid metabolites, cytokines, and a variety of neurotransmitters, into the extracellular matrix. The insult also activates Hageman factor as the first step in a series of reactions that result in the release of kinins. Complement is activated. The initial effects of these biologic mediators include vasoconstriction, increased microvascular permeability, attraction of cells to the site, and protection against invasion by oral microorganisms. The wound area is infused with platelets, and fibrin is deposited. Platelets attach to collagen fibrils of severed vessels and to one another, and together with fibrin form initial hemostatic plugs, or microthrombi. Fibrin filaments begin binding the wound edges together and provide an initial clot dressing. Moreover, the fibrin matrix facilitates eventual migration of cells into the wound area (Kurkinen et al., 1980).

The subsequent cellular inflammatory events begin with the entry of neutrophils into the wound site. The neutrophil serves as the primary defensive cell of the periodontium and may also participate in some enzymatic debridement of damaged tissue. However, in the absence of infection neutrophils do not appear to be essential in the wound repair process, as evidenced by the fact that fibroblastic phases of healing in severely neutropenic and normal animals are similar (Simpson and Ross, 1972). The cellular sequence continues with the entry of macrophages, which play a major role in successive phases of healing. In addition to wound debridement, macrophages elaborate growth factors that regulate fibroblasts, smooth muscle cells, and endothelial cells (Martin et al., 1981; Leibovich, 1984). The presence of macrophages appears critical to the wound-healing process, since experimental depletion of macrophages severely inhibits fibroplasia and ensuing wound repair (Leibovich and Ross, 1975). The final event in the cellular inflammatory response is the arrival of a lymphocytic infiltrate, the magnitude and character of which depend on the presence and nature of foreign material and microorganisms in the wound. Lymphokine release and antigen-antibody interaction will invoke a variety of mechanisms to control the spread of infection and further debride the wound.

In the fibroblastic and remodeling phases of healing, fibroblasts and endothelial cells are attracted to the wound from adjacent tissues. These cells proliferate to form granulation tissue. Fibroblasts produce several collagen types, fibronectin and other glycoproteins, and proteoglycans. Endothelial cells generate capillary sprouts that anastomose with existing blood vessels. The wound undergoes an extended transition in which there is a shift from highly cellular granulation tissue to relatively avascular and increasingly cross-linked connective tissue.

Cells that are responsible for regeneration of the attachment apparatus, including cementum, alveolar bone, and periodontal ligament, appear to arise from the periodontal ligament (Melcher, 1976). Extensive regeneration of the attachment apparatus occurs only under conditions that favor repopulation of the wound area adjacent to denuded root surfaces by periodontal ligament cells rather than by cells from the gingival connective tissue (Nyman et al., 1982a, 1982b). Conversely, experimental destruction of the periodontal ligament precludes restoration of the attachment apparatus and may lead to extensive root resorption and ankylosis.

REGULATION OF WOUND HEALING

The sequential entry of cells to the wound site and subsequent ordered phases of repair are characteristic features of wound healing. The regulatory mechanisms postulated for this cellular cascade include different migratory rates among cell types, changing conditions in the local wound microenvironment, and the sequential elaboration of specific chemoattractants and growth factors.

Varying rates of cell migration in response to the same set of stimuli may explain differences in the time that different cells require to appear at the wound site. Given a

mutually desirable chemoattractant, neutrophils would precede macrophages, and both these phagocytic cells would precede fibroblasts. The extent of epithelial as compared with connective tissue cell migration along the root surface after therapy has a major influence on periodontal healing. After excision of epithelial and connective tissue components of the periodontal pocket, the epithelium frequently migrates apically to approach its presurgical location. This epithelial lining appears to preclude the formation of a fibrous attachment. Retardation or exclusion of the epithelium such that the root surface is repopulated by gingival connective tissue results in some fibrous attachment, but also in extensive root resorption (Karring et al., 1980).

The microenvironment of the wound changes markedly from the edge of the healing tissue to fully mature, healed tissue (Hunt et al., 1967). At the edge of the healing tissue, macrophages and neutrophils function in an acidic environment with a low oxygen tension. Lactate levels are high, as are concentrations of potassium generated by dying phagocytes. Rapidly dividing fibroblasts are found deep to this area, where the first capillary arcades cause the oxygen tension to rise rapidly. Deeper into the more mature granulation tissue, oxygen gradients become flatter, lactate decreases, and glucose levels approach normal. Because many cells are differentially sensitive to the chemical nature of their surroundings, these microenvironments play a role in regulating cellular succession and metabolism. For example, angiogenesis can be experimentally inhibited by increasing the oxygen tension within the wound cavity (Knighton et al., 1981). Similarly, radical changes in the wound environment caused by infection can arrest the healing process.

Major progress has been made in defining chemical factors in the wound site that attract cells to the wound and regulate their subsequent cellular growth and metabolic activity. These chemical chemoattractants and growth factors are thought to have primary responsibility for the ordered entry of cells into the wound area and the ensuing predictable series of healing events. Many cells, including neutrophils, macrophages, fibroblasts, and endothelial cells, exhibit chemotaxis. The migration of these cells to the wound site is an essential and limiting step in the healing process (Grotendorst et al., 1984). Chemotactic factors for neutrophils and macrophages include microbial products (Ward et al., 1968; Van Dyke, 1984), products of clotting and complement cascades (Snyderman et al., 1970), and factors elaborated by platelets (Ross et al., 1986). Fibroblasts are attracted by collagen and collagen peptides, as well as by fibronectin fragments (Postlethwaite et al., 1981). Fibronectin may also be chemotactic for endothelial cells (Grinnell, 1984). Once cells are attracted to the wound site, a number of wound hormones, or growth factors, appear to stimulate proliferation and metabolic activity. The most thoroughly studied of these wound hormones is platelet-derived growth factor (PDGF) (Kohler and Lipton, 1974; Ross et al., 1974). PDGF has a wide range of biologic activity, including both chemotactic activity and induction of cell proliferation. In addition, PDGF stimulates fibroblasts and regulates the composition of the connective tissue matrix. In gingival fibroblasts, PDGF stimulates production of type V collagen and appears to regulate the relative synthesis of type III versus type IV collagen (Narayanan and Page, 1983). It also induces the production of collagenase from fibroblasts and smooth muscle cells (Bauer et al., 1985). Other growth factors with similar biologic properties have been isolated from a variety of cell types, including macrophages, fibroblasts, and endothelial cells (Gospodarowicz et al., 1986; Ross et al., 1986).

HISTOLOGIC PATTERNS OF PERIODONTAL HEALING

Wound healing after periodontal therapy can show one or more of six general histologic patterns:

1. No repair
2. Long junctional epithelial attachment to the root surface
3. Connective tissue attachment to the root surface
4. New bone separated from the root surface
5. New bone with root resorption and/or ankylosis to the root surface
6. New attachment apparatus

Factors that influence the relative contribution of each pattern to the healed wound include plaque control, the initial architecture of the osseous damage, the therapeutic

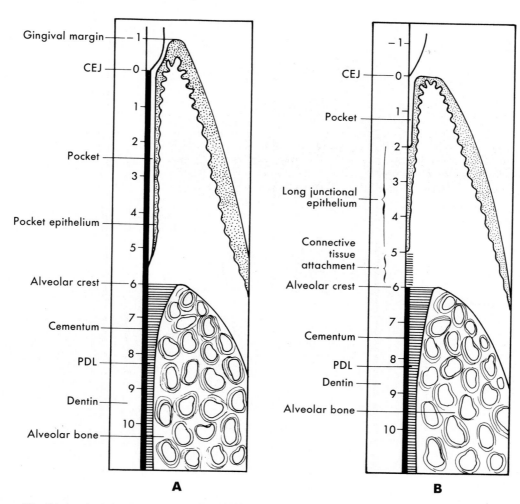

Fig. 31-1. A, Suprabony lesion before therapy. Gingival margin is located 1 mm coronal to cementoenamel junction *(CEJ)*. Pocket depth is approximately 6 mm, and attachment loss is approximately 5 mm, measured from apical termination of epithelium to gingival margin and CEJ, respectively. Four to 5 mm of alveolar bone and associated periodontal ligament *(PDL)* attachment to cementum have been lost. **B,** Example of healing in a suprabony lesion by long junctional epithelial and gingival connective tissue attachment to root surface.

approach employed, the source of cells that repopulate the wound, and postoperative maintenance care (Robertson, 1983; Ramfjord, 1984). Examples of these healing patterns are illustrated in suprabony lesions in Fig. 31-1 and infrabony lesions in Fig. 31-2.

The first pattern, failure of repair, has been related to insufficient control of infection, inadequate debridement of the lesion, and the absence of a long-term maintenance care program (Ramfjord, 1984).

Healing by a long junctional epithelial attachment to the root surface (Figs. 31-1, *B*, and 31-2, *B*) has been demonstrated in both suprabony and infrabony pockets (Caton and Nyman, 1980; Caton et al., 1980). Many studies have found that a long junctional epithelial attachment extending to the apical location of preexisting pocket epithelium was the primary pattern of healing after periodontal therapy.

Connective tissue attachment to the root surface is often termed *reattachment* and is illustrated apical to the junctional epithelium in Fig. 31-1, *B*. Two forms of this healing pattern have been postulated. The first is the insertion of collagen fibers into newly formed cementum in areas of the root surface that have not been affected by periodontitis. The second is splicing or interdigitation of gingival fibers with collagen fibers of the root surface that have been exposed by demineralization with citric acid (Register and Burdick, 1976; Ririe et al., 1980).

The last three patterns of healing involve the formation of new bone. New bone occurs primarily in infrabony defects and has been demonstrated both after careful debridement of the lesion (Prichard, 1983) and after placement of a variety of grafting materials (Schallhorn, 1980; Gara and Adams, 1981). A number of studies have suggested that the primary relationships of such new bone with the root

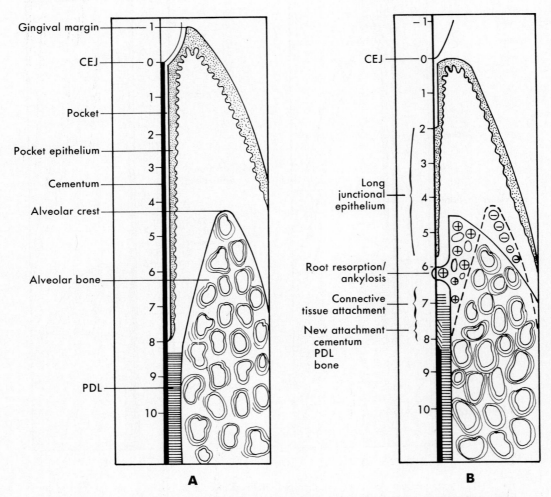

Fig. 31-2. A, Infrabony lesion before therapy. Gingival margin is located 1 mm coronal to CEJ. Pocket depth is approximately 9 mm, and attachment loss is approximately 8 mm. Horizontal component of alveolar bone loss is 2 to 3 mm, and pocket epithelium extends an additional 4 mm apically from alveolar crest. **B,** Example of healing in an infrabony pocket by long junctional epithelial attachment to root surface, new bone separated from root surface by epithelium, new bone with ankylosis to root surface, and regeneration of attachment apparatus.

surface is separation by epithelium in coronal areas and islands of ankylosis and root resorption in apical areas of the treated infrabony pockets. Demonstration of true regeneration of cementum, alveolar bone, and functionally attached periodontal ligament fibers has been confined to the most apical portions of treated lesions as illustrated in Fig. 31-2, *B*.

A number of studies have evaluated the histologic patterns of healing after various forms of periodontal therapy (Caton and Zander, 1976; Listgarten and Rosenburg, 1979; Caton and Nyman, 1980; Caton et al., 1980; Stahl and Froum, 1986; Froum and Stahl, 1987). Taken collectively, these investigations show that healing after most forms of periodontal therapy occurs by the formation of a long junctional epithelial attachment to the root surface and by limited areas of connective tissue attachment at the apical extent of the lesion. Most studies have failed to demonstrate new cementum or connective tissue attachment in coronal areas of root surfaces previously affected by periodontitis that were covered by gingival connective tissue. The results of studies that examined the use of citric acid to induce gingival connective tissue attachment have not been consistent (Crigger et al., 1978; Nyman et al., 1981; Marks and Mehta, 1986), and clinical use of demineralization techniques to achieve connective tissue attachment remains experimental. However, citric acid demineralization with coronally placed flaps appears promising in furcation defects (Gantes et al., 1988).

New bone formation is common in infrabony pockets, particularly after placing osseous grafts, or with procedures that favor regeneration from cells of the periodontal ligament. Some regeneration of the entire attachment apparatus appears possible in apical areas of the healing lesion with most forms of therapy. But the extent to which this healing represents new attachment or reattachment is unclear in many studies. This lack of certainty is a function of methods used to define, at the time of histologic examination, those areas of the root surface that were initially healthy or diseased. Examination of root surface areas that were initially healthy and subsequently healed by reattachment might be interpreted as new attachment. Many investigations have addressed the problem in suprabony pockets by placing a notch in the root surface before therapy to indicate the most apical extension of the pocket epithelium. New cementum, inserted connective tissue fibers, and bone observed coronal to the notch during histologic evaluation after therapy serve as an indication of new attachment. Such notches improve definition of previously healthy and diseased root surfaces. However, notches are mechanically difficult to place in infrabony pockets. In suprabony pockets, notches placed at the crest of the alveolar bone tend to overestimate the pretreatment apical extent of epithelium. Where possible, placing the notch at the most apical location of calculus is the most reliable reference point for studies of new attachment, since regeneration of the attachment apparatus coronal to the notch must have occurred on a previously diseased root surface.

Considerable insight into factors that favor a particular healing pattern has come from experiments in dogs and monkeys wherein teeth affected with experimental periodontitis were extracted and reimplanted into unaffected recipient sites (Gottlow et al., 1984; Isidor et al., 1986). Reimplantation procedures were designed such that cells repopulating the wound adjacent to the root surfaces were derived either from epithelium, from gingival connective tissue, from alveolar bone, or from the periodontal ligament. Where migration of epithelium was permitted, a long junctional epithelial attachment was formed. Where epithelium was excluded, roots in close contact with gingival connective tissue consistently showed root resorption, whereas roots apposed to bone showed both root resorption and ankylosis. In neither case was there formation of new cementum or new connective tissue attachment. Under these conditions, migrating epithelium appeared to function as a barrier to root resorption and ankylosis, but also prevented formation of a new attachment apparatus. However, true regeneration of cementum with entrapped periodontal ligament collagen fibers was demonstrated where cells from oral epithelium, gingival connective tissue, and bone were excluded and repopulating cells were derived from the periodontal ligament.

CLINICAL PATTERNS OF PERIODONTAL HEALING

Most studies of periodontal therapy have used clinical methods to evaluate healing. These have included periodontal probing, radiographic examination, and surgical reentry of the treated area. In general, these measurement techniques fail to define the histologic relationship between the tooth surface and other periodontal structures. The extent of penetration of the periodontal probe is influenced by the degree of gingival inflammation (Listgarten, 1980). Thus decreased penetration may reflect improved gingival health rather than the formation of new bone. Radiographic and reentry studies can identify newly formed bone but cannot define the relationship of that new bone with the root surface. Indeed, all of the healing patterns except no repair would be considered clinically successful, since long junctional epithelial and gingival connective tissue attachments to the root surface show decreased probing depth and are no more susceptible to recurrent attachment loss than are comparable nondiseased sites. Healing patterns with new bone formation show decreased probing depth, as well as radiographic and reentry evidence of increased osseous support.

Periodontal therapy usually consists of a series of individual procedures. These procedures may include supragingival plaque control, scaling and root planing, periodontal surgery, regeneration procedures, and periodontal maintenance.

Plaque control

Essentially all periodontal therapy includes instructional programs to establish excellent personal oral hygiene. Such programs may be supplemented by professional plaque removal at regular intervals (Axelsson and Lindhe, 1978) or by antimicrobial agents (Kornman, 1986). In patients with gingivitis, supragingival plaque removal is effective in resolving gingival inflammation. For example, subjects who developed experimental gingivitis coincident with abstention from all oral hygiene practices returned to baseline levels of excellent gingival health within 7 days after reinstitution of plaque control (Löe et al., 1965). However, oral hygiene procedures alone are much less effective in patients with periodontitis. Monkeys with ligature-induced periodontitis that received thrice-weekly tooth cleaning with a rubber cup and pumice for 6 weeks showed only minor changes in the Gingival Index, levels of attachment, and subgingival microflora (Siegrist and Kornman, 1982). Studies in humans also have suggested that plaque control alone in areas with deep periodontal pockets may have some beneficial effects on overt gingival inflammation but will not resolve gingivitis, significantly improve attachment levels, or effect major changes in the subgingival flora (Listgarten et al., 1978; Smulow et al., 1983).

Scaling and root planing

Like plaque control, scaling and root planing have long been considered an essential component of periodontal therapy. The rationale for the procedure is that it removes subgingival plaque and calculus, mechanically removes the remaining subgingival flora in and attached to the root surface, and eliminates toxic substances that have been incorporated into the root surface (O'Leary, 1986). Many studies have shown that scaling and root planing, combined with excellent plaque control, are effective in resolving both gingivitis and periodontitis (Axelsson and Lindhe, 1981; Pihlstrom et al., 1983; Badersten et al., 1987). However, both supragingival and subgingival debridement are required for resolution of periodontitis. Scaling and root planing performed every 6 months in the absence of other therapeutic components, including plaque control, were not effective in controlling naturally occurring periodontitis in dogs (Morrison et al., 1979).

Periodontal surgery

Surgical methods for the treatment of periodontal disease have been used for centuries. The primary rationale for periodontal surgery is to expose root surfaces that are inaccessible, such as those associated with deep pockets or furcations, in order to improve the efficiency of scaling and root planing (Ramfjord and Nissle, 1974). The extent of calculus removal by scaling and root planing with and without surgical access is similar in pockets less than 6 mm deep, but in pockets deeper than 6 mm, removal of calculus with hand instruments is significantly better when scaling and root planing are combined with access flaps (Buchanan and Robertson, 1987).

Differences among various surgical procedures are not always clear and in many instances represent technical variations of a previously established method. Indeed, in what Waerhaug (1971) called "the surgical fashion show," the popularity of particular procedures has often been based on force of personality rather than biologic insight. Beginning with the pioneering work of Ramfjord and colleagues (Ramfjord et al., 1968), a number of investigators have used controlled longitudinal studies to compare the ability of various surgical methods to restore damaged periodontal tissues and maintain periodontal health.

Investigations at the University of Michigan compared two procedures: scaling and root planing plus subgingival curettage versus scaling and root planing plus surgical pocket elimination either by gingivectomy or by apically positioned flaps with osseous surgery (Ramfjord et al., 1968). Subsequent studies included modified Widman flaps in the comparison (Ramfjord et al., 1973, 1980, 1982, 1987; Hill et al., 1981). These studies employed a split-mouth design whereby the procedures were performed in different areas of each patient's mouth. All teeth were evaluated. Using a similar design, Pihlstrom et al. (1983) compared scaling and root planing alone with scaling and root planing plus a modified Widman flap 4 years after these procedures were performed. In a 4-month trial, Zamet (1975) also used a split-mouth design to evaluate subgingival curettage, an apically positioned flap, and an envelope flap sutured near the presurgical position of the gingival margin.

Investigations begun at the University of Gotenburg in 1973 used five groups of patients to compare five procedures: scaling and root planing plus a modified Widman flap, with and without osseous surgery; apically positioned flaps, with and without osseous surgery; and gingivectomy (Lindhe and Nyman, 1975; Nyman et al., 1975; Rosling et al., 1976a, 1981). Clinical evaluation included incisors, canines, premolars, and the mesial surfaces of first molars. In addition, the modified Widman flap in single groups of patients was evaluated by Axelsson and Lindhe (1981) 6 years after surgery and by Raeste and Kilpinen (1981) 4 years after surgery. Yukna and Williams (1980) have reported results in a group of patients 5 years after the excisional new attachment procedure, a minimally reflected access flap.

A number of variations exist among these investigations, including initial disease severity, split-mouth versus group design, length of the postoperative evaluation period, degree of plaque control during the evaluation period, and specific tooth types studied. Despite these variations, clinical patterns of healing in all studies were similar. Gingival inflammation and pocket depths were reduced equally by all surgical procedures, and postsurgical gain or loss of attachment was not related to the degree of pocket reduction. Approximate changes in attachment levels in initially shallow, moderate, and deep pockets after various surgical procedures are shown in Fig. 31-3. In areas exhibiting initial pocket depths of 1 to 3 mm, all procedures were associated with some loss of attachment 2, 4, and 8 years after therapy. In moderate pockets, with initial depths of 4 to 6 mm, these procedures were equally effective in maintaining or improving postoperative attachment levels for up to 8 years after therapy. The greatest gain of attachment for all procedures was observed in pockets ini-

tially deeper than 6 mm. In general, flap procedures that included osseous surgery were no more effective in reducing pocket depths or improving attachment levels than were flap procedures that did not include osseous resection. Moreover, plaque and gingival index scores were essentially equal 24 months after modified Widman and apically positioned flap surgery regardless of whether bone recontouring was performed (Rosling et al., 1976a, 1976b).

Regeneration procedures

A number of studies have shown significant clinical gain of attachment and formation of new bone after gingival surgery (Ellegaard and Löe, 1971; Rosling et al., 1976b). As previously discussed, this clinical improvement probably results primarily from restoration of gingival health and from healing by a long junctional epithelial attachment to the root surface, which, in some areas, separates new bone from the root surface. Various graft materials have been inserted into the lesion in efforts to improve the amount of new bone formed and to encourage regeneration of the attachment apparatus. Osseous autografts and allografts are associated with significant new bone formation, particularly in infrabony pockets (Schallhorn, 1980). Other studies on the use of osseous grafts have been less encouraging (Renvert et al., 1985; Schrad and Tussing, 1986), and some reports have suggested that the long-term results of osseous grafting are not substantially different from those of nongrafted controls (Carraro et al., 1976). Osseous grafts do not appear to induce bone formation or to stimulate connective tissue attachment, and the long-term relationship of such grafts with the root surface remains a necessary area of future research using the time-honored, double-blind control, human trial (Egelberg, 1987).

In recent studies investigators have attempted to induce regeneration by placing various membranes over the denuded root surface such that cells from all periodontal tissues except the periodontal ligament were prevented from repopulating the wound area (Nyman et al., 1982a, 1982b; Pontoriero et al., 1988). The procedure has been termed *guided tissue regeneration.* Preliminary results in humans suggest that healing after guided tissue regeneration is characterized by extensive amounts of new attachment (Gottlow et al., 1986). Routine use of the procedure in periodontal therapy awaits controlled studies with improved membranes and refined surgical techniques for membrane placement, and an evaluation of possible adverse effects such as root resorption and ankylosis over time.

Periodontal maintenance

No matter what combination of procedures is used in periodontal therapy, the clinical success of healing depends on reinforcement of personal oral hygiene and main-

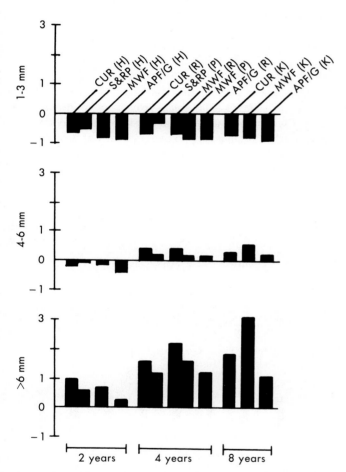

Fig. 31-3. Approximate values from four studies of periodontal therapy for gain or loss of attachment in areas with initial pocket depths of 1 to 3, 4 to 6, and greater than 6 mm. These values were obtained at 2, 4, and 8 years after subgingival curettage *(CUR)*, scaling and root planing *(S&RP)*, modified Widman flap *(MWF)*, and apically positioned flap or gingivectomy *(APF/G)*. For the latter, areas with initial pocket depths greater than 4 to 5 mm were treated by apically positioned flaps with osseous surgery. Note loss of 0.5 to 1 mm of peridontal attachment in sites with initially shallow pockets (1 to 3 mm), modest gain (<1 mm) in sites with 4 to 6 mm initial pocket depths, and gain of 1 to 3 mm of attachment in sites with initial pocket depths of >6 mm. *H,* Hill et al., 1981; *R,* Ramford et al., 1975; *P,* Pihlstrom et al., 1981; *K,* Knowles et al., 1979.

tenance of oral conditions consistent with plaque control. Considerable evidence suggests that rapid wound healing, improved measures of periodontal health, and prevention of further attachment loss require maintenance therapy at frequent intervals (Axelsson and Lindhe, 1981; Ramfjord et al., 1982). In fact, one series of studies has suggested that performing periodontal therapy in a plaque-infected dentition results in additional periodontal damage rather than resolution of the lesion (Nyman et al., 1977).

COMPLICATIONS AFTER PERIODONTAL THERAPY

Major immediate complications common to all surgery may include bleeding, swelling, infection, tissue necrosis, and severe pain. Grafting procedures pose an additional risk of sequestration and resorption of the root surface adjacent to the graft site. Gingival recession is the most common long-term problem after periodontal therapy. Recession increases the area of root surface susceptible to root caries. Other long-term complications may be associated with the use of electrosurgery.

Immediate complications of periodontal wound healing

For periodontal surgical procedures, the risks of immediate complications are extremely small. A recent survey (Curtis et al., 1985) of 304 surgical sessions that involved gingival surgery, osseous surgery, or osseous grafts showed a low percentage of cases with moderate to severe bleeding (1%), infection (1.3%), swelling (1%), and adverse tissue changes (3%). Minimal or no pain was reported by 51.3% of the patients. More severe pain was directly related to the duration and complexity of the procedure. In a retrospective study of 218 patients who had been treated with a variety of periodontal surgical procedures, the prevalence of postoperative infection, including swelling and progressive pain, was approximately 1%, and no difference in the occurrence of postoperative infection was observed between patients who had received prophylactic antibiotic coverage and those who had not. Mean pain scores, as measured on a visual analogue scale, of 20 patients who had been treated with periodontal surgery peaked at 4 to 6 hours and steadily returned to presurgical levels by 24 hours (Linden et al., 1986).

In addition to these immediate complications, graft procedures have been associated with postoperative sequestration of graft material and root resorption (Schallhorn, 1980). Sequestration of graft materials has been reported to begin immediately after surgery and to continue as long as 2 years after graft placement (Listgarten and Rosenberg, 1979). Root resorption has been observed after placement of a variety of osseous and synthetic graft materials (Schallhorn, 1972; Jaffin et al., 1985; Froum and Stahl, 1987). Resorption is a major feature of healing in studies in dogs and monkeys when gingival connective tissue or bone cells repopulate a diseased root surface (Nyman et

al., 1980). Root resorption appears to be less frequent after grafts in humans but may be a significant problem after placing fresh iliac marrow (Dragoo and Sullivan, 1973).

Periodontal dressings have long been advocated to prevent or minimize immediate problems after periodontal therapy. Comparisons of dressed and nondressed sites after therapy have not shown advantages for periodontal dressings in postoperative discomfort, bleeding, swelling, inflammation, or clinical resolution of the treated lesion (Allen and Caffesse, 1983). Moreover, periodontal dressings appear to favor microbial colonization of the wound. Periodontal dressings have a number of practical advantages that include preventing coronal displacement of flaps and protecting the wound site from mechanical injury, but in general, dressings neither prevent complications nor promote wound healing (Sachs et al., 1984).

Recession

Recession is the loss of gingiva over the root surface. Recession resulting from apical movement of the gingival margin is common after periodontal therapy and may be associated with the postoperative problems of thermal sensitivity, esthetics, phonetics, and interproximal food reten-

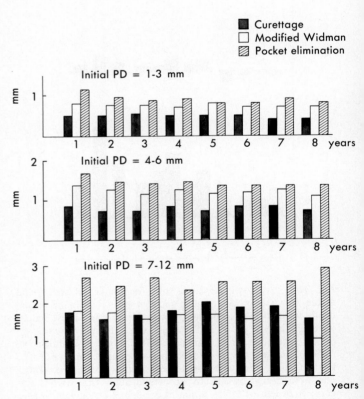

Fig. 31-4. Gingival recession measured 1 to 8 years after curettage, modified Widman flap, and pocket elimination surgery in sites with initial pocket depths of 1 to 3 mm, 4 to 7 mm, and 7 to 12 mm. (Data from Knowles JW et al: J Periodontol 50:225, 1979.)

tion. The extent of recession is influenced by the initial pocket depth and the type of therapy (Badersten et al., 1984). Values for recession derived from longitudinal studies of periodontal therapy (Knowles et al., 1979) are shown in Fig. 31-4. In areas with initially shallow pocket depths, average values for recession ranged from approximately 0.5 to 1 mm. Recession in areas with initial pocket depths of 4 to 6 mm averaged approximately 1 mm, whereas pockets 7 to 12 mm deep showed substantially greater recession, which approached 3 mm after pocket elimination surgery. For all initial pocket depths, recession was least after curettage and greatest after pocket elimination surgery. In general, the recession recorded 1 year after therapy remained constant for the remaining 7 years of the study regardless of initial pocket depth or treatment procedure.

Root carles

Root caries is usually seen as a shallow (less than 2 mm deep), softened area that is often discolored and is characterized by destruction of cementum and penetration of underlying dentin. As it progresses, it extends circumferentially rather than in depth. Undetected lesions on the proximal surface may ultimately involve the pulp (Newbrun, 1983).

A strong association between root caries and advanced periodontal disease has been reported in many human populations (Newbrun et al., 1984). It is clear that root caries causes the loss of teeth in patients with periodontal disease (Hamp et al., 1975). In one population with untreated moderate to severe periodontal disease, 58% of all patients had root caries, with an average of nearly four lesions per patient (Hix and O'Leary, 1976). Patients treated for periodontal disease and then seen once a year for maintenance care appeared to have less root caries: 45% of such patients had root surface lesions, with an average of two lesions per patient. In a prospective study of root caries in a group of treated periodontal patients who were being seen at 3- to 6-month intervals for maintenance care, approximately two thirds developed new root surface lesions during a 4-year observation period (Ravald and Hamp, 1981). However, in these patients the attack rate was low, and fewer than 5% of exposed root surfaces developed lesions.

Conditions, in addition to recession, that have been most strongly associated with root caries are microbial colonization of exposed root surfaces and low salivary secretion rates. Root caries is undoubtedly of microbial etiology. Bacteriologic sampling of human plaque covering caries of the root surface has yielded predominantly *A. viscosus*. Microbial sampling of softened human dentin from root caries has also revealed the presence of other species of the genus *Actinomyces (A. naeslundii, A. odontolyticus, A. eriksonii)*, as well as *Rothia dentocariosa, Nocardia, Streptococcus mutans*, and aerobic diphtheroidal organisms with characteristics similar to those of the genus *Ar-*throbacter (Sumney and Jordan, 1974; Syed et al., 1975). In general, however, neither a specific microorganism nor a consistent pattern of oral flora has been associated with the initiation and progression of root caries in humans. The host response must also play a major role in development of the lesion, since patients suffering from decreased or absent salivary secretion experience a dramatically increased rate of root caries. The problem is especially acute in patients with Sjogren's syndrome or radiation-induced xerostomia.

Caries-preventive treatment in patients at high risk for root caries may involve oral hygiene instruction and dietary advice, but the cornerstone of any preventive regimen for these patients includes some mode of topical fluoride therapy.

Electrosurgery

Electrosurgery has been suggested for resection of gingival tissues to facilitate making impressions and restoration of subgingival caries, increasing clinical crown length, and managing osseous and furcation problems associated with periodontitis (Oringer, 1975). Healing of gingival tissues after electrosurgery appears to be comparable with that of conventional surgery (Kalkwarf et al., 1981). However, some studies of the effects of electrosurgery on alveolar bone report normal repair and no tissue damage, whereas others report delayed healing, necrosis, and loss of attachment. This variability among reports of healing after electrosurgery has been attributed to differences in the current wave form, shape and size of the electrode, and speed of the electrode through the tissue (Williams, 1984). Electrosurgery that involves based or unbased cervical amalgam restorations often results in damage to the pulp and may cause resorption of cementum and alveolar bone in interadicular areas of multirooted teeth (Robertson et al., 1978; Spangberg et al., 1982). Thus electrosurgery that may involve alveolar bone or cervical restorations should be avoided, since it is often associated with an increased risk of postoperative complications.

REFERENCES

Allen DR and Caffesse RG: Comparison of results following modified Widman flap surgery with and without surgical dressing, J Periodontol 54:470, 1983.

Axelsson P and Lindhe J: Effect of controlled oral hygiene procedures on caries and periodontal disease in adults, J Clin Periodontol 5:133, 1978.

Axelsson P and Lindhe J: The significance of maintenance care in the treatment of periodontal disease, J Clin Periodontol 8:281, 1981.

Badersten A, Nilveus R, and Egelberg J: Four-year observations of basic periodontal therapy, J Clin Periodontol 14:438, 1987.

Badersten A et al: Effect of nonsurgical periodontal therapy. II. Severely advanced periodontitis, J Clin Periodontol 11:63, 1984.

Bauer EA et al: Stimulation of in vitro human skin collagenase expression by platelet-derived growth factor, Proc Natl Acad Sci USA 82:4132, 1985.

Buchanan SA and Robertson PB: Calculus removal by scaling/root planing with and without surgical access, J Periodontol 58:159, 1987.

Carraro JJ et al: Intraoral cancellous bone autografts in the treatment on infrabony pockets, J Clin Periodontol 3:104, 1976.

Caton J and Nyman S: Histometric evaluation of periodontal surgery. I. The modified Widman flap procedure, J Clin Periodontol 7:212, 1980.

Caton J and Zander H: Osseous repair of an infrabony pocket without new attachment of connective tissue, J Clin Periodontol 3:54, 1976.

Caton J et al: Histometric evaluation of periodontal surgery. II. Connective tissue attachment levels after four regenerative procedures, J Clin Periodontol 7:224, 1980.

Crigger M et al: The effect of topical citric acid application on the healing of experimental furcation defects in dogs, J Periodont Res 13:538, 1978.

Curtis JW, McLain JB, and Hutchinson RA: The incidence and severity of complications and pain following periodontal surgery, J Periodontol 56:597, 1985.

Dragoo MR and Sullivan HC: A clinical and histological evaluation of autogenous iliac bone grafts in humans. II. External root resorption, J Periodontol 44:614, 1973.

Egelberg J: Regeneration and repair of periodontal tissues, J Periodont Res 22:233, 1987.

Ellegaard B and Löe H: New attachment of periodontal tissues after treatment of intrabony lesions, J Periodontol 42:648, 1971.

Froum S and Stahl SS: Human intraosseous healing responses to the placement of tricalcium phosphate ceramic implants. II. 13 to 18 months, J Periodontol 58:103, 1987.

Gantes B et al: Treatment of periodontal furcation defects. II. Bone regeneration in mandibular Class II defects, J Clin Periodontol 15:232, 1988.

Gara GG and Adams DE: Implant therapy in human intrabony pockets: a review of the literature, J West Soc Periodont Periodont Abstr 2:1981.

Gospodarowicz D et al: Fibroblast growth factor, Mol Cell Endocrinol 46:187, 1986.

Gottlow J et al: New attachment formation as the result of contolled tissue regeneration, J Clin Periodontol 11:494, 1984.

Gottlow J et al: New attachment formation in the human periodontium by guided tissue regeneration case reports, J Clin Periodontol 13:604, 1986.

Grinnell F: Fibronectin and wound healing, J Cell Biochem 26:107, 1984.

Grotendorst GR et al: Molecular mediators of tissue repair. In Hunt TK et al, editors: Biological and clinical aspects of soft and hard tissue repair, New York, 1984, Praeger Publishers.

Hamp SE et al: Periodontal treatment of multirooted teeth: results after 5 years, J Clin Periodontol 2:126, 1975.

Hill RW et al: Four types of periodontal treatment compared over two years, J Periodontol 52:655, 1981.

Hix JO and O'Leary TJ: The relationship between cemental caries, oral hygiene status and fermentable carbohydrate intake, J Periodontol 47:398, 1976.

Hunt TK et al: Respiratory gas tensions and pH in healing wounds, Am J Surg 114:302, 1967.

Isidor F et al: The significance of coronal growth of periodontal ligament tissue for new attachment formation, J Clin Periodontol 13:145, 1986.

Jaffin R, Greenstein G, and Berman C: External root resorption associated with placement of Durapatite—case report, Periodont Case Rep 7:32, 1985.

Kalkwarf KL et al: Healing of electrosurgical incisions in gingiva: early histologic observations in adult men, J Prosthet Dent 46:662, 1981.

Karring T et al: Healing following implantation of periodontitis affected roots into bone tissue, J Clin Periodontol 7:96, 1980.

Knighton DR et al: Regulation of wound healing angiogenesis: effect of oxygen gradient and inspired oxygen concentration, Surgery 90:262, 1981.

Knowles JW et al: Results of periodontal treatment related to pocket depth and attachment level: eight years, J Periodontol 50:225, 1979.

Kohler N and Lipton A: Platelets as a source of fibroblast growth-promoting activity, Exp Cell Res 87:297, 1974.

Kornman KS: The role of supragingival plaque in the prevention and treatment of periodontal diseases: a review of current concepts, J Periodont Res 21:5, 1986.

Kurkinen M et al: Sequential appearance of fibronectin and collagen in experimental granulation tissue, Lab Invest 43:47, 1980.

Leibovich SJ: Mesenchymal cell proliferation in wound repair: the role of macrophages. In Hunt TK et al, editors: Biological and clinical aspects of soft and hard tissue repair, New York, 1984, Praeger Publishers.

Leibovich SJ and Ross R: The role of macrophages in wound repair: a study with hydrocortisone and antimacrophage serum, Am J Pathol 78:71, 1975.

Linden ET et al: A comparison of postoperative pain experience following periodontal surgery using two local anesthetic agents, J Periodontol 57:637, 1986.

Lindhe J and Nyman S: The effect of plaque control and surgical pocket elimination on the establishment and maintenance of periodontal health: a longitudinal study of periodontal therapy in cases of advanced disease, J Clin Periodontol 2:67, 1975.

Listgarten MA: Electron microscopic features of the newly formed epithelial attachment after gingival surgery, J Periodont Res 2:46, 1967.

Listgarten MA: Periodontal probing: what does it mean? J Periodontol 7:165, 1980.

Listgarten MA and Ellegaard B: Electron microscopic evidence of a cellular attachment between junctional epithelium and dental calculus, J Periodont Res 8:143, 1973.

Listgarten MA and Rosenberg MM: Histological study of repair following new attachment procedures in human periodontal lesions, J Periodontol 50:333, 1979.

Listgarten MA et al: Effect of tetracycline and/or scaling on human periodontol disease: clinical, microbiological and histological observation, J Clin Periodontol 5:246, 1978.

Löe H et al: Experimental gingivitis in man, J Periodontol 36:177, 1965.

Marks SC and Mehta NR: Lack of effect of citric acid treatment of root surfaces on the formation of new connective tissue attachment, J Clin Periodontol 13:109, 1986.

Martin BM et al: Stimulation of non-lymphoid mesenchymal cell proliferation by a macrophage-derived growth factor, J Immunol 126:1510, 1981.

Melcher AH: On the repair potential of periodontal tissues, J Periodontol 47:256, 1976.

Morrison EC et al: Effects of repeated scaling and root planing and/or controlled oral hygiene on the periodontal attachment level and pocket depth in beagle dogs, J Periodont Res 14:428, 1979.

Narayanan AS and Page RC: Biosynthesis and regulation of type V collagen in diploid human fibroblasts, J Biol Chem 258:11694, 1983.

Newbrun E: Cariology, ed 2, Baltimore, 1983, Williams & Wilkins.

Newbrun E et al: Root caries, CDA J:12:68, 1984.

Nyman S et al: Effect of professional tooth cleaning on healing after periodontal surgery, J Clin Periodontol 2:80, 1975.

Nyman S et al: Periodontal surgery in plaque-infected dentitions, J Clin Periodontol 4:240, 1977.

Nyman S et al: Healing following implantation of periodontitis-affected roots into gingival connective tissue, J Clin Periodontol 7:394, 1980.

Nyman S et al: Healing following surgical treatment and root demineralization in monkeys with periodontal disease, J Clin Periodontol 8:249, 1981.

Nyman S et al: New attachment following surgical treatment of human periodontal disease, J Clin Periodontol 9:290, 1982a.

Nyman S et al: The regenerative potential of the periodontal ligament: an experimental study in the monkey, J Clin Periodontol 9:157, 1982b.

O'Leary TJ: The impact of research on scaling and root planing, J Periodontol 57:69, 1986.

Oringer MJ: Electrosurgery in dentistry, Philadelphia, 1975, WB Saunders Co.

Pihlstrom BL et al: Comparison of surgical and nonsurgical treatment of periodontal disease: a review of current studies and additional results after 6½ years, J Clin Periodontol 10:524, 1983.

Pontoriero R et al: Guided tissue regeneration in degree II furcation–involved mandibular molars: a clinical study, J Clin Periodontol 15:247, 1988.

Postlethwaite AE et al: Induction of fibroblast chemotaxis by fibronectin: localization of the chemotactic region to a 140,000 molecular weight non-gelatin binding fragment, J Exp Med 153:494, 1981.

Prichard JF: The diagnosis and management of vertical bony defects, J Periodontol 54:29, 1983.

Raeste AM and Kilpinen E: Clinical and radiographic long-term study of teeth with periodontal destruction treated by modified Widman flap operation, J Clin Periodontol 8:415, 1981.

Ramfjórd SP: Changing concepts in periodontics, J Prosthet Dent 52:781, 1984.

Ramfjord SP and Nissle RR: The modified Widman flap, J Periodontol 45:601, 1974.

Ramfjord SP et al: Subgingival curettage versus surgical elimination of periodontal pockets, J Periodontol 39:167, 1968.

Ramfjord SP et al: Longitudinal study of periodontal therapy, J Periodontol 44:66, 1973.

Ramfjord SP et al: Results of periodontal therapy related to tooth type, J Periodontol 51:270, 1980.

Ramfjord SP et al: Oral hygiene and maintenance of periodontal support, J Periodontol 53:26, 1982.

Ramfjord SP et al: Four modalities of periodontal treatment compared over 5 years, J Clin Periodontol 14:445, 1987.

Ravald N and Hamp SE: Prediction of root surface caries in patients treated for advanced periodontal disease, J Clin Periodontol 8:400, 1981.

Register AA and Burdick FA: Accelerated reattachment with cementogenesis to dentin, demineralized in situ. II. Defect repair, J Periodontol 47:497, 1976.

Renvert S et al: Healing after treatment of periodontal intraosseous defects. III. Effect of osseous grafting and citric acid conditioning, J Clin Periodontol 12:441, 1985.

Ririe CM et al: Healing of periodontal connective tissue following surgical wounding and application of citric acid in dogs, J Clin Periodontol 15:314, 1980.

Robertson PB: Surgical periodontal therapy: indications, selection and limitations, Int Dent J 33:137, 1983.

Robertson PB et al: Pulpal and periodontal effects of electrosurgery involving cervical metallic restorations, Oral Surg 46:702, 1978.

Rosling B et al: The healing potential of periodontal tissues following different techniques of periodontal surgery in plaque free dentitions, J Clin Periodontol 3:233, 1976a.

Rosling B et al: The effect of systematic plaque control on bone regeneration in infrabony pockets, J Clin Periodontol 3:38, 1976b.

Rosling B et al: Longitudinal study of surgical treatment of periodontal disease: results after 6 years, J Dent Res 60A:644, 1981.

Ross R et al: A platelet-dependent serum factor that stimulates the proliferation of arterial smooth muscle cells in vitro, Proc Natl Acad Sci USA 71:1207, 1974.

Ross R et al: The biology of platelet-derived growth factor, Cell 46:155, 1986.

Sachs HA et al: Current status of periodontal dressings, J Periodontol 55:689, 1984.

Schallhorn RG: Postoperative problems associated with iliac transplants, J Periodontol 43:3, 1972.

Schallhorn RG: Long term evaluation of osseous grafts in periodontal therapy, Int Dent J 30:101, 1980.

Schrad SG and Tussing GJ: Human allografts of iliac bone and marrow in periodontal osseous defects, J Periodontol 57:205, 1986.

Siegrist BE and Kornman KS: The effect of supragingival plaque control on the composition of the subgingival microbial flora in ligature induced periodontitis in the monkey, J Dent Res 61:936, 1982.

Simpson D and Ross R: The neutrophilic leukocyte in wound repair: a study with anti-neutrophil serum, J Clin Invest 51:2009, 1972.

Smulow JB et al: The effect of supragingival plaque removal on anaerobic bacteria in deep periodontal pockets, J Am Dent Assoc 107:737, 1983.

Snyderman R et al: Polymorphonuclear leukocyte chemotactic activity in rabbit serum and guinea pig serum treated with immune complexes: evidence for C5a as the major chemotactic factor, Infect Immun 1:521, 1970.

Spangberg L et al: Pulpal effects of electrosurgery involving based and unbased cervical amalgam restoration, Oral Surg Oral Med Oral Pathol 54:678, 1982.

Stahl SS and Froum S: Histological evaluation of human intraosseous healing responses to the placement of tricalcium phosphate ceramic implants. I. Three to eight months, J Periodontol 57:211, 1986.

Sumney DL and Jordan HV: Characterization of bacteria isolated from human root surface carious lesions, J Dent Res 53:343, 1974.

Syed SA et al: Predominant cultivable flora isolated from human root surface plaque, Infect Immun 11:727, 1975.

Takata T et al: Ultrastructure of regenerated junctional epithelium after surgery of rat molar gingiva, J Periodontol 57:776, 1986.

Taylor AC and Campbell MM: Reattachment of gingival epithelium to the tooth, J Periodontol 43:281, 1972.

Thilander H and Hugoson A: The border zone tooth-enamel and epithelium after periodontal treatment, Acta Odontol Scand 28:147, 1970.

Van Dyke TE: Neutrophil receptor modulation in the pathogenesis of periodontal diseases, J Dent Res 63:452, 1984.

Waerhaug J: Role of periodontal surgery, J Dent Res 50:219, 1971.

Ward PA et al: Bacterial factors chemotactic for polymorphonuclear leukocytes, Am J Pathol 52:725, 1968.

Williams VD: Electrosurgery and wound healing: a review of the literature, J Am Dent Assoc 108:220, 1984.

Yukna RA and Williams RA: Five year evaluation of the excisional new attachment procedure, J Periodontol 51:382, 1980.

Zamet JS: A comparative clinical study of three periodontal surgical techniques, J Clin Periodontol 2:87, 1975.

Chapter 32

GENERAL PRINCIPLES OF ANTIINFECTIVE THERAPY

Joseph M. Mylotte

Polymicrobial nature of periodontal disease
Antibiotics used to treat periodontal disease
    Antibiotic susceptibility
    Toxicity of antibiotics
    Pharmacokinetic considerations
Factors affecting response to therapy
    Route of drug administration
    Dose and duration of therapy
    Duration and extent of infection
    Bacteriostatic versus bactericidal agents
    Host factors
Summary

In this chapter general aspects of the use of antibiotics as they pertain to periodontal disease are addressed. To understand therapeutic approaches with antibiotics, the practitioner must keep in mind that one is dealing with a mixed or polymicrobial infection in periodontal disease. Furthermore, this infection can be located in a relatively closed space (i.e., the periodontal pocket). Thus the pathology of periodontal disease has dictated the major approach to therapy: adequate drainage and removal of infected and necrotic tissue. Presently, the use of antibiotics must be considered adjunctive therapy and not a substitute for drainage, root debridement, and other accepted periodontal procedures.

In the remainder of this chapter the polymicrobial nature of periodontal infection is discussed briefly, followed by a general discussion of the antibiotics used to treat periodontal disease, pharmacokinetic considerations, and factors that may affect the response to therapy.

POLYMICROBIAL NATURE OF PERIODONTAL DISEASE

The use of antibiotics as part of the therapy for periodontol disease is based on the following observations: (1) differences in the microflora of those with and without periodontal disease (Socransky, 1977; Slots, 1979; Slots and Genco, 1984) or in active as compared with inactive sites in patients with periodontitis (Dzink et al., 1988); (2) isolation of the same organism or group of organisms from a large number of patients with the same periodontal disease; and (3) a detectable antibody response to specific bacterial strains in those with periodontal disease (Genco and Slots, 1984).

These various aspects are discussed in detail in other parts of this text. Suffice it to note that the organisms isolated are predominantly anaerobic or microaerophilic, and that multiple organisms are frequently isolated from a single lesion. Table 32-1 lists the bacteria commonly isolated from various forms of periodontal disease.

An important question is which organism(s) isolated from a periodontal lesion is responsible for specific types of periodontal disease. Certain organisms may be more important than others in producing periodontal disease. One of these groups is the black-pigmented *Bacteroides* strains (Slots and Genco, 1984). It is of interest that other *Bacteroides* species have been found to be important in the pathogenesis of infections at other body sites, notably encapsulated *Bacteroides fragilis* in experimental intraabdominal infection (Onderdonk et al., 1977). Thus, although multiple organisms may be isolated from periodontal lesions, there may be specific species responsible for initiating or propagating the process. This has important

Table 32-1. Predominant culturable flora of common periodontal diseases

Disease	Organism
Gingivitis	*Actinomyces* species
	Bacteroides intermedius
	Fusobacterium nucleatum
	Veillonella parvula
	Treponema species
Adult periodontitis	*Actinobacillus actinomycetemcomitans*
	Bacteroides gingivalis
	Bacteroides intermedius
	Bacteroides forsythus
	Eikenella corrodens
	Eubacterium species
	Fusobacterium nucleatum
	Spirochetes
	Wolinella recta
Juvenile periodontitis	*Actinobacillus actinomycetemcomitans*
	Capnocytophaga species
	Eikenella corrodens

therapeutic implications, as pointed out by Socransky (1977). If one can use antibiotic therapy directed against certain species of bacteria, it might improve the treatment of periodontal disease and possibly lessen adverse reactions associated with broad-spectrum antibiotic therapy.

Attempts have been made to evaluate the importance of a specific bacterial species in periodontal disease by creating monomicrobial infections in gnotobiotic animals. Many bacterial species tested in this manner have produced infection. However, Socransky (1977) noted that such models are somewhat artificial and may not be an accurate representation of human disease. He suggested using antibiotics with selective (versus broad-spectrum) activity as probes such that only susceptible organisms are eliminated and determine if this impacts on the disease process. No such studies have been done as yet. This is primarily because the antibiotics evaluated, such as penicillin, tetracycline, and their derivatives, have activity against most isolates as noted in Chapter 12, Table 12-1. However, erythromycin and metronidazole are not active against all periodontopathic organisms; in addition, organisms resistant to one of these agents are not, in general, resistant to the other. Thus these antibiotics would appear to be likely candidates to use in a comparative trial to determine the importance of certain organisms in periodontal disease.

In summary, multiple organisms, predominantly gram-negative anaerobes and microaerophilic bacteria, have been isolated in association with periodontal disease. This has led to the notion that periodontal infection is polymicrobial. However, certain organisms, such as black-pigmented *Bacteroides* and *Actinobacillus actinomycetemcomitans,* may be more important than others in the patho-genesis of periodontal infection. Thus, in terms of antimicrobial therapy for periodontal infection, one must consider agents with activity against the prominent pathogens, as well as a variety of other potentially pathogenic organisms, that have overgrown after repeated and unsuccessful treatments.

ANTIBIOTICS USED TO TREAT PERIODONTAL DISEASE

The choice of an antibiotic in the treatment of any infection must take into consideration several factors: the most likely organism(s) causing a particular infection, the antibiotic susceptibility of the infecting organism(s), comparative toxicities of appropriate antibiotic agents, and antibiotic pharmacokinetics. The first factor, the most likely organism(s) causing periodontal infection, has been discussed briefly in the previous section, and more detailed discussion of this important topic can be found in subsequent chapters dealing with specific periodontal infections. In this section the remaining factors listed above are discussed in a general way to give the dental practitioner insight into an approach to using antibiotic therapy in periodontal infection. One can find more detailed information on the use of antibiotics in periodontal disease in Chapter 12.

Antibiotic susceptibility

A limited number of antibiotics have been used to treat periodontal disease. These are listed in Chapter 12, Table 12-1, along with the susceptibility of periodontopathic bacteria to those antibiotics obtained from the published literature (Sutter et al., 1983; Baker et al., 1985). Based on susceptibility testing of a large number of isolates, both penicillin G and tetracycline and its derivatives (doxycycline and minocycline) would appear to be well suited for the treatment of periodontal infections. As a result of this type of susceptibility data, penicillin G and tetracycline have been the most frequently used agents to treat periodontal infection. Recently, however, there have been reports of beta-lactamase production by some oral *Bacteroides* strains (Murray and Rosenblatt, 1977). Beta-lactamase is an enzyme that degrades penicillin G and some of its derivatives to an inactive form; tetracyclines are not altered by this enzyme. Those organisms capable of producing beta-lactamase are resistant to killing by penicillin G, and this has caused concern for the use of penicillin G empirically to treat periodontal infection. Nevertheless, the actual prevalence of penicillin resistance among certain periodontopathic bacteria is not known at present.

Other agents have been used to treat periodontal infection, but each has some drawbacks from the point of view of susceptibility testing. Erythromycin is often used as an alternative to penicillin G in the penicillin-allergic individual. Periodontopathic bacteria are often resistant to erythromycin, as noted in Table 32-2. Therefore one must be

Table 32-2. Major toxicity of antibiotics currently used in treatment of periodontal disease

Antibiotic	Major toxic reaction
Penicillin	One of the least toxic antibiotics, but commonly causes hypersensitivity reactions of two types: (A) anaphylactic reactions with a prevalence of 0.004% to 0.04% of penicillin-treated patients and a mortality of 10% (especially with procaine-penicillin G); (B) serum sickness occurs in 1% to 7% of patients treated with penicillin; characterized by fever, malaise, urticaria, joint pains, lymphadenopathy, angioneurotic edema, and exfoliative dermatitis.
Clindamycin	Gastrointestinal side effects, including nausea, vomiting, abdominal cramps, and diarrhea. Diarrhea (often watery) varies from 0.3% to 21% and *Pseudomonas colitis* from 1.9% to 10%.
Erythromycin	Gastrointestinal side effects, including nausea, vomiting, and diarrhea.
Metronidazole	Gastrointestinal side effects, including unpleasant taste, furred tongue, nausea, and abdominal pain. Mutagenicity and carcinogenecity have been reported in bacteria and rats, respectively.
Tetracycline	Gastrointestinal side effects, including nausea, heartburn, epigastric pain, vomiting, and diarrhea. *Pseudomonas colitis* rarely occurs. *Candida albicans* superinfection, especially in debilitated patients. Photosensitivity and staphylococcal enterocolitis reported. Tooth pigmentation and delayed fontanelle closure seen in children; avoid use during pregnancy and in children up to 6 or 7 years old.
Minocycline	In general, the side effects seen with tetracycline can be seen with minocycline; in addition, minocycline can cause vestibular disturbances, characterized by vertigo, reversible dizziness, ataxia, and tinnitis associated with weakness.

From Genco RJ: J Periodontol 52:545, 1981.

cautious when prescribing erythromycin empirically to treat periodontal infection. Metronidazole has been evaluated recently in the treatment of periodontal disease (Loesche et al., 1981; Lindhe et al., 1982; Lekovic et al., 1983.) Although metronidazole has excellent activity against *Bacteroides* species and other obligate anaerobes, it is not effective against some important microaerophilic periodontal pathogens.

In summary, on the basis of antibiotic susceptibility testing of likely periodontal pathogens alone, tetracycline remains a good first choice for treatment of most patients with periodontal disease; however, it may not be optimal. One must then go on to refine the antibiotic choice by considering adverse effects of the antibiotics and their pharmacokinetics. Also, one must keep in mind the age of the patient in regard to these latter factors.

Toxicity of antibiotics

With a plethora of antibiotics now available, the issue of drug toxicity has assumed more importance in the process of choosing one agent over others. In regard to periodontal infection, only a limited number of agents have been used, and the adverse effects of these agents are well defined. The major adverse effects of antibiotics used to treat periodontal infection are given in Table 32-2. On the basis of drug toxicity alone (excluding the risk of hypersensitivity), penicillin would be the most acceptable agent. All the other agents listed can produce various adverse, nonallergic reactions. Thus, in prescribing an antibiotic, the practitioner must consider the issue of side effects. The risk of such effects may be greater than the benefits of the antimicrobial effect in some situations. Likewise, the practitioner is obligated to communicate to the patient the possible side effects of any agent prescribed.

Pharmacokinetic considerations

The principles of antibiotic tissue penetration and pharmacokinetic analysis of antibiotics form a highly complex and controversial area. Schentag and Gengo (1982) have reviewed this area and pointed out the pitfalls of this literature. Most important of many factors are the concentration and activity of an antibiotic at the infection site. In turn, multiple factors are involved in determining the concentration of an antibiotic at a tissue infection site, including the antibiotic serum concentration achieved, serum protein binding of the antibiotic, blood flow to the infection site, penetration of the antibiotic from the serum to the tissue infection site, and effects of underlying disease or infection on all these factors (Schentag and Gengo, 1982). It is not within the scope of this chapter to delve into these areas in detail. However, these issues are brought to the attention of the reader to emphasize that subsequent comments in this section are an oversimplification of complex interactions that have not been adequately studied.

In periodontal disease the gingival crevice/periodontal pocket is the usual infection site. There is recent evidence that the underlying connective tissue and alveolar bone may also be invaded by bacteria in some individuals (Saglie et al., 1982; Christersson et al., 1987a, 1987b). Therefore the "ideal" antibiotic for treatment of periodontal infection would be one that could penetrate into the gingival crevice/periodontal pocket, underlying connective tissue, and alveolar bone and achieve concentrations at those sites that would effectively kill or inhibit the growth of invading or penetrating bacteria.

Gingival crevicular fluid concentrations have been measured for only a few antibiotics: tetracycline (Gordon et al., 1981), minocycline (Ciancio, 1980), and metronidazole (Britt and Pohlod, 1986). The tetracyclines and metronidazole penetrate extremely well into the gingival crevicular fluid. The propensity of tetracycline to penetrate into bone is also well known. There is, however, little or no data on other commonly used antibiotics. This lack of studies has hindered evaluation of the minimal effective dose of various antibiotics and the best way to administer antibiotics for periodontal infection (Genco, 1981).

The issue of the antimicrobial activity of an agent at the tissue infection site must be considered separately from antibiotic penetration into the site. Such factors as pH, availability of oxygen, and oxidation-reduction potential may influence the antimicrobial activity of certain agents at infected tissue sites. Aminoglycoside antibiotics have markedly reduced activity against susceptible organisms at a pH of less than 7 (Barber and Waterworth, 1966). The activity of penicillins and cephalosporins is not affected by pH in the range of 5.5 to 8. Metronidazole is an example of an agent that not only penetrates well into infection sites such as abscesses but also retains excellent antibacterial activity in this environment (Joiner et al., 1982). These factors, along with the antimicrobial spectrum and ease of administration of metronidazole, have led to the recent interest in using this agent in the treatment of periodontal infection. Similarly, clindamycin can also penetrate into abscesses and retain its antimicrobial activity, but to a lesser extent than metronidazole (Joiner et al., 1982). Tetracycline and its derivatives are lipid soluble and penetrate well into most tissues. The activity of tetracycline at infection sites has not been studied to any great extent. However, numerous clinical studies attest to the value of tetracyclines in the treatment of bacterial infections.

Despite the extensive use of antibiotics for over 40 years, there is still a lack of knowledge concerning the optimal concentration of an antibiotic that must be achieved at an infection site. There is a general opinion that the antibiotic tissue concentration must be equal to or greater than the minimal inhibitory concentration (MIC) of an antibiotic (as measured in broth culture) for a given organism (Kunin, 1981). The duration of time during a dosing interval that the tissue concentration should exceed the MIC is not clear but is being actively investigated (Schumacher, 1982; Schentag et al., 1985; Moore et al., 1987). Until more information is available to clarify these issues, dosing of antibiotics will be based primarily on pharmacokinetic parameters rather than also taking into consideration antimicrobial activity.

• • •

In this section the factors that should be taken into consideration in choosing an antibiotic to treat periodontal infection have been discussed, including (1) the polymicrobial etiology of periodontal infection, (2) the antibiotic susceptibility of various periodontopathic organisms, (3) the toxicity of various antibiotics, and (4) antibiotic pene-

tration and activity at the infection site. When all these factors are used to evaluate various antibiotics in the treatment of periodontal infection, tetracycline and its derivatives appear to be the "best" choice for many patients at present. As more studies are performed, other agents may be found that are less toxic but at least as efficacious as the tetracyclines. Regardless of which agents are used in the future, the factors noted above will continue to be used to evaluate and select antibiotics for treatment of periodontal infection.

FACTORS AFFECTING RESPONSE TO THERAPY

Multiple factors can affect the response to antimicrobial therapy. Some of these have been discussed in previous sections, including the spectrum of activity of an antibacterial agent, resistance to antibacterial agents, and concentrations of the antibiotic at the site of infection. Other factors affecting the response to therapy are discussed in this section.

Route of drug administration

In many cases oral administration of antibiotics is used to treat periodontal disease. It should be emphasized that gastrointestinal absorption of various drugs given orally differs considerably and can be altered by the presence of food or gastric pH. Penicillin G is acid labile and should not be administered within 1 to 2 hours before or after a meal. The absorption of tetracycline given orally is decreased in the presence of dairy products and certain cation-containing antacids. On the other hand, clindamycin and certain formulations of erythromycin can be absorbed adequately in the presence of food.

Dose and duration of therapy

For all antibiotics, whether given orally or parenterally, standard dosing regimens are developed prior to marketing. Thus it should be uncommon to prescribe an inadequate dose of a particular drug. A more common problem is the use of excessive doses of antibiotics. Such prescribing is based on the fallacy that "if a little is good, a lot must be better." Adverse reactions of some antibiotics (e.g., erythromycin and tetracycline) more commonly occur with excessive doses.

On the other hand, the optimal duration of treatment for periodontal infection is not known. (Unfortunately, this is also true for most other types of bacterial infections.) As a general rule, one usually continues antimicrobial therapy for 48 hours beyond the time when symptoms and signs of infection abate. Most periodontal infections can probably be effectively treated with 14 days or less of antibiotic therapy (along with standard periodontal procedures) with good patient compliance. One must rely, however, on clinical judgment to determine the exact duration of therapy.

Duration and extent of infection

Consideration of the duration and extent of infection as factors impacting on the response to therapy have their basis in common sense and clinical experience more so than in scientific fact. Infections that have persisted for days or weeks will usually take longer to respond to therapy than those present for short periods of time prior to treatment. Development of an abscess, a localized collection of bacteria, inflammatory cells, and necrotic tissue, is at one extreme of the spectrum of bacterial infection. Treatment of bacterial infection with abscess formation requires not only antibiotic therapy but, more important, surgical intervention. Bacterial infection of bone also poses a problem in regard to therapy. The presence of abscess formation or bone infection usually indicates a need to prolong the duration of antibiotic therapy beyond the usual 14 days of therapy for periodontal infection.

Bacteriostatic versus bactericidal agents

A bactericidal antibiotic is one that in vitro produces killing of bacteria as measured by the reduction of viable bacterial counts during a defined period of exposure. In contrast, a bacteriostatic agent is one that does not allow a susceptible bacterial strain to grow, but also does not reduce the viable bacterial counts during a period of exposure, even at antibiotic concentrations well above the MIC. As a general rule, penicillins, cephalosporins, and metronidazole are bactericidal agents; erythromycin, clindamycin, and tetracyclines are bacteriostatic (however, these latter three agents may be bactericidal in vitro, depending on the specific organism and antibiotic concentration tested).

For most infections, including periodontal infections, it would appear that bacteriostatic agents will suffice if host response is intact. There are, however, certain infections in which bactericidal therapy appears to be required, and these include bacterial endocarditis, bacterial meningitis, and infections in the granulocytopenic patient. In these latter situations limitations of host response, antibiotic penetration, or both, mandate bactericidal therapy. In the individual patient with periodontal infection, if there is concern about host response, it would seem prudent to choose a bactericidal agent or combinations of agents.

Host factors

As already discussed, multiple factors are important in producing a "cure" with antibiotic therapy. The most important factor, however, in the response to treatment of an infection is the ability of the infected person to galvanize various host defense mechanisms into action against the infection. Without this host response, antibiotic therapy will usually not be effective. The inadequacy of antibiotic therapy alone in the treatment of infection in patients with impaired host defenses is exemplified best by two patient populations: patients with acute leukemia and granulocy-

topenia and patients with acquired immunodeficiency syndrome. Such underlying diseases markedly affect the response to treatment of infection. Other diseases affecting host defense mechanisms that may manifest periodontal infection are discussed in other parts of this text. The practitioner caring for the patient with periodontal infection and an underlying disease that may limit host defense must be aware that the response to therapy will not be the same as in the "normal" host. Again, there are no specific guidelines to use to determine the dose of antibiotic or duration of therapy. One must rely on clinical judgment and common sense.

The age of the patient is also an important consideration in predicting response to therapy. It appears that host defenses are diminished as one gets older (Gardner, 1980). Thus one should not expect the same response to therapy in the 65-year-old as in the 25-year-old. Finally, one must always be concerned about pregnancy when treating women of childbearing age with periodontal disease. Drugs such as tetracycline, which are highly effective for periodontal infection, may have adverse effects on the fetus. Thus one must resort to penicillin or erythromycin in this setting, since these agents are known to be relatively safe to administer to the pregnant patient.

SUMMARY

A general approach to antibiotic therapy for periodontal infection has been discussed that has emphasized the polymicrobial nature of this process. Although research studies have used very careful culture techniques to identify anaerobes, such techniques are impractical in the day-to-day care of patients. Therefore considerable reliance must be placed on research studies that define the bacteriology of various periodontal infections. These studies are described in subsequent chapters. This information, along with a sound knowledge base of the commonly used antibiotics in the treatment of periodontal disease, should allow the practitioner to make rational choices in prescribing antibiotics.

REFERENCES

Baker PS et al: Antibiotic susceptibility of anaerobic bacteria from the human oral cavity, J Dent Res 64:1233, 1985.

Barber M and Waterworth PM: Activity of gentamicin against pseudomonas and hospital staphylococci, Br Med J 1:203, 1966.

Britt MR and Pohlod DJ: Serum and crevicular fluid concentrations after a single oral dose of metronidazole, J Periodontol 57:104, 1986.

Christersson LA et al.: Tissue localization of *Actinobacillus actinomycetemcomitans* in human periodontitis. I. Light, immunofluorescence and electron microscopic studies, J Periodontol 58:529, 1987a.

Christersson LA et al: Tissue localization of *Actinobacillus actinomycetemcomitans* in human periodontitis. II. Correlation between immunofluorescence and culture techniques, J Periodontol 58:540, 1987b.

Ciancio SG: Chemotherapeutics in periodontics, Dent Clin North Am 24:813, 1980.

Dzink JL et al: The predominant cultivable microbiota of active and inactive periodontal lesions, J Clin Periodontol 15:316, 1988.

Gardner ID: The effect of age on susceptibility to infection, Rev Infect Dis 2:801, 1980.

Genco RJ: Antibiotics in the treatment of human periodontal diseases, J Periodontol 52:545, 1981.

Genco RJ and Slots S: Host responses in periodontal disease, J Dent Res 63:441, 1984.

Gordon JM et al: Tetracycline levels achievable in gingival crevice fluid and in vitro effect on subgingival organisms, I, J Periodontol 52:609, 1981.

Joiner K et al: Comparative efficacy of 10 antimicrobial agents in experimental infections with *Bacteroides fragilis,* J Infect Dis 145:561, 1982.

Kunin CM: Dosage schedules of antimicrobial agents: a historical review, Rev Infect Dis 3:4, 1981.

Lekovic V et al: The effect of metronidazole on human periodontal disease: a clinical and bacteriologic study, J Periodontol 54:476, 1983.

Lindhe J et al: The effect of metronidazole therapy on human periodontal disease, J Periodont Res 17:534, 1982.

Loesche WJ et al: Treatment of periodontal infections due to anaerobic bacteria with short-term metronidazole, J Clin Periodontol 8:29, 1981.

Moore RD et al: Clinical response to aminoglycoside therapy: importance of the ratio of peak concentration to minimal inhibitory concentration, J Infect Dis 155:93, 1987.

Murray PR and Rosenblatt JE: Penicillin resistance and penicillinase pro-duction in clinical isolates of *Bacteroides melaninogenicus,* Antimicrob Agents Chemother 11:605, 1977.

Onderdonk AB et al: The capsular polysaccharide of *Bacteroides fragilis* as a virulence factor: comparison of the pathogenic potential of encapsulated and unencapsulated strains, J Infect Dis 136:82, 1977.

Saglie R et al: Bacterial invasion of gingiva in advanced periodontitis in humans, J Periodontol 53:217, 1982.

Schentag JJ and Gengo FM: Principles of antibiotic tissue penetration and guidelines for pharmacokinetic analysis, Med Clin North Am 66:39, 1982.

Schentag JJ et al: Dual individualization: antibiotic dosage calculation from the integration of in vitro pharmacokinetics and in vivo pharmacokinetics, J Antimicrob Chemother 15(suppl A):47, 1985.

Schumacher GE: Pharmacokinetic and microbiologic evaluation of antibiotic dosage regimens, Clin Pharm 1:66, 1982.

Slots J.: Subgingival microflora and periodontal disease, J Clin Periodontol 6:351, 1979.

Slots J and Genco RJ: Black-pigmented *Bacteroides* species, *Capnocytophaga* species, and *Actinobacillus actinomycetemcomitans* in human periodontal disease: virulence factors in colonization, survival, and tissue destruction, J Dent Res 63:412, 1984.

Socransky SS: Microbiology of periodontal disease: present status and future considerations, J Periodontol 48:497, 1977.

Sutter VL et al: Antimicrobial susceptibilities of bacteria associated with periodontal disease, Antimicrob Agents Chemother 23:483, 1983.

Chapter 33

SCALING AND ROOT PLANING
Removal of calculus and subgingival organisms

D. Walter Cohen
Lindsey A. Sherwood

Current research has put in question the rationale for many traditional resective surgical procedures and is reestablishing the importance of the roles of scaling and root planing as definitive periodontal treatment modalities. The techniques of scaling and root planing are considered basic in the treatment of periodontal diseases, with the primary objective being to restore the gingival tissues to health by removing the etiologic factors of plaque, calculus, and contaminated cementum. Although scaling and root planing are fundamental procedures in the treatment of periodontitis, they are also among the most difficult techniques to perform in all of clinical dentistry (Kakehashi and Parakkal, 1982).

RATIONALE FOR THERAPY

Scaling is a necessary treatment procedure to remove hard and soft deposits from the tooth surface coronal to the junctional epithelium. Scaling alone is sufficient to completely remove calculus from the enamel surface. The treatment of patients with periodontal disease also requires root planing. Proper root planing results in a biologically acceptable root surface and involves removal of the microbial flora, bacterial toxins, calculus, and diseased cementum and dentin by meticulous hand or ultrasonic instrumentation. Root planing requires removal of the root surface cementum and dentin, since calculus may be in cracks and fissures of the root surface. In addition, the root surface of periodontally infected teeth may act as a reservoir for periodontopathic bacteria that are in resorption lacunae and have penetrated the dentinal tubules to varying depths (Adriaens et al., 1988a, 1988b).

Scaling and root planing should not be considered separate procedures. The difference between scaling and root planing is only a matter of degree; root planing is a definitive, more thorough procedure, directed to the radicular surfaces exposed by periodontal disease (Pattison and Pat-

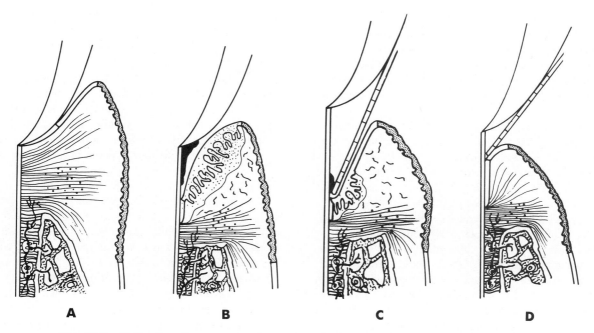

Fig. 33-1. If bleeding does not occur from base of pocket, given adequate wound healing over time, one may assume that pocket area is biologically acceptable. If bleeding or suppuration does occur from base of pocket, given adequate wound healing over time, there is a strong possibility that plaque and calculus still remain in apical portion of root surface area of pocket. **A,** Normal periodontium. **B,** Inflamed gingival unit with bone loss. **C,** Wound healing with plaque and calculus remaining. **D,** Wound healing with biologically acceptable root.

tison, 1979). Scaling alone is often inadequate to effectively remove local etiologic factors responsible for gingival inflammation.

Producing smooth root surfaces by the technique of root planing has long been the most popular means by which the therapist determines adequate root preparation. This means of assessment must be questioned, since it is physically impossible for one to clinically determine tactilely the presence of microscopic deposits of calculus, absorbed toxic by-products, or residual microorganisms on and in root surfaces that have been reported to be barriers to proper wound healing (Aleo et al., 1974; Jones and O'Leary, 1978).

There are several methods of assessing adequate root preparation. A clinician must not rely solely on tactile acuity during instrumentation, but must also use auditory and visual clues to aid in root preparation. The most decisive clinical parameters available to the operator at present are the ability to determine accurately the periodontal status of the patient in a site-specific fashion and to possess a keen knowledge of how to evaluate soft tissue response of wound healing over time. In most instances the absence of bleeding or suppuration from the base of the pocket after adequate wound healing and evidence of elimination of the pathogenic periodontal microflora should be the main criteria for assessing the effectiveness of root planing (Fig.

33-1). Monitoring the suppression or eradication of the pathogenic periodontal microbiota after scaling and root planing is proving to be a valuable adjunct as an end point in periodontal therapy, in general, as well as in root planing.

OBJECTIVES OF THERAPY

The principal objectives of scaling and root planing are:
1. Suppression or elimination of the pathogenic periodontal microflora and replacement with the sparce flora found in health
2. Conversion of inflamed, bleeding, or suppurative pathologic pockets to healthy gingival tissue
3. Shrinkage of the deepened pathologic pocket to a shallow, healthy gingival sulcus
4. Providing a root surface compatible with reestablishment of a healthy connective tissue and epithelial attachment as evidenced by maintenance of, or coronal gain in, the probing attachment level

These objectives cannot always be achieved by closed scaling and root-planing procedures; local or systemic antimicrobial therapy or access flaps may be necessary.

INSTRUMENTATION

The rationale for the selection of instruments for scaling and root planing is based on the objectives of therapy, which are to produce biologically acceptable root surfaces by removing plaque, calculus, and contaminated cementum and dentin, which results in the reversal of the inflamed periodontal tissues to health. The main factor to be considered in the selection of a specific instrument is efficacy; however, ease of sharpening and sterilization are also important.

The design of periodontal instruments used in scaling and root planing should allow for effective and efficient calculus removal and root preparation. In addition, it should provide operator comfort, minimize muscle fatigue, and increase tactile sensitivity. Tactile sensitivity is greatest with instruments with the tip, shank, and handle as one solid piece. The hand instruments suited for these procedures are sickle scalers, hoes, files, and curettes. Sonic and ultrasonic instruments are also available for scaling and root planing and, in general, show clinical results comparable to those of hand instruments. In addition, there are chemical treatments of the root surface using decalcifying agents such as citric acid, tetracycline, or EDTA; detergents; and antimicrobial agents such as iodine. These chemical agents may prepare the mechanically root-planed surfaces for healing by removing toxins, by exposing collagen and other root surface components that promote healing, and by removing the smear layer. However, whatever agents are used, prior or concomitant thorough scaling and root planing are necessary.

Use of anesthesia

The commonly used hand instruments are described below. Since calculus, the pathogenic periodontal microbiota, and the infected root surface extend to the bottom of the pocket, it is necessary to fully instrument the entire root surface facing the pocket. This almost always is painful and requires local anesthesia. In general, supragingival scaling can be accomplished without anesthesia; however, proper subgingival scaling and root planing, even when done as closed procedures without access flaps, most often require local anesthesia.

Sickle scalers

When calculus accumulates not only interproximally but also on the buccal and lingual surfaces of the clinical crowns of teeth, sickle scalers with varied angular shafts may be used because of their strength and ability to assimilate rather heavy stress. These instruments are thin and triangular in cross section, and they taper to a point. They have two cutting edges: the corners at the base of the triangle. Because of their size, their use is generally limited to coronal and supragingival scaling.

Hoes

Because of its design, the hoe is a powerful instrument. Its shaft may be bent in many angles to reach all surfaces of all teeth. It has a short blade extending no more than 1

mm from the shaft. The short blade must be held flat on the root surface in order that the sharp corners will not gouge the root (gouging may be prevented by rounding the sharp corners of the tip of the hoe). The hoe may be placed subgingivally but cannot be expected to reach the root surface at the apical border of the pocket. It can often be inserted in the pocket to a point apical to the calculus deposits, and with a sharp, steady pull stroke of only a few millimeters, the deposit may be removed. The instrument must rest on the tooth for the entire length of the stroke.

Files

The file is an instrument designed for a pull stroke as well as for a push-and-pull stroke. Files are similar to hoes of very short lengths, and in those designed for a pull stroke, the blades, which are triangular, are set with their bases at right angles to the shank. The push-and-pull type has many small teeth set closely together, thus allowing the instrument to cut in both directions. In deep, constricted pockets files may be used to free the roots of granular deposits, but otherwise they have a restricted use. The file, like the hoe, cannot reach the apical portion of the pocket in most instances.

Curettes

Periodontal curettes are efficient and can be used to perform the bulk of the root-planing procedure. Curettes can be used on flat, concave, and convex surfaces or roots, in wide furcations, and the tips can be used to clean cementoenamel junction (CEJ) regions. The instrument is com-

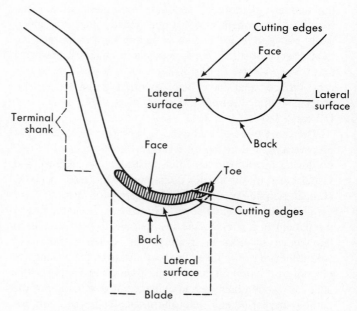

Fig. 33-2. Blade components and terminal shank.

posed of three parts: the handle, shank, and working end, which includes the blade (see Fig. 45-1).

Curettes are usually double ended, having working ends paired so that each end is a mirror image of the other. The blade of the periodontal curette often has two cutting edges, which meet to form a rounded tip or toe. The cutting edges are formed by the junction of the face and the curved sides or lateral surfaces. The lateral surfaces extend from the cutting edge to form the rounded bottom or back of the blade. The posterior portion of the blade narrows to form the terminal aspect of the shank (Fig. 33-2).

Two types of periodontal curettes are commonly used in scaling, root planing, and gingival curettage. These are the universal curette series and the Gracey curette series (Fig. 33-3). Universal curettes can be used throughout the mouth, although there are often root surfaces that they are

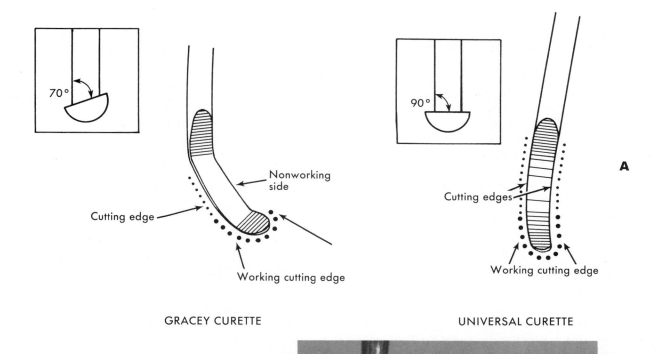

GRACEY CURETTE   UNIVERSAL CURETTE

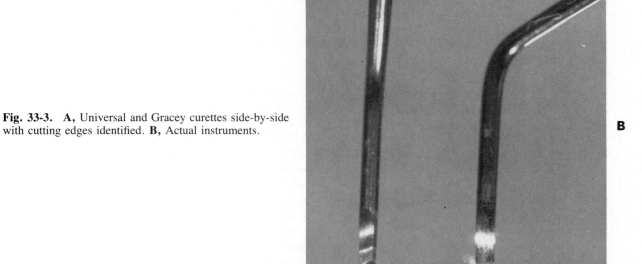

Fig. 33-3.   A, Universal and Gracey curettes side-by-side with cutting edges identified. **B,** Actual instruments.

not able to reach. The distinguishing characteristic of the universal curette is that the face is offset 80 to 90 degrees to the terminal shank. Both cutting edges and the tip of one working end are used. Gracey curettes are specific to certain areas of the mouth. The face of the Gracey curette is offset 60 to 70 degrees to the terminal shank. Only the lower or outside cutting edge and tip are actually used.

OPERATOR POSITIONING

The operator must see the field of operation clearly without having to assume body positions that are uncomfortable if held over long periods of time (Wilkins, 1983).

The patient is placed in the chair, and the operator is seated so that the mouth is at the same level as the elbows of the operator. The open mouth should form a V, with the apex directed to the floor. The operator's forearms are more or less parallel with the floor when in use.

In a patient who has supragingival calculus and plaque, the first one or two appointments are often used for gross supragingival debridement and the initial oral hygiene instructions. At a series of subsequent appointments, subgingival scalings and root planings are then carried out.

Depending on the severity of the disease, the depth of the pockets, the tortuousness of the pockets, and the skill of the operator, a session of subgingival scaling and root planing usually involves no more than four to six teeth and is done with the patient under local anesthesia. The diseased site is probed to determine the depth of the pocket, root conformations, whether or not furcations are involved, and the extent of calculus accumulation.

The curette is inserted into the pocket using a modified pen grasp with a finger rest; usually the fourth or third finger rests on adjacent teeth or the other hand, which is on the teeth of the opposite jaw, or on the opposite jaw itself. The finger rest acts as a fulcrum for the movement of the blade of the instrument. It also permits optimal angulation of the blade. In general, the finger rest should be as close as possible to the root surface selected for treatment to enable careful instrumentation. The face of the blade is parallel and only in light contact with the root surface as the tip is guided apically to the base of the pocket. Once the base of the pocket has been reached, the instrument is turned to a cutting position for root planing. Force between the cutting edge and root surface is increased, and the working stroke is begun in a coronal direction. Several overlapping vertical strokes, repeating the above motions, are performed to plane the root surface, which is easily reached in this position.

The operator position should allow for comfortable achievement of these motions during scaling and root planing. In general, the shoulders should be parallel with the floor, the forearm at the level of the mouth and parallel to the floor, and the back as straight as possible during these procedures. In the standing position, both feet should be on the floor with equal weight on the balls of the feet. Typical positions are as follows:

Position	Areas of the mouth	Vision access
7:30 (Fig. 33-4)	Lingual mandibular anterior sextant	Direct or indirect
	Labial maxillary anterior sextant	Direct
	Palatal maxillary anterior sextant	Indirect
9-10 o'clock (Fig. 33-4)	Buccal mandibular right posterior sextant	Direct
	Lingual mandibular right posterior sextant	Direct or indirect
	Buccal mandibular left posterior sextant	Direct or indirect
	Lingual mandibular left posterior sextant	Direct
	Buccal maxillary right posterior sextant	Direct
	Palatal maxillary right posterior sextant	Direct or indirect
	Buccal maxillary left posterior sextant	Direct or indirect
	Palatal maxillary left posterior sextant	Direct or indirect
11-12 o'clock (Fig. 33-4)	Labial mandibular anterior sextant	Direct
	Labial maxillary anterior sextant (optional)	Direct
	Palatal maxillary left posterior sextant	Direct or indirect
	Lingual mandibular right posterior sextant	Direct or indirect

BASIC TECHNIQUES
Grasp

The recommended way of holding a periodontal curette is with the modified pen grasp (Fig. 33-5). Note that the pad of the middle finger is in contact with the shank of the instrument rather than supporting the instrument with the side of the finger as in a conventional pen grasp. The modified pen grasp improves tactile sensitivity, blade adaptation, and pressure control. Instrument adaptation is controlled because the thumb can be used to roll the instrument against the middle and index fingers in precise degrees to adapt the blade to the slightest changes in tooth contour. Using a finger rest (fulcrum) enhances control in order to reduce the possibility of inadvertent slippage of the curette.

Posterior section

The working end of a universal curette in the posterior section of the mouth is determined by placing the face of the blade parallel to the occlusal plane of the teeth with the tip directed interproximally and the handle coming out of the front of the mouth (Fig. 33-6).

Insertion. On initial placement at the orifice of the pocket, the face of the blade is oriented parallel to the root surface. The curette is inserted to the base of the pocket using a light exploratory stroke. This exploratory stroke should give the operator some notion of pocket topography and location and the amount of calculus in the pocket.

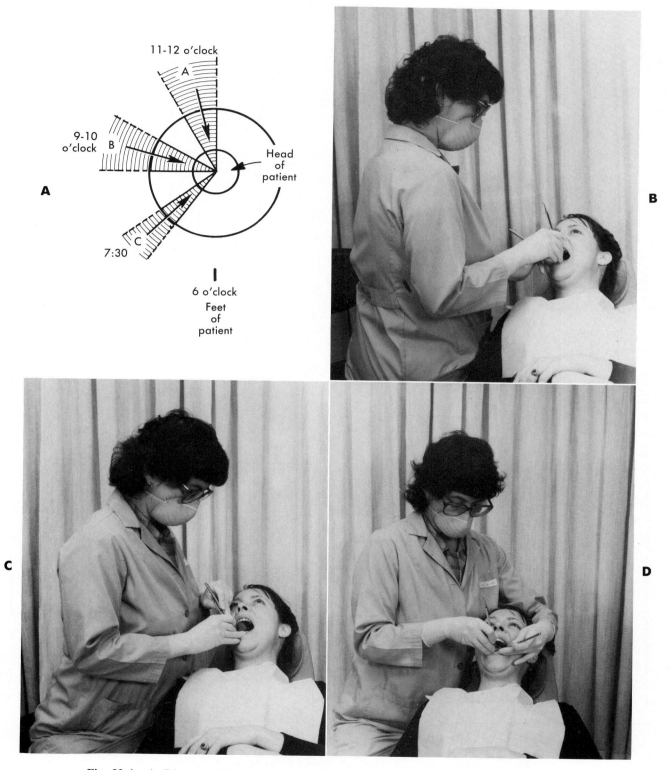

Fig. 33-4. A, Diagram of operator positions. **B,** Operator in 7:30 position. **C,** Operator in 9:00 to 10:30 position. **D,** Operator in 11 to 12 o'clock position.

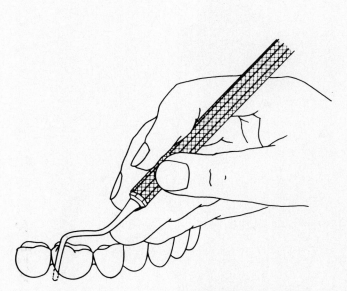

Fig. 33-5. Modified pen grasp; note also finger rest as close as possible to working area.

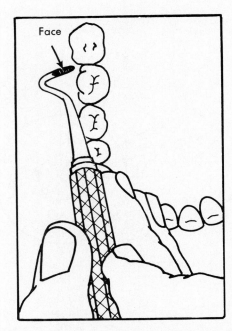

Fig. 33-6. Working end—posterior section of mouth.

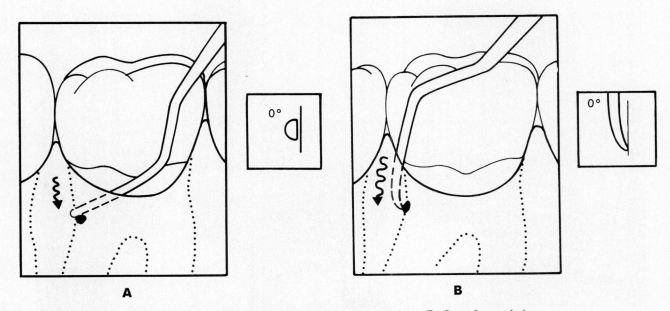

Fig. 33-7. Insertion 0 degrees. **A,** Traditional technique. **B,** Open-face technique.

Traditional technique (Fig. 33-7, *A*).   The traditional method of determining the proper working end of a universal curette in the posterior section of the mouth is to use the mirrored partner (opposite end) of the working end as illustrated in Fig. 33-6. The face of the blade is positioned parallel to the root surface, with the lateral surface of the blade negotiating the most apical portion of the pocket.

Open-face technique (Fig. 33-7, *B*).   The open-face method of determining the proper working end of a univer-

sal curette in the posterior section of the mouth is to use the working end as illustrated in Fig. 33-6. The face of the blade is positioned parallel to the root surface, with the tip of the blade negotiating the most apical portion of the pocket.

NOTE: Gaining access to the most apical portion of the periodontal pocket is necessary for proper removal of all deposits and root planing. The open-face technique may prove to be more effective in removing root surface contaminants at the most apical portion of the pocket, since it facilitates placement of the tip, which contains a cutting edge in this critical apical area.

Angulation and adaptation (Fig. 33-8).   For the working angulation in scaling and root planing, the face of the blade is positioned at 45 to 90 degrees to the tooth surface. Proper adaptation of a universal curette uses only the anterior third and tip of the blade.

Distal aspect, vertical stroke

Traditional technique.   For scaling and root planing, the curette is directed in a series of vertical, oblique, and horizontal overlapping strokes. Fig. 33-9, *A*, illustrates activation of the universal curette in the posterior section of the mouth.

A vertical stroke is performed in interproximal and deep pocket areas. With a vertical stroke, a wrist-rock motion is used while the fingers simultaneously rotate the instrument to adapt to the natural contours of the tooth.

Open-face technique.   The open-face technique employs the working end as illustrated in Fig. 33-9, *B*. Vertical strokes used should be short to moderate in length and overlap each other.

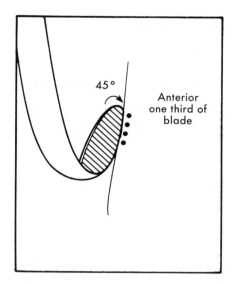

Fig. 33-8.   Angulation and adaptation.

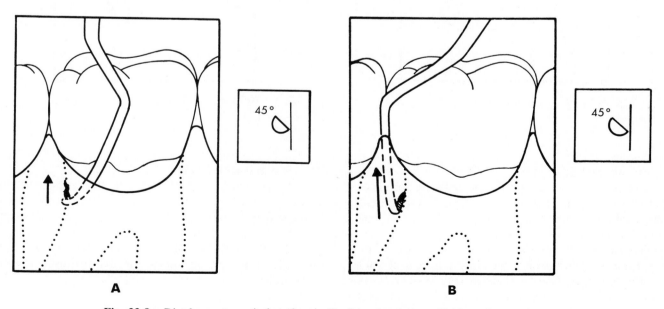

A   **B**

Fig. 33-9.   Distal aspect, vertical stroke. **A,** Traditional technique. **B,** Open-face technique.

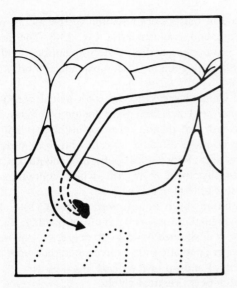

Fig. 33-10.   Distobuccal line angle, oblique stroke.

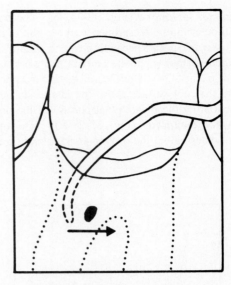

Fig. 33-11.   Buccal aspect, horizontal stroke.

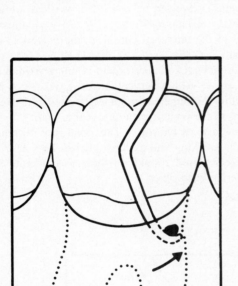

Fig. 33-12.   Mesiobuccal line angle, oblique stroke.

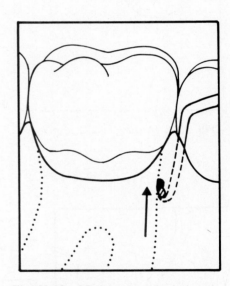

Fig. 33-13.   Mesial aspect, vertical stroke.

Distobuccal line angle

Oblique stroke (Fig. 33-10).   An oblique stroke is used for transitional line angles. When moving from the interproximal areas, the blade is rotated so the tip is pointed apically. The anterior third of the opposite cutting edge is then moved mesially in an oblique direction, instrumenting the distobuccal line angle to the facial surface of the tooth.

Buccal aspect, horizontal stroke (Fig. 33-11).   A horizontal stroke is used on facial and oral surfaces of the teeth.

Mesiobuccal line angle

Oblique stroke (Fig. 33-12).   As the operator negotiates the mesiobuccal line angle of the tooth, the face of the curette blade is rotated to 45 to 90 degrees, and an oblique stroke is then used.

Mesial aspect, vertical stroke (Fig. 33-13).   The mesial aspect of the tooth will be instrumented using a vertical stroke.

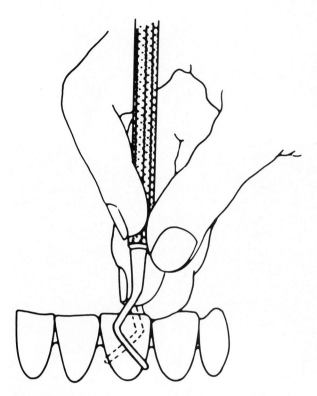

Fig. 33-14. Universal curette as used in anterior section.

Anterior section

For the anterior teeth, the universal curette is positioned with the handle parallel to the long axis of the tooth (Fig. 33-14). The anterior third of the face of the blade is placed against the surface to be instrumented. The curette is activated with the face of the blade at 45 to 90 degrees to the tooth. Vertical strokes are used for mesial and distal surfaces. A short horizontal stroke is used for midfacial and lingual surfaces. The instrument is reversed (mirror end), and the technique is repeated to instrument the opposite side of the tooth.

Gracey series

The Gracey series of periodontal curettes is specific to certain areas of the mouth. Gracey curettes can be used for refining aspects of root planing and negotiating difficult access areas (e.g., deep tortuous pockets and furcation invasions). Curettes such as the Columbia 13/14 can be used for most scaling and root-planing procedures.

For activation of all Gracey instruments, the lower cutting edge is first identified. The anterior third of the blade is placed against the tooth. When the terminal shank is parallel to the surface of the tooth being instrumented, proper angulation of the blade is attained.

The Gracey series suggested are:
Gracey 3/4 (anterior teeth) (Fig. 33-15, *A*)
Gracey 7/8 (lateral surfaces of posterior teeth) (Fig. 33-15, *B*)
Gracey 11/12 (mesial and lateral surfaces of posterior teeth) (Fig. 33-15, *C*)
Gracey 13/14 (distal surfaces of posterior teeth) (Fig. 33-15, *D*)

Furcations

The most difficult areas of the mouth to instrument are furcations. A knowledge of root morphology and pocket topography is paramount for negotiating the limited-access areas encountered in the closed root-planing approach. Intraoral radiographs, furcation probes, sharp curettes, or cow-horn explorers are useful in determining the location and extent of furcation invasions. Information from radiographic interpretation and probing will aid instrument selection to gain optimum access to the problem areas in furcations.

Curettes such as the Columbia 13/14 or the finer-tipped M23 (Deppeler) posterior curette may be used to negotiate most maxillary and mandibular furcations (Figs. 33-16 and 33-17). When scaling and root planing furcations, one uses a vertical stroke on the lateral aspects of the root surfaces and a "scooping" motion with the curette tip in the trunk area.

A Gracey 11/12 curette is used to root plane the mesiopalatal aspect of a furcation of a maxillary molar from a mesiopalatal approach (Fig. 33-18). The distopalatal furcation root may be planed with a Gracey 13/14 curette from a distopalatal approach. The palatal groove of the palatal root of a maxillary molar is instrumented with a Gracey 13/14 curette from a distopalatal approach (Figs. 33-19 and 33-20). Finally, root planing of the distal furcation of a maxillary molar is completed by using a Gracey 13/14 curette from a buccal approach to overlap the strokes from the distopalatal approach (Fig. 33-21).

Open furcations, especially Class III and Class II involvements, often present irregularities such as grooves, narrow V-shaped root junctions, a concave furcation roof, or ridges that preclude complete calculus removal and root planing. Careful odontoplasty of such furcations with fine diamonds and fluted burs may be necessary for access and complete debridement.

Tray setup

A prearranged sterile tray setup for scaling, root planing, and gingival curettage should include a mouth mirror; explorers; a straight periodontal probe; a furcation probe; universal scalers such as the GX-2 (Deppeler); curettes such as the universal Columbia 13/14, Goldman-Fox 3, the posterior Columbia 4R/4L, or the anterior Columbia 2R/2L; and curettes for specific regions such as the Gracey series 3/4, 7/8, 11/12, and 13/14. Also important is a hand-

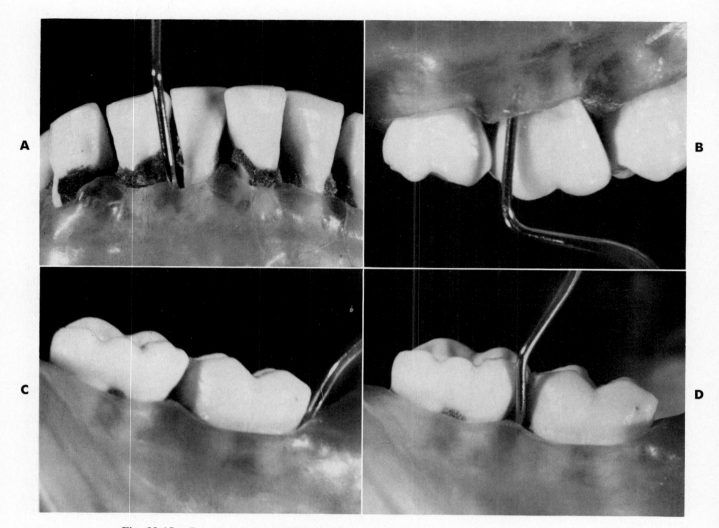

Fig. 33-15. Gracey series of curettes. **A,** Gracey 3/4 (anterior teeth). **B,** Gracey 7/8 (lateral surfaces of posterior teeth). **C,** Gracey 11/12 (mesial and lateral surfaces of posterior teeth). **D,** Gracey 13/14 (distal surfaces of posterior teeth).

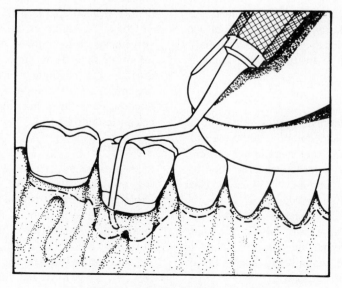

Fig. 33-16. Curette negotiating furcation.

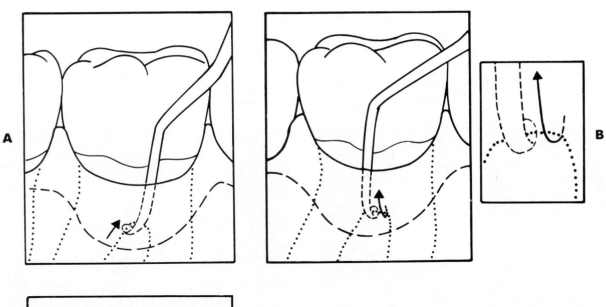

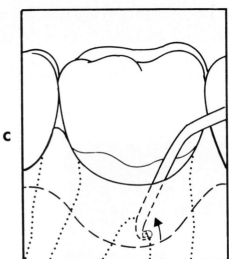

Fig. 33-17. **A,** Universal curette in position to root plane mesial aspect of distal root. **B,** Curette in position to root plane trunk of furcation. **C,** Curette in position to root plane distal aspect of mesial root.

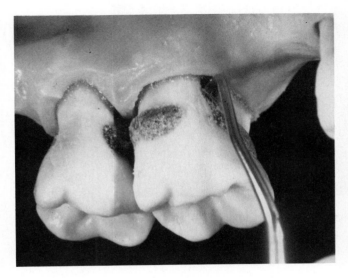

Fig. 33-18. Gracey 11/12 curette in position to root plane mesiopalatal aspect of a maxillary molar from a mesiopalatal approach.

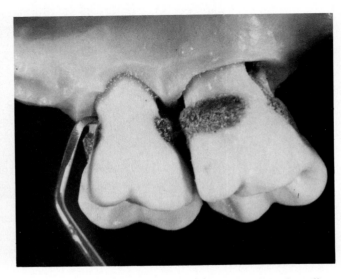

Fig. 33-19. Gracey 13/14 curette in position to root plane distopalatal aspect of a furcation of a maxillary molar from a distopalatal approach.

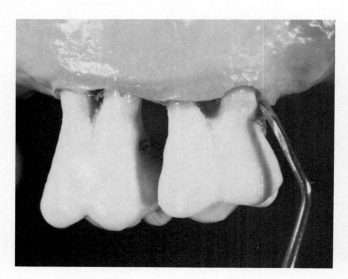

Fig. 33-20.   Gracey 13/14 curette in position to root plane palatal root of a maxillary molar from a distopalatal approach.

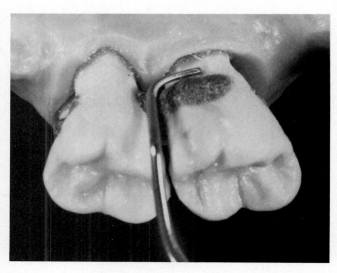

Fig. 33-21.   Gracey 13/14 curette in position to root plane distal furcation of a maxillary molar from a buccal approach.

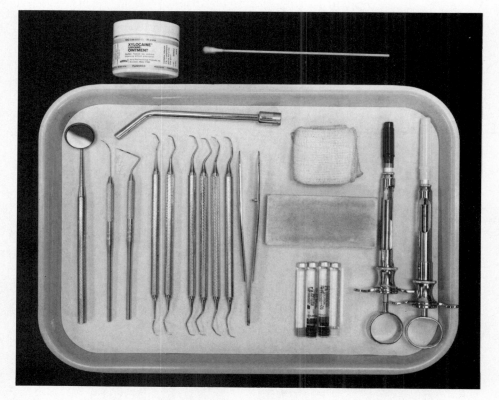

Fig. 33-22.   Sterile tray setup for scaling, root planing, and gingival curettage.

sized fine Arkansas stone, sterile lubricant, aspirating tip, cotton pliers, topical anesthetic, syringe needles and capules for local anesthesia, maxillary and mandibular irrigating syringes, and sterile gauze pads (Fig. 33-22).

CASE MANAGEMENT

Before the procedures of scaling and root planing are initiated, it is necessary to accurately assess the levels of periodontal disease. All patients should receive a thorough, systematic periodontal examination. This should include a medical and dental history and a clinical and radiographic examination. The following information is essential in developing a diagnosis of periodontal health, gingivitis (case type I), early periodontitis (case type II), moderate periodontitis (case type III), or advanced periodontitis (case type IV):

1. Gross periodontal pathosis—evaluation of the topography of the gingiva and related structures
2. Existence and degree of gingival inflammation
3. Periodontal probing depth to assess pocket depths and attachment levels, and to provide information on the health of the subgingival area (e.g., the presence of bleeding or purulent exudate)
4. Presence and distribution of bacterial plaque and calculus, and assessment of periodontal bacteria
5. Condition of tooth proximal contact relationships
6. Degree of mobility of teeth
7. Presence of malocclusion
8. Condition of existing dental restorations and prosthetic appliances
9. Interpretation of a satisfactory number of diagnostic-quality periapical and bitewing radiographs

TREATMENT PLANNING

Treatment planning for accomplishing the objectives of scaling and root planing should include a proper sequence of treatment that involves careful evaluation of the level of periodontal disease and accurate determination of the degree of difficulty of each case. The overall plan should include:

1. The periodontal procedures to be performed
2. Treatment that may be performed by others (e.g., endodontic therapy)
3. Provisions for reevaluation during and after active periodontal therapy
4. A consideration of adjunctive restorative and prosthetic treatment
5. A recall program of supportive periodontal treatment for type III and type IV cases

SEQUENCE OF THERAPY

Definitive root planing in most cases is performed over many treatment hours (Lindhe et al., 1982). Each visit should include oral hygiene instructions and motivation in addition to treatment of a given area of the mouth. The following aspects of treatment should serve as a guideline in developing a workable sequence of therapy.

First, select the areas of the mouth to be treated and estimate the number of visits.

The gross debridement phase of treatment involves either ultrasonic or hand instrumentation. It is typical to debride the entire mouth, concentrating on supragingival calculus and plaque removal, to achieve as much resolution as possible in the inflamed gingival tissues prior to definitive root planing. Ultrasonic instrumentation may expedite the removal of most supragingival and easily accessible subgingival deposits. However, definitive subgingival root planing should be accomplished as separate procedures, with the patient under local anesthesia, for four to six teeth at a time over several appointments. Healing occurs between each appointment, resulting in gingival recession with exposure of remnants of subgingival deposits. Also, as inflammation subsides, there is less bleeding. Ultrasonic instruments, when properly used, can be a valuable adjunct to scaling with hand instruments (Rosling et al., 1986).

Selected areas of the mouth to be root planed may fall in the following ranges:

Sextants: Difficult access areas (e.g., furcations or advanced levels of disease).

Quadrants: Most typical division of mouth areas; used for moderate to advanced levels of disease.

Half mouth: Beginning to moderate levels of disease; patient difficulty in making multiple visit appointments. NOTE: When treating the patient in half-mouth sessions, work in the maxillary and mandibular quadrants on the same side of the mouth for postoperative patient comfort.

Full mouth: Beginning levels of disease usually involving one or two visits. In exceptional cases requiring full-mouth treatment in moderate to advanced levels of disease, treatment is performed with the patient under local or general anesthesia. This approach is very restricted when it is employed for advanced levels of disease.

LOCAL ANESTHESIA

The use of local anesthesia is generally required when scaling and root planing areas of the mouth that are inflamed, involved with moderate to advanced levels of disease, or have root hypersensitivity. Certain sites in the mouth may have some or all of the above problems. Local anesthesia provides for control of pain in the operating site and hemostasis in the adjacent soft tissues (provided there are no contraindications to epinephrine). The operator may decide where to administer local anesthesia depending on the levels of disease around the teeth or tooth surfaces and on how sensitive the roots are to repeated subgingival instrumentation. Periodontal lesions are site specific, and local anesthesia should be used to help maximize the com-

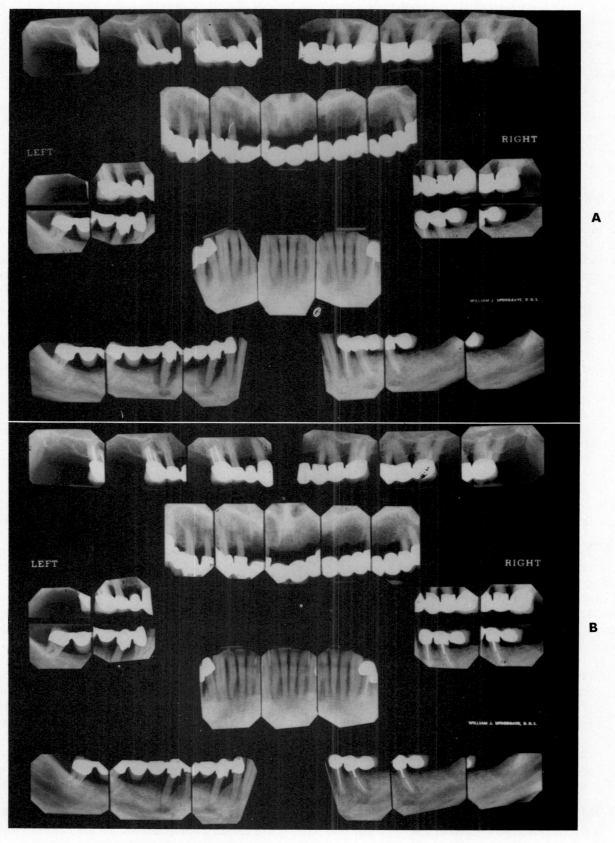

Fig. 33-23. **A,** Full-mouth pretreatment radiographs of a 56-year-old man who had had advanced restorative therapy approximately 5 years previously. Note severe periodontal lesion on mandibular left second premolar. **B,** Full-mouth posttreatment radiographs of same patient seen in **A.** Treatment consisted of scaling, instruction in personal oral hygiene, root planing, curettage, and occlusal adjustment by selective grinding. Note repair about mandibular left second premolar without any flap or surgical procedure. This tooth is vital.

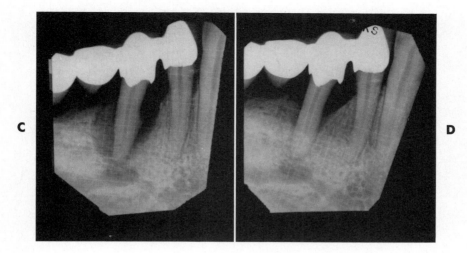

Fig. 33-23, cont'd. C and **D,** High-power radiographs of mandibular left second premolar seen in **A** and **B. C** is pretreatment film, and **D** was taken 1 year later. Treatment was delivered in collaboration with periodontal cotherapists V. Deaver and L. Sherwood.

fort of the patient and the efficiency and effectiveness of the operator. Often complete root planing results in dissection of the labial or lingual papillae, or detachment of other areas of the gingiva. When this occurs, the area may be sutured, and local anesthesia again is necessary for proper suturing.

PERIODONTAL DRESSING

The areas of subgingival instrumentation may be protected with a surgical dressing. The use of chlorhexidine mouth rinse twice daily aids in reducing the plaque accumulation in areas that are too sore for proper mechanical oral hygiene. The patient is instructed not to eat or drink anything hot for 2 hours, and not to brush or chew on that side for 48 hours.

The patient is advised to watch for bleeding. A "pinkish" tint in the saliva is acceptable; however, a deep red pooling of blood in the bottom of the mouth or the formation of large purple clots indicates hemorrhage and should be treated. A moist tea bag applied with pressure to the area for no less than 10 minutes may help as a first attempt to stop bleeding. If the bleeding persists, the operator should be notified. Within 4 to 5 days the patient may remove the dressing and resume oral hygiene in that area.

Sutures should be placed if the soft tissues, especially gingival papillae, are retractible after subgingival root planing or a possibility of heavy postoperative bleeding is anticipated.

EVALUATION OF WOUND HEALING

For the procedures of scaling and root planing to be considered effective treatment modalities, the patient must be able to be maintained at a level of periodontal health that will prevent reinfection with periodontal pathogens.

For the objectives of therapy to be met, the clinician must know what is a realistic maintainable end point to active therapy and be able to make a decision if further definitive treatment is needed to achieve those objectives. At present, the most accurate way of determining a maintainable end point is to assess wound healing over time (see Fig. 33-1).

The criteria for assessing proper wound healing over time following scaling and root planing are as follows:
A. One to two weeks after root planing
   1. Resolution of edema
   2. Shrinkage of the gingival margin
   3. Color is about normal
   4. Moderate pocket depth may be present, but there is little or no bleeding from the base of the pocket when probed
   5. No suppuration can be expressed after pressing on the gingiva or on deep probing
   6. No obvious calculus is present
   7. Oral hygiene is excellent
   8. Histologically, epithelialization is about complete
B. Two to three weeks after root planing
   1. Color is normal
   2. Consistency is firm
   3. No bleeding from the base of the pocket
   4. Tooth mobility may decrease
   5. Subgingival flora is free from periodontal pathogens, and organisms should be the same as seen in healthy sites
   6. Histologically, connective tissue maturation continues for 21 to 28 days, and final gingival contours may not be seen for 3 to 6 months

Since periodontal disease is often site specific (Goodson et al, 1982; Haffajee, 1983), each tooth or tooth surface

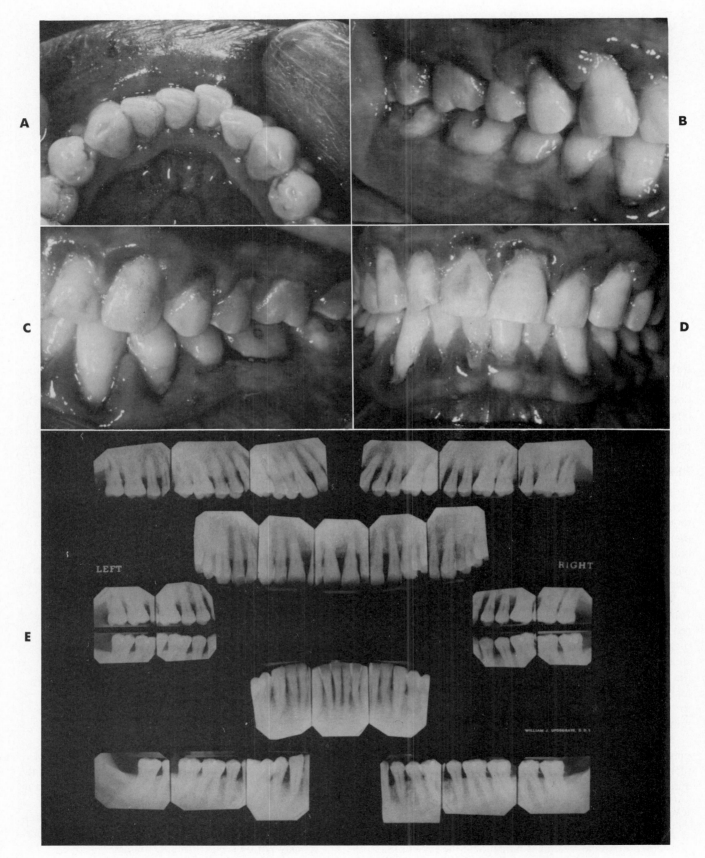

Fig. 33-24. A to **D,** This 56-year-old man exhibited heavy plaque and calculus deposits, which resulted in severe gingival inflammation. **E,** Pretreatment radiographs of same patient. Note heavy deposits, alveolar resorption, and thickening of periodontal ligament space. Diagnosis was periodontitis with occlusal traumatism.

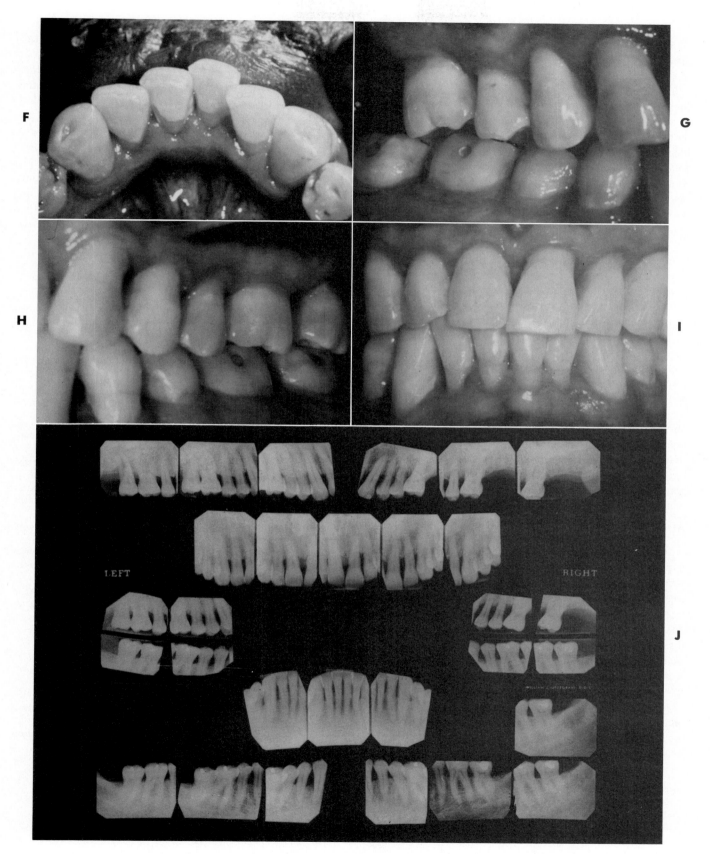

Fig. 33-24, cont'd. F to **I,** Same patient 2 years later after scaling, root planing, instruction in personal oral hygiene, and occlusal adjustment. Maxillary right second molar had to be extracted. Treatment was delivered in collaboration with periodontal cotherapist L. Sherwood. **J,** Two-year posttreatment radiographs show repair in ligament spaces and alveolar bone.

should be evaluated for proper wound healing. If a treated lesion still elicits bleeding on probing after adequate wound healing, an assessment of the nature of the bleeding is helpful in deciding on the next step in therapy. If bleeding occurs from the margin of the gingiva at reevaluation, newly formed plaque may be the reason, and reinforcement of oral hygiene may resolve the inflammation. If bleeding occurs from the base of the pocket (2 to 3 weeks following root planing), there is a good possibility that the root is not biologically acceptable, because of residual deposits on the root surface or a residual pathogenic flora in the pocket. These should be removed.

A decision must be made as to whether the active lesion should be reinstrumented with a closed root-planing procedure or with an open-flap entry technique for access to the contaminated root surface and infiltrate. Badersten et al. (1981, 1984a, 1984b) suggest moderate careful, conservative periodontal therapy before surgical intervention is considered. Current research has demonstrated that the clinical severity of periodontitis is reduced significantly 1 month following the conservative phase of periodontal therapy and that the need for surgical pocket treatment cannot be assessed properly until the completion of the conservative phase of treatment (Morrison et al., 1980). If the periodontal pathogens persist and repeated attempts have been made to mechanically debride the site or sites that bleed or suppurate on probing, a course of antibiotics may be given. Systemic tetracycline, penicillin, metronidazole, or ampicillin and metronidazole given until pathogens are eliminated often is successful in resolving inflammation.

BENEFITS OF ROOT PLANING*

The 1950s saw a marked proliferation of surgical techniques in the treatment of osseous and soft lesions observed in individuals suffering from periodontal disease. Many of these procedures were introduced without adequate testing in animal or human studies, and as a result later investigations showed some of the hazards of using these methods on the supporting structures of the dentition. In the 1970s and 1980s several longitudinal studies were conducted which clearly help the clinician understand the efficacy of certain approaches to treatment. The result of these clinical investigations is that many surgical phases are being reserved for later periods in the treatment plan or are being postponed indefinitely in cases where no major restorative treatment is needed.

*Text in this section and Figs. 33-23 and 33-24 are from Cohen DW: Periodontics 1985—reflections and projections, Quintessence Int 4:271, 1985.

Clinical studies have also demonstrated that dental hygienists can be trained to be very skillful in using root planing and curettage in the initial phases of periodontal treatment. Certain programs such as those started at the University of Pennsylvania in 1969-1970 to give expanded functions to dental hygienists in the area of periodontics have resulted in the term *periodontal cotherapists* for these personnel, who have become extremely valuable members of the dental team treating periodontal diseases (Figs. 33-23 and 33-24). Some of the most popular participation forms of continuing education courses being presented today are those that help hygienists and dentists enhance their skills in root-planing techniques. If more hygienists receive this training, it will add a greater dimension to the general practice that wishes to expand its activities in the treatment of periodontal disease.

REFERENCES

Adriaens PA, De Boever JA, and Loesche WJ: Bacterial invasion in root cementum and radicular dentin of periodontally diseased teeth in humans—a reservoir of periodontopathic bacteria, J Periodontol 59:222, 1988a.

Adriaens PA et al: Ultrastructural observations on bacterial invasion in cementum and radicular dentin of periodontally diseased human teeth, J Periodontol 59:493, 1988b.

Aleo JJ et al: The presence and biologic activity of cementum bound endotoxin, J Periodontol 45:672, 1974.

Badersten A, Nilveus R, and Egelberg J: Effect on non-surgical periodontal therapy. I. Moderately advanced periodontitis, J Clin Periodontol 8:52, 1981.

Badersten A, Nilveus R, and Egelberg J: Effect on non-surgical therapy. II. Severely advanced periodontitis, J Clin Periodontol 11:63 1984.

Badersten A, Nilveus R, and Egelberg J: Effect of non-surgical periodontal therapy. III. Single versus repeated instrumentations. J Clin Periodontol 11:114, 1984b.

Goodson JM et al: Patterning progress of progression and regression of periodontal disease, J Clin Periodontol 9:472, 1982.

Haffajee AD, Socransky SS, and Goodson JM: Comparison of different data anaylsis for detecting changes in attachment level, J Clin Periodontol 10:298, 1983.

Jones WA and O'Leary TJ: The effectiveness of in vivo root planing in removing bacterial endotoxin from the roots of periodontally involved teeth, J Periodontol 49:337, 1978.

Kakehashi S and Parakkal PF: Proceedings from the state-of-the-art workshop on surgical therapy for periodontitis, J Periodontol 53:475, 1982.

Lindhe J et al: Healing following surgical/non-surgical treatment of periodontal disease: a clinical study, J Clin Periodontol 9:115, 1982.

Morrison EC, Ramfjord SC, and Hill RW: Short term effects of initial, non-surgical periodontal treatment (hygienic phase), J Clin Periodontol 7:199, 1980.

Pattison G and Pattison AM: Periodontal instrumentation, a clinical manual, Reston, Va, 1979, Reston Publishing Co.

Rosling BG et al: Topical antimicrobial therapy and diagnosis of subgingival bacteria in the management of inflammatory periodontal disease, J Clin Periodontol 13:975, 1986.

Wilkins EM: Clinical practice of the dental hygienist, ed 5, Philadelphia, 1983, Lea & Febiger.

Chapter 34

REMOVAL OF PLAQUE RETENTION AREAS

Beatrice E. Siegrist
Niklaus P. Lang

Removal of overhanging fillings
Removal of overcontoured and inadequate crown margins
Reshaping of inadequate pontics
Elimination of iatrogenic plaque retention areas by replacing reconstructions
Removal of "hopeless" teeth

The key role of plaque-retaining factors in the etiology and pathogenesis of dental plaque infections is well established. Therefore, not only is the goal of therapy bioacceptability of root surfaces through effective scaling and root planing, but also dental restorations must be incorporated so that periodontal tissues are not damaged and do not provide areas for plaque retention and colonization by a pathogenic microbiota. Furthermore, dental restorations should not severely impinge on the patient's ability to perform optimal oral hygiene.

If iatrogenic plaque retention areas are present in patients with periodontal diseases, they must be removed during the early antiinfective phase of periodontal therapy, at the time that subgingival scaling and root planing are carried out. In removing plaque-retaining areas, the microbiologic ecosystem of these sites is affected favorably and the establishment of a more health-associated microbiota results (Lang et al., 1983).

Removal of plaque-retaining factors includes elimination of:
1. Overhanging fillings
2. Overcontoured and inadequate crown margins
3. Convex pontic surfaces in close contact with the underlying gingival tissue
4. Portions of removable prostheses that impinge on the gingiva or otherwise contribute to periodontal inflammation and plaque accumulation

Often the elimination of these iatrogenic factors requires the replacement of existing restorations by more biologically acceptable reconstructions. If the morphology of the roots is ignored, especially in multirooted teeth, overcontouring frequently results. Hence an area leading to alteration in the composition of the plaque microbiota is provided, resulting in an environment that encourages the establishment of a pathogenic microbiota and maybe calculus formation.

REMOVAL OF OVERHANGING FILLINGS

The goal of this procedure is to provide smooth surfaces on roots and fillings, especially in the transition area between dental materials and natural tooth substance. Gaps, shoulders, and other ecologic niches for plaque maturation must be avoided. Furthermore, these areas of marginal adaptation of dental reconstructions must be accessible for oral hygiene aids. Generally, it is not the overhanging reconstruction per se, but the inaccessibility of this area to oral hygiene procedures that is detrimental to periodontal health and disturbing to the integrity of a tooth surface by allowing the development of root surface caries.

Overhanging margins of amalgam or composite fillings may be removed using fine flame-shaped diamond points combined with sufficient irrigating spray. Also, abrasive diamond strips (GC-Fuji) or paper strips (3M) have been

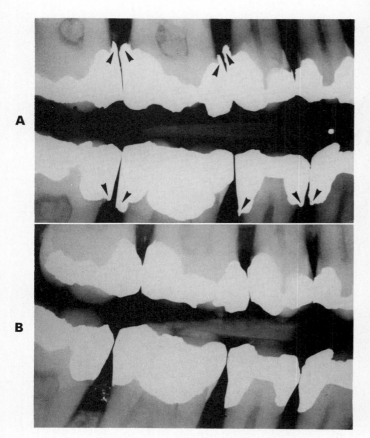

Fig. 34-1. Radiographic demonstration of removal of overhanging amalgam fillings using diamond points and abrasive strips. **A,** Before removal. **B,** After removal. (Courtesy Dr. A. Grendelmeier, Olten, Switzerland.)

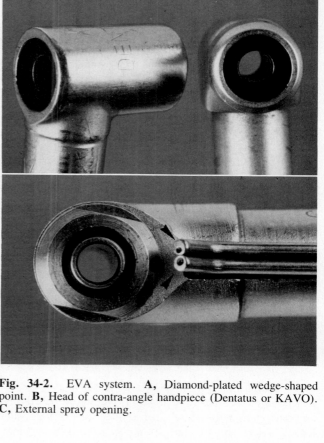

Fig. 34-2. EVA system. **A,** Diamond-plated wedge-shaped point. **B,** Head of contra-angle handpiece (Dentatus or KAVO). **C,** External spray opening.

advocated for polishing interproximal surfaces after iatrogenic factors are removed (Fig. 34-1).

In recent years, the EVA system* (Axelsson, 1969) has gained great popularity for these time-consuming procedures (Fig. 34-2). A wedge-shaped diamond-plated point (Fig. 34-2, *A*) may be fixed by friction in a specially designed head (Fig. 34-2, *B*) fitted to a contra-angle handpiece. Sufficient waterspray (Fig. 34-2, *C*) is used during the filing motions of these points. The development of the Proxoshape system† (Lutz et al., 1981) further improved the possibilities of the EVA system not only in removing overhanging margins, but also in finishing and polishing all interproximal fillings, whether amalgam or composite

*Dentatus, Sweden, or KAVO, Germany.
†W. Hubschmid & Son, Lugano, Switzerland.

(Fig. 34-3). Very thin diamond-plated steel wedges with 75, 40, or 15 μm diamonds (Fig. 34-3, *A*) allow for a stepwise procedure to achieve optimal smoothness in the interdental area of filling margins (Lutz et al., 1981). Fig. 34-4 documents the successful removal of several amalgam filling overhangs using the EVA system in combination with the Proxoshape diamond points.

REMOVAL OF OVERCONTOURED AND INADEQUATE CROWN MARGINS

Since inadequate restorations often go unreplaced because of financial or socioeconomic aspects, overcontoured crown margins must be removed during the hygienic phase of periodontal therapy. In Fig. 34-5, *A*, a reconstruction from teeth Nos. 11 and 12 to 14, replacing No. 13 with a pontic, severely jeopardized the periodontal health on the mesial aspect of tooth No. 12. The removal

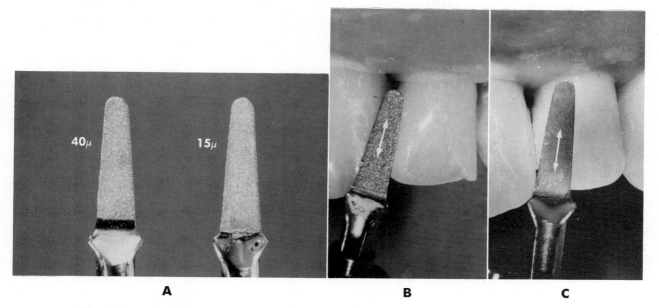

Fig. 34-3. Proxoshape system. **A,** Wedge-shaped steel blades with diamond plating of 40 and 15 μm, respectively. **B,** Composite filling overhang before removal. **C,** Composite filling overhang after using Proxoshape system. (Courtesy Dr. M. Gygax, Zofingen, Switzerland.)

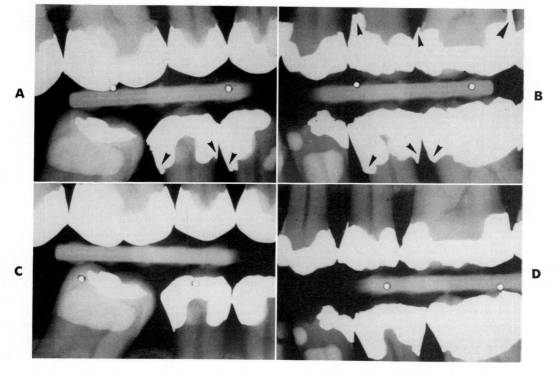

Fig. 34-4. Radiographic demonstration of removal of several overhanging filling margins *(arrows).* **A** and **B,** Before removal. **C** and **D,** After removal with EVA and Proxoshape systems.

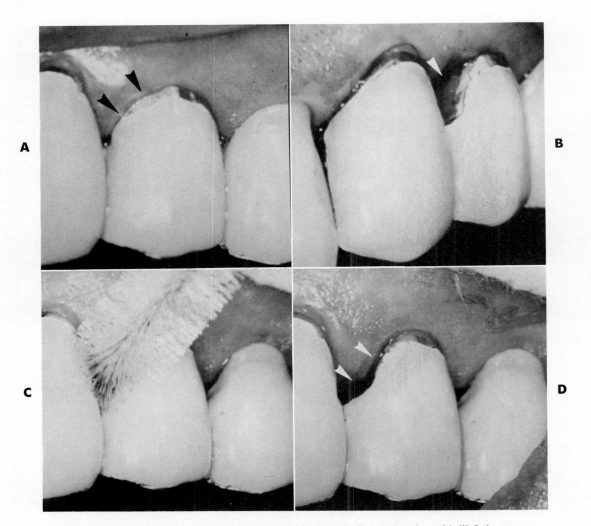

Fig. 34-5. Reconstruction of teeth Nos. 11 and 12 to 14. **A,** Reconstruction with ill-fitting crown margin on mesial aspect of No. 12 *(arrows)*. **B,** Appearance following removal with a flame-shaped diamond. **C,** Oral hygiene practices. **D,** Appearance 3 weeks following removal.

of the ill-fitting crown margin using flame-shaped diamond points (Fig. 34-5, *B*) resulted in improved accessibility for interdental brushes in the interdental space between Nos. 11 and 12 (Fig. 34-5, *C*). Regular and effective oral hygiene led to gingival health in the course of 3 weeks (Fig. 34-5, *D*).

Quite often the interdental spaces of reconstructions are overcontoured and hence inaccessible for effective oral hygiene. If the reconstruction must be retained, the interdental spaces should be opened and made accessible for toothpicks or interdental brushes even if crown margins have to be shortened during this procedure (Fig. 34-6).

Old ill-fitting crown margins may require circumferen-

tial removal (Fig. 34-7) to allow a healing of the gingival tissues and accessibility of the crown margin to oral hygiene (Lang, 1978). The procedure to remove these margins is outlined in Fig. 34-8. A groove is placed circumferentially approximately 1 to 2 mm supragingivally using a high-speed bur (Fig. 34-8, *A*). The inadequate or ill-fitting margin may then be removed totally or in increments (Fig. 34-8, *B*). The trimmed crown margin is then finished using the EVA and Proxoshape systems, as well as finishing diamond points (Fig. 34-8, *C*). The accessibility of the crown margin to oral hygiene results in gingival and dental health, which can be seen in Fig. 34-8, *D*, taken 6 years after the removal of the ill-fitting margin.

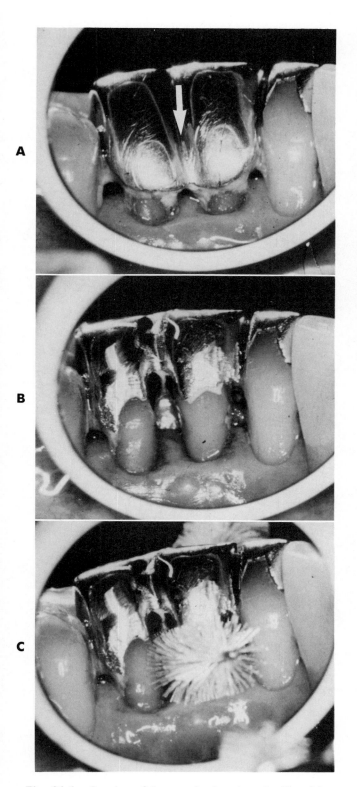

Fig. 34-6. Opening of interproximal region. **A,** Closed interproximal area of a mandibular front reconstruction *(arrow).* **B,** Appearance after opening using a diamond point. **C,** Placement of interdental brushes.

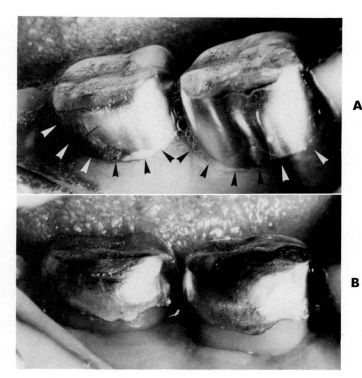

Fig. 34-7. **A,** Circumferentially ill-fitting crown margins of gold band reconstructions. **B,** Gingival health after removal of ill-fitting margins.

RESHAPING OF INADEQUATE PONTICS

If pontics show concave surfaces combined with intimate contact with the underlying mucosal surface, ulcerations may be expected, usually because a more pathogenic ecosystem is created for microbial plaque (Gusberti et al., 1985). Although these pathologic alterations may be affected by vigorous and complete regular plaque removal (Silness et al., 1982), reshaping of the pontic may be necessary to provide easy accessibility for oral hygiene aids. Since the optimal design of a pontic closely resembles an egg shape with no concavities and very subtle pinpoint contacts with the mucosa, this design should be kept in mind during reshaping procedures.

ELIMINATION OF IATROGENIC PLAQUE RETENTION AREAS BY REPLACING RECONSTRUCTIONS

A prosthetic reconstruction must never jeopardize the patient's efforts for optimal oral hygiene. All margins of fillings and crowns must be accessible to oral hygiene aids, such as interdental toothpicks and brushes. If this goal cannot be met by the elimination of plaque-retaining areas using conservative methods, replacement of the re-

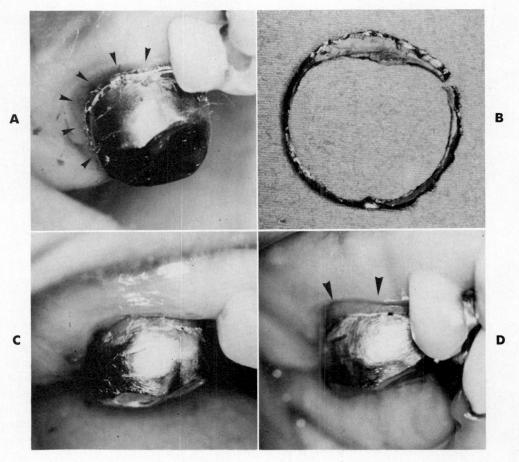

Fig. 34-8. Removal procedure for ill-fitting crown margins. **A,** Circumferential groove, 1 to 2 mm supragingivally *(arrows)*. **B,** Removal of ill-fitting crown margin. Ring is filled with bacterial plaque. **C,** Appearance immediately following finishing of margin using Proxoshape system. **D,** Gingival health 6 years following removal of ill-fitting margin.

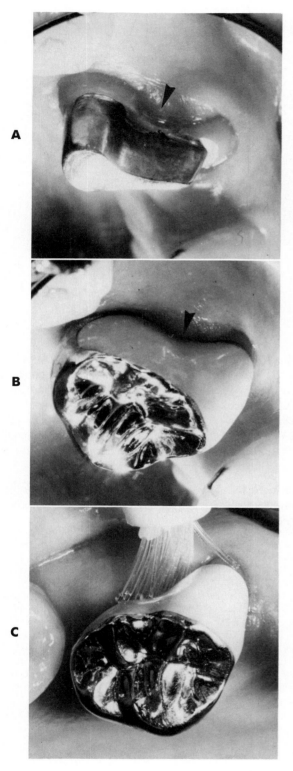

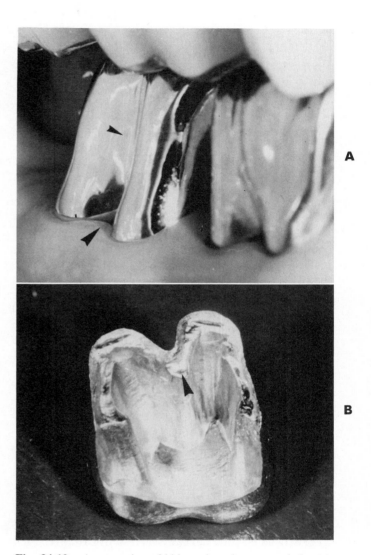

Fig. 34-10. Accentuation of kidney-shaped root morphology in a lower molar with a treated furcation involvement. **A,** Transferring root contour to crown (undercontouring). **B,** Deliberate exaggeration of furcation contour.

Fig. 34-9. Replacement of overcontoured reconstruction. **A,** Accentuation of tooth morphology with post and core placement. **B,** Avoidance of plaque-retaining areas. **C,** Accessibility for oral hygiene brushes.

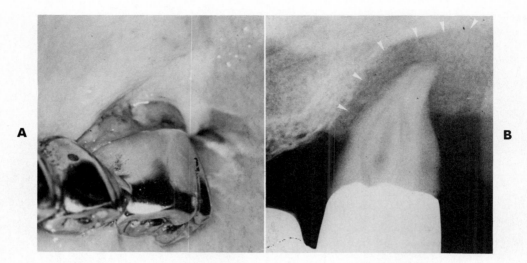

Fig. 34-11. Extraction of "hopeless teeth" constituting plaque retention areas, **A**, and having completely lost their periodontal support, **B**.

construction becomes inevitable. In such cases, mostly multirooted teeth demonstrate altered morphologic features that, if ignored, may lead to new plaque-retaining areas. These include atypical root morphology following the amputation of roots, root malformations, and retained lingual grooves. To avoid overcontouring these areas, the altered morphologic features of the teeth must be accentuated (Fig. 34-9), especially in furcation areas involved in periodontal diseases. Periodontal therapy often results in reduced height of the supporting apparatus below the level of the furcation entrance. To ensure optimal oral hygiene in this area and minimize risks for plaque retention, furcation areas must be transferred to the crown contours in reconstructions of teeth with treated furcation involvements (Fig. 34-10).

REMOVAL OF "HOPELESS" TEETH

Teeth that have completely lost their function to periodontal infection from the marginal to the periapical region may no longer be treated successfully. They represent plaque-retaining areas completely inaccessible to oral hygiene. Since therapy for a periodontal infection includes elimination of all plaque-retaining factors and elimination

or suppression of the pathogenic periodontal microflora, these hopeless teeth should be extracted during the hygienic phase of periodontal therapy (Fig. 34-11) to remove potential sources for reinfection of the dentition.

The decision for extraction of teeth or only single roots should always follow a carefully performed examination and treatment planning. Special consideration must be given to strategically important teeth.

REFERENCES

Axelsson P: EVA-systemet: ett nytt hjälpmedel för approximal rengöring, puts och polering, Swed Dent J 61:1086, 1969.

Gusberti FA, Finger M, and Lang NP: Scanning electron microscope study of 48-hour plaque on different bridge pontics designs, Schweiz Monatsschr Zahnmed 95:539, 1985.

Lang NP: Die Vorbehandlung in der Parodontaltherapie, Dtsch Zahnarztl Z 33:3, 1978.

Lang NP, Kiel RA, and Anderhalden K: Clinical and microbiological effects of subgingival restorations with overhanging or clinically perfect margins, J Clin Periodontol 10:563, 1983.

Lutz F, Curilovic Z, and Mörmann W: Interdentale Restorationsüberhänge—rationelle Entfernung, mit neuentwickelten Maschinen und Instrumenten, Schweiz Monatsschr Zahnheilkd 91:969, 1981.

Silness J, Gustavsen F, and Maugersnes, K: The relationship between pontic hygiene and mucosal inflammation in fixed-bridge recipients, J Periodont Res 17:434, 1982.

Chapter 35

ANTIINFECTIVE THERAPY FOR GINGIVITIS AND PERIODONTITIS

Robert J. Genco
Lars A. Christersson

Antiinfective therapy consists of those procedures that counteract or control disease-causing microorganisms. For many systemic infections emphasis is placed on the use of antimicrobial drugs; however, for localized infections, such as periodontal diseases, antiinfective therapy often consists of a combination of mechanical debridement and antimicrobial agents. It is clear that the mainstay of antiinfective therapy for gingivitis and periodontitis consists of professionally applied mechanical debridement, including scaling and root planing, as well as personal oral hygiene, including regular supragingival plaque removal. Several studies have shown that mechanical debridement proce-

dures to remove the bulk of the infection are effective in the treatment of gingivitis and most mild to moderate forms of periodontitis in adults (Badersten et al., 1981; Ramfjord, 1987). While antiinfective therapy is adequate for patients with mild to moderate periodontitis, periodontal surgery is often necessary for patients with advanced periodontitis and deep pockets to provide access for complete root debridement (see Antczak-Boukoms and Weinstein, 1987, for a review of the literature supporting these conclusions). The use of antimicrobial agents, particularly systemic antibiotics in conjunction with mechanical therapy, is often necessary for less common forms of periodontal disease, including localized juvenile periodontitis and periodontitis that is refractory to debridement therapy.

Antiinfective therapy is applicable to all forms of periodontal diseases, including those associated with systemic disorders such as diabetes and acquired immunodeficiency syndrome (AIDS). The underlying rationale indicates elimination of the bacterial cause of these forms of periodontal disease. Contraindications are specific, such as precautions for mechanical debridement in hemophiliac patients and the use of particular agents in subjects with allergies or hypersensitivities.

The general effectiveness of antiinfective therapy, including mechanical debridement and successful oral hygiene, in the management of periodontal disease is well established in the literature and has met the test of success in clinical practice for most cases of gingivitis and mild to moderate periodontitis in adults (Badersten et al., 1981; Ramfjord, 1987).

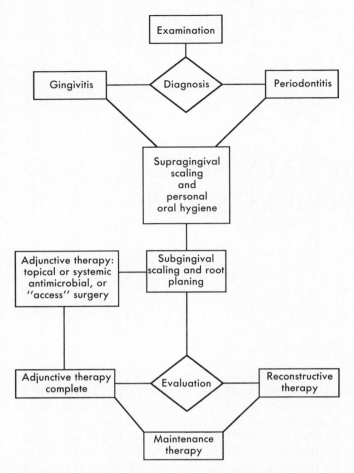

Fig. 35-1. Sequence of antiinfective, reconstructive, and maintenance therapy.

INTEGRATION OF ANTIINFECTIVE THERAPY WITH OTHER MODES OF THERAPY

The treatment of most patients suffering from periodontal disease and dental caries consists of three major phases (Fig. 35-1). The first is *antiinfective therapy* in which the infections causing periodontal diseases and caries are treated to suppress the pathogenic organisms. The second is *reconstructive therapy* in which structures and tissues lost to the ravages of caries and periodontal disease are restored as necessary. The third is *maintenance therapy* in which prevention of recurrence of disease and monitoring of plaque control by the patient are carried out.

OBJECTIVES OF ANTIINFECTIVE THERAPY

The overall goals of antiinfective therapy are to suppress the bacteria associated with periodontal disease and to resolve inflammation in the periodontal tissues. Specifically, the aims of the antiinfective phase of therapy are:

1. To remove all supragingival and subgingival calculus

2. To eliminate or reduce levels of the specific pathogenic periodontal microflora
3. To remove or eliminate plaque retention areas such as overhanging restorations, ill-fitting crowns, and root abnormalities
4. To teach the patient how to perform personal oral hygiene
5. To motivate the patient to maintain low levels of plaque and a periodontal pathogen–free dentition

Antiinfective therapy in patients suffering from caries and periodontal disease is often integrated with strategic extraction of hopeless teeth, endodontic therapy, restorative and prosthetic therapy, and orthodontic therapy. The ultimate goal of antiinfective therapy combined with other modes of dental therapy is to provide an esthetic, comfortable, and functional dentition able to be maintained disease-free for a lifetime.

PROCEDURES FOR ANTIINFECTIVE THERAPY

The specific procedures used for antiinfective therapy described here have been in use for many years and have been evaluated in research clinical trials demonstrating their usefulness and limitations (Genco, 1981; Rosling, et al., 1983; Slots and Rosling, 1983; Christersson et al., 1985; Rosling et al., 1986; Zambon et al., 1986).

A treatment plan incorporating antifective therapy is given in the box on p. 429. The listing of procedures serves to illustrate the framework for a treatment plan necessary for patients with advanced dental disease who require multiple modes of therapy, including antiinfective periodontal therapy.

For purposes of clarity, *the antiinfective phase of periodontal therapy* is described in detail below. This therapy is often adequate periodontal therapy for patients who suffer only from gingivitis and mild or moderate periodontitis. Those suffering from advanced periodontitis or those who require other modes of therapy must be treated by these antiinfective procedures integrated with those other therapies.

Examination

The examination should gather information to determine the nature and extent of the periodontal disease. The initial examination provides baseline measurements of probing pocket depths, probing attachment levels, gingival recession, mucogingival abnormalities, gingival inflammation, bleeding on probing, suppuration, the presence of periodontal pathogens, and tooth mobility. This provides the basis for an accurate diagnosis, a rational treatment plan, and a baseline for assessment of treatment progress or of further disease progression. It also provides the basis for case presentation to the patient, which begins the educational process; allows proper consent to be obtained; and helps ensure patient cooperation with all phases of therapy.

Treatment plan for patients with advanced dental disease requiring periodontal therapy and other forms of dental treatment

Procedures	*Appointments necessary*
Examination, medical history, dental history, charting, radiographs, models, microbiologic tests, systemic tests as indicated, consultation, and presentation of findings and proposed treatment to patient	1-3
Palliative procedures: extractions, endodontics, and transitional restorations or prostheses as needed	0-4
ANTIINFECTIVE THERAPY	
Supragingival scaling, removal of plaque retention areas, and personal oral hygiene training	1-3
Subgingival scaling and root planing, access flaps, and closed curettage, including topical antimicrobial and/or adjunctive systemic antibiotic therapy, as necessary	2-4
Evaluation of the effects of therapy on resolution of inflammation, pocket reduction, establishment of oral hygiene, reduction of tooth mobility, and suppression of pathogenic microflora	1-2
Additional therapy after evaluation may include ultrasonic bactericidal debridement, antimicrobials, revision of oral hygiene, occlusal adjustment and temporary splinting for progressive mobility, and periodontal surgery	Variable
Temporary or provisional prostheses: further extractions or orthodontics if necessary	Variable
Reconstructive periodontal procedures: periodontal surgery including access flaps, closed curettage, root planing, free grafts, tooth lengthening, periodontal regenerative procedures, gingival augmentation, esthetic recontouring of gingiva or pontic areas, or other surgical procedures as necessary for esthetics, access for oral hygiene, or prosthetics.	1-4
Implant surgical procedures: install implants and attach abutments	2-4, separated by 3-6 months
FINAL RESTORATIONS AND PROSTHESES	Variable
MAINTENANCE THERAPY	
Maintenance recall: evaluate periodontal inflammation, pocket depth, attachment levels, furcations, recurrent or new caries, microbiologic tests, and radiographs as necessary; evaluate prosthesis and occlusion; evaluate esthetics; update medical history; and administer regular prophylaxis, fluoride treatments, and retreatment as indicated	1 visit every 3-6 months

---

Personal oral hygiene, and scaling and root planing

Personal oral hygiene instruction and sugragingival scaling usually require two to three appointments of 1 hour each. Supragingival scaling is often carried out with ultrasonic instruments and is directed to removing accessible plaque accumulations and supragingival calculus. Subgingival scaling may also begin at this time. During this phase of treatment, open carious lesions are excavated and appropriate fillings placed. Also, plaque retention areas, including overhanging margins of restorations, open margins of restorations, and ill-fitting restorations, are replaced or repaired (for details on removal of plaque retention areas, see Chapter 34). Anatomic plaque retention areas, such as retained developmental grooves, open furcations, and malposed teeth, are identified, and specific oral hygiene aids and instructions are given for these areas. Correction of some of these anatomic defects may be possible by recontouring of grooves and odontoplasty.

Oral hygiene instruction and motivational discussion should begin early. However, if there are large amounts of plaque and calculus, and excessive gingival swelling and bleeding, oral hygiene instruction may be given after removal of the gross debris and partial resolution of the gingival inflammation.

Details of preventive procedures for individuals are given in Chapters 28 and 44. Below we describe personal hygiene procedures in a practical manner, as they are incorporated with the scaling and root-planing appointments. They are designed to allow the periodontal patient to practice effective personal oral hygiene with few traumatic side effects.

Personal oral hygiene instruction

Oral hygiene practices are those practices employed personally or professionally to prevent establishment in the oral cavity of pathogenic flora or their disease-causing products, with the ultimate objective of preventing disease initiation, progression, or recurrence (Löe and Kleinman, 1985).

It is clearly recognized that periodic removal of supragingival plaque is essential to the maintenance of periodontal health, but the individual response to different levels of plaque may vary dramatically. Hence for clinical use, the monitoring of disease variables, such as gingival bleeding, is more valid than the monitoring of plaque accumulation only. The practical goal of oral hygiene practices for each individual is to obtain the level of plaque control required for the maintenance of gingival health.

Clinicians are often discouraged by the patient's response to oral hygiene instruction, and many patients are inaccurately labeled as uncooperative. However, every patient who seeks dental care on a regular basis has to be considered cooperative and an individual who will most likely assume the role of cotherapist.

Professional cleaning of the teeth and oral hygiene instruction typically have only a short and transitional effect on the gingival status. Patients often lapse into their previous behavior with return of plaque to the original levels, unless they are carefully and repeatedly motivated (Fig. 35-2).

Patients with periodontal disease often exhibit poor oral hygiene; however, most patients indicate that they use oral hygiene aids once or twice a day. One should not blame the patient for the insufficient level of oral hygiene; the patient is often *performing* oral hygiene measures several times a day; however, the *effectiveness* of these measures is inadequate.

There is no convincing evidence that any specific toothbrush type and design or toothbrushing method is substantially superior at removing plaque. As a clinician, one might have to instruct patients in the use of several different approaches, depending on the needs and preferences of the patient. However, a single regimen for oral hygiene taught and reinforced by all members of the office team is most likely to be used by the patient on a long-term basis.

Mechanical plaque removal

Toothbrushes. Toothbrushes are available in a variety of shapes, sizes, forms, and materials. Nylon is the preferred bristle material, since it can be standardized, is easier to keep clean, and will not retain moisture. Good toothbrushes have the following specifications:

1. The bristles are typically 10 mm long.
2. The bristles have a diameter of approximately 0.2 mm.
3. The bristles are soft, and the ends rounded.
4. The bristles are arranged on a relatively small head (eg., 30 × 10 mm).
5. Individual bristles are multitufted with a straight trim for optimal overall cleaning effect.
6. The handle is wide and long with a long neck for easy grip, maneuverability, and access.

In Fig. 35-3 tufts of a commonly used toothbrush are shown, illustrating the straight trim and rounded ends. Studies have shown that nonrounded bristles can be twice as abrasive as rounded ends and can produce more gingival abrasions.

Electric toothbrushes. Several electric toothbrushes are available on the market. Generally, studies have shown that they are as effective as, or marginally more effective than, manual brushes (i.e., the buccal and lingual surfaces may become fully cleaned). However, the interproximal

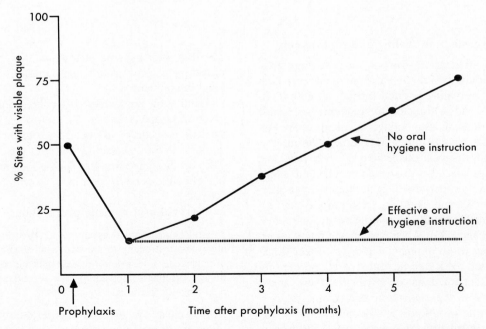

Fig. 35-2. Dental plaque accumulation after a single prophylaxis with no personal oral hygiene instructions as compared with little or no accumulation with proper personal and professional oral hygiene. (Idealized from data of our own studies.)

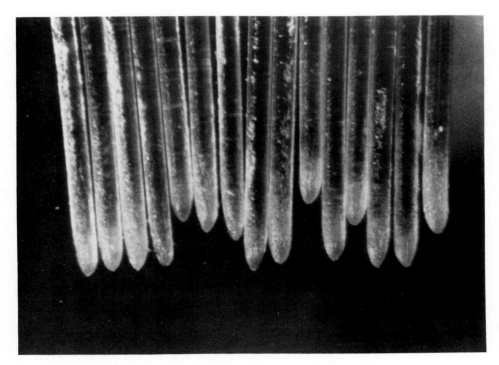

Fig. 35-3. Tufts from a modern nylon-bristled toothbrush. Note tapered and rounded ends, which are desirable for effective plaque removal with minimal abrasiveness for tooth or gingival surfaces. (Butler G-U-M No. 411; ×32; courtesy Bud Tarrson.)

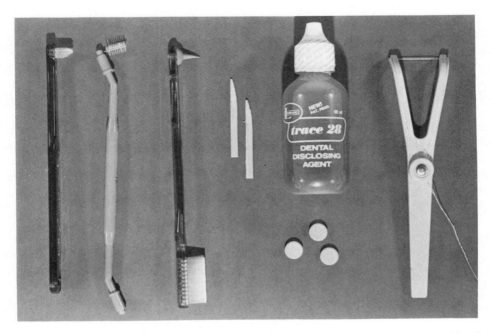

Fig. 35-4. Several aids for interproximal plaque control. *Left to right:* End-tufted toothbrush, interproximal brush, rubber tip, wooden interdental cleansers, disclosing agents for staining plaque, and dental floss in holder.

tooth surfaces are not adequately cleaned with either regular manual or electric toothbrushes. Individuals with specific needs for electric toothbrushes are handicapped and hospitalized patients.

Mechanical oral hygiene aids for interproximal surfaces. Interproximal tooth surfaces are generally not cleaned by toothbrushing alone. Furthermore, the interdental areas are often severely affected by periodontal disease and caries; hence effective removal of plaque from these surfaces is necessary. Fig. 35-4 illustrates several aids that are useful for interdental plaque control; at least one of these should be used daily by each patient.

Dental floss. Dental floss is available as waxed or unwaxed, flat or round floss and comes in several sizes. Its reported effectiveness for interproximal plaque removal varies, possibly because of the technique employed for its use. Floss is often maneuvered digitally; however, dental floss holders may make it easier to use.

Single-tufted brushes. These brushes are also called end-tufted toothbrushes and are useful for teeth separated by large diastemas or where a neighboring tooth is missing, in furcations, and for the distal surfaces of most posterior teeth.

Interproximal toothbrushes. These brushes are used for interproximal or interradicular cleaning.

Toothpicks and wooden interdental sticks. Toothpicks come in a variety of shapes and material choices; however, the recommended toothpick has a triangular cross section and is made of a moderately soft wood.

Rubber tips. Rubber tips are useful for cleaning interproximal regions and into shallow pockets. No therapeutic benefit of gingival massage per se has been shown.

Irrigation devices. Irrigation devices have little or no effect when used alone; hence there is no scientific justification for recommending their use except as an adjunct to mechanical plaque control in patients with orthodontic appliances or bridges. They have been shown to cause gingival abscesses and bacteremias, especially in patients with inflamed gingiva; hence they should be used with care when there is periodontal pocketing and gingival inflammation. However, they may decrease the time of lowered pH after a meal if used immediately after the intake of food and hence may play a role in reducing caries. Forced irrigation devices have recently gained renewed interest when used as a delivery system for antimicrobial drugs in solution, and this regimen may be useful during the maintenance phase of therapy to reduce the recurrence of gingivitis.

Dentifrices. Dentifrices are available in powder, paste, gel, and liquid forms. The main components of dentifrices include abrasives; detergents; humectants; thickening agents; flavoring agents; coloring agents; preservatives; therapeutic agents such as fluoride, antiplaque, or anticalculus agents; and water.

The single largest component is usually the abrasive, or polishing agent, making up 40% to 50% of the volume. Examples of abrasives are calcium hydroxide particles, silica, sodium bicarbonate, and acrylic spheres. Most patients expect a dentifrice to remove stain and hence prefer a dentifrice with a strong to moderate abrasive. One of the most beneficial effects of a dentifrice on plaque is the slower regrowth observed when subjects brush with a dentifrice as compared with when they brush with water alone.

Fluoride is the most important therapeutic and preventive ingredient in dentifrices. For populations where controlled fluoridation of water does not exist, fluoridated dentifrices are probably very important in the prevention of caries. Other ingredients of therapeutic nature include anticalculus agents, antiplaque agents, antimicrobial agents, oxygen-releasing agents, and desensitizing agents. Most often, the scientific value for the effectiveness of these agents is not clear, although dentifrices have a great potential to deliver such therapeutic agents.

Disclosing agents. The use of disclosing agents improves the ability of the patient to recognize plaque deposits, which often are not visible before staining. Also, disclosing agents improve the clinician's ability to demonstrate defective oral hygiene techniques and to monitor progress. Disclosing of dental plaque should become routine in oral hygiene instruction and monitoring.

Disclosing agents in the form of chewable tablets or solutions include simple dyes (FDA E28) that highlight plaque on the teeth by giving it an intense stain. Unfortunately, pellicle, mucosa, and gingiva also stain, which may make it offensive to some patients.

Oral hygiene techniques. Many different techniques for toothbrushing have been described; however, none has convincingly been shown to be superior in its ability to contribute to oral hygiene. The mode of action itself against the individual tooth is not the most important factor in toothbrushing. Most techniques, such as those of Bass, Charters, Stillmans, and others, have the capacity to clean the tooth. It is more important to recognize the limitations of each technique. The most important factor is that the brushing is employed on *all* surfaces in the oral cavity to which the technique is applicable.

To suggest a somewhat rigid regimen may be beneficial, especially if it is embraced and taught by the entire dental team in the office. This avoids confusion if two or more individuals of the dental team are involved in giving oral hygiene instructions to patients. For example, an office team may select a system such as the Bass technique as a basic procedure. In the Bass technique the bristles of a soft nylon brush are placed at the gingival margin at a 45-degree angle to the long axis of the tooth. The brush is rotated, addressing groups of teeth in a specific order; this can help achieve systematic cleaning with minimal gingival trauma.

Flossing techniques. Flossing is difficult to master;

Table 35-1. Adverse effects of improper oral hygiene

	Reversible	Irreversible
Tooth	Not applicable	Cervical defects, such as abrasion on root or enamel surfaces
Gingiva and peri-odontium	Ulceration, clefting	Gingival recession with attachment and alveolar bone loss

however, correctly exercised, it is an excellent technique for interproximal cleaning. The floss should be gently forced across the point of contact between two teeth and then moved coronally and apically—up and down—repeatedly. Individual attention should be given to the two tooth surfaces involved with an interproximal space by alternatively directing the floss against each tooth. Care should be taken not to use a "sawing" action, which may traumatize the gingival tissues. The use of a floss holder may dramatically increase the effectiveness of flossing.

Use of specialty aids. The technique for use of different additional aids varies from device to device, and no specific effort is made here to discuss in detail the use of these items. However, in general, it is best to minimize the number of aids and different paraphernalia that a patient uses. As a guideline, one brush and brushing technique, one interproximal cleaning aid, and one dentifrice may be recommended. If at subsequent appointments or after periodontal or prosthetic treatment, other aids would be more effective, they can be introduced later.

Adverse effects of oral hygiene. Oral hygiene aids can cause traumatic lesions such as gingival abrasions, gingival clefts, or cervical abrasion when used incorrectly (Table 35-1).

Gingival traumatization by a hard-bristled toothbrush or overzealous use of even a soft brush can result in painful mucosal or gingival ulcers. Gingival abrasion may occur shortly after a period of increased oral hygiene awareness. However, if carefully monitored and cared for, the lesion usually heals fully. Treatment usually includes changing or partially withholding oral hygiene efforts. If repeatedly traumatized, the gingiva may recede as a result of repeated ulcerations; such recession is often seen on the labial surface of teeth with prominent roots, such as maxillary canines. Other soft tissue lesions may occur, but these are usually the result of overuse or misuse of oral hygiene devices. The resulting clinical picture may include one or several of the following features: loss of tissue, recession, hypertrophy, keratinization, or ulceration.

Hard tissue lesions, including cervical abrasions, are mostly limited to the cementum and dentin and occur after or concomitantly with gingival recession. The lesion usu-

ally expresses a typical form, with approximately a 90-degree angle of the lesion to enamel coronally and a bevell-like shape tapering off apically. When deep, the lesions often contribute to increased sensitivity of the teeth. The occurrence of cervical abrasions has declined substantially over the last few decades, most likely because of the lower abrasiveness of dentifrices. Severe forms of abrasions are seldom seen today with the widespread use of gentle abrasives in dentifrices and soft toothbrushes.

Most traumatizing oral hygiene behavior leads to localized damage. However, occasionally patients may display a "pathologic" degree of oral hygiene concern and cause damage of a generalized nature with severe gingival recession and cervical abrasion.

Chemical plaque control: chlorhexidine. Chlorhexidine is an effective oral chemical antiplaque agent. The agent was first described as an antiplaque agent in 1970 (Löe and Schiött) and has since been widely used. Chlorhexidine was approved as a prescription drug in the United States in 1987 in a 0.12% solution. It is usually recommended for use as an adjunct to mechanical plaque removal after or along with periodontal procedures. Long-term use of chlorhexidine is not recommended, since the effects on oral mucosa and overall bacteriologic ecology are not fully understood. Also, even moderately extended use of chlorhexidine can cause severe tooth stain, and occasionally staining of the tongue, especially in patients who drink red wines and tea. A condition resembling "black hairy tongue" may develop as a result of the altered desquamation of epithelial cells on the dorsal surface of the tongue. In spite of these side effects, chlorhexidine is useful in periodontal therapy as an adjunct to, but not a substitute for, mechanical oral hygiene.

Other antiplaque rinses or dentifrices contain quaternary ammonium compounds, phenolic compounds, sanguinarine, and fluorides. In general, the costs and marginal effects of these agents may not warrant their use for long periods, since mechanical plaque control can be effective. The long-term use of chemical antiplaque and antigingivitis agents for patients with physical or mental handicaps may, however, be advantageous.

Individual oral hygiene program. To obtain successful cooperation and achieve the level of plaque control needed for each individual, cooperation between the patient and the dental care team is essential. Patients need to understand their responsibility and to acknowledge their important role in the care and prevention of dental diseases. It is important to develop an *individual* program for each patient, since the level of care and plaque control needed to fulfill the goals might vary dramatically from individual to individual.

For practical reasons, a two- or three-visit regimen for motivation and instruction in personal oral hygiene can be incorporated with supragingival and initial subgingival scaling appointments.

First visit:

1. Have the patient demonstrate his current method of oral hygiene. Keep the patient in an upright position; have the patient sit up or stand.

2. Introduce disclosing agents, possibly for both in-office and at-home use. Show the result with the use of a mirror. A fixed mirror is preferable, since it leaves both hands free.

3. Have the patient identify stained areas. Explain what is seen and discuss remedial techniques.

4. Have the patient brush again, restain, and check for improvements. Use this situation to actively indicate an alternative use of the regular toothbrush in an attempt to increase effectiveness.

5. Take the opportunity to introduce an aide for interproximal cleaning. However, do not rush. Give the patient a chance to ask for assistance in the interproximal area.

6. Perform scaling and professional tooth cleaning.

Second visit:

1. Apply a disclosing agent and have the patient evaluate the results of the oral hygiene performed between visits.

2. Discuss the results and, if indicated, introduce additional or alternative devices. Again, wait for the patient to absorb the information and ask for help.

3. Perform scaling and begin root planing.

Third visit:

1. Apply a disclosing agent and have the patient evaluate the results of the oral hygiene performed before the visit.

2. Discuss the results and evaluate the patient's perception of the situation. It is important to encourage the patient. However, the patient should perform oral hygiene to satisfy his own needs, not those of the clinician.

3. Perform scaling and root planing.

Additional visits may have to be devoted to training in oral hygiene techniques, and these can be incorporated with other periodontal treatments.

It has been well documented that the long-term success of definitive periodontal therapy is dependent on an intensive maintenance program consisting of frequent recall visits at which time professional tooth cleaning, along with reinstruction and remotivation in oral hygiene, is carried out. It is not clear to what extent each component contributes to the prevention of recurrence of periodontal attachment loss and the establishment of a healthy periodontium over a prolonged period of time. From a practical standpoint, all three—(1) *professional tooth cleaning,* (2) *reinstruction,* and (3) *remotivation*—are recommended for an effective maintenance program. The foundation for a successful maintenance program is laid and the initial personal oral hygiene habits established during active periodontal therapy.

Subgingival scaling and root planing. These procedures are described in detail in Chapter 43, and the instruments used for them are described in Chapter 56. Practical considerations for the role of subgingival scaling and root planing in antiinfective therapy include the following:

1. *Thorough subgingival scaling and root planing* in a patient who has years of accumulation of subgingival calculus is a painstaking procedure. Most often, this requires a series of two to four appointments after the supragingival (coronal) scaling and oral hygiene appointments described above. Different views exist with respect to how this is performed. Some perform the procedure by quadrants, with each quadrant being anesthetized at separate appointments. Others scale and root plane the whole mouth at each appointment with no anesthesia or with selective areas anesthetized as needed.

However accomplished, the objective of scaling and root planing should be to thoroughly remove all detectable vestiges of subgingival calculus and plaque from all root surfaces exposed by periodontal disease. The advantage of carrying out the procedure as a whole-mouth procedure over several appointments is that in areas where calculus and plaque remain from the previous procedure, there will be inflammation at subsequent appointments; this inflammation signals remnants that are then removed.

One can continue subgingival scaling and root planing over a number of appointments until pockets show little or no bleeding or suppuration on probing. However, scaling and root planing may be very painful, and the patient may require anesthesia. In such cases it may be easier for both the patient and the operator to complete a quadrant at a time with the patient under adequate local anesthesia, or at least to anesthetize the painful areas.

Complete freedom from bleeding on probing may be difficult to achieve; however, a desired end point of a series of subgingival scaling and root-planing appointments is freedom from suppuration. Exceptions may include areas with furcation involvement and deep pockets that reach or approach the tooth apex, or other sites where calculus cannot be removed by the blind scaling and root-planing procedure because of fluting and concavities of root surfaces or some other anatomic abnormality.

Scaling and root-planing procedures can be performed adequately by skilled dental hygienists under direct supervision. However, hygienists frequently require special training in the objectives and methods of scaling and root planing of patients with periodontitis.

At each subgingival scaling and root-planing appointment, the patient is evaluated for effectiveness of plaque control. If plaque control is poor, the opportunity is provided for the hygienist and supervising dentist to reinforce hygiene instructions or to alter the original hygiene instructions to provide for more efficient personal hygiene.

2. *Use of antimicrobial agents during the scaling and root-planing phase.* There is a strong body of evidence

that topical or systemic antimicrobial agents are useful adjuncts during scaling and root planing. The guidelines are as follows: if after establishment of good plaque control, observed over several appointments, and if after multiple scaling and root-planing sessions gingival inflammation or multiple areas of suppuration persist, adjunctive topical or systemic antibiotics are indicated.

In cases where *Actinobacillus actinomycetemcomitans* is detected, a course of systemic antibiotics will likely be necessary to resolve the inflammation and to stop further progression of periodontitis (Slots and Rosling, 1983; Haffajee et al., 1988; Listgarten, 1988; van Winkelhoff et al., 1989). When systemic antibiotics are used, microbiologic as well as clinical evaluation is important. If the periodontal pathogens *A. actinomycetemcomitans, Bacteroides gingivalis,* and *Bacteroides intermedius* are present, one is justified in using tetracycline, clindamycin, or metronidazole, or combinations of amoxicillin and metronidazole (van Winkelhoff, et al., 1989). The effectiveness of the latter combination is illustrated in Table 35-2. Persistent

suppuration after the course of systemic therapy is an indication for further therapy possibly requiring surgical access, as well as culture and antibiotic sensitivity assessment of the remaining pocket flora.

Compliance. A course of antibiotic therapy for a minimum of 1 to 2 weeks is usually necessary, and extraordinary efforts should be carried out to ensure that the patient will comply with the drugs prescribed. A positive, definitive attitude on the part of the dentist will help to ensure patient compliance. This should not be trial and error; the systemic antibiotic should be discussed initially as a possibility to be used based on the results of therapy and microbial testing. If the results, as mentioned above, show that antibiotics are needed, this should be a definitive part of the therapy, and the patient should be apprised of this and admonished to comply. The patient is then brought back 2 to 3 weeks after the course of antibiotics, at which time another subgingival scaling and root-planing session may be useful, since the gingiva may recede, exposing further areas of calculus. There is also less bleeding, and more de-

Table 35-2. Elimination of periodontal pathogens in patients with LJP or refractory periodontitis with a combination of adjunctive metronidazole and amoxicillin.

Patient No.	Age	Sex	Periodontal clinical diagnosis	Treatment history	Microbiology					
					Before treatment			After treatment*		
					A.a.	B.g.	B.i.	A.a.	B.g.	B.i.
1	17	F	LJP	R	+	−	+	−	−	+
2	14	M	LJP	None	+	−	−	−	−	+
3	14	M	LJP	R	+	−	+	−	−	−
4	14	F	LJP	None	+	−	−	−	−	−
5	20	M	LJP	IT + TTC	+	−	−	−	−	−†
6	20	F	LJP	IT + MIN	+	−	−	−	−	−
7	23	F	LJP	None	+	−	−	−	−	+
8	25	M	LJP	None	+	−	+	−	−	−
9	25	F	LJP	None	+	−	−	−	−	−
10	33	F	LJP	IT + S + DOX	+	−	−	−	−	−
11	38	F	LJP	None	+	+	+	+	+	−†
12	22	M	RP	IT + TTC + S + R	+	−	−	−	−	+
13	26	F	RP	IT	+	−	+	−	−	−
14	28	F	RP	IT + MIN	+	−	−	−	−	−
15	30	M	RPP	None	+	−	−	−	−	−
16	31	F	RP	IT + MIN	+	−	−	−	−	−
17	32	M	RP	IT + MIN	+	−	−	−	−	−
18	35	F	RP	IT	+	+	+	−	−	−
19	37	F	RPP	None	+	−	+	−	−	−
20	37	F	RP	IT	+	+	−	−	−	−
21	38	F	RP	S + R	+	+	+	−	−	+
22	44	M	RP	IT	+	−	+	−	−	+

From van Winkelhoff AJ et al: J Clin Periodontol, 16:128, 1989. © 1989 Munksgaard International Publishers, Ltd., Copenhagen, Denmark.
F, Female; *M*, male, *LJP*, localized juvenile periodontitis; *RP*, refractory periodontitis; *RPP*, rapidly progressive periodontitis; *IT*, initial treatment; *S*, periodontal surgery; *R*, recall; *TTC*, tetracycline hydrochloride; *MIN*, minocycline; *DOX*, doxycycline; *A.a.*, Actinobacillus actinomycetemcomitans; *B.g.*, Bacteroides gingivalis; *B.i.*, Bacteroides intermedius.
*Subgingival debridement including amoxicillin plus metronidazole.
†Severe diarrhea.

finitive scaling and root planing can be accomplished. At this point an evaluation of the patient's response to therapy should be done before proceeding with the next phase of treatment.

EVALUATION OF RESPONSE TO THERAPY

The appointment at which the patient's response to therapy is evaluated is extremely important, as it represents the end of the first part of antiinfective therapy: the scaling, root-planing, and oral hygiene phase. The effects of this first phase of antiinfective therapy are evaluated by assessing the following:

1. Resolution of gingivitis as assessed by a markedly decreased number of bleeding points on probing. Typically, before therapy 80% to 90% of gingival sites bleed on probing. After therapy 10% or fewer sites should bleed on deep probing.
2. Reduction in probing pocket depth through recession and gain in probing attachment level.
3. Gain in clinical attachment level. This may be modest and not detectable in the first few weeks after therapy, but when it is assessed 3 to 6 months later, it should be apparent.
4. Resolution of gingival inflammation. This should be dramatic in most sites. However, residual inflammation is sometimes seen along gingival margins in areas of gingival retraction by frenum, or in areas showing little or no attached gingiva. Most of the time after antiinfective therapy, these mucogingival defects show resolution of inflammation and require no further therapy. However, if they continue to be inflamed, or if progressive recession is measured, mucogingival surgery may be necessary (see Chapter 47).
5. Effectiveness of personal plaque control. This is evaluated again. There should be no tooth surfaces with continuous bands of gingival plaque; however, flecks of plaque on the crowns of some teeth may be present. Also, there should be no areas of residual plaque accumulation with inflammation at the same sites. Calculus should not be present.
6. Reduction of tooth mobility. Often, resolution of inflammation results in decreased horizontal tooth mobility. If either stability or reduction in mobility is noted, then mobility may not require further treatment. However, if progressive mobility is seen, if teeth are depressible, or if there is pain on occlusion, further occlusal therapy or extraction may be indicated.
7. Level of periodontal pathogenic organisms. If there is any indication of residual inflammation, such as bleeding on deep probing or suppuration, the level of periodontal pathogenic organisms is evaluated. Assessment of the common periodontal microbiota using rapid tests such as antibody-based tests, DNA

probes, or other tests for pathogens, including *A. actinomycetemcomitans, B. gingivalis,* and *B. intermedius,* will often be useful in assessing the completion of therapy. However, if the patient has used antibiotics and inflammation persists, the periodontal microflora should be assessed by cultural methods, since the flora may be altered and atypical organisms may be present. For example, the flora may be composed of opportunistic organisms such as *Candida albicans,* enterobacteria, or *Pseudomonas.* In this instance the flora should be cultured and antibiotic susceptibility tests carried out to aid in the selection of antibiotics.

Possible decisions after evaluation

No further therapy is needed if:

1. All areas of suppuration are resolved.
2. There is little or no residual bleeding on deep periodontal probing.
3. Oral hygiene has been established.
4. Previous mobile teeth are stable, or mobility is reduced.
5. All areas of mucogingival defects are free of inflammation and are stable.
6. The pathogenic periodontal microflora is suppressed or eliminated.

These objectives can often be achieved through thorough scaling and root planing, and the establishment of oral hygiene in patients with gingivitis or mild to moderate periodontitis. However, if there are deep pockets that bleed on probing, furcation areas that remain inflamed, areas of residual suppuration, or furcation openings impossible to keep plaque-free, *further antiinfective therapy, including ultrasonic bactericidal debridement (UBD) or access flaps, may be needed.* Also, there may be a need for other periodontal surgical procedures to provide for more attached gingiva, to recontour pontic areas, or to provide for regeneration of periodontal structures, including bone and connective tissue attachment.

PERIODONTAL SURGERY FOR DEFINITIVE ANTIINFECTIVE THERAPY

Modified Widman flaps, access flaps, or curettage and root-planing procedures, such as the UBD procedure, can be used for surgical access to root surfaces for definitive root planing and to eliminate periodontal pathogens (Rosling et al., 1986).

Ultrasonic bactericidal debridement procedure

The UBD procedure described by Rosling et al. (1986) has been shown to result in significant probing attachment gain. For example, a 3 mm gain in attachment was observed in pockets that were initially 7 mm or greater in depth. This can be compared with ultrasonic scaling and root planing with a saline placebo, which resulted in 2 mm

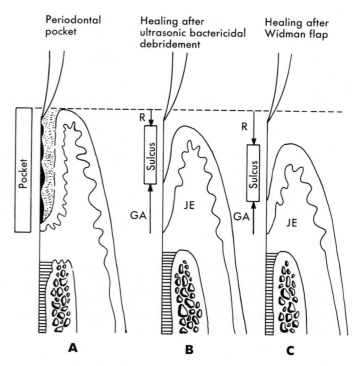

Fig. 35-5. Healing of deep pockets (≥7 mm) after antiinfective therapy, and comparison of UBD and Widman flap access procedure. Original pocket depth, **A,** is reduced to a healthy sulcus by recession of gingiva *(R)* and by gain in periodontal attachment *(GA).* Note long junctional epithelium *(JE)* and modest healing of alveolar crestal bone resulting from UBD, **B,** or Widman flap procedure, **C.** Note that residual sulcus depth is comparable with these procedures; however, UBD results in less recession and greater gain in probing attachment, and hence less root exposure, as compared with Widman flap procedure. (Data from Rosling et al: J Clin Periodontol 13:975, 1986.)

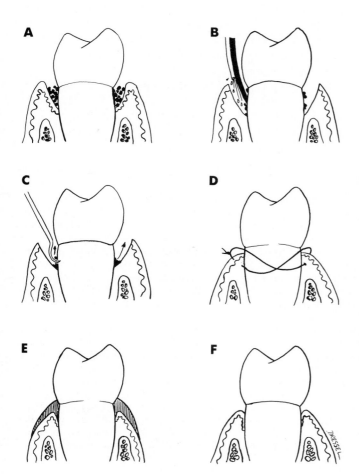

Fig. 35-6. UBD, antiinfective therapy of smooth surfaces of single-rooted teeth and flat surfaces of multirooted teeth. **A,** Pretreatment showing supracrestal pocket depths filled with subgingival flora and calculus on tooth surface. **B,** After anesthesia, ultrasonic curette with copious irrigation of 0.1% povidone-iodine is introduced to depths of pocket and removes subgingival flora and calculus, as well as pocket lining epithelium with its adherent bacteria and portions of underlying granulation tissue. **C,** After ultrasonic debridement, final hand root planing is carried out with sharp scalers and curettes. This removes remaining remnants of calculus and also outer surface of root where bacteria and bacterial products may have penetrated. **D,** In some instances where gingiva is inflamed, interproximal papillae may be dissected as part of procedure, and sutures are used to adapt gingiva to root surface. **E,** In most areas gingiva has sufficient rigidity such that adaptation with a periodontal dressing is adequate. In some instances, where there is very little detachment of gingiva, no dressing is used and chlorhexidine mouth rinse is recommended. **F,** Healing after procedure, showing restoration of normal sulcus depth, long junctional epithelium, and modest recession. For details on crevice depths, recession, and attachment gain to be expected in pockets ≥7 mm, see Fig. 35-5 and Rosling et al. (1986).

of attachment gain in pockets of 7 mm or greater depth (Fig. 35-5). In addition to giving greater attachment gain, other advantages of UBD include (1) minimal postoperative discomfort; (2) retention of attached gingiva; (3) good coverage of the alveolar bony process, reducing crestal resorption; and (4) simplicity of the procedure and ease of combination with other surgical procedures in the same sextant or quadrant.

It should be noted, however, that the method is a closed-flap procedure with limited visual access to root surfaces for root planing. Open-flap access procedures may offer better visual access and should be used if necessary to achieve thorough root planing. Open-flap access surgical procedures, such as the modified Widman flap and apically repositioned flaps, are discussed in detail in Chapters 46 and 47.

The UBD procedure has been remarkably successful and of general utility in treating mild to moderate periodontitis (usually American Dental Association types II and III) (Rosling et al., 1986). This procedure may also be useful in treating more severe cases of periodontitis where there are multiple infrabony defects and furcation involvement (Rosling et al., 1987). This procedure consists of debridement of the root surface with a high-frequency (42,000 c/s) ultrasonic scaler while irrigating with 0.1% povidone-iodine (Fig. 35-6). The operative procedure follows:

1. The procedure is carried out by sextant, quadrant, or half mouth, and the areas are anesthetized with 2% lidocaine (Xylocaine) and 1:50,000 epinephrine.
2. The subgingival area is curetted, and the root surfaces planed thoroughly to the alveolar crest with an ultrasonic scaler. During the entire procedure, irrigation is carried out with a 0.1% povidone-iodine solution. Each surface is carefully debrided with deliberate removal of the pocket epithelium, the junctional epithelium, and the granulation tissue. The root is then thoroughly root planed with the ultrasonic instrument. Detachment of the epithelium and of some of the connective tissue attachment is inevitable, as is removal of most of the pocket epithelium and underlying granulation tissue; hence this procedure must be carried out with the patient under local anesthesia.
3. The area is then thoroughly scaled with hand scalers and curettes, using overlapping strokes until the root surfaces are clean and smooth.
4. The subgingival area is then flushed and root planed with an ultrasonic scaler that has a circular tip motion, which leaves the root surface relatively smooth. Good aspiration is required to remove the excess fluids.

The procedure takes 1 to 2 hours per quadrant. Often the interdental papillae are dissected with the UBD procedure. If this happens, the granulation tissue is trimmed from the inner surface of the flap and the papillae are sutured to fully cover the interproximal bone.

In cases where there are deep infrabony pockets, access flaps or mesial or distal wedges may be necessary to gain access to the roots in the areas of deep pocketing (Fig. 35-7). The gingiva is then sutured to cover the bone as completely as possible. This procedure can also be combined with gingivectomy or gingivoplasty on the maxillary or mandibular labial areas where bulbous fibrotic gingiva is unesthetic or impairs oral hygiene. In fact, UBD can be combined with almost any periodontal surgical procedure. The combined procedures must be planned in advance to ensure that they are compatible and practical (e.g., the use of iodine on exposed bone surfaces should be minimized, since it may inhibit healing).

Fig. 35-7. A, Moderate to severe periodontitis; copious amounts of plaque and calculus are seen supragingivally, and subgingival areas are populated with high levels of *B. gingivalis* and *B. intermedius*. **B,** Appearance after four sessions of supragingival scaling, removal of overhangs, restoration of supragingival carious lesion, and establishment of oral hygiene. **C,** Maxillary left quadrant after supragingival scalings and establishment of oral hygiene. Note calculus on root surface mesial to first premolar and distal to canine with swollen interdental papillae, suggestive of continuing infection. Also note recession and Class II furcation on buccal surface of molar. **D,** Maxillary left quadrant was subjected to access flap using Widman approach. Conservative scalloping incisions were made on buccal and palatal surfaces (not shown). **E,** Flap was reflected sufficiently to expose margin of bone, and entire surface was root planed, with concentration on removing all debris from roots and instrumenting in furcation and root concavities. **F,** Gingiva readapted to root surfaces and interproximal areas and positioned by suturing. **G,** Appearance 2 weeks after healing. Note adaptation of gingiva to interproximal areas and staining from use of chlorhexidine during postoperative healing state. **H,** Appearance 2 years postoperatively. Note there is little or no evidence of inflammation of gingiva, except labial surface of No. 24, where calculus has accumulated. Patient has been on 3-month recall schedule and forms calculus rapidly, especially around lower anteriors. However, in general, there are no pocket depths greater than 4 mm, no bleeding on probing, no suppuration, and patient is free of periodontal pathogens. For explanation of healing see Fig. 35-5, which shows that in an average 7 to 8 mm pocket, about 3½ mm of gingival sulcus will remain after therapy; this results from 2 mm of recession and 2 mm of periodontal regeneration after Widman access flap procedure.

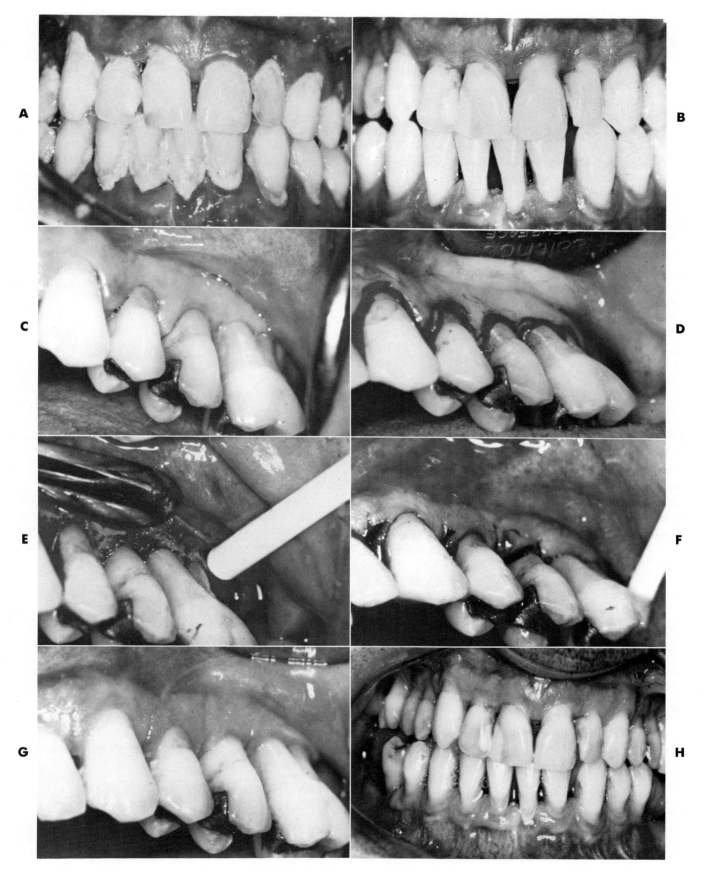

Fig. 35-7. For legend see opposite page.

Furcations.   Class I and shallow, wide Class II furcations often can be treated with UBD as long as the furcation openings and all involved root surfaces are accessible to the ultrasonic curette or the hand instruments. The root surfaces, including all aspects of the furcation, including the roof, should be thoroughly smoothed and root planed. If access to the furcation cannot be achieved because of a narrow or V-shaped furcal roof, odontoplasty using a fine rotating diamond can be carried out to open the furcation roof for access. Also, if there are enamel projections into the furcation, they can be removed by odontoplasty. For treatment of deep Class II and Class III furcations, tunnel operations by root resection (see Chapter 47) or regenerative therapy may be required (see Chapter 48).

Suturing.   When the interdental papillae have been dissected, or if access flaps or mesial or distal wedges are made for definitive scaling and root planing, these should be sutured to provide maximum coverage of the alveolar process. Otherwise, sutures are not required for UBD procedures that result in gingival coverage of the bone.

Dressing.   If gingivoplasty has been carried out, or if gingivectomy or wedges have been performed, these may be covered with a dressing for patient comfort. However, a dressing may not be necessary, since with the use of 0.12% chlorhexidine postoperatively, surgically treated areas often heal rapidly.

Postoperative instructions.   It is important to treat the UBD procedure as any other surgical procedure, with proper attention given to pain control and plaque control after the procedure. The use of chlorhexidine mouth rinse (0.12%) is recommended for at least 2 weeks. The use of postoperative antibiotics is often unnecessary unless the patient has a systemic disorder such as diabetes and there is a need to control the spread of infection that might have been induced by the surgical procedure. In these cases the patient should be started on a regimen of antibiotics the day before the procedure and continued on the regimen for at least 2 weeks after the procedure.

Patients should be seen after 5 to 7 days for suture and dressing removal. After 1 to 2 weeks of further healing, the patient can have other quadrants treated. It is thought best to complete this phase of therapy for the whole mouth in as short a time as possible to minimize cross-contamination of treated areas with flora from untreated areas.

Reconstructive therapy

In some patients further treatment, including prosthetics and special periodontal surgical procedures, is necessary. This phase of therapy is referred to as reconstructive therapy.

Periodontal surgery in the reconstructive phase includes:

1. Regenerative procedures such as guided tissue regeneration (see Chapter 48)
2. Preprosthetic periodontal surgical procedures (see Chapter 51)
3. Mucogingival and cosmetic procedures (see Chapter 47)

Regenerative procedures

It is clear that before regenerative procedures are contemplated, maximum healing achievable with diligent antiinfective therapy should be sought. The suggestion is to proceed through all stages of antiinfective therapy, including access flap or ultrasonic debridement, for complete resolution of inflammation and suppuration, and also for eradication or suppression of the periodontal pathogens. Once this has been achieved (i.e., after final evaluation), regenerative procedures might be indicated. The indications for regenerative periodontal surgical procedures are:

1. Open furcations where the tooth in question needs additional support, or the furcation has a low probability of being maintained by the patient
2. Deep infrabony pockets that are unesthetic or jeopardize the function of the tooth, or markedly compromise the ability of the patient to perform oral hygiene in that area

In these instances, which are uncommon except in patients with advanced periodontitis, regenerative therapy should be carried out, and the procedure should be done at this time in the surgical therapy phase.

Finishing procedures and reevaluation at the completion of antiinfective and surgical periodontal therapy

After all antiinfective and reconstructive procedures, including temporary or provisional prosthetic and surgical periodontal procedures, are completed, the patient is seen for a final series of periodontal visits at which time healing is evaluated.

At this point, all stain and calculus that might have formed during the periodontal procedures is removed. The periodontium is again checked carefully for gingival inflammation as assessed by bleeding on probing, suppuration, pocket depths, attachment level changes, and contours of the gingiva. If inflammation is still present, microbiologic tests are indicated. If systemic antibiotics were used and the disease refractory, culture with isolation of the organism and sensitivity testing, and a course of antimicrobial therapy based on the sensitivity testing may be attempted again. After completion of this phase of therapy, the patient is ready for final prostheses, if necessary, or for maintenance therapy.

POSSIBLE OUTCOMES OF ANTIINFECTIVE THERAPY

There are several possible outcomes of antiinfective therapy, including the following:

1. *Active periodontal therapy is completed.* The patient has proper oral hygiene, few or no areas of gingival bleeding, no areas of suppuration, and no areas of persistent plaque accumulation; the teeth do not show progressive mobility; and function and esthetics are adequate. When these conditions are met, therapy is complete. This occurs in the majority of patients who are treated with antiinfective therapy and, if needed, periodontal surgery. These patients should then be put on a maintenance therapy program to prevent recurrence of periodontitis.

2. *Further therapy is needed, but oral hygiene is poor.* The patient has poor oral hygiene despite repeated instructions and successful antiinfective periodontal therapy. Such patients are often detected early and are poor candidates for periodontal surgery. These patients should be put on a maintenance program, and surgical periodontal therapy should be deferred. They may be brought to good oral hygiene with diligent effort, at which time surgical periodontal therapy can be carried out. These patients may be candidates for restorative treatment with the caution that they are prone to reinfection and must be maintained on a diligent maintenance therapy program. In such patients the therapy should be conservative, and extensive fixed prostheses or implants should not be attempted until good oral hygiene is demonstrated for a period of at least 1 to 2 years.

3. *Further therapy is needed, and oral hygiene is adequate.* These patients can be treated with needed periodontal surgery and final prostheses and implants as indicated. At the completion of all phases of therapy, they are then put on a maintenance therapy program, with maintenance of the prostheses and prevention of recurrent periodontitis.

REFERENCES

Antczak-Boukoms A and Weinstein M: Cost-effectiveness analysis of periodontal disease control, J Dent Res 66:1630, 1987.

Badersten A, Nilveus R, and Egelberg J: Effect of non-surgical periodontal therapy. I. Moderately advanced periodontitis, J Clin Periodontol 8:57, 1981.

Christersson LA et al: Microbiological and clinical effects of surgical treatment of localized juvenile periodontitis, J Clin Periodontol 12:465, 1985.

Löe H and Kleinman DV, editors: Dental plaque control measures and oral hygiene practices, Washington, DC, 1985, IRL Press.

Genco RJ: Antibiotics in the treatment of human periodontal diseases, J Periodontol 52:545, 1981.

Haffajee AD et al: Clinical, microbiologic, and immunologic features of subjects with refractory periodontal diseases, J Clin Periodontol 15:390, 1988.

Listgarten MA: A rationale for monitoring the periodontal microflora after periodontal treatment, J Periodontol 59:439, 1988.

Löe H and Schiött CR: The effect of mouthrinses and topical application of chlorhexidine on the development of dental plaque and gingivitis in man, J Periodont Res 5:79, 1970.

Ramfjord S: Surgical periodontal pocket elimination: still a justifiable objective? J Am Dent Assoc 114:37, 1987.

Rosling BG, Christersson LA, and Genco RJ: Unpublished data, 1987.

Rosling BG et al: The microbiological and clinical effects of topical subgingival antimicrobial treatment, J Clin Periodontol 10:487, 1983.

Rosling BG et al: Topical antimicrobial therapy and diagnosis of subgingival bacteria in the management of inflammatory periodontal disease, J Clin Periodontol 13:975, 1986.

Slots J and Rosling BG: Suppression of the periodontopathic microflora in localized juvenile periodontitis by systemic tetracycline, J Clin Periodontol 10:465, 1983.

van Winkelhoff AJ et al: Metronidazole plus amoxicillin in the treatment of *Actinobacillus actinomycetemcomitans*–associated periodontitis, J Clin Periodontol, 16:128, 1989.

Zambon JJ, Christersson LA, and Genco RJ: Diagnosis and treatment of localized juvenile periodontitis (periodontosis), J Am Dent Assoc 113:295, 1986.

Chapter 36

SURGICAL ACCESS PROCEDURES

Jay S. Seibert

RATIONALE FOR SURGICAL ACCESS PROCEDURES

The successful conversion of an infected periodontal pocket into a healthy gingival sulcus is determined to a great extent by the thoroughness of the debridement procedure used to remove periodontal pathogens from the root surface, the pocket, and the pocket epithelium. Complete debridement of infected root surfaces is a difficult, demanding, and time-consuming task, especially in deep, tortuous pockets or where there are grooves or other irregularities on the root surface. Incomplete removal of the pathogens results in partial resolution of inflammation; however, in a few months inflammation usually returns as the microbial organisms repopulate the subgingival area (Slots et al., 1979).

It is clear that prophylaxis is effective in treating gingivitis when pockets are less than 4 mm deep. Prophylaxis includes scaling and root planing where needed, supragingival plaque and calculus removal, coronal polishing, and oral hygiene instruction. In moderate periodontitis, where pockets are 4 to 6 mm deep, several studies have shown no differences in clinical results between scaling and root planing, and periodontal surgery (Badersten et al., 1981; Pihlstrom et al., 1983; Lindhe et al., 1984; Ramfjord et

al., 1987). However, access to deeper pockets (7 mm or deeper) is often difficult; hence periodontal surgery may be required to provide proper access for thorough scaling and root planing (National Institute of Dental Research, 1982; Ramfjord, 1987). This chapter is directed to a description of these access procedures.

Thorough subgingival scaling and root planing is technically a *surgical procedure,* since it results in removal of gingival soft tissue, as well as the outer surface of the root. The objective sought in subgingival scaling and root-planing procedures, regardless of the methods employed, is the conversion of an infected, physically/chemically altered root surface to a surface that is biologically acceptable to the gingival tissues. For a new attachment or reattachment of the periodontal tissues to occur, the pathogens remaining on the root surface and within the confines of the pocket area must be reduced to minimal or subcritical levels that will permit the defense mechanisms of the host to complete the task of removing them from the healing wound.

Developmental grooves, concavities, furcation areas, and overhanging restoration margins have been shown to retain plaque and calculus, reducing the chances for thorough root preparation (Caffesse et al., 1986; see also Chapter 13). Also, the chances for complete removal of calculus from the root surface in pockets 7 mm or greater in depth are often improved if visual and mechanical access is provided by using a surgical flap or gingivectomy procedure (National Institute of Dental Research, 1982; Caffesse et al., 1986; Matia et al., 1986). These surgical access procedures are indicated when thorough subgingival scaling and root planing with the patient under local anesthesia were attempted during the initial phases of antiinfective therapy and were not successful. They are also indicated when subgingival scaling and root planing, and systemic antibiotic therapy have not been successful in eliminating indicator organisms such as *Bacteroides gingivalis* or *Bacteroides intermedius* from subgingival sites. It has been amply documented that often if these initial attempts to reduce periodontal infections are unsuccessful, it is likely that residual subgingival calculus and/or plaque deposits remain and may require surgical access for complete removal.

CLOSED SUBGINGIVAL SCALING AND ROOT PLANING

Even in deep pockets, root surfaces can often be completely instrumented if sufficient time is devoted to the procedure. Tissue shrinkage aids in reducing pocket depth and providing greater access. In many cases deposits of calculus that were missed on the first round of subgingival scaling and root planing are removed during the second, third, or fourth scaling and root-planing visits. There are positive aspects from such closed ("nonsurgical") approaches. For example, patients who for medical or psychologic reasons cannot or will not tolerate having a surgical flap procedure done in their mouth can be treated by repeated root-planing procedures. Also, periodontal attachment is often lost by creating a surgical flap. This is especially the case on the radicular aspects of teeth where the investing bone and gingival tissues are thin (i.e., canine eminence). Also, interproximal bone in the lower anterior region may resorb after a flap procedure. If one can avoid the use of a surgical flap, it may aid in preventing further loss of attachment in these situations.

The benefits that can be gained from a nonflap approach to treatment must be balanced against some of the negative features of this technique, which include incomplete root preparation, especially in deep pockets on multirooted teeth; root damage due to blind overinstrumentation of root surfaces; and excessive time required to completely debride the root surfaces.

SPECIFIC PROCEDURES

The major advantage of using a surgical flap procedure (or gingivectomy procedure under certain limited conditions) for root preparation in deep pockets is visual and mechanical access. Nonsurgical root planing relies on the tactile sense to judge the thoroughness of the planing procedure. Surgical access procedures permit us to employ the more critical sense of sight in assessing the thoroughness of a root-planing procedure. Mechanical access is equally important. The working blade and tip of most periodontal curettes is very large in relation to the histologic space of the apical and lateral extent of a periodontal pocket (Figs. 36-1 and 36-2, *E*).

A clinical illustration of the apical extent of periodontal pockets and the relationship of the leading edge of the plaque-calculus front to the adjacent normal tissues is

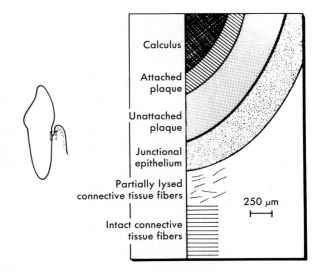

Fig. 36-1. Diagrammatic representation of bottom of a pocket. (From Carranza FA, Jr: Glickman's clinical periodontology, ed 6, Philadelphia, 1984, WB Saunders Co.)

shown in Fig. 36-3. The calculus deposits are found at the depths of the pockets but 1 to 2 mm from the alveolar bony margin, suggesting that closed debridement with the patient under local anesthesia and with scaling to the bony surface in suprabony pockets would be adequate to remove these deposits. However, in deep infrabony pockets the calculus deposits are often apical to the alveolar crest and difficult to remove, especially in narrow infrabony pockets. In either case, root planing to the bony surface will destroy the zone of intact connective tissue fibers located on the crestal surface of the bone (see Fig. 36-1).

Selection of surgical access techniques

Factors that influence the amount of access to root surfaces during subgingival scaling and root planing include the following:

1. Tissue type—thick fibrous tissue versus thin edematous tissue or combinations thereof
2. Pocket depth and pocket type—infrabony versus suprabony
3. Location of pockets on root surfaces (e.g., smooth surfaces versus concavities or furcations)
4. Number of root surfaces involved—single versus multiple surfaces
5. Root proximity
6. Tilt or malposition of teeth
7. Degree of mouth and jaw opening—constricted access versus easy access

Surgical flaps should not be used or made in tissue that is highly inflamed and edematous, since the tissue is likely to tear and is difficult to handle and suture. Edema should

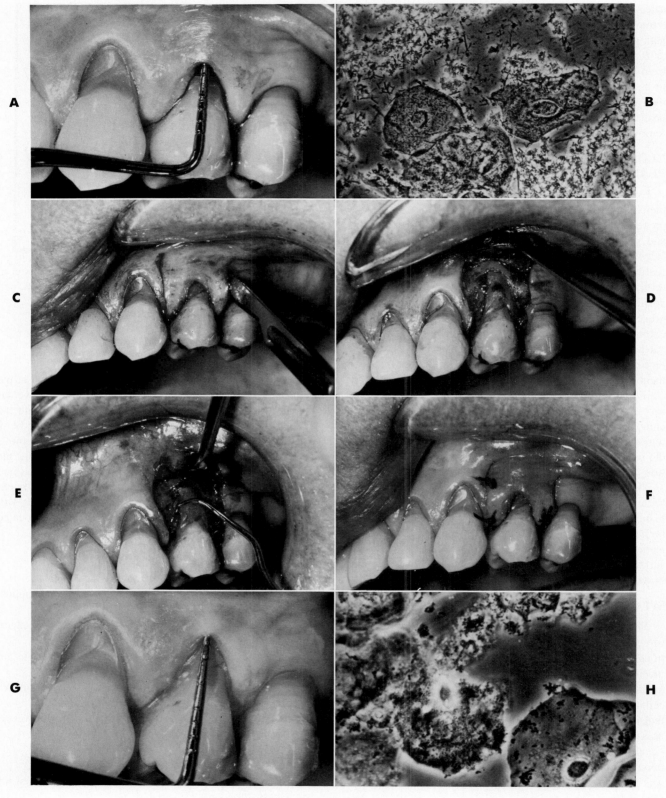

Fig. 36-2. For legend see opposite page.

Fig. 36-2. Flap used to gain access to calculus that was incompletely removed during a nonaccess root-planing procedure. **A,** Marginal and attached gingival tissues on buccal surface of first premolar remained inflamed 8 weeks after first nonaccess root-planing procedure had been done. Bleeding was easily produced on gentle probing. **B,** Photograph, taken through a phase-contrast microscope, of subgingival plaque obtained before area was probed. Numerous rod-shaped microorganisms can be seen surrounding desquamating epithelial cells. **C,** Scalpel used to make vertical and horizontal releasing incisions for a full mucoperiosteal flap. **D,** Flap was carefully elevated to expose dento-osseous junction. Note calculus that was not removed during root-planing procedure. **E,** Gracey 11/12 curette in position to plane root surface. This instrument has been sharpened many times, and working tip and blade are smaller than those of a new instrument. Note size of instrument in relation to normal tissue surrounding root surface of pocket. **F,** Flap has been stabilized in its former position with three interrupted sutures. **G,** Appearance 2 months after treatment. Pocket has been eliminated, and tissues are normal by all clinical criteria. **H,** Photograph of subgingival flora taken through a phase-contrast microscope. Plaque sample was taken before buccal crevice was probed. A sparse coccoid flora was noted surrounding and adhering to desquamating epithelial cells. (Treatment done in conjunction with Dr. Thomas R. Tempel, Brig./Gen., U.S. Army Dental Corps.)

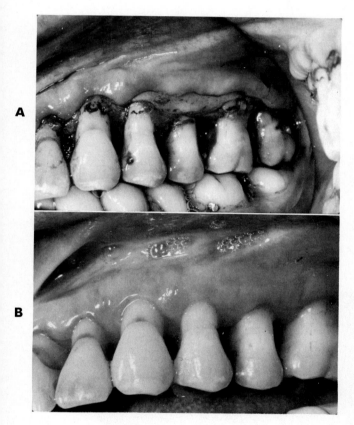

Fig. 36-3. Full-thickness internally beveled mucoperiosteal flap used to gain access to dento-osseous junction. **A,** Patient had not received any preventive maintenance treatment for 8 years. Note relationship of plaque and calculus to normal tissues at boundary of pocket. **B,** Appearance 2 months after treatment. A normal dentogingival junction was formed, and a shallow healthy sulcus exists about all of the teeth. Considerable recession existed prior to treatment.

be eliminated and tissue tonus regained by means of improved plaque-control measures, closed subgingival scaling and debridement procedures, and the use of topical or systemic antimicrobial agents. If inflammation persists, it is usually localized to one or a few tooth surfaces, and these are the areas that may require a surgical access procedure.

A variety of surgical procedures are available to gain access for root planing and odontoplasty, including full mucoperiosteal flaps either replaced or apically repositioned, modified Widman flaps, and gingivectomy. (See Figs. 36-4 and 36-5 for surgical access flap design.) Flap procedures provide the clinician with a wide range of surgical versatility.

Odontoplasty at the time of surgical access

Fig. 36-6 illustrates a deep developmental groove on the mesial surface of a mandibular premolar. A double periodontal ligament space, passing in an apicocoronal direction through the center of the root, can be seen on the radiograph. The histologic cross section that is shown was cut at the midlevel of the root. If a tooth of similar root morphology were involved with moderate to advanced bone loss, it would be easy to understand how or why plaque and calculus could be left in place in the depth of the groove. An access flap employed for root planing would allow removal or smoothening of this groove by curetting or by the use of rotating burs. Partially fused roots, furcations, and similar areas that limit visual and instrument access are usually incompletely prepared because of the inability of instruments to reach the pathogens on the root surface. In these cases surgical access and odontoplasty are often necessary.

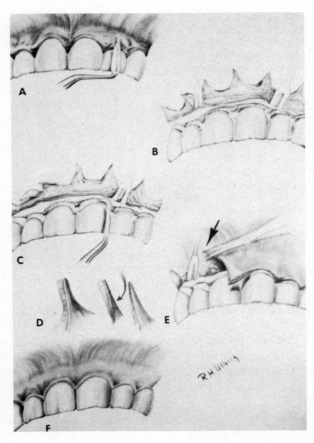

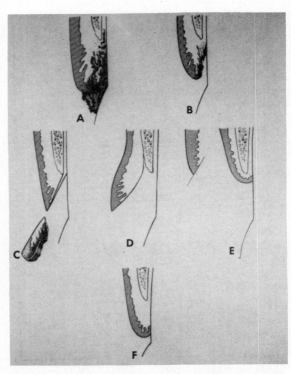

Fig. 36-4. Step-by-step procedure of debridement by means of flap method. **A,** Internally beveled incision is made; this is usually performed with a scalpel. **B,** Flap is raised. **C,** Entire tissue above bone is removed, and root surfaces are cleansed. **D** and **E,** Flap is thinned so that on readaptation it will completely cover alveolar crestal area. **F,** Healed gingival tissue and gingival attachment.

Fig. 36-5. Operative steps of debridement by means of flap procedure. **A,** Calculus occupying entire pocket; it is removed by scaling. **B,** Resultant gingival tissue is seen. Note that there is still an ulcerated pocket wall. **C,** An internal bevel is made, and excised section is removed. **D,** Flap is retracted, and tooth surface cleansed. **E** and **F,** Readaptation of flap. In **E,** gingival tissue is reduced and tightly placed over bone, whereas in **F,** adaptation is more coronal.

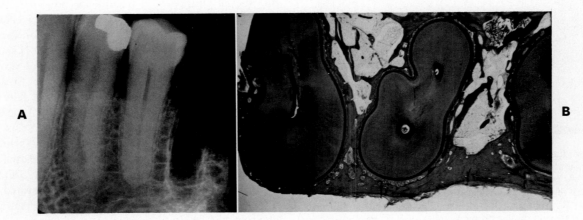

Fig. 36-6. Radiograph of block section of normal tissue on border of cancer area in molar region. **A,** Canine and premolar teeth had a normal periodontium. Note radiolucent image of periodontal ligament passing parallel to root canal vertically through long axis of first premolar. **B,** Photomicrograph of horizontal section of first premolar cut at level of midsection of root. Note deep developmental groove that exists on mesial surface of root. (Hematoxylin and eosin.)

General principles affecting the design of access flaps for root preparation

1. If a narrow zone of attached gingiva exists, the horizontal incision used to release the gingiva is usually made in the gingival sulcus.
2. If an ample zone of attached gingiva exists, the horizontal incision used to release the gingiva is usually started at the crest of the free gingival margin or slightly apical to the gingival margin on the lateral surface of the marginal or attached gingiva.
3. A full mucoperiosteal flap is reflected only enough to expose the alveolar margin. Extensive exposure of the alveolar bone is unnecessary and may lead to pain and excessive bony resorption. Reflection of the flap should be adequate for visual and mechanical access to the root surface so that adequate debridement can be accomplished.

Atraumatic reflection of the tissues with sufficient release of the tissues to permit gentle retracting forces to be used is desirable. This should provide sufficient visual and instrument access to accomplish the objectives of the surgical procedure: (1) total debridement of the root surface and (2) removal of grooves or enamel projections into furcations or other root abnormalities by odontoplasty.

The gingivectomy procedure can be used effectively in treating cases in which pseudopockets have been created by hyperplastic proliferation of the gingiva. Dense fibrotic gingival tissue that is overgrown, such as that found in phenytoin hyperplasia, will not shrink and return to normal physiologic architectural form on elimination of the irritants from the root surface. The tightly adapted excessive amount of dense gingival tissue limits instrument access to the root surface and forms a barrier that inhibits thorough root planing. The surgical excision of the gingival wall of the pocket facilitates root preparation while at the same time the tissues are recontoured to their former or normal dimensions. The percentage of cases requiring treatment by soft tissue resection are extremely low, and for this reason gingivectomy procedures are seldom used to gain access for root planing.

REFERENCES

Badersten A, Nilveus R, and Egelberg J: Effect of non-surgical periodontal therapy. I. Moderately advanced periodontitis, J Clin Periodontol 8:57, 1981.

Caffesse R, Sweeney P, and Smith B: Scaling and root planing with and without periodontal flap surgery, J Clin Periodontol 13:205, 1986.

Lindhe J et al: Long-term effect of surgical/non-surgical treatment of periodontal disease, J Clin Periodontol 11:448, 1984.

Matia JI et al: Efficiency of scaling the molar furcation area with and without surgical access, Int J Periodontics Restorative Dent 6:25, 1986.

National Institute of Dental Research: Proceedings from the state of the art workshop on surgical therapy for periodontitis, J Periodontol 53:475, 1982.

Pihlstrom B et al: Comparison of surgical and non-surgical treatment of periodontal disease: a review of current studies and additional results after six and one-half years, J Clin Periodontol 10:524, 1983.

Ramfjord S: Surgical periodontal pocket elimination: still a justifiable objective? J Am Dent Assoc 114:37, 1987.

Ramfjord S et al: Four modalities of periodontal treatment compared over five years, J Clin Periodontol 14:445, 1987.

Slots J et al: Periodontal therapy in humans. I. Microbiological and clinical effects of a single course of periodontal scaling and root planing and of adjunctive tetracycline therapy, J Periodontol 50:495, 1979.

Chapter 37

MICROBIAL DIAGNOSIS IN PERIODONTAL THERAPY

Joseph J. Zambon

Specific microorganisms have been implicated in the pathogenesis of the major oral infections. *Streptococcus mutans* and lactobacilli, for example, are the major microbial pathogens involved in the etiology of dental caries. For periodontal disease, a number of microbial species have been associated with the different forms of periodontitis. For some of these species, there is convincing evidence as to their importance in causing periodontal disease, whereas the role of other species is less clear. The evidence, for example, implicating *Actinobacillus actinomycetemcomitans, Bacteroides gingivalis,* and *Bacteroides intermedius* in the etiology of some forms of periodontitis is relatively strong (see Chapter 11). The role of other species such as *Fusobacterium nucleatum, Bacteroides forsythus,* and *Wolinella recta* is less clear; however, they are frequently detected at high levels in periodontal lesions undergoing breakdown.

PRINCIPLES OF ANTIINFECTIVE THERAPY

If one accepts that certain species are etiologic in the pathogenesis of periodontitis, then the use of clinical microbiologic and immunologic assays for these species is a reasonable and useful component of periodontal diagnosis and treatment. An analogy with the treatment of infections elsewhere in the body may be useful in demonstrating this point. Assume, for example, that a 14-year-old girl sees her physician complaining of a sore throat and slight fever of 3 days' duration. The physician notes the presence of bilateral submandibular lymphadenopathy, as well as erythema and edema in the oropharynx. Then a bacteriologic sample, a throat swab, is analyzed and reveals the presence of group A beta-hemolytic streptococci. Based on the patient history, the physical examination, and the bacteriologic findings, the disease is diagnosed as streptococcal pharyngitis, distinguishing it from pharyngitis caused by viruses or other bacteria. Appropriate antibiotic therapy is then instituted.

As this example points out, several steps are involved in the diagnosis of a disease of microbial etiology. These steps include (1) taking the patient history, (2) a thorough physical examination, and (3) microbiologic and other laboratory tests as indicated by data gathered in the previous two steps. Using the accumulated data, the clinician can then arrive at a diagnosis reflecting the microbial etiology. Subsequently, a course of treatment can be prescribed that is aimed at eliminating the microbial etiology; the efficacy of the treatment protocol can also be monitored by repeated bacteriologic testing.

Even though the importance of controlling dental plaque in the treatment of periodontal disease has been known for some time, identification of the role of specific microbial species in dental plaque is a relatively recent development. It now appears possible to treat certain periodontal diseases as specific infections in the same manner as for extraoral infections. For example, suppose that the same 14-year-old girl discussed above visits her dentist for a routine dental examination. During this examination, 6 to 7 mm periodontal pockets are discovered on the mesial surface of the first molar teeth. Subsequent radiographic examination reveals angular osseous defects on the mesial surface of these same teeth. Based on the clinical and radiographic data, the dentist arrives at the clinically descriptive diagnosis of localized juvenile periodontitis (LJP) and institutes treatment consisting of scaling and root planing, empirical antibiotic therapy, and, possibly, further periodontal surgery. The efficacy of the treatment is measured by repeated clinical examinations looking for elimination of gingival inflammation and reduction in probing pocket depth measurements. This approach, including a patient history and clinical and radiographic examination, is the traditional one used in the diagnosis and treatment of periodontal disease. All of this information is then used in the formulation of a clinically descriptive diagnosis. The traditional diagnosis and treatment of periodontal disease does not, therefore, involve the identification of the periodontal pathogen(s), because, until recently, they were unknown. However, useful tests for the microbiologic diagnosis and monitoring of periodontal disease are currently available. For example, the 14-year-old with LJP can be tested for subgingival pathogens. If *A. actinomycetemcomitans* is found, therapy can then be directed not only to resolution of the clinical signs of the disease, but also to elimination of the *A. actinomycetemcomitans*. This has been shown to correlate well with clinical success and is a good indicator that therapy is complete (Slots and Rosling, 1983; Kornman and Robertson, 1985; Mandell and Socransky, 1988).

In treating bacterial infections, there are a number of important factors to consider. First, the *identity of the infecting microorganism(s)* should be ascertained. This key step in the diagnosis of an infectious disease enables the clinician to arrive at a diagnosis based on the microbial etiology of the disease rather than solely on the clinical appearance. Identification of the infectious agent also suggests the most efficacious treatment. Second, clinical microbiology can serve as an *indication of the efficacy of the therapy*, and it will also enable the clinician to set an end point for treatment (i.e., elimination of the bacterial pathogen from the site of the infection). Third, the potential *utility of an antiinfective therapy* such as mechanical debri-

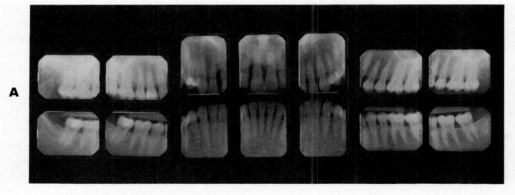

Patient No. 0335
34y, female
Pretreatment microbiology: 8/29/87

Results:

B

Individual sites	% Bacteroides gingivalis	% Bacteroides intermedius	% Actinobacillus actinomycetemcomitans
9D	0	0	2.9
9M	0	0	0.98
10M	0	0	2.5
14M	0	0	6.3

Fig. 37-1. A, Radiographs taken before treatment of a 34-year-old woman suffering from periodontitis. Note bone loss around maxillary anteriors. There was also a 7 mm pocket mesial to maxillary left first molar *(left side)*. Maxillary anterior segment bled on probing and was suppurative, and left center and lateral incisor were grade II mobility. Gingiva was slightly inflamed, with no patient discomfort. **B,** Subgingival flora assessed by immunofluorescence, expressed as percent of total flora shows infection with *A. actinomycetemcomitans*.

dement, an antibiotic, or a combination of both should be evaluated. The choice of an appropriate antibiotic should be based on both the susceptibility of the infecting organism(s) and the nature of the infection. Fourth, host factors such as *allergy* and other possible *adverse reactions* to chemotherapeutic agents should be taken into consideration.

INDICATIONS FOR MICROBIOLOGIC ASSAYS

1. *During initial diagnosis and treatment planning.* Clinical studies show that most adult periodontitis patients can be successfully treated by thorough mechanical debridement of the root surface or by means of topical adjunctive antimicrobials applied at the time of scaling and root planing. There are certain patients, however, who do not respond well to this local therapy. These patients include those with *refractory periodontitis, recurrent periodontitis, localized juvenile periodontitis, rapidly progressing periodontitis,* and *generalized juvenile periodontitis.* Microbiologic assays are often indicated in these patients as an adjunct to the usual clinical and radiographic examinations in the formulation of an etiology-based diagnosis.

The underlying indication for such microbiologic assays is that the detection of certain subgingival periodontal pathogens may indicate the need for systemic antimicrobial therapy to eliminate the infected periodontal tissues. For example, effective eradication of *A. actinomycetemcomitans* in localized juvenile periodontitis often requires a combination of mechanical debridement, surgery, and systemic antibiotic agents, since *A. actinomycetemcomitans* can invade the gingival tissues (Christersson et al., 1987a, 1987b).

An illustration of the usefulness of microbiologic tests in the initial diagnosis and treatment planning of two young patients with periodontal disease is shown in Figs. 37-1 and 37-2. The patient shown in Fig. 37-1 was a 34-year-old woman with bone loss around the maxillary incisors and an incipient lesion mesial to the maxillary left first molar (Fig. 37-1, *A*). The microbiologic analysis prior to treatment showed heavy infection of the affected sites with *A. actinomycetemcomitans* but no detectable *B. gingivalis* or *B. intermedius* (Fig. 37-1, *B*). Treatment therefore included systemic tetracycline along with conventional therapy, and this regimen was successful in eliminating the

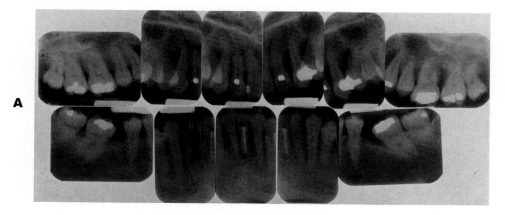

Patient No. 5587
25y, female
Pretreatment microbiology: 8/27/86

Results:

Individual sites	% Bacteroides gingivalis	% Actinobacillus actinomycetemcomitans
2M	27.3	Trace
3M	18.3	Trace
5M	24.7	0
11M	16.0	0
12M	2.2	0
14D	37.7	0
26M	0.97	Trace

Fig. 37-2. **A,** Radiographs taken before treatment of a 25-year-old woman suffering from periodontitis. Note extreme alveolar bone loss; gingiva was red and swollen, bled spontaneously, and was suppurative. Patient experienced foul oral odor, sore maxillary canines, and dull pain in maxillary first molar region. Lower molars were extracted 10 years earlier. **B,** Subgingival flora assessed by immunofluorence, expressed as percent of total flora. Selective culture was also done, and *A. actinomycetemcomitans* was not detectable; patient was infected with *B. gingivalis,* however.

infection and in resolving the inflammation. The patient was free of *A. actinomycetemcomitans, B. gingivalis,* and *B. intermedius* at 6 and 12 months after therapy.

In contrast, the 25-year-old woman shown in Fig. 37-2 had severe alveolar bone loss around most teeth (Fig. 37-2, *A*). She was heavily infected with *B. gingivalis* but had only traces of *A. actinomycetemcomitans* and no *B. intermedius* (Fig. 37-2, *B*). Treatment included mechanical debridement and open-flap curettage, which was successful in eliminating the infection and resolving the inflammation. She was free of detectable *B. gingivalis, B. intermedius,* and *A. actinomycetemcomitans* at 3, 6, and 12 months after therapy. In both cases the end points for periodontal therapy included eradication of the periodontal pathogens initially detected, as well as pocket elimination, reduction of bleeding on probing, freedom from suppuration, and radiographic evidence of remodeling with cortication of the interproximal alveolar bone.

Patients with *refractory* or *recurrent periodontitis* present a special problem. Often these patients have received extensive treatment, including periodontal surgery and multiple courses of systemic antibiotics, without improvement. Anaerobic culture and antibiotic susceptibility testing are often necessary in these patients, since microorganisms not normally associated with periodontitis may be involved in the etiology of their periodontal disease.

An appropriate clinical sample for microbiologic analysis at the time of initial diagnosis and treatment planning is one that is representative of the whole mouth. This could be subgingival plaque samples from several teeth, a mouth rinse, or a saliva sample. A rapid microbiologic assay is appropriate at this stage.

2. *To monitor treatment efficacy.* As demonstrated by the two young women with periodontitis discussed above, the treatment of an infectious disease such as periodontitis is greatly aided by the use of microbiologic assays after treatment to assess the efficacy of the therapy. The clinician is looking for objective measures to assess when therapy is completed, in addition to clinical indications such as a reduction in the probing attachment level and decrease in the number of bleeding points. Microbiologic assays can tell the clinician if the mechanical, surgical, and chemotherapeutic approach has been effective in eliminating the microbial etiology identified initially. Appropriate samples for monitoring treatment include pooled plaque or, if therapy has been directed to one or several involved and critical teeth, samples from these teeth. Reduction of inflammation coupled with suppression or elimination of specific periodontal pathogens, such as *A. actinomycetemcomitans* and the black-pigmented *Bacteroides,* especially *B. gingivalis,* can provide a convenient, meaningful end point for therapy (Zambon et al., 1985; Genco et al., 1986; Bragd et al., 1987; Listgarten, 1988).

3. *To select an appropriate recall interval.* After periodontal therapy has been completed, microbiologic tests using pooled plaque samples can be useful in determining the rate of reinfection, if any, by periodontal pathogens as an additional parameter to be assessed in determining an individual patient's optimum recall interval. If a patient is found to have become infected with high levels of periodontal pathogens at one recall interval, then more frequent recall may be necessary. Conversely, if a patient does not exhibit reinfection, longer recall intervals may be appropriate.

4. *To determine sites of "active" tissue destruction.* Related to the selection of an appropriate treatment or recall interval is the determination of which sites are subject to "active" tissue destruction. Clinically, these are determined by changes in probing attachment level measured using custom-fabricated acrylic stents or automated periodontal probes. The presence of several microbial species such as *A. actinomycetemcomitans, B. gingivalis, B. intermedius, B. forsythus, F. nucleatum,* and *W. recta* can be related to loss of probing attachment (Dzink et al., 1988). Therefore, if a causative agent is present in sufficient numbers, either the disease may be active in specific sites or these sites may be "at risk" for loss of attachment. Appropriate samples for analysis of site-specific tissue destruction include subgingival plaque from the site or tooth in question, and these can be analyzed by rapid tests targeted to specific periodontal pathogens. The clinician will be interested in determining if the patient has become reinfected with the same periodontal pathogen as was present during initial diagnosis. The failure to detect such a target species may necessitate the use of more complete microbiologic assays such as anaerobic culture.

5. *For prevention of periodontitis in persons "at risk" for either the initial onset of periodontal disease or for recurrent disease.* Patients in certain categories may be especially at risk for the development of periodontitis. For example, 30% to 50% of prepubertal siblings of LJP patients will develop this form of periodontal disease, especially if they have neutrophil chemotactic defects. Also, treated LJP patients or patients with refractory periodontitis are at increased risk for subsequent periodontal disease. Patients with diabetes mellitus, Down's syndrome, and neutrophil disorders are also susceptible to periodontal disease. Microbiologic monitoring of the subgingival flora in these patients may be useful in preventing initial or recurrent disease. A positive microbiologic test may indicate the need for antibiotic therapy to eliminate periodontal pathogens before signs of probing attachment loss occur. Pooled plaque samples and rapid microbiologic tests are likely to be useful in these high-risk patients.

SAMPLING DENTAL PLAQUE FOR MICROBIOLOGIC ANALYSIS

A key step in the analysis of dental plaque in the diagnosis and treatment of periodontal disease is sampling. What is desired is a sampling technique and microbiologic

Table 37-1. Possible outcomes for bacteriologic tests

Possible test result	Explanation
True positive	Patient sample contains target species, and microbiologic test is able to detect it
True negative	Patient sample does not contain target species, and microbiologic test is unable to detect it
False negative	Patient sample contains target species, but microbiologic test is unable to detect it
False positive	Patient sample does not contain target species, but microbiologic test is able to detect it

analysis, which leads to true positive or true negative results (Table 37-1). A *true positive* result is the finding of a target species by a microbiologic test in a patient who truly harbors that species. A *true negative* result is one in which the microbiologic test does not detect a target species in a sample that truly does not contain the species. A poorly taken patient sample or inadequate microbiologic test can lead to findings other than true positive or true negative findings (i.e., incorrect findings). The usual error is a *false negative* result occurring in a test with poor sensitivity. This is defined as the inability to detect a particular microorganism in a patient who in fact is infected with the species in question. In this error, the pathogenic microorganism will remain undetected and unknown. *False negative errors* can occur for several reasons related to sampling. For example, if not enough plaque is sampled, if the sample becomes contaminated with other material such as saliva, or if the sample is taken properly but is mishandled prior to the performance of the microbiologic test, then a false negative error may occur. *False positive errors*, on the other hand, occur less frequently. A false positive error can occur if the patient sample becomes contaminated from another source or if the test has poor specificity (i.e., falsely detects the organism in question when it is not present).

The goal in taking a patient sample is to provide a specimen for analysis that is representative of the lesion in question. In the case of plaque samples, subgingival plaque is most appropriate for analysis, since it is in close contact with the gingiva and epithelial attachment and is more likely than supragingival dental plaque to contain higher numbers and proportions of those microorganisms that are etiologic in periodontitis. Other materials that have been used as patient samples in determining periodontal status include supragingival dental plaque, scrappings from oral soft tissue surfaces, saliva, and gingival crevicular fluid. It is becoming clear that patients are often infected in several sites and that the pathogen spills over into

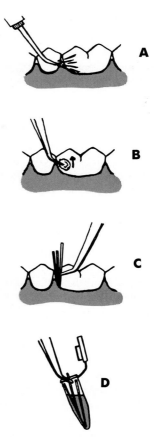

Fig. 37-3. Procedure for sampling subgingival flora. Samples may be put into transport media for culture, into preservative for immunofluorescence, shipped dry in a tube for DNA probe, or put into extracting solution for in-office tests. **A,** Site to be sampled is isolated with cotton rolls and air dried. **B,** Supragingival plaque is removed by rubbing tooth surface with a sterile cotton pellet from gingival margin coronally so as to avoid pushing supragingival plaque into periodontal pockets. **C,** Three paper points are placed into pocket interproximally with moderate pressure and directed so that tip of each paper point is in deepest portion of periodontal pocket directly underneath contact point. **D,** All three paper points are left in place for 10 seconds. All are removed at same time and immediately placed into tubes, making sure that each point is completely covered by solution. Cap is securely refastened and tube returned.

the saliva. Hence, saliva samples or oral wash samples may be useful in detecting infected patients.

Subgingival dental plaque can be sampled in several ways. One relatively expeditious and noninvasive method for sampling subgingival dental plaque involves the use of sterile endodontic paper points (Fig. 37-3). A site or sites of interest is selected. Selection of one diseased site per sextant may be useful during initial diagnosis of a new patient or during screening of large patient groups, since cross-sectional studies have shown that one half to two thirds of diseased sites harbor *A. actinomycetemcomitans*, *B. gingivalis*, or *B. intermedius* (Genco et al., 1986; Savitt et al., 1988). The selection of six sites in a patient is usually adequate to ensure detection of the pathogen. After therapy a site may be of interest by virtue of its failure to respond to conventional periodontal therapy as seen by continued loss of attachment, continued suppuration, or loss of alveolar bone.

Quadrants or sextants are isolated with cotton rolls to prevent contamination of the sample with bacteria in saliva and then air dried. Supragingival plaque is removed using either a sterile cotton pellet or a sterile curette. The instrument is moved in a coronal direction to avoid pushing supragingival plaque into the subgingival space. Three fine sterile paper points are then sequentially inserted to the depth of the gingival sulcus/periodontal pocket using firm pressure. If an interproximal site is being sampled, the paper points are directed in such a way that the tip of the paper points come to rest in the deepest point interproximally. At 10 seconds from the time the last paper point is placed, they are removed together and then placed into appropriate transport media for prompt shipment to the laboratory. Samples intended for analysis using DNA probes do not require the use of a transport medium. Samples for antibody assays are usually placed in an appropriate extracting/preservative solution.

Alternatively, subgingival plaque can be sampled using a sterile curette. Again, after the sample site has been isolated and the supragingival dental plaque removed as described above, a curette is placed to the depth of the gingival sulcus/periodontal pocket and moved coronally with firm lateral pressure against the root surface. The material is then dislodged from the curette tip into the transport medium, sterilized in a salt sterilizer, and then used to sample the next site. Some investigators advocate the use of nickel-plated curettes as a means of avoiding oxidation within the sample and the death of oxygen-intolerant anaerobic microorganisms.

Differences in proportions of various microorganisms sampled from subgingival sites has been found for the different sampling techniques. Subgingival plaque sampling using sterile paper points is thought to sample higher proportions of the loosely adherent dental plaque that may be present. This technique is relatively passive in that the bacteria are absorbed onto the dry paper. Samples taken using periodontal curettes are thought to include higher proportions of adherent dental plaque, since this technique involves scraping the plaque from the root surface.

TYPES OF MICROBIOLOGIC ASSAYS
Phase-contrast and darkfield microscopy

Phase-contrast and darkfield microscopy assays involve taking a sample of the patient's plaque and examining it with a microscope. The optics of phase-contrast and darkfield microscopes permit the visualization of living bacterial cells as opposed to conventional light microscopy, which necessitates the use of stains such as Gram's or Gi-

emsa stain in order to see the individual bacterial cells. Advocates of these microbiologic assays target their examinations toward certain indicator microorganisms such as motile species and spirochetes. The presence of the indicator microorganisms in a patient plaque sample then indicates the presence of a pathogenic microflora and the need for therapeutic intervention in order to eliminate the microbial pathogens. Clearly, phase-contrast and darkfield microscopy can detect motile rods and spirochetes that are often associated with periodontal disease—particularly chronic adult periodontitis. However, these microscopic techniques do not give information regarding particular bacterial species. There are, for example, at least three genera of microorganisms that exhibit a spirochetal form, and there are a large number of defined and undefined species within each genera. Neither light microscopy nor phase-contrast microscopy is able to give information beyond the size, shape, and motility of the bacterial species in patient plaque samples. By analogy, it would be inappropriate to take a throat swab and analyze it for the size, shape, and motility of the bacterial species present. For this test to be meaningful, it is necessary to assay for particular bacterial pathogens such as group A streptococci. Similarly, optimum microbiologic assays for periodontal disease should be based on identifying the bacterial species rather than a morphologic description of the bacteria in dental plaque. The phase-contrast enumeration of subgingival plaques does not readily distinguish between *periodontitis* and *gingivitis* and hence has severe limitations for routine clinical use (Wolff et al., 1985; Listgarten, 1988).

Bacterial culture

The definitive microbiologic assay is bacterial culture. If a species can be cultured from a lesion, there is usually no doubt that that microorganism is in fact infecting a particular site. For this reason, bacterial culture can be considered to be the "gold standard" against which other methods must be compared. In addition, bacterial culture of plaque microorganisms affords the opportunity to examine the antibiotic susceptibility of the pathogen to determine which antibiotic is most useful in eliminating the organism.

Bacterial culture is, however, time consuming and expensive; it requires considerable technical expertise; and certain periodontal organisms such as spirochetes and many motile rods are cultured only with difficulty or not at all with present methods. To culture, for example, *B. gingivalis* from a patient sample, approximately 1 week is required for the initial or "primary" culture. The agar plates must then be examined, and the black-pigmenting colonies must be subcultured. These subcultures must then incubate anaerobically for 5 to 7 days and may often require restreaking in order to achieve a pure culture. This pure culture is then inoculated into broth medium and subjected to several biochemical tests and analysis of metabolic acid end products by gas-liquid chromatography. The definitive identification of a single colony of *B. gingivalis* can therefore require 3 weeks or more from the time of initial sampling. All of the steps in the culture are performed by highly trained laboratory personnel, and the entire identification is expensive.

There are short-cut or "presumptive" identification schemes for bacterial isolates. These make certain assumptions about the patient sample and use those assumptions to shorten the list of tests that are used to identify an isolate. They can reduce the time and cost of bacterial culture; however, presumptive identification schemes result in increased levels of false positive and false negative findings. Other technical difficulties may also be associated with the anaerobic culture of patient plaque samples. These problems include the loss of viability during transport of the patient sample from the dental office to the laboratory. This loss of viability is of particular concern in samples shipped to a distant laboratory. As a general rule, anaerobic microorganisms will become less viable as the time between sampling and initial culture increase.

Antibody-based assays

While bacterial culture is the "gold standard," nonculture techniques of microbiologic analysis can be very useful in identifying the microorganisms present in a patient sample. These nonculture techniques include immunologic methods based on specific antibodies, DNA probes, and assays for specific bacterial enzymes. Each of these assays can provide rapid and relatively inexpensive identification of both cariogenic and periodontopathic microorganisms, and they can be used to screen large numbers of patients, as in epidemiologic studies. In clinical practice they can be used to more thoroughly characterize individual patients — to diagnose disease, to monitor the course of therapy, and to detect previously treated subjects who have become reinfected.

Rapid tests are generally validated by bacterial culture. It should be remembered, however, that bacterial culture does not exhibit 100% sensitivity or specificity. Bacterial culture, especially for anaerobic microorganisms such as *B. gingivalis,* may yield significant numbers of false negative results, especially when the organisms are present in small numbers or are not viable at the time of sampling. False positive results, although less likely, can also occur because of misidentification or cross-contamination.

Immunologic techniques such as immunofluorescence microscopy rely on antigen-antibody reactions and are more likely than bacterial culture to detect specific microorganisms in clinical samples, since these methods do not require cultivable (viable) bacterial cells. In addition to detecting the bacteria themselves, antibody-based assays can also be used to detect bacterial virulence factors such as toxins. In contrast to bacterial culture, however, rapid methods cannot currently be used to determine antibiotic susceptibility.

There are several immunologic methods that can be used to detect microbial pathogens, including immunofluorescence microscopy, latex and other particle agglutination assays, flow cytometry, and enzyme-linked immunosorbent assays (ELISA). Each of these methods uses polyclonal antisera or monoclonal antibodies specific for bacterial antigens or for microbial virulence factors, and each method offers certain advantages and disadvantages (Table 37-2). Flow cytometry, for example, takes only a few minutes, but the cost of the equipment and the technical expertise needed for operation and maintenance make it practical only in a reference laboratory. Latex agglutination is a rapid method requiring little equipment or technical expertise, which is useful in the examination of individual patient samples in a clinical setting. ELISA-based tests are becoming increasingly useful in the clinician's office and show great promise as inexpensive, sensitive, specific, rapid tests for the presence of periodontal pathogens in subgingival samples.

All immunologic methods require serologic reagents, either polyclonal antisera or monoclonal antibodies, which react only with the "target" bacterial species and not with the myriad of other bacteria that may be present in the same patient sample. The specificity of these reagents lies in the inherent specificity of antigen-antibody reactions. These serologic reagents can be used singly or in combination in various immunologic assays.

Immunofluorescence microscopy

Immunofluorescence microscopy for the detection of periodontal pathogens, particularly *A. actinomycetemcomitans* and *B. gingivalis,* has been used for the past several years for the routine clinical detection of these species in patient plaque samples. Using this method, patient samples are transported in a preservative to the laboratory, where they are mixed and a portion of the plaque suspension is placed on glass slides. The patient sample is then reacted with species-specific antisera or monoclonal antibody that is coupled to a fluorescent compound. The slides are then examined using a fluorescence microscope. The presence of the target bacteria in the patient sample can be seen as a bacterial cell of the same size and shape as what would be expected and that appears green as a result of labeling with the antibody. The test can be made quantitative, since the percent of stained organisms as compared with the total number observed in the same fields can be calculated. This is expressed as the percent of total organisms, and this percentage is often lower than that reported for culture, since culture results are often expressed as the percent of cultivable organisms.

In developing a "new" test such as immunofluorescence, determination of true positive, true negative, false positive, and false negative values is made using the "gold

Table 37-2. Comparison of nonculture techniques for identification of periodontal pathogens

Method	Performance site	Time required	Comments
Immunologic			
Flow cytometry	Reference laboratory	1-2 min, plus sample and report transit time	Expensive instrumentation Method not demonstrated for use in dental plaque
Latex agglutination	Office	5-10 min	Does not require any instrumentation and only minimal technical expertise
Enzyme-linked immunosorbent assay	Reference laboratory	1-2 hr plus sample and report transit time	Requires instrumentation but only minimal technical expertise
Enzyme-linked immunosorbent assay	Office	5-15 min	Office kits relatively easy to use by minimally trained personnel
Immunofluorescence microscopy	Reference laboratory or office	1-2 hr if in office plus sample and report transit time in reference lab	Moderately expensive instrumentation requires significant technical expertise
Nucleic acid hybridization			
DNA probes	Reference laboratory	1-2 days	Requires accurately performed laboratory techniques; equipment costs modest
RNA probes	Reference laboratory	1-2 days	Requires accurately performed laboratory techniques; equipment costs modest
Polymerase chain reaction	Reference laboratory	1-2 days	Extremely sensitive; requires significant technical expertise

Table 37-3. Comparison of immunofluorescence microscopy with bacterial culture for detection of *A. actinomycetemcomitans* and *B. gingivalis*

Microorganism	Immunofluorescent	Culture media	Sensitivity	Specificity
*A. actinomycetemcomitans**	Polyclonal antisera	Nonselective	100	88
	Polyclonal antisera	Selective	96 (77)[†]	92 (81)
	Monoclonal antibody	Nonselective	90	88
	Monoclonal antibody	Selective	82	92
B. gingivalis[‡]	Polyclonal antisera	Nonselective	100 (91)[†]	87 (80)
	Polyclonal antisera	Selective	92	87
	Monoclonal antibody	Nonselective	92	88
	Monoclonal antibody	Selective	91	89

*Data from Bonta et al. (1985).
[†]Data from Zambon et al. (1985).
[‡]Numbers in parentheses from Slots et al. (1985).

standard," in this case, bacterial culture. For immunofluorescence, for example, a true positive finding occurs when both bacterial culture and immunofluorescence tests are positive for the target species; a true negative finding occurs when both bacterial culture and immunofluorescence tests are negative for the target species; a false positive finding occurs when the immunofluorescence is positive but the culture is negative; and a false negative finding occurs when the culture is positive but the immunofluorescence is negative. Comparative studies indicate that the *sensitivity* of immunofluorescence ranges from 82% to 100% for detection of *A. actinomycetemcomitans* and from 91% to 100% for detection of *B. gingivalis,* with specificity values of 88% to 92% and 87% to 89%, respectively (Table 37-3).

Immunofluorescence also indicates that most people do not harbor periodontal pathogens. Of nearly 300 patients examined in a recent study (Zambon et al. 1986), the vast majority, 92%, demonstrated li le or no *A. actinomyce-temcomitans.* The overwhelming number of subjects, 87%, also demonstrated little or no *B. gingivalis.* There were in this group, however, some subjects who harbored this latter species. These latter subjects were found to be periodontitis patients.

Flow cytometry

Flow cytometry (cytofluorography) has been used routinely to characterize and analyze eukaryotic cells such as lymphocytes. Recently, however, flow cytometry has been used to study bacterial cells. For example, flow cytometry has been used to study the microbial growth and metabolism of *Escherichia coli,* to identify *Legionella pneumophilia,* and to differentiate bacterial species such as *E. coli, Klebsiella pneumoniae, Pseudomonas aeruginosa, Staphylococcus aureus, Streptococcus pneumoniae,* and *Streptococcus pyogenes* in clinical samples. Flow cytometry using polyclonal antibodies has been used to identify oral bacteria such as *Actinomyces viscosus, Streptococcus mutans,* and *B. gingivalis* (Kornman et al., 1984).

Very little has been written regarding the use of flow cytometry in patient plaque samples. This is probably because of the difficulties inherent in dispersing a bacterial plaque composed largely of cell clumps into a single-cell suspension suitable for analysis.

ELISA

Enzyme-linked immunosorbent assay (ELISA) for bacterial species involves binding the species-specific serologic reagent to the wells of polystyrene plates or to membranes placed on an absorbant base. The bacterial plaque sample is dispersed in a buffer with the addition of a detergent or other extractant, and an aliquot of the bacterial extract is added to the antibody-coated wells or on the membrane. Binding of the target microorganism can then be detected by the addition of a second antibody conjugated to an enzyme, followed by the addition of the substrate. These tests have been developed as tests for periodontal pathogens with a potential for use in the dental office.

Latex agglutination assays

Latex agglutination assays have potential for widespread use in the clinical detection of periodontal pathogens. These assays are used in both reference laboratories and clinics for the routine detection of a number of different bacterial pathogens. For example, traditional culture of throat swabs from pharyngitis patients is rapidly being supplanted by antibody-based tests, including latex agglutination assays, for streptococcal species. These assays involve the use of latex beads coated with the species-specific antibody. When these beads come in contact with microbial cell-surface antigens or antigen extracts, crosslinking occurs and visible clumps of beads are formed, usually within 2 to 5 minutes.

DNA probes

Techniques of molecular biology have been adapted to the diagnosis of infectious disease. Reference laboratory services are currently available that use DNA probe technology to detect certain bacterial species in patient plaque samples (Savitt et al., 1988). The key to these assays is the use of a probe DNA—a piece of DNA that will hybridize specifically to the target species in a manner analogous to antibody-antigen reactions in serologic assays. One way in which these probes are developed is to purify the bacterial DNA from a target species, such as *A. actinomycetemcomitans,* to fragment the bacterial DNA into small pieces using restriction endonucleases, and then to purify each different fragment of DNA. The DNA fragment is tagged, usually with a radioactive label, and then allowed to bind or hybridize with the bacterial DNA isolated from the same species and from a number of different species. The fragment of DNA reacts only with the target species and not appreciably with any of the other bacterial species under specific conditions of hybridization and washing. Hence it can then be used for the detection of that species in patient samples.

Patient samples sent to a reference laboratory for analysis by DNA probe are usually taken using sterile paper points and then placed into a plastic tube for shipment. At the laboratory the bacteria on the paper point are extracted to release the bacterial DNA, which is then bound to a filter. The labeled DNA probe is applied and allowed to hybridize. If the target species is present in the patient sample, the probe DNA will hybridize to the DNA bound to the filter. The hybridization can then be detected by exposing photographic film to the radioactive label. The darker the spot on the film, the more probe DNA is bound to the filter and the more target species was present in the original patient sample.

This technique holds great future promise for the sensitive detection of bacterial viruses and other pathogens in biologic samples (Tenover, 1988). Recent technologic advances using the polymerase chain reaction in which the DNA present in the patient sample is used as a template for multiple cycles of synthesis promises to greatly enhance the sensitivity of these DNA probe assays. Also, assays for microbial RNA offer great promise, since they, too, offer the possibility of greater sensitivity than DNA probes.

Enzyme assays

One factor in the pathogenesis of periodontitis is the production of various bacterial enzymes by the periodontal pathogens. These enzymes include collagenase and hyaluronidase, which can destroy gingival connective tissue; acid and alkaline phosphatase, RNAase, and DNAase; and various proteases and peptidases. Some of these enzymes are produced specifically by certain periodontal pathogens. For example, collagenase is produced by *A. actinomyce-*

Table 37-4. Summary of diagnosis of periodontal disease

	Gingival bleeding	Periodontal pockets or suppuration	Probing attachment	Radiographic alveolar bone loss	Bacteriology: *B. gingivalis*, and/or *B. intermedius* and/or *A. actinomycetemcomitans*
Health	−	−	−	−	−
Gingivitis	+	−	−	−	−
Periodontitis	±	+	+	+	+
Posttreatment (successful)	−	±	+	+	−
Posttreatment (recurrence)	±	±	+	+	+

temcomitans and *B. gingivalis,* and *B. gingivalis* produces a specific tripeptidase. Using these enzymatic markers as a key to the presence of these species, the corresponding bacteria can be detected in the patient sample by assaying for the enzyme. Toward this end, several methods are available to examine a patient sample for the presence of specfic enzymes. Tissue-derived enzymes have also been proposed as useful for the diagnosis and monitoring of periodontitis; however, none has been able to distinguish periodontitis from gingivitis.

CONCLUSIONS

A variety of methods are currently available for examining the subgingival microflora in periodontitis patients. These techniques should be incorporated into clinical practice in a scheme such as that presented in Table 37-4. Microbiologic tests can assist the clinician in making objective decisions regarding diagnosis, treatment planning, and monitoring of pockets. For example, patients who exhibit clinical signs and symptoms of gingival inflammation, without evidence of subgingival infection, and with a pathogenic periodontal flora may require less extensive treatment than a patient who harbors high numbers of periodontal pathogens in subgingival sites. Future improvements in immunologic tests, especially improvements that will enable clinicians to efficiently perform these tests in their offices, as well as the development of new tests, will enable clinical microbiology to become an integral part of clinical dentistry for the benefit of both the patient and the dental profession.

REFERENCES

Bonta Y et al: Rapid identification of periodontal pathogens in subgingival dental plaque: a comparison of indirect immunofluorescence microscopy with bacterial culture for detection of *Actinobacillus actinomycetemcomitans,* J Dent Res 64:693, 1985.

Bragd C et al: The capability of *Actinobacillus actinomycetemcomitans, Bacteroides gingivalis,* and *Bacteroides intermedius* to indicate pro-

gressive periodontitis: a retrospective study, J Clin Periodontol 14:95, 1987.

Christersson LA et al: Tissue localization of *Actinobacillus actinomycetemcomitans* in human periodontitis. I. Light, immunofluorescence and electron microscopic studies, J Periodontol 58:529, 1987a.

Christersson LA et al: Tissue localization of *Actinobacillus actinomycetemcomitans* in human periodontitis. II. Correlation between immunofluorescence and culture techniques, J Periodontol 58:540, 1987b.

Dzink JL, Socransky SS, and Haffajee AD: The predominant cultivable microbiota of active and inactive lesions of destructive periodontal disease, J Clin Periodontol 15:316, 1988.

Genco RJ, Zambon JJ, and Christersson LA: Use and interpretation of microbial assays in periodontal diseases, Oral Microbiol Immunol 1:73, 1986.

Kornman KS and Robertson PD: Clinical and microbiological evaluation of therapy for juvenile periodontitis, J Clin Periodontol 12:465, 1985.

Kornman KS et al: Detection and quantitation of *Bacteroides gingivalis* in bacterial mixtures by means of flow cytometry, J Periodont Res 19:570, 1984.

Listgarten M: A rationale for monitoring the periodontal microbiota after periodontal treatment, J Periodontol 59:439, 1988.

Mandell RL and Socransky SS: Microbiological and clinical effects of surgery plus doxycycline on juvenile periodontitis, J Periodontol 59:373, 1988.

Savitt ED et al: Comparison of cultural methods and DNA probe analysis for the detection of *Actinobacillus actinomycetemcomitans, Bacteroides gingivalis,* and *Bacteroides intermedius* in subgingival plaque samples, J Periodontol 59:431, 1988.

Slots J and Rosling BG: Suppression of the periodontopathic microflora in localized juvenile periodontitis by systemic tetracycline, J Clin Periodontol 10:465, 1983.

Slots J et al: Detection of *Actinobacillus actinomycetemcomitans* and *Bacteroides gingivalis* in subgingival smears by the indirect fluorescent-antibody technique, J Periodont Res 20:613, 1985.

Tenover FC: Diagnostic deoxyribonucleic acid probes for infectious diseases, Clin Microbiol Rev 1:82, 1988.

Wolff LF et al: Distinct categories of microbial forms associated with periodontal diseases, J Periodont Res 20:497, 1985.

Zambon JJ, Bochacki V, and Genco RJ: Immunological assays for putative periodontal pathogens, Oral Microbiol Immunol 1:39, 1986.

Zambon JJ et al: Rapid identification of periodontal pathogens in subgingival dental plaque: comparison of indirect immunofluorescence microscopy with bacterial culture for detection of *Bacteroides gingivalis,* J Periodontol (suppl), p 32, 1985.

Chapter 38

ACUTE NECROTIZING ULCERATIVE GINGIVITIS

Ronald B. Cogen

Acute necrotizing ulcerative gingivitis (ANUG) is an infectious disease that results in acute gingivitis and is characterized by ulceration and necrosis of the gingival margin and also by destruction of the interdental papillae. In the 1890s Plaut and Vincent suggested that ANUG was caused by a fusospirochetal microorganism. Approximately 60 years ago, during World War I, ANUG became important from an epidemiologic point of view because of its high prevalence among frontline soldiers engaged in trench warfare. It was popularly known as trench mouth, and because of its apparent occurrence within communities, it was considered contagious (Pickard, 1973). Today, although the condition is no longer considered communicable, the pathogenic mechanisms are still somewhat unclear, since ANUG is a complex disease and not a simple infectious process. The bacteria presently implicated in the etiology of ANUG—spirochetes (Loesche et al., 1982), fusiform bacteria, and *Bacteroides intermedius*—appear to function as opportunistic pathogens requiring underlying tissue changes to become pathogenic (Rosebury and Sonnenwirth, 1958; Listgarten, 1965). This view is supported by several observations (see box, above right):

Summary of important observations in ANUG

1. Epidemiology: young (17-35) in developed countries; under 10 in poor countries
2. Acute infection associated with common endogenous oral flora (fusiform bacilli; spirochetes, *Bacteroides intermedius*)
3. Host resistance key:
   A. High incidence in blood dyscrasias, malnutrition, Down's syndrome, terminal cancer, steroids
   B. Nontransferable in humans
4. Acute emotional stress and anxiety (war, exams, marital troubles) is thought to be a key predisposing factor
5. Easily diagnosable; easily treatable (scaling); short-lived (1-3 days)

---

1. Symptoms resolve rapidly following antibiotic therapy or simple mechanical debridement.
2. Researchers have been unable to transfer the infection to different hosts.
3. Microscopic and microbiologic findings indicate that the mouths of some subjects with gingivitis or periodontitis, and even the mouths of some healthy individuals (Johnson and Engel, 1986), harbor the organisms associated with ANUG and yet these persons do not have the disease.
4. The incidence of ANUG increases markedly in patients with diseases associated with depressed numbers or function of leukocytes.
5. Although poor dental hygiene (Giddon et al., 1964; Goldhaber and Giddon, 1964; Jiménez and Baer, 1975) and gingivitis (Pindborg, 1951) seem to pre-

dispose an individual to ANUG, these factors alone are not sufficient; many individuals with poor oral hygiene and generalized gingivitis or even periodontitis do not ever develop ANUG.

COMPREHENSIVE APPROACH TO THERAPY

The ANUG patient usually reports to the dental office or clinic because the condition is painful (Stevens et al., 1984). Frequently this is a first visit, and even when the individual is a patient of record, dental visits may have been infrequent or may have involved emergency therapy only. However, the approach to therapy requires a good medical history, dental history, and physical evaluation of the patient before the clinician proceeds with a diagnosis, treatment plan, therapy, and maintenance program.

The medical and dental history may be obtained by questionnaire, interview, or both. Special care should be exerted to determine whether there is any history of valvular heart disease, communicable diseases, bleeding disorders, present medications, recent medical or dental treatments, and allergic or adverse drug reactions. Also of importance is information regarding previous dental treatment, its nature, extent, and frequency.

ANUG is an acutely painful disease. Recurrences are common (Manson and Rand, 1961; Giddon et al., 1964; Jiménez and Baer, 1975), and often patients afflicted with ANUG stop treatment as soon as the symptoms are alleviated. Therefore information regarding the history of the present illness should be obtained. Attention should be paid especially to information regarding the nature (if any) of previous therapy for the present illness, how long ago the illness occurred, how many episodes the patient has experienced, and, very important, the patient's attitude toward therapy aimed at complete resolution of the condition.

In addition to the medical and dental history and the history of the present illness, useful information for proper management of the ANUG patient involves demographic information. This includes the patient's age, general socioeconomic status (education, employment, income) (Jiménez and Baer, 1975), general living habits (diet and nutritional status, sleep, smoking), recent physical or emotional stress, and any recent illness.

ANUG is an invasive periodontal infection that has a markedly increased incidence associated with some systemic illnesses. Moreover, it sometimes is one of the early signals of impending serious illness (Enwonwu, 1972). Also, although it is not the usual situation, ANUG is sometimes severe enough to cause systemic symptoms.

The systemic disorders associated with ANUG include physiologic and psychologic stress, malnutrition, endocrine imbalances, blood dyscrasias, side effects of chemotherapy and radiation therapy, AIDS, and Down's syndrome. It is therefore necessary to observe the general appearance of the patient, especially for pallor, weakness, lassitude, and apparent nutritional status. Also, the patient's temperature should be taken, and the submaxillary, submental, and cervical areas should be palpated to detect any enlarged lymph nodes. General malaise, anorexia, fever (Grupe and Wilder, 1956; Goldhaber and Giddon, 1964), and enlarged regional lymph nodes, although they do not usually occur in patients with ANUG, suggest systemic involvement if present.

DIAGNOSIS

The diagnosis of ANUG is not difficult if there is strict adherence to certain diagnostic criteria, listed in the box below. Three criteria are necessary for reliable diagnosis: (1) acute inflammation with necrosis and ulceration of interproximal papillae (typical crateriform or punched-out papillae), (2) gingival pain, and (3) gingival bleeding (either spontaneous or on slight provocation) (Emslie, 1963; Cogen et al., 1983). Other criteria, such as pseudomembrane, fever, abnormal sensations in the teeth, increased salivary flow, metallic taste, and "fetor oris," are often present and are additional signs and symptoms but are of themselves not diagnostic. Therefore, with strict adherence to the three required criteria, diagnostic accuracy can

---

Diagnostic features of ANUG

1. Interproximal necrosis and ulceration (punched-out cratered papillae)*
2. Painful gingivae*
3. Bleeding (spontaneous or on slight provocation)*
4. Pseudomembrane (fibrin, debris)
5. Fever, malaise, lymphadenopathy variable
6. "Fetor oris"

*Necessary diagnostic criteria.

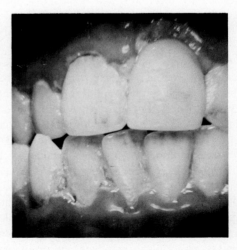

Fig. 38-1. Fairly typical appearance of a patient with ANUG. Note punched-out interdental papillae, many of which are covered by pseudomembrane. Since they were necrotic and ulcerated, papillae bled easily and were painful.

be extremely high (Stevens et al., 1984). These features are pictured in Fig. 38-1.

Several oral mucosal lesions may be confused with ANUG (Schluger, 1949), including desquamative gingivitis associated with hormonal imbalances of pregnancy, puberty, or menopause; benign mucous membrane pemphigoid; primary herpetic gingivostomatitis; and advanced marginal gingivitis. These conditions all may present with widespread redness that appears more severe than one would expect with chronic inflammatory periodontal diseases. However, none of these displays the necrosis of the crests of the papillae seen in ANUG, which results in the typical punched-out interproximal papillae.

The condition most frequently mistaken for ANUG is primary herpetic gingivostomatitis (Klotz, 1973). However, several features seem to differentiate ANUG from primary herpes. ANUG, except in underdeveloped countries (Emslie, 1963), mainly affects young adults (Stammers, 1946) within an age range of 17 to 35, whereas primary herpes occurs mostly in young children. ANUG is not usually characterized by a markedly elevated temperature (Grupe and Wilder, 1956; Goldhaber and Giddon,

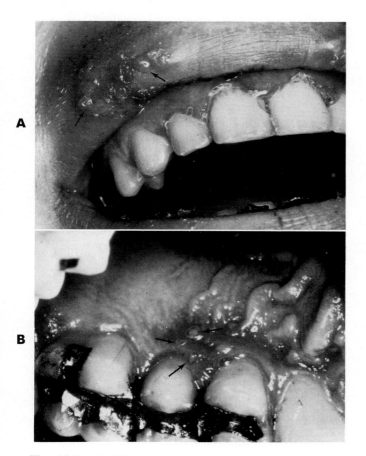

Fig. 38-2. A, Ulceration on gingiva may be confused with ANUG; however, note that there is no necrotic interproximal papillae, and note lesion on lip. **B,** Small ulcers on palate surrounded by erythematous halo is indicative of acute herpetic stomatitis.

1964) or malaise, whereas primary herpes is frequently accompanied by a high fever and general systemic illness. The lesions of primary herpetic gingivostomatitis usually begin as small vesicles that burst to form small ulcers surrounded by an inflammatory halo. These lesions, as can be seen in Fig. 38-2, almost always involve several of the oral mucous membranes, such as the lips, tongue, buccal mucosa, and palate, in addition to the gingiva. ANUG, on the other hand, is most often localized to the interdental papillae and sometimes to the marginal gingiva.

Although there is little doubt that the clinical manifestations of ANUG are caused by bacteria, several other factors are strongly associated with ANUG: (1) physical trauma or emotional stress, (2) smoking, (3) poor oral hygiene, and (4) gingivitis. It appears that these predisposing factors create conditions that allow the microorganisms to become pathogenic, thereby causing overt symptomatic disease.

STRESS AND OTHER HOST SUSCEPTIBILITY ISSUES

The most frequent systemic illnesses associated with ANUG are the blood dyscrasias (Barling, 1948; Levy and Schetman, 1961; Wintrobe, 1967). The incidence of ANUG is extremely high in patients afflicted with acute myelogenous leukemia. The ANUG infecting organisms may be superimposed on gingival tissues with weakened defense mechanisms resulting from the leukemia. It should be noted that there is no clear clinical distinction between ANUG in healthy individuals and in leukemic patients, except that the leukemic state is the underlying predisposing etiologic factor for the infection.

Other systemic diseases associated with ANUG are severe malnutrition (Miller and Greene, 1958; Pindborg et al., 1967; Enwonwu, 1972; Jiménez and Baer, 1975) and debilitating diseases (Listgarten, 1965), such as cancer, metal intoxication, AIDS, and advanced renal disease. It has become obvious that many of the predisposing systemic conditions associated with ANUG involve depression of leukocyte numbers or function (Barling, 1948; Cohen, 1960; Levy and Schetman, 1961; Johnson and Young, 1963; Wintrobe, 1967; Cogen et al., 1983; Claffey et al., 1986). The leukocyte most commonly involved is the neutrophil (polymorphonuclear leukocyte, PMN) (Cogen et al., 1983).

ANUG affects young adults (17 to 35) who otherwise are seemingly healthy. In these cases emotional stress may be the primary predisposing factor (Pindborg, 1951; Moulton et al., 1952; Giddon et al., 1964; Goldhaber and Giddon, 1964; Shannon et al., 1969; Formicola et al., 1970; Davis and Baer, 1971; Manhold et al., 1971; Maupin and Bell, 1975; Cohen-Cole et al., 1983). Frequently ANUG is closely associated with situations that are emotionally stressful or that result in acute anxiety (Cohen-Cole et al., 1983). There appears to be an interactive effect between the magnitude of the stressor and the individual's adaptive capacity that plays a part in host resistance (Rogers et al., 1979). Thus stress in an individual with ineffective coping response may result in depression of leukocyte function (Cogen et al., 1983). This may increase the host's susceptibility sufficiently, albeit temporarily, to enable an opportunistic infection such as ANUG to gain a foothold. This is an extremely complex process involving the interaction of many variables (social support etc.).

THERAPY

ANUG is an acute disease that usually runs a short and stormy course. Numerous treatment modalities have been tried, and most have worked or not worked equally well (Miller and Greene, 1958). The distinction between effective treatments and those that are merely palliative is difficult to make, since the disease is cyclic and tends to go into remission in a week or so. The quickest, safest, least eventful, and therefore best treatment of ANUG involves mechanical debridement to eliminate microbial accumulations to the greatest degree possible (Schluger, 1949; Goldberg, 1966). In general, the same guidelines used in the management of periodontal diseases apply in the treatment of ANUG: (1) scaling of gross deposits followed by careful root planing to eliminate plaque, (2) home care instruction and use of an antiplaque mouth rinse such as chlorhexidine to prevent plaque accumulation, (3) elimination of local contributing factors such as overhangs, (4) surgery to eliminate areas inaccessible to home cleansing procedures, (5) a good preventive program with periodic office recall visits, and (6) systemic antibiotics, especially penicillin or metronidazole (Loesche et al., 1982), if there is systemic involvement or if mechanical treatment cannot be instituted.

Beginning therapy

The most immediate need at the first visit is to alleviate the symptoms. Removal of calculus, bacteria, necrotic tissue, and other accumulations on the teeth should begin as quickly as possible. If it is done gently and carefully, the surest way to alleviate the pain is by mechanical debridement, even though the tissues are already tender. The entire dentition should be scaled coronally and subgingivally as thoroughly as possible. Ultrasonic scalers with copious water spray or antimicrobial irrigants used with an ultrasonic scaler are excellent for this initial scaling. In addition, patients should be instructed to rinse frequently (every 1 to 2 hours while awake) and forcibly with a bland mouth rinse. Warm water is effective, as are diluted oxygenating products such as 1 part 3% hydrogen peroxide to 1 part warm water, which has the added property of effervescence (Wennstrom et al., 1979). Patients should be instructed in oral hygiene procedures, with the importance of diligent performance stressed. If necessary for pain, analgesics such as acetaminophen, aspirin, or ibuprofen may

be prescribed, and the patient is instructed to return in 24 to 48 hours.

When the patient returns in 1 to 2 days, there is usually dramatic improvement as a result of the office debridement and home care. Root planing can now be initiated, although the need for good oral hygiene should continue to be emphasized. Rinsing frequency can be reduced, and analgesics are probably no longer needed. The patient should be instructed to return in approximately 5 days.

In most instances the acute inflammation will have subsided by the time the patient returns in 5 days, and pain, bleeding, and ulceration should no longer be present. If inflammation and pain are still present, a course of systemic antibiotics may provide relief (Emslie, 1971). The root planing can now be continued and completed, if possible. Oral hygiene measures should be reviewed at this visit, and rinsing can be terminated. The patient should be instructed to return to the office in 2 weeks.

At the 2-week return visit, root planing should be reviewed and refined to completion; also, any remaining local factors, such as restoration margins, should be corrected and thorough polishing performed. Evaluation of the patient's tissue response and oral hygiene at this or a subsequent visit will determine whether satisfactory resolution has occurred or if further treatment will be needed.

Systemic therapy for ANUG with antibiotics and/or nutritional supplements is rarely if ever necessary. Among the exceptions to this are when local therapy is not effective; when symptoms of ANUG include fever, malaise, lassitude, and enlarged regional lymph nodes; or when the patient's general health is affected (Libby, 1963; Emslie, 1971). One such situation might be when ANUG occurs secondary to acute myelogenous leukemia. In these cases antibiotics may be prescribed in addition to the local mechanical debridement and meticulous home care. In the absence of allergy, penicillin V, 250 mg every 6 hours for 5 days, is the drug of choice for ANUG. If there is a history of sensitivity to penicillin, then erythromycin, 250 mg, may be substituted. Metronidazole has been used effectively. In cases involving leukemia, consultation with the hematologist could result in the use of systemic antibiotics in conjunction with very gentle debridement and/or local irrigation.

Nutritional supplementation may be indicated in the rare instances when ANUG patients suffer such severe pain that ingestion of a normal diet is difficult or when ANUG is secondary to severe debilitating illness. This may lead to anorexia, which might cause malnutrition. Supplementation of nutritional elements and vitamins would probably be indicated in such cases.

Continuation of therapy

On thorough and complete debridement and institution of good home care procedures, as seen in Fig. 38-3, superficial to moderate cases of ANUG should resolve com-

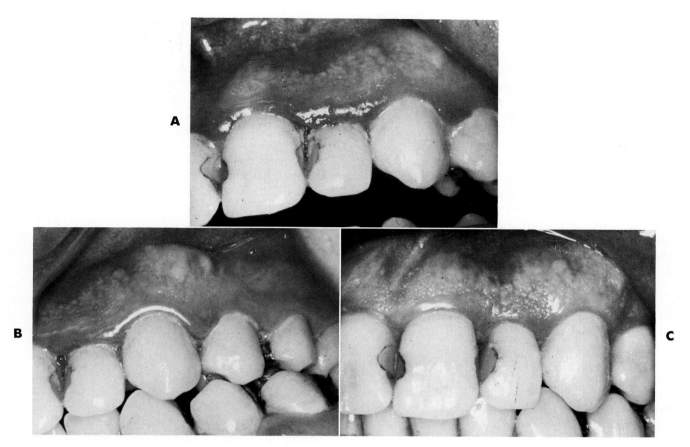

Fig. 38-3. **A,** ANUG patient at initial office visit. Note plaque in association with interproximal necrosis and acute inflammation. **B,** Same patient after gross mechanical debridement and home rinsing for several days. Note marked improvement and reduction in inflammation. **C,** Same patient after root planing and improved home care. Note reduction in plaque, and satisfactory resolution of ANUG and restoration of tissue form.

pletely. In some moderate and many advanced and recurrent cases in which tissue destruction has been severe, interproximal defects (Fig. 38-4) may remain even after the pain, bleeding, and necrosis of ANUG have resolved. These remaining interproximal craters frequently increase plaque retention and may make effective home care more difficult or virtually impossible. Eliminating such defects will greatly improve the conditions for home plaque-control procedures and possibly prevent recurrences (Pickard, 1973). The craters in such cases should be eliminated surgically. The defects are usually amenable to elimination by simple gingivectomy-gingivoplasty.

If the defects are more severe, flap surgery and/or mucoperiosteal procedures may be needed to achieve proper interproximal form and contour. Surgery should not be attempted until the local etiologic factors have been completely eliminated and inflammation has resolved. In addition, if the patient is not performing proper oral hygiene, then correction of deformities will probably not prevent recurrence of ANUG and/or progression of chronic inflam-

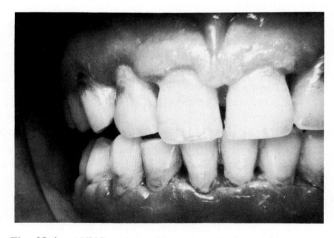

Fig. 38-4. ANUG patient with marked gingival deformities resulting from recurrent episodes. This is frequently observed after incomplete therapy.

matory periodontal disease; in these instances surgery is probably not indicated.

The dentist must eliminate all local etiologic factors in the treatment of ANUG. The organisms causing the disease must not multiply and gain a foothold. Dramatic reduction in bacterial plaque is urgent in the proper management of the ANUG patient, and local factors that contribute to plaque retention, such as rough tooth surfaces, overhangs, and poor contours, should be corrected.

As in chronic inflammatory periodontal diseases such as gingivitis and periodontitis, therapy for ANUG cannot be successful or complete unless meticulous attention is directed toward oral hygiene. Good oral hygiene cannot be emphasized too much, since it is crucial to the successful therapeutic outcome in periodontal diseases in general and ANUG in particular. Unfortunately, this is one of the more difficult phases in which to achieve success. Unquestionably, ANUG patients as a group present the therapist with difficult patient management problems. They frequently do not appear for their appointments, especially when they are no longer in pain, and it is particularly difficult to motivate them to participate in a program of oral hygiene. It is not unusual for them to cease oral hygiene, rinsing, and office maintenance procedures as soon as acute symptoms have subsided. In fact, on recurrent episodes of disease, many will self-medicate with antibiotics if they were previously treated with them, not understanding that in the absence of proper diagnosis, self-medication may be wrongfully instituted. The probability that many of these patients are emotionally disturbed adds greatly to the substantial patient motivation problems faced in the performance of adequate periodontal therapy (Cohen-Cole et al., 1983). Each office visit should be used to evaluate, motivate, and instruct the patient in proper home care procedures.

PREVENTION

Individuals engaged in periodontal therapy carry a substantial burden in terms of prevention of disease through patient education in home care procedures. Maintenance programs have become a major component of proper periodontal therapy.

A patient who has had ANUG should be considered at risk for recurrences. The disease is associated with the interplay of opportunistic bacteria with hosts susceptible because of their inability to cope with stressful life situations. It is virtually impossible to lessen stress or to improve coping ability, so plaque removal becomes the only major contributing factor that can be controlled. This is best accomplished by cooperation between the dentist and the patient in an adequate plaque-control program.

Most patients who have ANUG have preexisting gingivitis. However, it is also possible for ANUG to be superimposed on periodontitis. In either event the treatment and

patient management are similar to that used for other chronic inflammatory periodontal diseases, varying somewhat to accommodate the pain and bleeding of ANUG. Proper treatment for inflammatory periodontal diseases involves reversal of the etiologic conditions, oral hygiene instructions, patient motivation, functional therapy (when required), and surgical elimination of defects (when needed to aid plaque control).

In addition, a periodic recall system for follow-up of periodontal patients is necessary. This is designed for the long-term control of dental disease. For periodontal patients the maintenance phase should (1) be tailored to the needs of the individual patient; (2) include meticulous scaling and polishing; (3) include thorough review of oral hygiene; (4) include examination for the return of etiologic factors of periodontal disease, as well as documentation and treatment of these factors; and (5) include examination for loss of attachment or deepening pockets, increased tooth mobility, or other pathosis, recording and treating any that are observed. The maintenance phase is extremely important for the overall management of the periodontal patient.

SUMMARY

ANUG is an opportunistic bacterial infection of the gingivae that is associated with stress in individuals who cope poorly and that results in temporary depression of PMN function(s). It usually occurs in otherwise healthy young adults and is rapidly destructive. The most important symptoms are the typical necrotic and ulcerated interproximal papillae, bleeding, and pain. Proper treatment includes thorough mechanical debridement via subgingival scaling and root planing, oral irrigation at home, establishment of good oral hygiene, repair of remaining deformities, and a recall and maintenance program to prevent recurrences of ANUG, as well as other periodontal diseases.

The most difficult problem in the treatment of ANUG is not in recognition and treatment, but in patient management. Maintaining patient cooperation and participation beyond relief of pain is the most challenging part of ANUG therapy. Patients must understand that the high rate of disease recurrence results from patient neglect and that they must assume a major part of the responsibility for the outcome of the disease and its various sequelae.

REFERENCES

Barling B: Chronic cyclical granulopenia, Proc R Soc Med 41:653, 1948.
Claffey N, Russell R, and Shanley D: Peripheral blood phagocyte function in acute necrotizing ulcerative gingivitis, J Periodont Res 21:288, 1986.
Cogen RB et al: Leukocyte function in the etiology of acute necrotizing ulcerative gingivitis, J Periodontol 54:402, 1983.
Cohen MM: Periodontal disturbances in the mentally subnormal child, Dent Clin North Am, p 483, July 1960.
Cohen-Cole S et al: Psychosocial and endocrine aspects of acute necrotizing ulcerative gingivitis, Psychiatr Med 1:215, 1983.

Davis RK and Baer PN: Necrotic ulcerative gingivitis in drug addict patients being withdrawn from drugs, Oral Surg 31:200, 1971.

Emslie RD: Cancrum oris, Dent Pract 13:481, 1963.

Emslie RD: Clinical trials of treatment for acute periodontal diseases, Int Dent J 21:33, 1971.

Enwonwu CO: Epidemiological and biochemical studies of necrotizing ulcerative gingivitis and noma (cancrum oris) in Nigerian children, Arch Oral Biol 17:1357, 1972.

Formicola AJ, Witte ET, and Curran PM: A study of personality traits and acute necrotizing ulcerative gingivitis, J Periodontol 31:36, 1970.

Giddon DB, Zackin SJ, and Goldhaber P: Acute necrotizing ulcerative gingivitis in college students, J Am Dent Assoc 68:381, 1964.

Goldberg HJV: Acute necrotizing ulcerative gingivitis, J Oral Ther 2:451, 1966.

Goldhaber P and Giddon DB: Present concepts concerning the etiology and treatment of acute necrotizing ulcerative gingivitis, Int Dent J 14:468, 1964.

Grupe HE and Wilder LS: Observations of necrotizing gingivitis in 870 military trainees, J Periodontol 27:255, 1956.

Jiménez M and Baer PN: Necrotizing ulcerative gingivitis in children: a 9 year clinical study, J Periodontol 46:715, 1975.

Johnson BD and Engel D: Acute necrotizing ulcerative gingivitis: a review of diagnosis, etiology and treatment, J Periodontol 57:141, 1986.

Johnson MP and Young MA: Periodontal disease in Mongols, J Periodontol 34:41, 1963.

Klotz H: Differentiation between necrotic ulcerative gingivitis and primary herpetic gingivostomatitis, NY State Dent J 39:283, 1973.

Levy EJ and Schetman D: Cyclic neutropenia, Arch Dermatol 84:429, 1961.

Libby RH: The use of antibiotics in the treatment of necrotizing ulcerative gingivitis, J West Soc Periodont 10:27, 1963.

Listgarten MA: Electron microscopic observations on the bacterial flora of acute necrotizing ulcerative gingivitis, J Periodontol 36:328, 1965.

Loesche WJ et al: The bacteriology of acute necrotizing ulcerative gingivitis, J Periodontol 53:223, 1982.

Manhold JH, Doyle JC, and Weisinger EH: Effects of social stress on oral and other tissues. II. Results offering substance to a hypothesis for the mechanism of formation of periodontal pathology, J Periodontol 42:109, 1971.

Manson JD and Rand H: Recurrent Vincent's disease: a survey of 61 cases, Br Dent J 110:386, 1961.

Maupin CC and Bell WB: The relationship of 17-hydroxycorticosteroid to acute necrotizing ulcerative gingivitis, J Periodontol 46:721, 1975.

Miller SC and Greene HI: A worldwide survey of acute necrotizing ulcerative gingivitis: a preliminary report, J Dent Res 13:66, 1958.

Moulton R, Ewen S, and Thieman W: Emotional factors in periodontal disease, Oral Surg Oral Med Oral Pathol 5:833, 1952.

Pickard HM: Historical aspects of Vincent's disease, Proc R Soc Med 66:695, 1973.

Pindborg JJ: Gingivitis in military personnel with special reference to ulceromembranous gingivitis, Odontol Revy 59:407, 1951.

Pindborg JJ, Bhat M, and Roed-Petersen B: Oral changes in South Indian children with severe protein deficiency, J Periodontol 38:218, 1967.

Rogers MP, Dubey D, and Reich P: The influence of the psyche and the brain on immunity and disease susceptibility: a critical review, Psychosom Med 41:147, 1979.

Rosebury T and Sonnenwirth AC: Bacteria indigenous to man. In Dubos RJ, editor: Bacteria and mycotic infection in man, Philadelphia, 1958, JB Lippincott Co.

Schluger S: Necrotizing ulcerative gingivitis in the Army: incidence, communicability and treatment, J Am Dent Assoc 38:174, 1949.

Shannon IL, Kilgore WG, and O'Leary TJ: Stress as a predisposing factor in necrotizing gingivitis, J Periodontol 40:240, 1969.

Slots J: Importance of black-pigmented *Bacteroides* in human periodontal disease. In Genco RJ and Mergenhagen SE, editors: Host-parasite interactions in periodontal diseases, p 27, Washington, DC, 1982, American Society for Microbiology.

Stammers AT: Vincent's infection: observations on histopathology and their applications to clinical practice, Br Dent J 81:4, 1946.

Stevens AW et al: Demographic and clinical data associated with acute necrotizing ulcerative gingivitis in a dental school population, J Clin Periodontol 11:487, 1984.

Wennstrom J and Lindhe J: Effect of hydrogen peroxide on developing plaque and gingivitis in man, J Clin Periodontol 6:115, 1979.

Wintrobe MM: Clinical hematology, Philadelphia, 1967, Lea & Febiger.

Chapter 39

SPECIAL CONSIDERATIONS IN THE TREATMENT OF JUVENILE PERIODONTITIS

Lars A. Christersson

Periodontal diseases are not restricted to adults; they also affect children and adolescents, resulting in loss of teeth and subsequent functional and esthetic handicaps. Also, periodontal disease in the young may predispose the patient to adult forms of periodontitis.

The most common form of periodontal disease evident in younger age groups is *localized juvenile periodontitis* (LJP; formerly referred to as periodontosis). LJP has been defined as a disease occurring in otherwise healthy individuals, under age 30, with destructive periodontitis localized to the first permanent molars and incisors, and not involving more than two other teeth (Van Dyke et al., 1980). This disease is reported to affect 0.02% to 0.8% of children and teenagers, with the higher prevalence occurring in African-Caribbeans (Saxby, 1987).

This disease form was described by Gottlieb at the beginning of the twentieth century as a chronic, degenera-tive, noninflammatory disease of the periodontal tissues, which he referred to as "diffuse atrophy of alveolar bone" (Gottlieb, 1923). Gottlieb postulated that this disease was caused by systemic factors, a view supported by histologic studies reporting degeneration of the gingival connective tissue. However, more recent histopathologic studies have shown mainly inflammatory changes (Liljenberg and Lindhe, 1980).

Extensive periodontal destruction can be present in LJP even though in many cases little evidence of "local irri-tants"—dental plaque and calculus—is found around the affected teeth. Recently there has been a rapid accumula-tion of evidence that LJP is primarily the result of an in-fection with specific microorganisms, including *Actinoba-cillus actinomycetemcomitans,* in the subgingival flora.

Generalized juvenile periodontitis (GJP) has been de-fined as destructive periodontitis affecting more than 14 teeth in individuals under age 30 (i.e., it is generalized to an arch or an entire dentition) (Van Dyke et al., 1980). There is often marked inflammation of the gingiva and cal-culus formation. Whereas the localized form is clinically distinct and may represent a homogeneous disease, GJP most likely represents a collection of diseases that includes the localized form (LJP), which has become generalized; early-onset adult periodontitis of a generalized nature; and alveolar bone loss associated with recurrent acute necrotiz-ing ulcerative gingivitis (ANUG) (Genco et al., 1986).

Studies on the subgingival microbiota associated with juvenile forms of periodontitis have led to the current rec-ognition of *A. actinomycetemcomitans* as a key organism in the etiology and pathology of LJP. Other forms of periodontitis in juveniles have been associated with *A. actino-mycetemcomitans,* but these have also been associated with *Bacteroides gingivalis, Eikenella corrodens,* and other microorganisms that have been implicated as being important in adult forms of periodontitis (Zambon et al., 1986; Genco et al., 1988).

A number of systemic diseases in children and adolescents include periodontal disease as a complication. Most of these involve primary or secondary neutrophil disorders and are discussed in detail in Chapter 16. The primary neutrophil disorders associated with periodontal disease include neutropenia, Chédiak-Higashi syndrome, and leukocyte adherence abnormalities. Systemic diseases with secondary neutrophil disorders and periodontal disease complications include diabetes mellitus, Down's syndrome, Crohn's disease, Papillon-Lefèvre syndrome, and the preleukemic syndrome.

The near future may very well bring information allowing for a definitive classification of periodontal diseases based on biologic grounds (bacteriologic and/or host response factors), and we may see an end to the present multitude of arbitrarily designed classifications based mainly on clinical characteristics. However, presently it is convenient to classify periodontal diseases based on these clinical characteristics, as shown in the box below.

Periodontitis in systemically healthy individuals

1. Localized juvenile periodontitis (LJP; periodontosis)
2. Generalized juvenile periodontitis (GJP)
   a. GJP preceded by LJP
   b. Early-onset adult periodontitis
   c. Recurrent acute necrotizing ulcerative periodontitis (ANUG)

LOCALIZED JUVENILE PERIODONTITIS
Diagnosis

Clinically, LJP is characterized by alveolar bone loss most often affecting the permanent first molars and incisor teeth of adolescents and teenagers (Fig. 39-1). The disease becomes apparent at about the time of puberty, usually between the ages of 10 and 15 years. In a retrospective study of 17 LJP patients, however, it was found that all but 1 had radiographic evidence of bone loss in the primary teeth, suggesting an early onset for LJP (Sjödin et al., 1989). The localized pattern of alveolar bone loss often leads to a characteristic radiographic appearance of "mirror image" osseous defects on both sides of the dental arch. In contrast to previous clinical observations, dental plaque is present on the root surfaces in areas of periodontal pocket formation in LJP patients, although not always in the large amounts associated with patients with adult periodontitis. Subgingival calculus is, however, rare in LJP.

Bleeding on probing of the periodontal pockets is also evident, reflecting ulceration of the pocket epithelium. This has been confirmed by histologic examination of LJP lesions, which reveals numerous areas of chronic inflammation containing polymorphonuclear leukocytes, lymphocytes, and large numbers of plasma cells. Histologic evidence of inflammation is particularly prominent in the gingival epithelium and connective tissues near the base of the periodontal pocket. Gingival inflammation does not necessarily extend to the marginal gingiva or to the oral epithelium. This most likely accounts for the occasional lack of clinically apparent gingivitis even where the gingiva overlies areas of severe alveolar bone loss.

The subgingival microbial flora of LJP lesions is well described, and evidence has rapidly accumulated to indicate that this disease is caused by an infection with specific microorganisms (see Chapter 11). In LJP 60% to 70% of

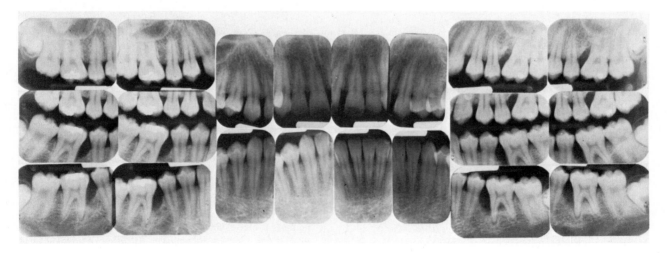

Fig. 39-1. Full-mouth radiographic examination of a 17-year-old girl showing severe bone loss at three (molars only) of the typical LJP predilection sites. Note that alveolar bone height at upper first right molar is intact.

the subgingival flora in periodontal lesions can be made up of *A. actinomycetemcomitans*. This organism is found in low prevalence and in low numbers in subgingival sites of normal juveniles and in patients with other forms of periodontal disease. For example, in studies by Zambon et al. (1983), 97% of LJP patients (28/29) were heavily infected with *A. actinomycetemcomitans*. This compared with fewer than 20% of periodontally healthy individuals (24/142), who harbored very small numbers of the organism.

A. actinomycetemcomitans is a human pathogen that can cause severe extraoral infections, including endocarditis, brain, facial and thyroid abscesses, osteomyelitis, meningitis, and urinary tract infections. It is often found in actinomycotic lesions along with *Actinomyces israelii* in the "sulfur granules," which is reflected in its name.

Several lines of evidence incriminate *A. actinomycetemcomitans* as a key etiologic agent in LJP and can be summarized as follows (Zambon et al., 1988):

1. The organism is found in high numbers in periodontal lesions in LJP patients, whereas it is either not present or is present in very low numbers in healthy sites in these same patients. It is found in a small proportion of, and in low numbers in, normal juveniles and normal adults.

2. Over 90% of LJP patients have high titers of serum IgG antibodies to *A. actinomycetemcomitans*. Often these antibodies show remarkable specificity and are directed to antigens of the *A. actinomycetemcomitans* serotype infecting the patient.

3. *A. actinomycetemcomitans* possesses several potent virulence factors. These include an endotoxin that can cause bone resorption, a leukotoxin that kills neutrophils, and a chemotaxis-inhibiting factor that can impair the migration of neutrophils to sites of infection. Also, *A. actinomycetemcomitans* can induce suppression of lymphocyte responses to mitogens and antigens and is very resistant to killing by serum bactericidal mechanisms.

4. Elimination of *A. actinomycetemcomitans* from periodontal lesions by therapeutic measures results in healing, whereas failure to eliminate the organism is associated with continuous periodontal attachment loss.

Treatment

LJP has been considered difficult to treat, and a number of modalities have been used in the treatment of this disease with varying degrees of success. Also, LJP lesions were thought to have a pronounced tendency to recur, and the long-term result was highly unpredictable.

Traditionally, a combination of meticulous scaling and root planing, periodontal surgery, systemic antibiotics, and tooth extraction has been used in the treatment of LJP. However, the disease often recurred or remained active in up to 25% of patients. A marked improvement in treatment success of LJP came with the recognition of the importance of *A. actinomycetemcomitans* in its etiology. Successful treatment of LJP now is based on the rationale of the elimination of this organism from subgingival locations (Slots and Rosling, 1983; Christersson et al., 1985; Mandell et al., 1986; Zambon et al., 1986; Mandell and Socransky, 1988).

Mechanical debridement of periodontal pockets by scaling and root planing is ineffective in suppressing *A. actinomycetemcomitans* in most periodontal pockets (Christersson et al., 1985) (Fig. 39-2). In fact, *local* therapy (mechanical and antibiotic) directed to suppressing the pocket flora may eliminate competing microorganisms from the periodontal pocket and often results in a subgingival flora dominated by *A. actinomycetemcomitans* (Slots and Rosling, 1983; Mandell et al., 1986).

Inability to eliminate *A. actinomycetemcomitans* from subgingival sites of LJP by mechanical treatment alone is most likely related to the ability of this microorganism to invade deep into the gingival connective tissues (Saglie et al., 1982, 1986; Christersson et al., 1987a, 1987b) (see Figs. 5-14 and 5-15). This is a key feature of LJP that is not generally seen in other types of periodontal disease. Apparently, *A. actinomycetemcomitans* can persist in soft

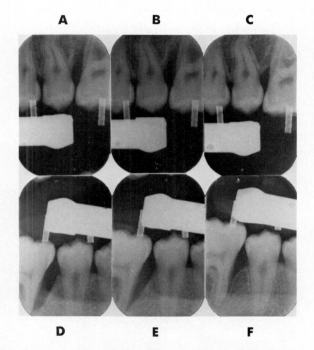

Fig. 39-2. Radiographs of upper left and lower right first molar defects in a 17-year-old girl. **A** and **D** show conditions before therapy. **B** and **E** show conditions 6 months after thorough scaling and root planing. Patient was still heavily infected by *A. actinomycetemcomitans* at this time. **C** and **F** show conditions 24 months following initial treatment, after additional treatment by a modified Widman flap procedure and systemic tetracycline hydrochloride.

tissues even after scaling and root planing or locally applied antibiotics have temporarily suppressed the flora of periodontal pockets and the root surfaces.

Periodontal surgical procedures have the potential for successful elimination of *A. actinomycetemcomitans;* however, the predictability is too low for it to be an acceptable routine treatment regimen. This is shown in a study in which excision of *A. actinomycetemcomitans*–infected gingival tissues by periodontal surgical procedures, such as the Widman flap procedure or gingival curettage, resulted in a reduction of the levels of this microorganism in sites involved by the surgical procedure (Christersson et al., 1985). However, small areas of infected tissue were found to remain unless large amounts of tissue were sacrificed. It is these "reservoirs" of remaining infection that are most likely to lead to the often-observed continued and recurrent disease (Christersson et al., 1985).

The optimal procedure for elimination of subgingival *A. actinomycetemcomitans* is a combination of systemic antibiotic therapy and mechanical local debridement of root surfaces and infected gingival tissues. This therapy results in successful treatment of LJP (Lindhe, 1982; Slots and Rosling, 1983; Christersson et al., 1989).

Systemic antibiotic therapy without concomitant mechanical debridement can eliminate subgingival *A. actinomycetemcomitans;* however, this treatment modality may require extended periods of antibiotic administration, depending on the choice of drug.

Meticulous scaling and root planing can remove most subgingival bacteria, including a large portion of *A. actinomycetemcomitans,* from accessible areas, leading to reduced total numbers of subgingival organisms. However, duced total numbers of subgingival organisms. However,

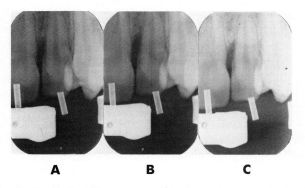

A **B** **C**

Fig. 39-3. Radiographs of upper left lateral of a 14-year-old girl diagnosed as having LJP. **A,** Conditions before therapy. **B,** Conditions 12 months after treatment with thorough scaling and root planing only. Patient tested positive for subgingival *A. actinomycetemcomitans* at all recall visits during this first year. Note increased loss of alveolar bone. **C,** Conditions 24 months after initiation of therapy. Patient now tested negative for subgingival *A. actinomycetemcomitans.* After 12-month evaluation patient was treated with additional scaling and root planing in conjunction with systemic tetracycline hydrochloride.

the proportion of *A. actinomycetemcomitans* in the subgingival plaque is often increased. Periodontal surgery can also reduce the numbers of *A. actinomycetemcomitans* by excision of the infected gingival tissues and, if successful, allow normal healing to occur. The addition of systemic antibiotic therapy to the treatment will eliminate the remaining *A. actinomycetemcomitans* (Slots and Rosling, 1983; Mandell and Socransky, 1988; Christersson et al., 1989). With the use of this regimen for the treatment of LJP, the bacterial etiology is eliminated. Such treatment will halt the progression of the disease, provide an environment for healing, and minimize the potential for recurrence (Fig. 39-3).

The systemic antibiotic should be given concomitantly with mechanical debridement to allow maximum effect and should be continued until the patient tests negative for *A. actinomycetemcomitans* in subgingival plaque samples. It is imperative that systemic antibiotic administration be administered beyond the point where *A. actinomycetemcomitans* is no longer detectable in the subgingival flora.

The choice of antibiotic is important; however, it is essential that clinical monitoring be carefully carried out, and if inflammation persists, microbiologic monitoring should be instituted to ensure successful therapy. Traditionally, tetracyclines have been used successfully (Lindhe, 1982; Slots and Rosling, 1983). Tetracycline's effect is bacteriostatic and therefore may not be ideal. Drugs with a bactericidal effect, such as amoxicillin, penicillin, and erythromycin, have also been used to treat LJP. Recently the combination of amoxicillin and metronidazole was demonstrated to be particularly effective in eliminating *A. actinomycetemcomitans.* The concomitant administration of the two drugs has had remarkable effectiveness in eliminating subgingival *A. actinomycetemcomitans,* not only in LJP, but also in patients with refractory adult periodontitis who harbor subgingival *A. actinomycetemcomitans* after repeated unsuccessful therapy (Christersson et al., 1989; van Winkelhoff et al., 1989) (Fig. 39-4).

Microbiologic monitoring of treatment of LJP patients is performed on a routine basis today because of the 25% failure rate in therapy that has been observed even with the use of antibiotics such as tetracycline (Lindhe, 1982; Slots and Rosling, 1983). On the other hand, microbiologic tests may not be necessary for diagnosis of LJP, since 97% of patients harbor *A. actinomycetemcomitans* and hence there is a high probability of finding *A. actinomycetemcomitans* in patients with classical first molar–incisor LJP.

Local delivery of antibiotics has recently become a popular alternative to systemic administration and is an attractive and effective approach for treatment of most adult forms of periodontal disease. However, local application of antimicrobial agents as an adjunct to mechanical debridement is ineffective in eradicating *A. actinomycetemcomitans* from heavily infected periodontal leions. So far, studies have failed to find a local chemical agent effective against *A. actinomycetemcomitans*. The reason may very well be that *A. actinomycetemcomitans* is protected from the effects of topical subgingival antimicrobial agents when the organism is located deep in the tissues.

A good example of the failure of local delivery of antibiotics in LJP is the poor to alarming results from a study using fibers for the delivery of tetracycline hydrochloride into the pockets (Mandell et al., 1986). The results of lo-

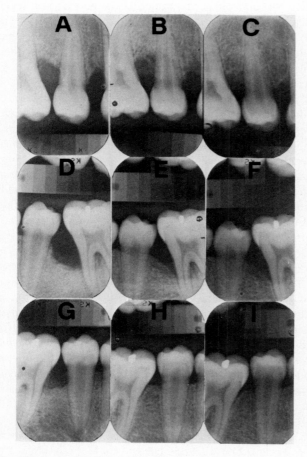

Fig. 39-4. Radiographs of upper first molar region, **A** to **C,** lower left first molar, **D** to **F,** and lower right first molar, **G** to **I,** of a 15-year-old boy with LJP. **A, D,** and **G** show initial conditions when treatment was initiated. Patient was at this time heavily infected with *A. actinomycetemcomitans* in all three subgingival areas. **B, E,** and **H** show conditions at 12 months postoperatively. Treatment consisted of initial preparation followed by periodontal surgery (modified Widman flap) and systemic tetracycline hydrochloride. Note that **E** and **H** show bone fill associated with clinical healing. However, **B** shows further loss of alveolar bone associated with remaining infection of *A. actinomycetemcomitans*. **C, F,** and **I** indicate clinical success with bone fill in all three original defects at 24 months following additional treatment by scaling and root planing in conjunction with concomitant systemic administration of amoxicillin and metronidazole. (From Christersson LA et al: J Dent Res 68, 1989 [abstract 128].)

cal drug delivery when employed on typical LJP defects are similar to those achieved by scaling and root planing alone. The treatment thoroughly depresses the main portion of the subgingival plaque without total eradication of *A. actinomycetemcomitans* and with a subsequent overgrowth of *A. actinomycetemcomitans*.

Local delivery of antiinfective drugs is not currently recommended for the treatment of LJP, either alone or in combination with mechanical procedures. Furthermore, caution should also be exercised in the use of topical subgingival antimicrobial therapy in adults who are infected with *A. actinomycetemcomitans*, since a similar overgrowth of *A. actinomycetemcomitans* after therapy has been observed.

Maintenance

LJP has generally been considered to recur easily. However, with the introduction of bacterial monitoring, the recurrence rate has been dramatically reduced. The maintenance for these patients can now be based on adjunctive microbiologic criteria rather than clinical characteristics alone. The fully treated LJP case (i.e., where clinical and radiologic evidence of active periodontal destruction are absent and *A. actinomycetemcomitans* has been successfully eradicated from subgingival sites) has a low tendency to recur. The recurrence rates are likely to be similar to or lower than those for adult forms of periodontal disease.

Prevention

Factors other than *A. actinomycetemcomitans* infection alone are likely to contribute to the initiation and development of LJP. *A. actinomycetemcomitans* is present in approximately 20% of the normal adult population, and LJP has a prevalence of 0.2% or less, suggesting other contributing factors for disease development. One candidate is reduced host resistance associated with neutrophil defects, which is seen in 70% of LJP patients (see Chapter 16).

LJP occurs only in children and adolescents; hence aging of the patient is a favorable factor in the maintenance of health. The typical age for LJP onset is between 10 and 20 years; thereafter, this disease rarely develops.

Recommendations for the prevention and maintenance of *A. actinomycetemcomitans*–associated periodontitis can be formulated as follows:

1. Institution of meticulous supragingival plaque control, since *A. actinomycetemcomitans* reinfection or infection by other periodontal pathogens may be enhanced by the accumulation of supragingival plaque and subsequent gingival changes. Also, typically, LJP patients may have several locations with "hard-to-reach" areas that need particular attention.
2. Careful clinical and microbiologic monitoring of family members or other close contacts of the LJP patient. Elimination of periodontal lesions harboring

A. actinomycetemcomitans from family members or contacts is likely to decrease interpersonal or intrafamilial transmission of this bacteria.

LJP has a marked tendency to occur among members of the same family, suggesting that genetic or hereditary factors may be involved in the pathogenesis of this disease (Cohen and Goldman, 1960). LJP is rare, affecting approximately 0.2% of the population. However, recent data indicate that an individual having a brother or sister with LJP may have a dramatically increased chance of also developing the disease (Van Dyke et al., 1985). Close to 25% of siblings in affected families develop the disease, and the risk for development of LJP in families with neutrophil chemotactic defects is 10 times greater than that in families with normal neutrophils (Van Dyke et al., 1985). The genetic component of LJP is also reflected in the fact that certain blood groups and major histocompatibility tissue antigens are found in higher prevalence in LJP patients than in periodontally normal control groups. However, these findings are controversial, and some groups have reported no differences in LJP as compared with controls.

A major contribution to our understanding of the familial and possible genetic link of LJP comes from the finding that in most families who suffer from this disease, both diseased and normal siblings have neutrophil function defects (Van Dyke et al., 1985). Hence it appears that at least two factors may be responsible for the familial nature of LJP: infection with *A. actinomycetemcomitans* and depressed host protective response.

Monitoring of *A. actinomycetemcomitans* in subgingival plaque is the most important means of preventing the development of the disease in the typical high-risk patient. The use of systemic antimicrobials should be considered justifiable here. At the first sign of significant infection with *A. actinomycetemcomitans* and with early signs of LJP, the high-risk patient should be treated with systemic antimicrobial therapy and debridement. Similarly, a previously treated patient should be given antibiotics and debridement at the first sign of reinfection. The choice of antibiotic includes tetracycline hydrochloride or the combination of amoxicillin and metronidazole, and these should be administered until *A. actinomycetemcomitans* is no longer detected in the subgingival flora.

A systematic community-based program for prevention of primary infection with LJP may not be cost-effective at this time. However, new techniques for rapid detection of periodontal pathogens and an increased understanding of their respective roles may lead to guidelines that warrant screenings of 10- to 12-year-olds, particularly if noninvasive techniques for detection of *A. actinomycetemcomitans* in saliva or oral washes can be employed. Hypothetically, a screening for pertinent pathogens such as *A. actinomycetemcomitans* combined with a screening for known host-related risk factors could form the basis for an effective targeted program to prevent periodontitis.

GENERALIZED JUVENILE PERIODONTITIS
Diagnosis

Clinically, GJP is diagnosed on the basis of the broad distribution of alveolar bone and attachment loss throughout the dentition. In contrast to the localized form, alveolar bone loss involves more than the first molars and incisors, extending to other molars, premolars, and canines.

The current theory is that most cases of GJP may result from spreading of the localized form. This has been suggested by cross-sectional studies indicating an age-related increase in the number of teeth involved in groups of juveniles with periodontal disease (Hørmand and Frandsen, 1979; Saxén and Murtomaa, 1986). It appears that at least this form of periodontitis is familial and a clinical variant of LJP. Support for this theory comes from the finding that GJP patients often have neutrophil defects resembling those found in LJP patients.

Generalized periodontal disease in juveniles may also result from early onset of adult periodontitis or from repeated episodes of ANUG that has progressed to periodontitis. The patient history is useful in distinguishing previous experience of ANUG from other forms of periodontitis, and the family history or previous dental radiographs can indicate GJP secondary to progression of LJP.

Studies of the microbial flora in GJP are limited to a description of one or a few cases in each study, since the disease is uncommon. In general, these reports show black-pigmented *Bacteroides* species and *A. actinomycetemcomitans* as prominent subgingival organisms associated with periodontal lesions (Wilson et al., 1985).

Much more work is needed to determine which microorganisms are responsible for periodontitis, including "rapidly aggressive periodontitis," in adolescents and young adults. Microbiologic studies may lead to the subdivision of non-LJP types of juvenile periodontitis into several distinct entities, each associated with different periodontal pathogens.

Treatment

Generally, the treatment of GJP follows the same guidelines as for LJP. Namely, the bacterial infection has to be eliminated, and therapy is chosen to suppress the pathogenic bacteria, as well as to eliminate inflammation (Fig. 39-5).

Particular attention should be given to systemically diseased patients such as diabetic patients and those with neutrophil disorders who suffer from periodontitis. Generally, the use of systemic antimicrobials in combination with debridement is indicated in these patients. The cautious approach of giving an initial regimen of a systemic antibiotic in combination with mechanical debridement is recommended. The systemically compromised host has a high tendency for treatment complications such as abscesses and other exacerbations. These events are largely avoided if the periodontal pathogens are suppressed. A combina-

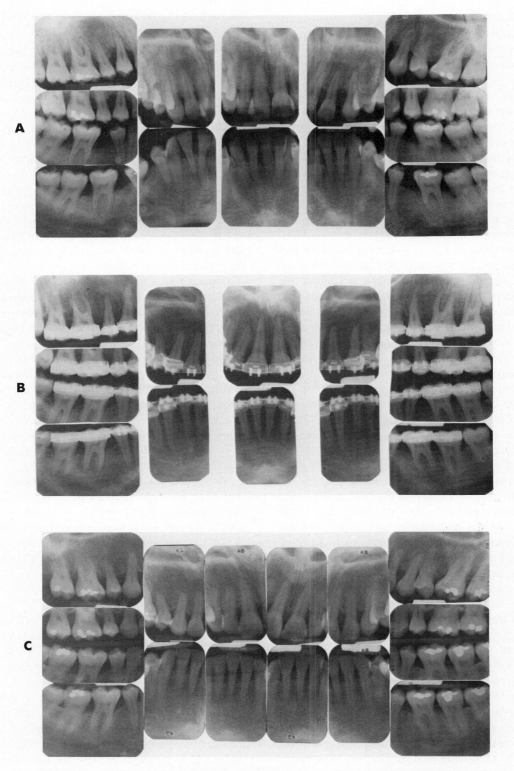

Fig. 39-5. **A,** Full-mouth radiographic examination of a 24-year-old woman showing severe bone loss around most teeth, qualifying patient for clinical diagnosis of GJP. Note that tooth migration has resulted in malpositioning and overlapping of teeth. **B,** Full-mouth radiographic examination of same patient 2 years after completion of comprehensive antiinfective treatment phase. Radiographs indicate use of orthodontic treatment to correct remaining malpositioning. **C,** Full-mouth radiographic examination 12 years after treatment. Note generally more favorable alveolar bone height indicating long-term successful elimination of periodontal infection.

tion of antibiotics supported by mechanical debridement and often repeated regimens of antibiotics may be necessary to resolve periodontitis in these systemically compromised patients.

The use of periodontal surgery should be kept to a minimum, since these patients, especially those with uncontrolled diabetes and those with neutrophil disorders, may have aberrations affecting wound healing, leading to excessive pain and/or unnecessary loss of supporting tissues.

Maintenance

The repeated use of antibiotics may be considered for GJP; however, culture and antibiotic sensitivity testing of the subgingival flora is often useful in selecting the antibiotics to be used to treat recurrences. Also, intermittent use of chlorhexidine mouth rinse is an effective aid in the maintenance of systemically compromised patients. Prolonged use may have certain disadvantages; however, a regimen of alternating 4 weeks of chlorhexidine rinse with 2 to 4 weeks without the rinse has been used successfully for long periods of time with no severe adverse effects.

JUVENILE PERIODONTITIS IN THE COMPROMISED HOST

Most individuals who suffer from localized (molar-incisor) or other forms of juvenile periodontitis are otherwise healthy and do not exhibit any obvious systemic disease. Destructive periodontitis may affect either or both the primary and permanent dentitions of children and young adults with systemic diseases.

It is generally recognized that periodontitis does not occur in young children before puberty, except as a manifestation of some other disease state. For example, periodontitis in patients before puberty has been found to be associated with neutropenia, Papillon-Lefèvre syndrome, and leukocyte adhesion deficiency.

There have been reports of prepubertal periodontal disease in apparently normal children; however, these children may have an undetected immune defect or systemic disease. It is therefore important that children with prepubertal periodontitis be carefully examined for systemic disease or a history of recurrent infections or chronic skin disorders (see Chapter 16).

The diagnosis, treatment, and maintenance of these patients is complex, and the periodontal condition is important in total patient management, especially in diabetic patients. Generally, treatment and maintenance approaches are similar to those advocated for GJP patients.

SUMMARY AND FUTURE DIRECTIONS

In the future, periodontal diagnosis, patient classification, and treatment will rely more on microbiologic findings than currently is common. Specifically, increased knowledge regarding the composition of subgingival plaque and the relative importance of individual or combinations of periodontal bacteria will be used in the classification of periodontal diseases. Furthermore, the use of antibiotics will become more sophisticated, with single drugs or drug combinations indicated for specific pathogens on the basis of their antimicrobial sensitivity pattern. This is perhaps best illustrated today in the diagnosis and treatment of LJP.

REFERENCES

Christersson LA et al: Microbiological and clinical effects of surgical treatment of localized juvenile periodontitis, J Clin Periodontol 12:465, 1985.

Christersson LA et al: Tissue localization of *Actinobacillus actinomycetemcomitans* in human periodontitis. I. Light, immunofluorescence and electron microscopic studies, J Periodontol 58:529, 1987a.

Christersson LA et al: Tissue localization of *Actinobacillus actinomycetemcomitans* in human periodontitis. II. Correlation between immunofluorescence and culture techniques, J Periodontol 58:540, 1987b.

Christersson LA et al: Systemic antibiotic combination therapy in recalcitrant and recurrent localized juvenile periodontitis, J Dent Res 68, 1989 (abstract 128).

Cohen DW and Goldman HM: Clinical observations on the modification of human oral tissue metabolism by local intraoral factors, Ann NY Acad Sci 85:68, March 1960.

Genco RJ, Christersson LA, and Zambon JJ: Juvenile periodontitis, Int Dent J 36:168, 1986.

Genco RJ, Zambon JJ, and Christersson LA: The origin of periodontal infections, Adv Dent Res 2(2):1, 1988.

Gottlieb B: Die diffuse Atrophie des Alveolarknochens: Weitere Beiträ zur Kenntnis des Alveolarschwundes und dessen Weidergutmachung durch Zementwachstum, Z Stomatol 21:195, 1923.

Hørmand J and Frandsen A: Juvenile periodontitis: localization of bone loss in relation to age, sex and teeth, J Clin Periodontol 6:407, 1979.

Liljenberg B and Lindhe J: Juvenile periodontitis: some microbiological, histopathological and clinical characteristics, J Clin Periodontol 7:48, 1980.

Lindhe J: Treatment of localized juvenile periodontitis. In Genco RJ and Mergenhagen SE, editors: Host parasite interactions in periodontal diseases, Washington, DC, 1982, ASM Publications.

Mandell RL and Socransky SS: Microbiological and clinical effects of surgery plus doxycycline on juvenile periodontitis, J Periodontol 59:373, 1988.

Mandell RL et al: The effect of treatment on *Actinobacillus actinomycetemcomitans* in localized juvenile periodontitis, J Periodontol 57:94, 1986.

Saglie FR et al: Identification of tissue-invading bacteria in human periodontal disease, J Periodont Res 17:452, 1982.

Saglie FR et al: The presence of bacteria in oral epithelium in periodontal disease. II. Immunohistochemical identification of bacteria, J Periodontol 57:492, 1986.

Saxby MS: Juvenile periodontitis: an epidemiologic study in west midlands of the United Kingdom, J Clin Periodontol 14:594, 1987.

Saxén L and Murtomaa H: Age-related expression of juvenile periodontitis, J Clin Periodontol 12:21, 1985.

Sjödin B et al: A retrospective radiographic study of alveolar bone loss in the primary dentition in patients with localized juvenile periodontitis, J Clin Periodontol 16:124, 1989.

Slots J and Rosling BG: Suppression of the periodontopathic microflora in localized juvenile periodontitis by systemic tetracycline, J Clin Periodontol 10:465, 1983.

Van Dyke TE et al: Neutrophil chemotaxis dysfunction in human periodontitis, Infect Immun 27(1):123, 1980.

Van Dyke TE et al: Neutrophil chemotaxis in families with localized juvenile periodontitis, J Periodont Res 20:503, 1985.

van Winkelhoff AJ et al: Metronidazole plus amoxicillin in the treatment of *Actinobacillus actinomycetemcomitans* associated periodontitis, J Clin Periodontol 16:128, 1989.

Wilson ME et al: Generalized juvenile periodontitis, defective neutrophil chemotaxis and *Bacteroides gingivalis* in a 13-year-old female: a case report, J Periodontol 56:457, 1985.

Zambon JJ, Christersson LA, and Genco RJ: Diagnosis and treatment of localized juvenile periodontitis, J Am Dent Assoc 113:295, 1986.

Zambon JJ, Christersson LA, and Slots J: *Actinobacillus actinomycetemcomitans* in human periodontal disease: prevalence in patient groups and distribution of biotypes and serotypes within families, J Peridontol 54:707, 1983.

Zambon JJ et al: *Actinobacillus actinomycetemcomitans* in the pathogenesis of human periodontal disease, Adv Dent Res 2(2): 269, 1988.

Chapter 40

TREATMENT OF PERIODONTAL ABSCESSES

William J. Killoy

Periodontal abscesses have been recognized as a distinct clinical entity since the latter part of the nineteenth century. The International Conference on Research in the Biology of Periodontal Disease in 1977 defined a *periodontal abscess* as "an acute, destructive process in the periodontium resulting in localized collections of pus communicating with the oral cavity through the gingival sulcus or other periodontal sites and not arising from the tooth pulp" (Ranney, 1977). Although reference is often made to a chronic form (Grant et al, 1972), chronic periodontal abscesses may be indistinguishable from lesions of chronic periodontitis, even when fistulation is present. When an abscess is confined to the marginal gingiva, it has been termed a *gingival abscess* (McFall, 1964; O'Brien, 1970).

In spite of their long historical recognition, periodontal abscesses often present a challenge in terms of diagnosis, etiology, treatment, and prognosis. An accurate diagnosis and effective treatment must be given immediately. The dentist must therefore have an established and effective treatment program based on recognition of the clinical symptoms, an accurate differential diagnosis, and an understanding of the etiologic factors.

CLINICAL FEATURES

The periodontal abscess is often associated with a pre-existing periodontal pocket. Some acute periodontal abscesses are associated with impaction of foreign objects—frequently seeds, corn kernels, or nut husks lodged in the gingival sulcus or pocket. As long as the pocket communicates with the oral cavity, infectious material within the pocket can drain. If the orifice of the pocket becomes occluded by impaction of a foreign object or by healing, purulent material within the pocket cannot drain. The infectious material then accumulates within the occluded pocket, resulting in many of the following clinical symptoms.

The most common symptom is pain. The patient is usually oblivious to most of the accompanying symptoms until pain becomes evident. Gingival and/or mucosal swelling is often seen in the area of pain. The swelling can vary from a small enlargement of the gingival unit to a diffuse swelling involving the gingiva, alveolar mucosa, and oral mucosa and may extend to the face and neck. The affected tissues will be red to reddish blue. The swelling and associated changes are usually adjacent to the tooth affected (Fig. 40-1). Occasionally the affected tooth may be one or two teeth distant from the swelling and color changes. The tooth or teeth affected by a periodontal abscess are usually tender on chewing and sensitive to percussion. Frequently the tooth is mobile and may even extrude from the alveolar socket and feel "high" to the occlusion. Occasionally the abscess may already be draining through one or more sinus tracts into the oral cavity. Purulent exudate can often be noted in the periodontal pocket around the affected tooth.

Often regional lymphadenopathy and occasionally slight elevation of body temperature accompany periodontal abscesses.

Dental radiographs are helpful in confirming the diagnosis. They frequently reveal a radiolucent area along the lateral aspect of the tooth involved. It is possible, however, if the abscess is located on the facial or lingual surfaces that the radiograph will not reveal its presence (Fig. 40-2).

ETIOLOGY

A periodontal abscess is a bacterial infection involving the periodontal tissues. Both environmental and microbio-

logic factors play an important role in the development, progression, and treatment of the infection.

Environmental factors

In most cases the periodontal abscess occurs in a preexisting periodontal pocket. The pocket is therefore a major factor in the etiology of the abscess. In both spontaneous remission and remission through partial treatment, healing occurs especially at the coronal aspect of the pocket. The epithelial tissues can reattach to the root of the tooth while bacteria and debris remain in the apical aspect of the pocket. With the coronal portion of the pocket occluded, drainage is impaired and an abscess may result (Fig. 40-3). The deeper, narrower, or more tortuous the pocket, the more likely the abscess is to occur after partial healing.

Other local factors may set the stage for abscess formation. When foreign material such as a popcorn husk, impacted food, fish bone, or even a toothbrush bristle is forced into the gingival tissue or occludes the pocket orifice, bacteria can proliferate, leading to an abscess. If this foreign material remains in the pocket, a bacterial infection may occur, and a gingival or periodontal abscess can result. A periodontal abscess can also occur with improper use of oral irrigating devices that introduce bacteria into the tissues.

Microbiologic factors

Thirty years ago Ludwig (1957) studied the microbiota of suppurative periodontal abscesses. He considered the abscess to be a mixed infection including such microorganisms as *Streptococcus viridans, Staphylococcus albus,* nonhemolytic streptococci, *Neisseria,* diphtheroids, and

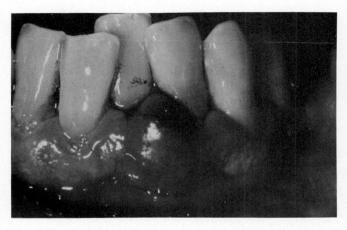

Fig. 40-1. Periodontal abscess between mandibular lateral and central incisors demonstrating gingival enlargement and discoloration.

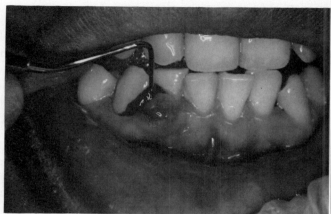

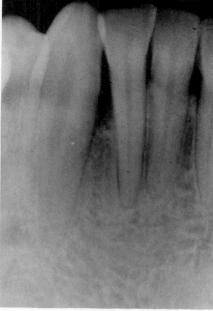

Fig. 40-2. A, Periodontal abscess probing 9 mm between mandibular canine and lateral incisor. Gingiva bled easily when probed. **B,** Radiograph shows loss of alveolar bone and loss of radiodensity between teeth. (Courtesy Dr. Phillip Parham.)

Escherichia coli. As late as 1972 (Merchant, 1972; Moore and Russell, 1972), *S. viridans* was still considered the predominant microorganism.

These findings are not surprising, considering the technology of the time. Sampling most often included healthy and diseased sites, as well as supragingival and subgingival microorganisms. These pooled samples often obscured differences. Laboratory technology was unable to cultivate oxygen-sensitive microorganisms, thereby leaving the impression that the primary etiologic agents were aerobic microorganisms (Newman and Sims, 1978).

Studies using continuous anaerobic culture techniques have shown anaerobes to be important in periodontal abscesses. For example, Newman and Sims (1978) found the microflora of periodontal abscesses to be predominantly gram-negative (66.2%) and anaerobic (65.2%), in contrast to the gram-positive (71.0%) and facultative (78.3%) microflora in healthy sites. They reported that the microorganisms most commonly found in periodontal abscesses were *Bacteroides melaninogenicus* subspecies, *Fusobacterium* species, "vibrio-corroders," *Capnocytophaga* species, *Peptococcus* species, and *Peptostreptococcus* spe-

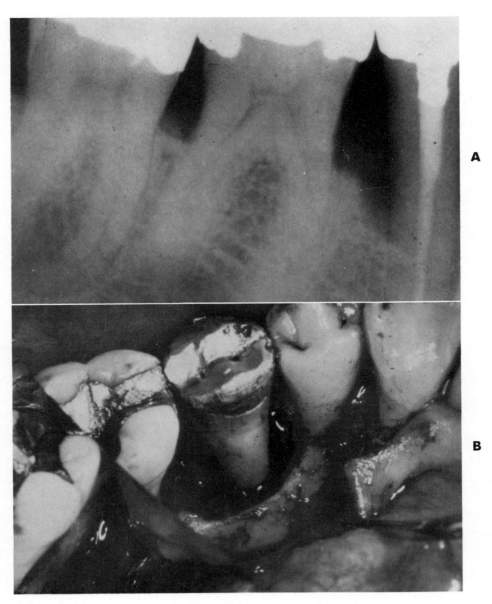

Fig. 40-3. A, Radiograph of periodontal abscess 1 week following "prophylaxis." **B,** On flap reflection, localized bone loss is present and calculus can be seen on root surface of second premolar.

cies. van Winkelhoff et al. (1985) found *Bacteroides gingivalis* and *Bacteroides intermedius* in all of the periodontal abscesses they cultured. DeWitt et al. (1985) noted the presence of bacteria and fungi in the connective tissue wall of 100% of the periodontal abscesses they studied (Fig. 40-4). Hence bacterial invasion of ulcerated and necrotic tissues observed was by predominantly gram-negative bacteria. The presence of fungi resembling *Candida* species in these periodontal abscesses was also observed. *Candida albicans* has also been found in abscesses of lung, heart, kidney, brain, and other organ systems. Since *Candida* is often a secondary invader in areas of preexisting infection, these organisms may play a role in the progression of the abscess.

DIFFERENTIAL DIAGNOSIS

Pain, swelling, color changes, mobility, extrusion, purulence, sinus tract, lymphadenopathy, fever, and radiolu-

cency, while symptoms of a periodontal abscess, are not always present, nor are they unique to this lesion. Since other dental infections and conditions share some or all of these symptoms, it is mandatory to make a differential diagnosis so that correct treatment procedures may be used.

1. *Gingival abscess.* This is a subgroup of the periodontal abscess. It usually occurs in a previously disease-free site and is confined to the marginal gingiva.

2. *Periapical abscess.* This is the most perplexing, since it shares most if not all of the symptoms of a periodontal abscess. Radiographically, a radiolucency often appears at the apex of the offending tooth. However, in an early periapical abscess there may be no radiographic changes evident.

A lack of pulpal vitality and the presence of deep carious lesions, deep fillings, and crowns are helpful when a periapical abscess is suspected, but are not specific to this disorder. Pain on palpation of the soft tissue at the apex of

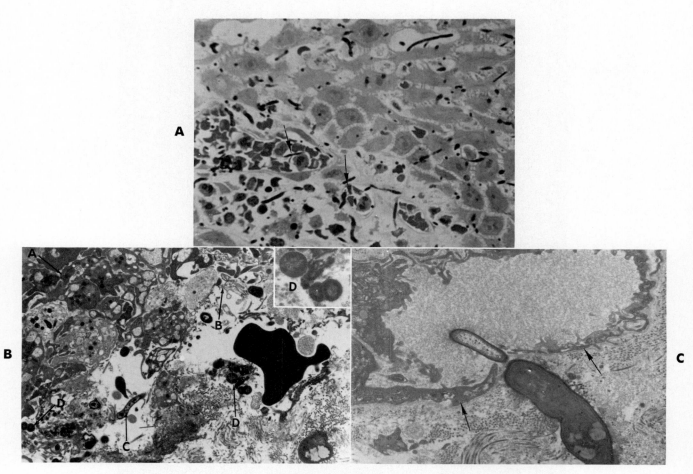

Fig. 40-4. A, Specimen of pocket epithelium and adjacent lamina propria showing extensive invasion of fungus elements. Note intracapillary penetration *(arrows).* (Original magnification ×400.) **B,** Central abscess area exhibiting neutrophil infiltrate *(A-arrow),* generalized cell debris *(B-arrow),* fungus invasion *(C-arrow),* and bacterial penetration *(D-arrows; inset at upper right).* (Original magnification ×5600.) **C,** Fungal hypha penetration of normal-appearing capillary wall *(arrows).* (Original magnification ×6800.) (Courtesy Dr. Charles M. Cobb.)

the tooth can be evidence of periapical infection. The periodontal abscess usually occurs in a preexisting pocket. Probing will identify a communication between the gingival margin and the abscess area.

Pain itself may be the most helpful symptom in differentiating between a periapical and a periodontal abscess. In a periapical abscess the pain is sharp, intermittent, severe, and diffuse. The patient may not be able to locate the offending tooth. In a periodontal abscess, on the other hand, the pain is dull, constant, and less severe but localized. The patient can easily identify the affected tooth. Pain on percussion is very severe in a periapical abscess. While a periodontal abscess exhibits pain following percussion, it is less severe. This severe reaction to percussion is considered by many experienced clinicians to be pathognomonic of pulpal infection.

3. *Acute pulpitis.* Acute pulpitis lacks most of the symptoms of a periodontal abscess except pain. The pain is diffuse, like that of a periapical abscess, and may affect the entire side of the face. It is common for the patient to have pain in the opposite arch. The pain can be affected by thermal changes.

4. *Incomplete tooth fracture.* A cracked tooth often poses a diagnostic dilemma for the dentist. The patient has very real symptoms, but clinically the fracture is often difficult to detect. Endodontically treated teeth are especially prone to vertical fractures. The most common symptoms are pain or sensitivity on biting and sensitivity to cold. Heat seldom causes discomfort. Pressure on individual cusps may elicit the pain. This can be done by having the patient bite on a rubber wheel or rubber anesthetic stopper. While occlusal adjustment will temporarily eliminate the pain, the tooth is better treated with a restoration providing cuspal protection. If the fracture extends into the root, there is often colonization by microorganisms through the fracture line into the periodontal ligament, resulting in a persistent periodontal abscess or a deep, narrow, draining periodontal pocket along the fracture line.

5. *Pericoronitis.* This is an acute infection occurring around the crown of a partially erupted tooth. The mandibular third molars are most frequently involved.

6. *Periodontal cyst.* The radiographic appearance of a periodontal cyst is a well-defined oval radiolucency on the lateral surface of the root. It has a predilection for the mandibular canine-premolar region but can occur at other locations (Fig. 40-5). If periodontitis extends apically to a preexisting periodontal cyst, the cyst will become infected and clinically indistinguishable from a lateral periodontal abscess.

7. *Osteomyelitis.* This serious infection of the bone and bone marrow tends to spread. It has a rapid onset, with pain being the only symptom, and is without radiographic evidence. Rapid diffuse bone destruction may occur within a few days, extending a significant distance from the original site of infection. The radiographic picture then may show an indistinct trabeculation and disappearance of the lamina dura. As this infection increases, lymphadenopathy, fever, and malaise are common symptoms.

8. *Manifestation of systemic disease.* Any time the patient's defense mechanism is significantly lowered, an existing periodontitis can develop into one or several periodontal abscesses. Systemic disease should be suspected in any patient with multiple abscesses or who is having repeated recurrences of periodontal abscesses. Diabetes mellitus is the most common systemic disease presenting with periodontal abscesses, which are often multiple.

TREATMENT

Periodontal abscesses most often present as a painful emergency. The patient should be treated immediately to relieve pain and resolve the infection, which may spread and lead to periodontal attachment loss. After a thorough clinical examination, the symptoms are assessed and a differential diagnosis is reviewed to eliminate unlikely diag-

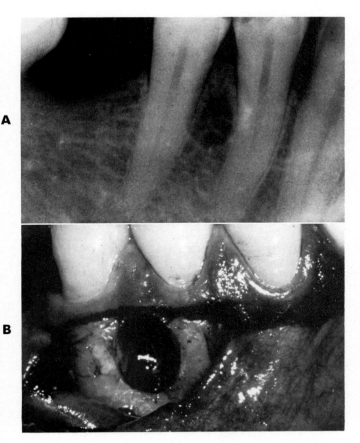

Fig. 40-5. A, Periodontal cyst between mandibular premolars. Radiograph shows a well-defined oval lesion subcrestally. Sulcus did not communicate with osseous defect. **B,** Diagnosis was confirmed following a periosteal flap and biopsy. (Courtesy Wilford Hall, USAF Medical Center.)

noses. Additional observations, radiographs, and clinical tests will hopefully narrow the choices to a single diagnosis. Familiarity with all aspects of a periodontal abscess enables the dentist to perform the diagnosis rather rapidly. It should be noted that in most clinics treating a broad range of dental patients, about 85% of toothaches are pulpal in origin and about 15% are due to periodontal abscesses. This percentage will vary markedly, however, according to the nature of the population served.

Treatment of the periodontal abscess should include drainage through an incision or through the gingival crevice or pocket orifice, as well as the use of antimicrobial agents.

Repair potential

A periodontal abscess usually results in considerable bone loss during its acute phase; in turn, this lesion has an excellent potential for repair following adequate treatment. The dentist should therefore consider treatment of the acutely affected tooth, even though there seems to be little remaining periodontal support, since remarkable regeneration of lost periodontal attachment may occur. The location and shape of the osseous destruction, as well as its degree of activity, appear to affect the prognosis of the periodontal abscess. Nabers et al. (1964) noted that acute abscesses repaired more completely than similar chronic lesions. They also concluded that narrow infrabony lesions had a better repair potential than wide lesions without bony walls.

Earlier methods of treatment (Trott, 1959) recommended that the abscess be incised and drained to reduce the acute phase and that the chronic phase be corrected by periodontal flaps and osseous correction. In view of the improved repair potential of an acute abscess, it would seem more logical today to definitively treat during the acute phase. The selection of treatment methods should always consider this repair potential.

Closed approach

Incision and drainage are often best obtained through the pocket. While drainage may be accomplished by directly incising into the surface of the fluctuant abscess, root planing is still required. Following adequate local anesthesia, the pocket is opened with a sharp curette to the depth of the abscess. Immediate drainage and hemorrhage are often obtained. The root surface is then thoroughly root planed to remove plaque and calculus deposits. During this root planing the occluded pocket is further opened, and drainage is enhanced. Irrigation with 0.1% povidone-iodine and 3% hydrogen peroxide aids in debridement and elimination of bacteria. In the absence of systemic symptoms, antibiotic therapy is seldom necessary. If, however, the patient has lymphadenopathy, fever, and/or malaise, systemic antibiotics should be considered.

Open approach

The dentist should attempt to maximize the repair potential of the periodontal abscess by definitively treating the abscess during the acute phase. This requires that in addition to establishing drainage, the diseased root surface must be free of all deposits and the surface of the root planed to remove infected dentin and cementum. Full access to the diseased root may in some instances be best obtained with a full-thickness access mucoperiosteal flap on both the facial and the lingual surfaces with sufficient reflection to completely visualize the infected root surface. The initial internal beveled incision can be made intrasulcularly or close to the gingival margin to preserve as much keratinized gingiva as possible. This incision should be continued laterally to allow for flap displacement for adequate visualization and access. If necessary for access, vertical incisions can be made over intact alveolar bone at the line angles of the adjacent noninvolved teeth.

The attached gingival tissue can now be reflected with a blunt tissue elevator. The reflection should be adequate to thoroughly visualize the entire infected root surface. With the aid of good light (the use of fiber optics is ideal) and sharp curettes, all visible bacterial deposits, both hard and soft, must be planed from the root surface. All of the root surface thought to have been exposed to a preexisting periodontal pocket should also be thoroughly root planed. The exposed bone can also be carefully debrided to remove soft tissue from the osseous defect (Figs. 40-6 to 40-8).

Following thorough root planing, the flaps are replaced and sutured. The patient should rinse with a plaque inhibitor such as chlorhexidine twice a day for at least 1 week.

Use of antibiotics

The goal of the open approach is to maximize healing and to gain new attachment of the periodontal tissues to

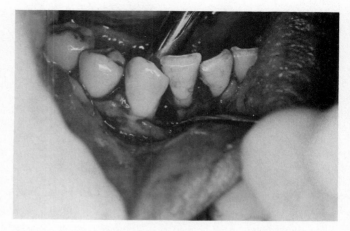

Fig. 40-6. Periodontal abscess shown in Fig. 40-2 treated with internal bevel flap; root was thoroughly root planed (detoxified), and osseous defect was debrided. (Courtesy Dr. Phillip Parham.)

Fig. 40-7. **A,** Periodontal abscess shown in Figs. 40-2 and 40-6 postoperatively after probing only 3 mm. Tissue contours are markedly improved. **B,** Radiograph shows improvement in radiodensity between involved teeth. Crestal bone height is only slightly improved. (Courtesy Dr. Phillip Parham.)

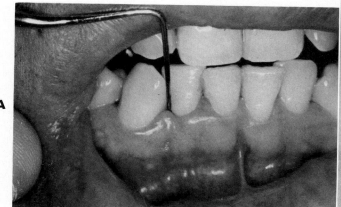

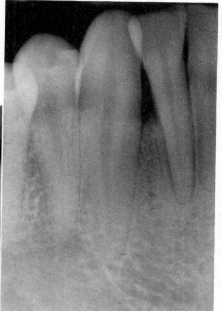

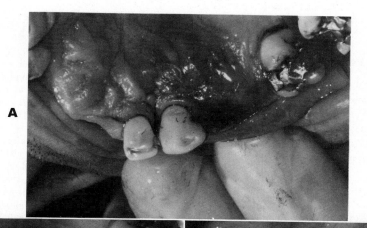

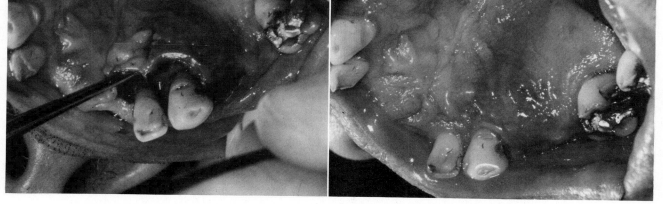

Fig. 40-8. **A,** Periodontal abscess between and palatal to maxillary canine and lateral incisor. Severe discoloration of palatal tissue can be noted. **B,** Area was treated with an internal bevel flap, roots were planed (detoxified), and osseous defect was debrided. **C,** Tissue is markedly improved 10 days postoperatively.

the previously diseased root surface. It is therefore desirable to give the patient a systemic antibiotic that is appropriate to treat the acute infection.

Based on early aerobic microbiologic studies, penicillin became the systemic therapy of choice. However, Goldberg (1970) cultured periapical and periodontal infections and found that 26% of these infecting bacteria were resistant to penicillin. He also noted a high number of gram-negative rods that were resistant to the antibiotics tested.

The best method to determine the appropriate antibiotic is to obtain a culture and to test for sensitivity. Since the causative microorganisms are usually anaerobic, anaerobic culturing should be requested in addition to aerobic culturing. While waiting for the result of culture and sensitivity testing, it is prudent to begin antibiotic therapy, selecting a systemic antibiotic that usually satisfies treatment goals. Tetracycline hydrochloride is a relatively safe, broad-spectrum antibiotic with a concentration in the gingival crevicular fluid two to four times that in serum (Gordon et al., 1981). Tetracycline usually reaches those microorganisms thought to cause the abscess, as well as those thought to cause periodontitis (Walker et al., 1981). A typical treatment program would be 250 mg four times a day for 10 days. Once the results of the culture and sensitivity testing are known, the appropriate antibiotic can be selected and prescribed.

COMPLICATIONS AND POSTOPERATIVE CARE

Occasionally a periodontal abscess will spread to involve other facial tissues, resulting in a cellulitis. The cellulitis may result in serious systemic symptoms, endanger the airway, or threaten a cavernous sinus infection. In these severe and generalized cases penicillin is preferred until the results of culture and sensitivity testing are obtained.

Postoperative care is important for the successful treatment of a periodontal abscess. The patient should be seen in 2 days and again at weekly intervals if necessary to evaluate resolution of the abscess. The area should be thoroughly debrided and all calculus, plaque, and stain removed. Since periodontal abscesses most often occur in patients with periodontitis, a full examination of the patient for evidence of periodontal disease is appropriate 1 or 2 weeks after the abscess has healed. If periodontitis is diagnosed, then the treatment plan should be formulated to allow for definitive treatment of the abscess area if necessary.

REFERENCES

DeWitt GV, Cobb CM, and Killoy WJ: The acute periodontal abscess: microbial penetration of the soft tissue wall, Int J Periodontics Restorative Dent 5:39, 1985.

Goldberg MH: The changing biologic nature of acute dental infection, J Am Dent Assoc 80:1048, 1970.

Gordon JM et al: Tetracycline: levels achievable in gingival crevice fluid and *in vitro* effect on subgingival organisms. I. Concentrations in crevicular fluid after repeated doses, J Periodontol 52:609, 1981.

Grant DA, Stern IB, and Everett EG: Orban's periodontics, ed 4, St Louis, 1972, The CV Mosby Co.

Ludwig TG: An investigation of the oral flora of suppurative oral swellings, Aust Dent J 2:259, 1957.

McFall WT: The periodontal abscess, J NC Dent Soc 47:34, 1964.

Merchant NE: Infections related to the jaws, Practitioner 209:679, 1972.

Moore JR and Russell C: Bacteriological investigation of dental abscesses, Dent Pract Dent Rec 22:390, 1972.

Nabers JM et al: Chronology, an important factor in the repair of osseous defects, Periodontics 2:304, 1964.

Newman MG and Sims TN: The predominant cultivable microbiota of the periodontal abscess, J Periodontol 50:350, 1978.

O'Brien TJ: Diagnosis and treatment of periodontal and gingival abscesses, J Ontario Dent Assoc 47:16, 1970.

Ranney RR: Pathogenesis of periodontal disease: position report and review of literature, International Conference on Research in the Biology of Periodontal Disease, Chicago, 1977.

Trott JR: The acute periodontal abscess, J Can Dent Assoc 25:601, 1959.

van Winkelhoff AJ, Carlee AW, and De Graaff J: *Bacteroides endodontalis* and other black-pigmented *Bacteroides* species in odontogenic abscesses, Infect Immun 49:494, 1985.

Walker CB et al: Tetracycline: levels achievable in gingival crevice fluid and in vitro effect on subgingival organisms. II. Susceptibilities of periodontal bacteria, J Periodontol 52:613, 1981.

Chapter 41

MAINTENANCE THERAPY
Preventing recurrence of periodontal diseases

Raul G. Caffesse

The practice of periodontics within the context of dentistry encompasses three different phases:

1. Prevention of initial periodontal diseases
2. Treatment of periodontal diseases
3. Maintenance, or prevention of recurrence of periodontal diseases

Chronic periodontitis, like most other chronic infections, requires supervision and maintenance over time after treatment is completed in order to assure long-term stability of results and to minimize recurrence.

Maintenance therapy after active treatment includes not only the care the patient receives through personal oral hygiene, but also recalls and reevaluations by the dental team. Maintenance therapy is often supportive in nature; however, it also may require more involvement, with early detection and prompt treatment of recurrent periodontal diseases. It is also called supportive treatment.

NEED FOR LONG-TERM MAINTENANCE

The overall goal of dentistry is the maintenance of the dentition in health and function for a lifetime. Periodontal therapy, including maintenance, is often required to achieve that goal. Over the years many clinical studies have shown that to maintain the results achieved with the active phase of periodontal therapy, patients need to be followed with frequent recalls. Retrospective studies have stressed that with good maintenance, periodontal patients can retain their dentitions for a long period of time (Hirschfeld and Wasserman, 1978; McFall, 1982; Meador et al., 1985). Furthermore, prospective longitudinal studies have shown the effectiveness of different approaches to therapy, both nonsurgical and surgical (Knowles et al., 1979; Pihlstrom et al., 1983; Badersten et al., 1984; Lindhe and Nyman, 1984; Lindhe et al., 1984; Ramfjord et al., 1987). Stability of results obtained with both nonsurgical and various surgical therapies was achieved on the basis of a regular program, with regular professional maintenance ranging from initially every 2 weeks to later every 3 to 4 months. Studies have shown the benefits of proper maintenance in posttreatment results (Rosling et al., 1976b, Nyman et al., 1977). In these studies periodontitis patients treated with different surgical techniques were assigned to two different maintenance groups: a well-maintained group with professional tooth cleanings every other week (plaque-free dentition) and a poorly maintained group with professional cleanings once a year (plaque-infected dentitions). After 2 years, the well-maintained patients maintained the initial gains in clinical attachment ir-

483

respective of the surgical technique employed. On the other hand, the poorly maintained patients with plaque-reinfected dentitions lost clinical attachment irrespective of the surgical technique employed.

Evaluations performed in a private practice setting again showed the benefits of proper maintenance (Becker et al., 1984a, 1984b). A group of 95 patients who followed routine maintenance were evaluated from 1.6 to 9.7 years after treatment. Similarly, a group of 44 patients who stopped maintenance after completion were evaluated (average time, 5.25 years). Tooth loss and bone loss doubled in the unmaintained group. Treatment without maintenance was of limited value.

It is evident that the current literature strongly supports the need for maintenance therapy as part of periodontal treatment. As with many other chronic infections, control of the levels of infection and of recurrent infections after a course of successful active therapy may require regular professional as well as personal oral hygiene for a lifetime for most patients.

OBJECTIVES OF MAINTENANCE THERAPY

Maintenance therapy is directed at maintaining the dentition for a lifetime following periodontal treatment. Whether or not this goal can be successfully reached depends on the severity of the initial lesion, the host response to therapy, and the commitment of the patient to maintenance. In essence, maintenance attempts to fulfill the following objectives:

1. *Preservation of alveolar bone support.* Maintenance of alveolar bone height, as evaluated with radiographs, represents one of the most important parameters clinicians have to assess long-term results of therapy. Bone height may not only be maintained but also improved when proper maintenance is provided after periodontal therapy (Rosling et al., 1976a). Special radiographic techniques can be used; however, good-quality radiographs taken with the long-cone paralleling technique can also be evaluated accurately using computer-assisted digitizing analysis (Diederich et al., 1987).

2. *Maintenance of stable clinical attachment levels.* De-

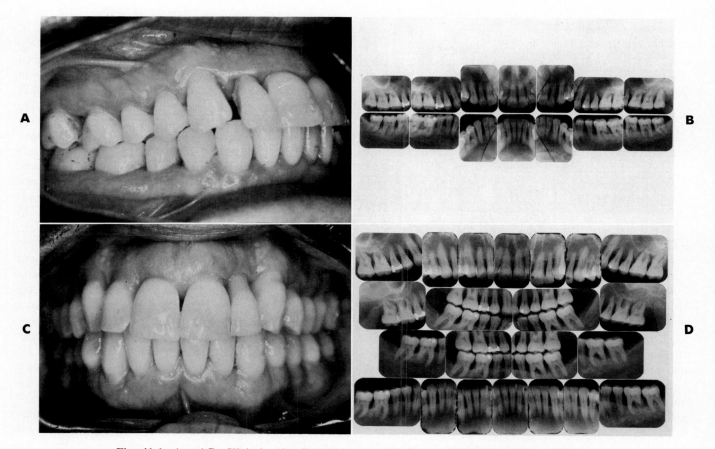

Fig. 41-1. **A** and **B,** Clinical and radiographic appearance of an advanced case of periodontitis treated in one of the Michigan Longitudinal Studies. **C** and **D,** Clinical and radiographic images recorded 10 years after treatment. Patient was maintained on a 3-month recall schedule.

spite all the variability associated with clinical measurements, maintenance of stable clinical attachment levels represents a reasonable clinical indicator to evaluate the stability of results (Haffajee et al., 1983). Longitudinal studies have shown consistently that clinical attachment levels can be improved by treatment and maintained over time (Fig. 41-1). In general, the more severe the initial lesion, the more clinical attachment can be gained (Knowles et al., 1979; Lindhe and Nyman, 1984). To evaluate changes over time, it is imperative to accurately record the level of clinical attachment loss at baseline, after treatment, and at yearly intervals. Use of automatic probing devices may in the future offer the possibility of monitoring smaller changes in pocket depth and attachment level, which will provide early warning of recurrence. Also, monitoring for the reappearance of periodontal pathogens such as *Bacteroides gingivalis* may offer hope for early detection of recurrent disease.

3. *Control of inflammation.* Without proper maintenance dental plaque will reaccumulate, and inflammation will be reestablished in periodontal tissues (Nyman et al., 1977). On the contrary, well-maintained patients will have low levels of inflammation after therapy (Rosling et al., 1976b). This low level of inflammation often correlates with gains in clinical attachment and reductions in probing depth. Six-month recalls are not considered conducive to the maintenance of stable results based on recurrence of inflammation (Olsen et al., 1985). However, increased marginal inflammation does not necessarily mean loss of clinical attachment. When patients who had been maintained for 5 years on a 3-month recall schedule (Ramfjord et al., 1987) were placed into 3- and 6-month recall groups for 2 additional years, it was found that although gingivitis increased, there were no changes in clinical attachment level (Caffesse et al., 1987). Within the frame-

work of the study, it was evident that increased levels of gingivitis did not necessarily correspond to greater attachment loss. This corroborates the clinical finding that in many instances patients who do not perform adequate home care will manifest variable levels of gingivitis but no reestablishment of periodontitis (Morrison et al., 1982) (Fig. 41-2). It is clear that present measurments of gingival inflammation are not good indications of recurrent periodontitis. However, it is also clear that in an inflammation-free dentition, recurrence of periodontitis is rare.

4. *Reevaluation and reinforcement of proper home care.* Proper home care must be reevaluated and, if necessary, reinforced each time the patient is seen for maintenance. Although 3- to 4-month recalls seem to compensate for improper plaque control as far as its effects on clinical attachment levels (Ramfjord et al., 1982), the better the oral hygiene the patient performs, the better the possibilities of maintaining stable results. With training and positive reinforcement the level of plaque control can be improved in most patients; however, it may take several sessions with some patients.

5. *Maintenance of a healthy and functional oral environment.* In addition to the evaluation of the periodontal parameters, the mouth and dentition should be thoroughly inspected and assessed for changes over time. This may require consultations with other specialists and/or treatment. Evaluation and treatment of new or recurrent caries, hypersensitive dentin, occlusal factors, endodontic treatment, and restorations, as well as soft tissue lesions, must be performed during maintenance. Any patient concerns or complaints should be addressed by the dental team during these visits. Also, the regular maintenance visits should be used to monitor general health and habits, and the extent to which this is done depends on the knowledge and interest of the clinician.

SEQUENCE OF A MAINTENANCE VISIT

Recall visits, on the average, last 1 hour if no disease is detected. This is sufficient time for the dental team to fulfill the objectives of this important phase of therapy in most patients. During a typical maintenance visit the following steps should be covered:

1. *Review of the medical and dental history.* Briefly, any necessary update on the record should be made regarding changes in the medical or dental status of the patient. If the medical status has changed, appropriate action including referral to a physician should be taken.

2. *Oral examination.* A systematic oral examination must be performed at each recall visit to screen for any possible oral or dental lesions that might have developed. Both soft and hard tissues must be inspected.

3. *Plaque-control evaluation.* The effectiveness of the patient's oral hygiene must be evaluated, not only to assess the patient's ability to remove plaque throughout the

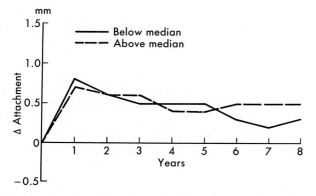

Fig. 41-2. Effect of level of oral hygiene on gain in clinical attachment in patients maintained on a 3-month recall schedule. Initial pockets were 4 to 12 mm. Observe that there is no difference in average gain of clinical attachment over the years.

existing dentition, but also as a reinforcement for the patient. A disclosing solution may be used to enable the patient to see the plaque that has accumulated. It is highly advisable to use an index system to quantify the plaque present. This is again important for patient reinforcement as well as for record-keeping purposes, since it describes clearly the level of oral hygiene of a particular patient at a particular time and permits comparisons over time. The plaque and gingival indices described in Chapter 6 can be adapted to the practice setting and performed by auxiliaries if they are well trained and monitored. It is also important to evaluate the cleanliness of any removable appliances that may be present.

Monitoring of suspected infected periodontal patients for pathogenic periodontal flora may be advisable using local laboratories or microbiologic detection services. In-office assessment of the periodontal microflora may also be possible in diagnosis of recurrent periodontal disease, especially when clinical signs of inflammation such as bleeding on probing, suppuration, deepened pockets, or progression of bone loss on radiographs is noted.

4. *Periodontal examination.* All periodontal tissues must be evaluated to determine the presence or absence of inflammation and to determine if reinfection has occurred. Inspection of the tissues will evaluate changes in color, texture, and consistency. Probing will explore the sulcular areas to assess bleeding tendency, suppuration, probing pocket depth, and clinical attachment levels. Furcation areas, especially if previously involved, deserve special attention at this time. During maintenance the stability of results is of critical importance. Consequently, the practitioner is interested in identifying sites or areas where clinically increased loss of attachment or deepened pockets are noticed. Although charting of these recordings every 3 to 4 months is not necessary, changes from previous chartings must be recorded, and a new charting should be performed once a year. Areas of recession must be assessed and compared with previous values to determine their progression or stability. The use of pressure on the gingiva permits evaluation of the presence of exudates within the pocket. During probing, an assessment is also made of the presence and distribution of subgingival plaque and subgingival calculus. Occlusal examination is performed to assess the functional impact, if any, on the periodontium. The pattern of tooth mobility is checked and compared with previous recordings. The development of separations or diastemas, as well as tooth migration, is considered. A functional analysis of those with evidence of trauma from occlusion, including increasing tooth mobility, pathologic migration of teeth, or pain on occlusion, should be carried out. This includes the detection of centric prematurities; the presence, direction, and extent of a centric slide; the final impact of closure; balancing or heavy-working interferences; and the development of heavy wear facets.

5. *Radiographic evaluation.* For safety reasons, full-mouth radiographs are generally taken only when there is a specific indication for them. However, vertical bitewing radiographs can be taken every year or so if indicated, and periapical radiographs of isolated areas of concern to the practitioner can certainly be taken more often. Whenever films are available, they must be thoroughly evaluated and compared with previous radiographs for signs of improvement or deterioration. Examination should include the bone, the tooth, and the periodontal space. When a patient is evaluated for periodontal maintenance, the most recent set of radiographs should be in sight on the view box, to be evaluated and compared with clinical findings.

6. *Scaling, root planing, and polishing.* In terms of its impact on prevention and treatment, this is the most important step within the sequence of the maintenance visit. It is intended to achieve the deplaquing of the teeth and the detoxification of the roots, thereby creating an environment that will continue to be biologically acceptable to the surrounding tissues. How much scaling and root planing is necessary varies with each patient, each tooth, and each pocket; it depends on how much instrumentation is needed to remove all the existing supragingival and subgingival deposits from the tooth surfaces. What every patient will need at each maintenance visit is a thorough prophylaxis for deplaquing, using a rubber cup, and interproximally, using either floss or an EVA prophylaxis system. It should be remembered that the objective of the prophylaxis is to thoroughly remove plaque and pellicle. It has been shown that all prophylaxis pastes tend to roughen the root surfaces (Roulet and Roulet-Mehrens, 1982; Walters et al., 1984). However, this increased roughness does not seem to be of clinical significance (Gartner et al., 1987). Polishing pastes that will roughen the root surface the least must be chosen for these routine prophylaxes.

If *recurrent periodontitis is detected, retreatment* should be undertaken in a series of appointments after maintenance to ensure adequate and complete retreatment. Several studies have shown that most recurrent periodontal disease occurs in a few patients, the "downhill patients," ranging from 4% to 8% of those treated. They may also be refractory, responding poorly to therapy (Haffajee et al., 1988).

7. *Application of fluorides.* Routine application of fluorides after maintenance prophylaxes seems advantageous, since it may reduce root hypersensitivity, minimize the possibilities for root caries, and promote remineralization. Topical fluorides at high concentrations may have some antibacterial properties, decreasing plaque accumulation (Brudevold et al., 1961; Loesche, 1976; Mazza et al., 1981). Care should be exercised when treating patients with porcelain restorations, since it has been shown that certain acidulated phosphate fluoride gels and stannous fluoride preparations can potentially etch the porcelain (Wunderlich and Yaman, 1986).

8. *Recommendations for further treatment needs and/or*

referrals. At the end of the maintenance visit, the dentist should recommend to the patient the course of action for any additional treatment needs he might have. These recommendations should also include any modifications in the frequency of maintenance recalls (either more or less frequent recall visits), prompt treatment of sites of recurrent periodontal disease, as well as referral to other specialists for evaluation and/or treatment of specific needs.

REEVALUATION DURING MAINTENANCE

The most crucial decision that must be made during maintenance is whether or not the result of treatment is stable and, if it is not stable, what degree of retreatment is necessary. Increased clinical attachment loss constitutes the most important criterion available to assess disease progression (Haffajee et al., 1983). However, once the loss of clinical attachment is detected, the damage has already taken place. It has been stated that no other clinical parameter can predict loss of attachment (Haffajee et al., 1983). For example, inflammation may be present in the tissues without promoting loss of attachment over time. Consequently, from a pragmatic standpoint inflamed areas need treatment not only because they do not represent a state of health, but also because they may lead to loss of attachment.

Longitudinal clinical studies already cited have shown repeatedly and convincingly that pockets do not need to be eliminated to maintain stable results after treatment. Consequently, pocket depth alone is a parameter that cannot be used to evaluate results. The long-term evaluation has to be determined clinically by the changes in the clinical attachment level and radiographically by the changes in the alveolar bone support. The assessment of whether there is inflammation present or not, at a particular maintenance recall, has to be done by evaluation of the response of the tissues to probing.

The following should therefore be considered:

1. *Clinical inflammation*. Assessment of clinical changes in the area based on color, form, and consistency of the tissue. If suppuration or bleeding on deep probing is present, microbiologic tests may help establish the diagnosis of recurrent disease.

2. *Ease of probing*. If resistance to probing is experienced, the marginal tissues are firmly adapted to the tooth, and there is a junctional epithelium of variable length. If, on the contrary, the probe does not find any resistance to penetration, inflammation is probably present in the gingival connective tissue and junctional epithelium.

3. *Bleeding on probing*. Although false negative results are always possible, research suggests that the more times a site bleeds during maintenance, the greater the chance that the site will lose attachment over time (Chaves et al., 1986; Lang et al., 1986) (Table 41-1). Furthermore, bleeding indicates that inflammation is present and must be controlled. Consequently, significant emphasis is placed on

Table 41-1. Number of sites experiencing clinical attachment loss in relation to the frequency of bleeding on probing during yearly examinations

Bleeding on probing frequency	No attachment loss after 5 years	Attachment loss after 5 years	
≥2	814	222	(21.4%)
≥3	497	161	(24.5%)
≥4	258	103	(28.5%)
=5	93	46	(33.1%)

Table 41-2. Number of sites experiencing clinical attachment loss in relation to the frequency of exudate during yearly examinations

Exudate frequency	No attachment loss after 5 years	Attachment loss after 5 years	
≥1	162	73	(31.1%)
≥2	44	29	(39.7%)
≥3	12	12	(50.0%)
=4	2	5	(71.4%)

repeated bleeding on probing during reevaluation of the tissues after therapy.

4. *Exudate*. The use of a ball burnisher or the handle of an instrument pressed against the gingival margins allows for the evaluation of exudates emanating from the crevice. Exudate also indicates an inflammatory process; and as with bleeding, although not all sites losing attachment show exudate, a high percentage of sites where exudate is present repeatedly, lose attachment over time (Chaves et al., 1986) (Table 41-2).

5. *Subgingival plaque*. If during exploration of the crevices, the probe removes plaque from the subgingival area, the area is already repopulated by bacteria, and subgingival flora has been reestablished following therapy.

6. *Subgingival calculus*. When subgingival calculus is detected with the probe or the explorer (No. 3 cowhorn), subgingival plaque has accumulated and calcified in the area or calculus has not been completely removed. Areas where subgingival calculus is present may show suppuration and bleed on probing.

7. *Changes over time*. Finally, comparisons of probing depth and clinical attachment levels with those recorded previously give a clear indication of the improvement or deterioration of the case over time.

All the clinical criteria allow the practitioner to evaluate tissue response. If clinically the tissues look inflamed, if they show no resistance to the penetration of the probe, if they bleed on probing or show exudate, and/or if subgingival plaque and calculus are present, the marginal seal has been broken and active disease is likely to be present. This diagnosed disease needs to be treated whether or not it is progressive.

The assessment of subgingival plaque samples by phase-contrast or darkfield microscopy has also been suggested as a means to predict and evaluate the presence of recurrent disease (Keyes et al., 1978). However, quantitation of plaque bacteria based on morphologic criteria is not a good predictor of loss of attachment when patients maintain a regular recall system (Listgarten et al., 1986).

Cultural analysis of bacterial plaque, looking for specific pathogenic bacteria, may be effective in predicting loss of attachment (Slots, 1986; Listgarten, 1988). Several laboratories offer the service on samples taken at chairside and brought or mailed to the central reference laboratory. Rapid tests are being designed to detect specific bacterial pathogens chairside. Laboratories can detect periodontal bacteria by indirect immunofluorescence (Zambon et al., 1985) or by DNA probes (Chen et al., 1986; Savitt et al., 1988).

RETREATMENT DURING MAINTENANCE

When areas of active disease are detected with or without loss of attachment, the area may require further treatment. Recurrence is most often localized, affecting one or a few sites. However, generalized recurrence may occur, especially if the patient has not been on a maintenance program. Retreatment is often initiated by performing scaling and root planing (Ramfjord et al., 1987). The difficulties of thorough calculus removal during scaling and planing have been stressed (Rabbani et al., 1981); however, thorough scaling and root planing may be effective, especially in early recurrent lesions. Scaling and root planing should be the first retreatment attempted in most lesions and may require several sessions per patient, as well as local anesthesia. If this fails, a course of antibiotics or scaling using flap accessibility may be applied. The results in terms of residual calculus will be improved if the area is surgically opened (Caffesse et al., 1986). The decision to do surgery is based on many factors, including the following:

1. *Accessibility.* This is in relation to the depth and type of the defect, as well as its location in the arch. Furcations are of special consideration.

2. *Previous surgery.* If surgery was performed previously, how long ago was it done? In general, no area should be reoperated during the first year following treatment.

3. *Spread of inflammation.* Inflammation can be generalized or localized to a specific area. If it is generalized and surgery was performed previously, a second round of surgery may be contraindicated. Antimicrobial therapy with systemic antibiotics (tetracycline, metronidazole, clindamycin, amoxicillin, or amoxicillin/metronidazole

combination), may be the treatment of choice. Bacterial culturing and sensitivity testing may be useful in selecting the antibiotic of choice, especially if retreatment is not successful.

4. *Cooperation of the patient with home maintenance.* If persistent inflammation is due to the patient's poor cooperation with home care, surgery is certainly contraindicated, since it will not solve the basic problem.

In essence, when retreatment is needed, it should start with several sessions of thorough scaling and root planing of the area by the practitioner, followed by assessment of tissue response 1 to 2 months later. If no positive response is found at this point, microbiologic monitoring, use of the appropriate antibiotic, surgery, or referral can be considered.

DETERMINATION OF THE MAINTENANCE RECALL INTERVAL

Based on studies of human periodontal treatment, it is recommended that the patient be seen initially for recall treatment 4 weeks following treatment. After three or four sessions, the interval can be extended to 3 months. The immediate posttreatment recall may be markedly affected by the use of chlorhexidine. However, the practitioner must determine what interval best suits the needs of the particular patient. Evidence indicates, however, that 3 to 4 months is the interval best suited for most patients in the first 4 to 5 years following therapy.

Factors to be considered in determining the recall interval include the following:

1. *Severity of the disease.* The more severe the disease, the more frequently the patient may need to be seen.

2. *Effectiveness of home care.* The better the home care, the less frequently the patient needs to be recalled.

3. *Age of the patient.* Given an equal degree of destruction, a younger patient requires more supervision to achieve stable results over a long life span than does an older patient.

4. *Degree of control of inflammation achieved.* The closer the results approach total health, the less frequent the recalls may have to be. However, it is evident that in many instances, especially where the disease is far advanced, total health cannot be restored and the goal of treatment should be to restore health as close to the ideal as possible. In such instances, the patient should be seen more frequently for recalls.

5. *Host response.* Maintenance is constantly involved with the balance of the host-bacterial interaction. In any case where systemic factors may be negatively affecting the host response, the recall interval should be reduced to try to restore the host-bacterial balance by better controlling plaque accumulation. A good example is in poorly controlled diabetes, wherein recurrence of periodontal disease is closely related to poor diabetes control. However, meticulous plaque control, both professionally and person-

ally applied, will minimize periodontal disease even in diabetics.

In essence, in the presence of unfavorable conditions the practitioner may decide to start seeing the patient every 2 months at the beginning, to observe the stability of the results obtained, and then move the recall interval to 3 months.

Since the core of the maintenance visit is reevaluation, it is evident that every time the professional assesses the condition and establishes the further course of action, he may very well reduce or increase the recall interval, according to the evaluation. Although guidelines can be given, the recall maintenance regimen must be customized for each patient after thorough evaluation of the results of therapy.

DETERMINATION OF THE PROVIDER OF MAINTENANCE

Although many periodontists prefer to maintain complete control of the recall of the patients they treat, in most instances it becomes a combined responsibility of the periodontist and the referring dentist.

As a guideline, if stable results have not been achieved and the patient exhibits poor oral hygiene or has other systemic complicating factors, the patient should be recalled by the periodontist every 3 months or more frequently, until stable results are obtained. If stable results are obtained and the patient has achieved good oral hygiene with little or no marginal gingival inflammation, maintenance can be carried out by the referring dentist every 3 months. In such an instance the periodontist should see the patient at least once a year, or sooner if the referring dentist detects deterioration of the results. One very workable arrangement is that the periodontist and the referring dentist share the recalls, with the patient alternating 6-month visits between them so that the patient is seen every 3 months.

When the referring dentist is totally or partially responsible for maintenance, it is imperative that the generalist recognize that the most important issue is proper assessment of periodontal health. Dentists and hygienists must be able to evaluate tissue health and assess stability. They must also be trained in proper treatment when needed if they elect not to refer the patient back to the periodontist. Evidence indicates that the periodontal condition deteriorates after several years in patients who have been totally maintained by general practitioners (Axelsson and Lindhe, 1981; Burgett et al., 1986). Dentists and hygienists who are involved in maintenance must develop the knowledge and skills to provide stable results. If, despite their efforts, the condition of a patient continues to deteriorate in isolated or generalized areas, the patient should be referred back to the periodontist immediately for evaluation and treatment.

Dental hygienists fulfill a fundamental role during the maintenance therapy, since most of the preliminary evaluation and treatment relies on them. The dentist or periodontist must routinely supervise the patient, diagnose, perform whatever treatment is required beyond what the hygienist has done, and recommend the future course of therapy.

SIGNIFICANCE OF MAINTENANCE

The overall objective of long-term therapy is to provide supervised control for the patient in order to maintain a healthy and functional natural dentition for life. Although realistically this goal cannot be guaranteed, it is only with proper maintenance, including early detection and treatment of recurrent periodontal diseases, that such an objective becomes achievable.

Overwhelming evidence indicates that clinical attachment levels and alveolar bone height can be maintained with good levels of personal and professional oral hygiene.

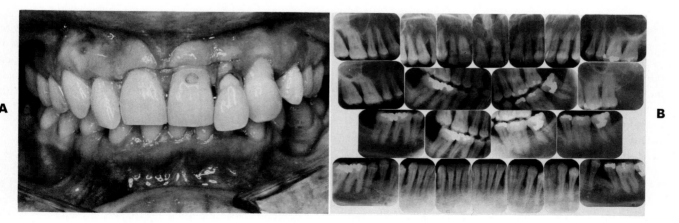

Fig. 41-3. Patient treated as part of the Michigan Longitudinal Study in 1974. **A,** Clinical appearance. **B,** Radiographs.
Continued.

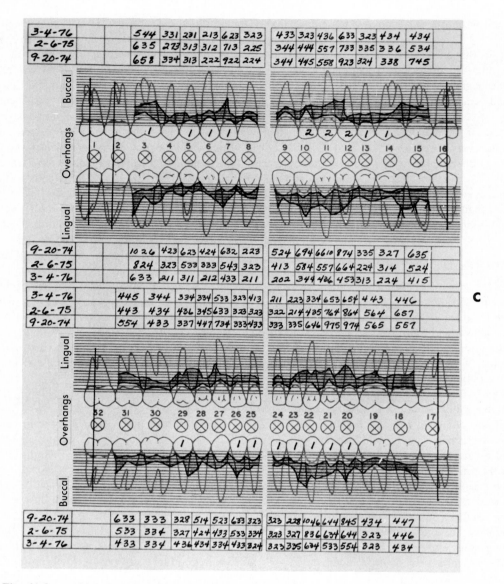

C

Fig. 41-3, cont'd. C, Initial charting, showing also the values for clinical attachment levels recorded after treatment and 1 year postoperatively.

Marginal gingival inflammation will also be controlled to the extent that if present, it may not affect clinical attachment values, when professional recalls are performed periodically (Fig. 41-3). Overall, tooth mortality can be reduced, which certainly attests to the benefits of an effective recall system. Again, it must be emphasized that in periodontitis, as well as in any other chronic disease, maintenance supervision is a must, and retreatment may be indicated during periodic evaluations. Furthermore, with a continuous supervision program it is feasible to monitor the patient over time to prevent, or to treat at an early date, not only recurrent periodontal diseases but also some of the complications, such as root hypersensitivity and root caries, that may arise from periodontal destruction not reversed by therapy. Regular professional care will not only remove the plaque thoroughly, but may also promote remineralization by the repeated application of fluorides on the exposed roots and hence reduce or prevent root caries.

The advantages of long-term therapy have been widely documented, to the point that periodontal treatment without maintenance must be considered of little value in achieving periodontal health.

CONCLUSIONS

Based on current knowledge, it can be concluded that:
1. Long-term maintenance therapy is imperative to maintain stable periodontal health.
2. The most important parameters presently available to evaluate stability are clinical attachment levels and radiographic alveolar bone height.

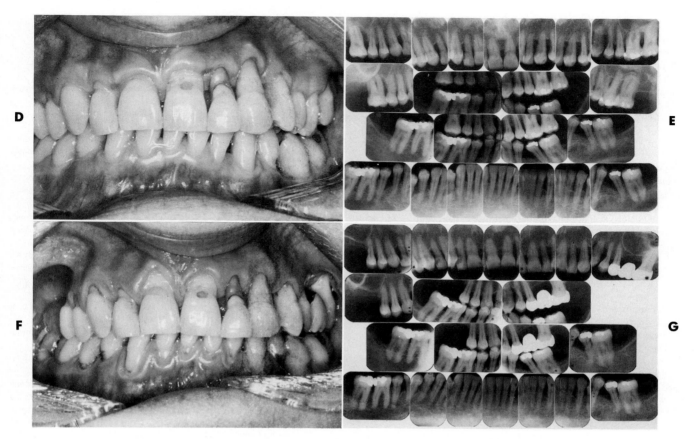

Fig. 41-3, cont'd.   D and **E,** Clinical and radiographic appearance 5 years after treatment. Upper right quadrant was treated with curettage, upper left with pocket elimination surgery, lower left with modified Widman flap, and lower right with scaling and root planing. Number 18 was lost 3 years after treatment because of an endodontic complication. Patient was maintained on a 3-month recall schedule. **F** and **G,** Same patient 10 years after treatment. Teeth Nos. 3 and 14 were lost. Remaining dentition shows stable results.

3. Maintenance is a lifetime responsibility shared by the patient and the dental team.
4. The maintenance recall interval must be customized for the individual patient; however, an interval of 3 to 4 months seems to be optimal for most patients with treated periodontitis.
5. Constant evaluation of tissue response is mandatory during maintenance.
6. Retreatment must be considered part of maintenance therapy.
7. A stable periodontium is more the rule than the exception after treatment when proper maintenance is provided.

REFERENCES

Axelsson P and Lindhe J: The significance of maintenance care in the treatment of periodontal disease, J Clin Periodontol 8:281, 1981.

Badersten A, Nilveus R, and Egelberg J: Effects of non-surgical periodontal therapy. II. Severely advanced periodontitis, J Clin Periodontol 11:63, 1984.

Becker W, Becker B, and Berg L: Periodontal treatment without maintenance, J Periodontol 55:505, 1984a.

Becker W, Berg L, and Becker B: Long-term evaluation of periodontal treatment and maintenance in 95 patients, Int J Periodontics Restorative Dent 4(2):55, 1984b.

Brudevold F, Amdur B, and Messer A: Factors involved in remineralization of carious lesions, Arch Oral Biol 6:304, 1961.

Burgett F, Morrison E, and Ramfjord S: Accelerated attachment loss after cessation of controlled maintenance care, J Dent Res 65:227, 1986 (abstract).

Caffesse RG, Sweeney P, and Smith B: Scaling and root planing with and without periodontal flap surgery, J Clin Periodontol 13:205, 1986.

Caffesse RG et al: Three and six month's maintenance care, J Dent Res 66:281, 1987 (abstact).

Chaves E, Caffesse R, and Stults D: Diagnostic discrimination of bleeding and exudate during maintenance periodontal therapy, J Dent Res 65:227, 1986 (abstract).

Chen M et al: Development of DNA probes for oral microorganisms, J Dent Res 65:352, 1986 (abstract).

Diederich RG et al: Computer analysis of non-standardized radiographs from periodontal patients, J Dent Res 63:285, 1984 (abstract).

Gartner B et al: Effect of polishing on plaque accumulation: an in vivo model, J Dent Res 66:361, 1987 (abstract).

Haffajee AD, Socransky S, and Goodson M: Clinical parameters as predictors of destructive periodontal disease activity, J Clin Periodontol 10:257, 1983.

Haffajee AD et al: Clinical, microbiological and immunologic features of subjects with refractory periodontal diseases, J Clin Periodontol 15:390, 1988.

Hirschfeld L and Wasserman B: A long term survey of tooth loss in 600 treated periodontal patients, J Periodontol 49:225, 1978.

Keyes P, Wright W, and Howard S: The use of phase-contrast microscopy and chemotherapy in the diagnosis and treatment of periodontal lesions—an initial report, Quintessence Int 9:69, 1978.

Knowles J et al: Results of periodontal treatment related to pocket depth and attachment level: eight years, J Periodontol 50:225, 1979.

Lang N et al: Bleeding on probing: a predictor for the progression of periodontal disease? J Clin Periodontol 13:590, 1986.

Lindhe J and Nyman S: Long-term maintenance of patients treated for advanced periodontal disease, J Clin Periodontol 11:504, 1984.

Lindhe J et al: Long term effect of surgical/non-surgical treatment of periodontal disease, J Clin Periodontol 11:548, 1984.

Listgarten MA: A rationale for monitoring the periodontal microflora after periodontal treatment, J Periodontol 59:439, 1988.

Listgarten MA et al: Failure of a microbial assay to reliably predict disease recurrence in a treated periodontitis population receiving regularly scheduled prophylaxes, J Clin Periodontol 13:768, 1986.

Loesche W: Chemotherapy of plaque infections, Oral Sci Rev 9:65, 1976.

Mazza J, Newman M, and Sims T: Clinical and antimicrobial effect of stannous fluoride on periodontics, J Clin Periodontol 8:203, 1981.

McFall W: Tooth loss in 100 patients with periodontal disease—a long term study, J Periodontol 53:539, 1982.

Meader H, Love J, and Suddick P: The long term effectiveness of periodontal therapy in a clinical practice, J Periodontol 56:253, 1985.

Morrison E et al: The significance of gingivitis during the maintenance phase of periodontal treatment, J Periodontol 53:31, 1982.

Nyman S, Lindhe J, and Rosling B: Periodontal surgery in plaque-infected dentitions, J Clin Periodontol 4:240, 1977.

Olsen C, Ammons W, and van Belle G: A longitudinal study comparing apically repositioned flaps with and without osseous surgery, Int J Periodontics Restorative Dent 5(4):11, 1985.

Pihlstrom B et al: Comparison of surgical and non-surgical treatment of periodontal disease: a review of current studies and additional results after 6½ years, J Clin Periodontol 10:524, 1983.

Rabbini G, Ash M, and Caffesse R: The effectiveness of subgingival scaling and root planing in calculus removal, J Periodontol 52:119, 1981.

Ramfjord S et al: Oral hygiene and maintenance of periodontal support, J Periodontol 53:26, 1982.

Ramfjord S et al: Four modalities of periodontal treatment compared over five years, J Clin Periodontol 14:445, 1987.

Rosling B, Nyman S, and Lindhe J: The effect of systematic plaque control on bone regeneration in infrabony pockets, J Clin Periodontol 3:38, 1976a.

Rosling B et al: The healing potential of the periodontal tissues following different techniques of periodontal surgery in plaque free dentitions: a 2-year clinical study, J Clin Periodontol 3:233, 1976b.

Roulet J and Roulet-Mehrens T: The surface roughness of restorative materials and dental tissues after polishing with prophylaxis and polishing pastes, J Periodontol 53:257, 1982.

Savitt ED et al: Comparison of cultural methods and DNA probe analyses for the detection of *Actinobacillus actinomycetemcomitans, Bacteroides gingivalis,* and *Bacteroides intermedius* in subgingival plaque samples, J Periodontol 59:431, 1988.

Slots J: Bacterial specificity in adult periodontitis: a survey of recent work, J Clin Periodontol 13:912, 1986.

Theilade E: The non-specific theory in microbial etiology of inflammatory periodontal diseases, J Clin Periodontol 13:905, 1986.

Walters C et al: In vitro root roughness following use of different polishing pastes, J Dent Res 63:204, 1984 (abstract).

Wunderlich R and Yaman P: In vitro effect of topical fluoride on dental porcelain, J Prosthet Dent 55:385, 1986.

Zambon J et al: Rapid identification of periodontal pathogens in subgingival dental plaque: comparison of indirect immunofluorescence microscopy with bacterial culture for detection of *Bacteroides gingivalis,* J Periodontol 56:(Nov suppl)32, 1985.

SUGGESTED READING

McFall WT: Supportive treatment. In American Academy of Periodontology: Proceedings of the World Workshop in Clinical Periodontics, Chicago, 1989, The Academy.

Chapter 42

OCCLUSAL THERAPY

Arnold S. Weisgold
Harold S. Baumgarten

Based on recent clinical research, certain features about trauma from occlusion, its relationship to infective periodontal diseases, and its modes of therapy seem to agree in large measure with long-term clinical observations. These characteristics of occlusal trauma can be listed as follows:

1. Both human and animal experiments demonstrate that trauma from occlusion does not cause pathologic changes in the supraalveolar connective tissue or junctional epithelium. For example, several studies have demonstrated that when "jiggling" force experiments are performed on animals with a normal periodontium, the supraalveolar connective tissue is *not* influenced by the occlusal forces, even though changes do occur in the periodontal ligament and alveolar process.

2. Once the periodontal space has increased in width to compensate for occlusal forces, the ligament tissue will usually show no signs of increased vascularity or exudation. Mobility will no longer be progressive in nature. Therefore the clinician must distinguish between *increased* mobility, which is greater than normal, and *increasing* mobility, which gets progressively worse over time.

3. Trauma from occlusion can cause resorption of the alveolar bone. This resorption can be reversed by eliminating or tempering the occlusal forces by means of occlusal adjustment. It has been demonstrated that with removal of the forces causing the trauma, bone tissue is deposited along the walls of the alveolus and on the bone crest area. This results in narrowing of the increased periodontal space. Stated another way, when tooth mobility be increased because of trauma, resulting in an increased width of the periodontal ligament, occlusal adjustment is an effective mode of therapy to reduce tooth mobility.

4. With continuing plaque-associated infective periodontal disease, trauma from occlusion, under certain circumstances, enhances the rate of progression of the disease. Recent findings appear to show, however, that the progression of plaque-associated lesions seems to be unrelated to the width of the periodontal ligament space.

5. Both a healthy periodontium with reduced height and a healthy periodontium with normal height appear to react similarly in their adaptation to excessive occlusal forces.

6. In the presence of reduced alveolar bone height in a healthy periodontium with a normal width of the periodontal ligament, tooth mobility can be accepted and splinting avoided if mastication is not impaired and the patient is comfortable.

7. Splinting is an indicated mode of therapy when the alveolar bone height is so compromised that tooth mobility

increases over time and mastication is impaired, or the patient is uncomfortable.

There are many definitions for the term *trauma from occlusion*. There is general agreement that it signifies pressure on the teeth capable of causing pathologic changes or adaptive alterations in the surrounding periodontium. The lesions of primary and secondary occlusal trauma are the same; however, primary origins of trauma may play a far more significant role in the pathologic changes because they are of greater intensity and more sustained in nature.

In treating patients with both infective periodontitis and trauma from occlusion, it is clear that initial therapy should be directed primarily toward control of plaque-associated etiology. Elimination or reduction of excessive occlusal forces may decrease tooth mobility but will not arrest the destruction of the periodontium associated with periodontal infection. *It is of paramount importance that tooth mobility be carefully monitored over a reasonable period of time to determine whether it is increased and stable or progressively increasing.*

THERAPEUTIC OCCLUSION

Once the clinician decides that there are rational reasons for altering an existing occlusion, it is important to outline the objectives of occlusal therapy to achieve a therapeutic occlusion that is consistent with health. The occlusion resulting after therapy may not conform to our preconceived concept of an ideal occlusion and often represents an acceptable compromise.

The basic objectives of any form of occlusal therapy should be:

1. Establishment or maintenance of a stable, reproducible intercuspal position
2. Freedom of movement to and from the intercuspal position
3. Development of an occlusion not noticeable to the patient
4. Maintenance of the newly established occlusal scheme over a reasonable period of time
5. Establishment of an occlusion with acceptable phonation, mastication, and esthetics

1. *Establishment or maintenance of a stable, reproducible, intercuspal position.* The posterior teeth should intercuspate in such a manner that forces will be directed along the long axes of the teeth. There is disagreement as to where the mandible should be when the teeth intercuspate. The prevailing concepts include the following: (1) all occlusal therapy should be done with the mandible in the intercuspal position; (2) the teeth should be made to articulate in the retruded path of the mandible; (3) the teeth should articulate in the retruded path, but allowance should be made for the mandible to move forward a certain distance to another intercuspal relationship; and (4) only the initial interference in the retruded path should be removed without changing the original intercuspal rela-

tionship. These ideas are often confusing to the clinician because it is difficult, if not impossible, to document on a statistical basis that one position is better than another. What appears to be of singular importance is that there should be a position where the teeth intercuspate.

In the naturally occurring healthy occlusion, postural position, occlusal vertical dimension, postural vertical dimension, and free-way space are of academic interest only. If the occlusion is healthy and all its parts are functioning to maintain it, then there is no need to alter the occlusal vertical dimension. However, in situations where, through loss, migration, or wear of teeth, the occlusal vertical dimension is less than would be found normally, change in this dimension may be necessary. It is here that occlusal vertical dimension and free-way space become significant to the clinician.

Free-way space measured in the premolar area is generally found to be in the range of 3 to 5 mm. However, any projected change in this dimension—either increase or decrease—should be approached with extreme caution, and a reasonable trial period should be instituted prior to the insertion of the completed prosthesis.

In developing a therapeutically established intercuspal relationship, the concept of *centric relation* is important. Although this term is relatively easy to define (it has at least 20 different definitions), it appears that centric relation is most difficult to find, at least from the standpoint that so many groups disagree on where it should be. Amsterdam (1974) has defined it as "the most favorable maxillo-mandibular relation at which position we would like to establish the maximum intercuspation of the teeth—whether by using full dentures, or occlusal adjustment of the natural dentition by selective grinding, orthodontics, restorative dentistry—including fixed and removable prosthesis, as well as periodontal prosthesis." The essential ingredients of centric relation are terminal condyle positioning, bilateral simultaneous neuromuscular activity, and maximum intercuspal relationship occurring at an occlusal vertical dimension that will allow for an adequate free-way space.

In altering the existing occlusion, at least two major objectives should be achieved: first, the new relationship must be physiologically acceptable to the patient, and second, it should be reproducible. Patient acceptability should include adequate mastication, phonation, and esthetics and can often be evaluated in a provisional prosthesis. Reproducibility of the new occlusion has two components: first, it should be reproducible for us to solve our transfer and adjustment techniques, and second and more important, it should be reproducible for the patient in that the mandible should be able to assume this position without any patient awareness of a change in position. It has been observed clinically that if the posterior teeth are made to intercuspate simultaneously at an occlusal vertical dimension that does not infringe on interdental clearance (i.e., free-way space), the patient is able to assume the position without an awareness of a change in the position.

2. *Freedom of movement to and from the intercuspal position.* The mandible must be able to move in all directions out of the intercuspal position without impediment. If the mandible is restrained in these movements, usually the teeth will either become mobile, wear excessively, or myofascial pain dysfunction will develop. A problem sometimes noted in extensive restorative dentistry is that the occlusal vertical is increased too much. As a result, the anterior overjet is increased, thereby making the anterior incisal guidance ineffectual. The mandible is then restrained from moving freely from the newly established intercuspal relationship.

3. *Development of an occlusion not noticeable to the patient.* The healthy functioning masticatory system is one in which the patient is totally unaware of the occlusion, being unaware of where the jaw is, of how the teeth articulate, and of the vertical dimension. The newly established occlusion should meet the same criteria.

4. *Maintenance of the newly established occlusal scheme over a reasonable period of time.* The therapist must evaluate and decide whether the teeth will maintain the occlusal relationship or require some adjunctive aid such as splinting.

5. *Establishment of an occlusion with acceptable phonation, mastication, and esthetics.* These are all subjective judgments made by the patient. The dentist, of course, can influence the patient's judgment as to the adequacy of these items; however, eventually the patient must be satisfied.

To review, then, the therapeutic occlusion is a man-made one. It should be based not on preconceived ideas, but on our knowledge of the system as it functions in health and those factors that can affect it adversely. A major decision of the therapist should be whether the occlusal problems can be solved or at least altered in the original intercuspal position or must be changed to such a degree that another mandibular position should be used.

DIFFICULTIES IN OCCLUSAL THERAPY

Most clinical concepts of occlusal therapy are applicable mainly to the Angle Class I, fairly intact dentition. Unfortunately, many patients with periodontal disease and occlusal trauma have missing teeth and skeletal and/or dental malocclusions. Provisions must be made for the occlusal management of these patients.

Form and function of the masticatory system

The forces on various groups of teeth differ. For example, only the posterior teeth and the mandibular anterior teeth should have functional forces placed along their long axes. Forces on the maxillary anterior teeth are directed primarily facially. Since teeth best withstand forces delivered along to their long axes (calling on the greatest number of periodontal ligament fibers—the oblique group), it is reasonable to expect that the posterior teeth as a group function to support the occlusal vertical dimension. The anterior teeth as a group are not suited to supporting the occlusal vertical dimension. Instead, they serve to disarticulate the posterior teeth during excursive movements of the mandible.

Thus it is not surprising that many patients with loss of posterior teeth have flared anterior teeth and a decreased occlusal vertical dimension. The anterior teeth, called on to support the occlusal vertical dimension, and which are actually in occlusal trauma, have responded by migrating to a new position.

In many situations, the anterior teeth are not positioned to provide their function of disarticulating the posterior teeth during mandibular excursions. A common clinical situation in which functional anterior guidance is not present is the non–orthodontically corrected Angle Class II, division 1. These situations can be treated by changing the form of the anterior teeth so that they may better fulfill their role in disarticulating the posterior teeth in excursive functions.

Altered canine form (Fig. 42-1)

Altering the palatal form of the maxillary canine (or all of the maxillary anterior teeth, if necessary) by providing a centric stop on an accentuated cingulum is indicated in the following situations:

1. Distal extension cases—allows the anterior teeth to function more like posterior teeth in supporting the occlusal dimension
2. Non–orthodontically corrected Angle Class II, division 1—provides anterior guidance where the teeth are not positioned to provide this function
3. Severe periodontal involvement of the posterior teeth—adds an additional vertical supporting stop

A commonly held misconception is that one must change a canine into a premolar. If this in fact were done, its lingual cusp would be a balancing interference. Our goal is to provide a platform on the palatal surface of the canine. This occlusal surface of the platform should be perpendicular to the long axes of the mandibular anterior teeth at the newly established occlusal vertical dimension.

In Angle Class II, division 1 malocclusions, placing the platform on the anterior teeth will allow the maxillary and mandibular teeth to contact. This will provide for immediate disarticulation of the posterior teeth when the mandible moves in excursions.

OCCLUSAL APPLIANCES

Occlusal appliances are used in dentistry in the diagnosis and treatment of a variety of dental disorders. Tooth hypermobility, myofascial pain dysfunction syndrome (MPDS), and disorders of the condyle-disk assembly are just a few situations where appliances are often quite

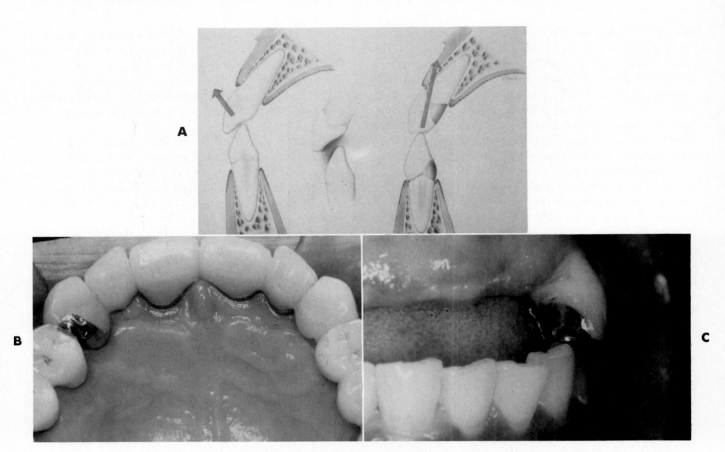

Fig. 42-1. A, *Left,* Normal anterior relationship. Note anterior direction of force on maxillary canine. *Center,* Restoring lost vertical dimension and using centric relation as preferred jaw position opens some interarch space. *Right,* Canine restored with altered canine form. Note redirection of force on maxillary canine. **B,** Lingual form of all anterior teeth has been modified in treatment of nonorthodontically corrected Angle Class II, division 1. Anterior guidance has been established. **C,** Various restorative materials may be used to alter lingual form of anterior teeth. Depicted is an etched cast metal retainer, bonded to a maxillary canine. Rest preparations have been placed to accept a removable partial denture. (**A** courtesy Dr. M. Amsterdam, Philadelphia.)

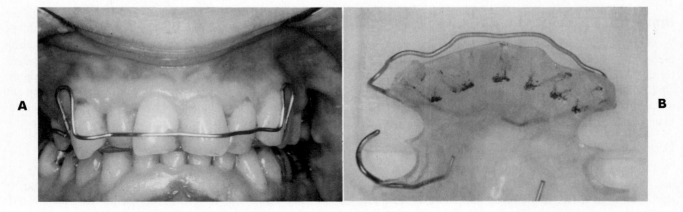

Fig. 42-2. A, Modified Hawley bite plane. Component parts include anterior bite plane, labial bow, and "C" clasps on most posterior abutment teeth. **B,** Properly adjusted modified Hawley bite plane—"Gothic arch" tracings from excursive contacts of each opposing tooth.

useful. When they are properly used, great benefit can be realized.

Classification

1. *Sectorial appliances.* These appliances contact a sector or group of teeth as opposed to all of the teeth. An example of this type of appliance is the modified Hawley bite plane (Fig. 42-2).
2. *Full-coverage appliances.* These appliances contact all of the teeth. An example of this type of appliance is the maxillary full-occlusal splint (night guard) (Fig. 42-3).

Use of sectorial appliances

Since sectorial appliances do not touch all of the teeth, these devices provide less control of the occlusal changes that may occur. The modified Hawley anterior bite plane, for example, disarticulates the posterior teeth. As a result, the posterior teeth are free to erupt. This can be beneficial if desired. However, eruption of the posterior teeth in an anterior open-bite case will make matters worse.

Other sectorial appliances include the Sved appliance, the mandibular orthopedic repositioning appliance (MORA), the pivot, and flexible athletic mouthguards.

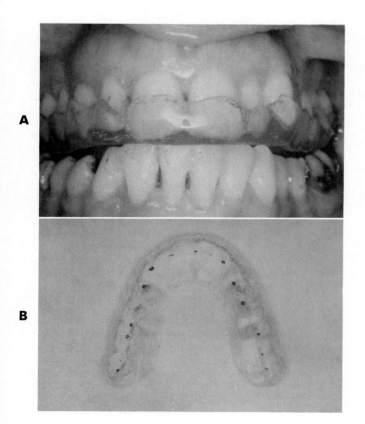

Fig. 42-3. A, Maxillary full occlusal splint. Occluding surface is flat, with as little guidance as can be tolerated. **B,** Each opposing tooth touches occluding surface of night guard with at least one contacting point.

Use of full-coverage appliances

Full-coverage appliances are used very often in clinical practice. They provide a tremendous amount of control in the sense that, assuming they fit well and are properly adjusted, very few untoward effects should be anticipated. Full-coverage appliances in general, the night guard in particular, are most commonly used for long-term nocturnal habit-control therapy and long-term mandibular repositioning.

Guidelines in the use of occlusal appliances

1. An assessment must be made of the patient's skeletal dental-muscular relationship. The muscular pattern may be either strong, weak, or average. The skeletal pattern may be classified as either dolichocephalic, brachiocephalic, or normocephalic. This can be determined by examining the patient in profile. If the mandibular plane is extended posteriorly and passes through the occiput, the patient is considered to be dolichocephalic and have a skeletal open-bite pattern. These patients often have a short ramus, an obtuse gonial angle, antegonial notching, and weak musculature. If the mandibular plane passes inferior to the occiput, the patient is brachiocephalic and displays a skeletal deep-bite tendency. These patients tend to have a square acute gonial angle, short lower face, and strong musculature. A normocephalic or average skeletal pattern is one in which the mandibular plane passes just below or crosses the base of the occiput.

A sectorial appliance that disarticulates the posterior teeth should be used with the utmost caution in patients with an anterior open-bite tendency. A sectorial appliance that disarticulates the anterior teeth should be used cautiously in patients with a deep-bite tendency—dolichocephalic patients. There is a greater propensity for these patients to intrude their posterior teeth, resulting in a posterior bite.

In all cases the teeth should occlude on smooth acrylic planes that allow freedom of movement into and out of a maximum intercuspal position. Furthermore, the appliance should be thin enough so that the free-way space is not interfered with.

2. Accuracy of fit of the appliance is as important as its design. The appliance should seat completely and be stable. If the slightest instability is noted, the appliance should be relined or remade. Only after the tooth/tissue fit is assured is the occlusion adjusted.

3. Occlusal appliances often enhance plaque and calculus development. Patients must be made aware of the need to clean the appliance and the covered teeth.

4. Side effects such as dental pain and induced MPDS are possible with even the most benign of appliances. It is the clinician's responsibility to carefully evaluate the patient at regular intervals (e.g., monthly) during the entire time the appliance is worn. This includes the maintenance phase of therapy. Any adverse effects must be noted and treated promptly.

OCCLUSAL ADJUSTMENT
Retruded position

Although the issue is controversial in its philosophy, we believe there are times when occlusal adjustment to the retruded position warrants consideration. For an occlusion to mechanically free itself from the intercuspal position, the anterior incisal guidance, posterior cusp height, and occlusal vertical dimension must be coordinated. For example, if the anterior incisal guidance is too shallow relative to the posterior cusp height, these cusps will probably clash in excursive movements of the mandible. Another example involves extruded posterior teeth, which may result in an effective cusp height too steep for the anterior incisal guidance.

A common example of the loss of harmony between anterior incisal guidance, posterior cusp height, and occlusal vertical dimension occurs when some posterior teeth have been previously lost and the remaining posterior teeth migrate, resulting in a decrease in the occlusal vertical dimension. Often this causes excessive overloading of the maxillary anterior teeth with labial migration and diastema formation. Often in these situations the remaining posterior teeth, especially the maxillary molars, have extruded, making their effective posterior cusp height greater than originally. As a result of these complex adaptive movements, cusps interfere in excursive movements. This results from the fact that their effective cusp heights are steeper and that there is an increase in the effectiveness of the anterior incisal guidance associated with anterior flaring. The problem, simply stated, is an anterior incisal guidance, posterior cusp height, and occlusal vertical dimension that are not in concert with each other. This is a situation wherein occlusal adjustment to the retruded position may be effective.

General considerations. When properly executed, occlusal adjustment procedures that establish a new intercuspal relation in the retruded path of closure can be a sound and rational approach to occlusal management of certain cases of occlusal trauma. Prior to instituting this therapy, it is important to determine definitively whether the objectives of occlusal stability and freedom of mandibular movement can be obtained in this new position. Certain severe malocclusions (such as the Class II, division I) often cannot be managed solely by selective grinding and require orthodontic procedures; they may also require prosthetic placement of the occlusal surfaces.

Of major importance, but often overlooked, is the amount of tooth structure available for adjustment. The occlusion with flat, worn cusps is generally not as amenable to selective grinding as that with steeper cusps. Also, the type and degree of discrepancy between the retruded position and the intercuspal position must be considered prior to therapy. For obvious mechanical reasons, the discrepancy with a more vertical component is usually easier to manage than the one with primarily a horizontal compo-

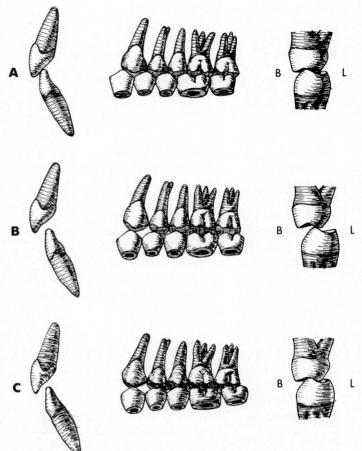

Fig. 42-4. A, "Normal" relationships of teeth in intercuspal position. Note anterior overbite and overjet, mesiodistal landmarks of teeth, and buccolingual landmarks. **B,** "Usual" relationships of teeth when mandible is in retruded contact position. Note decrease in anterior overbite and increase in overjet, mandibular buccoclusal line lingual to maxillary central fossa line, and mandibular buccal cusp tips distal to opposing marginal ridge areas. **C,** "Unusual" relationships of teeth when mandible is in retruded contact position. Note increase in anterior overjet with little or no decrease in overbite, mandibular buccoclusal line in central fossa line (not lingual to it), and mandibular buccal cusp tips distal to opposing marginal ridge areas. (From Weisgold A and Rosenberg E: Occlusal therapy. In Goldman H et al, editors: Current therapy in dentistry, vol 6, St Louis, 1977, The CV Mosby Co.)

nent (Fig. 42-4). Weinberg (1975) has investigated and compared the type and degree of discrepancy between the retruded contact position and the intercuspal position. He noted:

The amount of change in vertical dimension that accompanies the anterior slide will be inversely proportioned to the expected degree of anterior condylar displacement. The more change in vertical dimension that exists in proportion to the anterior slide, the less anterior condylar displacement we should expect. When the change in vertical dimension is almost as great as the amount of anterior slide, then little anterior condylar displacement should be expected. When the change in vertical dimension approaches one third of the anterior slide, then maximum anterior condylar displacement is produced with normal TMJ function . . . a deflective slide in centric relation to centric occlusion does not necessarily mean anterior condylar displacement. Its diagnosis and treatment depend on the correlation of three factors: the direction and magnitude of the slide from centric relation to centric occlusion, the change in vertical dimension of occlusion during the slide, and the position of the condyles in the fossae when the teeth are in maximum occlusion (centric occlusion).

Generally, when the mandible is placed in the retruded path of closure, the buccoclusal line angle of the mandibular posterior teeth relate lingually to (instead of directly into) the maxillary central fossa line. This is because of the disparity in size and shape of the mandible relative to the maxilla. Hence, when retruded, the narrower anterior part of the mandible (and its teeth) relates lingually to a wider part of the maxilla (and its teeth). When this occurs, the clinician is often able to reshape the cusp tips and inclines to better relate the mandibular and maxillary teeth. The advantage to this method is that cusp height can be decreased but the vertical dimension of occlusion is not compromised, since the condyles are in a more posterior and superior position. In fact, it is not uncommon to note an increase in anterior overjet and decrease in overbite after performing this type of adjustment, which has advantages.

There is a particular occlusal type that often is not treatable by selective grinding, and the therapist must take extreme precautions not to upset the original intercuspal relationship. Patients with this occlusal type often come for treatment with a complaint that a dentist "just adjusted one tooth or cusp and ruined my entire bite." Examination will frequently reveal a moderate overbite, greater than normal overjet, relatively stable intercuspal position, moderate to flat posterior cuspal form, worn mandibular incisal edges, and at times posterior tooth contacts in excursive movements. On further examination one notes a rather significant discrepancy (greater than 4 mm) between the intercuspal position and retruded contact position. This discrepancy is primarily horizontal in nature. Temporomandibular radiography also shows a horizontal discrepancy between these two positions, and the study casts reveal arches that are similar in size and shape, as opposed to the commonly occurring situation of a disparity in size and shape.

In this occlusal type, when the mandible is retruded, the mandibular buccoclusal line angle does not relate lingually to the maxillary central fossa line, but in the central fossa line. The mandibular teeth are merely more distal, but not lingual. However, what has happened is that the cusp tips in a mesiodistal position are no longer in opposing marginal ridge areas but now appose each other. The mandible is now restrained from leaving the intercuspal position. Furthermore, since the mandible is more distally placed, the anterior incisal guidance is not as effectual as previously noted, and this further complicates mandibular glide patterns. Since the cusp heights were minimal to begin with, it is difficult, if not impossible, to reduce them. As stated, it is most wise to do little or no grinding whatsoever to avoid changing the intercuspal relationship. Often all that the clinician can do for this type of occlusal problem is to try to reassure the patient, use muscle relaxants and/or exercises, and employ an occlusal appliance such as the full maxillary night guard. The modified Hawley bite plane, on the other hand, must be used with great care, for if the posterior teeth are left out of contact over a long period of time, they may erupt to further complicate and aggravate the situation. If the Hawley appliance is used, the posterior teeth should be kept in contact slightly and the anterior bite plane employed to provide for the loss of incisal guidance.

Use of selective grinding. Selective grinding is often indicated when there is evidence of trauma from occlusion or MPDS of known occlusal etiology, and/or prior to restorative or prosthetic dentistry. A very common indication for this therapeutic approach is in cases of primary occlusal traumatism. An approach to selective grinding whereby the entire occlusal scheme is altered is discussed in the following paragraphs. This technique should be employed only when the therapist realizes that the occlusal disorder cannot be managed solely by adjusting the original intercuspal relationship (i.e., when there are multiple nonworking interferences, inadequate anterior overjet, trauma to the maxillary anterior teeth, and/or an overawareness of the occlusion).

The procedure is carried out in three steps.

Step 1. Correction of the landmark relationships of the teeth in the retruded position of the mandible. The objectives of this step are to bring into simultaneous contact the supporting inclines of the posterior teeth, to close the occlusal vertical dimension sufficiently to provide for as effectual incisal guidance as possible, and also to have the mandibular functional outer aspect areas positioned properly. An additional advantage often will be gained because often the inclines that will have to be adjusted are the same ones that interfere on the nonworking side. In other words, completing this step properly will often eliminate some or all of the nonworking interferences.

As mentioned previously, when the mandible is placed in the retruded path of closure, the mandibular buccoclusal line angles will be lingual to the maxillary central fossae. Similarly, the maxillary linguoclusal line angles will be buccal to the mandibular central fossae. This will necessitate broadening the inner aspects of the mandibular buccal cusps and maxillary lingual cusps to position the cusp tips into their respective fossae.

Sometimes, however, the occlusal discrepancy is such that the mandibular buccoclusal line angle is buccal to the maxillary central fossae. In this situation narrowing of inclines would be indicated.

Step 2. Definition of the functional outer aspect (FOA) areas. The mandibular FOA may function to contact the maxillary guiding cusps during glide movements of the mandible. Once step 1 is essentially completed, a marking medium (e.g., articulating paper) is placed between the teeth and the patient is instructed to move the mandible from side to side (in effect creating horizontal glide movements). Grinding is now done by removing all markings on the outer aspects of the 1 mm band of FOA. Optimally, once completed, the dentist should be able to see a 1 mm ribbon on the outer aspects of all the teeth; this is the "functional outer aspect." Often, however, because of tooth position and limitations of grinding, this will not be

a perfect 1 mm line. As a general rule, once the FOA is established, it usually will not be altered.

Step 3. Adjustment of the guiding inclines. The guiding cusps are those that have the potential for contact only in glide movements. Step 3 is generally accomplished by having the patient move the mandible forward and also to the side. An impediment to mandibular movement should be managed by adjusting the guiding inclines of the maxillary teeth (i.e., inner aspects of buccal cusps and lingual of anterior teeth). If major adjustments must be made on the maxillary anterior teeth, the patient should be notified of this and his permission granted before proceeding (Fig. 42-5).

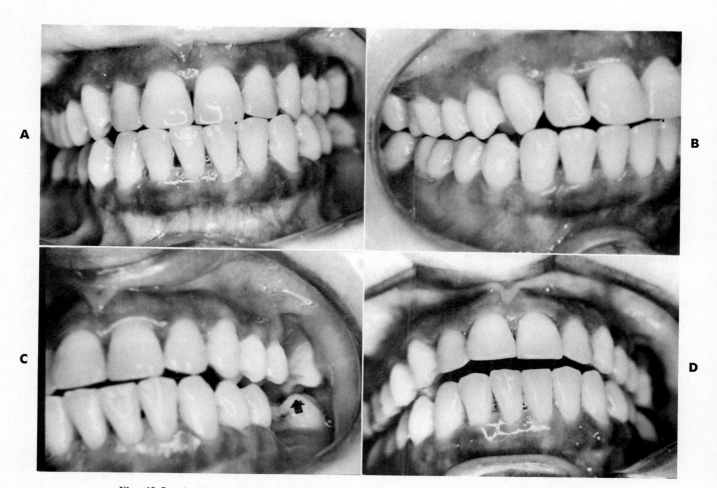

Fig. 42-5. **A,** Maximum intercuspal position. Note edge-to-edge relationship of anterior teeth, steep posterior cuspal form, and midline discrepancy. **B,** Right working movement. **C,** Left nonworking movement. Note nonworking interferences on molars and premolars. Arrow indicates nonworking interference occurring between $\underline{7}$ and $\overline{7}$. **D,** Retruded contact position. Note anterior "open bite" and landmark relationships of posterior teeth on right and left sides. (From Weisgold A and Laudenbach K.: Alpha Omegan 69:60, Dec 1976.)

An effort should be made at this time to eliminate all cross-tooth interferences. Cross-tooth interferences are those that occur in a working movement and will be located on the inner aspects of the mandibular lingual cusps and outer aspects of maxillary lingual cusps. Since the adjustment during step 3 will be made on the guiding inclines of the maxillary teeth, there is always the possibility of inadvertently decreasing the working side rise. In effect, this can result in the generation of working and nonworking interferences. The same problem can develop if grinding of the maxillary anterior teeth is overzealous. The clinician must check all excursive movements thoroughly at the completion of this phase of adjustment and remove working and nonworking interferences that were newly created.

Finally, polishing all tooth surfaces is extremely important at the completion of selective grinding. If inclines are left rough, the patient will often concentrate on this area or find the sound disturbing.

At the completion of therapy using the above approach, no discrepancy should be discernible between the retruded position and the intercuspal position. In other words, the teeth will have been reshaped to articulate in the retruded path of closure. There should be no "centric slip." How-

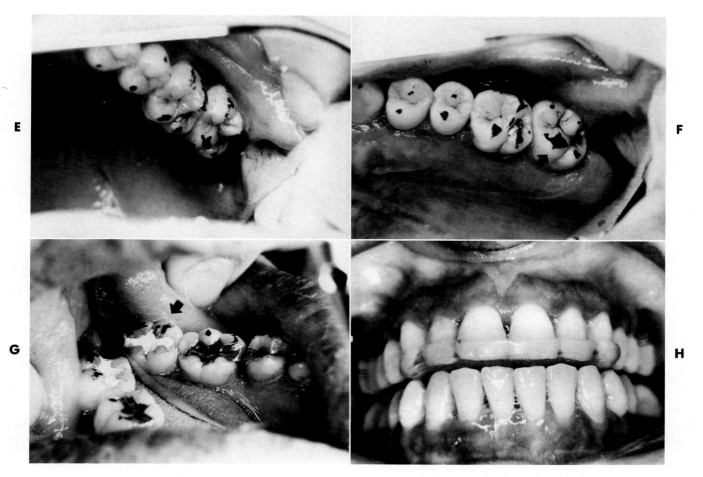

Fig. 42-5, cont'd. E, Occlusal view of maxillary right side. Markings were made in mandible's retruded path of closure. Note intitial interference *(largest marking)* occurring on mesiolingual cusp of maxillary second molar *(arrow)*. **F,** Occlusal view of maxillary right side. These markings were made as a result of mandible moving to opposite (i.e., left) side. This is a right-sided nonworking interference that is occurring on mesiolingual cusp of maxillary second molar. Direction of nonworking interference is oblique and runs in a mesiolingual to distobuccal path *(arrow)*. Note also that in this particular patient, same cusps that interfered in retruded path also interfered on nonworking side. **G,** Mirror view of mandibular right side. Note markings on second molar. Because this tooth is extruded beyond occlusal plane, it interferes both in retruded position and on nonworking side. Arrow indicates nonworking interferences on buccal cusps of ⟨7⟩ . **H,** Maxillary Hawley bite plane inserted. *Continued.*

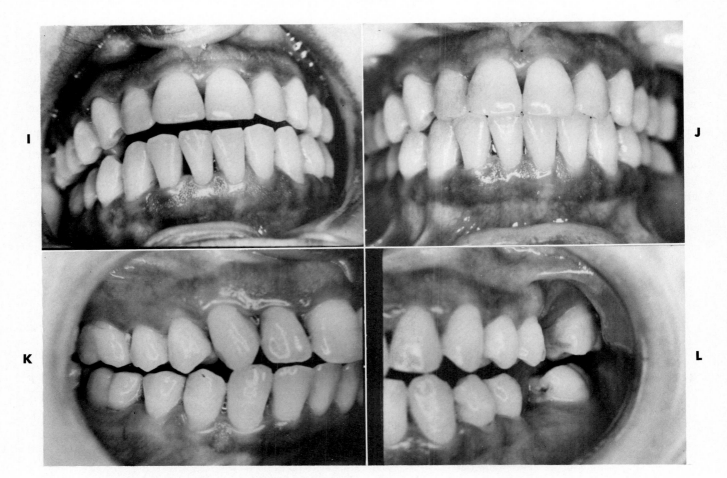

Fig. 42-5, cont'd. I. Appearance of patient after wearing appliance for 4 weeks while sleeping. Note anterior tooth relationship in retruded path of closure, buccolingual relationships of posterior teeth, and midline. Patient has been comfortable during this period of time. **J,** Appearance after selective grinding. Note midline and degree of anterior overbite and overjet (compare with **A**). **K,** Appearance after selective grinding—right working movement (compare with **B**). **L,** Appearance after selective grinding—left nonworking movement (compare with **C**).

ever, our observations have shown that in time a discrepancy generally appears and usually measures approximately 1 mm. Why has this occurred? Explanations that have been offered to the profession are that the mandible is seeking to return to its original position or some form of condylar remodeling has occurred. These are plausible explanations, but another possibility is that a tooth (or possibly a pair of teeth) has moved slightly. Now when the mandible is placed in the retruded position, the teeth that interfere are those that have moved; then the mandible slides forward into the intercuspal position—not the one that the patient originally had, but the one that was therapeutically developed by the dentist. Further investigations will hopefully give us a better insight into this perplexing problem.

Management of the nonworking interference. This interference is probably the most destructive: once it is operational, the teeth strike each other off their axes, generating lateral forces destructive to the periodontium. Because of its importance, various techniques are mentioned as follows:

1. *Elimination of interference during adjustment of step 1.* This is discussed earlier in the chapter.
2. *Channeling or "trolley-tracking."* The nonworking interference is marked on the mandibular tooth, and a groove is created on the inner aspect of the tooth so that the maxillary lingual cusp can move through it without interference.
3. *Shallowing the opposing fossa.* A restoration is placed in an opposing central fossa area, thereby

making it more shallow. In maximum intercuspation the opposing cusp tip may now be in premature contact. If so, the opposing cusp tip is shortened to obtain correct contact. In doing so, the nonworking interference is eliminated while tooth contact is retained during intercuspation.

4. *Increasing the opposite side working guidance.* This increase is usually accomplished by restorative dentistry.

5. *Extraction.* Often an unopposed mandibular third molar will erupt in such a direction that it will interfere on the nonworking side. Extraction of the third molar is often the best treatment.

Use of selective grinding and restorative or prosthetic dentistry. The objectives and technique for this form of adjustment are the same as those for selective grinding alone, differing only in the extent of therapy. Restorative or prosthetic dentistry is warranted when the therapist has decided that the objectives cannot be achieved and maintained solely by selective grinding. Generally, the occlusion is adjusted to remove interferences in the retruded path of closure, and the quadrants opposing the edentulous spaces are reshaped to create a functional occlusal environment. It is extremely important that *the remaining natural teeth support the vertical dimension when a removable prosthesis is being used.* Otherwise, the removable prosthesis will settle and the natural teeth will in fact support centric occlusion.

Adjusting the existing occlusion

Adjusting the existing occlusion is a very common way of treating occlusal problems; however, correction of the existing intercuspal position should be undertaken only after careful evaluation of the occlusion. Selection of the intercuspal position as the jaw position of choice limits the therapist, since all the factors of occlusion should now be considered fixed. In other words, cusp height, incisal guidance, and occlusal vertical dimension cannot be altered, which makes this form of adjustment difficult. Also, if occlusal grinding is to be extensive and is done in this position, there is a good possibility that either the occlusal vertical dimension will be closed or the cusps that originally supported this position will be altered, causing a change in jaw relationships.

If in spite of the limitations, the clinician can predict achievement of the objectives by correcting the occlusion in the intercuspal position, there is little reason not to use it.

Splinting. Aside from being a means of replacing missing teeth, splinting is an indicated mode of therapy when the alveolar bone height is so compromised that tooth mobility is increasing, mastication is difficult, and the patient is unable to use the dentition in a comfortable manner:

I. Temporary splints
  A. Extracoronal type
    1. Wire ligation
    2. Orthodontic bands
    3. Removable acrylic appliances
    4. Removable cast appliances
    5. Bonded metal mesh
    6. Light-cured composite
    7. Combinations of the above
  B. Intracoronal type
    1. Wire and acrylic
    2. Wire and amalgam
    3. Wire and light-cured composite
    4. Wire, amalgam, and acrylic
    5. Cast chrome cobalt bars with amalgam, acrylic, or both
    6. Combinations of the above
II. Provisional splints
  A. All acrylic
  B. Adapted metal band and acrylic
III. Permanent splints
  A. Etched bonded metal retainer
  B. Partial-coverage fixed prosthodontics
  C. Full-coverage fixed prosthodontics

Temporary splints are usually placed during active periodontal therapy. They are not as durable as permanent splints and often must be repaired periodically. *Provisional splints* are splints that are fabricated as part of a restorative dentistry program, such as full-coverage provisional splints. They are used to evaluate a new occlusal scheme, as well as to provide temporary coverage prior to insertion of the final prosthesis. The *permanent splint* is the final prosthesis; however, the term *permanent splint* is a misnomer. Almost nothing is permanent in dentistry or in any other discipline. Unfortunately, the term seems to be with us to stay.

DISEASES RELATED TO PATHOLOGIC OCCLUSION

Tooth hypermobility and retrograde wear are two of the major symptoms of pathologic occlusion. In many instances a pathologic occlusion may manifest itself with the appearance of extraoral symptoms. These extraoral diseases have traditionally been placed in the catchall category of *temporomandibular joint syndrome.* Recent advances in diagnosis and treatment have resulted in their being renamed to more accurately describe their cause.

Myofascial pain dysfunction syndrome

In MPDS, pain is caused by spasm of the muscles of mastication and/or the cervical musculature. The causes of the muscle spasm can be varied, and there is often a strong psychologic component. Before we modify the patient's occlusion in the treatment of MPDS, we must be able to unequivocally indict the occlusion as a causative factor in the disease. As an aid, occlusal appliances are often used to determine if the occlusion is a contributing factor in the disease. Insertion of a well-fitting, noninterfering, full-coverage maxillary night guard as an initial diagnostic/therapeutic aid in patients with MPDS is often successful in relieving symptoms. If this is the case, subsequent adjustment of the occlusion may give long-lasting relief from MPDS.

Disorders of the condyle-disk assembly

In the normal temporomandibular joint, the meniscus is interposed between the condyle and the articular eminence. Aberrations in the positions of these parts or abnormalities of the individual parts (i.e., meniscus dislocations or perforations) are termed *disorders of the condyle-disk assembly*. There is much disagreement as to the cause of these problems. Many investigators believe that the occlusion is a causative factor. Others believe that muscular or local intracapsular factors are the cause. Treatment of these disorders often involves the use of occlusal appliances. They function to relax the muscles of mastication, to unload the temporomandibular joint, and very often to reposition the mandible in order to recapture a dislocated meniscus.

CONCLUSIONS

The research data as to the efficacy of occlusal adjustment are sparse as of this time. Clinical observations over long periods of time give us the strong impression that minimizing forces on the teeth is beneficial to the periodontium, especially if it is compromised as a result of infectious periodontitis and occlusal traumatic lesions combined.

REFERENCES

Amsterdam M: Periodontal prosthesis—twenty-five years in retrospect, Alpha Omegan 67:9, Dec 1974.

Weinberg L: Anterior condylar displacement: its diagnosis and treatment, J Prosthet Dent 34:195, 1975.

SUGGESTED READINGS

Anderson D: Measurement of stress in mastication, II, J Dent Res 35:671, 1956.

Apes T and McIlwain JE Jr: The multiple uses of acid etch techniques, Dent Surv 50:25, 1974.

Baumgarten HS and Garber D: The use and abuses of occlusal appliances, Alpha Omegan 78:57, 1985.

Ericsson I and Lindhe J: Lack of effect of trauma from occlusion on the recurrence of experimental periodontitis, J Clin Periodontol 4:115, 1977.

Ericsson I and Lindhe J: The effect of long standing jiggling on experimental marginal periodontitis in the beagle dog, J Clin Periodontol 9:497, 1982.

Ericsson I and Lindhe J: Lack of significance of increased tooth mobility in experimental periodontitis, J Periodontol 55:447, 1984.

Farrar WB and McCarty WL: A clinical outline of temporomandibular joint diagnosis and treatment, ed 7, Montgomery, Ala, 1983, Normandie Study Group for TMJ Dysfunction.

Goodman P, Greene C, and Laskin D: Response of patients with myofascial pain-dysfunction syndrome to mock equilibration, J Am Dent Assoc 92:755, 1976.

Kayne B: Criteria for occlusal alteration in the management of craniomandibular dysfunction, Alpha Omegan 78:47, 1985.

Kegel W, Selipsky H, and Phillips C: The effect of splinting on tooth mobility. I. During initial therapy, J Clin Periodontol 6:45, 1979.

Lindhe J and Nyman S: Occlusal therapy. In Lindhe J, editor: Textbook of clinical periodontology, Copenhagen, 1984, Munksgaard.

Lindhe J, Nyman S, and Ericsson I: Trauma from occlusion. In Lindhe J, editor: Textbook of periodontology, Copenhagen, 1984, Munksgaard.

Miller GM and Kreuzer DW: The modified Hawley appliance, III, Int J Periodontics Restorative Dent 2:55, 1982.

Mohl NP et al: Textbook of occlusion, Chicago, 1988, Quintessence Publishing Co, Inc.

Nyman S et al: The significance of alveolar bone in periodontal disease, J Periodont Res 19:520, 1984.

Pihlstrom B et al: Association between signs of trauma from occlusion and periodontitis, J Periodontol 57:1, 1986.

Polson AM, Meitner SW, and Zander HA: Trauma and progression of marginal periodontitis in squirrel monkeys. IV. Reversibility of bone loss due to trauma alone and trauma superimposed upon periodontitis, J Periodont Res 11:290, 1976.

Potashnick S and Abrams L: The significance of occlusal adjustment in peridontal therapy, Alpha Omegan 78:25, 1985.

Rosling B, Nyman S, and Lindhe J: The effect of systemic plaque control on bone regeneration in infrabony pockets, J Clin Periodontol 3:38, 1976.

Sved A: Changing the occlusal level and a new method of retention, Am J Orthod 30:527, 1944.

Weisgold A: A review of the various concepts of occlusion: a historical perspective, Alpha Omegan 66:9, Dec 1973.

Weisgold A and Laudenbach K: Occlusal etiology and management of disorders of the temporomandibular joint and related structures, Alpha Omegan 69:60, Dec 1976.

Weisgold A and Rosenberg E: Occlusal therapy. In Goldman H et al, editors: Current therapy in dentistry, vol 6, St Louis, 1977, The CV Mosby Co.

Chapter 43

TOOTH MOVEMENT AS AN ADJUNCT TO PERIODONTAL THERAPY

Robert L. Vanarsdall, Jr.

As described in other chapters, there are many different forms of periodontitis, and each disease is quite different from the others. Moreover, periodontal disease for an individual may present itself differently from the disease description drawn from the pooled data of population groups, in which individual responses have been statistically masked. It is agreed, however, that periodontal diseases are infectious processes of bacterial origin. Not only does the disease exhibit cyclic episodes with periods of quiescence followed by acute exacerbation, but the rate of breakdown varies greatly. The disease may exhibit an enhanced rate of breakdown when associated with trauma from occlusion. Animal (beagle) studies have demonstrated that jiggling occlusal forces can aggravate an active periodontitis lesion and may accelerate loss of connective tissue attachment (Svanberg and Lindhe, 1974; Ericsson and Lindhe, 1982). In addition, an active periodontitis with superimposed trauma has been shown to produce more bone loss than periodontitis only (Kantor et al., 1976). Rapid loss of attachment has been observed in clinical patients with inflammatory disease who experience increased mobility during orthodontic tooth movement (Fig. 43-1). Therefore progression or attachment loss can be accelerated by occlusal forces that are beyond the adaptive capacity of the individual patient.

Evidence has revealed that during active disease episodes increased numbers of gram-negative, anaerobic bacterial flora are present. Clinical experience, as well as research, has shown that there are specific dental areas that are susceptible to the disease process.

The critical question involves why the disease process exhibits site/area specificity. Why does it occur on very specific surfaces of individual teeth? In furcation areas, for example, the maxillary molars are the first teeth to be lost because of periodontal disease. Mandibular molars, as well, exhibit bone loss in furcation areas. Tilted, malposed, overlapped, and crowded teeth allow for inaccessible embrasures and plaque retention. Areas inaccessible for patient cleaning or natural self-cleaning aspects of tooth surfaces may be rendered ineffective; this therefore partially explains site specificity. This disease characteristic, then, can be attributed to some degree to local environmental and anatomic relationships (Fig. 43-2, *A* to *E*). Root fissures, grooves, and concavities, as well as tooth and root position, allow for anatomic relationships conducive to rapid bone loss and pocket depth.

Periodontal care should be directed toward elimination of the bacterial infection and prevention of reinfection. This involves creating an environment more self-cleaning and less conducive to harboring pathogenic bacteria. Obviously, appropriate therapy for each individual depends on the type, severity, and morphology created by the specific disease, but patient compliance is also a factor. Areas ac-

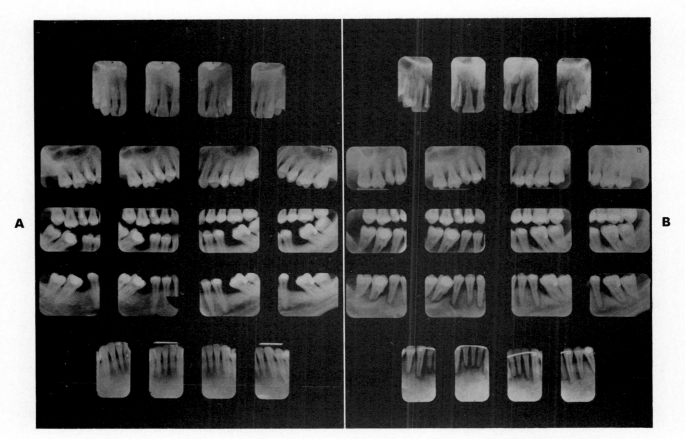

Fig. 43-1. **A,** Preorthodontic radiographs of a woman with mild to moderate periodontitis. **B,** Postorthodontic radiographs 3 years later reveal evidence of significant bone loss, root resorption, and radiographic signs of occlusal trauma. With good inflammatory and occlusal control, these hazards can be prevented. (**A** from Vanarsdall RL: Orthodontics and periodontics: interrelationships to maximize treatment results. In Graber LW, editor: Orthodontics: state of the art, essence of the science, St Louis, 1986, The CV Mosby Co.)

cessible for plaque removal by one person may not allow for effective oral hygiene by a less motivated individual. Regardless, elimination of as many plaque retentive areas as possible should be an objective. Large numbers of teeth are extracted in an effort to eliminate periodontal defects (defects that represent bacterial reservoirs) that could be corrected by simple tooth eruption (Fig. 43-3).

Our objectives in therapy must be realistic. Oral hygiene measures used alone have been ineffective in the removal of inflammation in deeper diseased sites of periodontal pockets. In addition, clinical trials have shown that regular- and short-interval prophylaxis by a hygienist

may lead to the prevention of disease. Unfortunately, large groups of patients are not always as compliant with suggested or recommended maintenance schedules as the study patient groups that have been reported (Wilson et al., 1987). Idealistic oral hygiene demands may not be realistic for many patient groups. Those less motivated diseased individuals can be cared for and treated in a fashion that would best prevent or minimize the chances of reinfection as much as possible. Overtreatment for one patient might be considered negligent care if not provided for another, depending on demands, needs, and personal circumstances.

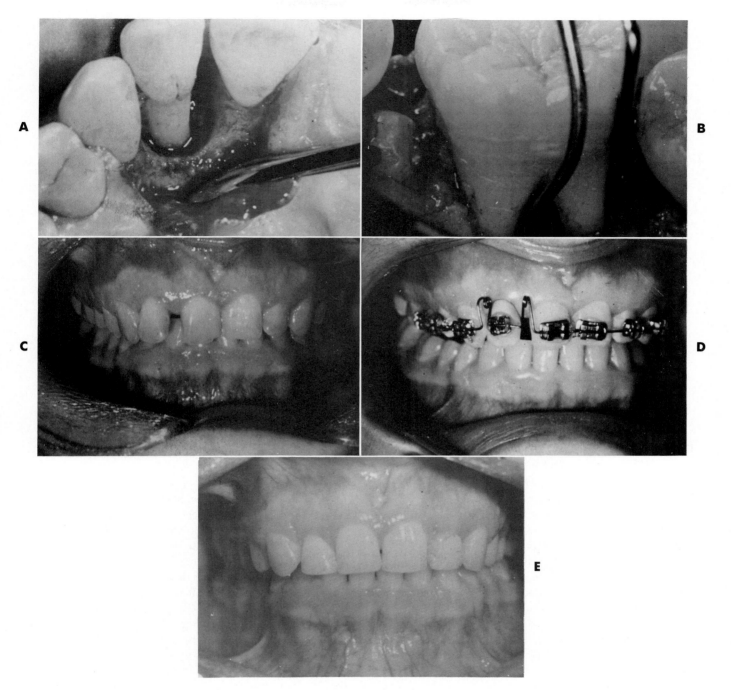

Fig. 43-2. A, Open curettage to allow a plaque-retentive palatogingival groove to be removed from root surface below cervical area of labially positioned right lateral incisor. Localized osseous defect is commonly associated with this developmental anomaly. **B,** Open furcation on lingual aspect of lower molar accumulates plaque and frequently demonstrates a site for progressive loss of attachment. **C,** Maxillary right lateral incisor is labially displaced as a result of severe palatal inflammation associated with a palatogingival groove. Isolated lesion is only bone loss exhibited in patient's dentition. **D,** After root planing to remove palatogingival groove and curettage to correct inflammation, tooth was extruded and retracted. Incisal edge and palatal aspect of anatomic crown were reduced with high-speed diamond to prevent trauma and to improve crown-to-root ratio. **E,** Five-years after treatment, lateral incisor remains firm with no recurrence of periodontal disease. *Continued.*

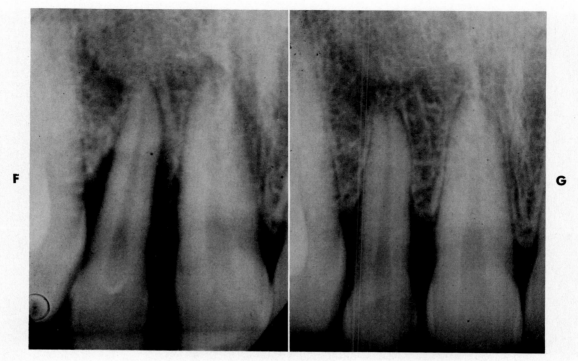

Fig. 43-2, cont'd. F, Preorthodontic radiograph of right lateral incisor. **G,** Five-year postoperative radiograph following retraction and extrusion. Tooth is stable with no recurrent disease.

INDICATIONS FOR AND CONTRAINDICATIONS TO TOOTH MOVEMENT

One of the most dramatic means available to improve local environmental factors is through tooth movement (Fig. 43-4). Tooth movement can be used to modify site specificity of the disease process and enhance the potential for long-term maintenance (see Figs. 43-2 and 43-3).

Periodontally susceptible patients who have experienced shifting, migration, extrusion, flaring, and lost teeth can benefit from tooth movement to correct local etiologic factors, predisposing malpositions, and certain bony and periodontal pockets. Solutions to occlusal problems may require repositioning teeth to establish buccolingual landmarks, eliminate interferences, reestablish incisal guidance, and correct loss of vertical dimension. Clearly delineated treatment objectives should be established before any appliances are placed. The most common indications and contraindications involving adjunctive tooth movement are as listed in the box on p. 511.

For patients with advanced disease and large numbers of deep pockets, surgery (ostectomy) may be contraindicated. Eruption of individual teeth can reduce pocket depth, provide physiologic gingival and osseous topography, preserve the maximum amount of attachment apparatus, and prepare a patient for long-term maintenance (Fig. 43-5).

Prior to irreversible tooth replacement and restorative dentistry procedures, tooth movement can allow for proper tooth preparation and parallel abutments, create pontic spaces, improve crown-to-root ratios, correct mucogingival and osseous defects, establish occlusal landmark relationships, provide proper embrasure spaces, and achieve the most favorable distribution of teeth (Vanarsdall and Musich, 1985). Furcation-involved abutments for restorative dentistry are considered to have a guarded or poor prognosis. Abnormal tooth position for the highly periodontally susceptible patient needing restorative care may create inaccessible areas, poor gingival contour, and other adverse local etiologic factors. Distobuccal root contacts with adjacent teeth can be repositioned for enhanced plaque control and reduced possibility of furcation caries.

Improved self-maintenance of soft tissue health is noted in patients following correction of accentuated mesial drift (Fig. 43-6) and bite collapse.

Once the teeth have been aligned, the tissue demonstrates less tendency to bleed on gentle probing and therefore may require less frequent root planing and curettage to control or prevent further periodontal breakdown. A recent study shows more plaque accumulation on malposed teeth as compared with contralateral well-aligned teeth (Griffiths and Addy, 1981). An acceptable level of mechanical plaque control requires an oral environment that enables the patient to remove plaque.

Uprighting abutment teeth improves osseous and soft

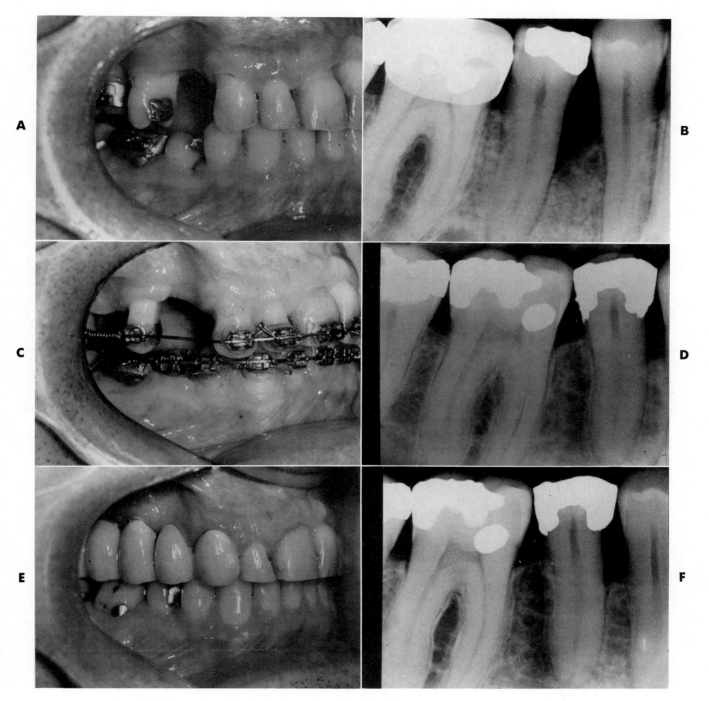

Fig. 43-3. A, Lower right second premolar was planned for extraction because of mesial infrabony defect. Observe mesial bleeding on gentle probing. **B,** Preeruption radiograph of lower right second premolar exhibiting mesial osseous defect. **C,** Instead of extraction, a fixed appliance was used to erupt second premolar relative to adjacent molar and first premolar. Note occlusal movement of gingival margin following eruption. **D,** Posteruption radiograph. Observe change in osseous topography on mesial and distal aspects of second premolar. **E,** Observe second premolar several years after eruption. **F,** Eight-year follow-up radiograph does not reveal any evidence of disease recurrence.

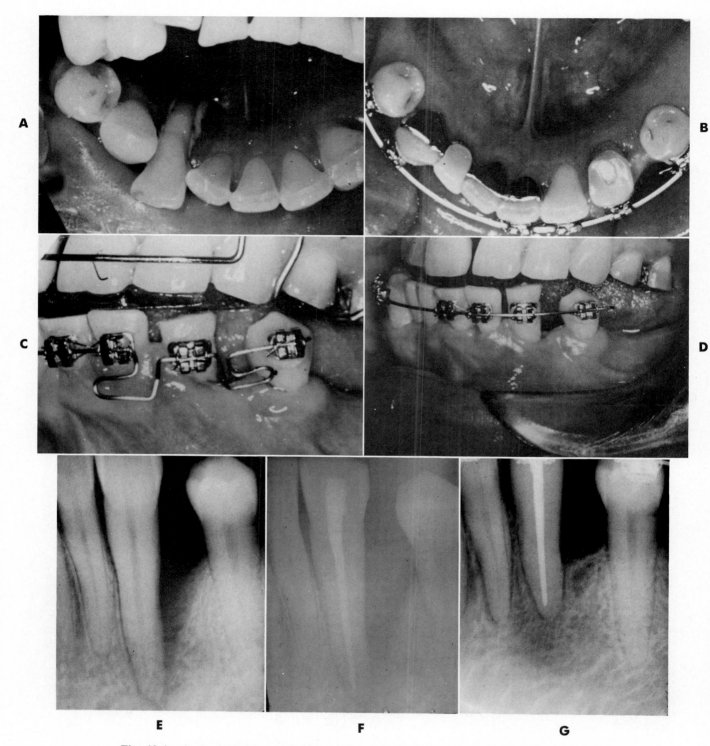

Fig. 43-4. **A,** Occlusal view of lower anterior teeth. Right lateral incisor is hopeless, with only labial soft tissue attachment remaining. Mandibular arch has only first premolar to first premolar remaining. Molars have been extracted because of periodontal disease. **B,** Occlusal view following removal and replacement of right lateral incisor with bonded cast Vitallium splint to act as anchorage. Lower left canine is devitalized to allow for eruption to modify distal osseous defect. Plan is to move lower left first premolar distally to serve as abutment to prevent need for a distal extension partial denture. **C,** Eruption and distal movement of first premolar. **D,** View following eruption and reflection of tissue on mesial aspect of canine to level attachment between left canine and lateral incisor. **E,** Preoperative radiograph of lower left canine. **F,** Radiograph 2 months after completion of endodontic treatment on canine and following scaling and root planing. **G,** Radiograph at completion of eruption after tissue procedure to level mesial attachment.

Adjunctive tooth movement: indications/contraindications

Indications	*Appliance and tooth movement*
1. Adverse gingival topography, root proximity, embrassure space, open contacts, lack of parallelism, poor distribution of abutments	Fixed appliance: alignment, tipping, translation
2. Flared anterior tooth, lip incompetency, lack of incisal guidance	Fixed and removable appliances: retraction, tipping, torque
3. Buccolingual landmark discrepancy preventing selective grinding for stability and redistribution of force	Fixed and removable appliances: tipping, translation
4. Severe curve of Spee and locked-in occlusal scheme with occlusal trauma or restorative needs	Fixed appliance: leveling occlusal plane
5. Severely tipped teeth	Fixed appliance: uprighting, tipping
6. Occlusal trauma with pseudo–Class III anterior crossbite, posterior crossbite, primary contact in centric relation	Fixed appliance: retraction, tipping
7. Improvement in gingival and osseous defects, poor crown-to-root ratio, unlevel bone between teeth	Fixed appliance: eruption, tipping, intrusion
8. Anterior deep bites and occlusal trauma with gingival trauma, retrograde wear, locked bites	Fixed appliance: intrusion
9. Anterior open bites and occlusal trauma with lack of incisal guidance	Fixed and removable appliances: eruption, retraction
10. Severe occlusal trauma/excessive mobility, muscle spasm, severe retruded contact (RC) position, maximum intercuspal (IC) position discrepancy, need to establish vertical dimension, need for selective grinding	Hawley bite plane for occlusal eruption, rest, and reduction of muscle hyperactivity

Contraindications

1. Lack of inflammatory control prior to, or lack of maintenance of periodontal health during, tooth movement
2. Lack of occlusal control (occlusal traumatism, parafunctional habits) for periodontally susceptible individuals

3. Short roots or idiopathic root resorption
4. Inability to retain individual teeth following movement or to secure a restorative commitment in cases of mutilation, severe skeletal dysplasias, or muscular habit problems

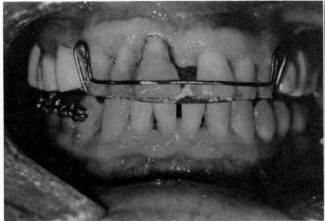 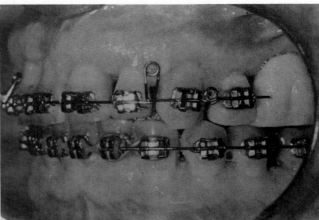

A   B

Fig. 43-5. A, Posterior alignment accomplished by sectional arch wires with posterior segments disarticulated by Hawley bite plane. Maxillary posterior provisional restorations were placed bilaterally to provide tooth placement and occlusal stability. **B,** Once posterior occlusion was established, anterior teeth were retracted to achieve lip competency and incisal guidance.

Continued.

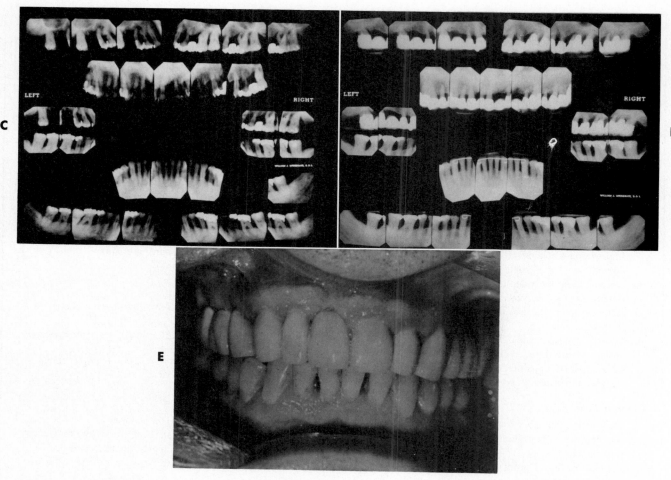

Fig. 43-5, cont'd. C, Pretreatment radiographs illustrate advanced bone loss for a 48-year-old man. **D,** Six-year postoperative radiographs. Although a bonded 3-to-3 retainer remains, splinting of lower posterior teeth was not necessary. **E,** Final maxillary restoration.

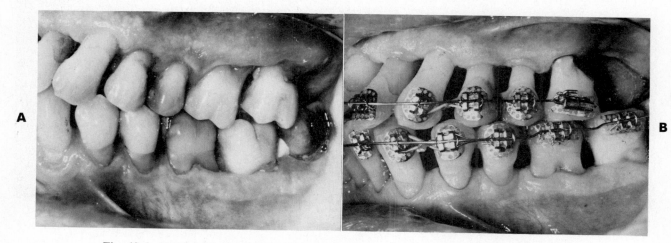

Fig. 43-6. A, Note gingival form with bite collapse and accentuated mesial drift in a 58-year-old man after scaling and root planing. **B,** Observe improved gingival topography as teeth are axially positioned. Control of gingival inflammation is easier once teeth are properly positioned.

tissue topography (Brown, 1973) (Fig. 43-7). Leveling the bone between individual teeth and correction of osseous defects can be done by active appliances or through disarticulation, selective grinding, and allowing natural tooth eruption to reduce or eliminate associated aberrant topography. Forced eruption has been reported to reduce osseous defects and to help in the management of fractured teeth (Ingber, 1974, 1978) (Fig. 43-8). For periodontal patients with bone loss on individual teeth, the clinical crown can be reduced with a high-speed handpiece; and as the tooth is erupted orthodontically (the same amount of bone will remain on the clinical root), the crown-to-root ratio will be made more favorable. Tooth movement in dogs resulting in *intrusion* has been shown to shift a supragingival plaque into a subgingival position, thereby changing a crevicular epithelium into a pocket epithelium and causing loss of attachment (Ericsson et al., 1977). However, in spite of rapid and extreme *extrusion* in the presence of periodontal inflammation in dogs, increased crestal bone levels were found, along with reduced bleeding on probing, a shallow sulcus depth, and less gingival inflammation (Van Venrooy and Yukna, 1985). This reduction in gingival inflammation with orthodontic extrusion is probably due to a shift from disease-associated microorganisms to flora found in gingival health (Van Venrooy and Vanarsdall, 1987).

Moving a tooth into a periodontal defect has been shown in monkeys to create a long epithelial attachment rather than new attachment (Polson et al., 1984).

Tooth movement may be necessary to allow for correction of occlusal problems. Deep bites can cause periodontal trauma to the gingiva (Fig. 43-9) and excessive force or retrograde wear on anterior segments. Patients with anterior open bites or severe Class II, division I malocclusions have ineffective incisal guidance, allowing for cross-tooth interferences and excessive forces. Correction of discrep-

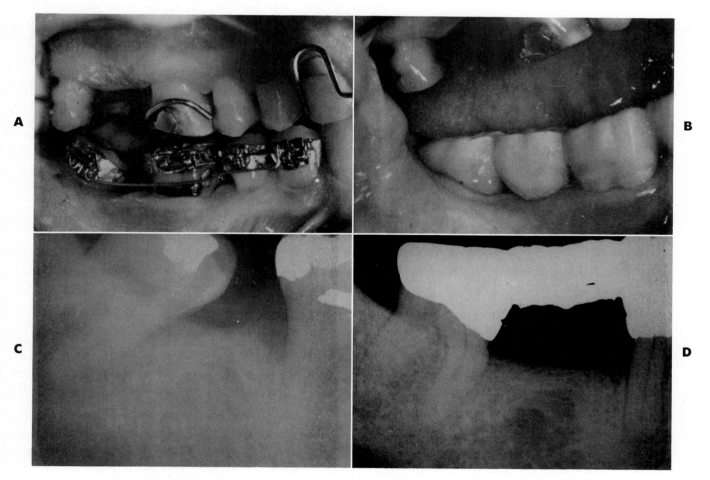

Fig. 43-7. A, Mandibular third molar uprighted to serve as distal abutment. **B,** Once molar is repositioned, a provisional restoration is placed. **C,** Pretreatment radiograph exhibiting mesial osseous defect on third molar and distal defect on first molar. **D,** Note radiographic evidence of favorable change in osseous topography on 8-year posttreatment film.   *Continued.*

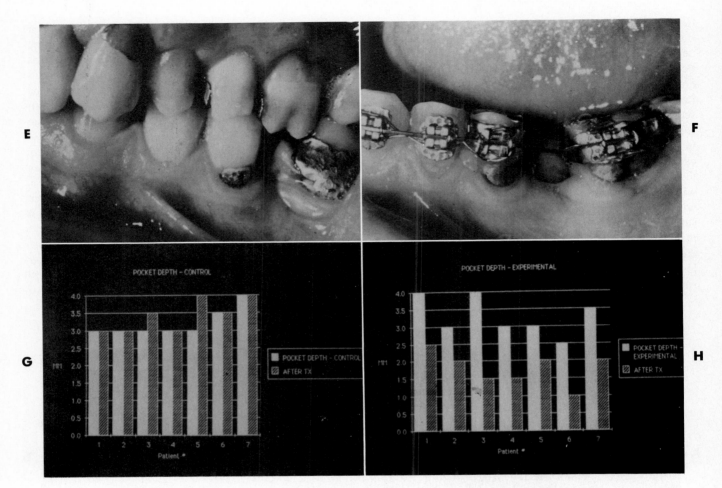

Fig. 43-7, cont'd. E, Observe mesial pseudopocket and characteristic rolled gingival tissue on mesially inclined second molar. **F,** Note change in form and resolution of mesial soft tissue depth with uprighting. **G,** Bar graph for mesially inclined molars that served as controls in seven patients for several months during molar-uprighting study at University of Pennsylvania, Department of Orthodontics. Control teeth (not moved) and experimental teeth (uprighted) did not receive scaling and root planing. Note teeth of patients 3 and 5 experienced increase in pocket depth. **H,** Bar graph for experimental teeth (mesially inclined molars that were uprighted) shows that all teeth in all seven patients exhibited reduction in pocket depth from 1 to 2.5 mm without scaling and root planing as they were axially positioned.

ancies between retruded contact (RC) position and inter-cuspal (IC) position and lateral interferences may require tooth movement to line up buccolingual landmarks and regain incisal guidance.

Though clinicians have used tooth movement to help stabilize the occlusion and selective grinding to reduce trauma and mobility, not all studies have been able to relate malocclusion to periodontal disease (Geiger et al., 1972; Shaw et al., 1980). Not only have clinical studies been conflicting and comparison of results difficult, but clinicians have been reluctant to accept that occlusion has any relationship to the pathogenesis of periodontal diseases. This has possibly been due to a limited ability to correct or have corrected certain types of occlusal etiology. For example, selective grinding (the most frequently

used form of periodontal occlusal therapy) as a definitive technique can best be used in a Class I skeletal pattern with an intact dentition and sufficient enamel present to accomplish the "take-away" procedure. Very few periodontally involved patients have these three clinical prerequisites. The child with Class II, division I malocclusion who has been corrected orthodontically to a Class I skeletal/dental relationship can be more successfully and conservatively managed occlusally as an adult, should occlusal therapy be required for periodontal reasons. This finding is an important factor in adult patients who develop significant periodontal disease and require occlusal therapy.

Complete orthodontic treatment or limited tooth movement can be an adjunct to prevent or intercept disease progression and even be therapeutic from a periodontal stand-

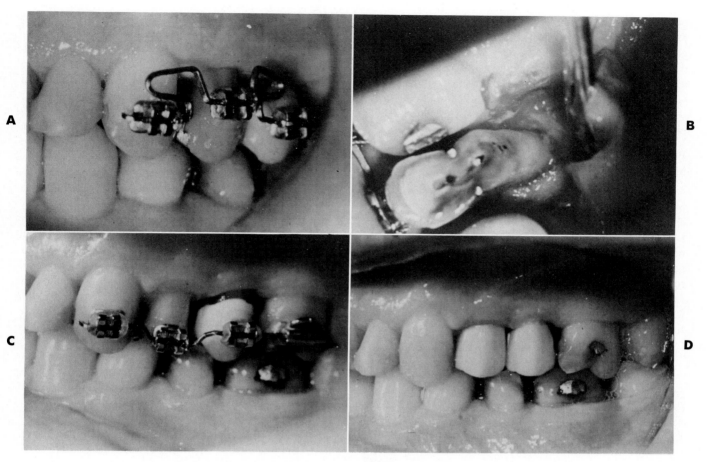

Fig. 43-8.   A, Initial wire to erupt maxillary first premolar because of fractured palatal cusp. Fracture line has extended subgingivally. **B,** Occlusal view of first premolar during palatal exposure for sound tooth structure on completion of eruption. **C,** After several millimeters of eruption and exposure of sound tooth structure, observe that most of anatomic crown has been removed. **D,** Premolar provisional restorations after soft tissue maturation. Following surgical procedure, premolar has not relapsed apically.

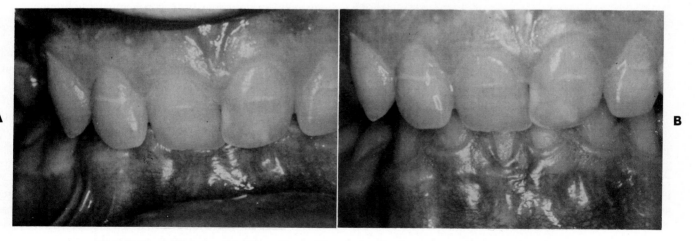

Fig. 43-9.   A, Anterior deep bite with maxillary incisor impingement on lower anterior gingival tissue. **B,** Facial recession caused by periodontal trauma will stop, and gingival margin will creep or migrate incisally on correction of physical trauma by maxillary central incisor.

point. However, to obtain these benefits from "properly executed" tooth movement, the periodontium must be properly prepared. Disease activity should be reduced with thorough root planing and curettage as indicated in the following section. Regular intervals for periodontal maintenance should be continued as necessary throughout orthodontic therapy, and attachment levels and bleeding on probing should be monitored.

PERIODONTAL AND OCCLUSAL MANAGEMENT DURING MOVEMENT

Uncontrolled inflammation during tooth movement for a periodontally susceptible patient can result in irreversible crestal bone loss, possibly causing more harm than benefit for the patient (Fig. 43-10). Therefore, before tooth movement is begun, meticulous root planing and curettage must be done to eliminate inflammation. Calculus removal and root surface preparation must be complete for all teeth and furcation areas (aberrant root surface or fluting). To achieve this level of root preparation, it may be necessary for direct vision to perform open-flap curettage (Rateit-

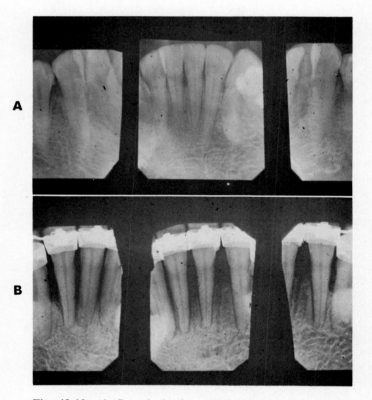

Fig. 43-10. A, Preorthodontic periapical radiographs just prior to placement of orthodontic appliance. Note lack of crestal dura and evidence of fine calculus present. **B,** Note radiographic evidence of loss of attachment after several months of tooth movement without inflammatory or occlusal control. Incisors were severely mobile even with arch wire in place. Loss of attachment could be prevented with strict inflammatory and occlusal control.

achak et al., 1985). Naturally, the patient should be required to maintain effective plaque control. Unfortunately, this may be impossible to achieve on tilted or severely crowded teeth. Therefore the clinician must accept the responsibility for adequate oral physiotherapy and mechanical maintenance of gingival health in the deep pocket areas. This is achieved by root planing, tooth polishing, and curettage throughout tooth movement on as frequent a basis as necessary to keep the area free of significant inflammation. Root planing and curettage should not be done overzealously. If the epithelial attachment is infringed on by instrumentation during this routine procedure, irreversible crestal bone loss can occur.

Bleeding on gentle instrumentation or probing is the most reliable index of significant inflammation. As the sulcular epithelium is removed during root planing, only slight hemorrhage should occur. If, during curettage, blood pools in the gingival margin area surrounding the tooth, too much inflammation will be present to do tooth movement for a periodontally susceptible patient. The frequency of visits during tooth movement will be determined not by orthodontic adjustments but by the necessity to control soft tissue inflammation during appliance therapy. This may be necessary on a weekly basis. Crestal bone loss *should not occur* during proper orthodontic therapy.

Occlusal parafunction

In addition to controlling soft tissue inflammation, it is necessary to prevent occlusal trauma during tooth movement. Unfortunately, whether or not the patient was a bruxer or clencher before orthodontic therapy, as soon as tooth movement begins and a prematurity develops, the patient may unconsciously begin to clench and/or grind. These parafunctional habits may not only slow movement, but can also traumatize the attachment. This trauma can be prevented by a combination of selective grinding and posterior disarticulation with a modified Hawley bite plane appliance (Amsterdam, 1974) worn particularly at night.

SUMMARY

No effort has been made to describe specific types of orthodontic appliances or techniques (Vanarsdall and Swartz, 1980). The critical decision is to establish specific treatment goals and use an appliance to deliver the type of movement that can efficiently and predictably resolve the periodontal or aggravating occlusal problem. A combination of fixed (preferably bonded attachments) and removable appliances will be required to treat adult mutilated dentitions with periodontal problems (Fig. 43-11).

Not all patients will tolerate the discomfort and expense of correcting severe malalignment and occlusal problems with orthodontic treatment. But those who are willing may not only minimize the amount of dental therapy necessary to solve certain periodontal problems, but may also be choosing the more conservative approach.

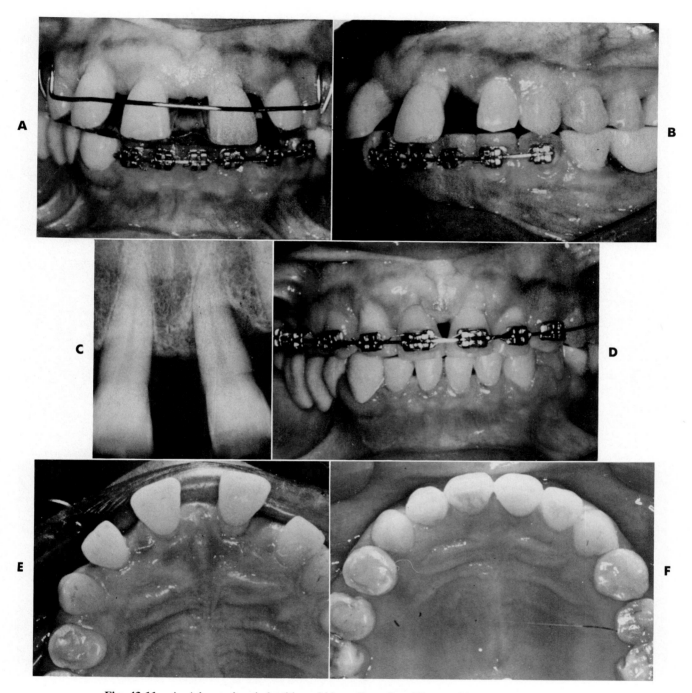

Fig. 43-11. A, Advanced periodontitis and bite collapse in a 57-year-old woman. Following establishment of posterior occlusion, anterior teeth can be consolidated and retracted. **B,** Hawley bite plane is removed once lower posterior teeth are stabilized with provisional restorations (tooth replacement). **C,** Maxillary central incisor radiograph prior to retraction. **D,** View on completion of maxillary anterior retraction. **E,** Preretraction maxillary occlusal view. **F,** Postretraction maxillary occlusal view.

Continued.

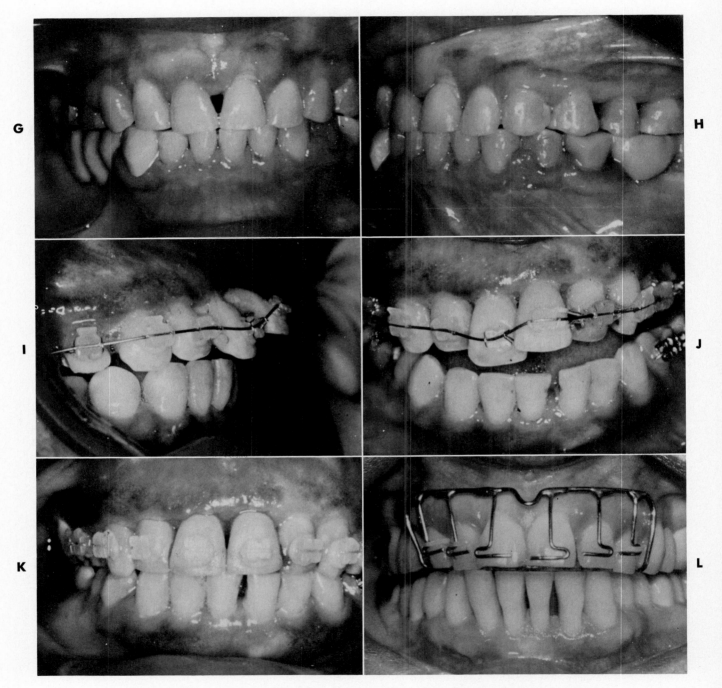

Fig. 43-11, cont'd.   G, Incisal guidance and lip competency on completion of tooth movement to reestablish posterior support. **H,** Left lateral view following tooth movement. Maxillary anterior teeth do not need to be stablized. **I,** View prior to retraction with porcelain brackets. **J,** Alignment of incisors with porcelain attachments is more esthetically acceptable to adult patients. **K,** View following alignment and retraction of periodontally involved maxillary anterior teeth. **L,** Example of a high labial removable appliance that provides controlled anterior retraction.

Clinical evidence is overwhelming that changing local environmental factors can improve periodontal health and maintenance. One of the most fruitful areas for growth in dentistry is periodontal/orthodontic interrelationships. Specialists are compelled to seek consultations in order to deliver optimal dental care. Solutions to advanced periodontal disease with malocclusion should involve a multidisciplinary approach—hygienist, generalist, periodontist, orthodontist, oral surgeon, etc. No clinician can remain an "island" or be a self-sufficient provider of care.

REFERENCES

Amsterdam M: Periodontal prosthesis: twenty-five years in retrospect, Alpha Omegan, Dec 1974.

Brown IS: The effect of orthodontic therapy on certain types of periodontal defects. I. Clinical findings, J Periodontol 44:742, 1973.

Ericsson I and Lindhe J: Effect of longstanding jiggling on experimental periodontitis in the beagle dog, J Clin Periodontol 9:497, 1982.

Ericsson I et al: The effect of orthodontic tilting movements on the periodontal tissues of infected and non-infected dentitions in dogs, J Clin Periodontol 4:278, 1977.

Geiger AM et al: Relationship of occlusion and periodontal disease. V. Relation of classification of occlusion to periodontal status and gingival inflammation, J Periodontol 43:554, 1972.

Griffiths GS and Addy M: Effects of malalignment of teeth in the anterior segments on plaque accumulation, J Clin Periodontol 8:481, 1981.

Ingber J: Forced eruption: a method of treating isolated one and two wall intrabony osseous defects, J Periodontol 45:199, 1974.

Ingber J: Forced eruption: a method of treatment of non-restorable teeth; periodontal and restorative considerations, J Periodontol 47:203, 1978.

Kantor M, Polson A, and Zander HA: Alveolar bone regeneration after removal of inflammatory and traumatic factors, J Periodontol 47:687, 1976.

Polson A et al: Periodontal response after tooth movement into intrabony defects, J Periodontol 55:197, 1984.

Rateitachak KH et al: Color atlas of periodontology, Stuttgart, 1985, Georg Thieme Verlag.

Shaw WC, Addy M, and Ray C: Dental and social effects of malocclusion and effectiveness of orthodontic treatment, Am Community Dent Oral Epidemiol 8:36, 1980.

Svanberg G and Lindhe J: Vascular reactions in the periodontal ligament incident to trauma from occlusion, J Clin Periodontol 1:58, 1974.

Van Venrooy JR and Vanarsdall RL: Tooth eruption: correlation of histologic and radiographic findings in the animal model with clinical and radiographic findings in humans, Int J Adult Orthod Orthognathic Surg 4:235, 1987.

Van Venrooy JR and Yukna RA: Orthodontic extrusion of single-rooted teeth affected with advanced periodontal disease, Am J Orthod 87:67, 1985.

Vanarsdall RL and Musich DR: Adult orthodontics: diagnosis and treatment. In Graber TM and Swain BF, editors: Orthodontics: current principles and techniques, St Louis, 1985, The CV Mosby Co.

Vanarsdall RL and Swartz ML: Adjunctive orthodontics for general practitioner molar uprighting, Glendora, Calif, 1980, ORMCO Corp.

Wilson TG et al: Tooth loss in maintenance patients in a private periodontal practice, J Periodontol 58:231, 1987.

Chapter 44

ACHIEVING PATIENT COOPERATION

Irene R. Woodall

Regardless of the technical and pharmacologic advances in treating and preventing periodontal disease, successful outcomes still hinge on the cooperation of the patient and the clinician. Skills in diagnosis, treatment planning, and instrumentation are not enough to ensure a good outcome. Disease will likely recur if a personal oral hygiene program to prevent periodontal disease is not followed on a daily basis (Waerhaug, 1978; Axelsson and Lindhe, 1981; Lindhe et al., 1982).

A successful clinician must be able to communicate effectively with patients and should be able to identify what motivators will help a patient adhere to a good oral hygiene program and place a high value on dental health. In some cases a simple demonstration of what to do, along with a series of warnings about what could happen if instructions are not followed, will be sufficient for the patient to change the amount of time and effort put into oral hygiene. In most cases, however, this is insufficient to bring about lasting change.

DEVELOPING A STRATEGY FOR COOPERATION

If "getting patients to cooperate" involves more than a demonstration and a warning, what components must be present for the desired change to occur? In an age when many consumers believe they have the right to question, to challenge, to doubt, and to seek a second opinion, most prospective patients are less likely to accept a clinician's statements as absolute truth. They are also likely to expect to be treated as equals in terms of intelligence and decision making. They expect to be informed and not treated as objects to be manipulated. People who believe that their lifestyle and habits affect their health also tend to see the advice and care of a physician or dentist as only one component necessary to achieve and maintain health. Patients often reject the idea that health care providers control their health (Wallston et al., 1978; Seeman and Seeman, 1983; Pill and Stott, 1985).

If the clinician communicates a false sense of superiority, the power differential that is created breaks down communication (Brown and Keller, 1973). The patient may be less willing to ask questions, to work to master skills, and to reappear for care. While the patient may work to improve oral hygiene out of fear of being mocked or chastised (Heszen-Klemens and Lapinska, 1984), it is unlikely that the patient will continue self-care after the relationship with such a clinician has ended. In any case, the dentist-patient relationship may undermine the likelihood of good oral hygiene compliance if it does not actively encourage patients to share in the responsibility for decision making and to recognize the limited role health professionals play in ensuring long-term health (Cockerham et al., 1986).

One key to promoting better self-care is to have the patient develop well-founded personal goals for improvement (Schou, 1985). The clinician's hopes for the patient need to be transformed into the patient's goals. The patient needs to acquire a strong sense of ownership of the need to change and improve oral hygiene and to appear as scheduled for treatment and maintenance evaluations. If patients believe that they share control over the effectiveness of treatment and long-term outcomes, they may be more willing to enlist in the care program (Kegeles and Lund, 1984).

How does the patient learn ownership and commitment? First, the patient should be involved in the initial assessment of oral conditions. The patient can be given a guided tour of his oral conditions, with the clinician explaining in simple terms what signs and symptoms are apparent. The patient should be observing the intraoral examination while the clinician explains what is being palpated, inspected, and discovered. For a patient with a periodontal problem, it is important that the signs of disease—especially signs that can be monitored at home—be observed (Glavind and Attstrom, 1979; Baab and Weinstein, 1983). Bleeding, redness, swelling, exudate, and mobility are signs that patients can see if they learn what to look for. The clinician can point out these signs and symptoms while the patient observes them, using a hand mirror, a mirror attached to the unit light, or an intraoral video unit that allows a magnified image of the oral condition to be visualized.

Patients often ask questions during the examination regarding what the bleeding or probing depths mean. The clinician can promote good communication early in the relationship by treating the patient with respect and allowing ample time for questions and clear answers in nontechnical terms. Information should be offered as the patient is interested in it. It should be offered in small parcels and will have more meaning if it accompanies the oral examination and is directly related to what the patient is seeing in the mirror.

Many clinicians use a phase-contrast or darkfield microscope to assess the percentages of cocci, motile rods, and spirochetes in a subgingival plaque sample. Using a video screen, the clinician can show the patient what the plaque mass looks like at the initial visit and then at subsequent ones as treatment and good oral hygiene progress. For some patients this may have motivational value (Tedesco et al., 1985).

During the case presentation the clinician can refer to radiographic signs and relate them to the signs the patient saw at the clinical examination, using simple descriptions. Again, there are opportunities for questions and for reinforcing the information offered earlier. The patient is ready for a first step in commitment when he asks: "What can you do about all this? What do I need?"

In general, the more active the patient is during assessment gathering and the case presentation, the more likely it is that patient acceptance will occur (Heszen-Klemens and Lapinska, 1984). The next step is mutual decision making. The clinician can explain the possible alternatives in treatment and what each alternative offers in terms of possible success and risk factors. While meeting the legal requirements of informed consent, the clinician helps the patient to learn about options and participate in decisions. The clinician and the patient discuss and agree to treatment goals and the overall treatment plan. In some cases the treatment agreed on will reflect considerable input from the patient.

A second phase of decision making involves introducing the idea that professional treatment is insufficient. Long-term success depends on what the patient is willing to do between visits on a daily basis. A willingness to adopt new ways of caring for one's teeth and gums is essential to a good treatment outcome and to prevent disease recurrence. The commitment becomes a partnership agreement that the clinician will provide necessary treatment and that the patient will work to maintain good oral hygiene.

Typically, the first treatment appointment in periodontal antiinfective therapy is supragingival debridement. At this appointment the patient should be shown the condition of the soft tissue prior to the debridement and be shown a modification of current brushing that enhances cleansing at the gingival margin. Method, duration of brushing, and use of disclosants can be introduced. The patient can be shown how to floss the teeth and instructed in other interdental and gingival crevice cleansing procedures. The clinician should let the patient practice the brushing strokes, flossing, and other techniques and can offer suggestions for improving methods.

National surveys in the United States (Chen and Rubinson, 1982) and in Scandinavia (Frandsen, 1985) have shown that toothbrushing is the most popular method of oral hygiene, with 48.1% to 65.7% of Americans and 80% of Scandinavians brushing daily. Only about 20% of American women floss daily, with men and children showing even lower percentages. Better compliance, as well as more thorough methods used for oral hygiene, can probably be adopted by the majority of patients seen in a general or periodontics practice. Thus it is important to assess the procedures they are using and stress thorough daily cleaning. It is reasonable for clinicians to expect that all of their patients will brush daily and will also floss and use other oral hygiene aids daily.

The next appointment should begin with the clinician showing the patient how the soft tissue has changed since the last visit, since often the initial debridement brings about remarkable reduction in gingival bleeding. There should be dramatic improvement in most cases. The point should be made that the changes are due to the joint efforts of the clinician and the patient's efforts at home. As the treatment sequence continues, the patient can introduce flossing to the newly cleaned areas and can monitor clinical results by observing tissue changes almost on a daily basis by close inspection with a mirror and by determining where bleeding occurs in response to flossing or to interproximal cleaning (Walsh et al., 1985). It is important, however, to resist overloading the patient with a series of time-consuming difficult procedures. In general, many procedures beyond brushing are abandoned by patients after a brief trial period (Johansson et al., 1984). It is important to introduce procedures only when signs indicate they are needed. The purpose of each step in oral hygiene must be clear to the patient, and the patient must be able to observe the positive benefits of each step.

Areas that persistently bleed or otherwise appear inflamed may require additional instrumentation or perhaps surgical intervention. The patient will be able to recognize obvious signs of slow healing if shown what to look for as each area is evaluated; thus the patient may be better prepared to understand why a treatment plan may need to be modified or extended.

At each appointment, healing and the presence of plaque deposits should be evaluated. Additional aids such as interdental brushes, rubber tips, toothpicks, or an oral irrigator can be introduced as needed to help the patient reach all areas and control plaque formation. Only those aids that are really needed should be suggested. Each additional step asks the patient to devote additional time each day to oral hygiene, even if it is only 5 more minutes.

Ideally, the patient will make successful efforts to control plaque and maintain healthy soft tissue.

FACTORS AFFECTING COMPLIANCE

Even when great attention is given to oral hygiene instruction and careful efforts are made to involve the patient in decision making, some patients seem to do poorly in helping keep a clean oral environment. In a review of compliance data in one periodontal practice, out of 961 patients only 16% complied with recommended maintenance schedules (Wilson et al., 1984). Why does this happen?

Mager and Pipe (1970) have listed possible reasons for this apparent failure to comply:

1. The patient does not know how to perform the recommended procedures, possibly reflecting a skill deficiency. This problem is remedied through a review of procedures and perhaps greater attention given to how the brush is placed and how the floss is wrapped around the tooth.

2. The patient may not see any benefit or reward in taking more time or being more careful in brushing, flossing, and irrigating. The evidence of improvement may not be obvious enough. Research has shown that people will be less likely to alter health behaviors if they do not believe they have control over their health. If the patient believes that poor dental health is inevitable, is a matter of luck, or is "up to the doctor," the compliance level will be much lower (Ludenia and Donham, 1983; Pill and Stott, 1985; Slenker et al., 1985). Such patients exhibit what is termed "external locus of control." They may not see a clear connection between the preventive health behavior suggested and improvement in the condition (Kristiansen, 1985).

Other patients exhibit "internal locus of control,"

wherein they believe that what they do is important in staying healthy. However, some patients, in spite of a strong "internal locus of control," may not place much value on periodontal health per se (Wallston et al., 1983), or they may believe that they simply are not capable of performing the behavior (Chen and Tatsuoka, 1984; Maddux et al., 1986).

Patients may believe that the procedures are unnecessary if they believe the disease is not serious. One study has suggested that people who believe a disease is highly prevalent also tend to believe it is less serious than diseases that are not so prevalent; also, those who discover that they have a particular malady tend to believe, at least at first, that it is not threatening (Jemmott et al., 1986). Even if they believe it is prevalent and serious, they may not believe they are susceptible (Brady, 1984). They may be less inclined to follow a strict regimen of oral hygiene. Identification of these attitudes is important in overcoming them to help achieve good patient cooperation.

3. Performing the desired procedures may actually be punishing to the patient. Flossing may be difficult and unpleasant. Brushing carefully may seem to take forever. Looking at the gum tissue for bleeding or redness may be unappealing. If a particular antiplaque agent is recommended, it may taste bad or seem to stain the teeth.

4. The patient may not see things getting any worse by not complying. If no one comments that the tissue looks worse or that the plaque seems to be working against healing, the patient may think it harmless to omit flossing or to brush only once a day. Some patients are less able to feel a difference between a plaque-ridden dentition and a clean one. If they do not look for changes or fail to see subtle changes in the early stages of healing, they may doubt that the new regimen is helpful.

5. Roadblocks may impede the patient's ability to perform. The floss may be missing from the drawer; the new toothbrush may have been used by a small child to brush a doll's hair. The irrigator may not reach from the electrical outlet to the sink, or there may be little space to store it conveniently. The oral hygiene regimen may make such a mess at the sink that others in the family may object to the routine. A tight bathroom schedule in the morning may make it difficult for any one person to take a few more minutes for oral hygiene.

An additional roadblock may be the interpretation of the information the clinician has shared with the patient. The patient may be able to express accurately the facts of the discussion but may have misinterpreted or forgotten what steps were most important or valuable. It may not be memory as much as the inability to actively interpret and evaluate the doctor's views. Including time to discuss differing points of view and to ask for the patient's understanding of the instructions and their importance may help minimize this roadblock to performance (Tuckett et al., 1985).

Another factor that apparently affects compliance is the patient's reaction to the materials provided or prescribed. For instance, the noncompliance rate for prescription medications is reported to be as poor as 72%, with a portion of this failure to follow instructions attributed to the color and other characteristics of the medication (Buckalew and Sallis, 1986). This could affect the use of specific brushing aids, floss and holders, and other paraphernalia suggested to a patient. The patient simply may react negatively to the appearance or feel of the items.

ACTIONS TO IMPROVE COMPLIANCE

It is up to the clinician to help sort through these possible reasons for noncompliance, looking for the clues that signal how the patient can be helped. If the problem is a skill deficiency, remedial instruction is in order. Reinforcement of efforts, emphasizing the visible signs of oral hygiene (or the lack of it), may be the answer. Systematically identifying, with the help of the patient, exactly what impedes the patient's efforts can generate a list of factors that make following oral hygiene recommendations seem impossible.

The forces that influence a person to change can be understood in terms of Lewin's field theory (1935). For every driving force that motivates a person to adopt a change, there are restraining forces that keep the person from performing this change. If the restraining forces are eliminated or reduced in importance, change will progress. If the driving forces are heightened, change will progress. The key is to identify which forces are operative for a given individual and which can be affected.

Personal driving forces may be the need for lower dental bills or the possibility of not needing surgery. The patient may want to spend less time in the dental chair or to feel that the teeth are clean and the breath is pleasant. Induced forces that can enhance or detract from the patient's following proper recommendations include the dental professional's wishes. The clinician is inducing the patient to change habits. If the relationship is a mutually satisfying one built on respect and trust, this will encourage compliance. If the relationship is antagonistic or paternalistic, the patient may purposely rebel or ignore the reasons to adopt good oral hygiene procedures.

Impersonal forces, such as society's expectation for clean, intact teeth and an odor-free mouth, also will affect the patient's motivation.

Silversin and Kornacki (1984) have summarized these variables as falling into five general categories: "psychologic factors, face-to-face interactions between people, broad societal influences, information and the immediate surroundings, and reinforcement schemes."

The array of forces that apply to a given individual can be determined only through discussion and carefully listening to the patient. If there is a problem with noncompliance, more time should be spent listening than talking.

What motivates the patient? Does that person see changes? What keeps the patient from being able to follow through?

Listening

Ferreting out what a patient thinks and feels so that a clinician can understand what motivates or inhibits behavior requires finely tuned listening skills and patience. The clinician should speak very little—usually just to initiate the discussion with a statement or brief question or to reflect back what the clinician heard the patient say.

The key to listening is reflection. Simple active listening involves rephrasing what a patient has said and saying it back for clarification. For example:

Patient: I'm so tired at night after working all day and driving the children's carpool and fixing dinner and maybe doing a load or two of laundry that I just fall into bed. The last thing I feel like doing is spending 10 minutes flossing, brushing, and irrigating.

Clinician: It sounds like you are so tired at night that you just can't muster the energy to go through all those gyrations to get your teeth clean.

Using simple, active listening lets the patient know that the clinician is attending to what is being said. It also gives the patient an opportunity to hear whether what was said was correctly interpreted. If the active listening conveys a sense of warmth and respect for the patient, it will build trust, especially when the patient is revealing concerns or feelings. Active listening lessens the sense of vulnerability that accompanies such statements. It encourages the patient to continue on, offering insights into what the problems are and how that person feels about them. Is the person embarrassed? Flippant? Depressed?

A further step is to use reflective listening to comment on the feelings that seem apparent in the message. A reflective response to the above example of a patient's comment would be: "You really sound upset by not feeling up to an oral hygiene routine every night. It sounds as though you think you should brush and floss but that you feel unable to do it."

If the reflective comment is accurate, the patient will agree and usually add to that statement. As long as the clinician continues to reflect back the content of the message and (at times) the perceived feeling behind it and does not lead the patient off in a different direction with a question, the patient will continue with more information until all that needs to be said is said.

A nonlistening response to the patient's comment could be a lecture, an insult, a joke, a warning, reteaching how to brush and floss, or silence. Such a response usually serves to cut off the speaker.

In a good listening situation the reasons for noncompliance may be quickly revealed, or it may take several minutes or hours to discuss openly the various factors that affect that person's oral hygiene behavior. When the patient has nothing new to offer and the clinician has used listening skills to check the clinician's assumptions, it is time for the clinician to start helping the patient problem solve. Based on Mager and Pipe's five reasons for "a failure to perform" (1970), the clinician can identify which factors apply and work with the patient to identify solutions.

For instance, it may be more convenient for the patient to floss and irrigate at noontime or during a midmorning break than in the evening. It may be easier for the patient to use a toothpick while driving than to floss. A packet of Stim-u-dents or a perio aid with round toothpicks could be kept in the glove compartment for handy access while waiting for the carpool to assemble. The evening can be reserved for a simple brushing.

Experience with listening and with helping people solve their time and inconvenience problems will help develop an array of problem-solving suggestions. Often the patient will be able to come up with alternatives that are acceptable and that will work. The patient's ideas are more likely to work than are the clinician's because, once again, there is ownership of the idea and it is more likely to fit within the limits of a patient's willingness to comply.

SUMMARY

While learning the diagnostic and technical skills associated with preventive and surgical periodontics is a considerable challenge, acquiring the insight and skills to move people into a pattern of good, consistent oral hygiene is usually far more difficult. It relies on an understanding of people, relationships, beliefs, attitudes, perceptions, and interpersonal communications. Few people have that understanding. Still, the long-term success of professional care relies on it.

REFERENCES

Axelsson P and Lindhe J: Effect of controlled oral hygiene procedures on caries and periodontal disease in adults, J Clin Periodontol 8:239, 1981.

Baab D and Weinstein P: Oral hygiene instruction using a self inspection plaque index, Community Dent Oral Epidemiol 11:174, 1983.

Brady W: Periodontal disease awareness, J Am Dent Assoc 109:706, 1984.

Brown C and Keller P: Monologue to dialogue: an exploration of interpersonal communication, Englewood Cliffs, NJ, 1973, Prentice-Hall, Inc.

Buckalew L and Sallis R: Patient compliance and medication perception, J Clin Psychiatry 42:49, 1986.

Chen M and Rubinson R: Preventive dental behavior of white American families: a national dental health survey, J Am Dent Assoc 105:43, 1982.

Chen M and Tatsuoka M: The relationship between American women's preventive dental behavior and dental health beliefs, Soc Sci Med 19:971, 1984.

Cockerham W et al: Social stratification and self-management of health, J Health Soc Behav 27:1, 1986.

Frandsen A: Changing patterns of attitudes and oral health behaviour, Int Dent J 35:284, 1985.

Glavind L and Attstrom R: Periodontal self-examination: a motivational tool in periodontics, J Clin Periodontol 6:238, 1979.

Heszen-Klemens I and Lapinska E: Doctor-patient interaction, patients' health behavior and effects of treatment, Soc Sci Med 19:9, 1984.

Jemmott J, Ditto P, and Croyle R: Judging health status: effects of perceived prevalence and personal relevance, J Pers Soc Psychol 50:899, 1986.

Johansson L, Oster B, and Hamp S: Evaluation of cause-related periodontal therapy and compliance with maintenance care recommendations, J Clin Periodontol 11:689, 1984.

Kegeles S and Lund A: Adolescents' health beliefs and acceptance of a novel preventive dental activity: a further note, Soc Sci Med 19:979, 1984.

Kristiansen C: Value correlates of preventive health behavior, J Pers Soc Psychol 49:748, 1985.

Lewin K: A dynamic theory of personality, New York, 1935, McGraw-Hill Book Co.

Lindhe J et al: "Critical probing depths" in periodontal therapy, J Clin Periodontol 9:323, 1982.

Ludenia K and Donham G: Dental outpatients: health locus of control correlates, J Clin Psychol 39:854, 1983.

Maddux J, Norton L, and Stoltenberg C: Self-efficacy expectancy, outcome expectancy, and outcome value: relative effects on behavioral intentions, J Pers Soc Psychol 51:783, 1986.

Mager R and Pipe P: Analyzing performance problems, Belmont, Calif, 1970, Pitman Management and Training.

Pill R and Stott N: Choice or chance: further evidence on ideas of illness and responsibility for health, Soc Sci Med 20:981, 1985.

Schou L: Active-involvement principle in dental health education, Community Dent Oral Epidemiol 13:128, 1985.

Seeman M and Seeman T: Health behavior and personal autonomy: a longitudinal study of the sense of control in illness, J Health Soc Behav 24:144, 1983.

Slenker S, Price J, and O'Connell J: Health locus of control of joggers and nonexercisers, Percept Mot Skills 61:323, 1985.

Silversin J and Kornacki M: Acceptance of preventive measures by individuals, institutions and communities, Int Dent J 34:17, 1984.

Tedesco L et al: Using phase-contrast microscopy to change oral health beliefs and behaviors, Clin Prev Dent 7:26, 1985.

Tuckett D, Boulton M, and Olson C: A new approach to the measurement of patients' understanding of what they are told in medical consultations, J Health Soc Behav 26:27, 1985.

Waerhaug J: Healing of the dento-epithelial junction following subgingival plaque control. I. As observed in human biopsy material, J Periodontol 49:1, 1978.

Wallston K, Wallston B, and DeVellis, R: Development of the multidimensional health locus of control (MHLC) scales, Health Educ Monogr 6:161, 1978.

Wallston K et al: Expectancies about control over health: relationship to desire for control of health care, Pers Soc Psychol Bull 9:377, 1983.

Walsh M, Heckman B, and Moreau-Diettinger R: Use of gingival bleeding for reinforcement of oral home care behavior, Community Dent Oral Epidemiol 13:133, 1985.

Wilson T et al: Compliance with maintenance therapy in a private periodontal practice, J Periodontol 55:468, 1984.

Chapter 45

INSTRUMENTATION
Selection and care

Lucinda B. McKechnie

Increasing emphasis on exact root instrumentation has focused attention on the design, selection, and care of instruments. By knowing how to select appropriately designed instruments and maintain proper cutting edges, clinicians can significantly improve instrumentation skills, increase the quality of patient appointment time, and expend less energy. Since root preparation is considered a tedious task, any factors that contribute to the ease of the procedure will enhance clinical efficiency and patient acceptance.

This chapter discusses the design, selection, and care of instruments essential to effective periodontal therapy.

QUALITY DESIGN OF PERIODONTAL INSTRUMENTS
General characteristics

Essential to the mechanics of quality instrument design is an instrument that minimizes damage to the hard and soft tissues. The design should help prevent gouging and grooving of the root surface, as well as of the sulcular epithelium. It should provide the operator with the greatest opportunity to maximize dexterity and minimize fatigue. The composition of the instrument should promote longevity and maintenance of sharp cutting edges subsequent to sterilization. Carbon steel has been replaced by stainless steel as the common material used in periodontal instruments today.

Working end (Fig. 45-1). The *working end* refers to the functioning part of the instrument, and its design assists in determining the area of use. Instruments may be single ended, with only one working end, or double ended, with mirror-image working ends, one on each end of the handle. Rounded working ends allow for efficiency of usage and permit application of horizontal, circumferential, and vertical strokes. One of the most important design features for instruments used in scaling and root planing is instrument balance. Regardless of whether the instrument has a straight shank or contra-angle shank design, the cutting edges of the working end should be centered over the long axis of the handle to achieve instrument balance (Fig. 45-2). Proper balance design ensures that during instrumentation pressure exerted is transmitted directly from the

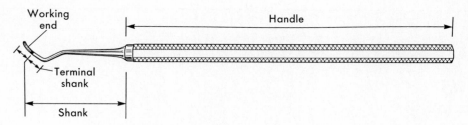

Fig. 45-1. Periodontal instrument design.

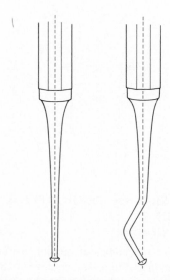

Fig. 45-2. Straight shank and contra-angle shank with cutting edges of blades centered over long axis of handle.

handle, through the shank, to the working end (Pattison and Pattison, 1979).

Shank (Fig. 45-1). The small shank of the instrument connects the working end to the handle. The angle of the shank may be specifically designed to allow access to particular surfaces of specific teeth. As a general rule, the more restricted the access to an area, the greater the number of shank bends or contra-angles required. Similarly, the simpler the shank, the more anterior the intended area of use. Anterior teeth, where there is minimal pocket depth or recession, can be adequately instrumented with a shorter, straighter shank. However, anterior teeth with pocket depth or recession demand a longer shank and possibly a contra-angle shank, depending on pocket topography. Posterior teeth require a longer shank, as well as a contra-angle design, to effectively negotiate posterior root morphology where apical migration of the junctional epithelium has occurred.

A thicker shank design is used for heavier, more tenacious calculus, whereas the thinner shank, since it is more tactilely perceptive, is used for removal of fine calculus and for root planing (Fig. 45-3).

Handle (Fig. 45-1). Instrument handles may be designed in various sizes and shapes. A handle design with a wider diameter allows for a comfortable grasp and will prevent muscle fatigue, particularly during prolonged instrumentation. The surface texture of the handle should be serrated or roughened, not smooth, in order to prevent slippage and contribute to a secure grasp. Hollow handles are preferred to solid handles, since they are lighter in weight and allow for transference of surface irregularities, thereby enhancing tactile sensitivity.

Thus mechanically well-designed instruments used in scaling and root planing should have the following characteristics:

1. Thick, roughened grip
2. Well-balanced handle
3. Working end centered with the long axis of the handle
4. Proper contra-angle shank construction

Sharp cutting edges

The quality of cutting edge sharpness for effective and efficient root planing cannot be overemphasized. Particular attention must be paid to the maintenance of the original working end design, hence its function, and the sharpness of the cutting edges. Root planing requires an ultrasharp blade to detect microscopic root surface irregularities and to cut efficiently.

SELECTION OF INSTRUMENTS USED FOR SCALING AND ROOT PLANING
Hand instruments

The goal of periodontal therapy is to produce a root surface biologically compatible with the maintenance of healthy periodontal tissue. The cytotoxicity of microbial by-products bound to the root interferes with the hard and soft tissue compatibility (Aleo et al., 1974, 1975). Elimination of causative factors by various techniques of root

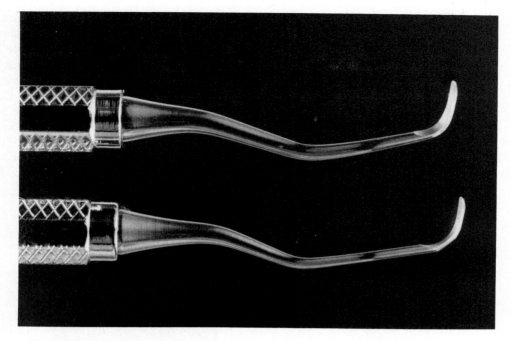

Fig. 45-3. Thicker-shanked rigid Gracey curette compared with a finishing Gracey curette.

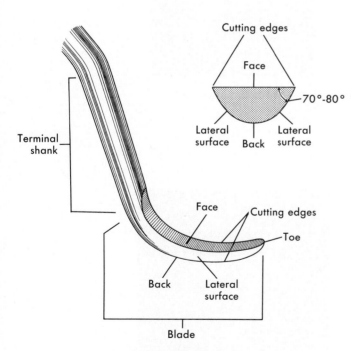

Fig. 45-4. Curette design.

preparation would help attain the goal of a root surface biologically acceptable to the healing tissue. Conventional means of root preparation are carried out with ultrasonic instruments supplemented by hand-activated curettes.

Curettes (Fig. 45-4).   There is general agreement that the curette is the most versatile instrument for use in root debridement procedures. Because of its rounded architecture, the curette tends to produce the least amount of trauma to the hard and soft tissues. There are two types of curettes: universal and area-specific.

Universal curettes.   The universal curette is described as one instrument designed to adapt to most tooth surfaces in most regions of the mouth. The curettes are usually double ended with mirror-turned blades. The facial surface of the blade is beveled at a 90-degree angle to the shank, creating two working cutting edges that curve up from the shank and are united by a rounded toe. The two cutting edges are straight and parallel (Fig. 45-5).

To determine the correct working end, select the blade that curves in the direction of the surface to be scaled. The position of the face of the blade should be close against the tooth and inserted at 0 degrees. To obtain a proper working angulation of 45 to 90 degrees, the lower shank is tilted slightly toward the tooth. Either cutting edge can be adapted in this manner.

Area-specific curettes.   Area-specific curettes (Gracey curettes) are designed to adapt to particular surfaces of specific teeth. The set includes the seven mirror-image pairs listed below:

Gracey 1/2	Anterior teeth
Gracey 3/4	
Gracey 5/6	Anterior and bicuspid teeth
Gracey 7/8	Posterior teeth—buccal and lingual surfaces
Gracey 9/10	
Gracey 11/12	Posterior teeth—mesial line angles and mesial surfaces
Gracey 13/14	Posterior teeth—distal line angles and distal surfaces

Although Dr. Clayton H. Gracey designed these instruments to be used in specific areas, it should be recognized that the instruments can be used in other areas as well, provided that the correct blade is applied to the tooth. For example, an anterior region where there is a deep, tortuous mesial pocket would be most effectively instrumented with a "posterior" Gracey 11/12 curette. The longer, contra-angle design of the Gracey 11/12 curette would enable adaptation to the depth of the pocket. Similarly, a Gracey 13/14 curette could be used in the distal aspect of an anterior region where there is considerable pocket depth. Replica-

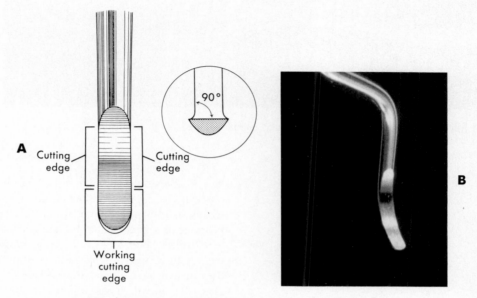

Fig. 45-5. **A,** Universal curette design. **B,** Actual instrument.

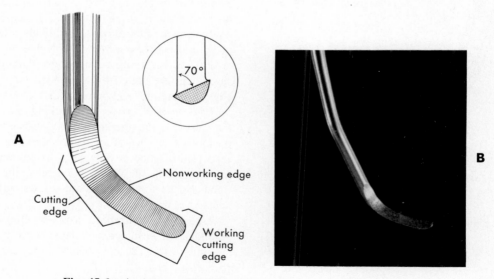

Fig. 45-6. **A,** Area-specific (Gracey) curette design. **B,** Actual instrument.

tion of shank design permits limiting the selection of Gracey curettes to only three or four to be included in the tray setup. The selection of Gracey 1/2, 7/8, 11/12, and 13/14, along with one or two universal curettes, will manage any area of the mouth and provide an efficient, uncluttered tray setup for root debridement procedures.

Unlike the universal curette, the Gracey curette has only one working cutting edge, created by a facial surface that is beveled at a 60- to 70-degree angle to the shank. This offset blade is the only one used during instrumentation. To determine the correct cutting edge, select the edge that is lower or farthest away from the shank (Fig. 45-6).

To obtain proper working angulation, position the terminal shank or last bend in the shank parallel to the tooth. This Gracey offset-blade feature provides an effective working angulation with minimal adjustment—a particular advantage in areas of difficult access. Like those of universal curettes, Gracey curette blades curve up from the shank to the toe, but also curve to the side. This blade curvature provides maximum blade adaptation when negotiating varying circumferential root contours (Fig. 45-7).

Sickles (Fig. 45-8). The working end of a sickle scaler is designed with either a straight or curved blade, which has a triangular cross section and two working cutting edges. Each of the two cutting edges is formed by the junction of the facial and lateral surfaces and terminate in a point. Both curved and straight-bladed sickles are available with angulated or straight shanks.

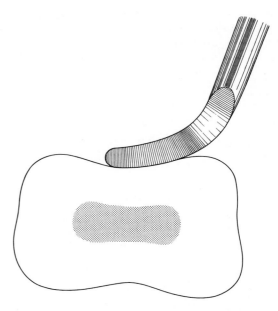

Fig. 45-7. Adaptation of curved Gracey curette blade to root concavity.

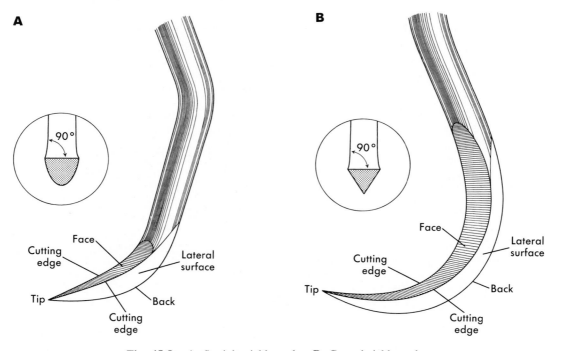

Fig. 45-8. A, Straight sickle scaler. **B,** Curved sickle scaler.

The relatively straight-cutting edges and pointed toe of the working end limit the sickle's usefulness. The instrument is used mainly for supragingival debridement or scaling in shallow pockets where the marginal tissue is soft, flexible, and easily displaced.

Effective instrumentation can be accomplished by positioning the blade so that it is less than 90 but more than 45 degrees to the tooth. Either cutting edge can be adapted in this manner.

Hoes (Fig. 45-9).   The hoe is an instrument that is used mainly for removal of large, accessible supramarginal calculus. It has only one cutting edge. The blade is turned at an angle of 99 to 100 degrees to the shank, and the cutting

edge is beveled at a 45-degree angle. The hoe is designed in sets of four working ends, one for each tooth surface: buccal, lingual, mesial, and distal.

Care must be taken to ensure that the entire cutting edge is adapted against the tooth; otherwise, gouging of the root surface and adjacent soft tissue may occur with the side edge of the hoe. Because of the blade size and design, adaptation to proximal surfaces is not possible. Therefore hoes are most effective when applied to buccal and lingual surfaces or to proximal surfaces adjacent to an edentulous area. The instrument is a heavy, bulky instrument lacking in tactile sensitivity that generally precedes additional scaling by curettes. Hoes can be considered an adjunctive instrument and may not be routinely included in a standard tray setup for scaling and root planing.

Files (Fig. 45-10).   The periodontal file has multiple cutting edges lined up as a series of miniature hoes on a round, oval, or rectangular base. Angulation of the blades in relation to the shank may be from 90 to 105 degrees. Like the hoe, the file is designed in sets of four working ends, one for each tooth surface: buccal, lingual, mesial, and distal.

The instrument is used mainly to crush and roughen heavy ledges of calculus so that remnants of calculus can be more easily removed with curettes. Smaller, flatter files provide the greatest access for planing root surfaces in furcation areas or narrow pockets, which may be inaccessible with other instruments. The instrument is best applied to buccal and lingual surfaces and to surfaces adjacent to edentuluous areas. As with the hoe, care must be taken to ensure that all cutting edges are well adapted against the tooth. Files can be considered adjunctive instruments and may not be routinely included in a standard tray setup for scaling and root planing.

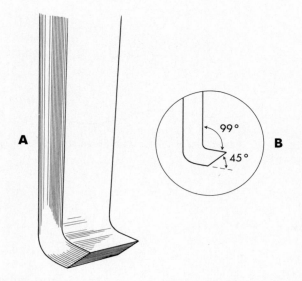

Fig. 45-9.   A, Hoe with its single cutting edge. **B,** Note position of cutting edge.

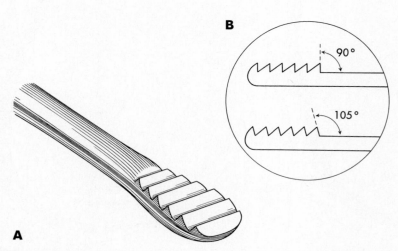

Fig. 45-10.   A, Periodontal file with its multiple cutting edges. **B,** Note position of cutting edges.

Chisels (Fig. 45-11). The chisel is used mainly for removal of heavy masses of calculus from the proximal and lingual surfaces of mandibular teeth. The instrument has a straight cutting edge, and the end of the blade is flat and beveled at a 45-degree angle. The blade is adapted against the proximal surfaces and used with a gentle, horizontal push stroke. Ultrasonic instrumentation has minimized the use of the chisel, since heavy, tenacious deposits can be removed more quickly and with less effort with ultrasonic instrumentation.

Ultrasonic instruments

Next to the hand-activated instruments, ultrasonic scaling devices are the most commonly used instruments for removal of plaque, gross deposits of calculus, and stains. The instrument serves as an excellent adjunct to hand instrumentation. Because of the ease of removal of calculus deposits by ultrasonic instrumentation, the time required is shorter and there is less patient discomfort and operator fatigue.

Ultrasonic instruments are mainly employed for gross removal of calculus and stain. They are particularly useful in the early phase of treatment when tissues are hemorrhagic. However, a combination of hand instrumentation and ultrasonic instrumentation may be implemented during periodontal therapy.

Ultrasonic instruments use high-frequency sound waves to fracture and dislodge deposits from teeth. The accompanying water supply is cavitated by the vibrating tip to effect flushing of the pocket (Fig. 45-12). The instrument tip vibrates approximately 25,000 cycles per second (c/s), with the water supply creating a fine mist surrounding the tip (Clark, 1969). The water lavage that accompanies calculus removal, along with coagulation of the pocket epithelium, allows for a favorable tissue response. Gentle manipulation of inflamed soft tissue makes this the instrument of choice for patients with acute necrotizing ulcerative gingivitis (ANUG). Caution is recommended when treating a patient with a pacemaker (Adams, 1982).

There is no need for a sharp cutting edge to engage calculus with the ultrasonic instrument tip. Since the motion of the activated tip fractures the deposit, the design of the instrument tip is blunted and dull. The side of the tip is kept in constant motion and must contact the deposit to dislodge it. Pressure applied on the tooth should be light, using short, rapid, vertical, or oblique strokes.

Scaling with an ultrasonic instrument may remove cementum and cause damage to the root surface if used improperly (Pameijer et al., 1972; Wilkinson and Maybury, 1973). When there is an undesirable surface alteration, it may be associated with the power setting of the unit, the pressure applied with the tip, or a tip that is not blunt. Stende and Schaffer (1961) reported that ultrasonic scaling was as effective as hand scaling for calculus removal but lacked the inherent capability (no cutting edge) to plane the root surface. Nishimine and O'Leary (1979) reported that ultrasonic scaling resulted in endotoxin values approximately eight times greater than those obtainable by hand-activated curettes. Loos et al. (1987) found no difference in the improvement of periodontal conditions between sites treated with sonic instruments and those treated with ultrasonic instruments. The sonic instruments produced vibrations in the range of 2300 to 6300 c/s, and the ultrasonic instruments caused vibrations of 26,000 to 46,000 c/s.

Ultrasonic instrumentation seems to leave a rougher surface than hand-activated curettes (VanVolkinburg et al., 1976; Meyer and Lie, 1977). It has therefore been suggested that ultrasonic instrumentation be supplemented

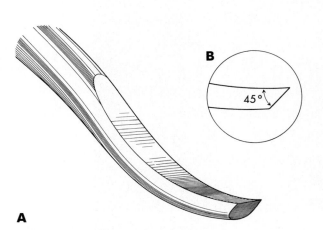

Fig. 45-11. **A,** Chisel with its single cutting edge. **B,** Note position of cutting edge.

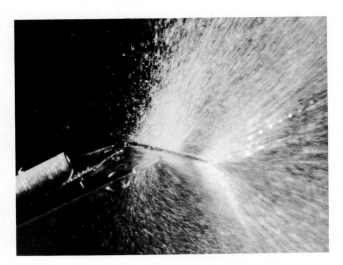

Fig. 45-12. Ultrasonic instrument tip showing spraying and cavitation of fluid. (From Grant DA, Stern IB, and Listgarten MA, editors: Periodontics in the tradition of Gottlieb and Orban, ed 6, St Louis, 1988, The CV Mosby Co.)

with hand-activated curettes to produce a smooth root surface (Björn and Lindhe, 1962). However, the relationship between root roughness, plaque accumulation, and gingival inflammation is not well established (Rosenberg and Ash, 1974).

Clinical studies have failed to demonstrate any significant differences between the effects of ultrasonic root debridement using instruments with a frequency of 26,000 c/s and hand instrumentation in the treatment of periodontal pockets 4 to 7 mm deep (Torafson et al., 1979; Badersten et al., 1981). These studies have suggested that debridement with ultrasonic instrumentation using the 26,000 c/s instruments is equally effective to that achieved with hand-activated curettes with regard to posttreatment pocket depths and attachment levels. Rosling et al. (1986) showed that scaling and root planing using an ultrasonic instrument operating at 46,000 c/s with a 0.1% povidone-iodine irrigant resulted in significantly more attachment gain in pockets initially ≥7 mm, suggesting that there is benefit from using the proper ultrasonic instrument in periodontal therapy.

Air-powder abrasive systems

Conventional periodontal therapy has focused on scaling and root planing with ultrasonic instruments and curettes. It has been customary to finish scaling, root planing, and plaque removal by polishing the exposed tooth surfaces. Until recently, polishing was accomplished with rubber cups in a slow-speed dental handpiece using an abrasive paste. Recently an air-powered device for removing stains and plaque has been introduced that uses a slurry of sodium bicarbonate and water. This unit has proved to be fast and effective in the removal of stains and plaque from grooves and crevices.

The device consists of a power unit and handpiece capable of emitting finely sieved particles of sodium bicarbonate through a stream of air surrounded by water. The resulting slurry is mechanically abrasive against surface stains and bacterial plaque.

Operation of the handpiece includes directing the slurry diagonally toward the tooth surface with the nozzle positioned approximately 4 to 5 mm from the tooth surface being cleaned. A light, circular motion is implemented to remove plaque and stain (Fig. 45-13).

The effects of the air-powder system on enamel compare favorably with those of the rubber cup and paste technique. However, the device roughened smooth enamel surfaces (Wilmann et al., 1980). Mishkin et al. (1986) compared the clinical effects of the air-powder abrasive device and the rubber cup and paste techniques on the gingiva. They reported no lasting difference in gingival trauma between the two methods in subjects with healthy gingiva or slight gingivitis. This is in agreement with previous reports by Weaks et al. (1984), who, although they observed some localized soft tissue trauma, reported that it was so minimal as to be undetectable after 6 days.

It should be recognized that the air-powder abrasive system can roughen restorative materials (Cooley et al., 1985).

Traditionally, use of the air-powder abrasive device (Dentsply Prophy-Jet Mark IV, C-100) has been restricted to removal of bacterial plaque and stain from enamel sur-

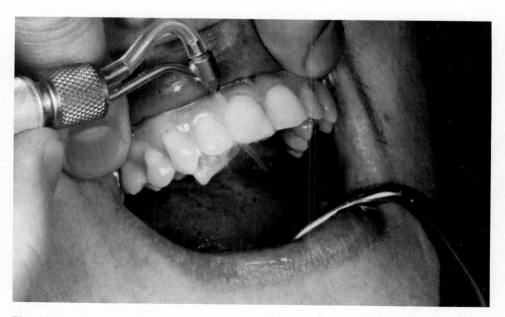

Fig. 45-13. Air-powder abrasive system nozzle showing slurry of sodium bicarbonate, air, and water.

faces. Several investigators have reported that conventional techniques (curettes, ultrasonics) frequently are incapable of completely eliminating bacterial plaque and their by-products, particularly in root surface irregularities (Walker and Ash, 1976; Waerhaug, 1978; Thornton and Garnick, 1982; Saglie et al., 1986). Supplemental treatment of root surfaces by air-powder abrasive devices may provide a more efficient method of producing a root surface biologically compatible with the soft tissue (Atkinson et al., 1984; Gilman and Maxey, 1986).

An advantage of the air-powder abrasive device in root preparation is that it allows cementum removal and potential detoxification in root surfaces of difficult access (i.e., flutes, defects, and lacunae) (Gilman and Maxey, 1986). Atkinson et al. (1984) reported both favorable and unfavorable effects on root surfaces. Favorable clinical results included the production of a uniformly smooth root surface texture, free of residue and debris. Daly et al. (1982) reported that following scaling and root planing with hand-activated curettes, the root surface was covered with debris. Toevs (1985) reported that the root topography produced with the air-powder abrasive system was significantly smoother than that produced with the curette or reciprocating contra-angle system. While root smoothness is clinically a goal in periodontal therapy, the biologic relationship between root roughness, plaque accumulation, and gingival inflammation is still a debatable point (Rosenberg and Ash, 1974).

It may be clinically significant to note the report by Atkinson et al. (1984), who described a relative lack of exposed dentinal tubules along the crater walls of root surfaces after use of the air-powder system, the presumption being that the slurry of sodium bicarbonate, air, and water functions to occlude or obliterate the tubule openings. Previous investigators (Clinical Research Associates, 1981) have suggested that this phenomena could possibly explain the decreased sensitivity noted during prophylaxis of hypersensitive root surfaces. Further investigation is necessary to determine the potential uses of the air-powder abrasive system in the treatment of periodontally diseased teeth. Until this occurs, instrument application should be limited to supragingival removal of bacterial plaque and stain.

SHARPENING PROCEDURES
Rationale and objectives

Greater control of the instrument with less pressure required on the tooth can be expected with sharp cutting edges. Since less pressure is required, the instrument does not have to be grasped as firmly. This results in increased tactile sensitivity, less patient discomfort, and less operator fatigue. Scaling with dull, rounded cutting edges frequently results in incomplete removal, as well as burnishing, of calculus. Walker and Ash (1976) observed that burnished calculus was not detectable from the surrounding root surface even with a sharpened No. 3 explorer.

Sharp cutting edges enable the operator to achieve the clinical impression of a root-planed surface. Without the fine line of a cutting edge, the hard, smooth, glasslike root surface will not be detected. Once root hardness and smoothness are obtained, the sharp blade will allow the operator to stop instrumentation when a properly root-planed surface is detected by touch. This improved tactile sense of a sharp instrument prevents overinstrumentation and excessive removal of root surface.

Principles of sharpening

Repeated sharpening procedures should not change the original geometry of the instrument (Project ACCORDE, 1976; Paquette and Levin, 1977; Pattison and Pattison, 1979). A blade angle between the facial and lateral surfaces of 70 to 80 degrees limits the amount of depth the curette can cut into the root structure. Carranza (1979) has suggested that this blade configuration is the most effective design for calculus removal and root planing. For this 70- to 80-degree internal angle to be maintained, the angle between the surface of the stone and the face of the blade must be between 100 and 110 degrees (Fig. 45-14).

Although it is possible to obtain sharp cutting edges by grinding on the facial surface, there is general agreement that lateral surface grinding may offer some advantage

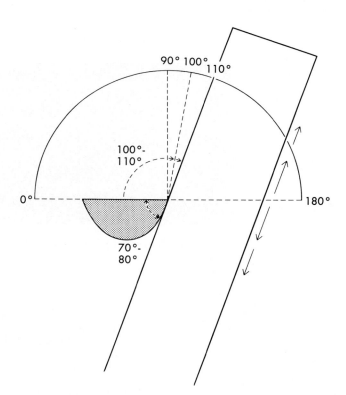

Fig. 45-14. Schematic representation of sharpening stone applied to lateral surface of a curette. Note that angle between face of blade and surface of stone is 100 to 110 degrees.

(Green, 1972; Paquette and Levin, 1977). Grinding on the lateral surface retains the original blade depth, hence strength of the blade, while narrowing the blade from side to side. This reduction in blade width is advantageous in instrumenting deep pockets where the marginal tissue is tight.

The Arkansas stone is the stone of choice for sharpening instruments used in scaling and root planing procedures. It is reputed to produce the smoothest, most linear, and finest line of a cutting edge. Although the India stone may be used for sharpening excessively dull instruments, the Arkansas stone should be applied for the finishing strokes (Fig. 45-15). The stones should be lubricated with a thin layer of oil or petroleum jelly. The lubricant acts as a slurry to gather up the metal shavings during sharpening. If "glazing" has occurred, the stone may be placed in the ultrasonic cleaner to shake loose the embedded metal particles, or the stone may be rubbed with emery paper. While the lubricant reduces frictional heat, it is recommended that excessive pressure be avoided during the sharpening procedure. Repeated autoclaving of stones may cause drying and breaking; therefore it is recommended that the stone be occasionally soaked in oil.

During the root debridement procedure the quality of the cutting edge must be controlled by testing it on an acrylic test stick (Fig. 45-16). A sterile sharpening stone and acrylic test stick should be considered a standard inclusion in the tray setup.

Sharpening curettes

The moving stone/stationary instrument method offers the advantage of accurate stone-to-instrument placement. Because of the grasp of the stone and instrument, the clinician can easily visualize the correct angle of the stone in relation to the facial surface of the instrument. This tech-

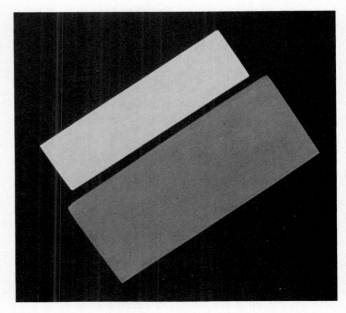

Fig. 45-15. Arkansas stone *(top)* and India stone *(bottom).*

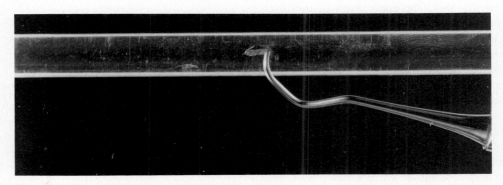

Fig. 45-16. Testing for sharpness with an acrylic test stick. Using light pressure, sharp cutting edges should immediately "grab."

Fig. 45-17. Sharpening of universal curette. **A,** Lubrication of stone. **B,** Stable grasp of stone and instrument off edge of cabinet top. **C,** Alternative method of stability by bracing elbows against body for support. **D,** Establishment of 90-degree angle between facial surface of instrument and surface of stone. Note that facial surface is parallel to floor. **E,** Position of stone rotated laterally 10 to 20 degrees to establish correct 100-degree angle. **F,** Movement of stone starting at heel, using short, overlapping up-and-down strokes. More pressure is applied to downstroke, since it is cutting stroke. This will minimize wire formation. **G,** Incremental sharpening of 10 to 12 cutting downstrokes from heel to toe side of opposite cutting edge. Angulation of 110-degree base is maintained throughout. **H,** Grasp of instrument for sharpening opposite cutting edge, starting at heel.

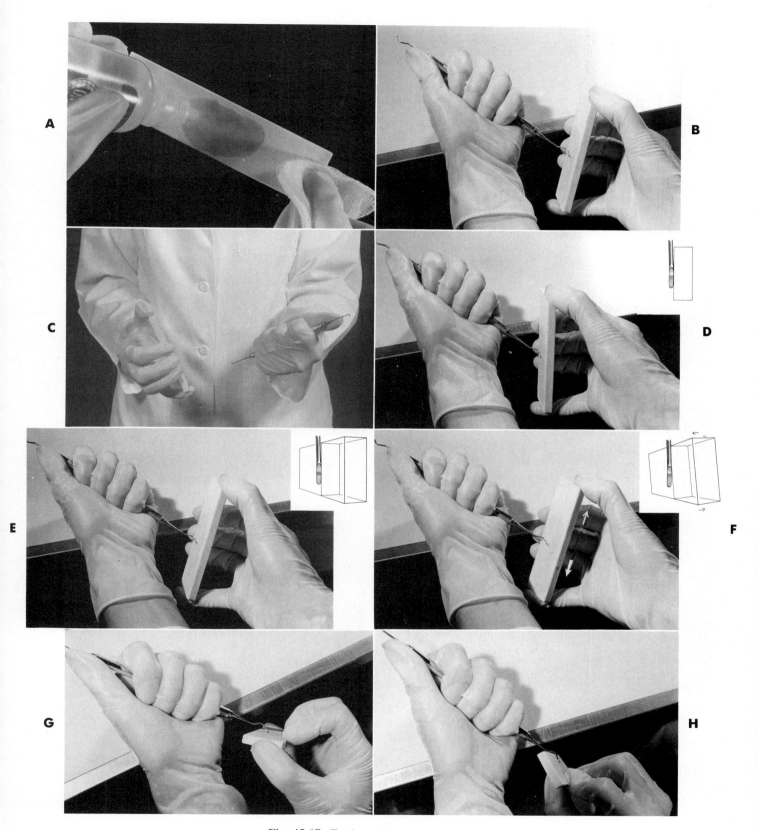

Fig. 45-17. For legend see opposite page.

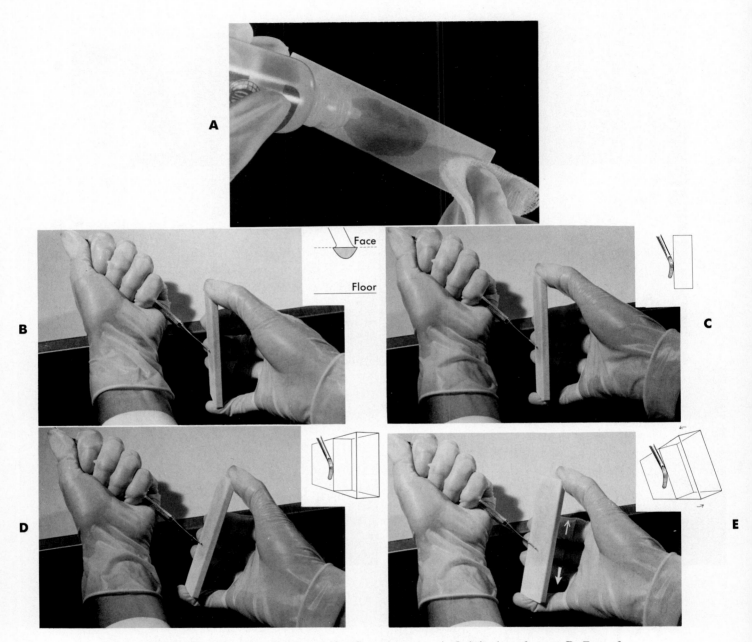

Fig. 45-18.   Sharpening of area-specific (Gracey) curette. **A,** Lubrication of stone. **B,** Face of Gracey curette must be parallel to floor. **C,** Establishment of 90-degree angle between facial surface of instrument and surface of stone. **D,** Position of stone rotated laterally 10 to 20 degrees to establish correct 110-degree angle. **E,** Movement of stone, starting at heel, using short overlapping up-and- down strokes. More pressure is applied to downstroke, since it is cutting stroke. This will minimize wire edge formation.

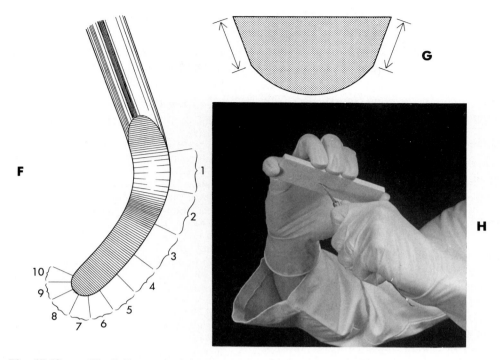

Fig. 45-18, cont'd. F, Incremental sharpening of 10 to 12 strokes from heel to toe, rotating stone on its long axis to accommodate and maintain Gracey curved blade. **G,** For both universal and Gracey curettes, sharpening on lateral surfaces will result in flat sides. **H,** Occasionally draw stone from heel to toe on lateral surface and back of blade to maintain original rounded contour.

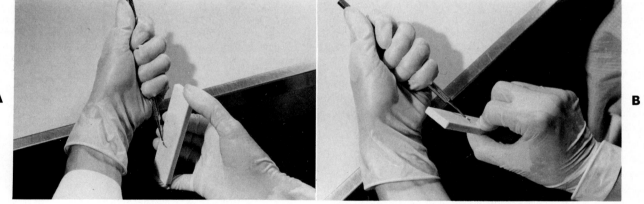

Fig. 45-19. A, Position of stone at same 110-degree angle established for curette. Begin at heel and work toward toe. There is no need to sharpen around toe. **B,** Position of stone on opposite cutting edge, starting at heel.

nique focuses primarily on lateral surface grinding.

Universal curettes (Fig. 45-17).   The universal curette has two working cutting edges. Both cutting edges will require sharpening.

Area-specific curettes (Fig. 45-18).   The area-specific (Gracey) curette has only one working cutting edge. Only the working cutting edge will require sharpening.

Sharpening sickle scalers (Fig. 45-19)

Like the universal curette, the sickle scaler has two working cutting edges. Both cutting edges will require sharpening.

Effects of repeated sterilization on cutting edges of curettes

For many years it was thought that repeated sterilization dulled the cutting edges of all scaling instruments. Recent clinical studies, however, have evaluated the effects of various methods of sterilization on the cutting edges of curettes. Parkes and Kolstad (1982) reported that saturated steam sterilization of carbon steel instruments produced oxidation and dulling of cutting edges. However, they observed that carbon steel blades were unaffected by dry heat or chemical vapor. Their study indicated that stainless steel blades retained their sharpness after repeated sterilization by dry heat, chemical vapor, and saturated steam sterilization. This is in agreement with Sasse (1987), who found no decrease in sharpness of the cutting edges of stainless steel curettes after repeated sterilization with steam under pressure and chemical vapor. Some stainless steel instruments contain specially tempered carbon and chromium, which allows for superior corrosion resistance and retention of blade sharpness and hardness. It appears that the material of choice for instruments used in periodontal scaling procedures would be stainless steel.

SUMMARY

Attention has been focused on the selection and maintenance of instruments used in complete root debridement. Without consideration of instrument design, function, and cutting edge characteristics, tactile sensitivity will be impaired. The result will be frustration and fatigue on the part of the clinician and inadequate elimination of the factors contributing to disease.

Superb instrumentation requires continuous assessment of instruments used in periodontal scaling. Clinicians should be concerned, on a microscopic level, with the quality of the cutting edge vis-à-vis the final root-planed product. Instrument selection and care is therefore critical to the success of periodontal therapy.

ACKNOWLEDGMENT

In the preparation of this chapter I gratefully acknowledge the help of Mr. Wing M. Woon, Director of Medical Photography, and Mr. Gary J. Nelson, medical illustrator, both of the University of Vermont College of Medicine.

REFERENCES

Adams D: The cardiac pacemaker and ultrasonic scaler, Br Dent J 152(5):171, 1982.

Aleo JJ, Farber PA, and Varboncoeur AP: The presence and biological activity of cementum-bound endotoxin, J Periodontol 45:672, 1974.

Aleo JJ et al: In vitro attachment of human gingival fibroblasts to root surfaces, J Periodontol 46:639, 1975.

Atkinson DR, Cobb CM, and Killoy WJ: The effect of an air-powder abrasive system on in vitro root surfaces, J Periodontol 55:1, 1984.

Badersten A, Nilveus R, and Egelberg J: Effect of non-surgical periodontal therapy. I. Moderately advanced periodontitis, J Clin Periodontol 8:57, 1981.

Björn H and Lindhe J: The influence of periodontal instruments on the tooth surface, Odontol Revy 13:355, 1962.

Carranza FA: Glickman's clinical periodontology, ed 5, Philadelphia, 1979, WB Saunders Co.

Clark SM: The ultrasonic dental unit: a guide for the clinical application of ultrasonics in dentistry and dental hygiene, J Periodontol 40:621, 1969.

Clinical Research Associates: Subject: oral prophylaxis; Prophy-Jet, Clinical Research Associates Newsletter 5:1, 1981.

Cooley RL, Lubow RM, and Young JM: Effect of Prophy-Jet on restorative materials, J Dent Res 64(special issue):186, 1985 (abstract 69).

Daly CG et al: Histological assessment of periodontally involved cementum, J Clin Periodontol 9:266, 1982.

Gilman RS and Maxey BR: The effect of root detoxification on human gingival fibroblasts, J Periodontol 57:436, 1986.

Green E and Seyer PC: Sharpening curets and sickle scalers, San Francisco, 1972, Praxis Publishing Co.

Loos B, Kiger R, and Egelberg J: An evaluation of basic periodontal therapy using sonic and ultrasonic scalers, J Clin Periodontol 14:29, 1987.

Meyer K and Lie T: Root surface roughness in response to periodontal instrumentation by combined use of microroughness measurements and scanning electron microscopy, J Clin Periodontol 4:77, 1977.

Mishkin DJ et al: A clinical comparison of the effect on the gingiva of the Prophy-Jet and the rubber cup and paste techniques, J Periodontol 57:151, 1986.

Nishimine D and O'Leary TJ: Hand instrumentation vs. ultrasonics in the removal of endotoxins from root surfaces, J Periodontol 50:345, 1979.

Pameijer CH, Stallard RE, and Hiep N: Surface characteristics of teeth following periodontal instrumentation: a scanning electron microscopic study, J Periodontol 43:628, 1972.

Paquette OE and Levin MP: The sharpening of scaling instruments. I. An examination of principles, J Periodontol 48:163, 1977.

Paquette OE and Levin MP: The sharpening of scaling instruments. II. A preferred technique, J Periodontol 48:169, 1977.

Parkes RB and Kolstad RA: Effects of sterilization on periodontal scaling instruments, J Periodontol 53:434, 1982.

Pattison GL and Pattison AM: Periodontal instrumentation, Reston, Va, 1979, Reston Publishing Co, Inc.

Project ACCORDE: Instrument sharpening, Castro Valley, Calif, 1976, Querus Corp.

Rosenberg RM and Ash M: The effect of root roughness on plaque accumulation and gingival inflammation, J Periodontol 45:146, 1974.

Rosling BG et al: Topical antimicrobial therapy and diagnosis of subgingival bacteria in the management of inflammatory periodontal disease, J Clin Periodontol 13:975, 1986.

Saglie FR, Johansen JR, and Feo MF: Tooth surfaces after scaling and root planing: stereomicroscopic and scanning electron microscope studies, Compend Contin Educ Dent 7:494, 1986.

Sasse J: Cutting edges of curets: effect of repeated sterilization, Dent Hyg 61:14, 1987.

Stende GW and Schaeffer EM: A comparison of ultrasonic and hand scaling, J Periodontol 32:312, 1961.

Thornton S and Garnick J: Comparison of ultrasonic to hand instruments in the removal of subgingival plaque, J Periodontol 53:35, 1982.

Toevs SE: Root topography following instrumentation: a SEM study, Dent Hyg 59:350, 1985.

Torafson T et al: Clinical improvement of gingival conditions following ultrasonic versus hand instrumentation of periodontal pockets, J Clin Periodontol 6:165, 1979.

VanVolkinburg JW, Green E, and Armitage GC: The nature of root surfaces after curette, Cavitron, and Alphasonic instrumentation, J Periodont Res 11:374, 1976.

Waerhaug J: Healing of the dentoepithelial junction following subgingival plaque control. II. As observed on extracted teeth, J Periodontol 49:119, 1978.

Walker SL and Ash MM: A study of root planing by scanning electron microscopy, Dent Hyg 50:109, 1976.

Weaks LM: Clinical evaluation of the Prophy-Jet as an instrument for routine removal of tooth stain and plaque, J Periodontol 55:486, 1984.

Wilkinson RF and Mayberry JE: Scanning electron microscopy of the root surface following instrumentation, J Periodontol 44:559, 1973.

Wilmann DE, Norling BK, and Johnson NN: A new prophylaxis instrument: effect on enamel alterations, J Am Dent Assoc 101:923, 1980.

SUGGESTED READINGS

Wilkins EM: Clinical practice of the dental hygienist, ed 4, Philadelphia, 1976, Lea & Febiger.

Woodall IR: Comprehensive dental hygiene care, St Louis, 1973, The CV Mosby Co.

Part III

Management of Advanced Periodontal Diseases

Chapter 46

GENERAL PRINCIPLES OF SURGICAL THERAPY

Peter J. Robinson
Charles H. Goodman

Case selection
Preoperative information
   Medical history
   Contraindications
   Consent
Intraoperative considerations
   Monitoring presurgical data
   Vascular supply and hydration
Surgical anatomy
   Attached gingiva
   Maxillary buccal and facial aspects
   Palate
   Mandible
   Lingual nerve and artery
   Retromolar regions
Complications
   Hemorrhage
   Infection
   Pain
Postoperative care

Adherence to basic general surgical principles during periodontal surgery may prevent lost flaps, excessive marginal necrosis, delayed healing, aberrant healing patterns, or excessive postoperative complications. However, a sufficient number of situations are unique to periodontal surgery and require amplification of many of the general principles of surgery. For example, a notable variation exists in the type of wound closure approach used, depending on whether periodontal pocket reduction is attempted by a new attachment procedure, a repositioned flap, or an apically positioned flap. In turn, deciding which approach to use for achieving this goal depends on such factors as the patient's expectations and attitude, local anatomic limitations, the overall treatment plan, and the probable maintenance schedule. This chapter focuses on the nuances in periodontal surgery that require amplification and/or modification of the basic rules.

CASE SELECTION

Because of the wide range of approaches (both surgical and nonsurgical) available in the treatment of soft tissue and bony periodontal defects, consideration must be given to the most appropriate approach for each involved site in each case. Unsatisfactory and unrestorable results often result if the therapeutic approaches are not coordinated in the design stage.

The following key factors should be addressed in determining the appropriate therapeutic approach:
1. Patient's expectations and desires
2. Goal of the surgical procedure
3. Maintenance program
4. Effect on adjacent teeth and optimization of retained attachment
5. Restorative treatment plan
6. Optimization of attachment
7. Infection control

1. *Patient's expectations and desires.* Knowing and understanding the patient's expectations and desires are paramount to designing an appropriate surgical treatment plan. Too often the patient's goals are ignored, leading to results that please the surgeon but displease the patient. Communication is critical. By paying close attention to the patient, listening to and observing the patient with great care,

the clinician can avoid choosing a treatment that appears technically ideal but does not achieve the patient's goals. Therefore the therapist should establish, prior to the initiation of definitive treatment, which clinical approach can both achieve a significant therapeutic improvement and satisfy the patient's goals of function, esthetics, and comfort. The limitations of the surgical approach, expected results, and a description of the possible complications should be effectively communicated back to the patient.

2. *Goal of the surgical procedure.* Once the patient's overall goals have been established, the specific purpose or purposes of the surgical procedure must be determined. The goal of the procedure may be to provide for complete antiinfective therapy, including access for root debridement, soft tissue excision, soft tissue replacement, or gaining new attachment.

Since no single design or technique is appropriate treatment for all periodontal defects, the surgeon must possess a repertoire of knowledge and technical skill to select and execute the appropriate procedure. Specific surgical designs and selection of specific surgical techniques for specific periodontal problems are discussed in Chapters 36, 47, and 48.

3. *Maintenance program.* Even the most careful preoperative surgical plan combined with a technically effective procedure will quickly fail without a reasonable postoperative maintenance program. Loss of attachment depth occurs at an accelerated rate in surgically treated cases without postoperative maintenance and is greater than in untreated cases (Nyman et al., 1975, 1977). Therefore it must be determined before surgery whether the bacterial plaque can be properly controlled through patient cooperation combined with an effective recall program, and whether the course of periodontal therapy chosen will result in suppression of the pathogenic microbiota and reduction of inflammation. Patients should be considered poor candidates for periodontal procedures if they are unable to maintain a favorable level of plaque control. Poor plaque control may result from either an inadequate response to attempts at behavioral modification or a handicap that impairs the patient's ability to practice plaque control. The long-term success of periodontal therapy is in serious jeopardy if an effective recall program cannot be maintained, since periodontal diseases have a marked tendency to recur in the absence of effective personal and professional oral hygiene after therapy. Only through careful long-term postoperative monitoring of the patient by an effective recall system can the maintenance of a treated patient be assured. The frequency of the recall program and the type of monitoring required are dictated by the patient's maintenance ability, the type of procedures performed, and the nature of the disease treated.

4. *Effect on adjacent teeth and optimization of retained attachment.* Since it has been reasonably well established that periodontitis is often severe in some sites that may be adjacent to healthy sites, it is critical to determine the effect the proposed surgical treatment will have on adjacent noninvolved teeth, as well as on the involved sites and teeth. A procedure is generally contraindicated if it compromises the remaining alveolar support of the teeth adjacent to the involved sites and should be carefully considered if it has the potential to jeopardize the alveolar support of the involved tooth or teeth. Zamet (1975) and Rosling et al. (1976) have demonstrated that with effective maintenance, surgical procedures designed specifically to conserve support are more effective in the long-term maintenance of attachment levels than are resective surgical procedures on single-rooted teeth. Therefore, resection of alveolar bone and soft tissue should likely be limited to the removal of soft or hard tissue enlargements (i.e., phenytoin enlargements, familial gingival hyperplasia, exostosis), crown-lengthening procedures, and facilitation of proper flap adaptation on single-rooted teeth. The effects of osseous resection procedures on multirooted teeth, especially those with furcation involvements, await thorough study. Regenerative procedures using barrier techniques and root surface demineralization techniques are being developed and show promise in the treatment of intrabony defects in molars. These procedures do not involve resection of the alveolar osseous structures.

5. *Restorative treatment plan.* Loss of soft tissue and/or bony support frequently follows periodontal surgical procedures on teeth severely involved with periodontitis. This resultant decrease in tooth stability of a single tooth or multiple teeth may have a dramatic effect on the restorative treatment plan. It is therefore crucial to coordinate the restorative and periodontal surgical treatment plans. Certain surgical plans may preclude specific restorative treatment plans, and vice versa. Coincidentally, it should be decided which teeth are strategic in the combined periodontal/restorative treatment plans. Judgment on a tooth-by-tooth basis, considering the alternate periodontal and restorative approaches, must be made before instituting any surgical procedures.

6. *Optimization of attachment.* The concern for retaining or improving tooth stability for restorative treatment goals also relates closely to selecting surgical procedures that optimize the amount of attachment retained and/or gained. In a simple, logical fashion the therapist should review each option, ranging from root planing alone, through various types of access flap approaches, to more complex reconstructive surgical procedures. Then the simplest and most predictable approach that can satisfy the therapeutic goals and needs should be selected.

7. *Infection control.* Prior to the scheduling of patients for nonemergency periodontal surgical procedures, the infectious aspects of the disease should be controlled by thorough scaling, root planing, establishment of oral hygiene, removal of all plaque retention areas, and antimicrobial therapy if necessary. Only after thorough antiinfec-

tive therapy is completed should surgical therapy be attempted. It may, of course, be necessary to complete antiinfective therapy by providing access to infected pockets for esthetics, for prosthetic reasons, or for regenerative therapy. Operating in an actively infected site frequently results in excessive operative bleeding, aberrant healing patterns, and loss of attachment (Nyman et al., 1977). Appropriate use of patient behavior modification in plaque control, root planing for root detoxification, and systemic antimicrobial therapy should be effectively instituted as an essential component of therapy. Nothing close to a sterile presurgical site can be achieved by these measures; however, by monitoring the involved sites with simple bleeding and plaque indices, and by evaluation of the level of pathogenic flora, an acceptable level of infection should be reached prior to the initiation of any surgical procedure. This level of infection control often requires several months of treatment, with four to six sessions of scaling, root planing, plaque retention area removal, and oral hygiene instruction.

PREOPERATIVE INFORMATION
Medical history

Well before scheduling an anticipated operation, the surgeon should determine if specific preoperative modifications are indicated because of the patient's medical history or current physical condition. Also, knowledge of the patient's current medications or drug allergy, if any, will dictate alterations in the type of anesthetic agent, analgesic, or prophylactic antibiotic considered.

Contraindications

Periodontal surgery is generally an elective procedure. Therefore, if the patient is medically compromised, the benefits versus the risks of the surgical procedure should be carefully weighed before committing the patient to the procedure. In addition, if the patient cannot maintain effective supragingival plaque control, considerable doubt is raised about proceeding with surgery. A presurgical reevaluation of the plaque and gingival indices will aid in making this decision.

Consent

The preoperative workup should ensure that the patient is fully informed about the details of the operation, what expectations are realistic, and possible complications. It is prudent to have the patient indicate agreement to the procedure both with an oral statement and by signing a consent form.

INTRAOPERATIVE CONSIDERATIONS
Monitoring presurgical data

Once the goal of the surgical procedure has been established (access for antiinfective therapy, crown lengthening, new attachment, or a cosmetic procedure), a specific surgical technique should be selected to best achieve the goals within the local anatomic limitations. The data necessary to select the appropriate surgical procedure include periapical radiographs, study casts, and a probing chart. The radiographs enable the clinician to determine the length, morphology, and proximity of the roots, as well as the location of anatomic landmarks such as the maxillary sinus. The study casts provide further information on anatomic landmarks, such as the presence of exostosis, the position of the internal and external oblique ridges, and the shape of the palatal vault, as well as serving as a template to outline the flap design. An accurate probing chart guides the surgeon to the approximate position and depth of the bony defects. However, only on surgical exposure can the actual size and morphology of a bony defect be determined. Therefore contingency surgical plans should be part of the overall design to allow proper adjustments during the operation if the therapist finds atypical anatomic variations in size or location of a bony defect.

Vascular supply and hydration

During the surgery the therapist must ensure maintenance of sufficient blood flow in the flaps and proper hydration of both the flaps and the surgical site. The base of the flap should be of ample width to provide adequate blood flow to support the edges of the flap and of sufficient thickness to include a suitable proportion of vascular connective tissue to support the avascular epithelium.

Very thin flaps, especially "split flaps," with very stylized scalloped architecture, providing "attractive" marginal adaptation, often slough as a result of inadequate vascular supply. This results in considerable postoperative pain and excessive loss of attachment and marginal alveolar bone. Likewise, flaps frequently undergo necrosis within the first several postoperative days if rough instrumentation has caused ischemia or if dehydration of the flaps has occurred during the operation. Dehydration can and should be avoided by ensuring that the flaps remain moist during the entire operation and by carefully limiting the amount of time the flap is reflected.

Hemorrhage control. The amount of hemorrhage should be carefully monitored and controlled during the operation. Judicious use of vasoconstrictors aids significantly in reducing the amount of operative bleeding (Buckley et al., 1984). Hemorrhage reduction also frequently follows the removal of diseased soft tissues; infected granulomatous tissue found at the base of periodontal pockets is typically highly vascular (Appelgren et al., 1979). Thorough antiinfective treatment prior to the surgical procedure should minimize residual inflamed granulation tissue and markedly reduce surgical bleeding. Additional sources of excessive bleeding can be small tears or partially cut vessels that continue to ooze rather than functionally collapse (often the result of rough dissection and/or ineffectively incised flaps). Unavoidably, sometimes in well-designed and well-executed operations, small vessels continue to profusely bleed, even following the cautious use of vasoconstrictors. These vessels should be effectively tied off before proceeding.

Avoiding dead spaces. When preparing for flap closure, the surgeon should seek hemostasis as completely as possible, since a large blood clot is an excellent medium for bacterial growth and hinders effective healing. In addition, if hemorrhage continues when the operative site is sutured, flap necrosis often follows because the blood clot causes a dead space to form, resulting in ischemia and infection of the flap margins.

Wound closure. Selecting the proper suture material is an important consideration, but an even greater requirement is the proper suturing technique. Since sutures function to approximate tissues, the spacing of sutures, the depth of the bite taken, and the tension applied on tying should accomplish approximation without strangulation. Firm closure with good approximation, full coverage of the alveolar bone, close adaptation to the tooth, and a thin fibrin clot should be the goal. This avoids flap ischemia caused by excessively tight and improperly placed sutures, reduces marginal alveolar bone loss, and provides an environment that enhances the chances for periodontal regeneration in the depths of infrabony pockets.

SURGICAL ANATOMY

Before beginning any periodontal surgical procedure, the clinician must have a thorough understanding of surgical anatomy (Clark and Bueltmann, 1971; Hunt, 1976). Fortunately, relatively few vital structures are at risk during routine periodontal surgery. However, knowledge of the location of nerves and vessels, as well as an understanding of the bony structures, minimizes the risk of surgical complications.

In addition to minimizing risks, knowledge of anatomic considerations can influence the surgical approach, allowing the surgeon to understand the limitations on what may be achieved in different regions of the oral cavity. This section describes anatomic features directly associated with periodontal surgery rather than providing a detailed overview of oral anatomy.

Attached gingiva

An important consideration before beginning any periodontal flap is the amount of attached gingiva present.

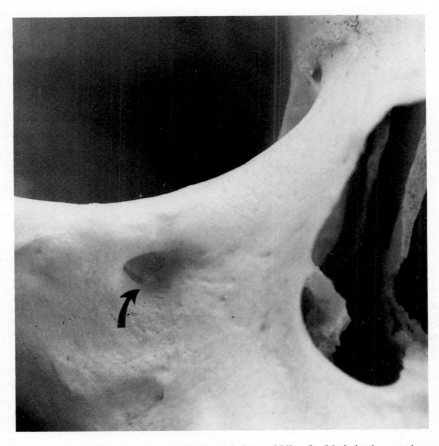

Fig. 46-1. Infraorbital foramen *(arrow)* is found below middle of orbital rim in superior portion of canine fossa.

The preservation of attached gingiva is an important surgical principle that strongly influences the incision design. The zone of attached gingiva varies in width on the buccal and labial surfaces of each tooth. This has been described in some detail by Bowers (1963). However, such great individual variation exists that the design of the initial incision relative to the amount of attached gingiva must be established on a case-by-case basis.

Maxillary buccal and facial aspects

No significant vessels or nerves are present in the anterior or posterior facial regions of the maxillary arch. The infraorbital nerve and vessels emerge through the infraorbital foramen, which is situated approximately 5 to 8 mm below the middle part of the inferior orbital rim (Fig. 46-1). The infraorbital nerve and vessels can only be disrupted during periodontal surgery if the caninus muscle attachment is lifted from the canine fossa.

On the lateral surface of the maxilla is the zygomaticoalveolar crest (Fig. 46-2). This bony structure originates from the zygomatic process and extends to the alveolar process in the region of the first molar. The shape of the ridge and its relationship to the alveolar process will determine the depth of the vestibule in the maxillary molar region. If the zygomaticoalveolar crest attaches close to the alveolar crest, it may interfere with flap reflection and placement. The zygomatic process could attach high enough on the alveolar crest to interfere with osseous recontouring or apical positioning of the tissue.

The maxillary sinus often extends into the alveolar process (Fig. 46-3). Frequently no cancellous bone is present

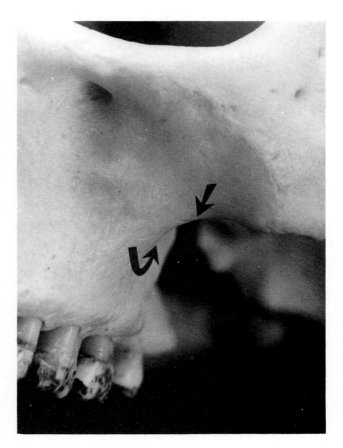

Fig. 46-2. Location of zygomaticoalveolar crest *(arrows)* with respect to alveolar process determines vestibular depth in maxillary molar region.

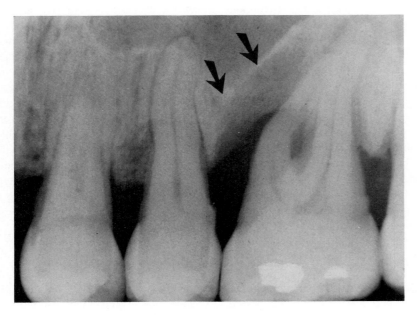

Fig. 46-3. Note thin cortical bone separating maxillary sinus from base of this large intrabony defect *(arrows)* on mesial aspect of molar.

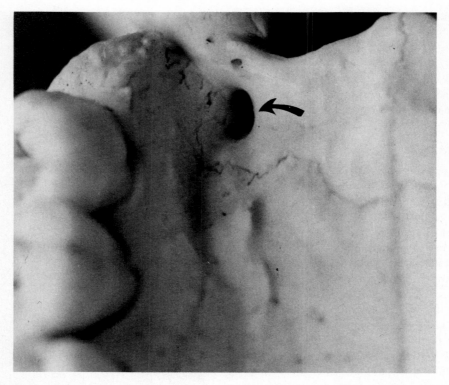

Fig. 46-4. Greater palatine foramen *(arrow)* is typically found at junction of alveolar and palatine processes.

between the cortical bone of the tooth socket and the sinus in the regions of the maxillary molars and premolars. The sinus may therefore become a complicating factor in osseous recontouring of intrabony pockets that approach the floor of the sinus or when osseous ramping of edentulous ridges is being performed.

Palate

Greater palatine nerve and artery. The palate contains several anatomic features of importance in periodontal surgery. Important structures encountered in this region are the greater palatine nerve and artery. The greater palatine foramen is located approximately 3 to 4 mm anterior to the posterior border of the hard palate and is typically found at the junction of the alveolar and palatine processes (Fig. 46-4). The greater palatine nerve and vessels course anteriorly in the submucosa of the hard palate to supply the mucous membranes and glands of the hard palate and the gingiva of the palatal surfaces of the maxillary alveolar process up to the canine region.

Palatal flap procedures should rarely involve the foramen itself. However, the greater palatine nerve and vessels may be encountered when surgery is performed along their course in the palate. The nerve and vessels are seldom damaged when a full-thickness flap is raised that fully con-

tains the structures. However, the thinning of palatal flaps too close to the midline may sever branches of the artery, resulting in excessive hemorrhage. In addition, donor tissue for free gingival grafts taken in an improper location or too deeply may also involve branches of the greater palatine artery.

Nasopalatine nerve and artery. The nasopalatine nerve and vessels enter the oral cavity via the incisive foramen located directly behind the maxillary central incisor teeth (Fig. 46-5). These structures supply the palatal gingiva of the incisor and canine region. Surgery to eliminate periodontal pockets in this area very often requires undermining of the incisive papilla, which may sever the nasopalatine nerve and artery. As an infrequently encountered consequence, patients may experience temporary parasthesia to the area supplied. Hemorrhage is rarely of any consequence, since the artery passing through the incisive foramen is only a small, terminal branch of the greater palatine artery.

Mandible

Anterior facial region. The primary concern in this region is the location of the mentalis muscle attachment. A high muscle attachment results in a very shallow vestibule. Elevation of the muscle attachment to gain adequate access

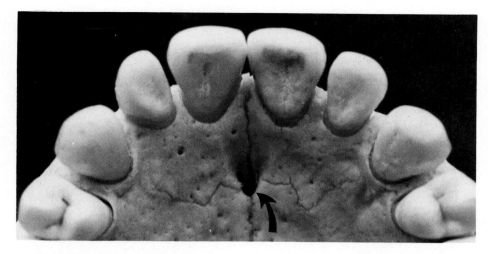

Fig. 46-5. Nasopalatine foramen *(arrow)* is located behind maxillary central incisors.

during flap surgery exposes the submental space, which may lead to infection originating in this space with the potential to spread posteriorly into the lateral pharyngeal space.

Posterior facial region. The mental foramen is typically located halfway between the alveolar crest and the lower mandibular border between the first and second premolars (Fig. 46-6). However, variations in location do exist, and location of the mental foramen prior to surgery in this region can prevent traumatization of the mental nerve, which can result in temporary or permanent parasthesia of the lip and gingiva. Also, severing of the mental artery results in excessive hemorrhage. These structures become important when mucogingival surgery or an apically positioned flap in the premolar region is being considered. Long releasing incisions should be avoided in the premolar area to reduce the potential trauma to these structures.

The location and degree of prominence of the external oblique ridge determines the depth of the vestibule in the molar area (Fig. 46-7). Particularly flat and broad external oblique ridges can complicate periodontal surgery in the mandibular posterior region. Because of the shelflike prominence, the ridge can hinder the performance of mucogingival procedures or apically positioned flaps. If intrabony defects extend below the level of the ridge, osseous resection to eliminate the defects may require excessive bone removal, which is contraindicated. Procedures in which barrier membranes or coronally repositioned flaps are used to achieve regeneration of the periodontium in buccal furcations on lower molars offer great promise for treating these regions (Gantes et al., 1988; Pontoriero, et al., 1988).

The temporal crest and anterior border of the ramus of the mandible often closely approximates the terminal man-

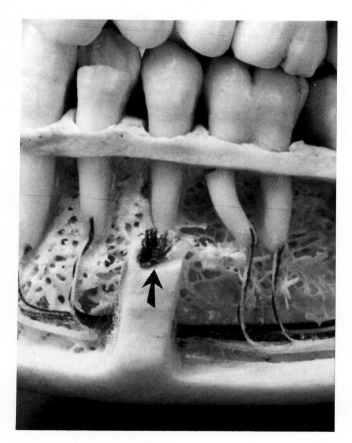

Fig. 46-6. Mental foramen *(arrow)* is typically located midway between alveolar crest and lower border of mandible in premolar region.

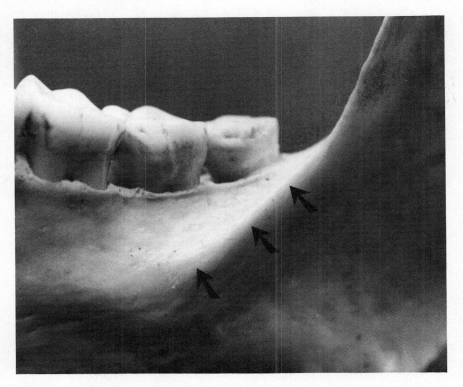

Fig. 46-7. Proximity of external oblique ridge *(arrows)* to molars may limit surgical access.

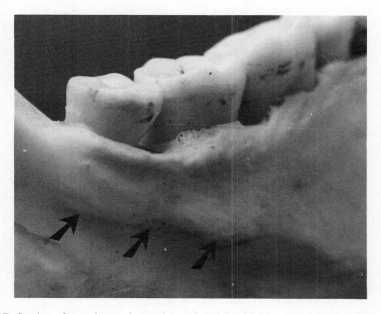

Fig. 46-8. Reflection of muscle attachment beyond mylohyoid ridge *(arrows)* provides entry into sublingual space.

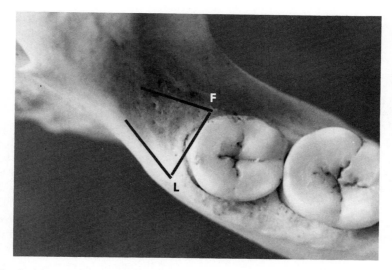

Fig. 46-9. Incisions performed distal to terminal molar must be confined to over bony ridge in retromolar triangle.

dibular molar. Because of these structures, intrabony defects distal to the second or third molar may not lend themselves to bone-recontouring procedures. As with intrabony defects associated with the external oblique ridge, these lesions are often best treated by open-flap debridement or bone replacement techniques rather than by a resective approach to achieve pocket reduction.

Mandibular lingual area

Anterior aspect. The only specific area of concern in the anterior lingual region involves the presence of an unusually high genial tubercle on which several muscles associated with movements of the tongue attach. Elevation of a flap past the tubercle provides access to the sublingual space. An infection in this region can communicate posteriorly with the parapharyngeal space.

Posterior aspect. Bony prominences, or exostoses, may often be found along the body of the mandible. The most common location for mandibular tori is along the lingual aspect of the mandible, superior to the mylohyoid muscle, in the region of the canines and premolars. The decision to remove these tori is dictated by their size, approximation to the alveolar crest, and prosthetic considerations. Large mandibular tori can interfere with flap placement or the correction of intrabony defects through osseous recontouring. The tissue overlying these tori can be very thin and easily torn during flap reflection.

Also, located on the inner surface of the mandibular body is the mylohyoid ridge on which the mylohyoid muscle attaches (Fig. 46-8). If this muscle is inserted high on the mandibular body or if there are deeper osseous defects, it may be necessary to reflect the lingual flap past the mylohyoid muscle attachment. While this is not necessarily contraindicated, detachment of this muscle provides access into the submandibular facial spaces. An infection in this region has free access directly into the neck.

Lingual nerve and artery

The major precaution in performing periodontal surgery on the lingual surface of the mandible is to avoid trauma to the lingual nerve and artery, which lie close to the mucosal surface in the region of the second and third molars. The nerve and artery are safe from trauma if full-thickness mucoperiosteal flaps are used and blunt rather than sharp dissection is employed. Releasing incisions on the lingual surface should be limited to the attached gingiva.

Retromolar region

In the mandible the retromolar pad is often created by a mass of glandular and loose areolar tissue. Attempts to reduce pockets in this area by a distal wedge incision are often frustrated by the loose character of the tissue. Before any incision is performed in this region, careful palpation of the mandibular ramus should be done to ensure that the incision is made over bone and not toward the lingual aspect, which could endanger the lingual nerve and artery (Fig. 46-9).

COMPLICATIONS

There are primarily three complications associated with periodontal surgery: hemorrhage, infection, and postoperative pain.

Hemorrhage

The risk of serious hemorrhage can be avoided by thoroughly understanding the local anatomy of the surgical site. The risk of traumatizing larger arteries or their branches will then be minimized. However, involvement of smaller arterioles and capillary bleeding are common and often unavoidable during periodontal surgery.

Control of bleeding sites within soft tissue may be approached in several ways. Identification of the source of

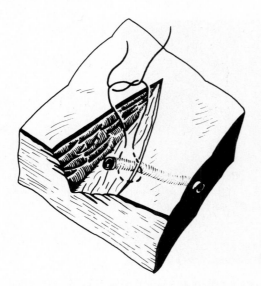

Fig. 46-10. Use of ligation suture for application of compression to severed arteriole.

bleeding is the first step to establishing control. Careful suctioning and local pressure applied with gauze sponges aid in this process. Once the bleeding site is identified, judicious injection of a vasoconstrictor combined with continued application of pressure encourages clot formation. If this is not effective, an artificial clot may be induced by use of an oxidized cellulose or microfibrillar collagen product. This approach is particularly useful on palatal donor sites used for free gingival grafts. In addition, electrocoagulation can be effective for capillary bleeding sites and small arterioles.

Large arteriole bleeding sites, which do not respond to pressure, vasocontrictors, or clot-enhancing gels, can be controlled by placing a suture in the soft tissue lateral to the free end of the vessel. The knot is drawn tight to occlude the vessel by compression from the surrounding tissue (Fig. 46-10).

Bleeding from intraosseous sites may require a different approach. Often, excessive bleeding from interproximal and intrabony lesions results from inadequate degranulation. Residual granulomatous tissue is a common source of hemorrhage, since it is composed largely of capillaries. Thorough degranulation often results in clean, nonbleeding bone margins. Oozing from narrow spaces or nutrient canals can be controlled by a combination of pressure and use of a vasoconstrictor. Bone wax (beeswax and salicylic acid) may be used to occlude bony canals that contain hemorrhaging vessels.

Several steps should be taken to minimize postsurgical bleeding. Prior to approximation of the flaps, all areas should be rinsed free of clots and the surgical site checked again for bleeding. Pressure should be applied to the flaps to encourage a minimal clot thickness. Good closure with tight flap approximation discourages postsurgical hemorrhage. Particular attention should be directed toward ensuring good closure of distal wedge and edentulous ridge sites, since these areas can be a source of postoperative bleeding if not well approximated.

Infection

Despite the fact that periodontal surgery is performed in a highly unsterile environment, the prevalence of postsurgical infection is very low when adequate infection-control procedures are used (Pack and Haber, 1983; Curtis et al., 1985). In addition, several studies have suggested that the routine use of postsurgical antibiotics is of little or no value in preventing postoperative infections if adequate infection control is observed during the procedures. Several studies (Karl et al., 1966) have shown that routine antibiotic therapy does not lower the prevalence of postoperative infection following general surgical procedures. Similar results have been observed in oral surgery (Curran et al., 1974; Yrastorza, 1976). Studies done on the use of antibiotics following periodontal surgery have indicated that this practice is ineffective in changing the prevalence of infection (Pack and Haber, 1983).

It has been suggested that patients tend to experience less pain during the first postoperative week when an antibiotic is prescribed (Kidd and Wade, 1974). The magnitude of the reduction is so small, however, that it does not justify using an antibiotic for this purpose. The routine use of antibiotics following periodontal surgery for control of postoperative sequelae is not supported. However, the clinician must weigh such factors as the medical status of the patient, the duration and extent of the surgery, and surgical entry into facial planes when considering antibiotic coverage in unique circumstances.

The use of antibiotics should be reserved mainly for instances when signs of infection occur. If an infection is diagnosed clinically, the patient should be given an antibiotic, and when practical, an antibiotic sensitivity test should be performed to guide the antibiotic selection.

Pain

The prevalence and severity of pain following periodontal surgery varies depending on such factors as the location, duration, and extent of surgery, as well as the skill with which the soft tissue and osseous tissues are manipulated during surgery. Psychologic considerations also play a role in pain perception. While some degree of discomfort is to be expected following any periodontal surgical procedure, gentle surgical technique and sincere concern for patient discomfort can minimize the discomfort. Curtis et al. (1985) found that in 304 periodontal surgical procedures, over 50% of the patients reported minimal or no pain; less than 5% experienced severe pain. Mucogingival surgery was found to be significantly related to pain, since it was three to five times more likely to cause pain than was osseous surgery and six times more likely to cause pain than were gingivectomies, distal wedge procedures, or internally beveled flaps.

POSTOPERATIVE CARE

Before release, the patient should be given both verbal and written instructions concerning postoperative care.

Slight oozing from the surgical site is normal for the first 24 hours. Patients should be given sterile gauze pads and instructed that if oozing persists, they can close firmly on moistened gauze for 30 to 60 minutes. The pressure will encourage hemostasis.

Swelling is handled by applying an ice pack to the face, alternating 20 minutes on and 20 minutes off, for several hours. However, swelling that progresses after the first 24 hours may indicate infection.

An analgesic should be prescribed. Minor procedures may require only the use of a nonsteroidal antiinflammatory agent such as acetaminophen or ibuprofen. More extensive procedures may dictate use of a narcotic analgesic such as a codeine-containing product. Clinical judgment and knowledge of the patient will aid in deciding on the appropriate analgesic to use.

As discussed earlier in this chapter, the routine use of an antibiotic for the prevention of infection is not indicated. However, patients should be instructed that persistent or progressive swelling combined with increasing pain and/or fever indicates infection. These signs and symptoms warrant evaluation by the therapist to determine if an antibiotic is needed.

The use of a periodontal dressing has been widespread for many years. Baer et al. (1969) stated that the main purpose of a periodontal dressing was to provide patient comfort and protect the wound from further injury during healing. However, the value of dressings and their effects on wound healing has been questioned.

It has been demonstrated that the use of a periodontal dressing does not improve the postoperative rate of healing (Stahl et al., 1969) or reduce the amount of pain and swelling (Greensmith and Wade, 1974). In addition, periodontal dressings do not improve clinically measured parameters such as the Gingival Index, pocket depth, or attachment levels postsurgically (Jones and Cassingham, 1979; Allen and Caffesse, 1983).

Therefore, based on recent studies, it appears that periodontal dressings do not improve postoperative healing and do not provide a greater degree of patient comfort. They do, however, contribute to plaque retention, and this may carry greater significance for final healing patterns. Well-adapted flaps may serve as a barrier to bacteria (Allen and Caffesse, 1983) and are thus more effective than any protection provided by a dressing. However, dressings still have selected indications; for example, if wound closure is inadequate or there are sites of exposed connective tissue or bone, coverage of the surgical site may be advantageous. Nevertheless, the routine use of dressings is decreasing significantly because current surgical techniques provide better wound closure and antimicrobial rinses are now available.

Rinsing with an effective antiplaque agent such as chlorhexidine reduces postoperative plaque accumulation and surgical inflammation. It has been demonstrated that rinsing with chlorhexidine is roughly equivalent to professional plaque control in postsurgical healing and is judged to be a viable alternative to mechanical plaque control in the first 3 months after therapy (Westfield et al., 1983).

REFERENCES

Allen DR and Caffesse RG: Comparison of results following modified Widman flap surgery with and without surgical dressing, J Periodontol 54:470, 1983.

Applegren R et al: Clinical and histologic correlations of gingivitis, J Periodontol 50:540, 1979.

Baer PM et al: Periodontal dressings, Dent Clin North Am 13:181, 1969.

Bowers GM: A study in the width of attached gingiva, J Periodontol 34:201, 1963.

Buckley JA et al: Efficacy of epinephrine concentration in local anesthesia during periodontal surgery, J Periodontol 55:653, 1984.

Clark MA and Bueltmann KW: Anatomical considerations in periodontal surgery, J Periodontol 42:610, 1971.

Curran JB et al: An assessment of the use of antibiotics in third molar surgery, Oral Surg 3:1, 1974.

Curtis JW et al: The incidence and severity of complications and pain following periodontal surgery, J Periodontol 56:197, 1985.

Gantes B et al: Treatment of periodontal furcation defects (II): bone regeneration in mandibular Class II defects, J Clin Periodontol 15:232, 1988.

Greensmith AL and Wade AB: Dressing after reverse bevel flap procedures, J Clin Periodontol 1:97, 1974.

Hunt PR: Safety aspects of mandibular lingual surgery, J Periodontol 47:224, 1976.

Jones TM and Cassingham RJ: Comparison of healing following periodontal surgery with and without dressings in humans, J Periodontol 50:387, 1979.

Karl RC et al: Prophylactic antimicrobial drugs in surgery, N Engl J Med 275:305, 1966.

Kidd EAM and Wade AM: Penicillin control of swelling and pain after periodontal osseous surgery, J Clin Periodontol 1:52, 1974.

Nyman S et al: Effect of professional tooth cleaning on healing after periodontal surgery, J Clin Periodontol 2:80, 1975.

Nyman S et al: Periodontal surgery in plaque-infected dentitions, J Clin Periodontol 4:240, 1977.

Pack PD and Haber J: The incidence of clinical infection after periodontal surgery: a retrospective study, J Periodontol 54:441, 1983.

Pontoriero R et al: Guided tissue regeneration in degree II furcation-involved mandibular molars: a clinical study, J Clin Periodontol 15:247, 1988.

Rosling B et al: The healing potential of the periodontal tissues following different techniques of periodontal surgery in plaque-free dentitions, J Clin Periodontol 3:233, 1976.

Stahl SS et al: Gingival healing. III. The effects of periodontal dressings on gingivectomy repair, J Periodontol 40:30, 1969.

Westfield E et al: Use of chlorhexidine as a plaque control measure following surgical treatment of periodontal disease, J Clin Periodontol 10:22, 1983.

Yrastorza JA: Indications for antibiotics in orthognathic surgery, Oral Surg 34:514, 1976.

Zamet JS: A comparative clinical study of three periodontal surgical techniques, J Clin Periodontol 2:87, 1975.

Chapter 47

PERIODONTAL SURGERY

Robert J. Genco
Edwin S. Rosenberg
Cyril Evian

Since periodontal diseases are bacterial infections, the mainstay of therapy is antiinfective procedures (i.e., procedures directed to removing the periodontal bacterial pathogens). Some periodontal surgical procedures are adjuncts to effective suppression of periodontal bacteria. There are also specific prosthetic and cosmetic indications for periodontal surgical procedures, as well as for most periodontal regenerative procedures.

Periodontal surgical procedures involve cutting or removal of soft or hard tissues of the supporting structures of the teeth. Many clinicians consider scaling and root planing to be surgical procedures, since they also involve cutting or removal of the root surface and often of periodontal tissues; however, scaling and root planing are often referred to as nonsurgical treatment of periodontal disease. The technical definition of surgery is "handwork."

OBJECTIVES OF PERIODONTAL SURGERY

Historically, periodontal surgical procedures were designed for excision of diseased tissue, elimination of periodontal pockets, and provision of "physiologic contours." Research in the last few decades has raised questions about these objectives as a rationale for periodontal surgery, and in fact many well-controlled clinical studies have compared various surgical methods for treating periodontal infections and have found little difference in the clinical results among these procedures. For example, clinical studies comparing gingivectomy and apically repositioned flaps, with and without osteoplasty (Rosling et al., 1976b; Knowles et al., 1979; Lindhe et al., 1982; Caffesse et al., 1987; Kaldahl et al., 1988) have shown only minor differences among these surgical procedures with regard to their effectiveness in pocket reduction, attachment gain, and reduction of gingivitis and plaque levels as long as 8 years after therapy. Furthermore, several studies have failed to show clinically significant differences between surgical procedures and "nonsurgical procedures" such as complete scaling and root planing for periodontal disease when carried out on single-rooted teeth or flat surfaces of molars (Rosling et al., 1976b; Lindhe et al., 1982; Pihlstrom et al., 1983).

There are, however, several clear reasons for performing periodontal surgery, all of which have to do with preservation of the periodontal tissues and, ultimately, the dentition.

In advanced periodontitis with deep pockets, periodontal surgery is often indicated for access to direct vision of the root surfaces for thorough debridement (see NIDR, 1982; also see a review of treatment literature by Antczak-Boukoms and Weinstein, 1987). Other indications for periodontal surgery include preparation for a prosthesis, regenerative therapy, and cosmetic reasons.

It cannot be emphasized enough that when periodontal treatment is completed, especially if periodontal surgical procedures are performed, a plaque-free dentition must be maintained; otherwise, periodontal disease may recur (Rosling et al., 1976a; Nyman et al., 1977; Westfelt et al., 1983). One way to help ensure that the patient will practice effective oral hygiene is to teach oral hygiene and establish effective plaque control for each patient before any periodontal surgical procedure is done. This can be conveniently carried out and monitored during the presurgical antiinfective phase of therapy (see Chapter 35).

At a recent World Workshop in Clinical Periodontics (American Academy of Periodontology, 1989) there was considerable controversy over the goals of resective periodontal surgery, and whether pocket reduction and physiologic contours per se were desirable goals of such therapy. Based on objective appraisal of over two decades of study of this problem (see review by Caffesse, 1989), we propose that there are several objectives of periodontal surgery.

The main objectives of periodontal surgery include one or more of the following:

1. *To gain surgical access* to deep or tortuous pockets for adequate cleaning and smoothening of the root surfaces. Surgical flaps, gingivectomy, and osseous contouring procedures are sometimes necessary to provide access for thorough debridement of the tooth surface under direct vision.

2. *To facilitate plaque control* by reduction or elimination of potential plaque retention areas. Some contours of the periodontal tissues, especially periodontal pockets, redundant gingiva, or bony ledges, remain after antiinfective therapy, and these may result in plaque retention areas. For example, hyperplastic, fibrous gingival tissue in the retromolar or tuberosity area distal to the last molar often represents a noninflamed area of probeable depth after antiinfective therapy. Since these residual probeable depths are potential plaque retention areas over the long term, resection may be necessary. Likewise, gingival hyperplasia results in "pseudopockets," which preclude good plaque control and lead to smooth surface caries and periodontal inflammation. In addition, shallow vestibules and frenal attachments close to or at the gingival margin may make oral hygiene difficult, necessitating surgical correction to facilitate the patient's plaque control. Periodontal surgical procedures can also be used to halt gingival recession and to cover denuded areas, resulting in better plaque control. Other potential plaque retention areas indicating periodontal surgery occur adjacent to root furcations, root depressions, and around crowded or malposed teeth.

3. *To provide an environment for an adequate prosthesis.* Preprosthetic surgical procedures such as crown lengthening; alveolar ridge alteration; and correction of mucogingival defects, including frenotomy, vestibule deepening, and increasing the amount of attached gingiva to resist abrasive forces, are often required. Also, soft and hard tissues of the periodontium may need to be removed to expose apical margins of subgingival carious lesions, to expose subgingival margins of crowns, to expose endodontic perforations, or to correct or expose other root abnormalities.

4. *For periodontal regenerative therapy.* To restore the lost functional attachment apparatus, reconstruction or regenerative surgical procedures may be necessary. Regeneration of new bone, cementum, and periodontal ligament may be desirable, particularly on teeth that are compromised or have deep infrabony pockets or open furcations.

5. *To correct cosmetic abnormalities.* The appearance of the gingiva, particularly the maxillary labial gingiva, which may be bulbous, receded, or have clefts, may not be acceptable to the patient. Also, the teeth may appear small or short if the gingiva has not receded, as occurs in altered passive eruption, and gingivectomy or gingivoplasty may be necessary to expose the crowns.

Surgical techniques for regeneration of lost periodontal tissue and other reconstructive periodontal surgical procedures are described in Chapter 48. Surgical access for root debridement is discussed in Chapter 36, and preprosthetic surgery in Chapter 51. The other surgical procedures are discussed here.

GENERAL PRINCIPLES

Most periodontal surgical procedures are performed only after antiinfective therapy has been completed; however, some surgical procedures provide access for antiinfective therapy and are used in the later stages of this phase of treatment. Antiinfective therapy, as described in detail in Chapter 35, consists of thorough scaling, root planing, removal of plaque retention areas, and the establishment of adequate oral hygiene. Also, systemic or topical antimicrobial agents *or surgical access procedures* may be necessary if the mechanical procedures are not adequate.

The end points of thorough antiinfective therapy are (1) *elimination of gingival inflammation,* (2) *elimination of supragingival and subgingival plaques and calculus,* and (3) *reduction or elimination of the periodontopathic subgingival flora.* Once these end points are achieved, periodontal surgical procedures may be necessary to meet the objectives mentioned in the preceding section.

Anesthesia

In general, most periodontal surgical procedures are done with the patient under local anesthesia; however, in certain circumstances, inhalation or intravenous analgesics may be used, or patients may be hospitalized and general anesthesia used. General anesthesia would be considered, for example, in patients who suffer from neurologic damage and are unable to tolerate a periodontal surgical procedure done on an outpatient basis. However, these are unusual cases, and most periodontal surgical procedures are done with local anesthesia on an outpatient basis.

Tissue management

In general, tissues should be handled carefully, and the minimum surgical trauma adequate to accomplish the objectives should be carried out. The oral cavity is highly vascular and highly innervated, and extensive surgical procedures may result in hemorrhage, paresthesia, fascial space infection, or excessive bone resorption. It is well established from dental implant research that heating of the bone to more than 47° C during bone reduction procedures will result in surface necrosis. Hence, slow-speed removal of bone (<2000 rpm) with sharp surgical burs and adequate cooling is necessary for optimal healing after osseous surgical procedures. Periodontal surgery should be carried out with the use of sterile surgical regimens that minimize introduction of new organisms into the oral cavity. For example, patients are draped, the oral cavity is rinsed with povidone-iodine or chlorhexidine, and surgeons and assistants wear gowns, gloves, head covers, and masks for all procedures.

Postoperative care

In general, postoperative care includes the following:
1. A dressing is placed as indicated for management of the tissue for hemostasis and patient comfort.
2. Antibiotic coverage may be used, depending on the history of the patient, the patient's general health, and the level of infectious periodontitis preceding the procedure. Universal antibiotic coverage after periodontal surgical procedures has not been documented to be effective and is discouraged.
3. Postoperative pain can often be controlled with minor analgesics such as ibuprofen or acetamide. More extensive procedures may require narcotics such as codeine. Aspirin should be avoided.

Postoperative complications are rare, but the patient should be made aware of the possibility of hemorrhage, infection, swelling and discoloration, and root sensitivity after periodontal surgery.

PERIODONTAL SURGERY IN THE TREATMENT PLAN

Periodontal surgical procedures should be carried out only after antiinfective therapy has been completed and adequate plaque control demonstrated. Also, elimination of acute occlusal trauma, gross occlusal discrepancies, carious lesions, and abscesses should be accomplished and all emergencies taken care of before periodontal surgery is undertaken. Root resection procedures or anticipated endodontic therapy should be completed, with amalgam fillings placed in the root(s) to be resected. If the root to be resected is not obvious, pulpectomy with calcium hydroxide filling of the canals should be done prior to surgery. If endodontic therapy is required for resolution of pulpal or periapical disease, this should be completed and an adequate interval allowed for evaluation of the success of the procedure before any periodontal surgical procedure is performed. If minor or major tooth movement is to be carried out, this should be completed and the patient placed in retentive appliances before the performance of any periodontal surgical procedure. In the case of extensive restorative dentistry, provisional or temporary restorations should be placed before the performance of any periodontal surgical procedure so that the gingival margin and the alveolar crest surrounding the restored tooth can be surgically positioned. This allows for an adequate width of epithelial and connective tissue attachment between the alveolar crest and the margin of the restoration.

CONTRAINDICATIONS

Periodontal surgical procedures should be delayed or not performed under the following circumstances:

1. *Patients who do not exhibit good plaque control.* Evaluation of the effectiveness of personal oral hygiene can be accomplished during the antiinfective phase of therapy during which plaque-control procedures are taught and their effectiveness monitored over several months. If supragingival plaque control is not adequate or supragingival calculus deposits form rapidly, periodontal surgery should be delayed until adequate control is achieved by the patient. The periodontal surgery should be delayed indefinitely if plaque control is not achievable. Often such patients can benefit from closely spaced scaling and root-planing sessions, and occasionally after a period of months or even years such patients "convert" to good plaque control and become candidates for surgery.

2. *Uncontrolled or progressive systemic diseases.* In general, most systemic diseases that are controlled are not contraindications to periodontal therapy. However, the following should be noted:
   a. Patients who have had recent myocardial infarctions should not be subjected to periodontal surgery until well after cardiac rehabilitation.
   b. Patients receiving anticoagulant therapy have the potential for bleeding after surgical procedures. This includes patients taking aspirin as a prophylaxis for heart disease, and such patients should stop taking aspirin temporarily before undergoing periodontal surgery.

c. Patients suffering from leukemia, neutrophil disorders such as neutropenia, or severe granulomatous disease should not be subjected to periodontal surgery unless they are in remission.

d. Patients with anemia may have lowered resistance to infection, and periodontal surgery should be performed only after correction of the anemia. However, mild and treated anemias are not necessarily contraindications to therapy.

e. Diabetes mellitus is often associated with delayed wound healing and lowered resistance to infection, and patients with diabetes mellitus should not be surgically treated until their diabetes is well controlled. Diabetic patients under good metabolic control may be subjected to periodontal surgery; however, the surgery should be timed so that it does not interfere with the diet or medication regimens. It may be that these regimens should be altered; for example, an increase in insulin may be required before the surgical procedure.

f. Patients taking large doses of corticosteroids (i.e., patients with Addison's disease or those with adrenal dysfunction) may have reduced resistance to stress associated with surgery. These patients may require adjustment of their corticosteroid regimen before and after periodontal surgery.

g. Patients with severe neurologic disorders, such as multiple sclerosis and Parkinson's disease, may make periodontal surgical procedures difficult as in-office procedures; thus these patients should be considered for treatment in a hospital. Patients with epilepsy are often taking phenytoin (Dilantin), and these patients may be subjected to periodontal surgery for gingival hyperplasia as indicated.

h. Patients with imminent terminal disease who are debilitated are not candidates for surgery.

i. Advanced cases where patients have not agreed to a restorative treatment plan after the surgical procedures should have surgery deferred until a restorative commitment is made.

In general, then, patients with systemic diseases should have these diseases well under control before undergoing periodontal surgery. It is best to monitor the patient for control of systemic diseases. This can be done during the antiinfective phase of therapy, which often takes several months to accomplish adequately.

• • •

Surgical procedures that are used to achieve the goals of periodontal therapy are divided into five categories as outlined below. A general definition of the most important types of periodontal surgical procedures; the specific objectives, indications, contraindications, advantages, and disadvantages of each procedure; and a step-by-step de-

scription of the procedure follow the outline.

  I. Gingival surgical procedures
     A. Curettage
        1. Open curettage with root planing
        2. Subgingival curettage
        3. Excisional new attachment procedures
        4. Chemical curettage
     B. Gingivectomy
     C. Gingivoplasty
     D. Tuberosity and retromolar reduction
        1. Wedges
        2. Gingival resection
 II. Periodontal flaps and alveolar osseous surgical procedures
     A. Modified Widman flap
     B. Repositioned flaps
        1. Apically repositioned
        2. Laterally repositioned
        3. Coronally repositioned
     C. Osseous surgery
        1. Osteoplasty
        2. Ostectomy
        3. Regenerative procedures (see Chapter 48)
III. Mucogingival surgical procedures
     A. Frenotomy and frenectomy
     B. Vestibuloplasty
     C. Grafts
        1. Free gingival grafts
        2. Coronal repositioning after a free gingival graft
        3. Subepithelial or interpositional connective tissue grafts
 IV. Surgical procedures for treatment of teeth with furcation involvement
     A. Odontoplasty or furcationplasty
     B. Root tunneling
     C. Root resection, or hemisection of mandibular molar
     D. Regenerative procedures (see Chapter 48)
  V. Combined surgical procedures
     A. Flap and osseous surgery
     B. Palatal gingivectomy (and palatal flap) with a buccal flap
     C. Flap and wedge incisions
     D. Flap and infrabony implant
     E. Flap and regenerative procedures
     F. Flap and root resection
     G. Flap and tooth extraction
     H. Flap with gingivectomy or gingivoplasty

GINGIVAL SURGICAL PROCEDURES
Curettage

Curettage is a surgical procedure directed to removal of the pocket epithelium and underlying granulation tissue. Gingival and subgingival curettage are often distinguished on the basis of the extent of gingival disease apical or coronal to the alveolar crest. Gingival curettage is used when the gingival pocket is supracrestal, whereas subgingival curettage is used when the procedure involves the subcrestal tissues or infrabony pockets. Curettage can be accomplished as an open procedure with a gingival incision, followed by root planing, or it may be carried out as a closed procedure with a sharp curette. Curettage also may be performed with an ultrasonic curette or chemically with a compound such as sodium hypochlorite.

The specific objectives of curettage are to eliminate or reduce pocket depths by shrinkage following tissue removal. Open curettage facilitates root planing and debridement by providing direct vision of the tooth surface.

Indications for curettage are shallow pocket depths with an adequate width and thickness of gingival tissue; treatment of patients when more extensive surgery is contraindicated; treatment of isolated infrabony pockets, especially in furcations; and shrinkage of localized areas of gingiva, particularly interdental papillae, which are bulbous and lead to plaque retention or accumulation.

Contraindications to gingival curettage include the presence of acute infection, such as acute necrotizing ulcerative gingivitis (ANUG), or acute lesions as found in periodontitis in patients with acquired immunodeficiency syndrome (AIDS); fibrous epithelial enlargement of the gingiva as found in phenytoin hyperplasia; frenal pull on the gingival margin; and extension of the base of the pocket apical to the mucogingival junction.

Advantages of curettage include the possibility for complete removal of infected crevicular epithelium and underlying connective tissue (e.g., in localized juvenile periodontitis [LJP] where the tissue is infected with *Actinobacillus*). There is minimal discomfort to the patient and minimal hemorrhage, although these procedures have to be done with the patient under local anesthesia. A further advantage is that healing is often uneventful.

A major disadvantage of curettage is that often limited access can be obtained, particularly if there are deep, tortuous pockets or if the pockets are infrabony or extend beyond the mucogingival junction.

The basic principle of this procedure is complete removal of the crevicular or pocket epithelium, including the junctional or attachment epithelium, and removal of the underlying inflamed connective tissue. This can be done with a sharp instrument, such as a curette (Fig. 47-1). This procedure can also be carried out with ultrasonic instruments or by chemicals such as sodium hypochlorite.

In the excisional new attachment procedure (ENAP), the gingiva is removed by an incision through the gingival crevice and the excised tissue is removed with a scaler or curette. After curettage that exposes the alveolar process, the gingiva should be sutured back close to the margin of the tooth to encourage healing by primary intention and to protect the alveolar process. There is no good evidence that ENAP actually leads to new connective tissue attachment. However, a related procedure, transseptal fiberotomy, with removal of transseptal fibers, is useful to prevent orthodontic relapse.

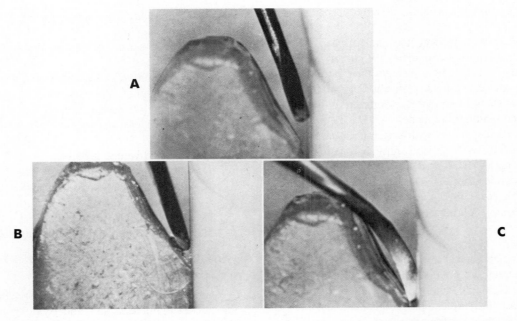

Fig. 47-1. Location of curette in position for, **A,** root planing, **B,** gingival curettage, and **C,** removal of epithelial attachment.

Operative procedure. The area is anesthetized by local injection of 2% lidocaine (Xylocaine) containing 1:50,000 epinephrine or another appropriate anesthetic. The curette is inserted to the bottom of the pocket, and pressure is applied to the soft tissue. Several overlapping strokes are used to completely remove the epithelium and underlying granulation tissue. Finger pressure against the oral surface of the gingiva can be used to facilitate the curettage. Root planing is performed next, since the gingiva can be pushed aside, allowing visual access to the root surface. The gingival tissues are then adapted to the tooth surface and sutured with single interproximal sutures if necessary. A periodontal dressing may be placed over the lesion for 1 week, or the patient may use a chlorhexidine mouth rinse for 2 weeks for postoperative plaque control with no dressing (Fig. 47-2).

Chemical curettage. The operative procedure for chemical curettage is very similar with the exception that after anesthesia the area to be treated is isolated with cotton rolls and a solution of sodium hypochlorite (100 ml sodium hypochlorite bleach, 7.8 g sodium hydroxide, and 19 g sodium carbonate) is placed into the pocket with the tip of an instrument until the pocket area is just filled. The sodium hypochlorite is allowed to remain in the pocket area for 1 minute, with care being taken to prevent contact of the adjacent tissues with the caustic material. Next, a 5% citric acid solution is introduced into the pocket for 1 minute to neutralize the sodium hypochlorite. The coagulated tissue is then removed with a curette, and the pocket is flushed with sterile saline to remove the remnants of the connective tissue. After this, the roots are often exposed and can be root planed. The tissues are sutured if neces-

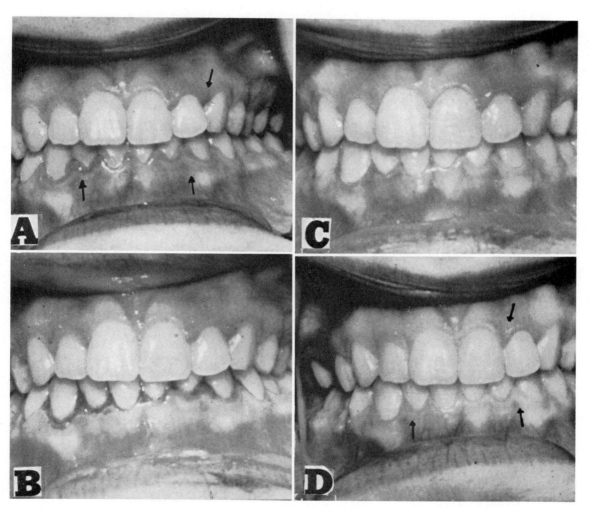

Fig. 47-2. Resolution of gingival inflammation in a 19-year-old patient treated with curettage. **A,** Preoperative appearance. Note soft edematous interdental papillae *(arrows).* **B,** Appearance immediately after gingival curettage. **C,** Appearance 3 weeks later. **D,** Appearance 3 months later. Arrows show return of papillae to normal form.

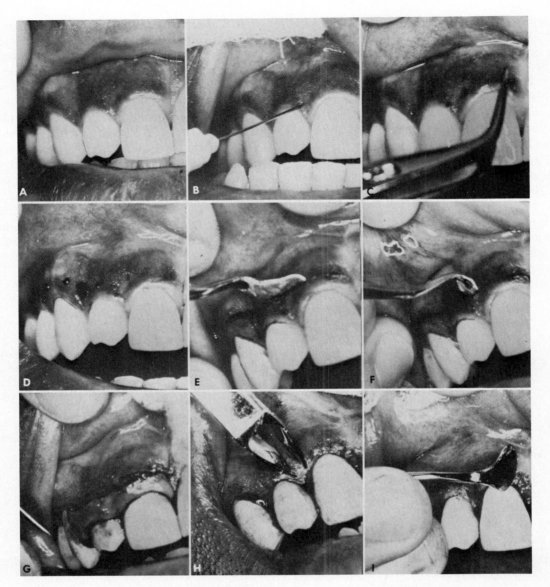

Fig. 47-3. Step-by-step procedure for gingivectomy. A local anesthetic has been injected into mucogingival area, resulting in anesthesia of area. Anesthetic fluid is also injected into palatal area corresponding to mucogingival site. **A,** Appearance before anesthetic. **B,** Injection of anesthetic into buccal peaks; this is also done in palatal peaks. By doing so, tissue becomes firmer and thus easier to contour. **C,** Pocket marking is then performed. Beaks of pocket marker must be parallel to root surface. Markings are made on mesial, central marginal, and distal aspects. **D,** Markings are then surveyed to ascertain relative levels of resultant gingival margins after resection of tissue. **E,** Initial cut is made; knife is held at an angle of approximately 45 degrees. It is made on a continuous line guided by markings. Cut starts apical to markings, since it must end slightly apical to them. Cut must be made firmly and extend down to teeth. **F,** Interdental cut is then made. Knife (No. 11 Goldman-Fox) is inserted into primary incision and extended interdentally as far as possible. **G,** If cuts are complete, tissue will lift off easily. Surgical surface is then inspected carefully. Teeth are dried to see if any calculus is present and scaled if necessary. Gingival topography usually needs further correction, and tissue tabs must be removed. For this, nippers, **H,** scraping with No. 7 Goldman-Fox knife, **I,** and a curette, **J,** are useful. Resultant surface should be smooth and clean, **K and M.** Use of dental tape will release any loosened tissue. Gingival margin should be thin and beveled. Interdental tissue should be pyramidally shaped. Operator must probe each margin to ascertain that all detached tissue has been removed. Same procedure is performed on palatal aspect. **T,** Interdental tissue must be left smooth. **N to S,** Step-by-step procedures for palatal aspect. Use of a diamond stone to shape gingival tissue is seen in **Q.** Interdental sluiceways are easily produced by this method. **L and U,** Gingival area is then covered with a Coe-pack periodontal dressing.

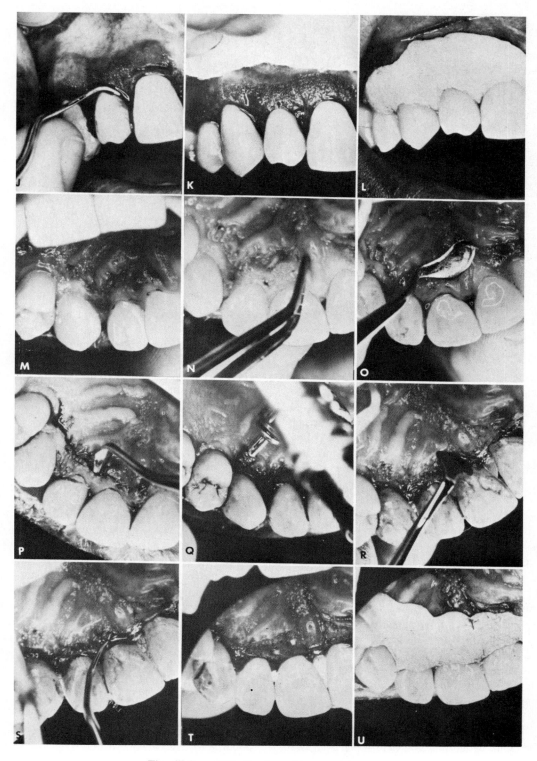

Fig. 47-3, cont'd. For legend see opposite page.

Continued.

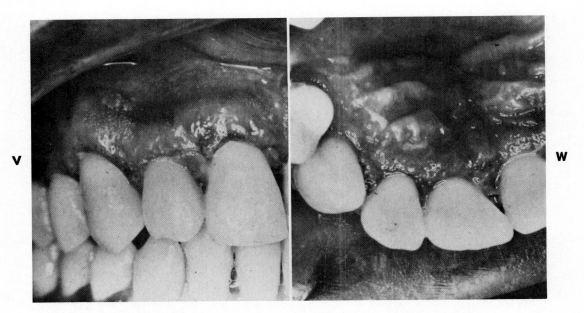

Fig. 47-3, cont'd. **V** and **W,** Appearance of gingival tissue 1 week postoperatively.

sary, and periodontal dressings placed. Postoperative oral hygiene using chlorhexidine oral rinses is indicated.

Gingivectomy

Gingivectomy is a procedure in which the soft tissue walls of supracrestal pockets are eliminated by excision. Since most often only a portion of the gingiva is removed, the procedure is not technically a gingivectomy (which denotes complete removal of the gingiva) but a gingivotomy. However, the common term *gingivectomy* is being used here for incisional procedures that remove the gingiva. *Gingivoplasty,* on the other hand, refers to surgical recontouring or modeling of the oral surface of the gingiva, and little or none of the pocket or crevicular epithelium is removed. Gingivectomy is usually carried out to remove the entire soft tissue wall of the periodontal pocket by an external bevel incision that leaves a cut surface exposed to the oral cavity. The specific objectives of gingivectomy and gingivoplasty are to eliminate suprabony pockets and/or to recontour overgrown, redundant fibrotic gingiva.

Indications for gingivectomy include gingival enlargement or overgrowth such as seen in phenytoin hyperplasia, pseudopockets that are coronal to the alveolar crest where there is adequate attached gingiva, idiopathic gingival fibromatosis, late or altered passive eruption, and the need to increase the length of the clinical crown to gain added retention for restorative purposes or crown lengthening for esthetics.

Contraindications include areas where there is little or no attached gingiva, where the bottom of the pocket is at or apical to the mucogingival junction, where there are infrabony pockets, where there is thickening or ledging of the marginal alveolar bone, and where osseous surgery is indicated; as well as labial areas where removal of gingiva may lead to unsightly, long clinical crowns.

The advantages of gingivectomy and gingivoplasty include their technical simplicity, with good visual access, especially on the labial aspect. Gingivectomy can lead to complete pocket elimination, and the morphologic result of both gingivectomy and gingivoplasty is predictable for cosmetic objectives or to eliminate plaque retention areas.

Disadvantages include the danger of exposing bone with subsequent resorption of alveolar crestal support. Gingivectomy may also result in loss of attached gingiva, and there may be exposure of cervical areas of the teeth, with increased root sensitivity, increased root surface caries, and unsightly lengthening of the teeth. When the procedure is carried out in the palatal region, there may be interference with speech.

Operative procedure. The gingivectomy is carried out with a continuous incision directed coronally at a 45-degree angle to the long axis of the tooth, ending on the tooth at the base of the pocket (Fig. 47-3). After local infiltration with 2% lidocaine containing 1:50,000 epinephrine, pocket depths are measured and the level of the base of the pocket is transferred to the external surface of the gingiva with the pocket marker or with a periodontal probe. The bleeding points indicate the base of the pocket. An initial incision is made slightly apical to the bleeding points with a broad-blade gingivectomy knife inclined at about a 45-degree angle to the long axis of the tooth in a coronal direction. After the first incision is made, a spear-shaped interproximal gingivectomy knife is placed in the incision and followed along to the base of the pockets, extending interproximally as far as possible. When this is done, the tissue is generally loosened and can be easily removed using a scaler or curette. The edge of the incision is then thinned with scissors, a rotary instrument, nippers, or the edge of the gingivectomy knife to make a smooth contour. Often the root surfaces will be exposed, and root planing can be carried out at this time. A periodontal dressing is placed over the entire surgical area, primarily for patient comfort.

Gingivoplasty

Gingivoplasty is a variant of gingivectomy in which the attached mucosa surrounding the teeth is reshaped to provide more esthetic or more functional contours. Gingivoplasty can be carried out with tissue nippers, rotary instruments, or electrosurgical tips (Fig. 47-3, *H, I,* and *Q*). If the electrosurgical instrument is used, care should be taken not to contact the bone, since heating will lead to necrosis and possible sequestration of devitalized bone. Gingivoplasty has also been carried out experimentally with cryosurgical instruments and with lasers; however, no significant advantages of these methods over the more traditional methods have been established.

Healing after gingivectomy or gingivoplasty

Epithelialization of the gingivectomy wound begins within a few days after the procedure and is usually complete within 7 to 14 days (Engler et al., 1966). Regeneration of the supraalveolar connective tissue then occurs, resulting in a gingival unit that has the characteristics of the normal free gingiva (Hamp et al., 1975). A new free gingival unit is established by coronal regrowth of tissue from the original incision level, and hence it can be expected that approximately one half of the coronal-apical height of tissue removed will return after gingivectomy. Total gingivectomy healing takes place in about 4 to 5 weeks, and remodeling of the alveolar bony crest has been shown to occur during this phase. Gingivoplasty wounds often heal faster than gingivectomy wounds.

Tuberosity and retromolar reduction

Tuberosity and retromolar reduction are used to remove the redundant or excessive soft tissue distal to the last molars in the maxilla or mandible. This extra soft tissue forms the soft tissue wall of a deep probeable area, which sometimes makes plaque control in this area difficult. There are two basic approaches to the removal of excessive tissue distal to the tuberosity or in the retromolar area: gingivectomy or various flap or wedge approaches.

The specific objective of these procedures is to remove fibrous tissue on the distal surfaces of molars in the tuberosity or retromolar area. Specifically, these procedures are directed to eliminating the fibrous tissue associated with these distal "pockets" and to enhancing oral hygiene pro-

cedures in these areas. These pockets should be carefully evaluated during the antiinfective phase of therapy before surgery to determine if they are truly plaque retention areas. Often patients are able to keep these areas relatively free of subgingival plaque without surgery. Surgery should be done only if necessary, since resection may leave a distal root surface exposed to plaque accumulation and root surface caries.

Gingivectomy is indicated when the retromolar or tuberosity pad areas are small and gingivectomy would remove the fibrous wall of the pocket without creating a large surgical wound. Gingivectomy is also indicated when there is adequate keratinized tissue present. The flap or wedge approach is indicated when the gingivectomy would expose a large surgical wound, when there is not sufficient keratinized tissue in the surgical area, and when access to underlying alveolar bone or to distal infrabony pockets or furcation openings is needed.

Both gingivectomy and the flap or wedge approach are contraindicated when there is little or no attached gingiva distal to the last molars. This sometimes happens in the retromolar area where loose alveolar mucosa abuts the distal surface of the tooth.

Gingivectomy has an advantage over the flap or wedge approach in that it is technically simple. The wedge approach has an advantage over gingivectomy in that it allows better access to infrabony pockets or furcation involvement of the molars.

As already stated, the general principle of gingivectomy and the flap or wedge approach is to remove the excess gingival tissue that forms the soft tissue wall of a probeable defect distal to the last molars (Robinson, 1966). These resective procedures can also be used where a pocket or redundant gingiva exists mesial or distal to a tooth bordering an edentulous region. After anesthesia, in the gingivectomy approach the depth of the pocket is marked with bleeding points, and the gingivectomy knife is placed apical to the bleeding points and directed as much as possible in a 45-degree angle coronally; an incision is then made to the base of the pocket. The collar of tissue is removed around the distal aspect, extending to the buccal and lingual aspects of the last tooth in the arch. That tissue is then removed, and root planing can be performed as necessary.

There are various distal flap approaches used for tuberosity or retromolar reduction (Figs. 47-4 and 47-5). The simplest is the distal wedge. In the distal wedge procedure a broad-based straight or angled blade is used to make a V-shaped incision, with the apex of the V at the most distal point. The excised tissue is then removed by undermining with a gingivectomy knife, and the two cut edges are approximated with sutures. Various H-shaped or rectangular flaps have also been used for this procedure. Distal tissue reduction is often done in combination with mucoperi-

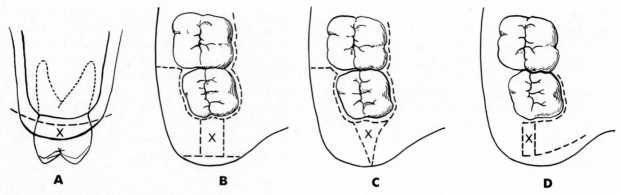

Fig. 47-4. Maxillary tuberosity soft tissue reduction procedures. **A,** Tuberosity reduction by gingivectomy. Removal of excess tissue by external bevel incision made along dotted line. Tissue marked with *X* is removed, and site is covered with a dressing. **B,** Tuberosity reduction by flap approach. Soft tissue, and if necessary hard tissue, of tuberosity may be removed via an H-shaped flap (parallel wedge). Releasing incisions are made to bone, along dotted line, and tissue marked with *X* is removed. Distal flaps are then apposed and sutured. **C,** Distal wedge procedure for removal of soft tissue and access to bone and furcation on distal aspect of last molar. Incisions follow dotted lines, and tissue marked with *X* is removed. Edges of distal wedge flaps are apposed and sutured. **D,** Palatal flap for tuberosity reduction. Incisions are made along dotted lines, tissue is undermined toward palatal aspect, and wedge marked *X* is removed. For any of these approaches, margins of flaps are adapted and sutured after treatment of distal root surface and alveolar tuberosity reduction are carried out as necessary.

osteal flaps, both buccal and lingual. The flap incision is extended straight distally to the retromolar or tuberosity area, and a vertical incision is made at the distal extent of the incisions. The flaps are then undermined, the intervening tissue removed, and the edges approximated; if necessary, the overlapping margins are excised. After suturing, a dressing is placed for patient comfort, or if adequate closure is obtained, these areas need not be dressed. An antiplaque rinse, such as chlorhexidine, can be used during the healing phase.

PERIODONTAL FLAPS AND ALVEOLAR OSSEOUS SURGICAL PROCEDURES

Flap procedures are the most commonly used of all periodontal surgical techniques. Often the purpose of making a periodontal flap is to reflect the soft tissue to gain access to the deeper periodontal structures or to reposition the gingiva. The most commonly used flaps are full-thickness mucoperiosteal flaps that are designed so that the vascular supply is minimally interrupted to provide the potential for optimal healing. With a full-thickness flap the entire gingival soft tissue complex, including gingiva, alveolar mucosa, and periosteum, is reflected from the root and alveolar bone surfaces. Partial full-thickness flaps are used where the underlying periosteum is to be preserved, such as in preparation of recipient sites for free gingival grafts. Full-thickness flap types include the Widman flap, apically repositioned flaps, and laterally and coronally repositioned flaps. These are discussed separately, since the specific ob-

jectives, indications, contraindications, advantages, and disadvantages are unique for each.

Modified Widman flap

The original detailed description of a flap procedure for pocket elimination was published by Widman in 1920. This flap procedure has been modified by Newman and also by Kirkland, but perhaps the most commonly used modification today is that described by Ramfjord and Nissle (1974), which is described here. The modified Widman flap is an open-flap technique and does not include apical displacement of the flap and osseous recontouring in order to obtain pocket elimination (as did the original Widman flap). The general purpose of the modified Widman flap is to remove the soft tissue adjacent to the pocket wall to allow for visualization of the root surface coronal to the alveolar crest, with the flap replaced to completely cover the alveolar bone. It is designed to maintain as much of the interdental papillae as possible in order to ensure healing by primary closure. The specific objectives are to gain access to the underlying bone and root surfaces, to reduce pocket depth by establishing new attachment at a more coronal level, to preserve an adequate zone of attached gingiva, and to provide an environment for healing by primary closure.

Indications for the Widman flap include pockets where the bases are located coronal to the mucogingival junction, where there is little or no thickening of the marginal bone. The Widman flap is also indicated when shallow to mod-

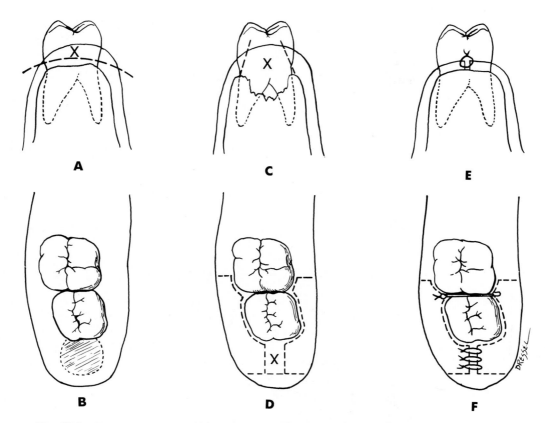

Fig. 47-5. Retromolar pad area reduction. **A** and **B,** Retromolar pad reduction by gingivectomy. Distal redundant tissue is removed with a gingivectomy knife using an external bevel incision (along dotted line), allowing access to distal surface of root. Furthermore, distal soft tissue wall of pocket is removed. Adequate attached gingiva must be present to do this. **C** and **D,** Incision for distal molar pad reduction using buccal and lingual flaps in retromolar pad area. Incision is made along dotted line in directions indicated, and tissue marked with *X* is removed. **E** and **F,** Buccal and lingual flaps shown are apposed and sutured together. A variant of this procedure is a distal wedge that involves removal of a pie-shaped wedge of tissue in retromolar area with buccal and lingual incisions meeting at a point several millimeters distal to distal surface of molar, comparable to that shown in Fig. 47-4, *C.*

erate pocket depths can be reduced and where esthetics is important, such as in the anterior region of patients with a high smile line.

The Widman flap is contraindicated when there is pronounced gingival enlargement or overgrowth, which is handled more efficiently by means of a gingivectomy or gingivoplasty, or when there is little or no attached gingiva. It is also contraindicated when there are large bony thickenings or exostoses to be removed.

Widman flap procedures, in general, have advantages over closed curettage, root-planing, and gingivectomy procedures, since they facilitate subgingival scaling and root planing to the base of deeper pockets with direct vision. Widman flap procedures also allow complete removal of the pocket epithelium, and the flaps can be replaced at the original location to encourage healing by primary intention. There is minimal tissue trauma during surgery, and

the Widman flap is often esthetically superior to gingivectomy or apically repositioned flaps.

Operative procedure. After adequate anesthesia, an initial incision is made with a small broad-based blade held parallel to the long axis of the tooth (Fig. 47-6). If the pockets are more than 2 mm deep, the incision is placed approximately 1 mm from the gingival margin. If the pockets are less than 2 mm deep or if esthetic considerations are important, this first incision can be made within the crevice or pocket. The incision is scalloped and should be extended as far as possible interproximally to minimize the amount of interdental tissue removed. A similar incision can be used on the lingual or palatal aspect; however, on the palatal aspect the scalloped outline of the initial incision may be accentuated by placing the knife 2 to 3 mm from the midpalatal surface of the teeth. A second incision is then made through the gingival crevice, meeting the first

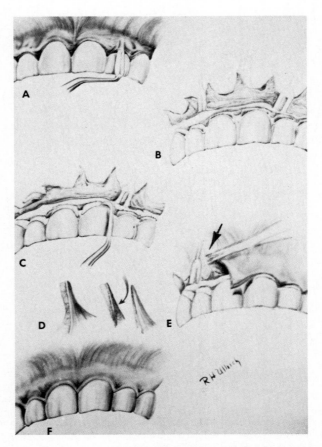

Fig. 47-6. Step-by-step procedure of debridement via modified Widman flap method. **A,** Inverse incision is made; this is usually performed with a scalpel. **B,** Flap is raised. **C,** Entire tissue above bone is removed, and root surfaces are cleansed. **D** and **E,** Flap is thinned so that on readaptation it will tautly cover alveolar crestal area. **F,** Healed gingival tissue and gingival attachment.

incision at the crest of the alveolar bone. The intervening tissue cuff is often loose and can be removed; however, sometimes a third incision is made horizontally, close to the alveolar crest to free the tissue cuff. This results in freeing of the pocket epithelium and infrabony granulation tissue, which then can be removed with curettes. The exposed roots are then scaled and root planed. All of the soft tissue from angular bony defects is removed with curettes.

After scaling, root planing, and curettage, the flaps are trimmed and adjusted to the alveolar bone to obtain as complete coverage of the interproximal bone as possible. Osteoplasty of marginal crestal ledges may be necessary for adaptation of the flap with complete coverage of the alveolar process. The flaps are sutured together with individual interproximal sutures to approximate the edge of the flaps to the teeth and to each other interproximally, which will encourage healing by primary intention. A surgical dressing is then placed to help maintain close adaptation of the flaps to the alveolar bone and root surfaces. The dressing and sutures are removed after 1 week. Chlorhexidine mouth rinse is used during the healing phase for 3 to 6 months.

Healing. The modified Widman flap procedure is routinely associated with excellent long-term results and reasonable gain of attachment in infrabony defects (Knowles et al., 1979). If the modified Widman flap is carried out in an area with deep infrabony lesions, bone repair may occur within the confines of the lesion (Rosling et al., 1976b). Also, a small amount of crestal resorption may be seen. The amount of bone fill is dependent on the anatomy of the osseous defect, with more fill seen in three-walled defects than in single- or two-walled defects. Contrary to previous theories, resection of infrabony defects following modified Widman flap procedures failed to give better pocket reduction or attachment gain as compared with Widman flaps done in conjunction with curettage of the infrabony defects and no osseous surgery (Westfelt et al., 1983, Caffesse et al., 1987). In one study in which patients with multiple infrabony defects were treated, there was greater attachment gain in pockets treated by modified

Widman flap and curettage as compared with modified Widman flap and osseous contouring of intrabony defects (Rosling et al., 1976b).

• • •

In summary, the modified Widman flap procedure, with removal of soft tissue from infrabony defects and osteoplasty limited to removing bony ledges to facilitate close flap adaption, is a mainstay of periodontal surgery on single-rooted tooth and on flat surfaces of molars affected by moderate pockets and infrabony defects.

Repositioned flaps

Mucoperiosteal or split-thickness flaps are used to reposition the gingiva. The gingiva can be repositioned apically to retain most, if not all, of the attached gingiva and to eliminate pockets; laterally to position gingiva over areas of recession; or coronally to replace gingiva in broad areas of recession. Each type of repositioned flap is discussed separately.

Apically repositioned flaps. The apically repositioned flap was described by Nabers (1954). Modifications were then described by Ariaudo and Tyrrell (1957) and by Friedman (1962). An apically repositioned flap is a full-thickness mucoperiosteal flap made with an internal bevel incision that is repositioned at or about at the level of the alveolar crest.

The main objective is to reposition the entire complex of excess soft tissue after osseous surgery so that pocketsdo not remain, and at the same time retain the entire attached gingiva. Hence the objective is to surgically eliminate deep pockets by positioning the flap apically while retaining the attached gingiva. The second main objective is surgical access for osseous surgery, treatment of infrabony pockets, and root planing.

The apically repositioned flap is used when there are moderate or deep pockets, especially those where the base is apical to the mucogingival junction; in treatment of furcation-involved teeth; and to lengthen crowns.

The apically repositioned flap is contraindicated for cosmetic reasons (e.g., on labial areas or anterior regions where tooth exposure would be unesthetic) and in patients at risk for root caries, since excessive root surfaces are often exposed.

Operative procedure. A reverse bevel incision from the gingival margin to the alveolar crest is made with a broad-based scalpel. The incision is made at varying distances from the margin of the gingiva, depending on the pocket depth, as well as the thickness and width of the gingiva. With thin gingiva and shallow pockets, the incision is made close to the tooth; with wide gingiva and/or deep pockets, the margin of the incision is made farther away. The incision is scalloped interproximally to ensure maximal coverage of the alveolar bone when the flap is re-

placed. This incision can be on the labial and buccal surfaces of the upper and lower jaws and on the lingual surfaces of the lower jaw. However, this incision is not useful on the palatal aspect, and a combination of reverse bevel and gingivectomy or reverse bevel and connective tissue excision is necessary to apically reposition palatal flaps. Vertical-release incisions extending into the alveolar mucosa are made at the ends of the reverse bevel incision, making possible the apical repositioning of the flap. Next, a full-thickness mucoperiosteal flap is raised, and the marginal collar of tissue is removed with curettes. It is often convenient to make a second incision in the gingival crevice or pocket that meets the first incision at the alveolar crest to facilitate removal of the gingival collar of tissue. The roots are planed, and granulation tissue is removed.

Often the bone is subjected to osseous recontouring after the flap is made, and this is a common combination of procedures used to treat severe periodontal disease (apically repositioned flap and osseous recontouring). However, as mentioned previously, there is little evidence to support the efficacy of the apically repositioned flap procedure coupled with osseous surgery over a less extensive procedure such as the modified Widman flap (Rosling et al., 1976b). The sacrifice of crestal alveolar process and supporting bone, and the extensive exposure of root surfaces are the main disadvantages of this procedure (Ramfjord and Costich, 1968; Karring et al., 1975).

Laterally repositioned flaps. A laterally repositioned flap is usually a full-thickness flap but may be a partial-thickness gingival flap that is attached at its base and transferred in the horizontal plane laterally to the adjacent recipient site. An objective of this procedure is to halt recession and to restore denuded areas cosmetically with attached gingiva. The laterally repositioned flap is indicated in areas where there is gingival recession that is narrow, adjacent to which a wide band of attached gingiva exists, which can be used as the donor site.

Contraindications include lack of sufficient donor gingiva adjacent to the area of recession, and dehiscence, fenestration, or thin alveolar bone at the donor site.

Advantages are considered in comparison with those of the free gingival graft, which is the alternative procedure that can be used. With a laterally sliding flap there is no wound in the palate from the recipient site.

Operative procedure. After anesthesia a V-shaped incision removing the gingival margin in the recipient site is made. The recipient flap is incised and dissected with a knife from the adjacent tooth. The flap is then rotated to the recipient root surface, which has been root planed. The flap is sutured into place on the recipient site, and surgical tinfoil or Telfa pads are placed over the recipient site to prevent the sutures from being incorporated into the periodontal dressing. The area is dressed and allowed to heal for 2 weeks. There are various modifications of the later-

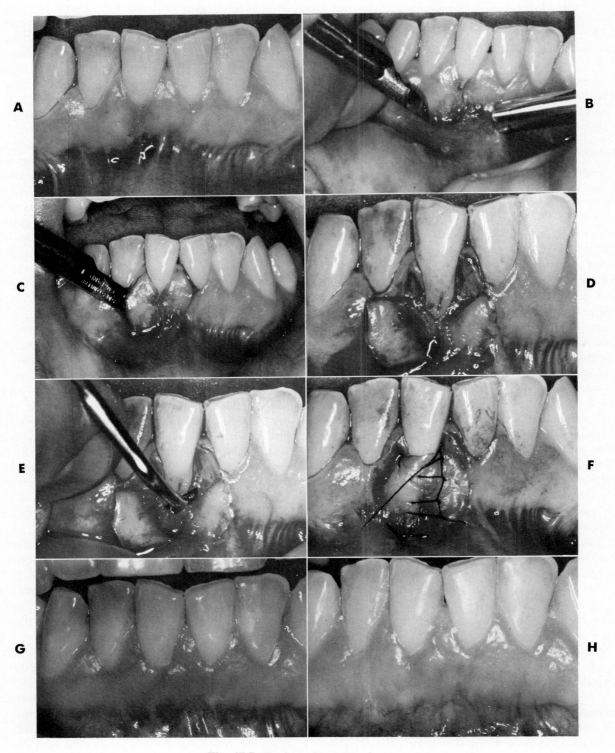

Fig. 47-7. For legend see opposite page.

Fig. 47-7. Correction of a gingival cleft in an area of persistent inflammation by a variant of the lateral sliding flap. the double papillae graft. **A,** Preoperative appearance. Note inflammation and clefting on labial aspect of lower right central incisor. This persisted for 6 months after antiinfective therapy was completed. **B,** Incisions made to release papillae distal and mesial to defect. **C,** Incisions completed. Note interdental papillae are preserved in marginal gingiva, and height of gingiva is maintained interproximally. **D,** Double papillae flaps (partial thickness) are dissected and displaced, revealing what appears to be a fissure on labial surface of root. **E,** Fissure is removed by root planing beyond depth of fissure. **F,** Flaps are sutured over radicular surface of root. **G,** Appearance 1 month after surgery. **H,** Appearance 5 years after surgery.

---

ally repositioned flap, including the double papillae flap (Cohen and Ross, 1968; Ross et al., 1986) in which the papillae on both the mesial and distal sides of the recipient tooth are sutured over the denuded area (Fig. 47-7). The donor site can vary from adjacent tooth to adjacent edentulous areas in which larger gingival flaps can be obtained.

Coronally repositioned flaps. A coronally repositioned flap is a mucoperiosteal flap that is repositioned in a coronal direction to cover exposed root surfaces. The main objective is to cover wide areas of gingival recession or multiple adjacent areas of gingival recession with attached gingiva for cosmetic reasons or to prevent further recession.

Wide or multiple areas of gingival recession are indications for this procedure. Areas where there is not an adequate amount of attached gingiva to coronally reposition or where the gingiva is extremely thin are contraindications.

Operative procedure. This procedure is often used after a free gingival graft to provide adequate attached gingiva for repositioning. The operative procedure for this is described later under Coronal Repositioning after a Free Gingival Graft. The operative procedures with and without a free gingival graft are similiar.

Osseous surgery

It was observed in the 1940s and 1950s that the gingival contour closely followed the contour of the alveolar bone, and from this observation it was reasoned that osseous recontouring of the alveolar process was necessary to provide physiologic contours of the gingiva (Schluger, 1949; Goldman, 1950). Hence the principles of osseous surgery were developed to reshape the bone and eliminate osseous craters and angular defects, to eliminate pockets, to provide access for root debridement, and to achieve optimal gingival contour after surgery. Osteoplasty and ostectomy are two types of periodontal surgery and as discussed here differ in intent from the minimal osteoplasty carried out to adapt the flaps in the modified Widman flap procedure.

The term *osteoplasty* as used by Friedman (1955) is a procedure wherein a physiologic form of the bone is created that is then adapted to the gingiva after healing. In general, then, osteoplasty involves thinning alveolar crestal ledges, removing the bony walls of interproximal craters, and eliminating the bony walls of circumferential de-

fects, as well as scalloping or contouring the interproximal and interradicular areas around the tooth.

The objectives of osseous surgery are to create contours that reduce bony ledges or irregular contours and to eliminate the bony walls of the pocket. This was thought to permit the patient to accomplish more effective plaque control. Several studies have shown, however, that alveolar osteoplasty should be used with caution. For example, from studies of surgical healing it is clear that all osseous surgery is followed by alveolar bone loss (Aeschlimann et al., 1979). It is also known that a repair phase often follows this bone loss, but the repair rarely restores all the bone lost by surgical injury (Wilderman et al., 1970). Also, the final alveolar bony contours may differ from those established by the osseous surgery (Pennel et al., 1967). Postsurgically the amount of alveolar crestal bone loss may be on the order of 0.5 to 1 mm (Wilderman et al., 1968); however, the loss may be up to 2.5 mm when there is a thin plate of bone over roots that are not completely covered with the flap. In addition, greater bone loss may result from overheating the bone (e.g., with the use of dull cutting instruments, high-speed handpieces, or inadequate cooling) (Costich et al., 1964; Boyne, 1966). The threshold level for heat-induced bone necrosis was found to be surprisingly low at 47° C for 1 minute (Eriksson and Albrektsson, 1983).

Another reason for critically reevaluating the need for osseous surgery in patients with severe periodontal disease is that there are several regenerative procedures available today that would not work if the alveolar process were markedly altered by osseous recontouring, resulting in loss of pocket walls. These procedures include procedures with the potential for repair of periodontal lesions, such as guided tissue regeneration, bony grafts (both of which are discussed in Chapter 48), resection and root amputation, orthodontic movement of teeth into infrabony pockets, strategic extraction, and maintenance by periodic curettage and root planing. However, there are specific indications for alveolar osteoplasty and ostectomy in periodontal therapy.

Osteoplasty. As indicated earlier, osteoplasy is the shaping of deformities in alveolar bone surrounding the teeth.

Specific indications for osteoplasty include the follow-

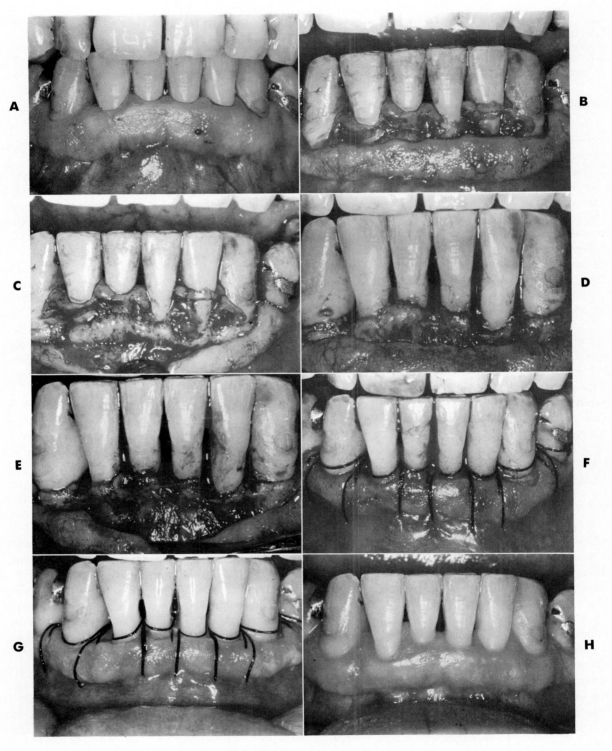

Fig. 47-8. For legend see opposite page.

Fig. 47-8. Osteoplasty to remove bony ledges that interfere with plaque control and lead to persistent infected periodontal pockets. **A,** Presurgical. Note bulbous gingiva, which bled on probing, even after multiple treatments by scaling and root planing. **B,** Initial flap incision is made. **C,** Flap is reflected, exposing ledging on labial aspect. Note protuberances over centrals and right lateral, and vertical lesion between left lateral and left central. **D,** Granulation tissue removed from infrabony defects and interproximally, revealing irregular bony margin. Full exposure of roots is obtained, and at this time definitive root planing is carried out. **E,** After osteoplasty note bony ledges have been removed. Bone was removed with sharp surgical steel burs rotating slowly with copious irrigation to prevent heat generation. **F,** Flap sutured to completely cover alveolar bone. **G,** Healing at 1 week postoperatively. **H,** Appearance 5 years postoperatively showing lack of inflammation and gingival recession at about same level as seen immediately postoperatively.

---

ing: (1) to aid in primary wound closure or flap adaptation by removing exostoses or alveolar marginal ledges; (2) to open furcations in tunneling procedures; (3) to contour alveolar ridges to make room for pontics; and (4) to remove extensive bony ledges or exostoses that interfere with plaque control and contribute to persistent pocket depths.

Osteoplasty is contraindicated when the bone is thin and excessive resorption may occur, or when a regenerative procedure is anticipated.

The removal of marginal ridges and exostoses for close flap adaptation gives a healing advantage over exposure of the interproximal bone to healing by secondary intention, which occurs with poor flap adaptation. Another advantage of osteoplasty is in preprosthetic preparation where pontic areas may be contoured so that adequately sized pontics can be used to replace missing teeth.

However, extensive flap reflection is often required, with potential exposure of alveolar dehiscences or fenestrations, and subsequent resorption of the radicular alveolar bone. Healing after extensive bony exposure and osteoplasty is often painful. Removal of alveolar bone may preclude healing of intrabony pockets after regenerative procedures, orthodontic movement, strategic extraction, or other procedures.

Operative procedure. After appropriate anesthesia and reflection of mucoperiosteal flaps to expose the area to be treated by osteoplasty, a slow-speed (2000 rpm) handpiece with a sharp carbide surgical steel bur is used to remove the alveolar bone (Fig. 47-8). Cooling with a copious spray of sterile saline is necessary so that the temperature of the bone is not raised beyond 47° C. Intermittent grinding also helps reduce heat generation. The root surface should not be touched with the bur, since this may lead to areas of root sensitivity or caries. After removal of the osseous tissue, the flap is adapted closely to cover the bone with the flap, which is then sutured in place. The area is dressed and followed postoperatively as for flap procedures.

Ostectomy. Ostectomy is removal of alveolar bone around the tooth, including the tooth-supporting bone. The supporting alveolar bone is that portion of the alveolar process with intact lamina dura and periodontal ligament connective tissue attached to the tooth.

Specific indications for this procedure include crown-lengthening procedures for esthetics, exposure of sound dentin apical to the caries or a fracture margin of a tooth that is to be restored, and opening of interradicular spaces for treatment of furcation involvement.

Contraindications include removal of bone on the affected tooth that would result in a sharp angle, jeopardizing the adjacent tooth, and removal of alveolar bone.

If the adjacent teeth are not jeopardized, ostectomy may expose sound dentin so that the tooth can be saved with a properly fitting restoration.

Operative procedure. The mucoperiosteal flap is reflected in the surgical area, with as much attached gingiva retained as possible (Fig. 47-9). The bone is removed with a chisel wherever possible; however, the initial bulk removal may be carried out with a slow-speed carbide surgical bur with saline irrigation. Saline irrigation should also be carried out during chiseling, since this also generates heat. Care should be taken not to notch the tooth with the chisel as it proceeds through the periodontal ligament space. Careful measurement should be made of the sound dentin so that approximately 2.5 to 3 mm is exposed coronal to the alveolar crest. This will allow for approximately 1 to 1.5 mm of gingival attachment and 1 to 1.5 mm of connective tissue attachment, a biologic width necessary for health. If the restorative margin is to be placed subgingivally, the alveolar crest need be only 1.5 to 2 mm from the margin of sound dentin. This will allow for adequate connective tissue and epithelial attachment; the rest of the crevicular epithelium will be on the subgingival margin of the restoration. The flap is sutured over the area, a dressing is placed, and the patient is followed postoperatively as with other flap procedures.

MUCOGINGIVAL SURGICAL PROCEDURES
Historical perspective

Mucogingival procedures were originally designed as treatment for gingival recession and high frenal attachments, and to extend the depth of the vestibular fornix. However, several studies have demonstrated that periodontal health can often be maintained regardless of the width of the attached gingiva or the depth of the fornix. It was originally thought that an inadequate zone of attached gin-

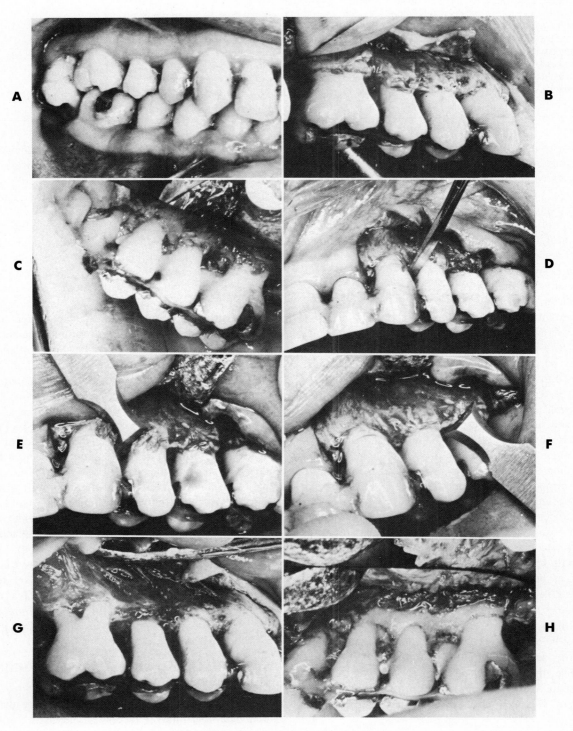

Fig. 47-9. For legend see opposite page.

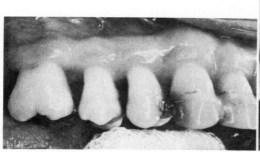 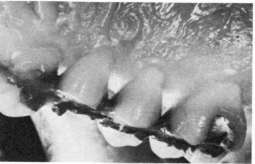

Fig. 47-9. Osseous surgical procedure combining ostectomy and osteoplasty. **A,** Pretreatment, buccal view. **B,** There is cratering on distal aspect of maxillary left molar and between premolars and molars (mirror view). **C,** Palatal exposure showing irregular osseous defects as well as granulation tissue invading mesial furca of first molar. Teeth are in secondary occlusal trauma and have been stabilized by means of intracoronal amalgam wire-and-acrylic A splint. **D,** No. 401 Wedelstadt chisel is used to eliminate interdental craters. **E and F,** Ochsenbein chisel enables ostectomy for correction of distal line angle of canine, interproximal rise between canine and first premolar, and radicular elliptic form on mesial aspect of first premolar. This chisel can cleave off irregular osseous margins. **G,** Completion of osseous surgery with elimination of all defects. Elastic connective tissue of submucosa has been removed, and an immobile base remains. **H,** Correction of palatal defects. Note mesial furca of molar has correct osseous configuration permitting an interproximal gingival rise and thus avoids return of interproximal pocket formation. **I and J,** One year after surgery, all pockets are eliminated. (Courtesy Dr. Herman Corn and Dr. Manuel H. Marks, Levittown, Pa.)

giva is important for the maintenance of gingival health and precludes loss of connective attachment (Carranza and Carraro, 1970; Matter, 1982). It was also suggested that in the absence of an attached gingival cuff, the nonkeratized alveolar mucosa was incapable of withstanding masticatory forces or dissipating the pull from the frena (Ochsenbein, 1960; Friedman and Levine, 1964). Controversy exists with respect to what should be considered an adequate width of gingiva, with proposals that 1 mm is sufficient (Bowers, 1963), whereas others believe that as much as 3 mm is required (Corn, 1962). These opinions regarding the necessity for various widths of attached gingiva are based on clinical opinions; however, several studies have addressed this question, and the findings can be summarized as follows.

Narrow bands of attached gingiva (e.g., 2 mm or less) never appear to be completely healthy and are red regardless of the amount of bacterial plaque, whereas thicker areas of gingiva appear healthy (Lang and Löe, 1972). In a dog study, Wennstrom et al. (1982) provided an explanation for this. They showed that the keratin layer of the oral epithelium covering the narrow zones of attached gingiva was thinner than the epithelium covering the wider zones. Hence the narrow zones, with their thinner epithelium, appeared red, but they were not more inflamed on the basis of histometric evaluation of the subgingival connective tissue.

A number of studies of the effects of grafting procedures have shown that they often result in a wider zone of attached marginal gingiva. However, there is no indication that this increase influences periodontal health. Also, resistance to further recession does not seem to be any more impeded by a wider band of attached gingiva than in the nongraft areas. For an example of these studies, see Dorfman et al. (1980), who found that there was approximately a 4 mm increase of attached gingiva at the sites after free gingival grafts, and that this was maintained for at least 2 years. The probing attachment level was also maintained throughout this period. In the control sites, where the width of attached gingiva was less than 2 mm, there was also no variation in the width of attached gingiva or in the attachment level over the 2-year period. Hence they concluded that a narrow zone of gingiva apparently has the same resistance to attachment loss as a wider zone. This conclusion is also supported by the studies of Hangorsky and Bissada (1980) and DeTery and Bernimoulin (1980).

Overall, then, clinical studies have suggested a limited use for mucogingival surgery. However, there are specific indications wherein mucogingival surgical procedures are necessary. For example, they are used to halt progressive gingival recession, to achieve creeping reattachment, to provide a widened band of marginal attached gingiva (Lang and Löe, 1972), and to deepen the buccal vestibule, which may enhance plaque control and resist the trauma of mastication (Carranza and Carraro, 1970). Mucogingival surgery is also used for esthetic reasons (e.g., to cover denuded roots or to provide more cosmetic gingival contours in patients who show labial gingiva during smiling).

The question of whether to provide attached gingiva over a tooth with no marginal gingiva prior to orthodontics is still open. Most studies show that although about one third of such sites show recession after orthodontic therapy, it is not possible to predict which sites will go on to recession and which will not.

Frenotomy and frenectomy

In frenotomy and frenectomy the fibers that radiate into and retract the marginal gingiva are excised. This can be accomplished by simply cutting through the frenum (frenotomy) or by excision of the entire fibrous tissue of the frenum (frenectomy). A high rate of frenum reformation is found, and free gingival grafts in the triangular wound created by the frenotomy or frenectomy are often used to prevent recurrence.

Frenotomy/frenectomy procedures are used to eliminate frena that radiate directly into the marginal gingiva, resulting in pull and retraction of the gingival margin, which often is associated with progressive localized recession.

Indications for these procedures include the need to remove frena whose fibers radiate into the marginal gingiva, where they produce gingival retraction and localized gingival recession. These procedures are also indicated when oral hygiene is hindered by vestibules caused by high frenal attachment, when prosthesis construction is hindered by high frenal attachments, or when the lingual frenum interferes with speech ("tongue tie").

Operative procedure.   The objective is to remove all of the frenal fibers down to the periosteum to minimize recurrence. After adequate anesthesia, the frenum is grasped with a hemostat to define its lateral, apical, and coronal extent. A broad surgical blade is used to incise the mucosa and to dissect the muscle fibers. This is carried out as a split-thickness procedure, leaving the periosteum on the labial bone. The mucosal (lip) extent of the incision is closed with sutures. The gingival extent is not closed and is allowed to heal by secondary intention, or the remaining triangular wound is covered with a free gingival graft. A dressing is placed over the surgical site. If increased attached gingiva is needed, often periosteal fenestration can be carried out with exposure of the alveolar bone, which then would allow for scar formation with the gingiva attached to the area of exposed alveolar bone (Fig. 47-10). It is very important to muscle trim the dressing; otherwise, considerable postoperative pain may ensue.

Vestibuloplasty

Vestibuloplasty is a procedure designed to extend the vestibular fornix. The specific objectives are to gain more retention for removable prosthetic appliances by expanding the prosthesis bed and to enhance plaque control by allow-

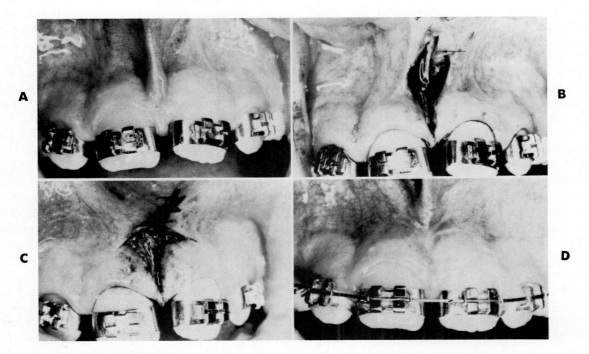

Fig. 47-10.   Frenectomy in an orthodontic patient. **A,** Papilla-penetrating frenum obscures presence of free gingival collars on mesial aspect of central incisors. **B,** Vertical incisions release frenum and reveal mesial marginal gingiva of central incisors. Arrow shows insertion of frenum prior to excision. **C,** Horizontal releasing incision and suturing. Note gingival collar present. **D,** Appearance 2 months postoperatively showing midline attached gingiva.

ing space for the effective nontraumatic use of plaque-control aids.

There are three basic procedures for extending the gingiva into the vestibule:

1. Gingival extension using a periosteal fenestration technique
2. Vestibuloplasty as a modified Edlan-Mejchar procedure
3. Gingival extension with a free gingival graft

The first two procedures are discussed here; the free gingival graft is discussed separately.

Historical perspective. Intraoral vestibular extension procedures in the past included removal of the soft tissue from the gingival margin to the fornix of the vestibule. A complete denudation technique was used in which all soft tissue, including the periosteum, was removed within the wound area, leaving the alveolar bone completely exposed (Ochsenbein, 1960; Corn, 1962). The complete denudation procedure was followed by some increase in the width of the attached gingiva; however, exposure of the alveolar bone produced severe bone resorption with permanent loss of alveolar bone height (Costich and Ramfjord, 1968). Severe recession of the marginal gingiva, alveolar bone resorption, and considerable postoperative pain after the denudation procedure have led to its demise. Next came the periosteal retention, or split-flap, procedure, in which only the superficial portion of the oral mucosa within the wound was removed, leaving the bone covered with periosteum (Staffileno et al., 1962; Pfeifer, 1965). Theoretically, covering the bone with periosteum should result in less crestal resorption; however, loss of crestal height also was observed following this procedure unless a relatively thick layer of connective tissue was retained on the bone surface (Costich and Ramfjord, 1968). Consequently, a modification of this procedure was devised and became known as the fenestration procedure (Robinson and Agnew, 1963). Although loss of alveolar height was minimal with the fenestration procedure, shrinkage of the attached gingiva and the tendency of muscle attachments to return to their original positions are limiting factors in vestibular extension (Spengler and Hayward, 1964; Pennel et al., 1965). However, often the periosteal fenestration procedure can produce deepening of the vestibule and increased attached gingiva.

Vestibular extension with periosteal fenestration. Indications for vestibular extension with periosteal fenestration include areas where a shallow vestibule puts tension on a broad region of the gingival margin, leading to progressive gingival recession. It is also indicated prior to construction of partial prostheses where expansion of the prosthesis bed is needed.

Operative procedure. After adequate local anesthesia, an incision is made at or near the mucogingival junction, retaining all of the attached gingiva from the mucogingival junction to the margin of the gingiva. A split-thickness flap is then reflected using a broad surgical blade, with reflection beginning at the mucogingival junction. The muscle fibers and tissue are sharply dissected from the periosteum, freeing the mucosal flap, which is then sutured in the depth of the vestibule using 4-0 silk or gut. Once the sutures are completed, a strip of the exposed periosteum is removed across the entire surgical area at the level of the original mucogingival junction, leaving a periosteal fenestration exposing bone. A dressing is placed over the surgical site to minimize patient discomfort. Following healing, the vestibular depth is maintained by scar tissue formed in the area of the fenestration.

Vestibuloplasty using the Edlan-Mejchar procedure. The Edlan-Mejchar procedure for vestibular deepening results in an increased width of attached mucosa extending into the fornix. No new attached gingiva develops from this procedure; however, it can provide a widened band of alveolar mucosa extending into the deepened vestibule and fixed to the underlying tissue.

Indications for this procedure include the need for expansion of the prosthesis bed and cases of generalized recession over a large arch segment. This procedure is also indicated for treatment of localized recession or for elimination of a broad, high frenum.

The Edlan-Mejchar procedure is contraindicated if a wide band of attached gingiva is needed to cover a recession area.

Operative procedure. Two vertical incisions are made from the gingival margin to outline the area of the operative field. This is followed by a horizontal incision 10 to 12 mm from the alveolar margin into the depth of the vestibule. A mucosal flap is elevated, exposing the periosteum. The periosteum is then separated from the bone beginning at the margin of the alveolar crest, including the muscle fibers. The periosteal flap is then transposed to the lip, and the margins of the flap are sutured to the margin of the incision on the lip. Next the mucosal flap is sutured at the depth of the vestibule. Caution should be exercised during incisions and flap reflection in the area of the mental foramen to prevent trauma to the mental nerve or severing the blood vessels in this region. To help adaptation of the mucosal flap to the denuded bone, a moist gauze square is applied to the flap and held for 3 to 5 minutes with gentle pressure. This will help control hemorrhage, reducing the chance of the flap being dislodged by a blood clot. A periodontal dressing is placed and carefully adapted to the vestibular contours.

Healing of the Edlan-Mejchar procedure is characterized by initial discoloration and swelling of the flap because of its compromised nutrition. However, revascularization is initiated from the base of the flap, and the normal tissue color of the flap returns within 1 week. Three to 4 weeks after the procedure, healing is complete, and the area apical to the mucosal flap is reepithelialized at this time. The new attached mucosa does not develop into gingiva.

• • •

Briefly, then, gingival extension or vestibuloplasty procedures are used rarely; however, when indicated, they are useful (e.g., in individuals with wide areas of recession that is progressive or when individual free gingival grafts, or lateral or coronal repositioning of the gingiva is not possible). Also, extension of the vestibule is often necessary for expanding the prosthesis bed.

Grafts

Vestibular extension procedures can also be carried out using grafts, including autogenous free gingival grafts and allografts of freeze-dried skin or freeze-dried dura mater. The objectives for these procedures are the same as for the Edlan-Mejchar and periosteal fenestration procedures. The free gingival graft provides an increased zone of attached gingiva.

The advantages of the allografts (either freeze-dried skin or freeze-dried dura mater) are that they eliminate the need for a donor site and that they provide abundant amounts of donor tissue for multiple extensive augmentation. A disadvantage of the allograft is the lower predictability of success with this procedure as compared with the free autogenous graft. Also, all allografts have the potential for transmission of disease such as hepatitis or AIDS from the donor, or for stimulating an adverse immune reaction that may compromise subsequent allografts, hence severely limiting their usefulness.

Free gingival grafts. The free gingival graft is used to halt gingival recession, to provide a cuff of abrasion-resistant gingiva around teeth and implants, and to provide esthetic and cosmetic coverage of denuded roots in patients with a high smile line. The free gingival graft is an autogenous graft of gingiva completely detached from its original site and blood supply and placed in a prepared recipient bed of periosteum and connective tissue covering the alveolar process. The gingival transplant is often taken from the palatal mucosa. Free gingival grafts offer reasonable predictability of success following treatment of areas with narrow gingival recession. The grafted tissues maintain their original characteristics after transplantation.

The general objectives are to create an increased attached zone of gingiva to correct gingival recession and improve esthetics, and to make mastication and plaque-control procedures less traumatic by providing attached epithelia around the necks of the teeth and implants.

Indications for free gingival grafts include the need to halt further recession in areas of localized gingival recession; free gingival grafts can be used in conjunction with frenotomy or frenectomy to prevent reformation of high frenal attachments and can be used in conjunction with vestibuloplasty.

Contraindications include wide and extensive denuded areas or areas of gingival recession that are not progressing or becoming larger. Alternate treatment options include laterally sliding repositioned flaps and coronal repositioning of flaps subsequent to free gingival grafts. Coronal repositioning subsequent to a free gingival graft shows the most promise in those situations where it is desirable to cover broad surfaces denuded by recession (Bernimoulin et al., 1975).

Operative procedure. After appropriate anesthesia, the recipient site is prepared by removing (with a broad surgical blade) all loose elastic connective tissue adhering to the underlying periosteum. The periosteum is left with a layer of connective tissue on the recipient site. The root surfaces are thoroughly root planed. The recipient site should be irrigated with sterile saline, and light pressure applied to control bleeding. A template of the recipient site is made with tinfoil or wax; however, the gingival graft should be at least 25% larger than the recipient site in all dimensions to allow for shrinkage that occurs postoperatively. The template is transferred to the donor site—usually the palate—and the outline of the donor tissue is made. The incision is begun, a corner of the donor tissue is undermined with the surgical blade, and a suture is placed in the released corner. The donor graft is then removed by dissection with light tension on the suture. The graft is put in place and sutured with 5-0 silk or gut. The superior border of the graft is sutured to the remaining coronal tissue. The apical border and body of the graft are held in place with a sling suture around the teeth as shown in Fig. 47-11. A layer of surgical tinfoil is placed over the graft to prevent the periodontal dressing from adhering to the sutures, and a periodontal dressing is then applied and muscle trimmed to make sure that it is not dislodged during healing. After approximately 1 week of healing, the dressing and sutures are carefully removed.

The healing of a free gingival graft placed on the connective tissue recipient bed can be divided into three phases (Oliver et al., 1968). The initial phase takes place during the first 3 days, during which time the grafted tissue survives decreasing nutrition by avascular plasmatic circulation from the recipient bed. The epithelium of the free graft degenerates early in this phase and subsequently becomes gray and desquamates. Since during this phase the graft receives its nourishment from the underlying bed, placing it over an avascular denuded root surface involves great risk of failure, particularly over the denuded root. Hence it is only relatively narrow gingival recession that can be treated successfuly with free gingival grafts. For this reason, coronal repositioning after a free gingival graft is the procedure of choice for coverage of moderate to wide denuded root surfaces.

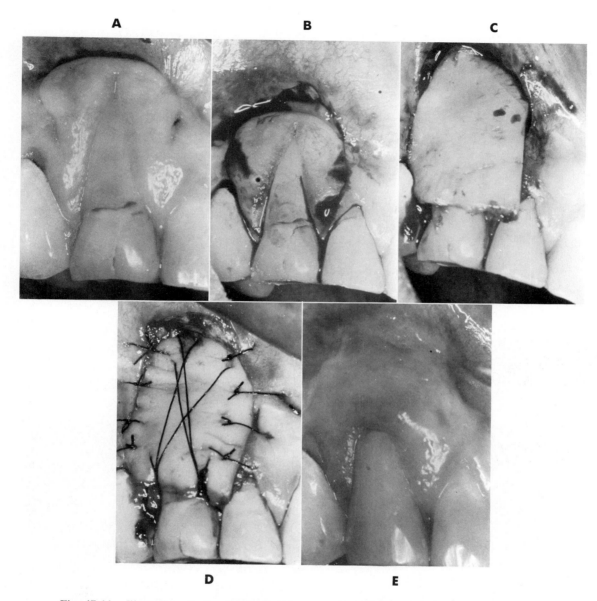

Fig. 47-11. Illustration of a free gingival graft to cover recession over a maxillary canine. Deep area of recession exists over maxillary canine, which is broad coronally and narrow apically and extends within 1 mm of mucogingival junction. **A,** Preoperative photograph. **B,** Initial incision prior to removing gingiva in interproximal areas mesial and distal to area of recession to prepare recipient bed. **C,** Graft (from palatal donor site of patient) is approximately one fourth to one third larger than area taken from gingival epithelium. **D,** Free gingival graft sutured into place over recipient bed and area of recession. **E,** Two-year postoperative view showing large band of attached gingiva covering approximately one half of original area of recession, resulting in an esthetic scallop matching that of adjacent teeth.

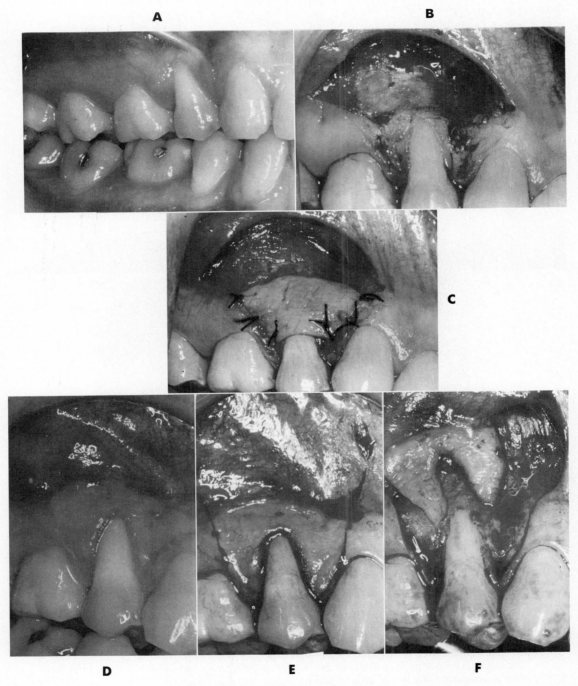

Fig. 47-12. For legend see opposite page.

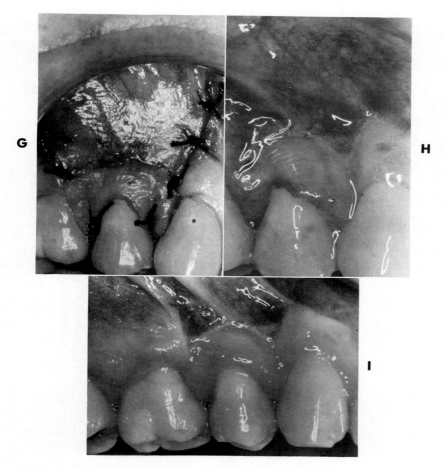

Fig. 47-12. Coronal repositioning of attached gingiva after free gingival graft. **A,** Preoperative photograph showing area of recession over radicular surface of maxillary right first premolar. Note attached gingiva close to mucogingival junction. **B,** Incision is made and split-thickness flap moved to expose recipient bed. Frenum attachment is dissected also. **C,** Free gingival graft material is taken from palate, and graft is placed over area of recession. **D,** Healing after 6 months. Note graft has healed, and 3 mm of attached gingiva is present on radicular surface, yet there still remains unesthetic recession. **E,** In second surgical procedure, incision is made beyond mucogingival junction. **F,** Split flap is raised, and entire flap is coronally repositioned such that margin is at or near cementoenamel junction of tooth in question. **G,** Flap is sutured in place. **H,** Appearance at 3 weeks. **I,** Stable and esthetic marginal gingiva seen 5 years after procedure.

In the second phase of healing, revascularization occurs during the second to fourteenth days. After 4 to 5 days of healing, anastomoses are established between the blood vessels of the recipient bed and those in the grafted tissue, establishing circulation in the preexisting blood vessels of the graft. Also, capillary proliferation and a fibrous union are established between the graft and the underlying connective tissue bed. Epithelialization of the graft occurs mainly by proliferation of epithelium from the borders of the adjacent tissues.

Next is the tissue maturation phase, which occurs from days 11 to 42. During this period the number of blood vessels in the transplant gradually becomes reduced, and after approximately 14 days the vascular supply of the graft is similar to that of normal attached gingiva. The epithelium matures, with formation of a keratin layer during the tissue maturation phase. After successful treatment of gingival recession by pedicle grafts or free grafts, it is still not clear whether there is establishment of a new connective attachment to the denuded root surface or a long junctional epithelium. It is possible that treatment of the root surface with citric acid or other agents may encourage connective attachment. However, it should be kept in mind that new connective attachment derived from gingival tissue often is associated with root resorption (Wikesjö et al., 1988); hence a long junctional epithelium may be a desirable response.

Coronal repositioning after a free gingival graft.

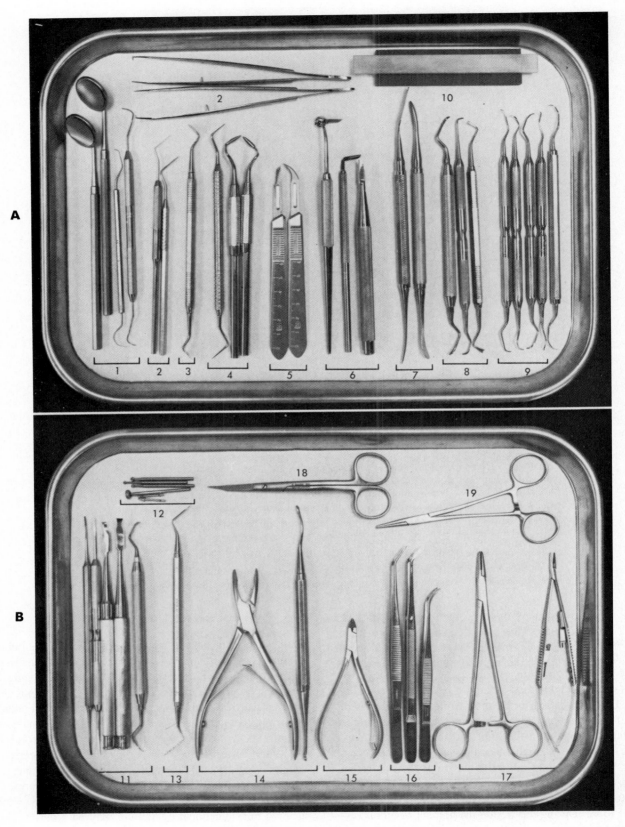

Fig. 47-13. For legend see opposite page.

Fig. 47-13. Examples of surgical tray setup. **A,** *1,* Mirrors, at least two large ones. Explorers, double-ended combination of Nos. 23 and 17 explorers, and double-ended cowhorn explorer for examination of furcation areas. *2,* Probe, thin Williams probe or Michigan type and Crane-Kaplan pocket markers. *3,* Knife, double-ended broad-blade, nondisposable knife. Examples are Goldman-Fox No. 7, Kirkland No. 14/15, and Buck No. 3/4. These knives may be used in various types of initial incisions, particularly in techniques that are basically involved in removal or dissection of soft tissues. Blades are angled for ease of access and sharpened on all sides, allowing operator to use a push or pull motion with any surface of blade. Major disadvantage is necessity of maintaining a refined surgical edge. Knife usually requires sharpening after each use. *4,* Knife, double-ended with a thin, pointed blade that is sharp on both edges. Examples are Goldman-Fox No. 11, Buck No. 5/6, and Sanders No. 4/5. These knives may be used to free interproximal tissue after initial incision, to thin and scallop flaps, or to make initial apically directed incisions during mucogingival surgery. Knives must also be sharpened to a fine surgical edge. Orban Nos. 1 and 2 are well designed for resection of mandibular lingual interproximal tissue. *5,* Disposable surgical blades with nondisposable Bard-Parker handles, Nos. 11, 12, 12B, and 15. No. 11 blade is long and pointed. It has one cutting edge and is useful in delicate sulcular incisions. Nos. 12 and 12B are curved "hawk-beak" blades. No. 12 blade is sharp on both surfaces of curve and may be used in a push or pull motion. No. 15 is most commonly used blade. It is a traditionally shaped surgical scalpel blade. Disposable blades are usually very sharp and are packaged as sterile. Disadvantages are limited shapes available and angulation of blade to handle, which makes access to many areas difficult. *6,* Special blade handles to overcome access problem, particularly in partial-thickness dissections of edentulous area of retromolar and tuberosity area. Examples are Blake handle (ash) and beaver handle. Blake handle can use usual disposable surgical blades and provides a 360-degree angle rotation for all areas of mouth. Two handles with blades are provided on surgical trays to enable access either buccally or lingually. Beaver handle (No. 3 KD) has a variety of stainless steel replaceable blades that can be used in gingivectomy and flap procedures. Castroviejo blade breaker is a handle that uses disposable razor blades. It is particularly useful for delicate graft dissections. *7,* Periosteal elevators; two are used on surgical tray. Examples are Prichard No. 3 and Allen No. 9 or Goldman-Fox. Goldman-Fox has sharp edges to aid in reflection of more delicate flaps. *8,* Instruments of various shapes for gross removal of hard deposits, granulation tissue, and tissue that remains attached to teeth following initial incision and reflection. Examples are Prichard Nos. 41 and 42 (large curettes), Goldman-Fox No. 10 (large surgical hoe), and Goldman-Fox No. 1 (Star) (large scaler). *9,* Curettes for definitive root planing and removal of remaining tissue fragments. Examples are Goldman-Fox Nos. 2, 3, and 4; Columbia Nos. 2R, 2L, 13, and 14; and Gracey Nos. 7, 8, 11, 12, 13, and 14. *10,* Stones for sharpening curettes. Examples are flat Arkansas No. 4 or Ivory No. 68, and Norton MB No. 4. **B,** Instruments that should be available for osseous and gingival reduction and contouring. *11,* Chisels; examples are Wedelstaedt (Hu-Friedy) Nos. 41 and 42, Schumacher No. 401, and Star Nos. 1 and 2. These are narrow-ended, side-cutting enamel chisels used for elimination of osseous craters and removal of interproximal hemiseptums. Ochsenbein Nos. 1 and 2 are excellent for removal of bone because of their shape and angulation. Rhodes chisel No. 36/37 is used for distal interproximal and radicular bony margin correction. Instrument is designed so that correct parabolic curve to osseous morphology can be achieved. Thodes No. 38/39 is used on mesial surfaces. *12,* Burs and diamonds for ultraspeed or slow-speed handpieces. Gingivoplasty diamonds, F-1, cone-shaped; F-2 (Star), small round; F-3 (Star), large doughnut Nos. 8, 10, and 12, round surgical burs. *13,* Interproximal file, Buck No. 11/12 (safe-sided). *14,* Rongeurs, useful in gross osseous reduction for obtaining osseous material for grafting. Examples are Cohen-Brenman (premier 5½-inch No. 4A) with small angled beak. Spoon curette, Miller No. 8 (Hu-Friedy), is ideal for developing correct osseous contour. *15,* Tissue nippers for removing elastic connective tissue fibers and for gingivoplasty. *16,* Pliers, serrated cotton pliers, Corn suture pliers, and tissue forceps (Hu-Friedy No. 34). *17,* Needle holder, diamond-jawed 6-inch Crile-Wood, designed for plastic surgery. It grasps very positively with minimum pressure to prevent flattening of small needles used in many periodontal surgical procedures. Castroviejo, small, delicate instrument that releases on continuous closure and lends itself to more delicate suturing. *18,* Scissors, Goldman-Fox, fine tissue scissors excellent for tissue tag removal; LaGrange (Banditt No. 905), double-curved scissors excellent in areas of difficult access. *19,* Mosquito hemostat, straight or curved 5-inch hemostat.

Coronal repositioning after a free gingival graft is a two-stage procedure in which a free gingival graft is placed as described above. It is suggested that at least 1 or 2 years be allowed for healing and creeping reattachment to occur after the graft is placed. Creeping reattachment or migration of the marginal gingiva coronally is not predictable after a free gingival graft; however, if it does not occur and there is still a denuded root surface exposed, the second stage of the procedure should be carried out with coronal repositioning of the attached gingiva to cover the area of recession. An example of this procedure is shown in Fig. 47-12.

Operative procedure.   In coronal repositioning, a scalloped incision is made on the labial surface, outlining the new interdental papillae. Two vertical incisions are then made at the extreme ends of the scalloped incision and extended into the vestibule to allow the flap to be coronally positioned, and a full mucoperiosteal flap is reflected into the vestibule. Next, a gingivectomy is performed to remove the epithelium of the papillae coronal to the horizontal incision. The root surface is thoroughly planed. The periosteum at the base of the flap is severed along the entire extent of the flap to allow coronal repositioning without flap tension. Care should be taken not to sever the flap or cut the blood vessels in the flap. The flap is then coronally repositioned and sutured tightly in place with interrupted sutures. A recession of about 50% may be expected (Bernimoulin et al., 1975). It cannot be expected that this will result in regeneration of a labial plate of bone; it most likely will result in attachment of the gingiva to the root surfaces via a long junctional epithelium.

Subepithelial connective tissue graft.   Subepithelial connective tissue grafts are covered in Chapter 51 on preprosthetic surgery.

SURGICAL PROCEDURES FOR TREATMENT OF TEETH WITH FURCATION INVOLVEMENT
Odontoplasty or furcationplasty

Treatment of teeth with furcation infections is one of the most challenging areas of periodontal therapy. Many procedures are available for treating Class I and shallow Class II furcations, including antiinfective therapy with scaling and root planing, or Widman flaps with osteoplasty to remove the marginal ledge of bone, allowing for flap adaptation. In more severe lesions such as the deep Class II or Class III furcations that do not respond to antiinfective therapy, regenerative procedures, including guided tissue regeneration (Chapter 48), tunneling procedures, or root resection, may be necessary.

The entrance to furcations may contain an enamel projection or, more rarely, an enamel pearl apical to the cementoenamel junction. These can be corrected by minor odontoplasty, making these plaque retention areas acceptable for hygiene and possible connective tissue reattachment. The overhanging enamel projection in the furcation is removed with a coarse diamond bur or an enamel shaver, followed by polishing with fine diamonds. These areas must then be carefully polished and treated with topical fluoride to prevent caries. Odontoplasty or furcationplasty often requires reflection of a mucoperiosteal flap for proper access and can be combined with osteoplasty and recontouring of the bony defects in the furcation area if indicated. Odontoplasty and osseous recontouring are indicated when the base of the furcation pocket is apical to the alveolar crest in the treatment of Class I and Class II furcation involvement. This treatment results in the establishment of soft tissue papillae that fill the furcation defect and cover the entrance to the furcation. Excessive recontouring of the tooth by grinding may result in hypersensitivity and be detrimental to the pulp, and it also enhances the risk for root surface caries; hence odontoplasty should be carried out with caution.

Root tunneling

Root tunneling involves exposure of the entire furcation from the buccal to lingual aspects on mandibular molars or the buccal to interproximal aspects on maxillary molars and is often used in Class III furcations that are probeable and not amenable to regenerative or root resection procedures.

Operative procedure.   After proper anesthesia, the buccal and lingual mucoperiosteal flaps are elevated, exposing the furcation. The root surfaces are scaled and root planed. Irregular alveolar bony crests are recontoured as necessary to allow for flap adaptation. The flaps are repositioned over the alveolar crest and sutured in this position. Dressing is applied, filling the furcation to prevent excessive granulation tissue formation in the furcation space during healing. This procedure is most often used on mandibular molars, although it can be successfully used on maxillary molars as well.

Disadvantages include the risk for development of caries on the denuded root surface within and adjacent to open furcations.

Root resection

Root resection, either by hemisection or root amputation of single roots of multirooted teeth with furcation infections, is often an effective treatment for teeth with Class III furcation involvement or if one root is severely diseased with little remaining alveolar support.

Indications are treatment of teeth that are needed for occlusion or for restorative abutments and that have one severely diseased root, or Class III or severe Class II infrabony defects that are not amenable to regenerative or other surgical procedures.

Contraindications include teeth with roots that are fused or teeth wherein the support of the root or roots remaining after amputation would be inadequate to maintain support of the tooth. Extraction is the treatment of choice in this situation.

Often an isolated tooth, such as a lower first molar, can be saved in an otherwise intact dentition by resecting the diseased mesial or distal root. The root area fills in with bone like an alveolar socket and can provide support to the adjacent tooth, as well as to the remaining root or roots. The crown can be recontoured to minimize the buccolingual width and reduce the occlusal stress on the tooth. Resected teeth can often be maintained for years and function as abutments or as occlusal stops for overdentures.

Operative procedure. Generally, endodontic treatment on teeth to be resected should be carried out before periodontal surgery. It may not be possible, especially in multirooted teeth with advanced destruction, to decide which root(s) will be removed. As an alternate to permanent filling of root canals with gutta-percha before surgery and placement of an amalgam plug in the root to be removed, a pulpectomy can be performed and the canals filled with calcium hydroxide. Each of the openings to the root canals is sealed with zinc oxide–eugenol cement, and root amputation can then be carried out without bacterial contamination of the remaining root canals. Permanent filling of these roots is performed after the periodontal surgery, and after an evaluation of the success of the root resection procedure.

The root to be amputated is selected on the basis of the amount of supporting tissue remaining. It is often easy to select the offending root; however, in cases where there is comparable bone loss around all roots, endodontic and prosthetic considerations should be the determining factor. Often the distobuccal root of the maxillary molars is the offending root, and distobuccal amputation is successful in retaining the molar.

On lower molars, root removal or hemisection of the tooth is indicated. The root is removed with a diamond bur and with care taken to remove the lip of the tooth structure overlying the alveolar crest in the furcation area. Careful smoothening of the remaining crown and root surface should be carried out to provide an environment conducive to good plaque control. Often a restoration is required to restore proper contour and occlusion.

COMBINED SURGICAL PROCEDURES

Often a quadrant or an arch will present multiple periodontal pathologic conditions that are amenable to treatment by a combination of two or more surgical procedures. Combined surgical procedures include the following:

1. Palatal gingivectomy (and palatal flap) with a buccal Widman flap
2. Modified Widman flap with a distal wedge or distal gingivectomy to remove fibrous tissue from the distal aspect of the last molars

3. Full mucoperiosteal flap and treatment of infrabony defects by infrabony grafts
4. Mucoperiosteal flap and regenerative procedures such as guided tissue regeneration
5. Mucoperiosteal flap with root resection
6. Flap with tooth extraction
7. Frenotomy with a free gingival graft
8. Gingivectomy (labial or lingual) with a modified Widman flap on the palatal aspect

• • •

Proper surgical instruments are essential to these procedures. A general purpose surgical tray is shown in Fig. 47-13, *A,* and instruments for osseous surgery are illustrated in Fig. 47-13, *B.*

It should be emphasized that different modalities of periodontal surgery, including those described here, are only part of the overall treatment of periodontal disease. It is clear that a high degree of plaque control must be maintained, particularly after periodontal surgery, to prevent recurrence of the disease.

REFERENCES

Aeschlimann CR, Robinson PJ, and Kaminski EJ: A short time evaluation of periodontal surgery, J Periodont Res 14:182, 1979.
Antczak-Boukoms A and Weinstein M: Cost-effectiveness analysis of periodontal disease control, J Dent Res 66:1630, 1987.
Ariaudo AA and Tyrrell HA: Repositioning and increasing the zone of attached gingiva, J Periodontol 28:106, 1957.
Bernimoulin JP, Luscher B, and Muhlemann HR: Coronally repositioned periodontal flap, J Clin Periodontol 2:1, 1975.
Bowers GM: A study of the width of attached gingiva, J Periodontol 34:201, 1963.
Boyne PJ: Histologic response of bone to sectioning by high-speed rotary instruments, J Dent Res 45:270, 1966.
Caffesse RG: Resective procedures. In American Academy of Periodontology: Proceedings of the World Workshop in Clinical Periodontics, Chicago, 1989, The Academy.
Caffesse RG et al: Cell proliferation after flap surgery, root conditioning and fibronectin application, J Periodontol 58:661, 1987.
Carranza FA and Carraro JJ: Mucogingival techniques in periodontal surgery, J Periodontol 41:294, 1970.
Cohen DW and Ross SE: The double papillae repositioned flap, J Periodontol 39:67, 1968.
Corn H: Periosteal separation—its clinical significance, J Periodontol 33:140, 1962.
Costich ER and Ramfjord SP: Healing after partial denudation of the alveolar process, J Periodontol 39:5, 1968.
Costich ER, Youngblood PA, and Walden JM: A study of the effects of high-speed rotary instruments on bone repair in dogs, Oral Surg Oral Med Oral Pathol 17:563, 1964.
DeTery E and Bernimoulin J: Influence of free gingival grafts on the health of the marginal gingiva, J Clin Periodontol 7:381, 1980.
Dorfman HS, Kennedy JE, and Bird WC: Longitudinal evaluation of free autogenous gingival grafts, J Clin Periodontol 7:316, 1980.
Engler WO, Ramfjord SP, and Hiniker AJ: Healing following simple gingivectomy: a tritiated thymidine radioautographic study. I. Epithelialization, J Periodontol 37:298, 1966.
Eriksson RA and Albrektsson T: Temperature threshold levels for heat-induced bone tissue injury: a vital-microscopic study in the rabbit, J Prosthet Dent 50:101, 1983.

Friedman N: Periodontal osseous surgery: osteoplasty and ostectomy, J Periodontol 26:257, 1955.

Friedman N: Mucogingival surgery: the apically repositioned flap, J Periodontol 33:328, 1962.

Friedman N and Levine HL: Mucogingival surgery: current status, J Periodontol 35:5, 1964.

Goldman HM: Development of physiologic gingival contours by gingivoplasty, Oral Surg Oral Med Oral Pathol 3:879, 1950.

Hamp SE, Rosling B, and Lindhe J: The effect of chlorhexidine on gingival wound healing in the dog: a histometric study, J Clin Periodontol 2:143, 1975.

Hangorsky U and Bissada NB: Clinical assessment of free gingival graft: effectiveness of maintenance on periodontal health, J Periodontol 51:274, 1980.

Kaldahl WB et al: Evaluation of four modalities of periodontal therapy, J Periodontol 59:783, 1988.

Karring T et al: The origin of granulation tissue and its impact on postoperative results of mucogingival surgery, J Periodontol 46:577, 1975.

Knowles J et al: Results of periodontal treatment related to pocket depth and attachment level, 8 years, J Periodontol 50:225, 1979.

Lang NP and Löe H: The relationships between the width of keratinized gingiva and gingival health, J Periodontol 43:623, 1972.

Lindhe J et al: Healing following surgical/non-surgical treatment of periodontal disease, J Clin Periodontol 9:115, 1982.

Matter J: Free gingival grafts for the treatment of gingival recession: a review of some techniques, J Clin Periodontol 9:103, 1982.

Nabers CL: Repositioning the attached gingiva, J Periodontol 25:38, 1954.

National Institute of Dental Research: Proceedings from the state of the art workshop on surgical therapy for periodontitis, J Periodontol 53:475, 1982.

Nyman S, Lindhe J, and Rosling B: Periodontal surgery in plaque-infected dentitions, J Clin Periodontol 4:240, 1977.

Ochsenbein C: Newer concept of mucogingival surgery, J Periodontol 31:175, 1960.

Oliver RG, Löe H, and Karring T: Microscopic evaluation of healing and revascularization of free gingival grafts, J Periodont Res 3:84, 1968.

Pennel BM et al: Retention of periosteum in mucogingival surgery, J Periodontol 36:39, 1965.

Pennel BM et al: Repair of alveolar processes following osseous surgery, J Periodontol 38:426, 1967.

Pfeifer JS: The reaction of alveolar bone to flap procedures in man, Periodontics 3:135, 1965.

Pihlstrom BL et al: Comparison of surgical and nonsurgical treatment of periodontal disease: a review of current studies and additional results after 6½ years, J Clin Periodontol 10:524, 1983.

Ramfjord SP and Costich ER: Healing after exposure of periosteum on the alveolar process, J Periodontol 38:199, 1968.

Ramfjord SP and Nissle RR: The modified Widman flap, J Periodontol 45:601, 1974.

Robinson RE: The distal wedge operation, Periodontics 4:256, 1966.

Robinson RE and Agnew RG: Periosteal fenestration at the mucogingival line, J Periodontol 34:503, 1963.

Rosling B, Nyman S, and Lindhe J: The effect of systematic plaque control on bone regeneration in infrabony pockets, J Clin Periodontol 3:38, 1976a.

Rosling B et al: The healing potential of the periodontal tissues following different techniques of periodontal surgery and plaque-free dentition, J Clin Periodontol 3:233, 1976b.

Ross S et al: The double papillae repositioned flap—an alternative: fourteen years in retrospect, Int J Periodontics Restorative Dent 6:47, 1986.

Schluger S: Osseous resection—a basic principle in periodontal surgery? Oral Surg Oral Med Oral Pathol 2:316, 1949.

Spengler DE and Hayward JR: Study of sulcus extension wound healing in dogs, J Oral Surg 22:413, 1964.

Staffileno H, Wentz F, and Orban B: Histologic study of healing of split thickness flap surgery in dogs, J Periodontol 33:56, 1962.

Wennstrom J, Lindhe J, and Nyman S: The role of keratinized gingiva in plaque-associated gingivitis in dogs, J Clin Periodontol 9:75, 1982.

Westfelt E et al: Significance of frequency of professional tooth cleaning for healing following periodontal surgery, J Clin Periodontol 10:148, 1983.

Widman L: The operative treatment of pyorrhea alveolarus: a new surgical method, Svensk Tandlakaretidskrift, 1918; reviewed in Br Dent J 1:293, 1920.

Wikesjö UME et al: Repair of periodontal furcation defects in beagle dogs following reconstructive surgery including root surface demineralization with tetracycline hydrochloride and topical fibronectin application, J Clin Periodontol 15:73, 1988.

Wilderman MN et al: Histogenesis and repair following osseous surgery, J Periodontol 41:551, 1970.

Wilderman PC, Ramfjord SP, and Nasjleti CE: Reverse bevel flaps in monkeys, J Periodontol 39:219, 1968.

Chapter 48

REGENERATIVE THERAPY IN PERIODONTICS

William H. Hiatt
Robert J. Genco

Since one of the end results of periodontal disease is loss of the periodontal attachment apparatus, including loss of tooth-supporting alveolar bone, regeneration of lost periodontal attachment is a reasonable goal of therapy. After thorough antiinfective therapy, including scaling, root planing with surgical access if necessary, and elimination of the subgingival pathogens, plaque, and plaque retention areas, some sites require additional periodontal treatment to either achieve additional tooth support or to provide contours that can be maintained in health. These include furcation lesions and other infrabony defects that jeopar-

dize the longevity of the tooth. Lesions on such teeth may persist, with pockets retained, and subgingival plaque and bleeding (Hiatt et al., 1986). Frequently, regenerative therapy offers a choice if such teeth are to be preserved. The end result is often improved function and the retention of teeth that serve to enhance the function of a prosthesis. *Regeneration,* defined as reconstitution of a lost part, differs from repair. *Repair* is healing of a wound by tissue that does not fully restore the architecture or function of the part. In addition to differentiating between regeneration and repair, it is also important to distinguish between new attachment and reattachment of the periodontium. *New attachment* refers to reunion of connective tissue to a root surface deprived of its periodontal ligament, usually by periodontitis. This reunion may occur by formation of new cementum with inserting collagen fibers. In contrast, *reattachment* refers to reunion of connective tissue and epithelium to a root surface on which viable periodontal tissue is present, and does not usually involve formation of new cementum. Periodontal regeneration, then, refers mainly to reconstitution of lost periodontium by formation of a new attachment apparatus, and hence histologic evidence is often presented to document its occurrence.

Regenerative therapy, as proposed over the years, includes the use of various grafts, guided tissue regeneration with barrier membranes, chemical root treatments, and coronally repositioned flaps. This chapter addresses the many facets of regenerative therapy, including reattachment to roots needing little or no preparation in some acute lesions and attachment to roots needing extensive preparation in chronic disease. New attachment is demonstrated on roots with and without new cementum formation.

Connective tissues form the primary attachment to the tooth, with a coronal seal of epithelium. Histologic sections shown in this chapter after various modes of periodontal therapy demonstrate Sharpey's fiber formation with new cementum and a new connective tissue attachment, or the formation of a long junctional epithelium and connective tissue formation with no new cementum.

New bone formation can occur adjacent to a long junctional epithelial attachment, as well as adjacent to a connective tissue attachment with new cementum formation and Sharpey's fiber attachment into the new cementum and bone. Root preparation and the management of the pocket tissue include curettage in both open and closed approaches. The nature of healing and the predictability of success for any treated lesion are not fully understood. However, the anatomy of the lesion is clearly important in the predictability of treatment success. Furthermore, recent developments in bone grafting and periodontal tissue regeneration with barrier membranes offer possibilities for greater predictability than in the past.

Graft materials emphasized in this chapter are those in current use and include biologic and synthetic materials. The role of grafts in the stimulation of cells to modulate in the direction of osteogenesis and the role of grafts in osteoconduction, or the "trellis effect" are explored. The fate of the graft during wound healing is observed.

Root resorption and ankylosis may occur with any regenerative procedure and, if severe, represent unacceptable side effects. Examples are drawn from nongraft and graft procedures. The significance and management of root resorption are discussed.

In this chapter, then, the long-term survival of periodontal lesions treated with various modes of regenerative therapy are discussed. These modes of therapy include closed- and open-flap curettage with root planing, root conditioning and coronal repositioning of flaps, "guided tissue regeneration," synthetic graft materials (alloplasts), autografts, and allografts. For recent reviews of this area see Hancock (1989) and Egelberg (1987).

CLOSED CURETTAGE WITH ROOT PLANING

Lesions that are treated without exposure by a surgical flap are approached in a closed environment. In these lesions it is usually not possible to visualize the root surface to the bottom of the pocket. Even so, success in closing the pocket by this method is often observed in deep acute lesions of short duration where only the coronal portion can be instrumented with accuracy and in chronic lesions where sequential sessions of scaling and root planing result in some pocket shrinkage, thus permitting more accurate instrumentation of the deeper root surfaces.

Acute lesions

Acute lesions of short duration often heal with regeneration of the periodontium (Hiatt, 1977). It has been specu-

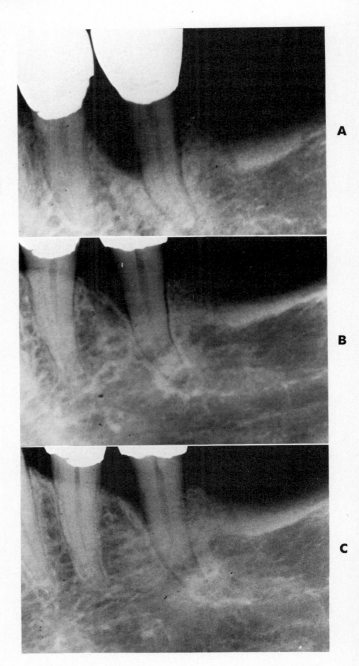

Fig. 48-1. Results of closed curettage and root planing. **A,** Pretreatment radiograph. **B,** Results 6 months after complete curettage and root planing. **C,** Results after 18 months.

lated that in acute cases the root has not had time to become infected, as it does in chronic periodontal disease.

The patient shown in Fig. 48-1 had a pocket of recent origin and was treated initially by curettage and root planing. The initial pocket reduction resulted from gingival shrinkage, and radiographic evidence of new bone formation was seen (Fig. 48-1, *B* and *C*). Pocket reduction by gingival shrinkage and reattachment following root planing

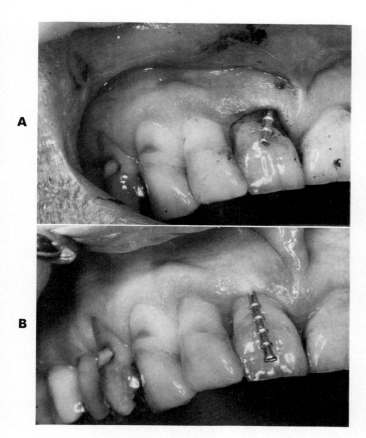

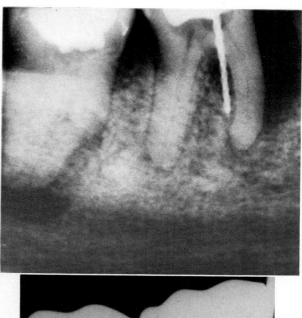

Fig. 48-2. Treatment of an acute abscess with pocket formation by root planing, topical iodine, and systemic antibiotics. **A,** Pretreatment appearance. **B,** Posttreatment appearance. Same metal point was used to mark pretreatment and posttreatment photographs. (From Hiatt WH: J Periodontol 48:598, 1977.)

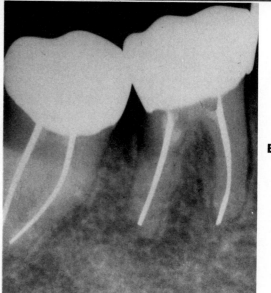

Fig. 48-3. Treatment of pulpal-periodontal lesions by combined endodontic and periodontal therapy. **A,** Pretreatment radiograph showing infrabony pocket on mesial aspect of both molars and periapical radiolucency around roots of second molar. Instrument could be placed in furcation of first molar. **B,** Six-month posttreatment radiograph showing evidence of bone fill around both molars. Note probe at osseous margin on first molar.

and curettage in a closed environment has been noted in a number of studies comparing various methods of treatment (see Chapters 35 and 47).

The patient shown in Fig. 48-2 had an acute abscess with pocket formation of short duration. Treatment consisted of root planing and medication with a topical iodine solution and systemic antibiotics. The metal point in the pocket demonstrates pocket depth before and after treatment.

In Fig. 48-3 the patient had developed a pocket on the mesial surface and in the furcation of a mandibular first molar. The lesion was probably of pulpal origin, and the pockets were associated with drainage pathways along the periodontal ligament space. In the second molar the retrograde lesion was narrow and can be seen radiographically in the apical half of the root, as well as in an angular defect at the coronal part of the lesion. Drainage, coronal root planing, systemic antibiotics, and endodontic therapy were started simultaneously. Healing of the lesion and reattachment of the pocket tissue were evident even during endodontic therapy, which was completed approximately 1

month after the beginning of therapy. Fig. 48-3, *B,* represents healing at 6 months.

OPEN-FLAP CURETTAGE WITH ROOT PLANING

The flap approach is done with surgical detachment of the gingiva and pocket tissue to obtain access, permitting visualization of the root surface and the bony defect. Variations of this procedure have been described as the exci-

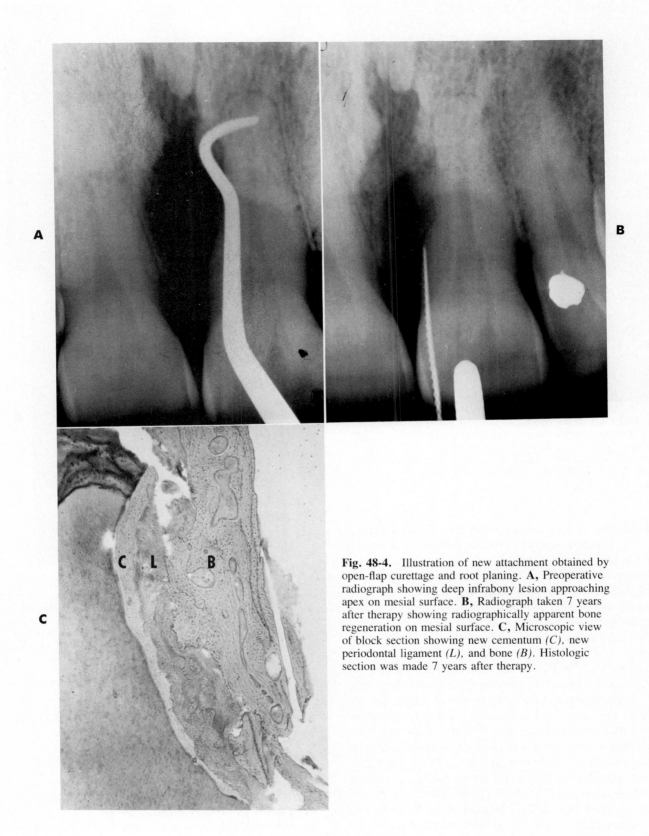

Fig. 48-4. Illustration of new attachment obtained by open-flap curettage and root planing. **A,** Preoperative radiograph showing deep infrabony lesion approaching apex on mesial surface. **B,** Radiograph taken 7 years after therapy showing radiographically apparent bone regeneration on mesial surface. **C,** Microscopic view of block section showing new cementum *(C)*, new periodontal ligament *(L)*, and bone *(B)*. Histologic section was made 7 years after therapy.

sional new attachment procedure (ENAP) by Yukna and Williams (1980), the infrabony approach by Goldman and Cohen (1958), the modified Widman flap by Ramfjord (1977), and the intrabony technique by Prichard (1957), and these are described in Chapter 47.

Fig. 48-4 illustrates a long-standing periodontal lesion with a pocket extending to the root apex. Treatment consisted of two open-flap procedures with root planing. The first procedure resulted in a narrowing of the lesion and new bone formation seen vertically. After the second procedure further new bone formation was seen. The tooth had to be removed because of trauma, and histologic evaluation demonstrated new cementum, ligament, and bone formation (Fig. 48-4, *C*).

Periodontal regeneration by root conditioning and coronal repositioning of flaps

Long-term follow-up of periodontal treatment suggests that most lesions in the majority of periodontal patients respond well to antiinfective therapy. However, on teeth with severe lesions, such as multirooted teeth with lesions that involve furcations, tooth mortality for periodontal reasons has been reported as 31% to 57% (Hirschfeld and Wasserman, 1978; McFall, 1982). This compares with the overall tooth mortality of 7% to 10% for all teeth treated by antiinfective therapy (Hirschfeld and Wasserman, 1978; McFall, 1982). The lower success rate of therapy in molars with multirooted teeth with furcation involvement may be explained in part by the difficulty in gaining access for oral hygiene or for instrumentation (Svardstrom and Wennstrom, 1988). It is clear that the prognosis of teeth, especially molars with Class II furcation lesions, may be improved with regenerative therapy, which may lead to closure of the defect (Martin et al., 1987). At least two relatively new approaches have been used to regenerate tissue in furcations. One involves root conditioning with acid, such as citric acid, followed by coronally positioned flaps, and the other involves guided tissue regeneration using barrier membranes.

Numerous animal experiments have shown that citric acid–conditioned root surfaces in Class II furcations in dogs will predictably regenerate (see Crigger et al., 1978; Nilveus and Egelberg, 1980). This approach has been applied with some success to the treatment of Class II furcation defects in humans (Gantes et al., 1988). About 40% of treated Class II defects were completely closed by bone fill when the root surfaces were etched with citric acid and coronal flaps were positioned over the furcations. The procedure consisted of reflecting a mucoperiosteal flap and debridement of the root surface, removing granulation tissue from the furcation, citric acid etching the exposed root surfaces, and coronally placing flaps with the margin of the flap at least 1 mm coronal to the opening of the furca-

tion. It is interesting that in this study half of the lesions were grafted with bone.* There was no difference in the bone fill of the grafted versus the nongrafted sites. This points to a reasonable success rate for root conditioning and coronal flap positioning.

Periodontal tissue regeneration with barrier membranes: the "guided tissue regeneration" procedure

Studies of dogs and monkeys, as well as trials in humans, have demonstrated that it is possible to enhance the regeneration of new connective tissue attachment to previously infected root surfaces through placement of a membrane between the gingiva and the root surface. This barrier membrane is thought to prevent gingival tissue, especially the epithelium, from contacting the root during healing. The barrier membrane thus appears to allow cells from the periodontal ligament and possibly marrow to repopulate the root surface, leading to regeneration of periodontal attachment.

The success rate of guided tissue regeneration appears to be high in Class II furcation–involved molars. For example, Pontoriero et al. (1988) found that more than 90% of sites treated with the guided tissue regeneration technique showed complete fill of the furcation when assessed by probing attachment measurements 6 months after surgery. The control sham-operated sites showed 20% fill.

Guided tissue regeneration appears less predictable for Class III mandibular molar furcations (Pontoriero et al., 1989). Also, it appears that success is achievable in two-to three-walled vertical defects; however, it is well known that many of these defects also fill with good antiinfective therapy. Guided tissue regeneration has also been used in complex lesions involving furcations, narrow interproximal defects, and very large defects along with bone grafting, with variable results and complication rates (Becker et al., 1985; Schallhorn and McClain, 1988).

Procedure. Before surgery, complete antiinfective therapy is performed. This includes the establishment of personal oral hygiene and complete resolution of inflammation by root planing and scaling as assessed by the elimination of areas of gingival bleeding on probing and the elimination of suppuration. However, deep lesions and furcations may not respond adequately to root planing and scaling even under the best conditions, given the difficulty in access to tortuous lesions or irregular furcation anatomy. Once antiinfective therapy has been completed and oral hygiene established, the Class II and Class III mandibular furcations, and possibly other lesions, are then amenable to guided tissue regeneration procedures.

---

*Freeze-dried, decalcified bone allografts.

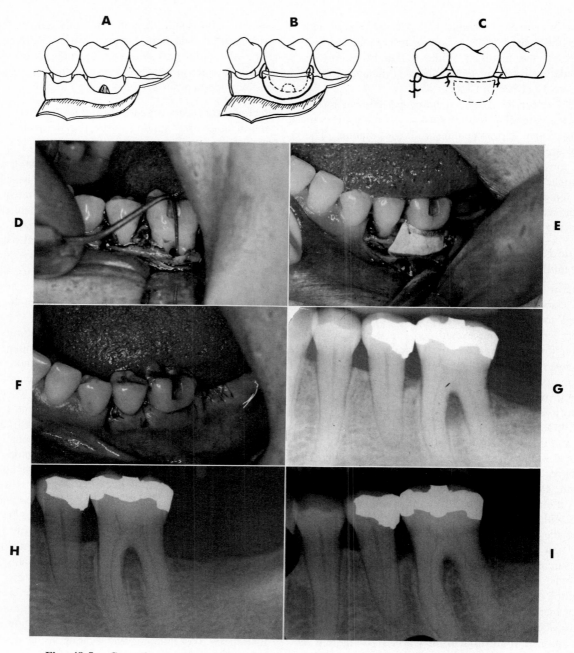

Fig. 48-5. General surgical procedure for placement of occlusive or barrier membranes for guided tissue regeneration. **A,** Initial incision is made through gingiva to periosteum with wide reflection mesial and distal to lesion to allow for placement of membrane. Note furcation lesion on first molar, which is to be treated. **B,** Placement of occlusive membrane to cover furcation lesion and margin of bone 3 to 4 mm in all dimensions, as well as root surface. **C,** Closure by suturing gingival flap. Note that coronal flap margin is coronal to margin of occlusive membrane, which is shown in dotted lines. For nonresorbable membranes such as Goretex removal using a similar but less extensive flap as indicated in **A** is carried out at 4 to 6 weeks. **D to I,** Clinical and radiographic documentation of treatment of a 54-year-old man with a buccal Class II mandibular molar furcation defect. **D,** Flap reflected showing a buccal Class II furcation 6 mm from osseous floor to furcation roof. **E,** Barrier membrane sutured in place. **F,** Mucoperiosteal flap sutured covering barrier membrane. **G,** Presurgical radiograph showing radiolucent area in furcation, as well as radiolucency mesial and distal to molar. **H,** Radiograph 9 months after surgery showing evidence of healing in furcation, as well as mesial and distal to molar. **I,** Nineteen-month postoperative radiograph showing further evidence of bony healing in furcation. Furcation probing in vertical or horizontal direction was 3 mm, suggesting reattachment, as well as bony fill of furcation. (**D to I** courtesy Dr. D. Conner.)

Surgical procedure. As shown in Fig. 48-5, an intrasulcular incision is made to preserve as much attached gingiva as possible, including the adjacent interdental papillae. Full-thickness flaps are then raised, and pocket epithelium and underlying granulation tissue is removed. Vertical relaxing incisions may be spaced mesial to the site being treated if necessary for access.

Defect preparation. The root surfaces are thoroughly scaled and root planed, and debridement is carried out to remove granulation tissue. Root planing of tortuous defects and of irregular furcations may require the use of diamonds or fluted burs to completely remove all diseased root surfaces. Also, enamel projections should be removed if they enter the furcation, since connective tissues cannot attach to enamel surfaces. The appropriate membrane is selected from among several membranes available. The use of nonresorbable Teflon membranes (expanded polytetrafluoroethylene, or e-PTFE) is discussed here, although the basic features of the procedure are likely to be useful for other materials, including resorbable membranes. The membrane is cut to size to totally cover the defect and extend over the defect margin at least 3 mm laterally and 3 to 5 mm apically. The membrane is sutured using a sling suture directly around the tooth, minimizing folds or overlaps of the material. Also, saliva and other contamination should be minimized. The flap is then placed over the barrier membrane covering, 2 to 3 mm apical to the flap margin. The interproximal incisions are then closed, after which the vertical incision is closed. Postoperatively the patient is covered with antibiotics and put on a chemical plaque-control regimen. Periodontal dressings are not suggested, and the patient should be seen every other week while the nonresorbable membrane is in place. The membrane (if nonresorbable) should be removed 4 to 6 weeks after placement. Beginning at 2 weeks, pieces of the membrane may be exposed.

Removal of the material. At 4 to 6 weeks after placement, or earlier if complications develop, nonresorbable membranes should be removed. The material is removed by making a sharp access incision for dissection of the material from the flap. The flap is then dissected from the membrane, and the membrane is removed. This may require a vertical incision on the mesial aspect for access. At this time, the sutures holding the membrane must be removed.

Complications. Infection, perforation, abscess formation, recession or flap sloughing, and gingival irregularities may occur. Abscesses occur in 6% to 10% of cases.

Membrane procedures using coronally repositioned flaps and root conditioning, or barrier membranes such as Teflon, collagen, or alloplastic membranes have shown promise in enhancing the regeneration of periodontal tissues in furcations and other severe infrabony lesions. Animal studies, however, have shown that when new periodontal attachment occurs, root resorption and ankylosis often result. The extent to which this occurs after guided tissue regeneration and coronally repositioned flap procedures in humans is unknown; hence ankylosis and root resorption remain a possible long-term adverse result of these procedures. However, short-term studies (1 to 2 years) in humans have not shown radiographically or clinically detectable root resorption (Fig. 48-5).

ROLE OF GRAFT MATERIALS

A search for the ideal graft material predates this century (Barth, 1895); however, only those materials in current use are discussed here. This includes various bone and marrow grafts, and synthetic materials such as hydroxyapatite and tricalcium phosphate.

The relative importance of the organic and inorganic phases of bone in regeneration was described by Glimcher and Krane (1968). Urist et al. (1967) described a preparation of decalcified bone that combined morphogenic proteins that actively induced new bone formation. They found that if bone reduced to appropriate particle size is demineralized, certain proteins are then available to induce new bone formation when the graft is in contact with the bone at the recipient site. Numerous studies have indicated that the bone marrow cells in cancellous bone and marrow grafts may either grow to form new bone or stimulate new bone formation.

Animal studies provide useful information inasmuch as they may indicate the potential of a graft to produce favorable results. About 75% of the studies performed over the past several decades comparing graft and nongraft procedures in artificially created periodontal osseous defects of animals have indicated that more favorable results are obtained with the placement of a bone graft than by leaving the defects alone. No nongraft control sites have been found to be superior to grafted sites when mean bone repair of the defect was compared (Hiatt, 1970; Ellegaard et al., 1974; Caton et al., 1980; Klinge et al., 1985; Blumenthal et al., 1986). However, all animal experiments must be viewed with a certain degree of caution, and the results may not be directly extrapolated to humans. Only when it is tested in controlled human clinical evaluations can the true potential of any bone graft material be objectively assessed.

The inductive effect of the various graft materials can be categorized under three headings. The first is *osteogenesis,* which occurs when cells of the graft survive the transplantation and contribute to the repair process. There is little evidence that this occurs in periodontal grafting, since most of the cells from the graft appear nonviable in subsequent histologic studies at 1 and 2 weeks.

Osteoinduction can be defined as occurring when two or more tissues of different nature or properties become intimately associated, resulting in alteration of the developmental course of the tissues. This effect has been observed with bone extracts, cells, bone, and even nonbone tissue such as kidney. Burwell (1985), in a review, concluded that marrow cells in the graft and in the surrounding host environment are important to the success of the graft. Urist et al. (1967) noted enhanced osteoinductive effects when bone was demineralized to expose the matrix proteins. The fact that cancellous bone grafts are better disposed to contribute to an active osteogenic effect may reflect their relatively greater surface relative to mass, rather than the action of any cellular components (Farley et al., 1982).

Osteoconduction, or the trellis effect, occurs with the ingrowth of capillaries in new connective tissue. The framework provided by the graft may occur with various bone grafts or nonbone grafts such as the synthetic materials. With bone grafts, this process is followed by simultaneous resorption of dead bone or of the synthetic trellis and the deposition of new bone lamellae.

The search to isolate inductive proteins or biologic response modifiers to be combined with filler material for grafts, using various materials and methods, continues. However, presently there are controlled studies showing

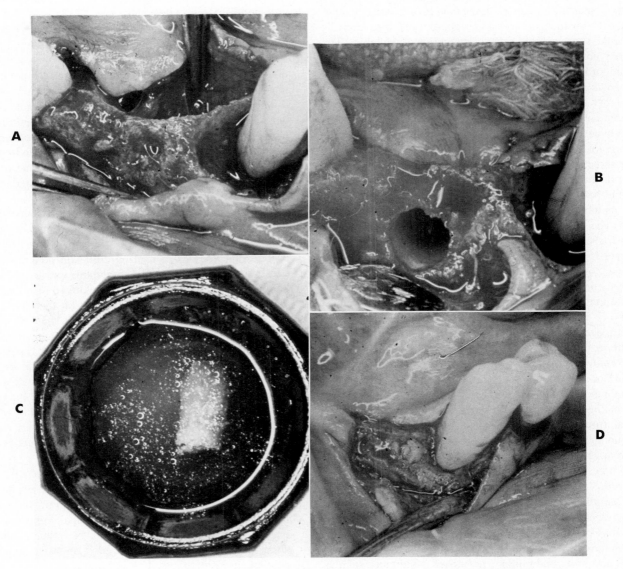

Fig. 48-6. Autograph of intraoral bone and marrow taken from adjacent edentulous ridge. **A,** Pretreatment clinical photograph showing circumferential defect on mesial aspect of canine. **B,** Core of bone and marrow taken with a trephine bur from edentulous ridge area of anterior mandible. **C,** Bone and marrow core after retrieval is placed in sterile saline. Core was cut into small pieces and placed into defect on mesial aspect of canine. **D,** Lesion area 1 year later showing bony fill on mesial aspect of canine. (Courtesy Dr. S. Kirsch.)

that bone-grafting materials do lead to better clinical results than do surgically debrided control sites. Biologic response modifiers may enhance these results.

Synthetic graft materials (alloplasts)

Research reports have demonstrated positive clinical results with synthetic ceramic graft materials similar in magnitude and frequency to those obtained with other graft materials. Defect fill has been shown with several types (Rabalais et al., 1981; Meffert et al., 1985), with no essential difference among them. Complete defect fills occur in about 10% of cases, whereas failures occur with about the same frequency. However, grafting of periodontal osseous defects with ceramic materials has not been predictably successful.

Surface-active biomaterials. Since the late 1960s synthetic surface-active materials that bond to bone have been described (Hench and Wilson, 1984). There are presently at least five major categories of surface-active materials, including dense hydroxyapatite ceramics, bioactive glasses, bioactive glass-ceramics, bioactive composites, and titanium. Most of these have found use in dental implants and in alveolar ridge augmentation. For example, ridge augmentation with particulate hydroxyapatite mixed with autogenous bone has been reported in 5-year human trials. However, particulate hydroxyapatite has not fulfilled its earlier promise in long-term applications in the treatment of periodontal defects. This lack of success may result from the soft tissue interface that often forms a capsule around the materials, with eventual movement and exfoliation through the gingiva. These materials have not demonstrated osteogenic potential. Future research on surface-active glass, glass-ceramic, or ceramic materials for use in periodontal lesions may lead to useful periodontal graft materials.

Bone marrow grafts. Pocket reduction, growth of alveolar bone, and gain in probing attachment level have commonly been observed with the use of bone grafts (Hiatt et al., 1986). True histologic new attachment appears to be less frequent and less predictable with ceramic graft materials (Froum et al., 1981) as compared with bone graft materials (Hiatt et al., 1978; Listgarten and Rosenberg, 1979).

Autografts

Intraoral sites. Intraoral sites for bone and marrow graft materials include the maxillary tuberosity and edentulous ridges. In the case illustrated in Fig. 48-6, a core of bone and marrow obtained from the edentulous ridge was grafted into an infrabony defect, and after 1 year the defect filled. Bone chip grafts may be procured during an osteoplasty or an osteoectomy when this procedure is done with hand instruments. Both bone and marrow, and the bone chip grafts are placed in a Dappen dish containing sterile saline on the surgical tray and reduced to size with scissors

prior to implantation in the infrabony pockets.

Osseous coagulum is generally obtained from denser bone, particularly when osseous contouring procedures are being performed with a bur or a stone in a handpiece. The resulting material is referred to as a coagulum, since it is mixed with blood as it is procured. This material differs from bone and marrow, or bone chip grafts in that fewer cells are present in the graft. Bone from intraoral sites is not procured under sterile conditions, and reliable methods of sterilizing such bone are not generally practical; therefore storage is not recommended.

Extraoral sites. Autograft material from extraoral sites may be obtained from either the anterior or the posterior iliac crest (Fig. 48-7). Red or hematopoietic marrow is obtained, along with cancellous bone, and is soft enough to be cut with scissors into 1 to 3 mm cubes. Procurement is usually done with special needles or coring devices by either a hematologist or an orthopedic surgeon.

Allografts

Allograft material is from cadaveric sources. Cortical bone is used from various sources, including ribs; it is ground into a bone powder, with particle sizes varying from 250 to 500 μm. Demineralization is often done to expose matrix proteins for greater inductivity. Packaging and storage is by a freeze-dried technique. Often freeze-dried bone is used as an extender for the more inductive autogenous bone and marrow.

Iliac and vertebral bone and marrow are also obtained from cadaveric sources and may be stored by freezing in special media with a cryopreservative agent, or may be irradiated for sterilization. Allograft materials often are

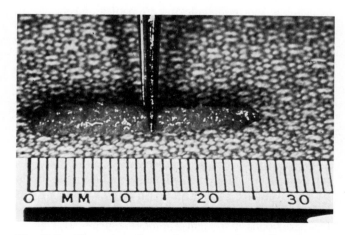

Fig. 48-7. Illustration of core of marrow and cancellous bone as autograft from iliac crest. Core can be cut into 1 to 3 mm segments and placed into infrabony defects. Allograft material obtained from iliac crest or vertebral column appear very similar and can be cut into segments for implantation into infrabony defects and sterilized. (Courtesy Dr. R.G. Schallhorn.)

freeze-dried. Clinical success with allografts in periodontal lesions has been documented. For example, an average of 4.8 mm (range 0 to 11 mm) bone fill in infrabony defects grafted with frozen allograft iliac crest material was reported (Hiatt et al., 1986). This is compared with an average of 0 mm gain (range −1 to +2 mm) in control lesions.

Some tissue banks procure under nonsterile conditions and depend on secondary sterilization by either irradiation or a gas—ethylene oxide. Because of the recognition of the possibility of transmission of viral diseases such as acquired immunodeficiency syndrome (AIDS) and hepatitis by allografts, some banks procure under sterile conditions, test for viruses and bacteria, and, in addition, employ a secondary sterilizing method, often 2.5 megarad of high-intensity gamma irradiation, which is adequate to kill HIV. This is the standard dose in secondary sterilization accepted by the Centers for Disease Control and the American Association of Tissue Banks. Ethylene oxide is also used for secondary sterilization; however, it may inactivate the bone-inducing potential of allografts. Also, ethylene oxide is a powerful mutagen; the Food and Drug Administration has decreased the acceptable level of residual gas and by-products several times in the past 5 years. Future developments should be noted, particularly in regard to nonsterile procurement, since the foreign proteins left by even dead bacteria may detract from the activity of the graft. Careful control of the source and processing of all allograft materials is essential to prevent inadvertent transmission of HIV, hepatitis, and other infectious agents to donors. Also, induction of immunity to the allograft, although apparently uncommon, especially with carefully prepared materials, is to be considered in the use of these materials (Schallhorn and Hiatt, 1972).

Caution in the use of allografts for periodontal therapy. It is clear that much progress has been made in understanding the tissue-inductive properties and the use of allografts in periodontal regenerative procedures. Caution is advised, however, in the selection of a tissue bank that is approved by a national agency. It is further suggested that one become familiar with their protocols for selection of donors and quality control of the graft materials.

SURGICAL PROCEDURES FOR REGENERATION BY GRAFTING
Preparation and fill of the graft site

Preparation of the graft site and selection of the donor site begin with the initial examination and diagnosis of the patient. Antiinfective therapy consisting of thorough scaling or root planing and adjunctive procedures to suppress the periodontal flora and eliminate inflammation is required to achieve as much healing as possible. If further regeneration of attachment is necessary, a graft may be attempted. Plaque-control techniques must be successfully accomplished early in the treatment, since the combination of instrumentation and plaque control permits an assess-

ment of tissue response, as well as an assessment of the ability of the patient to carry out maintenance care instructions. These are important predictors of ultimate success or failure in whatever treatment is suggested, since they measure attitudes and motor skills of the patient, as well as tissue response.

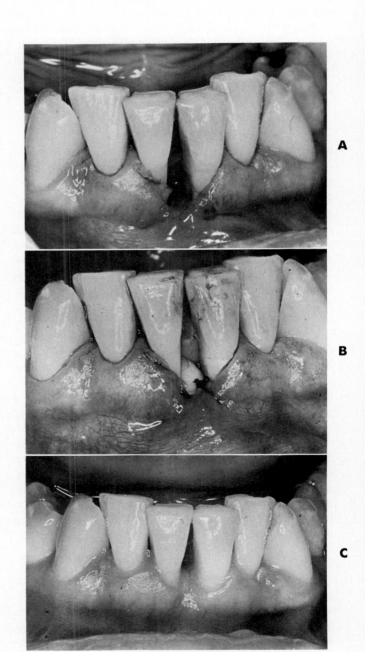

Fig. 48-8. Placement of a free gingival graft to cover an infrabony graft and adjacent alveolar crest. **A,** Initial incision made into mucosa covering area of infrabony defect. **B,** Free gingival graft placed over this region. **C,** Area healed with attached mucosa and stable marginal gingiva.

The objective in designing a flap is to preserve enough tissue to fully cover the graft and the alveolar bone. This could include an adjacent edentulous area or even a free gingival graft (Fig. 48-8). However, in most instances either a diagonal incision through the papilla to enhance coaptation or an incision between line angles of adjacent teeth having a wide interdental space is made. The benefit of an incision made perpendicular to the interdental space is that often the interdental position of the graft is fully covered by an uninterrupted flap with the sutures either on the facial or the lingual surface. A variety of suturing techniques are available; however, the interrupted vertical or horizontal mattress sutures function to keep the suture material away from the graft and are recommended to be used wherever possible.

Flap retraction should be adequate to expose the root for debridement and to expose the full extent of the osseous defect. With complete removal of the granulation tissue, the lesion can be visualized to permit definitive root planing. This must be done thoroughly to remove all remnants of calculus and any softened or demineralized root surface. Any pits or gross irregularities of the root surface should be planed thoroughly to reduce concavities, irregularities, or sharp convexities. Thorough debridement of the lesion also permits inspection of the osseous side of the defect. The graft material is then reduced to the appropriate size and is inserted into the prepared site as it is received from the bank. The flap is sutured into place. It is important to completely cover the site with the flap.

Predictability

Predictability is related to the number of walls of bone surrounding an infrabony lesion, the amount of root surface exposed, the flap coverage, and the elimination of root infection and deposits. One tooth wall surrounded by three osseous walls represents the ideal relationship in that it maximizes the vascularized osseous wall dimension versus the avascular tooth wall. For that reason, many graft

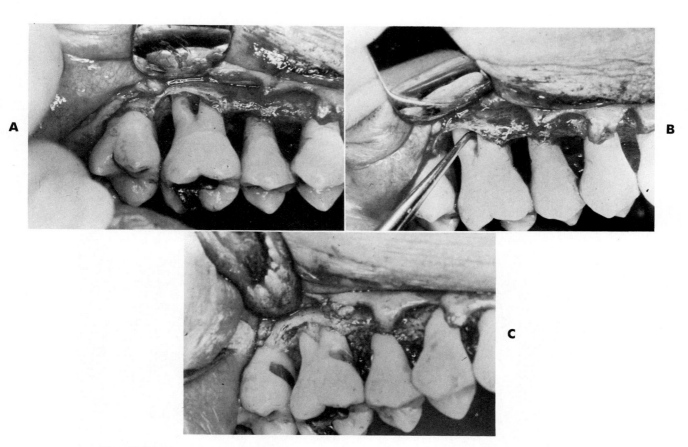

Fig. 48-9. Illustration of grafting in a trifurcation lesion on maxillary first molar. **A,** Surgical photograph at time of transplant showing open buccal furcation. **B,** Probe in buccal furcation extends to distal furcation. Bone and marrow extraoral autograft placed to fill trifurcation lesion after complete degranulation, root planing, and fenestration of bone into marrow. **C,** Appearance 1 year later showing bone fill in buccal furcation and leveling of alveolar crestal bone mesially and distally. (From Schallhorn RG and Hiatt WH: J Periodontol 43:67, 1972.)

procedures have been successfully demonstrated in this configuration; however, thorough debridement of these three-walled lesions is also successful with no graft. The worst case is when only one vascularized osseous wall faces three avascular tooth walls, as in a Class III furcation. In this situation healing with fill is rarely observed except in acute lesions of short duration.

Even though predictability remains to be demonstrated in all lesions, success has been observed. While bone and marrow have usually been used for grafts in these lesions, some newer graft materials have shown promise. The lesions presented here include trifurcation (Fig. 48-9); bifurcation; facial dehiscence; broad three-tooth, three–osseous wall lesions; cementoenamel relationship discrepancies; and teeth that have undergone root amputation procedures. Fig. 48-10 illustrates supracrestal bone fill and histologic new attachment after implantation of autograft bone and marrow in an infrabony defect that was overfilled. These cases illustrate the potential for bone and marrow to lead to new attachment in bony periodontal defects. For all re-

generative procedures, however, carefully controlled, double-blind studies are needed to establish the optimal combination of antiinfective and regenerative therapy necessary for predictable healing.

Free gingival graft and repositioned flap in periodontal regenerative therapy

The free gingival graft and repositioned flap are often appropriate when one root surface is exposed because of loss of bone and soft tissue covering. This can be accomplished with a lateral sliding flap or pedicle graft or, when such tissue is not available, often by coronal repositioning after a free gingival graft (see Chapter 47 for illustrations of these procedures).

POSTOPERATIVE MANAGEMENT

It is important that patients be thoroughly instructed in home care techniques before surgery if they are to be comfortable in continuing these practices in a sensitive postsurgical environment. It is also important that patients be seen

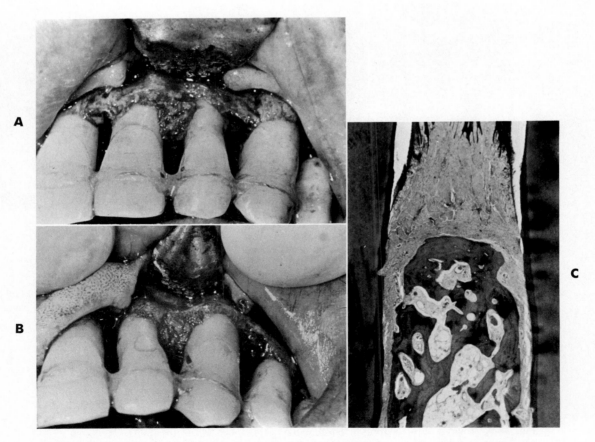

Fig. 48-10. Histologic evidence of new attachment in an infrabony lesion filled with extraoral bone and marrow. **A,** Presurgical photograph showing crestal lesion between canine and lateral incisor. **B,** Bone and marrow implanted to overfill lesion. **C,** Histologic evidence of supracrestal bone formation above notch that was placed at crestal extent of infrabony pocket. This illustrates new attachment apparatus formation supracrestally. (From Dragoo MR and Sullivan HC: J Periodontol 44:599, 1973.)

frequently during the first month postoperatively, usually once a week, so that they are encouraged to follow instructions. Use of chlorhexidine mouth rinses twice daily after 2 to 4 weeks will aid in this important healing phase. Human histologic observations have suggested that when bone and marrow are used, the marrow cells are replaced by new endothelial and connective tissue formation during the first 2 to 3 weeks. It has also been established that improved repair of the lesion occurs when the patient is protected by antibiotic therapy, such as tetracycline, during this period.

Ice and one of the antiinflammatory agents, including the nonsteroidal antiinflammatory agents, may be useful in reducing inflammation and in controlling pain and swelling. Often this regimen reduces the need for other pain medications.

WOUND HEALING

A series of cases are presented here to follow the events of wound healing from the day of grafting and initial healing, to the time when new cementum and bone form with a functional ligament, to a long-term 6½-year case. These histologic observations demonstrate new attachment, as well as healing by repair with a long junctional epithelium.

It is important to understand the histologic evidence for wound healing, which results in the return of hard and soft structures lost in the disease process. To date, histologic studies have been done on nearly 200 treated cases. Many of those cases treated by grafting showed evidence of new bone, ligament, and cementum formation. However, some of those treated by nongraft methods also showed new bone, ligament, and cementum formation.

It should be noted that in all comparative histologic studies to date, the results have strongly favored grafting. For example, in a study based on histologic evaluation of 100 human block sections and extracted teeth taken from sites treated with bone and marrow autografts and allograft and nongraft regenerative procedures, it was found that graft procedures resulted in new cementum formation in 86% of sites, whereas nongraft procedures resulted in new cementum in 33% of sites (Hiatt et al., 1986). Furthermore, new bone formation was observed in 85% of sites grafted and 33% of sites not grafted. It was concluded that the potential for regeneration of a functional attachment apparatus was qualitatively observed in autograft and allograft procedures and that no adverse tissue responses could be detected at the clinical or histologic level. Furthermore, there was no ankylosis or root resorption noted with fresh intraoral donor material or with frozen iliac, autograft, or allograft materials. However, root resorption was noted in 6% of sites treated with fresh iliac autograft material.

Some of the early events in healing of the periodontal lesion help the clinician by demonstrating the time involved and the structures seen in early attachment and suggest criteria for postoperative management and evaluation.

Some interesting highlights seen in 3 days are beginning revascularization and new connective tissue formation. After 1 week cell activity occurs at the decorticated area and empty lacunae are present in the graft material, suggesting death of the osteocytes (Fig. 48-11). At 2 weeks there is both osteoclastic and osteoblastic activity, with beginning cementogenesis and osteogenesis (Fig 48-11). At 3 weeks cementogenesis is noted, as well as osteogenesis adjacent to the marrow vascular spaces, suggesting primitive loose connective tissue differentiation into appropriate cell forms.

At 1 month (Fig. 48-11) remnants of the graft appear to be lining up beside a loose connective tissue attachment to the tooth. Reduced inflammation is noted at 1 and 2 months, and at 3 months (Fig. 48-11) new cementum appears, with fibers of the newly forming ligament embedded. At 3 months the ligament appears to be functionally oriented, attaching to both bone and cementum (Fig. 48-11).

In the autogenous bone and marrow case illustrated in Fig. 48-12, which was obtained for sectioning after 6½ years, several important features of regeneration by new attachment and repair are illustrated. Note the evidence of Sharpey's fiber penetration into new cementum, continuous apposition of cementum, and the connective tissue/long junctional epithelial attachment coronal to the new cementum formation. New bone formation at the base of the lesion, cementum formation, and repair to the root surface in the form of a connective tissue attachment to the planed dentin are demonstrated in this case. Also, at the most coronal portion of the lesion repair with a junctional epithelial attachment is observed.

Ankylosis and root resorption

Ankylosis has rarely been clinically observed in humans treated by regenerative therapy; however, ankylosis is difficult to assess clinically, especially if it occurs only in the region of the regeneration procedure. Root resorption is more commonly observed clinically and may even prepare the root in some instances for cementogenesis to follow. Root resorption was noted particularly in those instances where fresh iliac material was used without storage in the refrigerator for 3 to 5 days or without freezing. It was assumed that fresh iliac material is so highly inductive that both clast as well as blast activity was stimulated more than in other graft materials or in the same material used after storage. It has been observed clinically that frequent curettage of the resorbed area, particularly in the crestal areas of newly forming bone, often reverses the process (Dragoo and Sullivan, 1973). The occurrence of ankylosis and root resorption after root surface decalcification and flap procedures and after barrier membrane procedures is not known, since sufficient time has not elapsed to evaluate this potential complication.

Four cases of root resorption have been selected to il-

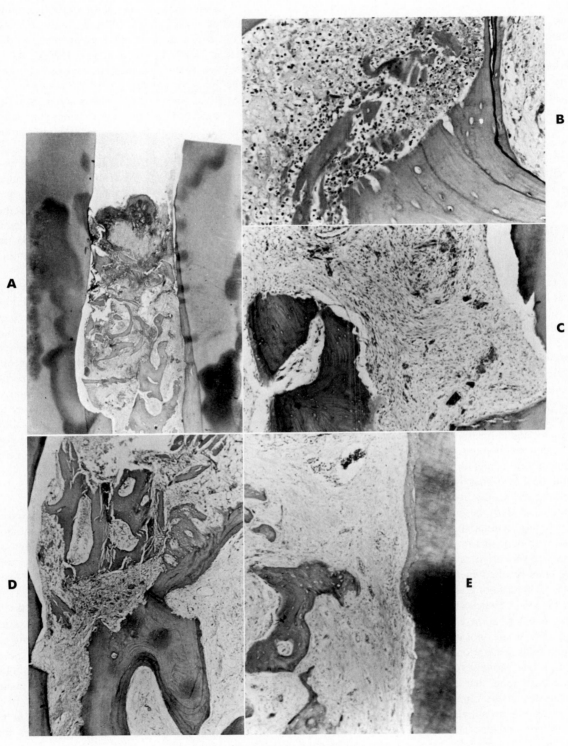

Fig. 48-11. For legend see opposite page.

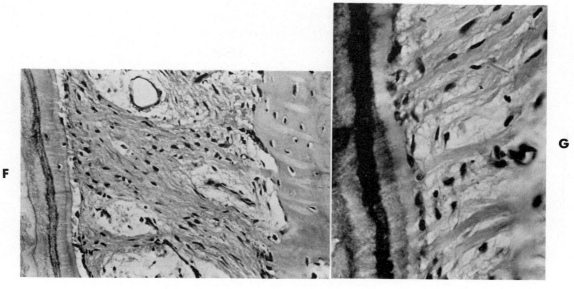

Fig. 48-11. Healing of infrabony lesions 1 week to 3 months after grafting with autogenous bone and marrow. **A,** Interproximal area 1 week after grafting. Note notch on tooth at left and graft material in area of notch. **B,** High-power view of graft and surrounding tissue at 1 week. Note empty lacunae in graft. **C,** View 3 weeks after graft. Note connective tissue in notch of tooth at right and resorption of graft material. **D,** Note remnant of graft at top and notch in tooth at bottom with loose connective tissue between the two. **E,** Healing after 56 days. Note persistence of remnants of graft and little or no inflammation. Also note resorption lacunae and new cementum on dentin at right. **F,** View 3 months after healing. Note new cementum on dentin at left and new periodontal ligament with fibers oriented in a horizontal manner from bone *(right)* to connective tissue. **G,** High-power view of healing at 3 months. Dentin with new cementum layer is at left. Sharpey's fibers are inserted in cementum, as well as into bone at right. All views are from material coronal to a notch in root made at apical portion of infrabony pocket and as such represent evidence for new attachment. (From Dragoo MR and Sullivan HC: J Periodontol 44:599, 1973.)

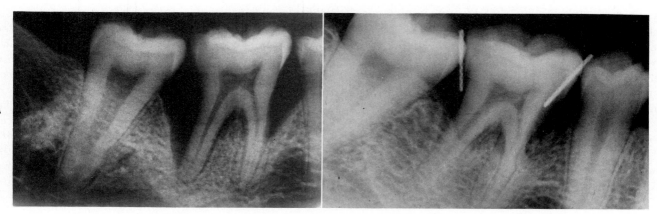

Fig. 48-12. Healing 6½ years after grafting with autogenous bone and marrow. **A,** Preoperative radiograph showing deep mesial and distal lesions with radiolucent furcation. **B,** Same area 6½ years later. Note partial bone fill of mesial and distal lesion with deep notching on surface of mesial root. (From Hiatt WH, Schallhorn RG, and Aaronian AJ: J Periodontol 49:495, 1978.)

Continued.

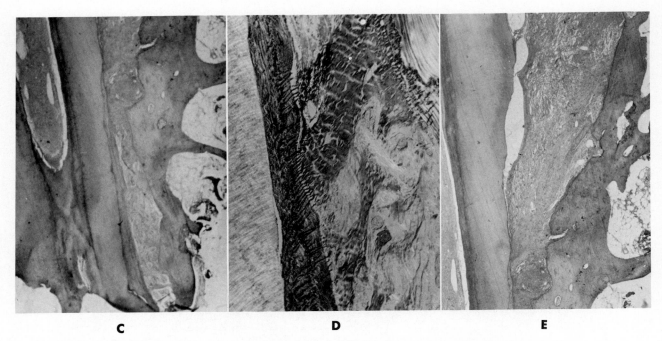

C   D   E

Fig. 48-12, cont'd. C, Section through distal root *(left)* and adjacent alveolar bone *(right)*. Note notch on bottom portion of distal root and bone fill of area adjacent and coronal to notch *(right)*. **D,** Silver stain of area (photographed with polarized light) 4 to 5 mm coronal to notch showing cementum layer with Sharpey's fibers inserted. **E,** New bone formation 2 mm above new ligament. Note connective tissue attachment to dentin and long junctional epithelium to cementoenamel junction.

lustrate the clinical course and radiographic appearance of this complication of regenerative therapy. The first (Fig. 48-13) shows resorption into the pulp chamber, followed by attempts to repair the defect through the formation of either new cementum or new bone formation and is referred to as osteocementum. Note that new cementum, ligament, and bone formed over the apical portion of the defect and that the resorption occurred at the most coronal portion.

The second case (Fig. 48-14) showing resorption into the pulp is a result of a nongraft regenerative procedure. A flap curettage procedure was done with excellent clinical

results, and 7 mm of new bone formation was achieved. Eight-and-one-half years later, resorption occurred into the pulp. It is not known whether the epithelialized granulation tissue found in the lesion produced the resorption or came after the fact. Ankylosis was not seen in this case or in over 100 human block sections.

The third and fourth cases occurred with fresh iliac material and were followed with careful maintenance procedures, including curettage of the healing defect (Fig. 48-15). In both instances the resorption appeared to be self-limiting and new bone formation occurred; both cases have been stable for over 20 years.

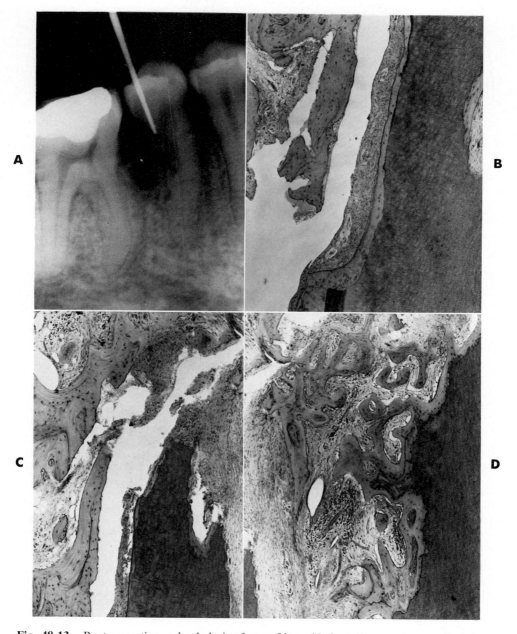

Fig. 48-13. Root resorption and ankylosis after grafting with fresh iliac crest autograft of bone and marrow. **A,** Radiograph of healed lesion 9 months after grafting demonstrating root resorption into pulp on distal aspect of second premolar. **B,** Histologic section with dentin at right and bone at left. Note termination of root planing and cellular cementum formation on root-planed root surface. **C,** Resorption into pulp *(left)*. Note extension of cellular cementum into root defect. **D,** Cellular cementum formation in pulp, with attachment to dentin surface. (From Hiatt WH, Schallhorn RG, and Aaronian AJ: J Periodontol 49: 495, 1978.)

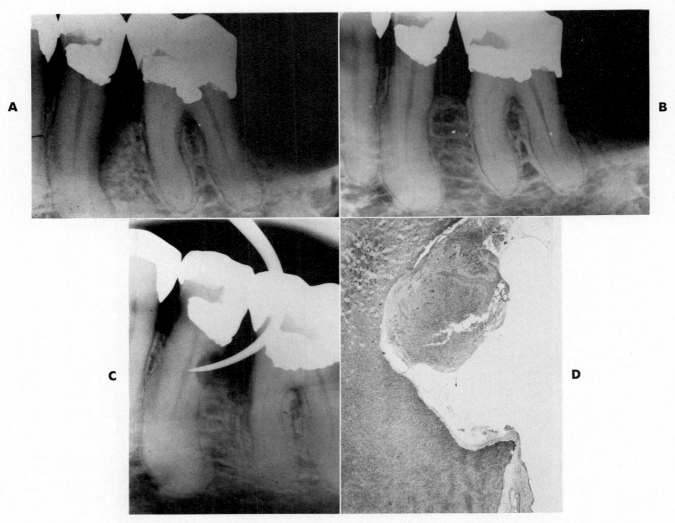

Fig. 48-14. Resorption and ankylosis of an infrabony pocket treated by Widman flap, curettage, and root planing. **A,** Pretreatment radiograph. Note vertical bony defect on distal aspect of second premolar. **B,** Posttreatment radiograph showing healing and radiographically apparent bone in area of original defect. **C,** Radiograph showing crestal root resorption on distal aspect of second premolar 8½ years after therapy. **D,** Histologic section of area of resorption with dentin at left. Note epithelium and granulation tissue in defect. (From Hiatt WH, Schallhorn RG, and Aaronian AJ: J Periodontol 49:495, 1978.)

SUMMARY

Most patients and most sites affected by periodontal disease are effectively treated by antiinfective measures directed to suppressing the pathogenic periodontal microflora and preparing the roots and gingival tissues for healing. However, some deep infrabony and furcation lesions are ideally treated with procedures designed to regenerate periodontal ligament and alveolar bone. These procedures include the use of various grafts, periodontal tissue regeneration with barrier membranes, various chemical root treatments, and coronally repositioned flaps. Many of these procedures have shown great promise in the treatment of severe periodontal lesions that jeopardize the longevity of the teeth.

Controlled, double-blind studies are needed to determine the predictability of periodontal regeneration; the prevalence and nature of adverse side effects, such as ankylosis and root resorption; and the relative efficacy of these regenerative procedures compared with alternate treatments. However, regenerative procedures hold great promise, since they are often more successful than scaling and root planing in deep infrabony pockets and furcation lesions.

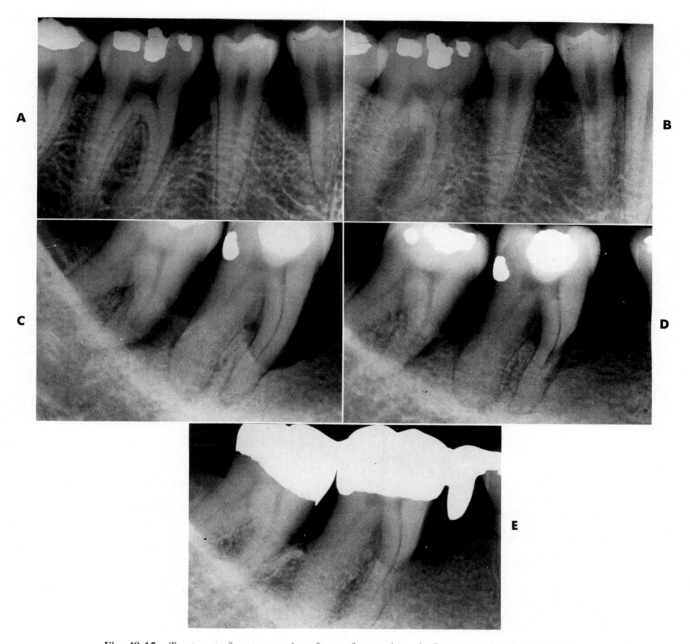

Fig. 48-15. Treatment of root resorption after graft procedure. **A,** Pretreatment radiograph showing mesial infrabony defect on molar and distal infrabony defect on first premolar. Both were treated with fresh iliac crest bone and marrow grafts. **B,** Radiograph 6 years after treatment. Note radiographically apparent bone fill of both lesions and repaired root resorption on distal aspect of premolar after root debridement. **C,** Pretreatment radiograph of another case in which mesial infrabony defects were treated with autogenous iliac crest bone and marrow grafts. **D,** Posttreatment radiograph showing evidence of bone fill of lesions and root resorption on mesial aspect of first molar. **E,** Radiograph 20 years postoperatively showing appearance of bone healed into mesial resorption area.

ACKNOWLEDGMENT

We wish to thank Dr. James Mellonig for his advice and assistance in preparing this chapter.

REFERENCES

Barth A: Histologische Untersuchungen über Knochenimplantationen, Beitr Pathol Anat 17:65, 1895.

Becker W et al: New attachment after treatment with root isolation procedures: report of treated Class III and Class II furcations and vertical osseous defects, Int J Periodontics Restorative Dent 5:9, 1985.

Blumenthal N, Sabet T, and Barrington E: Healing responses to grafting of combined collagen-decalcified bone in periodontal defects in dogs, J Periodontol 57:84, 1986.

Burwell RG: The function of bone marrow in the incorporation of a bone graft, Clin Orthop 200:125, 1985.

Caton J, Nyman S, and Zander H: Histometric evaluation of periodontal surgery. II. Connective tissue attachment levels after four regenerative procedures, J Clin Periodontol 7:224, 1980.

Crigger M et al: The effect of topical citric acid application on the healing of experimental furcation defects in dogs, J Periodont Res 13:538, 1978.

Dragoo MR and Sullivan HC: A clinical and histologic evaluation of autogenous iliac bone grafts in humans. I. Wound healing 2 to 8 months, J Periodontol 44:599, 1973.

Egelberg J: Regeneration and repair of periodontal tissues, J Periodont Res 22:233, 1987.

Ellegaard B et al: New attachment after treatment of intrabony defects in monkeys, J Periodontol 45:368, 1974.

Farley JR et al: Human skeletal growth factor: characterization of the mitogenic effect on bone cells in vitro, Biochemistry 21:3508, 1982.

Froum S et al: Human clinical and histological responses to durapatite implants in intraosseous lesions: case reports, J Periodontol 52:680, 1981.

Froum S et al: Osseous autografts. III. Comparison of osseous coagulum-bone blend implants with open curettage, J Periodontol 47:287, 1986.

Gantes B et al: Treatment of periodontal furcation defects. II. Bone regeneration in mandibular class II defects, J Clin Periodontol 15:232, 1988.

Glimcher MJ and Krane SM: The organization and structure of bone and the mechanism of calcification. In Gould BS, editor: A treatise on collagen, vol II, New York, 1968, Academic Press, Inc.

Goldman HM and Cohen DW: The infrabony pocket: classification and treatment, J Periodontol 29:272, 1958.

Hancock E: Regeneration procedures. In American Academy of Periodontology: Proceedings of World Workshop in Clinical Periodontics, Chicago, 1989, The Academy.

Hench LL and Wilson J: Surface-active biomaterials, Science 226:630, 1984.

Hiatt WH: The induction of new bone and cementum formation. III. Utilizing bone and marrow allografts in dogs, J Periodontol 41:596, 1970.

Hiatt WH: Pulpal periodontal disease, J Periodontol 48:598, 1977.

Hiatt WH, Schallhorn RG, and Aaronian, AJ: The induction of new bone and cementum formation. IV. Microscopic examination of the periodontium following human bone and marrow allograft, autograft, and non-graft periodontal regenerative procedures, J Periodontol 49:495, 1978.

Hiatt WH, Solomons CC, and Butler ED: The induction of new bone and cementum formation. II. Utilizing a collagen extract of ox bone, J Periodontol 41:273, 1970.

Hiatt WH et al: The induction of new bone and cementum formation. V. A comparison of graft and control sites in deep intrabony periodontal lesions, Int J Periodontics Restorative Dent 6:8, 1986.

Hirschfeld L and Wasserman BA: A long term survey of tooth loss in 600 treated periodontal patients, J Periodontol 49:495, 1978.

Klinge B, Nilveus R, and Boyle G: Effect of implants on healing of experimental furcation defects in dogs, J Clin Periodontol 12:321, 1985.

Listgarten MA and Rosenberg MM: Histological study of repair following new attachment procedures in human periodontal lesions, J Periodontol 50:333, 1979.

Martin M et al: Treatment of periodontal furcation defects. I. Review of the literature and description of a regenerative surgical technique, J Clin Periodontol 15:227, 1987.

McFall WT: Tooth loss in 100 treated patients with periodontal disease: a long term study, J Periodontol 53:539, 1982.

Meffert RM et al: Hydroxyapatite as an alloplastic graft in the treatment of human periodontal osseous defects, J Periodontol 56:63, 1985.

Nilveus R and Egelberg J: The effect of topical citric acid application on the healing of experimental furcation defects in dogs. III. The relative importance of coagulum support, flap design, and systemic antibiotics, J Periodont Res 15:551, 1980.

Pontoriero R et al: Guided tissue regeneration in degree II furcation–involved mandibular molars, J Clin Periodontol 15:247, 1988.

Pontoriero R et al: Guided tissue regeneration in the treatment of furcation defects in mandibular molars: a clinical study of degree III involvements, J Clin Periodontol 16:170, 1989.

Prichard J: The infrabony technique as a predictable procedure, J Periodontol 28:202, 1957.

Rabalais M, Yukna RA, and Mayer ET: Evaluation of durapatite ceramic as an alloplastic implant. I. Six-month results, J Periodontol 52:680, 1981.

Ramfjord SP: Present status of the modified Widman flap procedure, J Periodontol 48:9, 1977.

Schallhorn RG and Hiatt WH: Human allografts of iliac cancellous bone and marrow in periodontal osseous defects. II. Clinical observations, J Periodontol 43:67, 1972.

Schallhorn RG and McClain PK: Combined osseous composite grafting, root conditioning, and guided tissue regeneration, Int J Periodontics Restorative Dent 8:9, 1988.

Schrad SC and Tussing GJ: Human allografts of iliac bone and marrow in periodontal osseous defects, J Periodontol 57:205, 1986.

Svardstrom G and Wennstrom JL: Furcation topography of the maxillary and mandibular first molars, J Clin Periodontol 15:271, 1988.

Urist MR et al: The bone induction principle, Clin Orthop 53:243, 1967.

Yukna RA and Williams JE: Five year evaluation of the excisional new attachment procedures, J Periodontol 51:382, 1980.

Chapter 49

RELATIONSHIP BETWEEN PULPAL AND PERIODONTAL DISEASES

Louis E. Rossman

Diagnosis
    Pain
    Swelling
    Probing
    Mobility
    Tests
    Radiographs
Effects of pulpal diseases on the periodontium
    Fistulation
    Dentinal tubules
    Lateral canals
Effects of periodontal diseases on the pulp
    Atrophic changes
Microbiology
Classification of periodontal-endodontic problems
    Primary endodontic lesion
    Primary endodontic lesion with secondary periodontal
      involvement
    Primary periodontal lesion
    Primary periodontal lesion with secondary endodontic
      involvement
    True combined lesion

Inflammation of the supporting tissues with deep pockets along the side of the root, suppuration from these pockets, swelling and bleeding of the gingiva, fistula formation, tenderness to percussion, increased tooth mobility, and angular bone loss are most often associated with periodontitis, which begins at the margin of the gingiva and proceeds apically. However, these same signs and symptoms may be caused by pulpal infections that have entered the periodontal ligament either through the apical foramen or through the lateral canals. Pulpal irritants and infections cause lesions that are often difficult to distinguish from those caused by marginal periodontal infections. Differentiation of pulpal infections is possible, since pulpal infections most often produce severe pain that is localized to the tooth. Symptoms of plaque-associated infectious periodontitis are usually minor, and signs of disease are confined to the marginal periodontium. When these lesions occur as combined lesions (i.e., pulpal infection proceeding to periodontal infection), they are more difficult to diagnose. Furthermore, periodontal disease and periodontal treatment may cause pulpal changes, and proper diagnosis of these is also important.

In this chapter, the effects of pulpal disease on the periodontium, the effects of periodontal diseases on the pulp, classification of periodontal/endodontic problems, and their sequelae, treatment, and diagnosis are presented.

DIAGNOSIS

There are several signs and symptoms of pulpal and periodontal lesions that allow them to be distinguished. These include pain; swelling; periodontal probing; tooth mobility; percussion on palpation; pulp tests, including thermal, electric, and preparation of the test cavity; and radiographic interpretation.

Pain

Pain of endodontic origin is usually acute in onset and severe. It can occur spontaneously during the early stages of pulpal inflammation when there is poor localization, and the pain may be referred to other sites. Pain intensifies and localizes once the inflammation spreads to the periodontal ligament and surrounding osseous structures. Often, potent analgesics are not adequate to control endodontic pain, which can at times awaken the person from sleep. Endodontic pain can often be eliminated only by root canal treatment.

Pain of periodontal origin is chronic and usually mild or moderate, responding to mild analgesics. If an acute flare-up occurs, creating a periodontal abscess, pain can be severe. This severe pain often regresses following drainage. It does not awaken a patient from sleep.

Combined pulpal-periodontal infections usually exhibit minimal pain. Enough periodontal tissue loss occurs to open an avenue of drainage through the gingival sulcus, thereby minimizing pressure and pain.

Swelling

Swelling caused by endodontic infections often occurs in the mucobuccal fold or spreads to the facial planes. Muscle attachments and root length determine the route of drainage. Swelling associated with periodontal problems is characteristically found in the attached gingiva and rarely spreads beyond the mucogingival line, and most often no facial swelling is involved.

Probing

The presence of a sinus tract often allows a diagnosis of the problem. A radiograph taken with a gutta-percha point or fine wire threaded into the orifice of the fistula reveals the source. When the tracing goes to the apex of the tooth, the fistula is of endodontic origin. When the traced fistula goes to the midroot, furcation, or any other portion of the tooth, a lateral canal (Rossman et al., 1982) or periodontal problem is diagnosed (Fuss et al., 1986).

When endodontic problems develop into a periapical abscess, an escape route is made through a fistula. Therefore sulcular probing is always along a narrow single tract,

and conventional periodontal probes cannot determine the origin of the sinus tract. Periodontal problems, on the other hand, are more chronic, and the progressive bone loss from the margin to the apex creates periodontal ligament loss and often allows probing to the apex. Periodontal probing to the apex hence may not indicate a pulpal lesion (Fig. 49-1). The results of pulp testing are necessary to diagnose the origin of such lesions, since if the lesion is periodontal in origin, the pulp is most often vital.

Mobility

When mobility is present around one isolated tooth, the source of the problem can be either endodontic or periodontal. In the acute stage it is often of endodontic origin. Generalized mobility involving many teeth suggests a probable periodontal or occlusal origin.

Tests

Percussion and palpation.   Results of these tests are usually negative in an individual tooth with a periodontal problem. When a periodontal abscess is present, these clinical entities may be positive; however, other tests indicate a vital pulp. A tooth with an endodontic problem produces definite tenderness and pain on percussion and palpation.

Cold.   The normal response of a healthy pulp is immediate and disappears when the stimulus is removed. If there is no response or the pain lingers once the stimulus is removed, the pulp is necrotic or irreversibly inflamed. This is a one-time test because the pulp requires time to recover before it will respond again. Dichlorodifluoromethane (Frigident) should be used because it creates rapid fluid movement in the dentinal tubules better than any other cold substance (Fuss et al., 1986). This modality

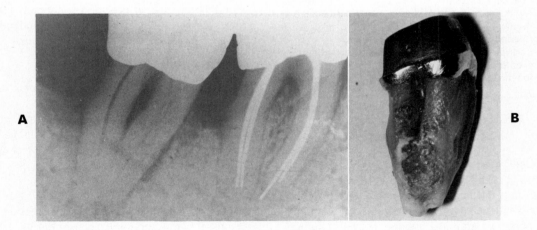

Fig. 49-1.   Primary periodontal lesion. **A,** Mandibular third molar with periapical radiolucency and minimal pain. Observe that borders of lesion are wider at gingival margin and that adjacent teeth have periodontal problems. Thermal testing and test cavity demonstrated pulp vitality. Periodontal probing to apex was done. **B,** Extraction of tooth revealed that source of periapical radiolucency was of periodontal origin—calculus formation secondary to a fused root and furcation breakdown. (Restorative therapy by Dr. M. Amsterdam.)

can also be used on teeth with metal crowns (Augsburger and Peters, 1981), and often it is effective with porcelain crowns.

Electric. This test is viewed as a yes or no response: there is vitality or no vitality. It does not indicate the status of the pulp (Seltzer and Bender, 1984). If there is no response, the pulp is necrotic and root canal therapy is required. However, one should not rely on one pulp test. Rubber gloves will not allow the passage of current, and the circuit will not be completed; hence electric pulp tests should be carried out with an ungloved hand (Cooley et al., 1984).

Heat. The normal response of a healthy pulp is pain that increases in intensity until the stimulus is removed. Once the heat is removed, the pain disappears immediately. Lingering pain indicates an irreversibly inflamed pulp. When pain persists after removal of the heat stimulus from periodontally involved teeth, pulpitis should be suspected (Seltzer and Bender, 1984). Hot gutta-percha should be applied to the tooth coated with petroleum jelly to prevent the material from sticking to the tooth surface. If a crown is present, a rotating rubber prophylaxis cup can be run on a dried tooth to create heat.

Test cavity. This test should be done without anesthesia. Access is made through a crown or through the enamel to determine whether vitality is present in the pulp. No response indicates necrosis of the pulp. This test does not give information as to the status of the pulp other than whether or not it is vital. These results are similar to the results obtained with the electric pulp test.

Radiographs

Periodontal and endodontic problems can radiographically mimic each other; therefore pulp testing and periodontal probing must be used along with the radiograph. If bone loss exists around one tooth in an otherwise periodontally healthy patient and pulp tests are negative, then this loss of bone may be of endodontic origin. The prognosis is excellent for regeneration of these structures. If there is a periapical radiolucency and the pulp tests necrotic, then the lesion may also be of endodontic origin.

Periodontally susceptible patients may exhibit lesions that appear to be of pulpal origin but are not. When bone loss exists in this situation and pulp test results are normal, the lesion is of periodontal origin. Periapical radiographic lesions can sometimes be of periodontal origin. These can occur with fused root or cementoenamel grooves (Fig. 49-1). Lesions of occlusal trauma can also be observed as radiolucencies around the apex of the tooth; however, the pulp will prove to be vital.

Radiographs are also helpful in determining the quality of a previous root canal treatment. If the etiology is questionable and there is any doubt as to the quality of previous root canal treatment, then retreatment should be considered.

EFFECTS OF PULPAL DISEASES ON THE PERIODONTIUM

The functions of the dental pulp include formative, protective, and reparative responses. The protective response is mediated by the neural and vascular elements of the pulp. Amsterdam (1974) has pointed out that the best root canal filling is healthy pulp tissue, and every effort should be made to preserve its integrity and to avoid unnecessary endodontic procedures.

Fistulation

A fistula, also called a sinus tract, is nature's way of allowing pus to escape when a chronic apical or lateral periodontitis is present. Pus seeks the easiest way out of the bone, with the resulting fistula usually appearing on either the buccal or lingual mucosa. The fistula often cannot be detected radiographically, because its path parallels the x-ray beam. When, however, the fistula occurs along the periodontal ligament, the radiographic appearance may mimic an infrabony defect or furcation involvement because the osseous lesion, created by the bone erosion that is not masked by the root, is perpendicular to the x-ray beam (Bender, 1982) (Fig. 49-2).

Pain is usually absent in the presence of a fistula, since it provides drainage. The diagnosis of its source can be aided by tracing the fistula with a gutta-percha point, fine orthodontic wire, or a silver point (Bender and Seltzer, 1961). A radiograph taken with the traced fistula reveals the source of the abscess. When the fistula is traced to the radiographic apex, the endodontic etiology can be confirmed by failure of the tooth to respond to electric or cold test procedures (Fuss et al., 1986). When the fistula is traced to the midroot, periodontal etiology or pulp necrosis in a lateral canal must be considered in the differential diagnosis (Rossman et al., 1982) (Fig. 49-3). When root canal treatment has already been performed, then an incomplete root fracture or a perforation must be suspected (Rossman and Rossman, 1981). The latter suspicion is aroused when there is overzealous instrumentation with marked enlargement of the root canal or a large post.

Periodontal abscesses can also drain through the gingival sulcus as a fistula. Tracing a fistula of periodontal origin usually demonstrates that the apex of the tooth is not involved. A positive response to pulp testing usually indicates vitality (Seltzer and Bender, 1984; Fuss et al., 1986).

Dentinal tubules

Dentinal tubules contain cytoplasmic extensions, the odontoblastic process, that extend from the odontoblasts at the pulpal dentin border to the dentinoenamel junction or dentinocementum junction. When dentin is cut, either by a bur or a curette, it reacts in the same manner as any other tissue in the body. There is an initial injury followed by an inflammatory response, concluding with a healing phase.

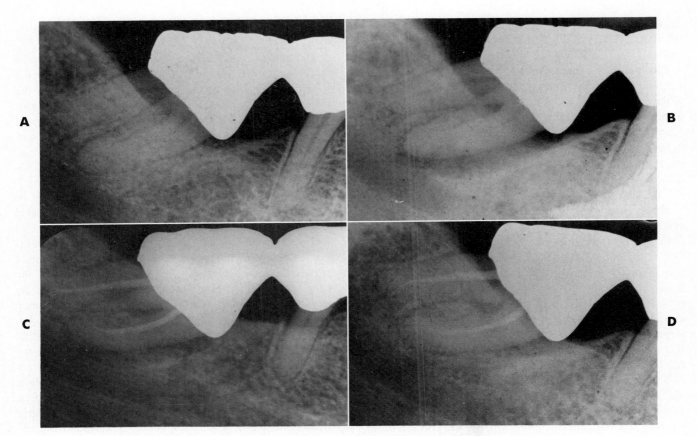

Fig. 49-2. Mandibular third molar. **A,** Postoperative radiograph following completion of posterior reconstruction. **B,** View 10 years later. Patient had drainage through a fistula and gingival swelling with periodontal probing to apex. Thermal testing and test cavity revealed no response. Note that radiographic appearance mimics an infrabony defect; however, adjacent teeth had no periodontal problems. **C,** Posttreatment view. Endodontic therapy alone was completed. No periodontal therapy and no root planing were performed. **D,** View at 8-year recall with complete osseous regeneration of mesial defect. (Restorative therapy by Dr. M. Amsterdam.)

Communication through dentinal tubules was demonstrated by Seltzer et al. (1967) in dogs and monkeys, in which interradicular changes in the periodontium were demonstrated following pulpotomy and placement of caustic agents in the pulp chamber. Communication in the other direction is demonstrated by the inflammatory reaction of the pulp to exposure of dentinal tubules after the protective layer of enamel or cementum has been removed with a bur or a curette (Trowbridge, 1981). The effect of periodontal disease on the dental pulp was first described by Turner and Drew in 1918. Cahn in 1927 and later Sicher (1936) described the presence of communicating channels, and these have been under active study ever since.

A pathologic condition that illustrates this intercommunication is inflammatory root resorption. This occurs following avulsion or replantation of the tooth because of injury to the periodontal ligament and necrosis of the pulp with the presence of bacteria in the root canal system (An-

dreasen, 1981). The result is quickly developing, large resorptive lacunae along the lateral aspect of the root despite the protection from the cementum. Experimental changes in the effects of pH on the root canal are limited to the dentinal tubules by the cementum (Tronstad et al., 1981). In immature teeth, with their wide dentinal tubules, removal of cementum facilitates rapid movement of bacterial products from the necrotic pulp to the periodontal ligament, resulting in inflammatory root resorption. In mature teeth, the tubules are much more narrow. If cementum is experimentally removed, a new basophilic layer can be formed (Andreasen, 1973).

Despite the damage to the periodontal ligament and the root surface during apical surgical or periodontal therapy, root resorption is seldom seen. Nyman et al. (1980) have shown that the downgrowth of a long junctional epithelium following reattachment procedures protects the damaged root surface. When this downgrowth is prevented, resorption and ankylosis often occur.

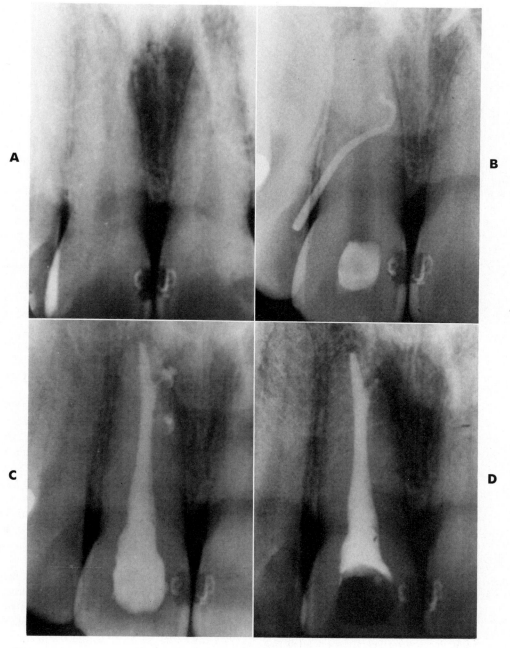

Fig. 49-3. Maxillary central incisor. **A,** Preoperative radiograph. **B,** Radiograph taken with fine gutta-percha point tracing a fistulous tract. Note origin of fistula at midpoint of root. No significant periodontal probing was observed. **C,** Posttreatment radiograph. Note bifurcated root canal and presence of lateral canal at midpoint of root. Root canal filling material now occupies apparent source of fistula. Fistula has completely healed. **D,** View at 2-year recall. Note disappearance of root canal sealer from lateral canal.

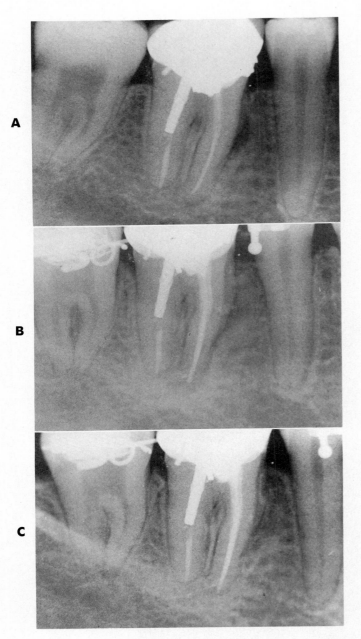

Fig. 49-4. Mandibular first molar. **A,** Pretreatment radiograph. Previous endodontic therapy was performed 3 years earlier by previous dentist. Note radiolucency on lateral aspect of mesial root, amalgam in chamber, post in distal canal, and inadequate biomechanical instrumentation of root canals. **B,** Posttreatment radiograph with root canal filling material forced into a lateral canal because tissue had become necrotic and created osseous breakdown. Distal canal was not treated conventionally, because of post. **C,** View at 7-month recall demonstrating complete regeneration of previous radiolucency.

The effect of direct dentinal communication can also be observed following free autogenous soft tissue grafts. The graft failure rate was higher when grafts were placed over untreated teeth with necrotic pulps than when they were placed over teeth with vital pulps or following successful root canal therapy (Takatsuka et al., 1984; Perlmutter et al., 1987). The bacteria and their toxins in the root canal system most likely adversely affect the ability of the soft tissue to reattach. Therefore careful assessment of pulpal status is critical for successful periodontal therapy. Another vivid example of the importance of dentinal tubules is hypersensitivity, in which the patient experiences pain to various stimuli such as cold and sweets. Pashley (1984) has suggested the use of a topical application of potassium oxylate solution that causes crystal formation within the dentinal tubules, thereby clogging these channels, to prevent fluid movement, which excites the sensory terminal nerve endings within the dentin-predentin region.

Lateral canals

The terms *lateral canal* and *accessory canal* are often used interchangeably. The glossary of the American Association of Endodontics (Cohen, 1984) makes the distinction that lateral canals run perpendicular to the main canal, whereas accessory canals branch off and run parallel to the main canal. The lateral canals are most often found in the apical third of the root and in the furcation area of multirooted teeth. Obliteration of these canals occurs naturally as part of the aging process as dentin and cementum are produced.

Rubach and Mitchell (1965) demonstrated that a large number of lateral canals exist in human teeth and showed that inflammation of the periodontal ligament can affect the dental pulp by way of these lateral canals. Weine (1984) pointed out that these lateral canals rarely cause endodontic therapy failure. Indeed, if the lateral canal contains vital tissue, it will not appear on the postendodontic radiograph. It is sometimes possible to force cement or a filling material into a lateral canal if the tissue in the canal has become necrotic and large enough to allow penetration of filling material.

When the concentration of contaminants in a necrotic lateral canal is great enough, pain or radiographic evidence of breakdown on the lateral surface of the root can occur (Fig. 49-4). When the pulp tests indicate necrosis and a sinus tract can be traced to the lateral portion of the root, a lateral canal might be the cause of an endodontic-periodontal fistula (Rossman et al., 1982). It is advisable to keep post preparations away from areas with demonstrated lateral canals to reduce the chance of leakage and contamination.

Lateral canals from the floor of the pulp chamber to the furcation area are responsible for the intraradicular bone loss seen when caustic compounds are placed in the chamber. This stresses the importance of sealing the floor of the pulp chamber following root canal therapy.

EFFECTS OF PERIODONTAL DISEASES ON THE PULP

Bender and Seltzer (1972) found that periodontally involved human teeth have a much higher incidence of pulpal inflammation and degeneration than intact human teeth with no periodontal disease. This correlation has not been noted in animal studies, most likely because they lack lateral canals (Seltzer et al., 1963; Seltzer and Bender, 1984). The teeth of rice rats and some monkeys, for example, do not demonstrate any lateral canals.

Atrophic changes

Bender and Seltzer (1972) found that teeth with caries or restorations that also suffer from periodontal disease have more atrophic pulps than teeth with caries or restorations but no periodontal disease. Histologically, they noticed a larger collagen content in the pulp with more dentin and dystrophic calcification. Radiographically, they observed that the canal space was markedly narrowed.

The cause of these atrophic changes is the disruption of blood flow through the lateral canals, which leads to localized areas of coagulation necrosis in the pulp. These areas eventually are walled off from the healthy pulp tissue by collagen and dystrophic mineralization.

Deep scaling and root planing have the same effect on the dental pulp and have been shown to increase the rate of reparative dentinogenesis (Hattler and Listgarten, 1984). One possible explanation for this is that blood vessels leading into lateral canals are severed, causing localized areas of pulpal necrosis. Another explanation is that the removal of the protective layer of cementum exposes dentinal tubules, providing an avenue for pulpal irritation with subsequent reparative dentin deposition.

In cases of slowly advancing periodontal disease, cementum deposition may act to obliterate a lateral canal before pulpal irritation occurs. This, along with the absence of lateral canals, may explain why not all periodontally involved teeth demonstrate pulpal atrophy and canal narrowing.

MICROBIOLOGY

Bacteria play an important role in the pathogenesis of both periodontal disease and caries. Trope et al. (1987) have suggested the use of darkfield microscopy as a diagnostic aid in the diagnosis of the combined endodontic-periodontal lesion. The routine periodontal problem has a greater percentage of spirochetes than the endodontic lesion draining through the sinus tract. Inflammatory changes in the pulp have been described following placement of lyophilized plaque on dentin (Bergenholtz and Lindhe, 1975). Trowbridge (1981) has described inflammation of the dental pulp due to bacterial products and toxins. When caries is removed, dead tracts that have been formed are sealed off by the remaining vital odontoblasts by elaborating reparative dentin. The dead tracts are not as highly mineralized as sclerotic dentin. In the presence of dead tracts, caries progresses more rapidly.

Given the right combination of periodontal and cariogenic pathogens, root caries develops, often rapidly. Endodontic complications with root caries include calcification at the level of the caries, thereby blocking access into the canal, and an inability to isolate the tooth and create a sterile operating environment. The most difficult problems occur when an acute or chronic apical periodontitis occurs as a result of pulpal necrosis.

Asymptomatic periapical areas around teeth with root caries are also often difficult to manage. Initiation of endodontic therapy can trigger an acute exacerbation of a chronic apical periodontitis, with pain and swelling. These abscesses are known as a recrudescent or "phoenix" abscess. The loss of pulpal vitality allows invading bacteria to penetrate the root canal and freely develop a periapical abscess. The future of endodontics in this area may be toward the development of an intracanal medicament to aid in the destruction of bacteria that have penetrated the dentinal tubules. The use of the ultrasonic instruments may also aid in the cleaning of these bacteria-laden canals.

CLASSIFICATION OF PERIODONTAL-ENDODONTIC PROBLEMS

Different systems have been developed for classification of endodontic and periodontal problems (Oliet and Pollock, 1968; Simon et al., 1972; Guldener, 1985; Mori, 1987; Whyman, 1988a, 1988b). When examining and treating the combined or individual problems in endodontics and periodontics, one must bear in mind that teeth are often in their terminal stage and that successful treatment depends on a correct diagnosis (Goldman and Schilder, 1988). Diagnosis and treatment methods are presented below.

Primary endodontic lesion

Sequelae. A primary endodontic lesion is one that manifests a necrotic pulp with a chronic apical periodontitis and a draining sinus tract. The sinus tract in these cases drains through the periodontal ligament of the furcation or the gingival sulcus. Usually the radiograph reveals an isolated periodontal problem around an individual tooth. There is no associated generalized periodontal disease, and osseous destruction involves this one tooth only (Fig. 49-5). If a buccal or lingual swelling appears, a lateral canal should be considered. Swelling in the mucobuccal fold is pathognomonic for endodontic disease.

Tests. Confirmation of the diagnosis comes from negative pulp vitality tests. The electric pulp test, thermal tests, and test cavity usually reveal no response. Periodontal probing is within normal limits throughout the patient's mouth. This type of lesion develops rapidly and presents a dramatic change, sometimes within a short period of time, even between regular dental appointments. Probing the gingival sulcus with a flexible probe, gutta-percha point, or fine silver point or wire often reveals the presence of a

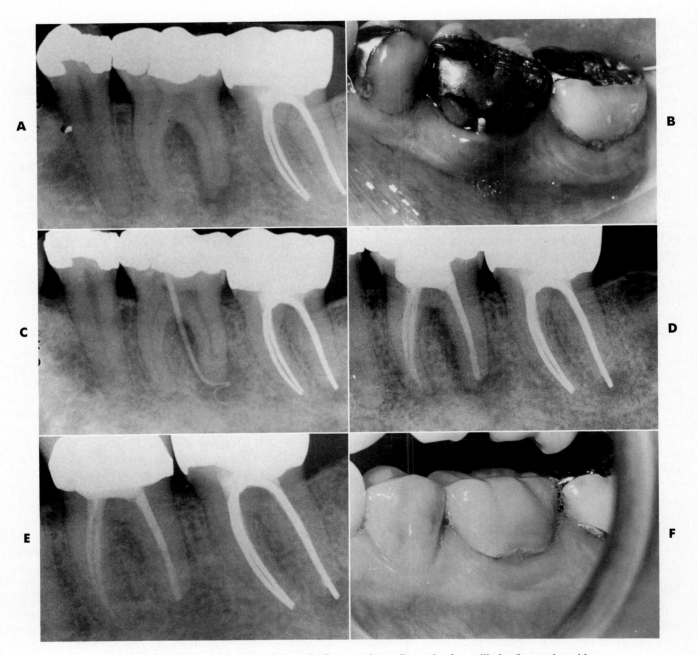

Fig. 49-5. Primary endodontic lesion. **A,** Preoperative radiograph of mandibular first molar with radiolucency along distal root, giving appearance of periodontal disease with osseous breakdown in furcation. **B,** Fine gutta-percha point placed into only probeable tract on direct buccal aspect. Thermal tests and test cavity confirmed necrotic pulp. **C,** Radiograph of fine gutta-percha point revealing root canal as source of draining abscess. Note that osseous destruction involves this one tooth. **D,** Posttreatment radiograph. No periodontal probing was obtained before obturation of root canals. No root planing was performed. **E,** View at 5½-year recall after endodontic therapy only. Furcation and surrounding osseous structures about distal root have regenerated. **F,** Appearance of gingival tissues and new restoration at 5½-year recall. (Restorative therapy by Dr. H. Silverstein.)

sinus tract. When the sinus tract is of endodontic origin, generally only one wire can be inserted, whereas if the lesion is of periodontal origin, multiple wires or diagnostic probes can be inserted. Conventional periodontal probes for this diagnosis are of limited value. Tracing the fistula often reveals that the origin is at the apex of the tooth. It also may go to the midroot, and a lateral canal may be involved. However, this region usually manifests a rarefied region.

Treatment.   Treatment consists of conservative or conventional root canal therapy. Root canal therapy should be performed with multiple appointments so that a reevaluation of the healing process between the completion of root canal debridement and obturation visits can be made. A fistulous tract usually heals following instrumentation and irrigation of the root canal. The closure of the tract and the elimination of probing depth indicate that the root canal has been properly cleansed, and the prognosis is excellent.

No root planing should be done when the fistulous tract is along the periodontal ligament. It is important to preserve these fibers so that reattachment can occur. If root planing and curettage are performed, the prognosis may be greatly reduced.

Prognosis.   The prognosis is excellent. The radiographic and clinical healing that occurs is rapid and quite spectacular. Healing is usually accomplished within 3 to 6 months.

Primary endodontic lesion with secondary periodontal involvement

Sequelae.   If the primary endodontic lesion with a sinus tract is not diagnosed and treated early, plaque and calculus often form in the draining fistulous tract, creating a secondary periodontal problem. This usually appears when healing with closure does not take place.

Tests.   Pulp vitality tests are negative. There is no response to the electric or thermal pulp test or test cavity. Probing the fistulous tract reveals the presence of plaque and calculus. Usually the coronal portion of the fistula resembles a more chronic periodontal problem such as is observed in a periodontal pocket.

Treatment.   Good, conservative endodontics must be performed. Periodontal therapy is necessary, usually in the form of root planing to eliminate the calculus and pathogenic flora. Root planing, however, should not be initiated until complete debridement of the root canal system has been performed. This will allow for maximal reattachment, and any remaining probing depth is usually a result of the periodontal flora and can be treated periodontally.

Prognosis.   The prognosis of the endodontic component is excellent, and regeneration of the attachment apparatus is limited by the periodontal prognosis. If root canal therapy alone is performed, only a limited healing capacity should be expected.

Primary periodontal lesion

Sequelae.   Primary periodontal lesions can sometimes mimic an endodontic problem both clinically and radiographically (Gold and Moskow, 1987). This problem, however, develops over a longer period. Periodontal problems that are chronic in nature can also often be observed on *other* teeth, as opposed to endodontic problems, which are isolated to individual teeth. The former lesion is usually observed as a progressive periodontal problem extending to the root apex. The borders of this lesion are usually wider at the gingival margin, whereas the endodontic lesion is usually wider at the root apex and narrower at the gingival margin. Minimal or no pain is usually experienced by the patient with periodontal disease.

Tests.   Periodontal probing may reach the apex of an involved tooth. The differential diagnosis is made when the results of thermal and electric pulp testing of these teeth are within normal limits (see Fig. 49-1). The pulp invariably manifests some vitality.

Treatment.   Periodontal therapy is indicated. Root canal therapy is not indicated, unless pulp vitality test results change. Reevaluation must be performed periodically after therapy to check for possible retrograde endodontic problems.

Prognosis.   The prognosis is entirely dependent on the periodontal therapy.

Primary periodontal lesion with secondary endodontic involvement

Sequelae.   When periodontal involvement extends to the apex of the tooth, retroinfection of the pulp tissue may occur, and the patient can sometimes experience severe pain. Infection of the pulp can also follow the path through a lateral canal. Dentinal abrasions and root planing can also contribute to the death of the pulp.

Tests.   The tests are similar to those used in primary endodontic and secondary periodontal lesions. There is generalized periodontal probing. Pulp vitality test results can sometimes be mixed. The pulp can be necrotic, or there may be partial necrosis with one or more vital canals, especially in multirooted teeth. When the original diagnosis is strictly periodontal disease and therapy produces no healing, pulp vitality tests should be repeated. Cold is the test of choice for vitality. There should be little if any response as compared with control teeth. When the pulp is inflamed, the application of cold produces an immediate response followed by a prolonged recovery phase. However, when the pulp is necrotic, there is no response.

Treatment.   Conservative root canal therapy is indicated. Periodontal therapy should already have been initiated and can proceed in conjunction with the endodontics.

Prognosis.   The prognosis is dependent on the periodontal therapy. The healing response of the periapical lesion is not predictable, because of the periodontal communication. A favorable endodontic prognosis is obtained only when the tooth is in a closed and protected environment (Evian et al., 1983). The periodontal problem that exists in these cases allows for a direct communication with the oral environment. Failures also occur when a periodontal problem develops along a cementoenamel groove or fused roots in posterior teeth. These areas become a haven for the accumulation of plaque and calculus and reduce the possibility for reattachment.

True combined lesion

Sequelae.   True combined endodontic-periodontal lesions are usually of periodontal origin. The lesion is formed when pulpal and periodontal pathoses develop independently and unite (Fig. 49-6). This problem is similar to the previously described secondary involvement on a preexisting primary lesion with clinical and radiographic evidence.

Differential diagnosis must include a vertical root fracture (Bender and Freedland, 1983a, 1983b; Luebke, 1984). Perforations and resorptive perforations can produce this true combined lesion. Aggressive instrumentation of the root canal can create perforation along the root canal, and this may initially mimic a lateral canal (Abou-Rass, 1986). If a perforation is created near the gingival sulcus, such as the furcation area, physical disruption of the periodontal ligament and adjacent alveolar bone results in an inflammatory response. Sulcular epithelium may migrate to this area, developing communication between the periodontal inflammation and the oral environment (Seltzer et al., 1970; Petersson et al., 1985; Beavers et al., 1986). The most severe reactions occur when perforations are not sealed, and the worst prognosis exists with perforations in the furcation region (Stromberg et al., 1972). These should be sealed as quickly as possible.

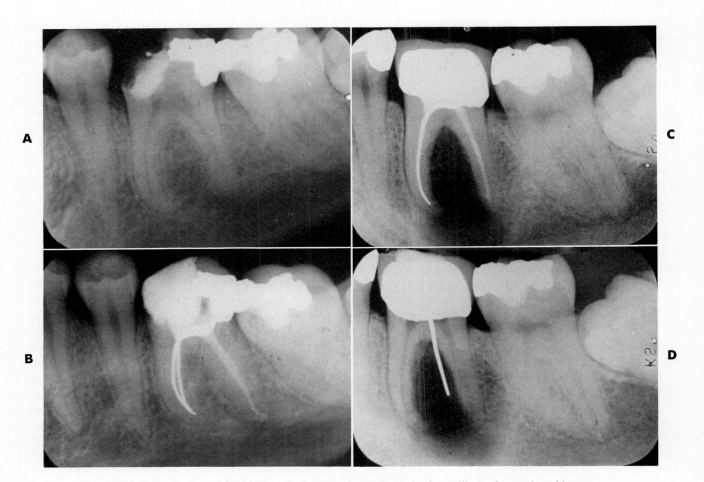

Fig. 49-6.   True combined lesion. **A,** Preoperative radiograph of mandibular first molar with caries necessitating endodontic therapy. **B,** Root canal therapy was performed using silver points in mesial canals and gutta-percha in distal canal. **C,** View at 10-year recall demonstrating severe periodontal and periapical breakdown. A primary endodontic lesion was suspected; however, no reduction in gingival probing was observed following root canal debridement. **D,** A silver point probe could still be placed anywhere along buccal or lingual surfaces following complete instrumentation. Note that probe did not go directly to root apex.

Tests.   In the combined lesion, pulp testing gives negative results. The tooth in question will have periodontal probing depths at numerous sites. Confirmation of the periodontal involvement of the apex of the tooth can be demonstrated with radiographs following the placement of a periodontal probe, multiple gutta-percha points, or silver points into the sulcus and tracing them to the apex. Multiple points, such as these, demonstrate the amount of periodontal destruction. If the probes are traced to any other area besides the apex, then it is possible that resorption, a perforation, or vertical root fracture is the source of the periodontal communication.

Another diagnostic technique is determining the percentage of spirochetes through darkfield microscopy

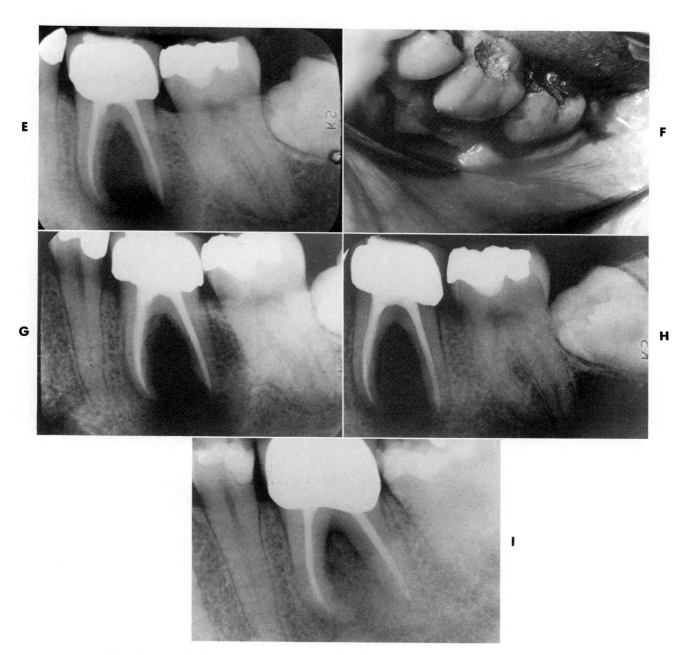

Fig. 49-6, cont'd.   E, Posttreatment radiograph following obturation of canals with gutta-percha. **F,** Severe osseous breakdown and a total lack of buccal bone revealed by a surgical flap. Note that crestal bone is still present. **G,** Postsurgical radiograph. **H,** View at 6-month recall. **I,** Radiograph at 8-year recall demonstrating excellent regeneration of osseous structures. (Periodontal therapy by Dr. D.W. Cohen.)

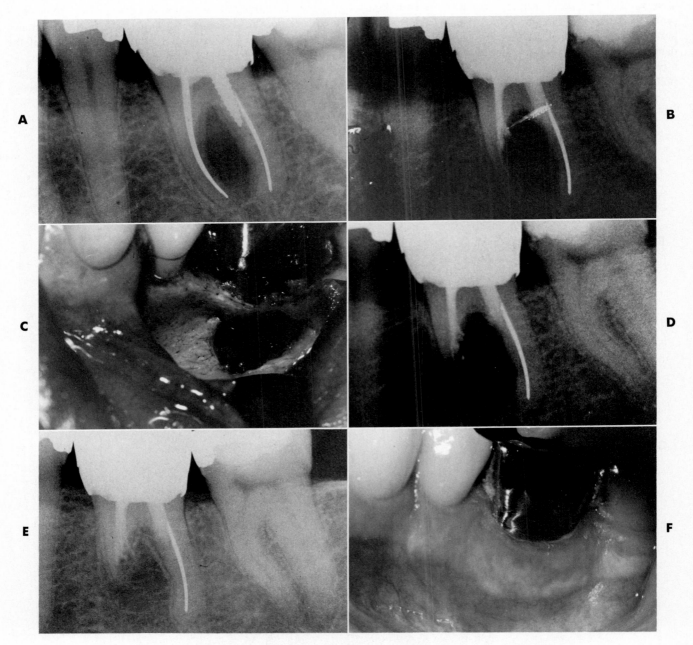

Fig. 49-7. Endodontic-periodontal advanced procedures. **A,** Radiograph of mandibular first molar. Previous root canal therapy was inadequately performed using silver points. Large screw-type post appears to have perforated mesial surface of distal root. Note apical resorption of distal surface of mesial root and severe osseous destruction. No significant periodontal probing was obtained. **B,** Presurgical radiograph following removal of post and mesial silver points, complete debridement of root canals, and obturation of root canals. Calcium hydroxide therapy was attempted with no success and no reduction of lesion over 6 months. **C,** A full-thickness flap revealed almost complete loss of buccal bone. Remaining crestal bone indicated that success was possible. **D,** Postsurgical radiograph following removal of partially resorbed apical half of mesial root. **E,** View at 4-year recall shows excellent regeneration of surrounding osseous structures. **F,** Appearance of soft tissue and previous gold crown at 4-year recall. Maintenance and preservation of arch integrity have been preserved.

(Trope et al., 1988). The routine periodontal problem has a greater percentage of spirochetes than the endodontic condition draining through the sinus tract. Pulpal status will then allow proper classification of this lesion.

A vertical root fracture can produce a "halo" effect around the tooth radiographically. Examination of the root surface should be done with a sharp explorer held perpendicular to the root surface to feel for any cracks. The fractured root can mimic the lesion of occlusal trauma (Amsterdam, 1974), with localized loss of lamina dura, altered trabecular pattern, and widened periodontal ligament.

Treatment. Treatment must not be initiated until the patient understands limitations on the prognosis. Good conservative endodontic treatment is performed to reduce the critical concentration of contaminants in the combined lesion. Periodontal therapy can be performed before, during, or immediately after the endodontic treatment.

A number of periodontal and endodontic clinical approaches may be required, including hemisection or root resection (Amsterdam and Rossman, 1968; Abrams and Trachtenberg, 1974; Langer et al., 1981; Saadoun, 1985; Eastman and Backmeyer, 1986). Advanced endodontic surgical intervention may produce a good result (Rossman et al., 1960; Skoglund and Persson, 1985). Any tissue that is surgically removed should be examined histologically (Baumann and Rossman, 1956).

Internal resorption, if detected radiographically, must be treated immediately by extirpating the pulpal tissue. The multinucleated giant cells must be removed before the resorptive process perforates the canal wall and establishes communication with the periodontal ligament. The prognosis decreases significantly if this communication is established. Treatment then involves the use of long-term calcium hydroxide therapy (Frank and Weine, 1973). External root resorption is a completely different clinical entity. It is usually not implicated in the combined lesion (Andreasen, 1985).

Fractures and complete bone loss are the two entities that condemn a tooth to extraction. Confirmation of the fracture can often be made through a surgical exploration (Rossman and Rossman, 1981). If the fracture line does not travel through the epithelial attachment at the base of the gingival sulcus and does not communicate with the oral environment, then surgical removal of the fractured segment may produce a good prognosis. This can be observed with oblique and apical fractures.

Perforations must be sealed immediately; various locations require different approaches. The important factor is to close off the perforation as quickly as possible and leave options open, treating this as a weak link. The location of the perforation and its size and duration often dictate the material of choice. Cavit, amalgam, gutta-percha, calcium hydroxide, and glass ionomer cements have all been used.

Prognosis. The prognosis in the combined endodontic and periodontal problem is dependent on the periodontal therapy. Obviously, the root canal therapy cannot be performed with any deviation from accepted standards. The greater the periodontal involvement, the poorer is the prognosis. Patients cannot be promised a favorable prognosis. As long as they understand this and are willing to undergo these procedures with the possibility of failure, advanced procedures can be tried (Fig. 49-7).

REFERENCES

Abou-Rass M: Endodontic preparation and filling procedures, San Francisco, 1986, California Dental Institute for Continuing Education.

Abrams L and Trachtenberg DI: Hemisection—technique and restoration, Dent Clin North Am 18:415, 1974.

Amsterdam M: Periodontal prosthesis: twenty-five years in retrospect, Alpha Omegan 67:7, 1974.

Amsterdam M and Rossman SR: Technique of hemisection of multi-rooted teeth, Alpha Omegan 53:4, 1968.

Andreasen JO: Cementum repair after apicoectomy in humans, Acta Odontol Scand 31:211, 1973.

Andreasen JO: Relationship between surface and inflammatory root resorption and changes in the pulp after replantation of permanent incisors in monkeys, J Endod 7:294, 1981.

Andreasen JO: External root resorption: its implications in dental traumatology, paedodontics, periodontics, orthodontics, and endodontics, Int Endod J 18:109, 1985.

Augsburger RA and Peters DD: In vitro effects of ice, skin refrigerant, and CO_2 snow on intrapulpal temperature, J Endod 7:110, 1981.

Baumann E and Rossman SR: Clinical, roentgenologic and histopathologic findings in teeth with apical radiolucent areas, Oral Surg 9:1330, 1956.

Beavers RA, Bergenholtz G, and Cox CF: Periodontal wound healing following intentional root perforations in permanent teeth of Macaca mulatta, Int Endod J 19:36, 1986.

Bender IB: Factors influencing the radiographic appearance of bony lesions, J Endod 8:161, 1982.

Bender IB and Freedland JB: Adult root fractures, J Am Dent Assoc 107:413, 1983a.

Bender IB and Freedland JB: Clinical considerations in the diagnosis and treatment of inter-alveolar root fractures, J Am Dent Assoc 107:595, 1983b.

Bender IB and Seltzer S: The oral fistula—its diagnosis and treatment, Oral Surg 14:1367, 1961.

Bender IB and Seltzer S: The effect of periodontal disease on the dental pulp, Oral Surg 33:458, 1972.

Bergenholtz G and Lindhe J: Effect of soluble plaque factors on inflammatory reactions in the dental pulp, Scand J Dent Res 83:153, 1975.

Cahn L: Pathology of pulps found in pyorrhetic teeth, Dent Items Interest 49:598, 1927.

Cohen S, editor: An annotated glossary of terms used in endodontics, ed 4, Chicago, 1984, American Association of Endodontics.

Cooley RL, Stilley J, and Lubow RM: Evaluation of a digital pulp tester, Oral Surg 58:437, 1984.

Eastman JR and Backmeyer J: A review of the periodontal, endodontic and the prosthetic considerations in odontogenous resection procedures, Int J Periodontics Restorative Dent 6:34, 1986.

Evian CI et al: The effect of submerging roots with periodontal defects, Compend Contin Educ Dent 4:37, 1983.

Frank A and Weine F: Nonsurgical therapy for perforative defect of internal resorption, J Am Dent Assoc 87:863, 1973.

Fuss Z, Bender IB, and Rickoff BD: An unusual periodontal abscess, Oral Surg 12:116, 1986a.

Fuss Z et al: Assessment of reliability of electric and thermal pulp testing procedures, J Endod 12:301, 1986b.

Gold SI and Moskow BS: Periodontal repair of periapical lesions: the borderland between pulpal and periodontal disease, J Clin Periodontol 14:251, 1987.

Goldman HM and Schilder H: Regeneration of attachment apparatus lost due to disease of endodontic origin, J Periodontol 59:609, 1988.

Guldener PHA: The relationship between periodontal and pulpal disease, Int Endont J 18:41, 1985.

Hattler AB and Listgarten MA: Pulpal response to root planing in a rat model, J Endod 10:471, 1984.

Langer B, Stein SD, and Wagenberg B: An evaluation of root resections: a ten year study, J Periodontol 52:719, 1981.

Luebke R: Vertical crown-root fractures in posterior teeth, Dent Clin North Am 28:883, 1984.

Mori K: Diagnosis and treatment of the dental pulp, Quintessence Int 6:43, 1987.

Nyman S et al: Healing following implantation of periodontitis affected roots into gingival connective tissue, J Clin Periodontol 7:394, 1980.

Oliet S and Pollock S: Classification and treatment of endo-perio involved teeth, Phila Co Dent Soc Bull 34:12, 1968.

Pashley DH: Smear layer: physiological considerations, Oper Dent 3:13, 1984.

Perlmutter S et al: Effect of the endodontic status of the tooth on experimental periodontal reattachment in baboons: a preliminary investigation, Oral Surg 63:232, 1987.

Petersson K, Hasselgren G, and Tronstad L: Endodontic treatment of experimental root perforations in dog teeth, Endod Dent Traumatol 1:22, 1985.

Rossman LE and Rossman SR: Endodontic surgery: diagnosis, considerations and technique, Compend Contin Educ Dent 2:18, 1981.

Rossman LE, Rossman SR, and Garber DA: The endodontic-periodontic fistula, Oral Surg 53:78, 1982.

Rossman S, Kaplowitz B, and Baldinger SR: Therapy of the endodontically and periodontally involved tooth, Oral Surg 13:361, 1960.

Rubach WC and Mitchell DF: Periodontal disease, accessory canals and pulp pathosis, J Periodontol 36:34, 1965.

Saadoun A: Management of furcation involvement, J West Soc Periodont Periodont Abstr 33:91, 1985.

Seltzer S and Bender IB: The dental pulp: the interrelationship of pulp and periodontal disease, ed 3, Philadelphia, 1984, JB Lippincott Co.

Seltzer S, Bender IB, and Ziontz M: The interrelationship of pulp and periodontal disease, Oral Surg 16:1474, 1963.

Seltzer S, Sinai I, and August D: Periodontal effects of root perforations before and during endodontic procedures, J Dent Res 49:332, 1970.

Seltzer S et al: Pulpitis induced interradicular periodontal changes in experimental animals, J Periodontol 38:124, 1967.

Sicher H: Über Pulpaerkrankungen als Folge von Paradontose, Z Stomatol 34:819, 1936.

Simon JH, Glick DH, and Frank AL: The relationship of endodontic-periodontic lesions, J Periodontol 43:202, 1972.

Skoglund A and Persson G: A follow-up of apicoectomized teeth with total loss of the buccal bone plate, Oral Surg 59:78, 1985.

Stromberg T, Hasselgren G, and Bergstedt H: Endodontic treatment of traumatic root perforations in man, Swed Dent J 65:457, 1972.

Takatsuka M et al: Effect of pulp vitality on periodontal reattachment following free autogenous gingival graft in dogs, Anat Anz 156:39, 1984.

Tronstad L et al: pH changes in dental tissues after root canal filling with calcium hydroxide, J Endod 7:17, 1981.

Trope M et al: Darkfield microscopy as a diagnostic aid in differentiating exudates from endodontic and periodontal abscesses, J Endod 14:35, 1988.

Trowbridge HO: Pathogenesis of pulpitis resulting from dental caries, J Endod 7:52, 1981.

Turner JH and Drew AH: Experimental injury into bacteriology of pyorrhea, Proc R Soc Med (Odontol) 12:104, 1919.

Weine FS: The enigma of the lateral canal, Dent Clin North Am 28:833, 1984.

Whyman RA: Endodontic-periodontic lesions. I. Prevalence, aetiology, and diagnosis, NZ Dent J 84:74, 1988a.

Whyman RA: Endodontic-periodontic lesions. II. Management, NZ Dent J 84:109, 1988b.

Chapter 50

PERIODONTAL CONSIDERATIONS IN RESTORATIVE DENTISTRY

Daniel P. Casullo

The periodontium and restorative dentistry
  Embrasure space
  Dental caries
  Gingival margin placement of restorations
  Full-coverage provisional restoration
  Root exposures, root caries, and restorative dentistry
Periodontal surgery for placement of restorations
  Free gingival graft and full-crown restoration
  Advantages of combined periodontal/restorative procedures
  Soft tissue and osseous reduction for exposing sound crown margins in areas of subgingival caries or root fractures
  Strategic extraction
  Surgical correction of a deformed edentulous ridge
The periodontium and excessive force: trauma from occlusion
  Primary occlusal trauma with gingivitis or periodontitis
  Primary occlusal trauma and tooth mobility
  Progressive mobility
  Secondary occlusal trauma
Summary

Periodontal health is critical for both the preservation of the natural dentition and the success of any restorative procedures. This chapter on periodontal considerations in restorative dentistry discusses adjunctive restorative and occlusal treatment modalities that may be combined or integrated with standard periodontal therapy (Fig. 50-1).

The following topics are discussed: (1) the relationship between the periodontium and restorative dentistry, (2) periodontal surgery for placement of restorations, (3) correction of a deformed edentulous ridge for health and es-

thetics, (4) the principle of strategic extraction for the maximum preservation of a functional dentition, and (5) the relationships among the periodontium (attachment apparatus), trauma from occlusion, and restorative dentistry.

THE PERIODONTIUM AND RESTORATIVE DENTISTRY

The marginal integrity, crown contours, proximal relationships, soft tissue–restoration interface, and occlusal morphology of dental restorations are critically important for long-term periodontal health.

Embrasure space

The gingival sulcus, the col, and interproximal soft tissue apical to contact areas of the teeth are common sites for the establishment of a pathogenic flora leading to periodontal disease. Often caries is found at or near the contact point. The gingival sulcus and interproximal col area (Fig. 50-2) are not fully keratinized and hence may have less inherent resistance and greater vulnerability to local infection.

Restorative procedures must allow for a healthy, nonulcerated sulcular lining, with space for adequate interdental gingiva to promote easy cleaning by the patient. The surfaces of proximal restorations should be flat or concave, and smooth and continuous with natural tooth structure, to meet the above requirements. The restoration of a tooth may result in alteration of the marginal ridges, crown contours, and interproximal contacts, which if incorrectly contoured will result in plaque retention, calculus formation, and inflammation. The resulting inflammatory response is evidenced clinically after placement of a defective restoration by sulcular bleeding and ulceration, gingival enlarge-

619

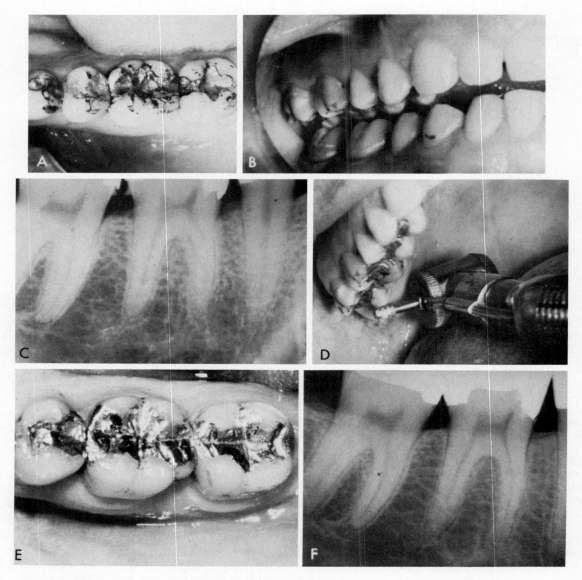

Fig. 50-1. Operative occlusal therapy. **A,** This 24-year-old patient's chief complaints were sensitivity to cold and pain on chewing, especially in mandibular first molar area. Amalgam restorations are cupped out, and first molar mesial-occlusal-distal (MOD) restoration is fractured. Soft tissue is edematous and bleeds on probing. **B,** In a left working movement, there are nonworking interferences associated with maxillary and mandibular first and second molars. **C,** Radiograph shows subgingival calculus, overhanging restorations, and dissolution of crestal bone. Treatment consisted of oral hygiene instruction and scaling and root planing to remove calculus and reduce soft tissue inflammation. **D,** Two weeks later, isolated occlusal adjustment was done in conjunction with placement of new amalgam restorations. Hanging palatal cusp associated with nonworking interference was adjusted first to remove interference. **E,** New amalgam restorations reduce depth of central fossae and are occluded with adjusted maxillary molars. **F,** Six-month postoperative radiograph shows healing of marginal bone. (From Morris AL, Bohannan HM, and Casullo DP, editors: The dental specialties in general practice, Philadelphia, 1983, WB Saunders Co.)

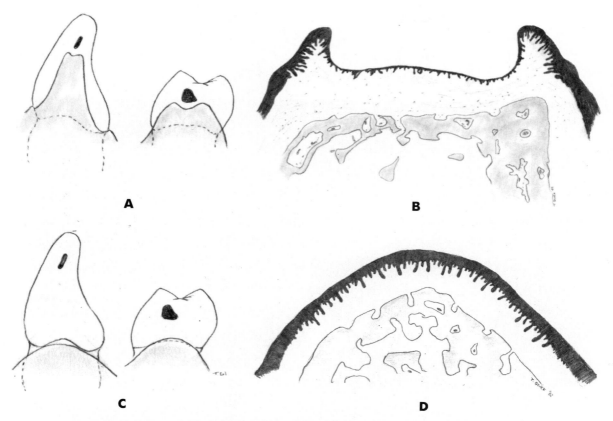

Fig. 50-2. Embrasure space and interproximal col. **A,** In a normal, ideal periodontium, depression of soft tissue below contact area (interproximal col area) is created by buccal and lingual papillae. **B,** This diagram represents histology of col area. Papillae are covered by keratinized epithelium, and interproximal col area is covered by a thin, nonkeratinized epithelium. **C,** Often after gingival recession or periodontal therapy, interproximal col area no longer exists. Soft tissue architecture of interproximal tissue is rounded or flat. **D,** This diagram represents histology of interproximal tissue after recession or surgery. It is now keratinized and similar to external gingival tissues. (From Morris AL, Bohannan HM, and Casullo DP, editors: The dental specialties in general practice, Philadelphia, 1983, WB Saunders Co.)

ment, detachment of the junctional epithelium, and the development of pocket depth, and radiographically by the dissolution of the crestal lamina dura. These changes occur within a few days to a few weeks after placement of a defective restoration, and the gingival inflammation may persist or worsen if the margin of the restoration is not able to be cleaned by the patient.

Dental caries

Dental caries is caused by the accumulation of cariogenic plaques. Caries destroys tooth structure, creating open contacts, poor embrasure form, and plunger cusps, all of which encourage food impaction, plaque formation, and periodontal disease. In the presence of debris and decay, the adjacent gingival soft tissue can become more inflamed and caries can extend deep into periodontal pockets, especially around defective restorations that suffer

from recurrent caries (Fig. 50-3).

The removal of dental caries and the restoration of sound tooth structure are necessary components of early treatment of a patient with periodontal disease. The reestablishment of marginal integrity with normal interproximal contacts and proper embrasure space will facilitate oral hygiene, prevent plaque accumulation, and create a local environment conducive to health. Restoration of dental caries should be as conservative as possible to maintain natural tooth structure and provide for gingival margins that are able to be kept plaque free by the patient if at all possible.

Gingival margin placement of restorations

The extent of the carious lesions and amount of remaining tooth structure in relation to the periodontium determines where the clinician must place a margin. Whenever

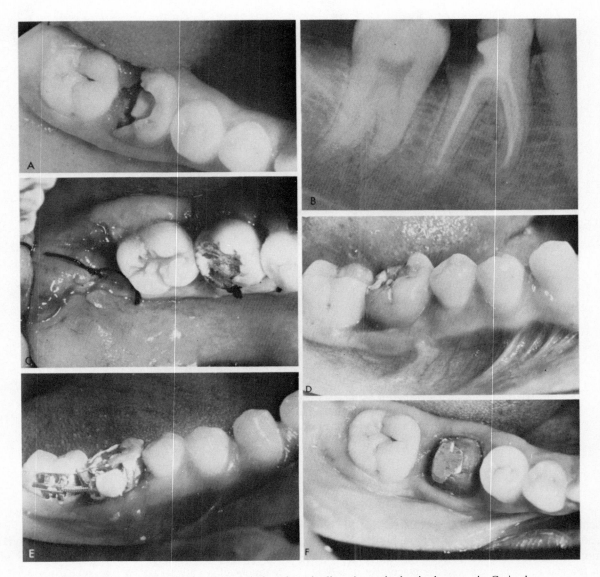

Fig. 50-3. Combined restorative, periodontal, and adjunctive orthodontic therapy. **A,** Caries has destroyed distal half of this first molar, with mesial drift of second molar. **B,** Note extensive caries with loss of crestal lamina dura, and mesial drift of second molar. Treatment consisted of scaling and root planing, tooth movement, and a full crown. **C,** Flaps allowed access to caries and reduced soft tissue enlargement. At this same visit, a temporary amalgam restoration was placed. **D,** Healing 4 weeks after procedure in **C. E,** An open-coil spring is placed. **F,** After orthodontic therapy, tooth is prepared for provisional full-crown restoration. (From Morris AL, Bohannan HM, and Casullo DP, editors: The dental specialties in general practice, Philadelphia, 1983, WB Saunders Co.)

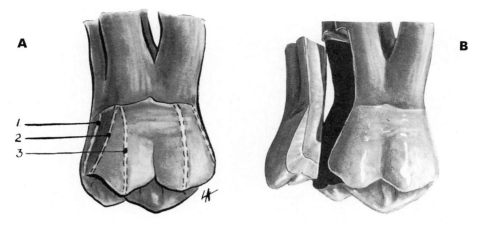

Fig. 50-4. Transitional line angle. **A,** Normal coronal contours of tooth can be divided into three areas: *1,* proximal surface—flat and in some instances concave; *2,* transitional line angle—also very flat; *3,* buccal surface—convex with height of convexity in gingival third of crown. **B,** Proximal section of tooth from transitional line angle to transitional line angle has been removed to emphasize flattened design of this area.

possible, all margins should be placed supragingivally. Subgingival margins are often difficult to cleanse and become plaque retention areas.

Partial-coverage restorations are the cast restorations of choice, since the margins can often be kept coronal to the periodontal tissues. This conservative approach, although ideal for the periodontium, may not always be possible, since full-coverage restorations may be needed to restore lost crown structure, for esthetics, and to better splint mobile teeth.

The full-crown restoration is a demanding and exacting restoration, since it can have the greatest adverse effect on the periodontium. The margin of the full-crown provisional and final restorations should be thin and placed supragingivally whenever possible. However, if it must be placed subgingivally, it should be placed into the sulcus short of the junctional epithelium. This position is preferred because it will (1) prevent recurring caries, (2) alleviate tooth sensitivity, (3) gain retention of broken-down teeth, (4) enhance appearance, and (5) establish optimal soft tissue crown contours.

Full-coverage provisional restoration

If dental caries extends close to the crest of bone and extensive tooth structure is lost, a cast restoration is required to replace lost tooth structure and reestablish proper occlusal form and function. A well-designed provisional restoration should be placed immediately to promote caries control, support the soft tissue, maintain arch integrity, create normal crown contours, and establish a normal occlusion.

Metal band and acrylic provisional restorations are preferred over all-acrylic provisional restorations because the metal band offers optimal strength in the gingival third of the crown, supporting the sulcular tissues and providing thin knifelike margins that minimize plaque accumulation. Once the bands are fitted, a reasonably well-adapted margin can be established. This metal margin serves as a guide for developing and refining the crown contours, especially those of the gingival third.

Crown contours. The proximal crown contours are generally flat or concave. This provides adequate embrasure space for the interdental gingiva and allows room for plaque removal. The facial and lingual surfaces are usually slightly convex to provide adequate support of the soft tissue and maintain harmony with the lips, cheek, and tongue. The transitional line angle (the area between the proximal surface and the facial or lingual surface) is also generally flat or concave to form the opening for the embrasure space and house the interdental tissue. The transitional line angle (Fig. 50-4) is an important consideration in tooth preparation and full-crown restoration, for if improperly established, it results in an overcontoured restoration that impinges on the gingiva.

Reevaluation. After the provisional restoration has been in place for 4 to 6 weeks and subgingival scaling and root planing have been completed with the establishment of good oral hygiene, the gingival tissues should be pink and firm with little or no bleeding. If ulceration and bleeding in the sulcus and col area and gingival enlargement have not been resolved, the adequacy of scaling and root planing, the patient's home care, caries control, and crown contours and margins must be reevaluated and corrected before further treatment (Fig. 50-5) is undertaken.

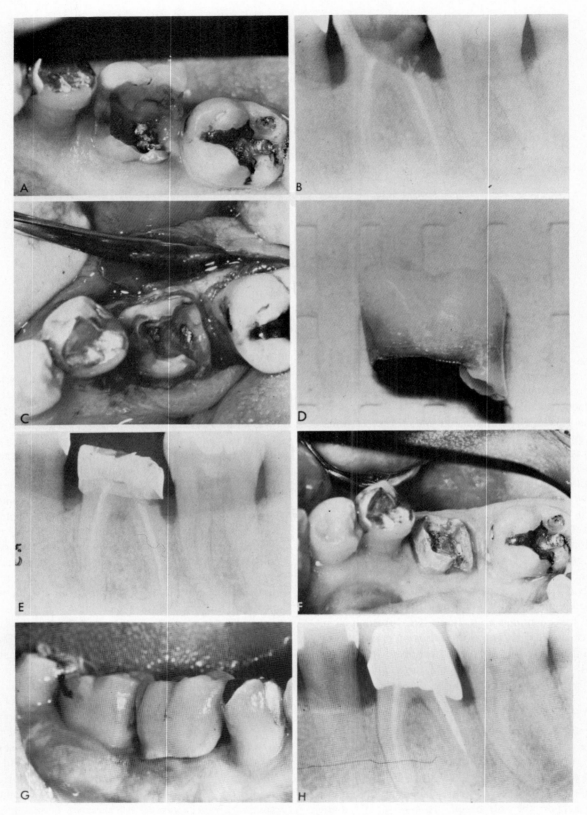

Fig. 50-5. For legend see opposite page.

Fig. 50-5. Concomitant provisional restoration to test and establish periodontal health. **A,** Mandibular first molar showing caries. **B,** Note caries extending to osseous crest on distal surface. Treatment included osseous surgery, fabrication of a provisional restoration, reevaluation, and a final post, core, and crown restoration. **C,** Metal band and acrylic provisional restoration placed. Flaps were raised to allow reduction of bone, and provisional restoration was relined. **D,** Relined provisional restoration. **E,** Provisional metal band and acrylic crown in place; note 3 to 4 mm of exposed distal tooth structure. **F,** Healing at 12 weeks. **G,** Final restoration. **H,** Final restoration radiograph. (From Morris AL, Bohannan HM, and Casullo DP, editors: The dental specialties in general practice, Philadelphia, 1983, WB Saunders Co.)

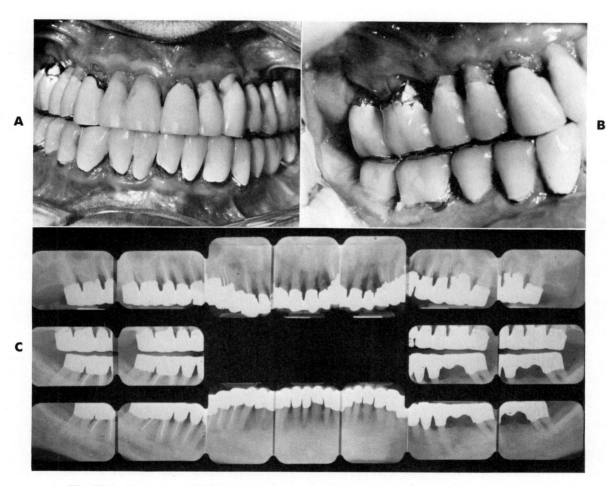

Fig. 50-6. Root caries. **A,** Complex restorative dentistry rendered in full-mouth reconstruction in this 54-year-old patient failed after 4 years. **B,** Right buccal view. **C,** Extensive disease is evidenced by advanced bone loss, periapical radiolucencies, and severe root caries. Complex restorative dentistry places an enormous burden on both patient and dental team to maintain health of dentition. Determination of cause of failure is critical in analysis of etiology and subsequent treatment. (From Morris AL, Bohannan HM, and Casullo DP, editors: The dental specialties in general practice, Philadelphia, 1983, WB Saunders Co.)

Root exposures, root caries, and restorative dentistry

The root exposure caused by periodontal disease is often characterized by a root surface with developmental depressions, undercuts, cul-de-sac areas, and furcation areas, all contributing to plaque retention and caries development (Fig. 50-6). Root caries in furcation areas should be treated with amalgam restorations, whereas buccal and lingual supragingival caries can best be treated by a combination of glass ionomers and dentin-bonding composite resin materials. When recession is extensive and aberrant root anatomy leads to plaque accumulation and periodontal disease, full-crown coverage may be necessary to change the anatomy of the exposed roots and openings to furcations. The full-crown preparation and restoration with subgingival margins controls the entrance of the furcation by either eliminating or at least minimizing the furcation involvement. It covers the exposed root structure, which is highly susceptible to caries and sensitivity. It establishes coronal contours that are conducive to the maintenance of gingival health by passively filling and smoothly exiting from the gingival sulcus. It can also modify the occlusal scheme in order to control force direction and dissipation, and often correct trauma from occlusion.

PERIODONTAL SURGERY FOR PLACEMENT OF RESTORATIONS

The mucogingival complex covers the attachment apparatus and extends to the root of the tooth. It comprises the keratinized masticatory mucosa or attached gingiva and the thin, friable, movable alveolar mucosa. In health, the masticatory mucosa adheres tightly to the tooth via the gingival fiber apparatus, connective tissue attachment, and the junctional epithelium. The nature of this soft tissue–crown interface allows for optimal oral hygiene and the protection of the underlying attachment apparatus.

When the masticatory mucosa is unattached or totally absent and the soft tissue–crown interface has been compromised by recession or inflammation, surgical augmentation to provide a collar of attached gingiva is often beneficial. When there is a small band of attached gingiva at the projected crown margin, evaluation with a provisional crown can often help in the decision as to whether surgical augmentation of the attached gingiva is necessary.

When no restorative therapy is indicated or supragingival margins are placed, any questionable or borderline mucogingival problems should be closely observed for evidence of inflammation and further recession. Gingival health may be maintained indefinitely; otherwise, surgery can be implemented when the need arises (Fig. 50-7).

When advanced restorative therapy involving the sulcular area is required in an area where it has been established that there is inadequate attached gingiva, the free gingival graft is a commonly used surgical procedure to provide the needed attached gingiva (see Chapter 47).

Free gingival graft and full-crown restoration

A free gingival graft may be placed after the response of the gingiva to a properly contoured provisional restoration has been observed. If it is decided that a free gingival graft is necessary, it can be placed at the final impression visit or at the coping or gold try-in visit. (If necessary, the tooth can be reprepared and the impressions retaken.) Moreover, by basing the decision on the marginal soft tissue response after placement of the provisional restoration, unnecessary surgery can be avoided (Fig. 50-7).

Advantages of combined periodontal/restorative procedures

There are distinct advantages to combining restorative and surgical procedures in the same visit. Executing the free gingival graft and preparing a tooth for the final impressions at the same visit minimizes treatment time, minimizes traumatic insult to the tissues, and improves overall patient comfort. Combining periodontal (free gingival graft) and restorative therapy is warranted when the following conditions have been met:

1. The mucogingival problem is isolated and easy to manage (any periodontal pockets, dehiscences, or fenestrations may be treated at the same visit).
2. All other periodontal therapy to control inflammatory disease has been completed, and the provisional restoration has been in place for an adequate amount of time to evaluate the need for greater attached gingiva.
3. The junctional epithelium has not been injured or destroyed, so there will be a band of tissue to separate the restoration and periodontium.

Soft tissue and osseous reduction for exposing sound crown margins in areas of subgingival caries or root fractures

When severe caries approaches or extends below the alveolar crest, a full-thickness flap extending to adjacent teeth and osseous reduction to gain sound tooth structure are required. During the procedure the attached mucosa must be preserved. The apically and laterally positioned flap is an excellent means of preserving and often of gaining attached gingiva (Fig. 50-8).

Soft tissue reduction by inverse bevel incisions and primary closure is generally the procedure of choice to preserve the attached gingiva, control the position of the tissues, and gain maximum access to the tooth structure and periodontium. During soft tissue retraction it can be determined if the amount of sound tooth structure is adequate for the placement of a full-crown restoration. Any restoration, especially a full-crown restoration, needs the biologic width of approximately 1 mm of tooth structure for connective tissue and 1 mm of tooth structure for the junctional epithelium, plus 1 to 2 mm of tooth structure for the

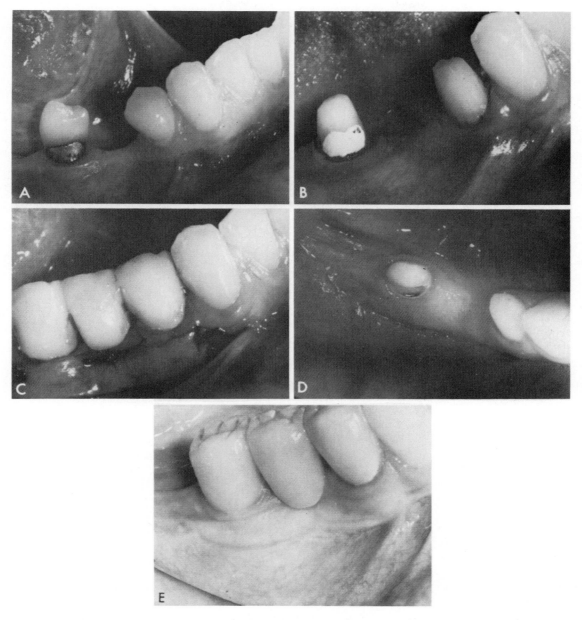

Fig. 50-7. Combined restorative and mucogingival surgery: free gingival graft. **A,** Treatment plan included a three-unit bridge, as well as a free gingival graft around abutment teeth and on edentulous ridge. **B,** Teeth were prepared for full-crown restorations, and final impressions were taken. **C,** Free gingival graft sutured in place, followed by cementation of provisional splint. **D,** Healing after 6 weeks. Note increased buccolingual dimension of edentulous ridge. **E,** Final restoration placed 12 weeks after surgery. (From Morris AL, Bohannan HM, and Casullo DP, editors: The dental specialties in general practice, Philadelphia, 1983, WB Saunders Co.)

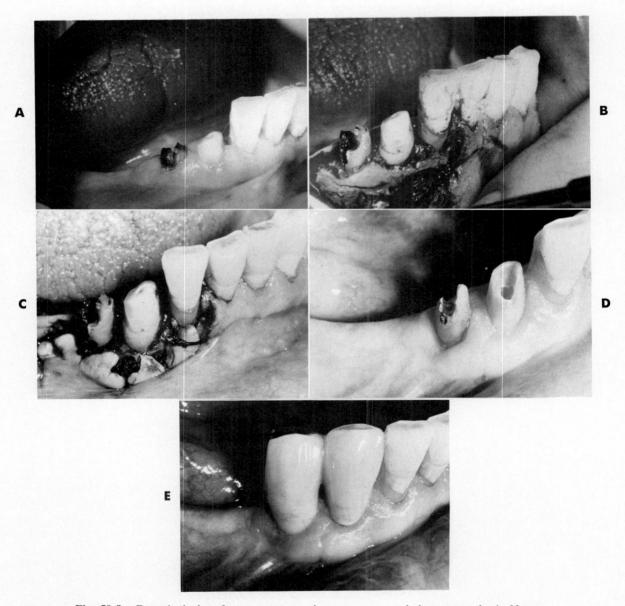

Fig. 50-8.   Free gingival graft to augment masticatory mucosa and abutment teeth. **A,** Note extensive decay approaching osseous crest on key abutments. **B,** Note fracture at distobuccal line angle of premolar where pin had been placed. Fracture extended below osseous crest and required osseous surgery to gain sound tooth structure. **C,** Masticatory mucosa was apically and laterally positioned to protect labial plate of bone and to maintain zone of attachment gingiva. **D,** Healing 3 months after surgery demonstrates adequate tooth structure for new restoration. **E,** Final restoration in place. (From Morris AL, Bohannan HM, and Casullo DP, editors: The dental specialties in general practice, Philadelphia, 1983, WB Saunders Co.)

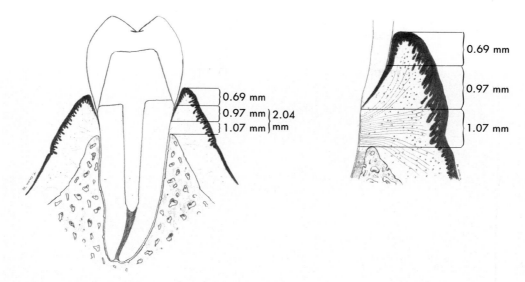

Fig. 50-9.   Biologic width. Biologic width is dimension from crest of aveolar bone to base of sulcus (2.04 mm) and includes connective tissue (1.07 mm) and epithelial (0.97 mm) attachments. (From Morris AL, Bohannan HM, and Casullo DP, editors: The dental specialties in general practice, Philadelphia, 1983, WB Saunders Co.)

crown margin placement and termination. Although inadequate tooth structure cannot be detected radiographically, it is often found when fractures and caries approach the alveolar crest. Ostectomy using burs and chisels is then needed to expose the requisite 3 to 4 mm of sound tooth structure 360 degrees around the root. The failure to expose the 3 to 4 mm of tooth structure may result in restorative infringement on the junctional epithelium and connective tissue attachment, which leads to bone loss and the apical migration of the soft tissue complex (Fig. 50-9).

The subgingival procedure to expose sound root structure involves a mucoperiosteal flap and ostectomy, with care taken not to nick the root structure. This procedure should precede placement of the provisional restoration.

Strategic extraction

Extraction may be the treatment of choice when the periodontal involvement of an individual tooth or root jeopardizes a contiguous tooth and there is unresolvable infrabony periodontal defects or caries extending apical to the osseous crest. Extraction often leads to the predictable healing of osseous structures by bridging the periodontally involved contiguous structures. The sectioning or extraction of roots may also help to establish adequate embrasure space, which is conducive to periodontal health (Fig. 50-10).

The importance of the involved tooth or root in relation to the rest of the dentition with respect to its esthetic function, its contribution to occlusal stability and function (especially masticatory efficiency), and its potential role as an abutment is considered in the decision to extract. Strategic extraction is chosen when removal of a root or tooth will improve the long-term, overall prognosis of the entire dentition. Strategic extraction is also indicated for teeth with untreatable defects, including those with root canals, fillings, vertical fractures, or perforations, or those with extensive internal or external root resorption (Fig. 50-11). Generally, the extracted tooth is then replaced with a fixed restoration to preserve arch integrity, stabilize lonestanding molars, maintain occlusal function, and establish optimal esthetics (Fig. 50-12).

Surgical correction of a deformed edentulous ridge

Inadequate or excessive alveolar ridges often compromise framework design, pontic form, pontic inclination, surface finish, and the pontic-ridge interface. These factors in turn can lead to accumulation of plaque and debris, inflammation, gingival hypertrophy, impeded oral hygiene, ridge resorption, mechanical instability, fractures, and flexure of solder joints of cast restorations. Poor esthetics with artificial teeth too short or too long in the maxillary anterior region also can result from poor ridge anatomy.

Pontic form.   The ideal pontic form has been described as being convex and ovate, and well adapted to a concave edentulous ridge. Such pontics require only simple prophylaxis to minimize plaque and food debris accumulation between the pontic and the edentulous ridge. For example, the convex form allows access for dental floss to clean the undersurface of the pontic.

Ridge deformities.   Two types of ridge deformities complicate restorative dentistry. The first, the *bulky ridge*, is usually associated with anodontia or early tooth loss

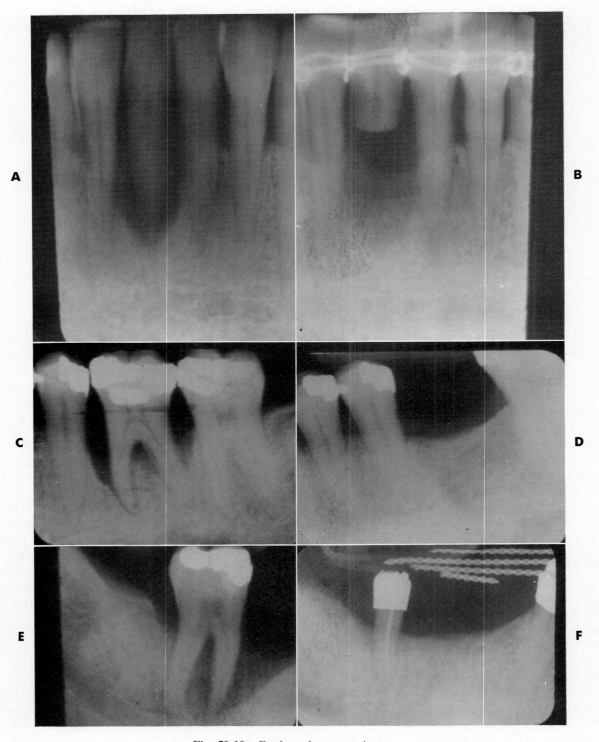

Fig. 50-10. For legend see opposite page.

Fig. 50-10. Strategic extraction for treatment of advanced periodontal disease. **A,** Radiograph of central incisor. **B,** After ligation of crown to adjacent teeth, root was extracted. **C,** Radiograph of mandibular first molar taken in 1973. **D,** Same area in 1980 demonstrating healing and maintenance of attachment apparatus. Patient underwent Hawley bite plane and periodontal therapy. **E,** Radiograph of mandibular second molar. Endodontic therapy was performed on distal root and stabilized provisional restoration. **F,** Same area as **E** 8 months after stabilization. (From Morris AL, Bohannan HM, and Casullo DP, editors: The dental specialties in general practice, Philadelphia, 1983, WB Saunders Co.)

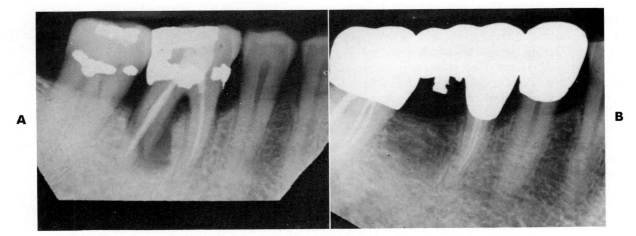

Fig. 50-11. Strategic extraction for treatment of fractured root. **A,** Distal root fracture of mandibular first molar. **B,** Distal root was extracted and osseous healing noted. (From Morris AL, Bohannan HM, and Casullo DP, editors: The dental specialties in general practice, Philadelphia, 1983, WB Saunders Co.)

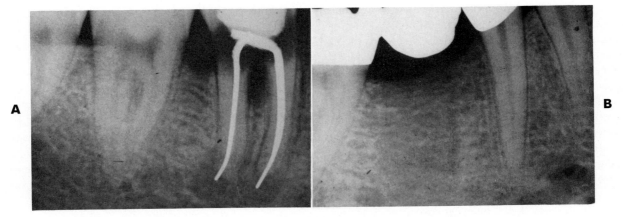

Fig. 50-12. Strategic extraction for treatment of caries. **A,** A 20-year-old patient had pain and swelling in mandibular first molar area. Internal aspects of roots were decayed. Surgical procedures were contraindicated. **B,** Tooth was extracted, bony socket healed, and supporting bone on adjacent teeth was preserved. A three-unit bridge was fabricated. (From Morris AL, Bohannan HM, and Casullo DP, editors: The dental specialties in general practice, Philadelphia, 1983, WB Saunders Co.)

(due to caries or avulsion) before the eruptive process was completed. The second, the *collapsed ridge*, is often associated with advanced periodontal disease, surgery, pulpal disease, surgical trauma during extraction, traumatic injuries, and trauma caused by ill-fitting removable prostheses. Surgical techniques can restore proper ridge form to both types.

Before surgical procedures are initiated, a provisional prosthesis is fabricated according to the dictates of the deformed ridge. It is placed in the mouth and used as a guide to determine the amount and location of tissue to be excised or added. During the surgery, the provisional restoration with its aberrant embrasure form and deformed pontic form, width, length, and inclination is corrected and adapted to the newly created ridge. If problems persist after surgery, the provisional restoration may be further adjusted (or the soft tissue further reduced or augmented).

The provisional restoration is also a valuable adjunct in treatment that involves the extraction of a tooth. Immediate placement of a well-designed provisional restoration serves as a guide in the healing and reformation of the tissues, resulting in an optimally shaped concave ridge form and obviating the need for future corrective surgery. Surgical techniques for correction of edentulous ridge abnormalities are described in Chapter 51.

THE PERIODONTIUM AND EXCESSIVE FORCE: TRAUMA FROM OCCLUSION

The periodontium has a great capacity to adapt to excessive force by movement of teeth into new positions or through repair and regeneration, commonly evidenced by radiographic signs of hyperfunction and increased density of the lamina dura (Fig. 50-13). However, repeated excessive force application by occlusal interferences, off-axis forces, and parafunctional habits can lead to forces that exceed the adapative capability of the tissues with widening of the periodontal ligament space, tooth mobility, and often root resorption. This dystrophic destruction of the attachment apparatus is known as trauma from occlusion.

Injury to the periodontal support results in qualitative and quantitative changes in the tissue that may be seen histologically as hemorrhage, thrombosis of the blood vessels, necrosis and hyalinization of the connective tissue of the periodontal ligament, and resorption of the bony wall of the alveolus.

Radiographic evidence of trauma from occlusion in the attachment apparatus includes a widened periodontal ligament space, loss of continuity of the lamina dura, loss of definition of the periodontal ligament space, root fractures, and root and osseous resorption. Clinical manifestations of occlusal trauma are increasing tooth mobility over time, visible tooth movement, fremitus (palpable tooth movement in function), and tooth migration. Symptoms often include tenderness, sensitivity, or pain, although lesions of trauma from occlusion may be free of symptoms.

When an adequate quantity of periodontal support re-

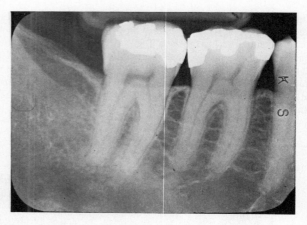

Fig. 50-13. Hyperfunction. Adaptive capacity of attachment apparatus to excessive forces is demonstrated by thickened lamina dura and yet a widened periodontal ligament space around second molar. This condition is most likely associated with an overcarved amalgam restoration and a nonworking interference. (From Morris AL, Bohannan HM, and Casullo DP, editors: The dental specialties in general practice, Philadelphia, 1983, WB Saunders Co.)

mains to withstand the normal forces of occlusion, yet excessive parafunctional forces exceed the adaptive capacity of the attachment apparatus, the disease process is referred to as *primary occlusal trauma* (Fig. 50-14). When the quantity of the remaining intact attachment apparatus has been compromised by periodontal disease and cannot withstand the normal forces of occlusion, the disease process is referred to as *secondary occlusal trauma*.

Primary occlusal trauma with gingivitis or periodontitis

In cases of primary occlusal trauma with gingivitis, the requisite treatment is simple and conservative. Occlusal trauma with gingivitis and occlusal trauma with periodontitis are separate diseases, and both may be reversible with minor therapy. Periodontal therapy involves scaling, root planing, and the establishment of oral hygiene to control inflammation. This is done first, and reduction of mobility may result. If mobility becomes progressively worse, or if there are other signs or symptoms of trauma from occlusion, occlusal therapy is justified. Occlusal therapy involves selective grinding to eliminate interferences and may include the use of a night guard to control nocturnal parafunctional activity.

Primary occlusal trauma and tooth mobility

Tooth mobility may be associated with inflammatory disease: gingivitis, incipient or moderate periodontitis, or pulpitis. Tooth mobility may also be associated with a readily identifiable occlusal etiology: an interference or parafunction, such as nocturnal bruxism, or an occlusal habit such as biting on a pipe stem or other hard object.

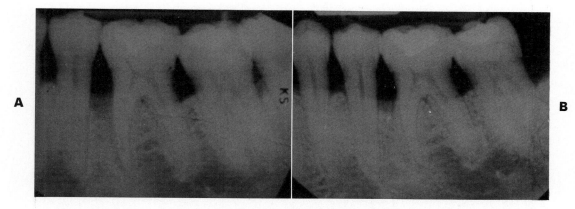

Fig. 50-14. Primary occlusal trauma. **A,** Radiographic signs of primary occlusal trauma include a widened periodontal ligament space, loss of continuity, and loss of definition of lamina dura (alveolar wall). In more advanced stages of primary occlusal trauma, radiographic manifestations are more extensive and severe. Note severe widened periodontal ligament space and bone loss on mesial aspect of first molar. **B,** Reversal of disease process is confirmed by absence of radiographic signs. (From Morris AL, Bohannan HM, and Casullo DP, editors: The dental specialties in general practice, Philadelphia, 1983, WB Saunders Co.)

Treatment of both the inflammatory condition and the occlusal etiology is often necessary for reduction of mobility and other signs or symptoms of primary occlusal trauma.

Progressive mobility

Soft tissue inflammation is controlled routinely in conjunction with occlusal therapy. If the mobility is generalized and associated with inflammatory periodontal disease, soft tissue management results in reduction of mobility and no further treatment is required. But if mobility persists or becomes more severe, the occlusion is carefully reexamined for changes in tooth position induced by the periodontal disease. If no interferences are discovered, undetectable nocturnal bruxism may be occurring and night guard therapy should be instituted.

When a patient manifests signs of wear or a widened periodontal ligament space or has symptoms of pain or impaired function of a tooth-to-tooth parafunction associated with progressive mobility, a night guard to control excessive force is often the treatment of choice. If progressive mobility is associated with missing teeth, the restoration of arch continuity and stability with a fixed prosthesis is implemented whenever possible.

Secondary occlusal trauma

Secondary occlusal trauma combined with periodontitis often requires extensive restorative treatment in addition to periodontal therapy (Fig. 50-15).

With secondary occlusal trauma, the quantity of the attachment apparatus may be diminished and teeth can no longer sustain force delivered even during normal function. Often the mobility is progressive, worsening over several months to a year, in spite of definitive scaling and root planing and the establishment of good plaque control. Hawley bite plane therapy may be useful after reduction of inflammation to evaluate the effects of reducing occlusal forces on the posterior teeth in assessing the need for more definitive occlusal therapy. If further occlusal therapy is needed, the following may be considered.

First, all teeth in secondary trauma may need stabilization. This may be difficult because of extreme mobility, excessive clinical crown length, loss of arch continuity, aberrations in occlusal form, such as a Class II, division 1 malocclusion, and severely distorted occlusal planes and curves. Hawley bite plane therapy, initiated in the first phase of treatment, may help reestablish arch integrity and stabilize the maxillary teeth. It also redirects occlusal forces to anterior teeth, disarticulates the posterior teeth, and aids in the control of parafunction. In addition, the posterior teeth may erupt, eliminating interferences and facilitating occlusal adjustment. Furthermore, this therapy may aid in locating the true terminal hinge axis, which can be used as a reference for the future occlusal pattern.

Splinting is a useful adjunct in the treatment of progressively mobile teeth in secondary trauma. It is used in conjunction with correction of the occlusal scheme, not as a substitute for poor occlusal relations. Splinting can also help stabilize weak teeth, maintain tooth position and relations after orthodontic therapy, prevent the eruption of unopposed teeth, and prevent open contacts and resulting food impaction.

Often, adjunctive orthodontics may be required to correct axial inclinations so that forces will be delivered vertically along the long axes of the teeth (see Fig. 50-3).

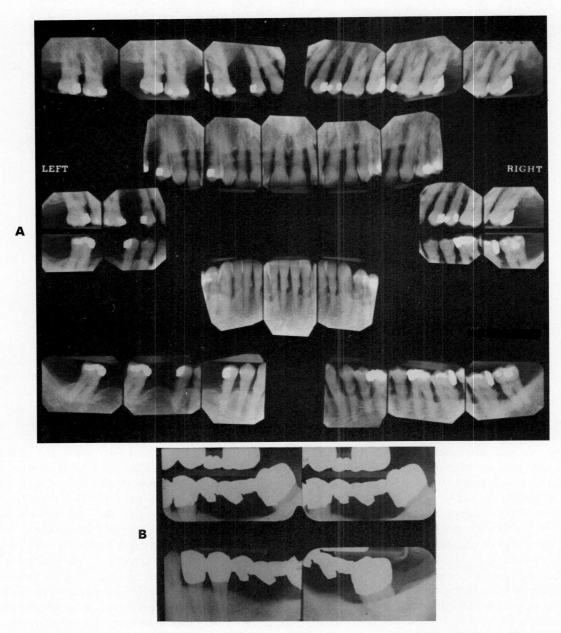

Fig. 50-15. Secondary occlusal trauma. **A,** This full set of radiographs is of mouth of a patient with secondary occlusal trauma. Like primary occlusal trauma, it is manifested by a widened periodontal ligament space and loss of continuity and definition of lamina dura. However, bone loss is much more extensive, and supporting structures are unable to sustain normal forces. **B,** In cases of secondary occlusal trauma, all radiographic signs of primary occlusal trauma are present, but bone loss is much more extensive. This mandibular second molar, restored in an extruded position, destroyed arch rhythmicity, resulting in interferences in protrusive and lateral protrusive movements. In addition to excessive occlusal forces associated with interference, horizontal forces were generated by parafunctional activity. To control occlusal forces, Hawley bite plane therapy and selective grinding were instituted in conjunction with antiinfective periodontal therapy.

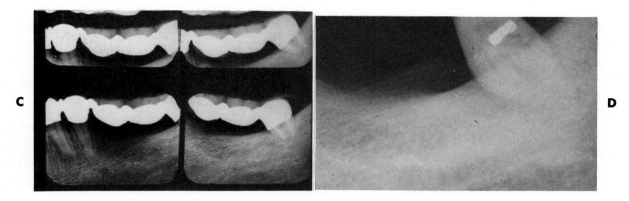

Fig. 50-15, cont'd.   C, This 6-month postoperative radiograph demonstrates healing of attachment apparatus. Intentional endodontic therapy was necessary to correct elevated plane of occlusion and exaggerated curve of Spee and transverse curve, thus eliminating interference. **D,** Final restoration is in place 2 years after treatment was initiated. (From Morris AL, Bohannan HM, and Casullo DP, editors: The dental specialties in general practice, Philadelphia, 1983, WB Saunders Co.)

Successful treatment of occlusal trauma is evidenced clinically by a decrease in mobility and fremitus and radiographically by a thinner, more distinct periodontal ligament space and a more continuous and distinct lamina dura. These changes occur because the actual injury to the attachment apparatus, caused by both primary and secondary occlusal trauma, is reversed when treated.

SUMMARY

Patients with occlusal trauma and advanced periodontitis often require advanced periodontal therapy, including root resection or strategic extraction, antiinfective therapy, and regenerative procedures, as well as adjunctive orthodontics, occlusal adjustment by selective grinding, and splinting for periodontal stabilization.

SUGGESTED READINGS

Abrams L: Augmentation of the deformed residual edentulous ridge for fixed prosthesis, Compend Contin Educ Dent 1(3):205, 1980.

Amsterdam M: Periodontal prosthesis—twenty-five years in retrospect, Alpha Omegan 67(3):8, 1974.

Casullo D: Diagnosis and treatment planning in general practice; Occlusion in general practice; Multidisciplinary approach to therapy. In Morris AL, Bohannan HM, and Casullo DP, editors: The dental specialties in general practice, Philadelphia, 1983, WB Saunders Co.

Corn H: Edentulous area pedicle grafts in mucogingival surgery, Periodontics 2:229, 1964.

Garber D and Rosenberg E: The edentulous ridge in fixed prosthodontics, Compend Contin Educ Dent 2(4):212, 1981.

Garguilo AW, Wentz FM, and Orban B: Dimensions of the dentogingival junction in humans, J Periodontol 32:261, 1961.

Löe H and Ainamo J: Anatomical characteristics of gingivae—a clinical and microscopic study of free and attached gingivae, J Periodontol 37:5, 1966.

Morris AL, Bohannan HM, and Casullo DP, editors: The dental specialties in general practice, Philadelphia, 1983, WB Saunders Co.

Nyman S and Lindhe J: Longitudinal study of combined periodontal and prosthetic treatment of patients with advanced periodontal disease, J Periodontol 50:163, 1979.

Nyman S, Lindhe J, and Lundgren D: The role of occlusion for the stability of fixed bridges in patients with reduced periodontal support, J Clin Periodontol 2:53, 1975.

Rosenberg E, Garber D, and Evian C: Tooth lengthening procedures, Compend Contin Educ Dent 1(3):61, 1980.

Stein RS: Pontic-residual ridge relationships: a research report, J Prosthet Dent 16:283, 1966.

Waerhaug J: Presence or absence of plaque on subgingival restorations, Scand J Dent Res 83:193, 1975.

Weisgold A: Contours of the full crown restoration, Alpha Omegan 70(3):77, 1977.

Weisgold A and Feder M: Tooth preparation in fixed prosthesis, I, Compend Contin Educ Dent 1(6)375, 1980.

Chapter 51

SURGICAL PREPARATION FOR FIXED AND REMOVABLE PROSTHESES

Jay S. Seibert

Prostheses are used to replace teeth that have been extracted, often because of periodontal disease. Furthermore, patients who require prosthetic replacement of teeth often require periodontal treatment. Coordination of periodontal and prosthetic procedures provides for optimal periodontal therapy, as well as optimal restorative therapy. This in-cludes coordination of periodontal surgical treatment procedures with those surgical procedures necessary for optimal prosthetic results. For example, periodontal access flaps may be carried out at the same time as root-lengthening procedures, as described in Chapter 47, or periodontal access procedures may be carried out at the same time as correction of ridge abnormalities prior to fixed or removable prosthetic treatment. The full treatment plan often includes initial antiinfective therapy, periodontal treatment involving surgical procedures for access or regeneration, preprosthetic surgery, prosthetic treatment involving fabrication of provisional prostheses, and final restorative procedures. Several newly developed procedures for correcting ridge deformities are presented in detail in this chapter.

EDENTULOUS RIDGE IN FIXED AND REMOVABLE PROSTHETIC TREATMENT
Normal ridge

The eminences that existed in the bone over the roots of teeth in prominent arch position usually disappear as bone remodels after healing of the extraction sockets. In fixed prosthetic therapy, a resorbed two- or three-tooth edentulous area may present major problems in the placement and arrangement of the pontic teeth. The teeth frequently look like they are resting on top of the smooth tissue of the ridge. For example, prominently placed pontic teeth lack a root eminence, marginal gingiva, and an interdental papilla. A dark triangle usually exists in the embrasure area between the abutment tooth and the pontic, or between the pontic teeth, even though the underlying ridge has maintained its former bulk. Patients dislike the lack of air seal, which affects phonetics and control of droplets of saliva while speaking. The spaces between or under the pontic teeth trap food particles.

A number of surgical implant and graft procedures have been developed to reconstruct the deformed partially edentulous ridge.

Deformed partially edentulous ridge in restoration cases with fixed prostheses

Etiology of ridge deformities. The loss of alveolar structures can result from many causes: clefts from birth defects, traumatic extractions, facial trauma from sports or automobile accidents, gunshot wounds or missle fragments, vertical fracture of endodontically treated teeth, advanced periodontal disease, abscess formation, removal of tumors, or implant failures. The resulting deformity in the healed, mature ridge is related to the volume of root structure and bone that is missing (cleft palate cases) or has been destroyed.

Classification of ridge defects. Ridge defects can be classified into three general categories (Seibert, 1983a):

Class I: Buccolingual loss of tissue with normal ridge height in an apicocoronal dimension

Class II: Apicocoronal loss of tissue with normal ridge width in a buccolingual dimension

Class III: Combination buccolingual and apicocoronal loss of tissue resulting in loss of normal height and width

This classification was made to improve communication among clinicians in describing ridge defects and to aid in the selection and sequence of therapeutic procedures to eliminate the various classes of defects. Success in therapy is dependent on an understanding of the various defects, their unique anatomy, blood supply to the area, and the wound healing involved. Often, different surgical techniques are required to correct the various defects.

Prevalence of ridge deformities. A number of studies have described techniques to treat the various forms of ridge defects *before the fabrication* of a prosthesis (Meltzer, 1979; Abrams, 1980a; Langer and Calagna, 1980, 1982; Seibert, 1980, 1983a, 1983b; Garber and Rosenberg, 1981; Kaldahl et al., 1982; McHenry et al., 1982; Allen et al., 1985; Miller, 1986; Seibert and Cohen, 1987).

Abrams et al. (1987) addressed the question of the prevalence of anterior ridge deformities in partially edentulous patients. They examined a random sample of 416 diagnostic casts at a university clinic, and 34 of the patients involved were found to be partially edentulous in the anterior region. Within this group of 34, 91% had some form of ridge defect, including 11 with Class I defects, 1 with a Class II defect, and 19 with Class III defects. This survey suggests that the number of patients with ridge defects may constitute a larger percentage of patients than was formerly believed to exist.

Traditional prosthetic treatment of ridge deformities. Dentists in the past have resorted to various prosthetic mechanical methods to restore normal contours in a deformed ridge. In an attempt to eliminate most Class I defects and less extensive Class II and III defects, the shape of pontic teeth has been modified by various means to make them contact the altered contours of the deformed ridge. The tissue surface of the pontics is frequently extended lingually, apically, or lingually and apically to bring them into contact with the ridge. Because of their adaptation to fit the ridge in this manner, the pontic teeth are usually longer in an apicocoronal dimension than the adjacent abutment teeth. If the patient has a high smile line and shows a considerable amount of gingiva above the teeth, the pontic teeth will often be disproportionately long, resulting in unacceptable esthetics.

Depending on the degree of concavity that exists in the pontic area or areas, the neck or cervical area of the pontic teeth is usually curved lingually in a smooth arc to bring this surface of the pontic into contact with the ridge. Abrams (1980a) has referred to this design as a "blended pontic" (Fig. 51-1). If a longer blended pontic is not acceptable and the pontic must be kept the same length as the contralateral abutment teeth, another problem is encountered. If the facial-cervical surfaces of the pontic teeth are not curved lingually in a gentle arc to contact the ridge, a plateau or ledge is created that acts as a food trap and impediment to normal movements of the upper lip.

The difficulties encountered in using longer blended pontics or normal-length pontics that have a ledge in the cervical area have frequently been avoided by using a flange of gingiva-colored plastic to fill the space between the pontic teeth and the surface of the ridge (Fig. 51-2).

Another concept used in treating larger defects has been

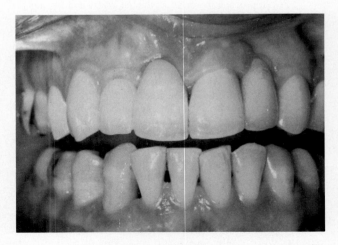

Fig. 51-1. Blended pontics. Facial contour in cervical one third of pontics replacing teeth Nos. 8 and 10 has been "blended" in a gradual arc to contact concavity in residual ridge. Pontics are longer than contralateral abutment teeth.

the combination of a fixed retainer and rectangular bar system that employs a clip-retained removable pontic and flange section (Andrew's bridge system). The clip device facilitates easy removal of the pontic section for hygiene, inspection, and servicing of the overall prosthesis (Fig. 51-3).

Various precision retainer systems have also been devised for multiple pontic spans for use with fixed and removable prosthetic appliances. The addition of a flange of simulated gum tissue can make a prosthesis look more lifelike. Air flow is also controlled, and phonetics may be improved. The major drawback to the *permanent* placement of such a pontic section is that it usually acts as a food trap and plaque retention area. The gingival and ridge tissues adjacent to the flange become inflamed and swollen, inducing periodontal disease or caries in the abutment teeth.

A flange prosthesis is a solution for certain large-volume ridge defects, since these devices provide the patient with acceptable esthetics and function. The treatment of these extensive maxillofacial defects is not within the scope of this chapter; however, a variety of predictable surgical procedures can be used successfully to augment ridge defects of *moderate dimensions,* and these are described here.

Types of pontics. It is useful to discuss pontic designs first, since they influence the surgical procedure. There are four pontic designs that have been used over the years:

1. Sanitary pontic
2. Total ridge lap pontic
3. Modified ridge lap pontic
4. Ovate pontic

The sanitary pontic may be used in the posterior sections of the mouth where esthetic considerations are not a concern. The convex tissue surface of the pontic is smooth in all dimensions and is kept well above the surface of the ridge. The wide, open space between the ridge and the pontic facilitates effective cleansing of the prosthesis and tissues. Many patients object to the space and the food trap it provides, or to the way the pontic feels against the tongue. For these reasons, the sanitary pontic design is seldom used.

The total ridge lap pontic (Fig. 51-4, *A*) was commonly used in the first half of this century. These pontics provide reasonably good esthetics, but to the trained eye they look as though they are resting on top of the tissue. The ridge lap pontic is designed to fit tightly against the ridge, and it eliminates the major part of the food trap problem experienced with the sanitary pontic. Retention of food debris against the teeth and tissues was formerly thought to be one of the major etiologic factors in the development of periodontal disease. As the plaque hypothesis supplanted the nonspecific irritant hypothesis in the causation of periodontal disease, it became obvious that microbial plaque could not easily be removed from the deeply concave tissue surfaces of total ridge lap pontics.

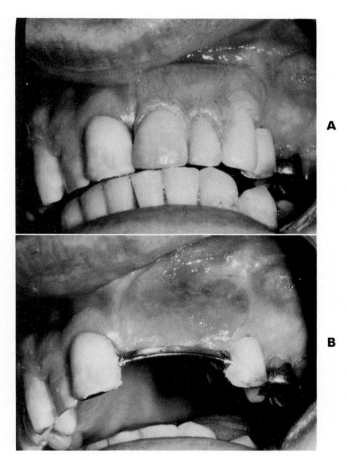

A

B

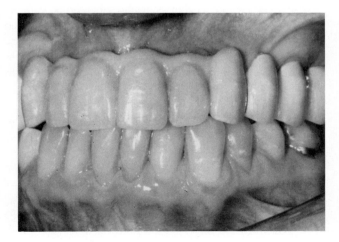

Fig. 51-2. Pontics with flange. To keep pontics in five-tooth span (teeth Nos. 7 to 11) from appearing too long, a flange of pink porcelain has been added to hide deformity in ridge. (Courtesy Dr. Leonard Abrams, Philadelphia.)

Fig. 51-3. Andrew's bridge system. **A,** Three-tooth facade with acrylic flange in position over supporting bar. **B,** Clip-retained removable section has been removed to show abutment crowns and supporting bar section of prosthesis.

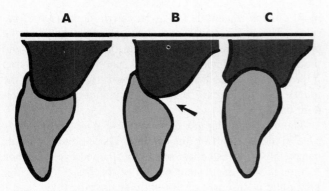

Fig. 51-4. Pontic designs. **A,** Total ridge lap. **B,** Modified ridge lap. **C,** Ovate. (From Garber D and Rosenberg E: The endentulous ridge in fixed prosthodontics, Compend Contin Educ Dent 2(4):212, 1981.)

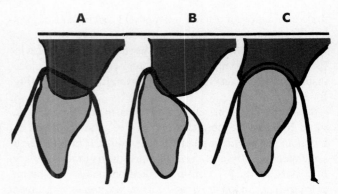

Fig. 51-5. Dental floss or similar cleansing materials cannot contact pontic tissue surface in concavity of total ridge lap pontic, **A.** While floss can contact more of tissue surface of modified ridge lap pontic, **B,** a concave area remains in center of tissue-contacting surface that cannot be cleaned. Floss can be brought into intimate contact with all of tissue-contacting surface of ovate pontic, **C.** (Courtesy Dr. David Garber, Atlanta.)

The modified ridge lap design (Fig. 51-4, *B*) was then developed, since it is easier to clean and may provoke less of an inflammatory response in the ridge tissues as compared with the total ridge lap pontic (Stein, 1966). The modified ridge lap pontic permits more of the tissue surface of the pontic to be contacted by dental floss or a similar type of mechanical cleansing device; however, there is usually a concave area in the center of the tissue surface that cannot be reached by dental floss. The floss spans the concave area, and plaque, calculus, and small food particles frequently can be found on this surface of the pontic (Fig. 51-5).

Other problems associated with modified ridge lap pontics include the following:

1. The triangular open area on the lingual-palatal surface traps food particles and may be annoying to the patient's tongue.
2. The pontic may not provide a sufficient air seal for correct speech.
3. The spaces that exist between pontic and abutment, pontic and pontic, or pontic and ridge may permit droplets of saliva to be forced through the spaces during speech, which may be annoying.

The ovate pontic (Fig. 51-4, *C*) was developed by Abrams (1980a) in an attempt to overcome the problems encountered with prostheses that incorporated pontics with total or modified ridge lap designs. The ovate pontic offers many advantages over the ridge lap pontics, including the following:

1. Good esthetics can be obtained in the final prosthesis. The ovate pontic is placed within the confines of the residual ridge. This makes the pontic look like it is emerging from the ridge rather than resting on top of it.

2. The placement of an ovate pontic into the ridge creates the illusion of a free gingival margin in the cervical area of the pontic that blends into the interdental papillae in the embrasure area.
3. The tissue-contacting surface is convex and can be reached and readily cleaned by dental floss.
4. The lingual third of the pontic can be contoured to the normal anatomic form of the tooth that is being replaced, including a cementoenamel junction (CEJ) and root form if desired.
5. A more effective air seal can be obtained, thereby eliminating air or saliva leakage.
6. The receptacle site of the ridge to receive the tissue surface of an ovate pontic creates "interdental papillae" (Fig. 51-6). This eliminates or minimizes the unesthetic dark triangles between the teeth.

The ovate pontic design is useful in treating patients who have a high smile line. Ovate pontics should not be used in or against a thin knife-edged ridge, since the ridge must have, or be capable of being augmented to, sufficient buccolingual thickness to contain the ovate pontic within the corpus of the ridge.

Deformed edentulous ridge in restoration cases with removable prostheses

A number of problems encountered in treating deformed partially or fully edentulous ridges that preprosthetic surgical procedures can correct are listed below.

Knife-edged ridge. Alveolar bone resorption after extractions frequently produces a thin, knife-edged edentulous ridge with inadequate attached gingiva, especially in the mandibular arch. If there is inadequate attached gingiva on which to place a denture, a tissue substitution procedure can be used to remove the alveolar mucosa on the

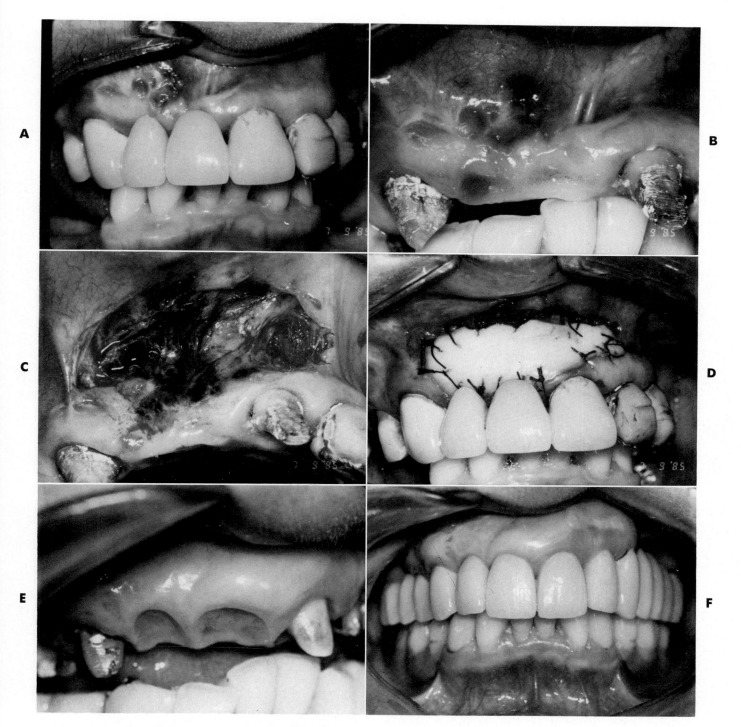

Fig. 51-6. Class I ridge deformity with amalgam tattoo resulting from an apicoectomy to treat former lateral and central incisior teeth. **A,** Pretreatment view with failing fixed prosthesis in position. Patient has had unsightly amalgam tattoo for 18 years. **B,** Pretreatment view with fixed prosthesis removed. **C,** Recipient site prepared to receive a free graft from palate. **D,** A thick free graft has been used to augment ridge and mask stained connective tissues. **E,** Gingivoplasty was used to create ovate receptacle sites in healed ridge. This view shows form and color of ridge tissues 20 months after surgical procedure. **F,** Final prosthesis has been placed. (Treatment in conjunction with Dr. Alex Koranyi, Toronto.)

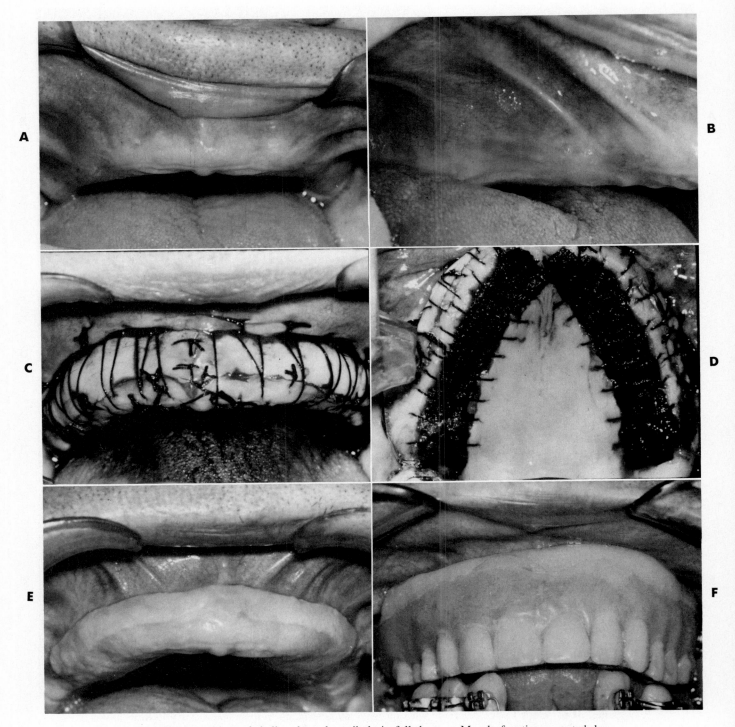

Fig. 51-7.   Problem of shallow buccal vestibule in full denture. Muscle function unseated denture. **A,** Ridge prior to treatment. Note muscle origins close to ridge crest. **B,** Pretreatment view of ridge showing multiple frena insertions close to ridge crest. **C,** Two free grafts sutured in place. **D,** Palatal donor site with Surgicel placed. **E,** Note vestibular extension and ridge augmentation obtained 7 weeks after procedure. **F,** Existing prosthesis has been relined, and denture is now stable during function. (Treatment in conjunction with Dr. Jeffrey Pearlman-Storch, Philadelphia.)

buccal (or lingual) side of the ridge and substitute in its place an equal zone of masticatory mucosa by employing a free graft of attached gingiva taken from the palate. The free graft procedure is also useful in providing attached gingiva over exostoses, for atrophic ridges, and for regaining vestibular extension in the area of the genial tubercles.

Elimination of ridge undercuts. To gain a path of insertion for the buccal flange of a prosthesis, a surgical flap and osseous resection procedures have been used to eliminate the bony projections that produce the undercut areas. This may still be the procedure of choice in many situations, especially if the bone projects laterally to an abnormal extent, creating a large undercut area. However, for slight, moderate, or deep undercuts on buccal ridge surfaces, bone can be preserved by eliminating the undercut with a free graft procedure that fills the concavity (McHenry et al., 1982).

Vestibular extension procedures. A shallow buccal or lingual vestibule frequently limits the placement of an adequate flange on a removable prosthesis. The masticatory mucosa of the palate functions as a special mucosa to withstand the forces of mastication. It can be used in place of skin in vestibular extension surgery. The major problem with using the palate as the donor site, as compared with skin, is the limitation in the amount of donor tissue that can be obtained during a single procedure (Fig. 51-7).

PREPROSTHETIC TREATMENT PLANNING: NEED FOR COORDINATION OF PROSTHETIC AND SURGICAL THERAPY

It is extremely important that the clinician who is to construct the prosthesis carefully coordinate the prosthetic procedures with the preprosthetic and periodontal surgical procedures to allow for proper healing and tissue remodeling prior to placement of the final prosthesis.

SURGICAL PROCEDURES FOR RECONSTRUCTION OF DEFORMED PARTIALLY EDENTULOUS RIDGES/PONTIC AREAS IN PREPARATION FOR FIXED PROSTHESES

The selection of a single surgical procedure or combination of several procedures staged over a period of months will depend on the nature of the ridge problems to be corrected. The indications, contraindications, predictability, and problems associated with the various surgical procedures are discussed below.

Deepithelized connective tissue pedicle graft or "roll procedure"

Surgical concept. The procedure involves the creation of a connective tissue pedicle that is placed into a subepithelial pouch (Fig. 51-8) and was developed by Abrams (1980b).

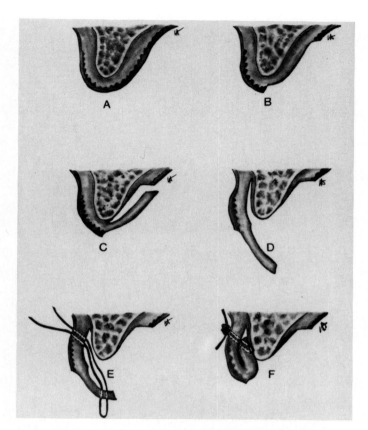

Fig. 51-8. Contiguous deepithelized pedicle graft. **A,** Cross section of residual edentulous ridge prior to procedure. **B,** Removal of epithelium. **C,** Elevation of pedicle. **D,** Creation of pouch. **E,** Sutures placed. **F,** Flap is secured, creating a convexity in ridge. (From Abrams L: Augmentation of the deformed residual edentulous ridge for fixed prosthodontics, Compend Contin Educ Dent 1(3):205, 1980.)

Indications. The procedure can be used to correct small to moderate Class I defects (Fig. 51-9). It will maintain the color and surface texture characteristics of the existing ridge tissue.

Contraindications. This procedure has limited usefulness in gaining ridge height and cannot be used to change the color or surface characteristics of the existing ridge. It is not suitable where the ridge tissue and adjacent palatal (or lingual) tissue is very thin.

Technique. The procedure requires the formation of a rectangular pedicle of connective tissue on the palatal side of the defect. The length of the pedicle to be created depends on the required amount of apicocoronal augmentation on the labial surface. This in turn is related to the high smile line and the amount of root prominence that exists on either side of the deformity. If a two- or three-tooth edentulous space is to be treated, separate pedicles are raised that will form the new root-cervical margin areas, and a space is left between the pedicles that will form the

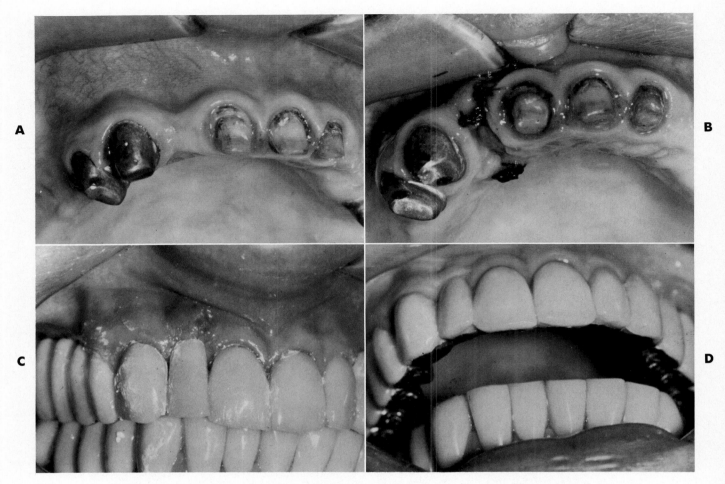

Fig. 51-9. A, Pretreatment view of Class I defect. Note marked concavity in ridge. **B,** Surgical site 1 week after use of a contiguous deepithelized pedicle graft procedure. **C,** Tissue surface of pontic relined. **D,** Final prosthesis in place. Note illusion of a root eminence and free gingival margin apical to lateral incisor pontic tooth. (Courtesy Dr. Leonard Abrams, Philadelphia.)

new interdental papillae between each of the pontics. When the pedicle flap is tucked into the pouch that will be created, it loses some of its length because of the U-shaped curve made as it is bent back on itself. It is advisable to make the pedicles 2 to 3 mm longer than the finished apicocoronal reconstruction to compensate for the length that will be lost when the pedicle is rolled into position.

The maximum amount of connective tissue that can be raised from the palate is elevated to make the pedicle. Sharp dissection is used to raise a split-thickness flap, with care taken to avoid denuding the bone. The void that is made in the donor site fills in with granulation tissue. The epithelium on the oral surface of the pedicle may be removed with a rotary diamond point, or by sharp dissection, prior to the elevation of the pedicle. Soehren et al. (1973) found that the epithelium in palatal free grafts

ranges in thickness from 0.1 to 0.6 mm. It is recommended that one cut approximately 1 mm into the surface (parallel to the surface) of the pedicle to ensure that all of the epithelium is removed. The epithelium may also be removed by sharp dissection after the pedicle is raised. The objective is to remove the epithelium and the *least amount* of connective tissue possible.

Caution must be exercised in dissecting the pedicle flap as the dissection approaches the labial surface. A concavity often exists on the labial surface in this area, instead of the usual convexity found in this area of a normal ridge. If the plane of dissection is not changed at the osseous line angle to follow the contour of the deformed ridge, the tissue may be perforated.

A pouch or tunnel is made on the labial surface of the ridge by extending the plane of dissection apically. A tunnel is made under the labial tissue; however, care is exercised not to make an exit opening at the apical border of the dissection. It is not necessary to raise the periosteum when making the pouch.

The next step is to tuck the loose pedicle into the space provided in the pouch. If the pouch is too short or too narrow, further dissection may be required. Once the pedicle fits as desired, it is sutured as shown in Fig. 51-8. To achieve the illusion of a root eminence, the entrance and exit of the suture material should be high in the vestibule near the mucobuccal fold. This enables the suture material to pull the pedicle to the apical end of the pouch. The provisional prosthesis is then placed in position, and the tissue surface of the pontic is examined to see how it contacts the deepithelized connective tissue surface of the pedicle.

Adjustment of pontic contours. It is desirable to maintain light positive pressure against the pedicle graft or implant surface by the tissue surface of the pontic. Autopolymerizing resin may be added to the cervical area and tissue surface of the pontic and allowed to cure until it reaches a doughlike state. The prosthesis is then seated, and the doughy consistency resin is pressed into the surface of the augmentation site and allowed to polymerize. The tissue surface of the pontic, cervical third, and embrasure areas are then carved to the shape that will be used in the final prosthesis and polished, and the provisional prosthesis is temporarily cemented.

Postoperative care and hygiene in the surgical area. A periodontal dressing is placed over the palatal donor site. The routine use of an appropriate prophylactic antibiotic is warranted.

Pouch procedures for subepithelial grafts and implants

Indications. These procedures are used to correct Class I defects. They will maintain the color and surface characteristics of the existing ridge tissue. The use of resorbable synthetic bone substitutes may aid in restoring arch contour in cases where larger-volume defects exist.

Contraindications. These procedures have limited usefulness in gaining ridge height and cannot be used to change the color or surface characteristics of the existing ridge.

Technique. Several pouch procedures have been designed to receive free grafts of connective tissue removed from the palate or synthetic bone substitutes. They vary only in the direction in which the entrance incision and plane of dissection is made (Langer and Calagna, 1980, 1982; Garber and Rosenberg, 1981; Kaldahl et al., 1982; Seibert, 1983a; Allen et al., 1985; Miller, 1986). A subepithelial pouch is created in the same manner as previously described for the deepithelized connective tissue pedicle graft procedure. Instead of rolling a pedicle of connective tissue into the pouch, a free graft of connective tissue that is taken from the palate, autogenous bone chips, or resorbable or nonresorbable synthetic bone material is placed

into the pouch. The graft or implant material is placed and molded to create the desired contour in the ridge, and the entrance incision is sutured (Fig. 51-10).

The entrance incision and plane of dissection may be made from an apical-to-coronal direction (Fig. 51-11) or laterally (Fig. 51-10).

Interpositional (wedge and inlay) procedures

Indications. These procedures are also used to correct Class I defects and small to moderate Class II defects. They aid in maintaining the color and surface characteristics of the existing ridge tissue.

Contraindications. The wedge and inlay procedures aid in gaining ridge height but are not as useful as onlay grafts for gaining ridge height. The wedge and inlay procedure cannot be used to change the color or surface characteristics of the existing ridge tissue.

Technique. These procedures differ slightly from the pouch procedures, in which a *subepithelial* (subconnective tissue) graft or implant is used. The opening of the pouch is not closed in this type of procedure. A pie-shaped free graft is removed from the palate, tuberosity area, or edentulous ridge and is inserted like a wedge into the opening of the pouch (Meltzer, 1979; Seibert, 1983a; Seibert and Cohen, 1987). The labial surface of the pouch is elevated bucally to eliminate the concavity in the ridge. The wedge-shaped graft is then placed into the space developed to maintain the labial surface of the pouch in the desired position. The epithelial surface of the wedge is positioned at the level of the surrounding epithelial surfaces, and the wedge is maintained in this position by sutures. If augmentation is required in an apicocoronal dimension as well as buccolingually, part of the wedge is positioned above the level of the surrounding tissues. This leaves a segment of the connective tissue of the graft exposed. The connective tissue in this design receives a flow of plasma and ingrowth of capillaries from the connective tissue *surrounding* the implanted tissue. The percentage of "take" or success with this technique is higher than that with thick onlay grafts that receive their nutritional supply from only one surface during wound healing (Fig. 51-12).

Onlay graft procedures

Indications. Onlay graft procedures are used to gain ridge height. They will also add bulk in the labial dimension and are therefore useful in treating Class III ridge defects. Onlay grafts can be used to replace undesirable pigmentation or amalgam tattoos in the tissue (see Fig. 51-6).

Contraindications. Onlay grafts are not well suited for use in areas where the blood supply to the recipient site is or has been compromised by scar formation from previous surgical procedures or trauma. Thick grafts require an abundant blood supply and rapid capillary proliferation, and if these needs cannot be met, the grafts may slough.

Text continued on p. 650.

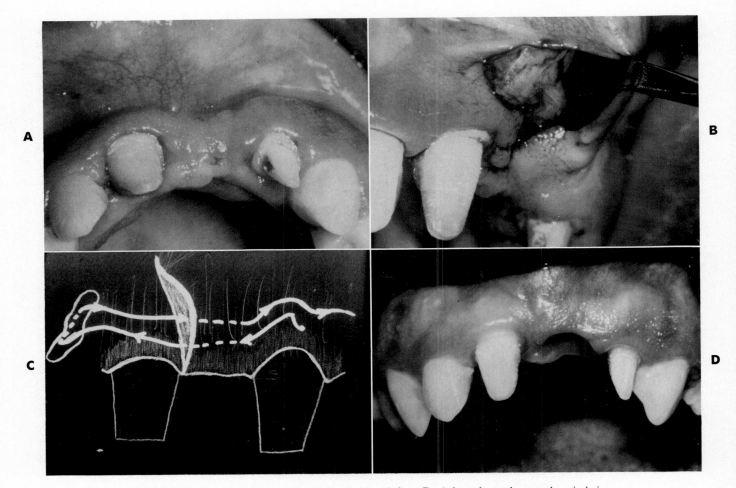

Fig. 51-10.   A, Pretreatment view, Class I ridge defect. **B,** A lateral pouch procedure is being used to augment ridge with connective tissue obtained from second molar–tuberosity area. **C,** Suturing to pull connective tissue into pouch. **D,** Two months after surgery, gingivoplasty was used to accentuate receptacle site for an ovate pontic. Note that concavity in ridge has been converted into a convexity and that ovate pontic will appear to be emerging or growing out of ridge. "Gingival margin" over pontic will match form of gingival margin on central incisor abutment tooth. (Courtesy Dr. David Garber, Atlanta.)

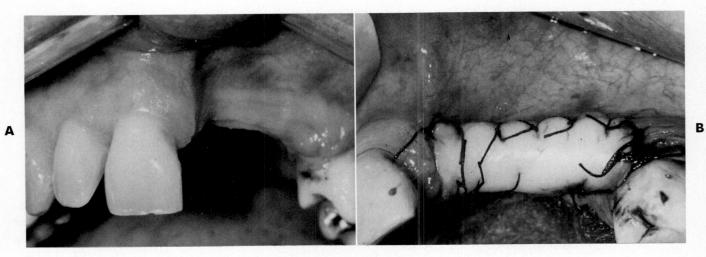

Fig 51-11.   For legend see opposite page.

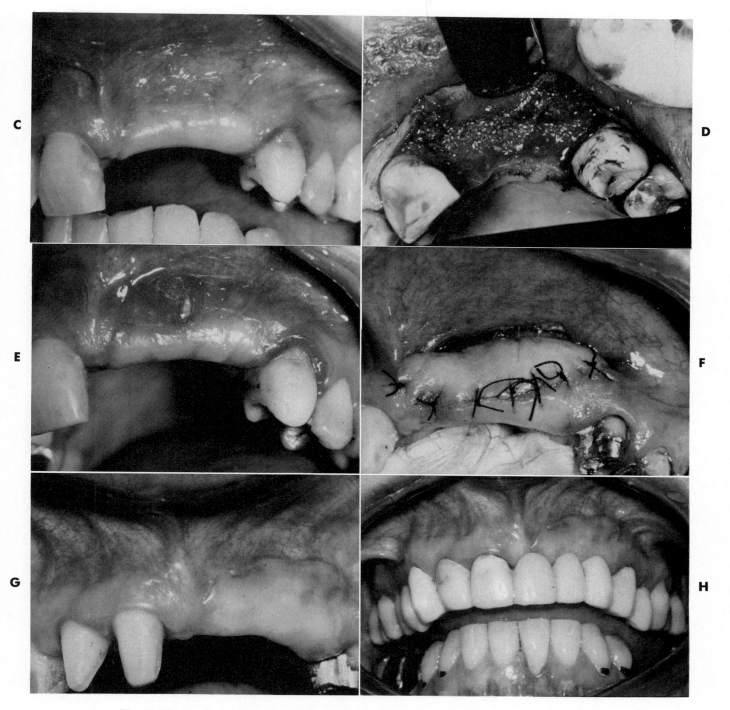

Fig. 51-11. **A,** Pretreatment view of extensive Class III ridge defect. Patient had worn a removable prosthesis for many years and wished to have a fixed prosthesis. **B,** Large, thick onlay graft sutured into position. **C,** Appearance 2 months after surgery. Onlay graft has gained ridge height. Second-stage procedure is needed to augment ridge further in a buccolingual dimension. **D,** A pouch has been created and small particles of hydroxyapatite implanted. **E,** Two weeks after second-stage procedure, pieces of hydroxyapatite can be seen emerging through a small perforation in flap just apical to mucogingival junction. **F,** A third-stage veneer type of free graft is being used to mask hydroxyapatite apical to mucogingival junction and gain a greater amount of augmentation in a buccolingual direction. **G,** Reconstructed ridge 2 months after third-stage grafting procedure. Compare contour of healed augmented ridge with that shown in **A. H,** Provisional prosthesis in place. Pontic teeth are shorter (apicocoronally) than contralateral abutment teeth and need to be lengthened to bring them into balance and symmetry with overall dental arch for better esthetics. (Prosthesis by Dr. Andrew Rosen, Media, Pa.)

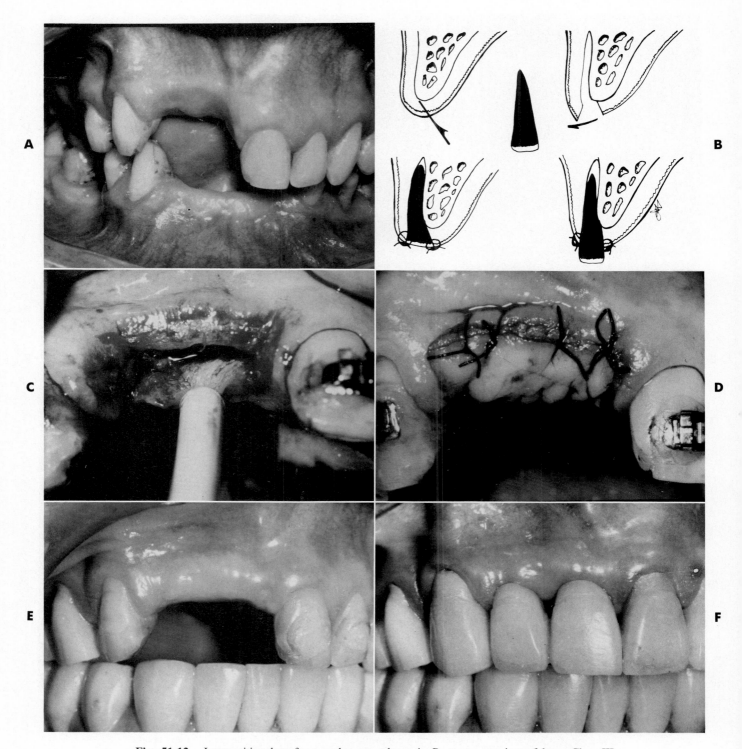

Fig. 51-12. Interpositional graft or wedge procedure. **A,** Pretreatment view of large Class III ridge defect requiring 18 months of orthodontic therapy to level plane of occlusion. **B,** Sequence of steps. First, a wedge-shaped section of connective tissue with its overlying epithelium is removed from palate and is inserted between elevated pouchlike flap and ridge. **C,** A midline incision has been made, after removal of epithelium from surrounding border area, to make a pouch to receive inlay-onlay graft. Small releasing incisions have been made at each end of midline incision (both labially and palatally), and labial tissues have been elevated to form a pouch. **D,** Part of wedge has been left above surface of surrounding tissue in an attempt to gain additional ridge height. **E** and **F,** Two months after surgery, note amount of ridge height obtained. A second-stage procedure will be done to gain more ridge height to fill in "dark triangle" in papillary area of lateral incisor and central incisor pontics.

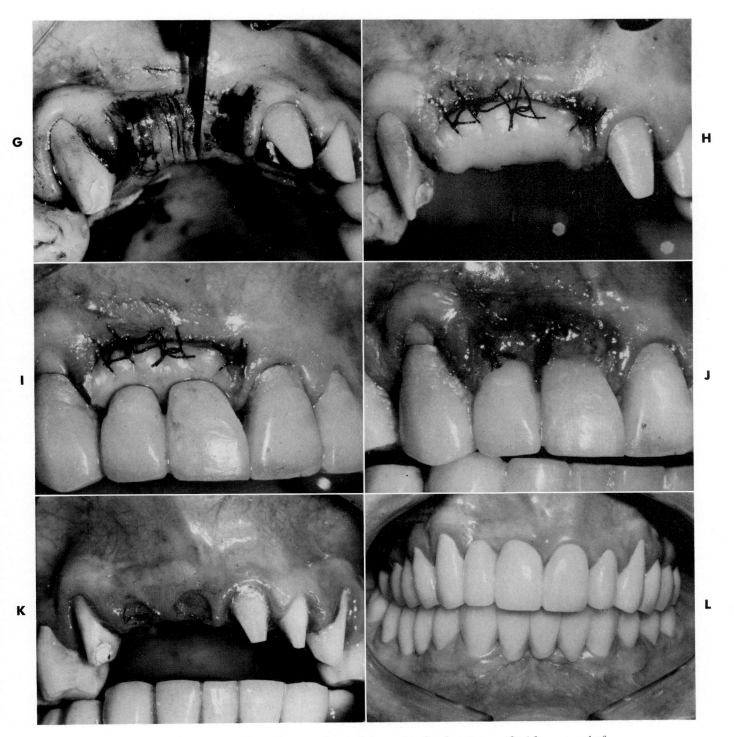

Fig. 51-12, cont'd. G, Second-stage onlay graft 2 months after first-stage graft. After removal of epithelium, striation cuts are made deep into underlying connective tissue. **H,** Second-stage onlay graft sutured into position. Graft is 1 mm thick at periphery and 5 mm thick in center. **I,** Pontics have been shortened and embrasure area opened to permit second-stage graft to adapt to contours of pontics. **J,** One week after surgery, epithelium has sloughed and connective tissue is adapting to contour of pontics. **K,** Two months after second-stage onlay graft procedure, receptacle sites are being prepared for ovate form of pontics. Note "interproximal papilla" that has resulted and that fills embrasures between pontic teeth. **L,** One year after surgery. (Prosthesis by Dr. P. Malpeso, New York.)

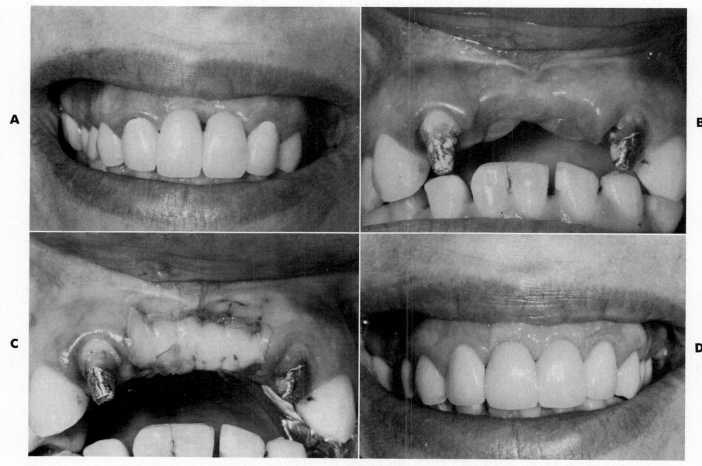

Fig. 51-13. **A,** Pretreatment. Patient disliked length of central incisor pontic teeth and dark triangle that existed between pontics. **B,** Pretreatment view of large-volume Class III ridge defect. **C,** Onlay graft sutured into position. Graft was 1 mm thick on its periphery and 6 mm thick in its central region. **D,** Two years after surgery, note augmentation that has been obtained and pleasing appearance and color match of tissues. Augmented tissue restored illusion of a midline papilla and permitted use of shorter pontic teeth, thereby improving overall esthetics. In addition, there was an improved air seal and phonetics. (Prosthesis by Dr. R. McClelland, Princeton, N.J.)

Technique. The onlay graft procedure was designed to augment ridge defects in the apicocoronal plane of space to gain ridge height (Seibert, 1980, 1983a, 1983b). This has been the most difficult problem to solve. Onlay grafts are thick "free gingival grafts," derived from the total or complete thickness of the palate. The amount of apicocoronal augmentation that can be obtained is directly related to the thickness of the graft that is used and the amount of connective tissue that "takes" or survives the grafting procedure (Figs. 51-12 and 51-13). The procedure can be repeated at 2-month intervals to build ridge height in successive increments.

Increasing the blood and plasma flow

An additional surgical maneuver has been devised that seems to aid in ensuring more rapid revascularization of the graft by increasing the amount of bleeding and plasma flow into the recipient site-graft interface. This last stage in the preparation of the recipient site is accomplished after the graft tissue has been obtained, tried in, and trimmed if necessary to fit the recipient site.

A series of parallel cuts are made deep into the exposed lamina propria of the defect (Fig. 51-12). A new scalpel blade is used to make the striations about 1 mm apart, parallel to one another and perpendicular to the general contour of the alveolar ridge. It has been observed that following the striation procedure, many of these full-thickness grafts actually increase in total volume. The swelling phenomenon is demonstrated in Fig. 51-12.

Variable secondary contraction has been observed in these full-thickness grafts at 3 to 6 months following surgery. After 4 to 6 months of healing, final contours of the prosthesis can be determined.

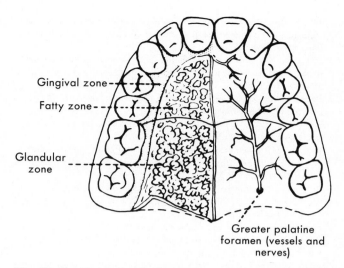

Gingival zone

Fatty zone

Glandular zone

Greater palatine foramen (vessels and nerves)

Fig. 51-14. Anatomic-histologic zones of palate. Note normal location of greater palatine foramen. It is usually located in palatal vault midway between midline raphe and gingival margin perpendicular to second molar tooth.

Selection and preparation of the donor site: anatomic considerations

The gingival zone and tuberosity areas of the palate are used most commonly as the donor sites for free grafts of masticatory mucosa because the lamina propria is thicker and more densely collagenized in these areas. Wedge procedures, inlay-onlay procedures, and onlay graft procedures require larger amounts of donor tissue than are removed during conventional free gingival grafting procedures. Free gingival grafts used to augment the zone of attached gingiva range in thickness from 0.75 to 1.75 mm. Sullivan and Atkins (1968) classified graft thickness in relationship to the thickness of the lamina propria. The lamina propria is rarely more than 2 mm thick, and then one encounters the submucosal zone of the palate. It was formerly believed that the inclusion of fatty or glandular submucosal tissue within a free graft would inhibit the flow of plasma and growth of new capillaries into the graft, thereby causing the graft to become necrotic and fail to take (Sullivan and Atkins, 1968). However, it has been shown that the full thickness of the palate may be used for grafting procedures and that the fatty and glandular components of the submucosal zone do not interfere with wound healing (Seibert, 1983a, 1983b).

The major palatine artery emerges from the palatine foramen, which is usually located adjacent to the distal surface of the maxillary second molar, midway between the midline raphe and the lingual surface of the second molar (Fig. 51-14). The artery passes in an anterior direction close to the surface of the palatal bone. It is important to avoid the second molar and third molar regions of the palate as donor sites for large-volume grafts. The tissue in the

palatal vault area opposite the premolars and first molar teeth is very thick and is the preferred site for large volume free grafts.

Planning the graft in three dimensions

The required surface pattern is measured on the palate and scribed lightly with a scalpel or sharp gingivectomy knife. The incision made into the palate to trace the outline of the graft should be only deep enough to produce light bleeding to define the surface borders of the graft.

Dissection of the donor tissue

The base of the graft frequently will be V or U shaped to match the shape of the defect in the ridge. The planes of incision deep into the palate will converge toward an area under the center or toward one edge of the graft. Various special scalpel blade holders are available that permit the blade to be positioned at various angles to the blade holder and permit one to cut with a back action anteriorly.

Treatment of the wound in the palate

The donor site should be inspected carefully for any signs of pulsatile or arterial bleeding. If such bleeding is observed, a circumferential suture should be placed around the vessel distal to the bleeding point.

The wound in the palate can be covered and dressed by many methods. An acrylic surgical stent can be made, a partial denture that covers only the posterior areas can be used, or a periodontal dressing can be applied. If a partial denture has an anterior flange, the partial denture will have to be placed in position at the termination of the procedure after the flange is shortened to fit lightly against the graft.

Wound healing in the donor area

Granulation tissue fills the donor area of the palate in the same manner as with any wound that produces a void within connective tissue. Initial healing in the palate is usually complete within 14 to 21 days after free grafts 1 to 1.25 mm in thickness are removed. When larger grafts are removed from the palate, it usually takes an additional 2 weeks for the surgical void to fill and reach the level of the surrounding tissues.

Wound healing in the recipient area

One should anticipate postoperative swelling during the first week following pouch, wedge, inlay-onlay, and onlay augmentation procedures. Periodontal dressings are not used to cover the grafted tissues. Part or all of the *epithelium* covering the donor tissue *may desquamate* during the first week of healing. This forms a gray or white film on the grafted tissue. Patients are informed that it is normal for the augmentation area to pass through a "white stage" of 4 to 7 days, since they frequently confuse the white appearance of the graft with infection and become unnecessarily alarmed.

The grafted tissue assumes its normal color as epithelization is completed and the epithelium thickens. Experience has shown that the grafts revert to the approximate size of the tissue implanted, or remain slightly larger in total volume, after the swelling subsides. Tissue form is stable after 2 months. However, from the second to fourth month variable shrinkage occurs; hence final restorative procedures should be delayed for 4 to 6 months to ensure that the tissues have reached their final form.

REFERENCES

Abrams H, Kopczyk R, and Kaplan AL: Incidence of anterior ridge deformities in partially edentulous patients, J Prosthet Dent 57:191, 1987.

Abrams L: Augmentation of the deformed residual edentulous ridge for fixed prosthesis, Compend Contin Educ Dent 1(3):205, 1980a.

Abrams L: Personal communication, 1980b.

Allen EP et al: Improved technique for localized ridge augmentation, J Periodontol 56:195, 1985.

Garber DA and Rosenberg ES: The edentulous ridge in fixed prosthodontics, Compend Contin Educ Dent 2:212, 1981.

Kaldahl WB et al: Achieving an esthetic appearance with a fixed prosthesis by submucosal grafts, J Am Dent Assoc 104:449, 1982.

Langer B and Calagna L: The subepithelial connective tissue graft, J Prosthet Dent 44:363, 1980.

Langer B and Calagna L: The subepithelial connective tissue graft: a new approach to the enhancement of anterior cosmetics, Int J Periodontics Restorative Dent 2:22, 1982.

McHenry K, Smutko G, and McMullen JA: Restructuring the topography of the mandibular ridge with gingival autographs, J Am Dent Assoc 104:478, 1982.

Meltzer JA: Edentulous area tissue graft correction of an esthetic defect: a case report, J Periodontol 50:320, 1979.

Miller PD Jr: Ridge augmentation under existing fixed prosthesis: simplified technique, J Periodontol 57:742, 1986.

Seibert JS: Soft tissue grafts in periodontics. In Robinson PJ and Guernsey, LH, editors: Clinical transplantation in dental specialities, St Louis, 1980, The CV Mosby Co.

Seibert JS: Reconstruction of deformed, partially edentulous ridges, using full thickness onlay grafts. I. Technique and wound healing, Compend Contin Educ Dent 4(5):437, 1983a.

Seibert JS: Reconstruction of deformed, partially edentulous ridges, using full thickness onlay grafts. II. Prosthetic/periodontal interrelationships, Compend Contin Educ Dent 4(6):549, 1983b.

Seibert JS and Cohen DW: Periodontal considerations in preparation for fixed and removable prosthodontics. In Full-mouth reconstruction: fixed removable, Dent Clin North Am 31(3):529, 1987.

Soehren SE et al: Clinical and histologic studies of donor tissues utilized for free grafts of masticatory mucosa, J Periodontol 44:727, 1973.

Stein RS: Pontic-residual ridge relationships: a research report, J Prosthet Dent 16:283, 1966.

Sullivan HC and Atkins JH: Free autogenous gingival grafts. I. Principles of successful grafting, Periodontics 6:121, 1968.

Chapter 52

DENTAL IMPLANTS

Vincent J. Iacono

Implant systems
Patient selection
Presurgical evaluation
Surgical techniques
Postsurgical problems, procedures, and maintenance
Summary and future directions

Man's search for the ideal replacement of missing teeth has been an elusive goal since antiquity. Implants of numerous designs and compositions have been tried, touted, and then discarded over the years. Unfortunately, for virtually all the implant systems, success has never been able to be predicted or guaranteed. Because of the numerous failures with implants and the paucity of well-controlled clinical studies of their survival, the use of implants was relegated to a small segment of the dental community. Since the late 1960s, however, significant basic and clinical research on a new and apparently successful implant system was performed by Brånemark and co-workers (Brånemark et al., 1977; Adell et al., 1981; Brånemark, 1983; Albrektsson et al., 1986).

The need for dental implants in the 1990s has been documented in a recent government study that indicated that there is a significant degree of edentulism in the U.S. population. According to this 1985 to 1986 national survey of the oral health of U.S. employed adults and senior citizens, conducted by the National Institute of Dental Research, 4% of persons 35 to 64 years old and 42% of those over 65 years of age are totally edentulous. Meskin and Brown (1988) compared these findings with the results of a 1971 national dental study (Harvey and Kelly, 1981) and found that total edentulism increased over a 15-year span from 19.9% in 1971 to 24.3% in 1985. In addition, per-

sons between 55 and 64 years of age with teeth had lost an average of 9 of 28 teeth, and dentate persons over 65 had lost an average of 10 of 28 teeth. Collectively, employed adults were missing 4.2 teeth (Meskin and Brown, 1988). These results indicate that for the next few decades there will be significant numbers of individuals with compromised dentitions for whom implants may be indicated. With the heightened health consciousness of our society and the increased availability of dental health insurance plans, implants will become a reasonable alternative to removable prosthetic appliances—an alternative that should enhance the quality of life during the senior years. It has been predicted that as many as 300,000 dental implants will be used on this population by 1992. However, it is also clear that tooth loss is very low in the younger population in the United States (e.g., only 4% of those 35 to 64 years of age were edentulous in the 1985 to 1986 U.S. survey). Hence in the distant future, 3 to 4 decades from now, there may be less need for implants.

The implant system developed by Brånemark is called tissue-integrated prostheses, and the term *osseointegration* was coined by him (Brånemark et al., 1985). *Osseointegration* is a histologic term defined as a direct structural and functional connection between ordered, living bone and the surface of a load-carrying implant as observed at the light microscopic level. In other words, no connective tissue or periodontal ligament-like interface is detectable at the light microscopic level (Fig. 52-1). An osseointegrated implant is analogous to a nonresorbing ankylosed tooth. An example of an osseointegrated implant is shown in Fig. 52-2. The positive bone response to implants of this type is significant. It is the firm implant bone anchorage of osseointegrated dental implants that has contributed to their long-term (20 years) success as shown in fully edentulous cases.

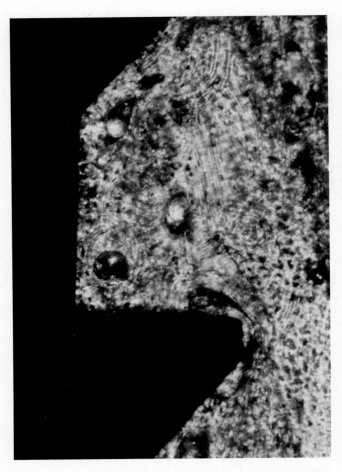

Fig. 52-1. Light microscopic view of osseointegrated implant fixture illustrating direct contact of bone with implant surface. (Courtesy O.R. Beirne, Seattle.)

Periodontists, because of the availability of successful implant systems, have become increasingly involved in implantology. Periodontists routinely treat and maintain partially edentulous patients, have an integral role in the restorative treatment-planning process, and are extensively trained in surgical procedures. As a result, the definition of periodontics has been changed to the following (American Academy of Periodontology):

Periodontics is that branch of dentistry which deals with the diagnosis and treatment of the supporting and surrounding tissues of the teeth or their substitutes and the implantation or transplantation of teeth or their substitutes. The maintenance of the health of these structures and tissues, achieved through periodontal procedures, is also considered to be the responsibility of the periodontist. Scope shall be limited to preclude permanent restorative care.

It can be reasonably predicted that implants will increasingly become a regular part of periodontal treatment plans for the partially edentulous patient. These patients often have remaining teeth that have significant amounts of attachment loss. Periodontists are being asked to develop treatment plans for these compromised dentitions, and the decision to extract or maintain individual teeth is usually being left to their judgment. More important, perhaps, periodontists are determining which teeth can serve as abutments and which should stand alone. Periodontists have therefore come to play a critical role in the treatment planning of the surgical phase of implant insertion and in the design of the final prosthesis. However, other dental practitioners have received special training in implant procedures and, either alone as generalists or in teams made up of surgeons and prosthodontists, are beginning to place implants. In any event, maintenance of the implant-supported prosthesis is becoming a necessary and regular part of the periodontal recall visit.

IMPLANT SYSTEMS

There are many implant systems available. These are classified according to their shape and position in the jaws. They include subperiosteal, transosteal, and endosseous implants.

Subperiosteal implants, which do not osseointegrate, are in the form of a metal framework made from casts of the patient's jaw bones. They are used in severely atrophic jaws when there is inadequate bone height to insert an endosseous fixture.

Transosteal implants, which are also nonosseointegrated, are essentially staple implants and are typically used in the mandibular anterior sextant as transmandibular implants.

The most common implants are *endosseous implants,* and these include many that osseointegrate. According to their shape, they may be pins (Fig. 52-3), blades (Fig. 52-4), cylindric screws (see Fig. 52-9), or basket-shaped cylinders (Fig. 52-5). Often early blade and other endosteal implants were inserted with high-speed drills, which generated a great deal of heat, and with traumatic seating instruments. As a result, they often became encapsulated with fibrous connective tissue, lacked a sufficient epithelial seal, and were prone to failure after 5 to 10 years (Armitage, 1980; Smithloff and Fritz, 1987).

A significant acceleration in implant loss over time appears to be characteristic of many implants and suggests caution in assessing early survival rates (Shulman, 1988). For example, the 5-year success rate of complete mandibular subperiosteal implants was as high as 93% but 10-year results have been reported to be no better than 64% (Bailey and Yanase, 1985; Bodine and Yanase, 1985). One should therefore take this into account when evaluating the 85% survival rate in the Veterans Administration's 3½-year blade implant study (Kapur, 1988) and the 83% success rate in the 3½-year Harvard blade study (Schnitman et al., 1988a, 1988b). The Brånemark system of osseointegration has dramatically affected implant suc-

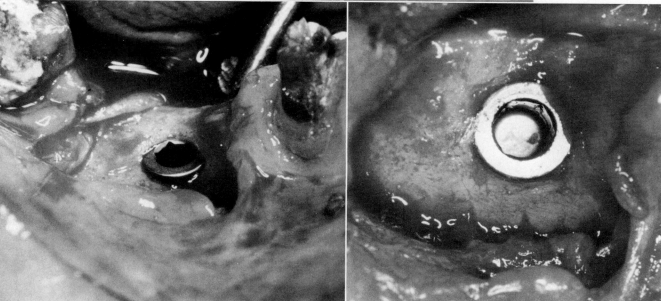

Fig. 52-2. A, Radiograph of osseointegrated fixture just prior to surgical exposure. Note lack of a radiolucent interface between implant and adjacent bone. **B,** Surgical exposure indicating bone growth over occlusal surface of implant. **C,** Exposed implant after removal of bone with rotary and hand instruments.

cess rates in fully edentulous cases. The criteria for success include not only maintenance of the implants but also fixture immobility and absence of periimplant radiolucency (Albrektsson et al., 1988). A 99% 5- to 8-year survival rate for mandibular fixtures and an 85% 5- to 7-year survival rate for maxillary fixtures have recently been reported for the Brånemark system (Albrektsson et al., 1988).

The data from partially edentulous cases are now being accumulated. Schnitman et al. (1988a, 1988b) have indicated that implants in partially edentulous patients are capable of 3-year survival rates above 90%, regardless of design or whether or not they are osseointegrated. However, as with studies of fully edentulous patients, caution should be used in assessing data from short-term studies. In addition, many of these studies have not considered the quality

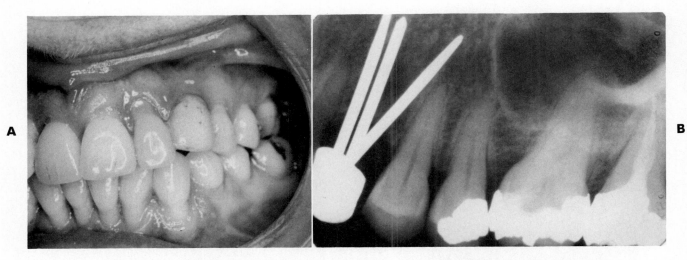

Fig. 52-3. **A,** Clinical appearance after 15 years of function of a tripod endosseous pin implant–supported maxillary left cuspid. **B,** Radiographic appearance of pin implant.

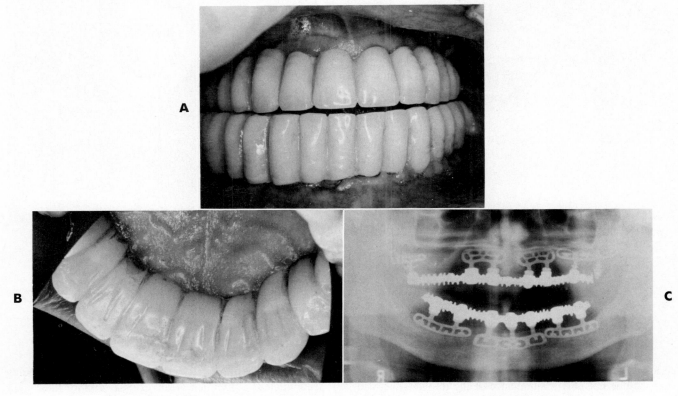

Fig. 52-4. **A,** Clinical appearance after 9 years of function of maxillary and mandibular endosseous blade-supported fixed bridges. **B,** Palatal view of maxillary bridge. **C,** Panoramic radiograph illustrating maxillary and mandibular blade implants.

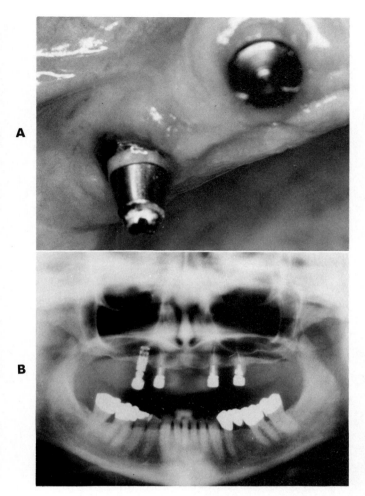

A

B

Fig. 52-5. A, Clinical view of basket-shaped endosseous implant overdenture abutment in maxillary right premolar region. **B,** Panoramic radiograph showing maxillary right implant. (Prosthetic appliance fabricated by Dr. Sherman Axinn, Stony Brook, N.Y.)

of the surviving implants (e.g., mobility and suppuration), and the studies have often been poorly designed with inadequate controls.

The success of osseointegration systems has been attributed to the strictly controlled manufacture of the implants from either titanium or an alloy of titanium, aluminum (6%), and vanadium (4%), coupled with a two-stage atraumatic insertion technique. Titanium is a tissue-tolerant material that on exposure to air instantly forms a titanium oxide surface layer that is hydrophilic, corrosion resistant, and not rejected by the host defense system (Albrektsson and Jacobsson, 1987). The importance of controlling heat generated by the surgical procedures of implant insertion has been demonstrated in animal and human studies (Eriksson and Albrektsson, 1983; Eriksson and Adell, 1986). Retarded bone growth occurred during experimental implant procedures by subjecting bone to as low as 47° C for 1 minute. The surgical techniques used in the various osseointegration systems have been designed to cause only minor and insignificant temperature elevations.

Osseointegrated implants may have as little as 20% to 25% of their surfaces in direct contact with bone, but they are clinically immobile (Roberts, 1988). The degree of osseointegration attained is a function of both the quality and the quantity of bone present at the fixture site. More cortical bone available results in a greater degree of fixture survival. This is why the greatest percentage of success occurs when implants are inserted in the mandibular anterior sextant in both fully and partially edentulous patients (Schnitman et al., 1988a, 1988b). The original Brånemark fixtures were originally designed to engage cortical areas at both their coronal and apical ends. A thin cortical plate would preclude success. Implants placed in the maxilla and distal to the mental foramen would therefore have lower survival rates than those placed in the mandibular anterior sextant. In areas lacking adequate cortical bone, modified basket-cylindric implants (e.g., Core-Vent fixtures) have been used. From a collective evaluation of all implant systems, the consensus would therefore be that there is no one ideal implant design. Implants of different design and shape are necessary to overcome the limitations imposed by inadequate residual bone morphology. The use of implants other than the original cylindric implant designed by Brånemark does not preclude osseointegration. Osseointegration appears to be a function of a relatively atraumatic insertion technique, the presence of a bioactive surface such as presented by titanium oxide or hydroxyapatite, and the fixture's ability to engage cortical bone.

There are several factors or qualities to consider when selecting an implant system. The efficacy of a feasible system, in terms of its record of success, is of primary importance. There are long-term studies that indicate that dental implants are effective for the fully edentulous patient (Albrektsson et al., 1988), but few are available for the partially edentulous patient (Schnitman et al., 1986, 1988a, 1988b). In addition, there has been a relative lack of randomized trials to compare different implant systems. However, the survival times for implants have been improving in recent years. In 1980 an implant system was considered successful if at least 75% of the implants survived 5 years (Schnitman and Shulman, 1980). At a more recent National Institutes of Health Concensus Development Conference on Dental Implants (Rizzo, 1988), a new definition of success was proposed: "Any implant system considered successful should carry an 85%-90%, 5- to 10-year statistical survival rate and leave the patient no worse off after removal, if necessary, than prior to placement" (Babbush, 1988). However, these figures are based on inconclusive studies, and further research is indicated.

A second factor to consider is the practicality of the system. This would include the initial costs of the equipment, maintenance, and the establishment of an operating room–like sterile environment. A third quality to consider is the prosthetic flexibility of the system. Most of the present Brånemark fixtures are only axially loaded, which limits the placement of crowns. Other systems that require nonaxial loading have not been shown to resist these lateral forces to the bone over time. Most of the osseointegrated endosseous implants require two surgical procedures. The first stage involves the insertion of the implant fixture in the jaw; the fixture is then isolated from the oral environment for several months to allow for osseointegration while it is not loaded. The second stage includes the surgical exposure of the fixture and the attachment of an abutment on which the prosthesis is fabricated.

Several implant systems have abutments of only one type and design, necessarily limiting their prosthetic applications. Conversely, other systems provide numerous alternative types of abutments that can be joined to the implants by several methods. An additional factor to consider is the retrievability of an implant should it fail or become symptomatic. Most of the available endosseous implants are designed to be recovered with minimal soft and hard tissue alteration. This is due to the availability of retrieval drills or trephines of slightly larger diameter than the failing implant. After the implant is removed, the area heals in the same manner as a typical extraction site.

PATIENT SELECTION

It is essential that a prospective implant patient be in good general health and not suffer from any disease that could adversely affect wound healing. Patients with serious disease must be assessed carefully. The most significant findings obtained from the medical history that have been suggested to have an adverse affect on implant survival include uncontrolled diabetes, alcoholism, and smoking. Age, on the other hand, is not an important factor that affects implant survival. However, it may be of considerable importance in treatment planning.

Patients should not have any psychologic illness and

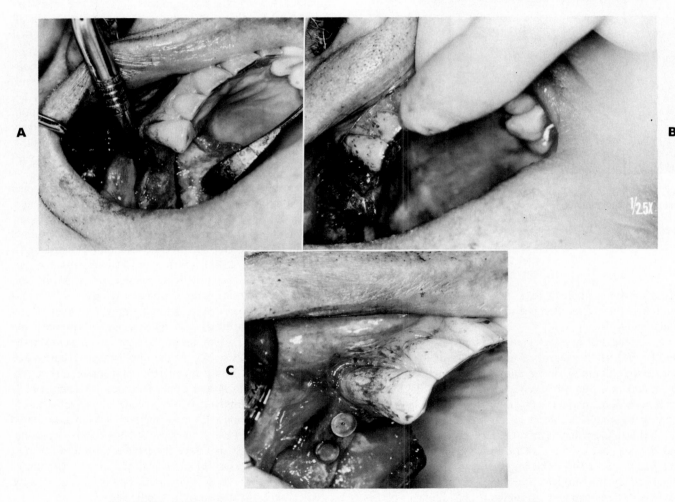

Fig. 52-6. **A,** Site prepared for insertion of two Screw-Vent implants in maxillary right premolar region. **B,** Processed acrylic stent used as a guide in preparation of properly aligned implant sites. **C,** Implants in place with their surgical inserts. (Stent fabricated by Dr. Charles Ullo, Stony Brook, N.Y.)

must be emotionally stable. They must be cooperative with the implant team and willing to keep the many presurgical, surgical, and recall visits. Their oral physiotherapy must be excellent. They must also be made to understand (and provide evidence of informed consent) that not all implants are successful; and that if an implant fails, a second implant or alternative procedure can be performed. Prospective patients must also be assured that after placement, osseointegrated implants do not present any proven health risks.

PRESURGICAL EVALUATION

Ideally, the team approach should be followed in diagnosing and formulating a treatment plan for a prospective implant patient. The restorative requirements must be established at the outset. The amount and quality of available bone and the location of edentulous areas need to be evaluated before implants are selected as a treatment alternative. Adequate radiographs, including panoramic lateral and occlusal views and periapical films, are necessary to determine the height of available bone for sizing of the fixtures and, of utmost importance, to determine the proximity of potential implant sites to the sinuses, mental foramen, mandibular canal, and adjacent teeth. The use of three-dimensional computed tomography (CT) scans is advocated when more accurate information regarding the topography of osseous structures is needed. For example, irregular, thin, or spiny osseous contours can be seen in CT images. In addition, the soft tissue contour and dimension, the continuity and density of the cortical plates, the vertical height of the residual alveolar ridges, and the density of the medullary space and basilar bone can be determined from CT scans (McGivney et al., 1986). Visual and manual examination of the oral tissues and residual ridge, in-

cluding bone sounding, should be done to assess the health of the oral tissues and the width of available bone, and in the determination of undercuts and exostoses.

After implant sites have been selected that optimize the benefits and minimize potential risks to vital structures, the restorative dentist should fabricate a stent that can be used as a guide to achieve ideal fixture alignment during the surgical phase (Fig. 52-6). It should be noted, however, that at the time of surgery, the provider may have to select an implant of different size and shape and insert the fixture at a different location because of unforeseen problems. On surgical exposure, at times, the buccolingual width of the alveolar ridge may be too narrow for the axial placement of a root-form implant. The implant would have to be inserted at an angle to the ridge, or an implant of different design and dimension would be used (e.g., blade implant). Another fairly common problem is the lack of adequate cortical bone to engage a classical Brånemark threaded fixture. In this situation, an IMZ implant, Screw-Vent, or self-tapping Nobelpharma fixture would be the implant of choice. The selection of different implants and the preparation of antiaxial receptor sites affect the prosthetic phase of treatment. Therefore, ideally, the restorative dentist should be present during the surgical phase.

If an implant is to be inserted in an extraction site, it is preferable to let the site heal for at least 6 months to 1 year before placing implants. Insertion of implants immediately after extraction is a questionable procedure, unless the implant has dimensions that are larger than the extraction site, allowing for its immediate mechanical fixation with bone (Shulman, 1988). However, there have been no published results of implantation to fresh extraction sites to date. Immobilization of the fixture at the time of insertion appears to be critical (Adell et al., 1985). The possibility

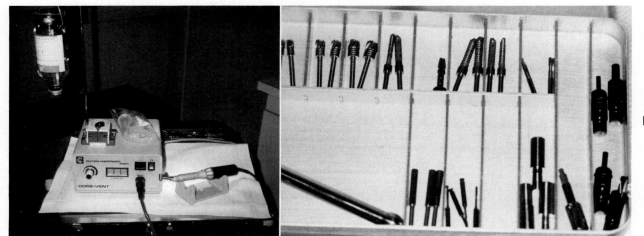

Fig. 52-7. **A,** Physiodispenser, micromotor, and electric handpiece used for low-speed preparation of implant sites with internally irrigated drills. **B,** Compartmentalized surgical tray holding various drills and trephines for Core-Vent, Screw-Vent, and Micro-Vent implants.

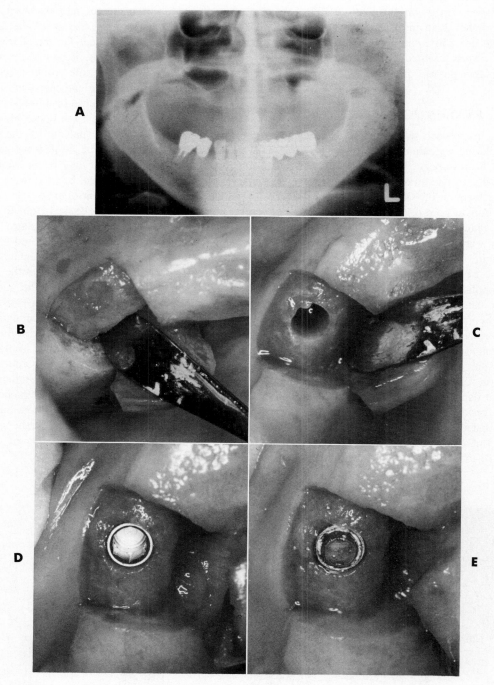

Fig. 52-8. **A,** Panoramic radiograph illustrating maxillary edentulous areas distal to remaining central incisor to be sites for four implants. **B** and **C,** Site preparation for most distal right implant. **D,** Implant in place. **E,** Implant with its surgical insert.

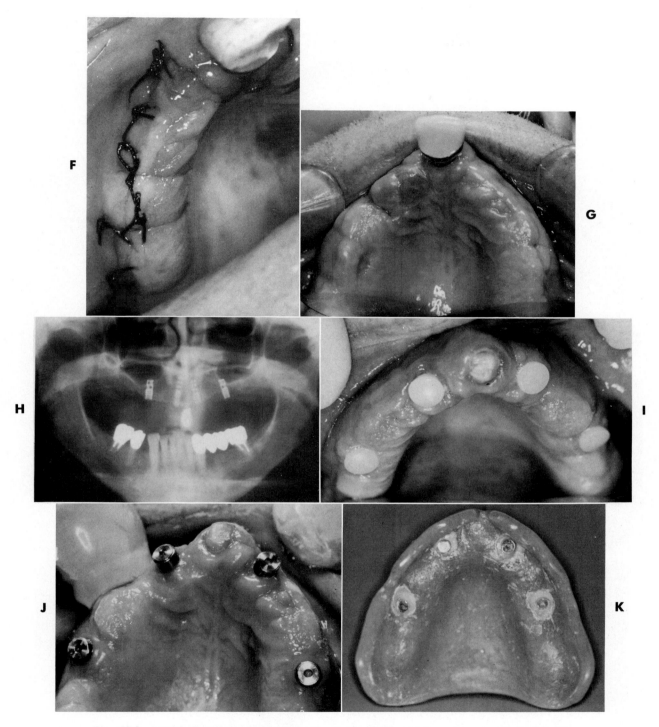

Fig. 52-8, cont'd. F, Flaps coapted and sutured. **G,** Healing at 2-week postsurgical visit. **H,** Panoramic radiograph illustrating the four osseointegrated implants. **I,** Exposed implants with their healing caps 10 months after insertion. **J,** Implants prepared as abutments for a maxillary overdenture. **K,** Maxillary implant-supported overdenture with magnets and full palatal coverage. (Prosthesis fabricated by Dr. Charles Ullo, Stony Brook, N.Y.)

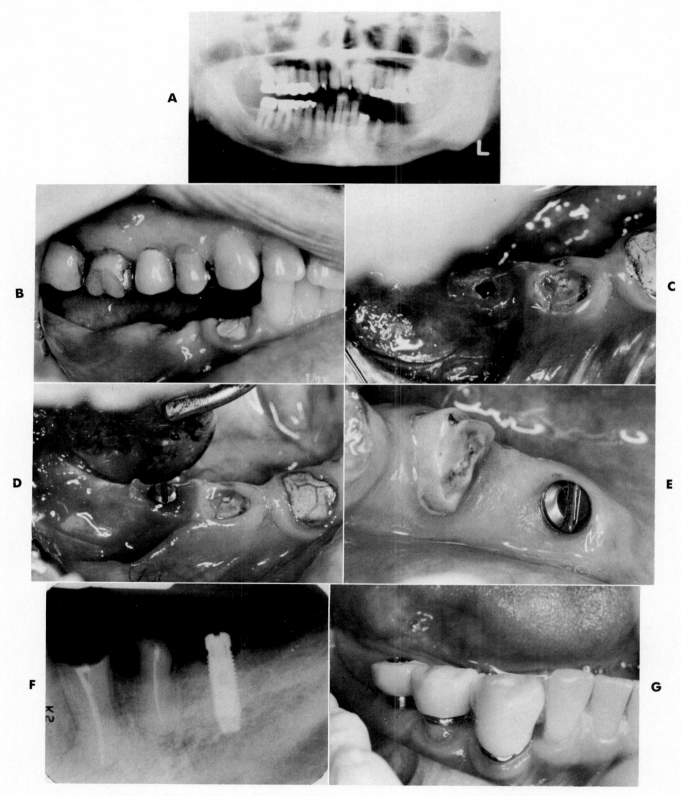

Fig. 52-9. **A,** Panoramic radiograph illustrating an edentulous area in mandibular left quadrant. **B,** Preoperative clinical view of implant site. **C,** Site prepared for insertion of a Screw-Vent implant. **D,** Implant in place with its cover screw. **E,** Exposed implant 6 months after insertion. **F,** Periapical radiograph illustrating osseointegrated implant. **G,** Implant–natural tooth–supported fixed prosthesis. (Prosthetic appliance fabricated by Dr. Sherman Axinn, Stony Brook, N.Y.)

of using various bone substitutes to coat implants and to fill voids between implants and surrounding bone is currently being investigated (Geesink et al., 1988).

SURGICAL TECHNIQUES

There are three important principles followed by virtually all endosseous osseointegrated implant systems. These include (1) surgical procedures that minimize thermal trauma to bone; (2) a primary healing period of 3 to 12 months, during which time the submerged endosseous implant is isolated from the oral environment; and (3) maintenance of an unloaded state during the healing period.

Thermal trauma to bone can be avoided by using copious irrigation and through the use of low-speed electric handpieces and a graded series of drills (Fig. 52-7). Low-speed (15 rpm) handpieces and titanium drills have also been designed to tap or thread fixture sites for cylindric screw-shaped implants. More recently, internally cooled trephines, as well as low-speed drills and self-tapping fixtures, have been developed (Figs. 52-7 to 52-9).

Shown in Figs. 52-8 to 52-10 are three series of surgi-

cal procedures illustrating the placement of modified hollow basket–screw-shaped implants in the maxillary arch to support an overdenture (Fig. 52-8), the placement of a cylindric screw-shaped implant in the mandibular left quadrant to serve as a distal abutment for a splint (Fig. 52-9), and the placement of two fixtures in the mandibular left quadrant to support a fixed bridge (Fig. 52-10).

The surgical procedures are done under aseptic conditions. Although suggested by some implantologists, a hospital operating room facility is unnecessary. The positioning of the patient on an operating room table, intubation, and the use of throat packs could hinder access to posterior sites in both the maxilla and the mandible. The procedures are usually done with the patient under local anesthesia with conscious sedation, if necessary.

At the selected sites mucoperiosteal flaps are prepared to achieve sufficient access for insertion of the implants. Incisions into the vestibular fold, which can eliminate the vestibule, should be avoided, particularly in the partially edentulous patient (Fig. 52-11). Otherwise, it is possible that vestibular extension procedures may have to be per-

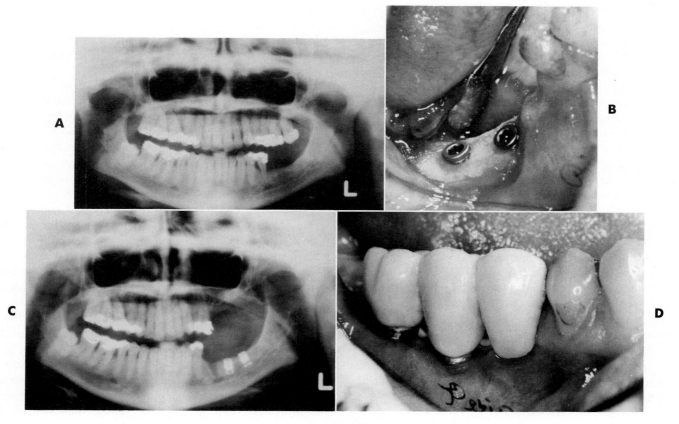

Fig. 52-10. **A,** Presurgical panoramic radiograph illustrating mandibular left edentulous area prior to extraction of left second premolar. **B,** Surgical placement of two fixtures. **C,** Panoramic radiograph showing the two osseointegrated fixtures prior to abutment connection. **D,** Implant-supported fixed bridge. (Prosthetic appliance fabricated by Dr. Sherman Axinn, Stony Brook, N.Y.)

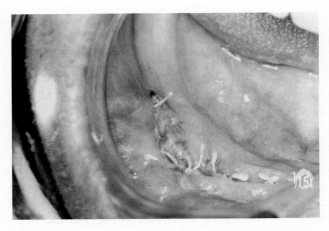

Fig. 52-11. Elimination of vestibule following a linear incision deep into vestibular fold during implant surgery.

formed after the final prosthesis has been inserted to allow the patient to follow an adequate oral hygiene regimen without traumatizing the alveolar mucosa. When implants are to be inserted in the maxillary arch, the flaps should be designed to be elevated from the labial and buccal aspects. When horizontal incisions are necessary, it is suggested that they be made buccal to the ridge. Horizontal palatal incisions should be avoided, since they may compromise the blood supply, resulting in necrosis of the flap.

Fixture sites are prepared in the exposed bone to the dimensions of the selected implants with either internally irrigated low-speed (less than 2000 rpm) trephines or a graded series of spiral drills. The implants are then slowly inserted by rotation with hex tools under profuse irrigation. It is essential that the implants are firmly adapted to bone. Any looseness or inadequate contact with cortical bone will adversely affect the degree to which the implant osseointegrates and may doom it to failure. Surgical inserts or cover screws are then placed into the inner hex hole or threaded site of the implants, and the flaps are coapted and sutured.

The patient is given prescriptions for an antibiotic and an appropriate analgesic, as well as an ice pack to control swelling, and is instructed to avoid the surgical area. Patients with removable appliances are not to use their dentures for the first 2 weeks to avoid premature loading of the implants and soft tissue perforations. Sutures are removed after 1 week.

The implants must remain submerged for as little as 3 months in the mandibular anterior sextant, where the site is generally composed of dense cortical bone, for 6 months in the maxillary anterior sextant, and for as long as 9 to 12 months in the maxillary posterior sextants, where the bone is virtually all cancellous.

At the second-stage procedure, or abutment connection step, the implants are exposed by a small surgical incision over the fixture sites. The surgical inserts, or cover screws, are removed, and the implants are evaluated for stability. Mobility at this stage indicates that the implant failed to osseointegrate, and the fixture should be removed. Healing caps are placed in the osseointegrated fixtures, and if necessary, the surgical wound is sutured. After 1 week, the site is reevaluated, and the sutures are removed. The patient is then referred to the restorative dentist for fabrication of the final prosthesis.

POSTSURGICAL PROBLEMS, PROCEDURES, AND MAINTENANCE

After implants are surgically exposed, gingival hyperplasia may occur around the abutments prior to fabrication of the final prosthesis (Fig. 52-12, *A*). This is readily corrected by a gingivectomy or gingivoplasty (Fig. 52-12, *B*). It is the restorative dentist's task to fabricate a prosthetic appliance that can be maintained by the patient (see Rizzo, 1988). Attention must be given to embrasures, subgingival extensions, labial veneers, and access to the abutments (Fig. 52-13). The implant-supported bridge or overdenture must be equilibrated in a functional occlusal relationship with the opposing teeth. It has been suggested, though not proved, that implant-supported fixed bridges may exacerbate alveolar ridge resorption under an opposing conventional denture. If this situation occurs, implants may be recommended for both arches.

Because osseointegrated endosseous cylindric fixtures were originally designed for the anterior sextants of fully edentulous patients, there has been a lack of data regarding the effects of splinting implants to natural teeth. Ericsson et al. (1986) reported that intrusion of splinted natural teeth and pronounced vertical bone loss around the implant abutments were potential sequelae, but the majority of patients evaluated in their study suffered no adverse effects. It is clear, however, that further studies are needed to evaluate splinting of osseointegrated implants to natural teeth in the partially edentulous patient.

The esthetics of the final prosthesis will depend on whether there is ideal fixture alignment, optimal abutment length, modified castable abutments, and the ability to use ceramics, as well as on the patient's facial and oral configuration. The presence of an ideal soft tissue environment may be of concern, but there are no data indicating that a lack of keratinized gingiva attached to the abutment or fixture will have an adverse effect on implant survival. Soft tissue grafting procedures to gain attached gingiva are not indicated unless they are necessary for optimal oral physiotherapy. In this regard, there is no evidence for the presence of an organized connective tissue interface between an implant or implant abutment and bone. Attached connective tissue probably plays little role in the stabilization and maintenance of an osseointegrated implant. It may actually contribute to the loss of an implant by failing to inhibit epithelial downgrowth with concomitant colonization by periodontopathic bacteria (Melcher, 1988). This break-

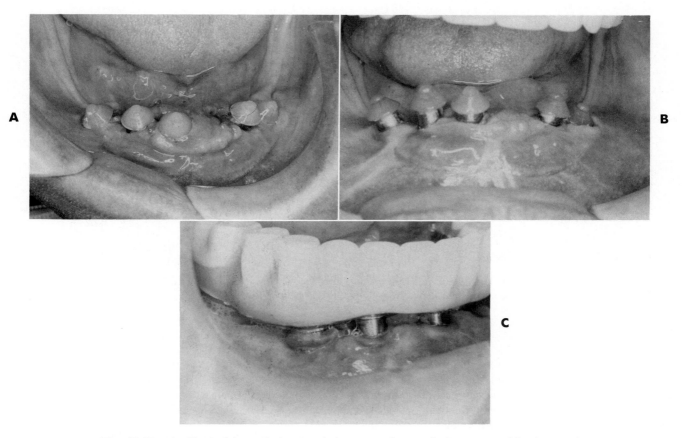

Fig. 52-12. A, Gingival hyperplasia around abutments after surgical exposure of implants and placement of healing caps. **B,** Exposed abutments after gingivectomy. **C,** Gingival hyperplasia around an abutment of an implant-supported fixed bridge.

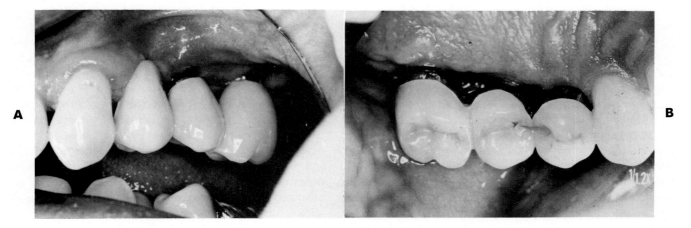

Fig. 52-13. A, Buccal view of maxillary three-unit implant–supported fixed bridge. First premolar is a pontic and second premolar and first molar are implant-supported abutments. **B,** Palatal view. (Bridge fabricated by Dr. Daniel Cunningham, Stony Brook, N.Y.)

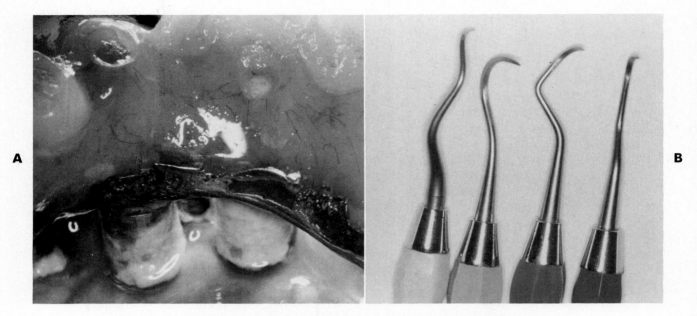

Fig. 52-14. **A,** Calculus accumulation around abutments of an implant-supported bridge. **B,** Titanium-plated curettes, which can be used to remove calculus from abutments.

down in "attachment" could be followed by occlusal trauma and adverse host-microbial interactions within the periimplant pocket. This latter aspect has yet to be documented, with the exception of ligature-induced breakdown in monkeys (Brandes et al., 1988). In that study implants were found to be more resistant than natural teeth subjected to the same environmental stresses.

The relative resistance of osseointegrated implants to plaque-mediated breakdown may be a function of anatomic relationships and the lack of a periodontal ligament. A hyperplastic gingival response, however, is not uncommon but is readily treatable (see Fig. 52-12, C).

Patients should be on a regular recall schedule to monitor the maintenance of the implant-supported prostheses and their plaque control. Maintenance programs, including radiographic evaluation, should be designed on an individual basis, because there is a lack of data detailing adequate recall intervals, methods of plaque and calculus removal, and appropriate antimicrobial agents. Calculus buildup occurs quite readily around titanium abutments (Fig. 52-14, A). It has been suggested that steel curettes not be used to remove calculus, because they may scratch the abutments, leading to further plaque accumulation. Titanium-tipped curettes have been developed (Fig. 52-14, B), but there are no studies of their effectiveness as compared with steel curettes on titanium surfaces. Plastic scalers are also available for calculus removal.

Osseointegrated implants rarely fail beyond the first year after clinical exposure (Albrektsson et al., 1988). However, if periodontitis develops around an implant, conventional periodontal therapy should be instituted. In the event that a fixture has to be removed, an alternative restorative treatment plan, including a second implant procedure, can be developed.

SUMMARY AND FUTURE DIRECTIONS

Osseointegrated dental implant systems have revolutionized the field of implantology. Implants are now routinely considered as an option in the treatment of partial or complete edentulism. Implant procedures are very technique sensitive and therefore should be done only by teams of adequately trained periodontists/surgeons and restorative dentists. Regardless of the implant system used, success is intrinsically dependent on the amount and quality of bone available at the implant site, the patient's health and cooperation, and the design of the prosthesis. Osseointegration per se, however, does not guarantee that an acceptable prosthesis can be fabricated. The number of fixtures that can be inserted, their location in the jaws, and potential alignment are all factors to consider in treatment planning for a prospective implant patient. The patient needs to be cooperative, well motivated, and free of any contraindications to implant surgery (e.g., uncontrolled diabetes, alcoholism, or a significant smoking habit).

Although the available implants are remarkably successful, there is no one ideal implant, and all current designs have their limitations. Concerns regarding edentulous sites with inadequate bone for cylindric fixtures, splinting of implants to natural teeth, long-term effects of microbial and occlusal stresses, and effects of implants on alveolar ridge maintenance need to be addressed. Research on implant design for narrow ridges and atrophic jaws is ongoing, with the possibility of osseointegrated subperiosteal and blade-form implants being developed. Interface studies at the molecular level are in progress regarding apatite coatings on titanium implants (Rivero et al., 1988). Some degree of coating may contribute to greater interfacial shear strength of the implant and may form very tight bonds with living bone (Geesink et al., 1988). This could enhance the fixation of implants at recent extraction sites and where there is porous bone.

Improvements in surgical techniques are being effected, such as the development of internally irrigated drills. Single-stage implant procedures are also being investigated for their efficacy in achieving predictable osseointegration. The expanding acceptance of implants has also seen the design of innovative prosthetic attachments and abutments for partially edentulous patients.

REFERENCES

Adell R, Lekholm U, and Brånemark PI: Surgical procedures. In Brånemark PI, Zarb G, and Albrektsson T, editors: Tissue integrated prostheses, Chicago, 1985, Quintessence Publishing Co, Inc.

Adell R et al: A 15-year study of osseointegrated implants in the treatment of the edentulous jaw, Int J Oral Surg 10:387, 1981.

Albrektsson T and Jacobsson M: Bone-metal interface in osseointegration, J Prosthet Dent 57:597, 1987.

Albrektsson T et al: The long-term efficacy of currently used dental implants: a review and proposed criteria of success, Int J Oral Maxillofac Implants 1:11, 1986.

Albrektsson T et al: Osseointegrated oral implants: a Swedish multicenter study of 8139 consecutively inserted Nobelpharma implants, J Periodontol 59:287, 1988.

American Academy of Periodontology Newsletter 20:1, 1985.

Armitage JE: Risk of blade implants. In Schnitman PA and Shulman LB, editors: Dental implants: benefit and risk, US Department of Health and Human Services Pub No 81-1531, 1980.

Babbush CA: Statement of the American Association of Oral and Maxillofacial Surgeons, J Dent Educ 52:768, 1988.

Bailey JH and Yanase RT: University of Southern California implant denture program—14-year study. Paper presented at the International Symposium on Preprosthetic Surgery, Palm Springs, Calif, May 16-18, 1985.

Bodine RL and Yanase RT: Thirty-year report on 28 implant dentures inserted between 1952 and 1959. Paper presented at the International Symposium on Preprosthetic Surgery, Palm Springs, Calif, May 16-18, 1985.

Brandes R et al: Clinical-microscopic observations of ligature-induced "periimplantitis" around osseointegrated implants, J Dent Res 67(special issue):287, 1988 (abstract 1397).

Brånemark PI: Osseointegration and its experimental background, J Prosthet Dent 50:399, 1983.

Brånemark PI, Zarb G, and Albrektsson T, editors: Tissue integrated prostheses: osseointegration in clinical dentistry, Chicago, 1985, Quintessence Publishing Co, Inc.

Brånemark PI et al: Osseointegrated implants in the treatment of the edentulous jaw: experience from a ten year period, Scand J Plast Reconstr Surg 11(suppl 16), 1977.

Ericsson I et al: A clinical evaluation of fixed bridge restorations supported by the combination of teeth and osseointegrated titanium implants, J Clin Periodontol 13:307, 1986.

Eriksson RA and Adell R: Temperatures during drilling for the placement of implants using the osseointegration technique, J Oral Maxillofac Surg 44:4, 1986.

Eriksson RA and Albrektsson T: Temperature threshold levels for heat-induced bone tissue injury: a vital-microscope study in the rabbit, J Prosthet Dent 50:101, 1983.

Geesink RGT, DeGroot K, and Klein CPAT: Bonding of bone to apatite-coated implants, J Bone Joint Surg (Br)1:17, 1988.

Harvey C and Kelly JE: Decayed, missing and filled teeth among persons 1-74 years, United States, Vital and health statistics, National Center for Health Statistics, US Department of Health and Human Services Pub No 81-1673, series 11, No 223, 1981.

Kapur KL: VA cooperative study on dental implants. In Weiss CM, editor: Current review of prospective studies on fibro-osteal integrated blade implants as compared to osteal integrated fixtures, Implantologist, Quintessence Int, 1988.

McGivney GP et al: A comparison of computer-assisted tomography and data-gathering modalities in prosthodontics, Int J Oral Maxillofac Implants 1:55, 1986.

Melcher AH: Summary of biological considerations, J Dent Educ 52:812, 1988.

Meskin LH and Brown LHJ: Prevalence and patterns of tooth loss in U.S. employed adult and senior populations, 1985-86, J Dent Educ 52:686, 1988.

Rivero DP et al: Calcium phosphate-coated porous titanium implants for enhanced skeletal fixation, J Biomed Mater Res 23:191, 1988.

Rizzo AA, editor: Proceedings of the Consensus Development Conference on Dental Implants, J Dent Educ 52(12):1988.

Roberts WE: Bone tissue interface, J Dent Educ 52:804, 1988.

Schnitman PA and Shulman LB, editors: Dental implants: benefits and risk, US Department of Health and Human Services Pub No 81-1531, 1980.

Schnitman PA et al: Implant prostheses: blade vs. cantilever—clinical trial, J Oral Implantol 12:449, 1986.

Schnitman PA et al: Implants for partial edentulism, J Dent Educ 52:725, 1988a.

Schnitman PA et al: Three-year survival results: blade implant vs. cantilever clinical trial, J Dent Res 67(special issue):345, 1988b.

Shulman LB: Surgical considerations in implant dentistry, J Dent Educ 52:712, 1988.

Smithloff M and Fritz ME: The use of blade implants in a selected population of partially edentulous adults: a 15-year report, J Periodontol 58:589, 1987.

Part IV

Future Directions and Controversial Questions in Periodontal Therapy

Chapter 53

FUTURE DIRECTIONS IN ANTIINFECTIVE THERAPY

Walter J. Loesche

Patient evaluation: whom to treat
Choice of agent
Mode of delivery
Duration of therapy
Retreatment
Summary

Periodontal disease results from bacterial growth on the tooth and root surface that induces an inflammatory cell response. Treatment has traditionally been antiinfective in nature but has relied mainly on root surface debridement as a means of obtaining a therapeutic effect. This, while clinically effective in the majority of patients, is labor intensive and time consuming, and often needs to be repeated at periodic intervals. It is not cost-effective, and for many individuals it is not affordable when surgical therapy is used. Yet, if bacteria are responsible for periodontal disease, their overgrowth on the tooth surfaces should somehow be controllable by the judicious use of chemical antimicrobial agents. The proper use of these agents requires knowledge of the bacterial etiology of periodontal disease.

The treatment of periodontal disease in the future will be based on the recognition that periodontal disease in its most advanced form is a specific, albeit chronic, bacterial infection due to the overgrowth or presence of one or more of the periodontopathogens (Loesche, 1976). Some of these bacteria, such as the spirochetes and black-pigmented bacteroides (BPB) such as *Bacteroides intermedius,* are acquired in early life, and their subsequent overgrowth is probably secondary to local changes in the plaque microenvironment due to poor oral hygiene (Löe et al., 1965), hormonal factors (Kornman and Loesche,

1980), or the placement of dental restorations (Lang et al., 1983). Periodontal infections due to this overgrowth of indigenous organisms have been classified as endogenous infections (Rosebury, 1982). Other periodontopathic microbes such as *Actinobacillus actinomycetemcomitans* and *Bacteroides gingivalis* (an asaccharolytic BPB) appear to be acquired later in life and may be considered as causing exogenous infections (Genco, 1987). Exogenous infections may be easier to prevent or control than the endogenous infections associated with organisms such as the spirochetes (Genco et al., 1988).

The demonstration of bacterial specificity in periodontal disease allows the clinician to direct therapy toward the elimination and/or suppression of the periodontopathogens. The classic questions of infectious disease control, somewhat modified to take into account the chronic and asymptomatic nature of most forms of periodontal disease, can now be asked. Namely:

Whom to treat
What agent to use
How to deliver the agent
How long to treat
When to retreat

The answers to these questions will determine the future direction of periodontal disease therapy. Enough is known now to expect that the use of antiinfective agents will profoundly change approaches to periodontal therapy.

PATIENT EVALUATION: WHOM TO TREAT

Many antimicrobial agents are so potent that they should not be used indiscriminately or for a prolonged period of time. Thus it is necessary that treatment be focused on those individuals with an infection (therapeutic) or those at risk for an infection (prophylactic). The decisions regarding whom to treat and whether to use a therapeutic or a prophylactic regimen should be based not only on the clinical appearance of the periodontium, but also on whether any of the known periodontopathogens are present in the plaque or have become dominant in the plaque. Thus the clinician must have some means of diagnosing a periodontopathic infection.

A limited number of bacterial species have been associated with the various forms of periodontitis, including *Treponema denticola, A. actinomycetemcomitans, B. gingivalis, B. intermedius, Bacteroides forsythus, Wolinella recta, Eikenella corrodens,* and *Fusobacterium nucleatum.* It is likely that future studies will discover yet others; however, it appears that among those listed, there are several good markers for periodontal disease. There are several methodologies that can, or will in the future, permit the identification and quantification of these marker periodontopathogens in the plaque. This information, when supplemented with the clinical appearance of the tissue and examiner judgment, should enable the clinician to make the correct diagnosis, to initiate the appropriate antiinfective therapy, and to determine the adequacy of treatment in eliminating and/or suppressing the periodontopathogens from the plaque.

Microscopic examination of plaque smears for the presence and levels of motile organisms and spirochetes is a simple procedure (Listgarten and Hellden, 1978). In plaques removed from diseased sites, the levels and proportions of spirochetes are significantly elevated as compared with values obtained from plaques removed from healthy sites or from successfully treated sites. However, since spirochetes are detectable in most plaques, including those from sites suffering from gingivitis, it is necessary to establish some critical value above which a diagnosis of a spirochetal infection can be made. Our experience suggests that ≥20% spirochetes in plaques removed from single pocket sites (Loesche et al., 1987b) and ≥15% spirochetes in plaques removed from multiple sites (Listgarten and Levin, 1981) are associated with periodontitis.

A microscopic examination cannot distinguish what species of bacteria are present unless one uses a staining reagent that is specific for the sought-after organism. For example, the levels of *B. gingivalis* in the plaque can be determined by staining with an antibody specific for a surface antigen(s) of *B. gingivalis.* If the antibody is coupled with a fluorescent dye, such as fluorescein, then in theory all the *B. gingivalis* cells will exhibit a green color when illuminated with ultraviolet light (direct fluorescent antibody test). In a modification of this procedure, the original antibody, which may have been made in a rabbit, is not labeled with fluorescein but, after binding to the *B. gingivalis* cells in the plaque, is itself stained with an antirabbit gamma globulin antibody that has the fluorescein label. This latter test, known as the indirect fluorescent antibody test, can detect *B. gingivalis, B. intermedius,* and *A. acti-*

nomycetemcomitans cells in the plaque when the appropriate antibody is used (Slots et al., 1985; Zambon et al., 1986.)

Cultural methods can be used to diagnose a periodontopathic infection. These methods will not detect most species of spirochetes but can, if the appropriate nonselective and selective media are used, provide a wealth of information concerning the nature of the other members of the pathogenic flora that are present. Also, the antibiotic sensitivities of the suspected periodontopathogens can be determined, which may be useful in certain instances (Slots, 1986).

Specific microbes can be demonstrated in plaque(s) by the use of DNA probes (French et al., 1986; Savitt et al., 1988). In this procedure the plaque bacteria must be lysed so as to release their DNA. This DNA is denatured into single strands and then reacted with a short segment (probe) of DNA that is derived from and highly specific for the sought-after organism(s). This probe DNA has either a radioactive label or an enzyme marker, so that if the probe recognizes a complementary segment of DNA in the plaque and is bound by that segment, the occurrence and magnitude of the interaction can be quantitated by counting radioactivity or measuring enzyme activity. The DNA probe technology is available as a reference laboratory test on samples taken by the dentist and then sent to a laboratory. Much effort is being expended on making such tests amenable to chairside use.

Other diagnostic procedures may rely on the detection of molecules such as hydroxyproline, a collagen degradation product (Svanberg, 1987), or prostaglandin, an inflammatory mediator (Offenbacher et al., 1986), or enzymes derived from either the host or the microbes. A trypsinlike enzyme is present in *T. denticola* (a spirochete), *B. gingivalis,* and *B. forsythus* and is absent from at least 20 other subgingival organisms (Loesche, 1986). A similar enzyme activity in subgingival plaque can be associated with a probing depth greater than 6 mm and with high levels and proportions of spirochetes (Loesche et al., 1987b) and may be a useful marker for disease.

Any one of these procedures may be used in the future as adjunctive diagnostic aids to enable the clinician to identify those patients or sites that require antiinfective therapy based on their level of infection.

CHOICE OF AGENT

The bacteriologic diagnosis and clinical appearance will in most cases dictate the choice of antiinfective agent and the delivery system to be used. This choice will be determined on the basis of whether the periodontal infection is due to anaerobic, microaerophilic, facultative, or aerobic organisms (Table 53-1).

In my opinion, in the majority of periodontitis cases an anaerobic infection due to spirochetes and/or bacteroides will be diagnosed, and the drug of choice will be metron-

Table 53-1. Drugs to consider for treating various periodontal infections

Bacterial diagnosis	Clinical diagnosis	Drugs to consider
Specific		
Anaerobic infection		Tetracycline
Spirochetes	Acute necrotizing ulcerative gingivitis	Metronidazole
Bacteroides gingivalis	Juvenile periodontitis	Clindamycin
Bacteroides forsythus	Adult periodontitis	Tetracycline
Bacteroides intermedius		Spiramycin
Fusobacterium nucleatum		Penicillin
Eubacterium sp.		
Microaerophilic infection		
Actinobacillus actinomycetemcomitans	Localized juvenile periodontitis	Tetracycline
Eikenella corrodens	Juvenile periodontitis	
Wolinella recta	Adult periodontitis	Erythromycin
Facultative or aerobic infection		
Pseudomonas sp.	Refractory periodontitis	Use antibiotic sensitivity pattern to make
Proteus sp.	Periodontal abscess	choice
Streptococcus faecalis		Nystatin
Candida		Amphotericin B
Nonspecific		
Plaque overgrowth	Gingivitis	Chlorhexidine

idazole because of its bactericidal activity against anaerobes, its safety (Roe, 1983), and its efficacy in treating anaerobic periodontal infections as shown in double-blind studies (Loesche et al., 1987a). Because clinical resistance to metronidazole is extremely rare, the failure of this agent to be effective will reflect either the wrong bacterial diagnosis (i.e., a microaerophilic or facultative infection) or patient noncompliance with drug usage. The other antibiotics listed in Table 53-1 have been reported to be of value in periodontitis. Of these, only clindamycin has been widely used in medicine against anaerobes.

Microaerophilic infections should be treated with agents other than metronidazole or clindamycin. Tetracycline in conjunction with debridement, surgery, and chlorhexidine has been used with success in the treatment of localized juvenile periodontitis (Zambon et al., 1986). Systemic tetracycline, but not topically delivered iodine, was able to suppress *A. actinomycetemcomitans* (Slots and Rosling, 1983). Penicillin would appear to be contraindicated, since penicillin-resistant strains of *A. actinomycetemcomitans* have been isolated from infective endocarditis (Zambon, 1985). Combinations of metronidazole and amoxicillin also show promise in the treatment of these infections.

Facultative and aerobic infections are sometimes observed in patients refractory to treatment and in periodontal abscesses (Newman and Sims, 1979). The organisms involved can be resistant to one or more antimicrobial agents; therefore antibiotic sensitivity tests should be performed in order to select an effective agent. If *Candida* organisms are diagnosed, then nystatin or amphotericin B should be used.

In general, the use of antibiotics or antimicrobial agents for treatment of periodontal diseases is done in conjunction with thorough scaling and root planing, and with monitoring of the flora to evaluate effectiveness based on suppression or elimination of the pathogenic microbiota.

MODE OF DELIVERY

Previously it was suggested that patient noncompliance could account for the failure of a clinical response to metronidazole when an anaerobic infection was diagnosed. Patient noncompliance, which is estimated to be greater than 40% when prescription medication is to be taken several times a day, can account for the failure of any systemic antimicrobial treatment in periodontal disease. Noncompliance can be reduced, if not eliminated, by the use of slow-release delivery systems. This slow-release methodology was developed initially for the delivery of tetracycline to the pocket (Goodson et al., 1983) but can be adapted to deliver agents such as chlorhexidine (Stabholz et al., 1986) or metronidazole (Addy and Langeroudi, 1984), among others.

The several delivery systems employed have in common the ability to release inhibitory levels of the selected agent to the pocket site for several days (Goodson et al., 1985; Stabholz et al., 1986). These inhibitory levels can be achieved with a great reduction in drug dosage (i.e., from 50- to 500-fold lower dosages than would be required if systemic medication were used).

In the case of locally delivered metronidazole, plaque levels and proportions of spirochetes were reduced beyond that which was observed with systemically delivered metronidazole (Loesche et al., 1987a).

There are several vehicles that can be used to deliver the antimicrobial agents. A thin, flexible ethylcellulose film can be placed subgingivally and be maintained there for several days (Stabholz et al., 1986). The thickness of the film and the initial concentration of the antimicrobial agent determine how long the agent will be released into the pocket microenvironment. We have found residual antimicrobial activity present in films containing 20% metronidazole that have been left in pockets for up to 7 days. The ethylcellulose film is not biodegradable and needs to be removed after the treatment effect has been achieved.

The antimicrobial agent can also be incorporated into a biodegradable polymer such as ethylene-vinyl ester. This polymer, containing tetracycline and fabricated in the form of a fiber, has been placed around diseased teeth or layered within a pocket. Tetracycline delivered in such a fashion leads to an apparent gain in attachment and reduced probing depths (Goodson et al., 1985).

Another delivery system designed for supragingival access involves the painting of ethanolic solutions of ethylcellulose containing chlorhexidine onto acrylic appliances of the Hawley type, which are then worn in vivo for several days (Friedman et al., 1985). In a modification of this system the chlorhexidine was painted onto the tooth surfaces in a varnish containing 10% to 20% chlorhexidine and benzoin. This therapeutic varnish was then covered with a polyurethane varnish so as to retard the release of the chlorhexidine from the tooth surfaces (Sandham et al., 1985). This varnish was designed for the suppression and/or elimination of *Streptococcus mutans* from the tooth surfaces, but the principle could be adapted for the control of periodontopathic infections, especially as it relates to prophylactic treatment of the supragingival surfaces. For example, if an individual were found to have *A. actinomycetemcomitans, B. gingivalis,* or *T. denticola* in his plaque in the absence of disease, topical application of varnishes containing an appropriate antimicrobial agent could eliminate or suppress these periodontopathogens before any disease occurred.

DURATION OF THERAPY

The use of any antimicrobial treatment in periodontal disease should be targeted on the suppression, if not elimination, of the pathogenic periodontal flora. The effective agent should have an immediate effect, and if the organism in question is persistent or remains elevated for more than 2 to 3 weeks, then treatment should be reevaluated. If compliance is assured, mechanical therapy may not have been adequate, or there may be another source of the infection, such as a pulpal infection or fractured root. If these are eliminated as a cause of failure, antibiotic therapy with another antibiotic, selected on the basis of sensitivity of the periodontopathogen, may be considered.

Thus antiinfective treatment with any particular agent should be of short duration, and its efficacy should be based on the suppression of the targeted periodontopathogen. The actual choice of agent and the dosages to be employed will be predicated on how quickly the chosen agent is able to suppress the periodontopathogen(s). The need for data obtained from double-blind clinical trials is currently a major priority in clinical research, and until this information is available, a cautionary note should be raised in regard to the immediate transfer of research findings to the private-practice sector. However, the development and refinement of slow-release delivery systems may facilitate this transfer.

RETREATMENT

If an antiinfective agent was effective in eliminating or suppressing a periodontopathogen in the plaque and if this effect coincided with an improvement or restoration of periodontal health, then one may conclude that the agent was effective and that the targeted organism was indeed periodontopathic. If over the succeeding months or years the periodontopathogens were to reappear or become dominant, then retreatment with the same or comparable agent that had been employed previously would be warranted. If the periodontopathogens were to reappear within weeks after initial treatment, then one might want to consider the use of a second agent or reuse the first agent but change the delivery system and/or increase the dosage and length of treatment of the first agent. In either case, retreatment is dependent on the reappearance or reemergence of the periodontopathogens in the plaque with one possible exception: if periodontal health is obvious, then the clinician might want to delay retreatment.

SUMMARY

This brief review indicates that antiinfective therapy will be important in the future. In particular, future developments in the monitoring of the pathogenic periodontal flora, in the selection of systemic antibiotics as adjuncts to mechanical therapy, and in the development and refinement of topical delivery systems will facilitate the use of antimicrobial agents.

REFERENCES

Addy M and Langeroudi M: Comparison of the immediate effects on the subgingival microflora of acrylic strips containing 40% chlorhexidine, metronidazole or tetracycline, J Clin Periodontol 11:379, 1984.

French CK et al: DNA probe detection of periodontal pathogens, Oral Microbiol Immunol 1:58, 1986.

Friedman M et al: Plaque inhibition by sustained release of chlorhexidine from removable appliances, J Dent Res 64:1319, 1985.

Genco RJ: Highlights of the conference and perspectives for the future: proceedings of the Seventh International Conference, J Periodont Res 22:164, 1987.

Genco RJ et al: The origin of periodontal infections, Adv Dent Res 2(2):245, 1988.

Goodson JM et al: Monolithic tetracycline containing fibers for controlled delivery to periodontal pockets, J Periodontol 54:575, 1983.

Goodson JM et al: Clinical responses following periodontal treatment by local drug delivery, J Periodontol 56(suppl 11):81, 1985.

Kornman KS and Loesche WJ: The subgingival microbial flora during pregnancy, J Periodont Res 15:111, 1980.

Kornman KS et al: Detection and quantitation of *Bacteroides gingivalis* in bacterial mixtures by means of flow cytometry, J Periodont Res 19:570, 1984.

Lang NP et al: Clinical and microbiological effects of subgingival restorations with overhanging or clinically perfect margins, J Clin Periodontol 10:563, 1983.

Lindhe J: Treatment of localized juvenile periodontitis. In Genco RJ and Mergenhagen SE, editors: Host-parasite interactions in periodontal diseases, Washington, DC, 1982, ASM Publications.

Listgarten MA and Hellden L: Relative distribution of bacteria at clinically healthy and periodontally diseased sites in humans, J Clin Periodontol 5:115, 1978.

Listgarten MA and Levin S: Positive correlation between the proportions of subgingival spirochetes and motile bacteria and susceptibility of human subjects to periodontal deterioration, J Clin Periodontol 8:122, 1981.

Loë HB et al: Experimental gingivitis in man, J Periodontol 36:177, 1965.

Loesche WJ: Chemotherapy of dental plaque infections, Oral Sci Rev 9:63, 1976.

Loesche WJ: The identification of bacteria associated with periodontal disease and dental caries by enzymatic methods, Oral Microbiol Immunol 1:65, 1986.

Loesche WJ et al: Metronidazole therapy for periodontitis, J Periodont Res 22:224, 1987a.

Loesche WJ et al: Trypsin-like activity in subgingival plaque: a diagnostic marker for spirochetes and periodontal disease? J Periodontol 58:266, 1987b.

Newman MG and Sims TN: The predominant cultivable microbiota of the periodontal abscess, J Periodontol 50:350, 1979.

Offenbacher S et al: The use of crevicular fluid prostaglandin E_2 levels as a predictor of periodontal attachment loss, J Periodont Res 21:101, 1986.

Roe FJC: Toxicologic evaluation of metronidazole with particular reference to carcinogenic, mutagenic and teratogenic potential, Surgery 93:158, 1983.

Rosebury T: Microorganisms indigenous to man, New York, 1982, McGraw-Hill Book Co, Chapter 10.

Sandham HJ et al: Clinical elimination of *S. mutans* with chlorzoin and polyurethane varnishes, J Dent Res 64:213, 1985 (abstract 343).

Savitt ED et al: Comparison of cultural methods and DNA probe analyses for the detection of *A. actinomycetemcomitans*, *Bacteroides gingivalis*, and *Bacteroides intermedius* in subgingival plaque samples, J Periodontol 59:431, 1988.

Slots J: Rapid identification of important periodontal microorganisms by cultivation, Oral Microbiol Immunol 1:48, 1986.

Slots J and Rosling BG: Suppression of the periodontopathic microflora in localized juvenile periodontitis by systemic tetracycline, J Clin Periodontol 10:465, 1983.

Slots J et al: Detection of *Actinobacillus actinomycetemcomitans* and *Bacteroides gingivalis* in subgingival smears by the indirect fluorescent-antibody technique, J Periodont Res 20:613, 1985.

Stabholz A et al: Clinical and microbiological effects of sustained release chlorhexidine in periodontal pockets, J Clin Periodontol 13:783, 1986.

Svanberg GK: Hydroxyproline titers in gingival crevicular fluid, J Periodont Res 22:212, 1987.

Zambon JJ: *Actinobacillus actinomycetemcomitans* in human periodontal disease, J Clin Periodontol 12:1, 1985.

Zambon JJ et al: Diagnosis and treatment of localized juvenile periodontitis, J Am Dent Assoc 113:295, 1986.

Chapter 54

RESEARCH DIRECTIONS IN REGENERATIVE THERAPY

Steven Garrett

DEFINITIONS AND PRINCIPLES

Regeneration therapy refers to those procedures used in the treatment of periodontal disease that are designed to achieve replacement of lost periodontal tissues. *New connective tissue attachment* is defined as reunion of connective tissue with a root surface that has been exposed pathologically. *Regeneration* is defined as restitution of lost supporting tissues, including new alveolar bone and a new periodontal ligament. *Bone fill* is defined as clinically present bone tissue in a previously treated periodontal defect. Bone fill does not address the presence or absence of histologic evidence of new connective tissue attachment or the formation of a new periodontal ligament.

With active periodontitis comes the loss of the tooth's support apparatus and eventually loss of the tooth itself. For teeth whose function requires additional periodontal support, or where elimination of the periodontal defect will enhance long-term survival, treatment involves not only prevention of further breakdown by eliminating periodontal infection, but also regeneration of the previously lost alveolar bone and periodontal ligament. With our cur-

rent knowledge it is difficult to produce the proper conditions in the healing periodontal surgical wound that lead to complete regeneration. Conclusive evidence that a certain amount of new connective tissue attachment may occur does exist (Cole et al., 1980; Bowers et al., 1985), but substantial regeneration is not a predictable outcome of most regenerative attempts regardless of the therapeutic modality employed (for review, see Egelberg, 1987).

Presently, the more promising research directions for developing predictable clinical procedures to achieve substantial periodontal regeneration seem to lie in two areas. The first area involves developing techniques to stabilize the healing wound at the root surface–blood clot interface and enhance the adhesion of the healing wound coagulum to the root surface. This will prevent apical migration of the epithelium and lead to connective tissue attachment to the root surface. The second area involves manipulating the cells that repopulate the wound-healing site to ensure that this repopulation includes cells that lead to regeneration. This is termed *guided cell repopulation* or *guided tissue regeneration*. It should be emphasized that these began as experimental procedures, but there is growing support for their use clinically.

STABILIZATION AND ENHANCEMENT OF THE ROOT SURFACE–BLOOD CLOT INTERFACE
Current techniques

To successfully regenerate a periodontal attachment apparatus, newly formed connective tissue must attach itself to the root surface. Traditionally, the root surface is prepared for this process by careful planing of the superficial portion that has been exposed to the pocket. We have little information about the healing events that will lead to new connective tissue attachment to this planed root surface. Conceptually, we have thought of this as a healing "race" between epithelium from the wound margin and connective tissue from within the wound, with the epithelium migrating apically along the root surface until it is stopped by connective tissue, which has adhered or attached itself to the root in some manner.

One of the most important aspects of this healing process may be the adhesion of the wound coagulum and/or granulation tissue to the root surface. Once this is accomplished, apical migration of the epithelium is not possible because of the barrier formed by the adherent connective tissue. It may be possible to improve this adhesion by altering the root surface in a way that will promote the formation of a more stable root surface–wound coagulum interface. One method to achieve this could be by treating the root surface by topical application of a demineralizing agent. Although many demineralizing agents have been

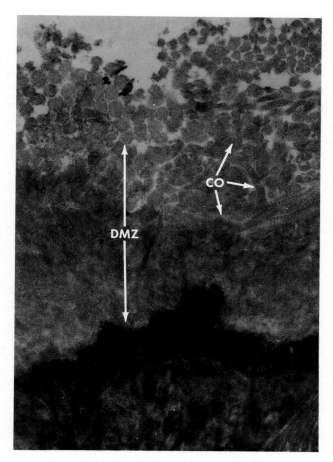

Fig. 54-1.   Citric acid–treated root surface showing a 3 μm zone of demineralization *(DMZ)* and exposed collagen fibers *(CO)*. (From Garrett JS, Crigger M, and Egelberg J: J Periodont Res 13:155, 1978. © 1978 Munksgaard International Publishers, Ltd., Copenhagen, Denmark.)

evaluated (see Egelberg, 1987), the agent used most often is citric acid (Register, 1973; Register and Burdick, 1975). Topical application of citric acid demineralizes the root-planed cementum and/or dentin to a depth of 1 to 5 μm, exposing the collagen fibrils in the cementum and/or dentin matrix (Fig. 54-1). Previously, this exposed collagen was thought to enhance new connective tissue attachment by allowing interdigitation of collagen fibrils from the healing wound and the exposed collagen fibers from the root surface (Ririe et al., 1980).

Presently, however, the focus is more on the early time points in healing and the effect of the exposed collagen fibers on the adhesion of the blood clot to the root surface. Studies by Polson and Proye (1983) have suggested that this exposed collagen enhances the linkage between the fibrin in the blood clot and the demineralized root surface. This initial fibrin linkage to acid-conditioned root surfaces is apparently stable and seems to prevent apical migration of the epithelium and promote new connective tissue attachment. Specimens that were not acid conditioned showed an initial fibrin linkage to the root surface. However, within 3 days this linkage seemed to break down and the epithelium had migrated apically, approaching the crest of the alveolar bone. In the acid-treated specimens the fibrin linkage was able to maintain itself, eventually resulting in connective tissue attachment (Fig. 54-2).

This technique of acid demineralization has been successful in promoting substantial new connective tissue attachment in both furcation and flat surface defects in animal models (Crigger et al., 1978; Klinge et al., 1981, 1985; Polson and Proye, 1982; Bogle et al., 1983). However, it has not been successful when applied to human periodontal disease, wherein only limited regeneration has been obtained in comparison with that achieved in the animal models (Stahl and Froum, 1977; Cole et al., 1981; Renvert and Egelberg, 1981). This difference may be related to the quality of initial wound closure. Immediate postoperative flap stability and wound closure would seem to be critical to protect the fragile root surface–fibrin interface and prevent tearing of this adhesion. Any such tear would obviate regeneration attempts by allowing epithelium to migrate on the granulation tissue and grow apically along the root surface. These tears will also allow salivary and bacterial contamination of the area, possibly resulting in additional breakdown of the root surface–wound coagulum interface. In the successful animal studies wound protection was achieved by coronally elevating the flap margins so that there was 4 to 5 mm of soft tissue wound coverage between the flap margin and the critical healing areas (Klinge et al., 1981). As an alternative to this extreme coronal repositioning of the flaps, in other studies, the flap margins were secured approximately 1 mm coronal to the cementoenamel junction with sutures attached to the crown with composite resins (Klinge et al., 1985). This technique may have stabilized the flap, preventing

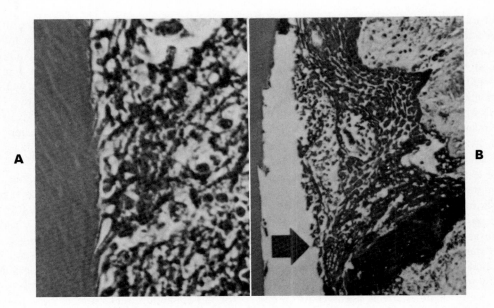

Fig. 54-2. A, Root placed with citric acid treatment (3-day specimen). Note interface between demineralized root surface and fibrin. No apical migration of epithelium has occurred. **B,** Root placed with no citric acid treatment (3-day specimen). Epithelium has migrated along root surface and terminates *(arrow)* at approximate level of alveolar bone. (From Polson AM and Proye MP: J Periodontol 54:141, 1983.)

flap recession and movement in the healing site. Both techniques resulted in connective tissue attachment.

Future directions

Future application of this working hypothesis concerning the importance of the root surface–wound coagulum interface in regenerative attempts requires the development of in vivo model systems that allow study of this concept. There is, to date, very little experimental evidence to support this hypothesis. The animal model used by Klinge et al. (1981, 1985) produces predictable new connective tissue attachment. Studies are under way, with this model, using techniques that interfere with the formation of the initial fibrin–root surface linkage. These studies should help to determine the importance of this concept of initial healing events in the formation of new connective tissue attachment. If results from this research support the hypothesis, studies attempting to identify methods to improve the stability of the interface between the root surface and wound coagulum should follow.

A possible application of this hypothesis in humans is Class II furcation lesions, especially those found in lower molars. These furcation defects cause significant destruction in the area between the roots of the tooth, but not completely through the intraradicular area. These are also areas that have not responded favorably to regenerative therapy in the past (for review see Martin et al., 1988). The anatomy seems to be suitable in terms of protection of the root surface–coagulum interface. The healing wound is protected by the adjacent root surfaces and bony walls of the furcation defect, the only opening being the one exposed furcation orifice. This furcation opening can be closed by coronally positioning the associated buccal or lingual flap margin and securing the flap with crown-attached sutures in a manner similar to the technique used in the animal model of Klinge et al. (1985).

Studies have indicated that the flap margin can be routinely elevated to a point approximately 3 mm coronal to the furcation orifice (Martin et al., 1988). Results from an initial study wherein Class II mandibular furcation defects were treated by surgical opening, root planing, citric acid demineralization, and closure with coronally positioned flaps showed a mean bone fill of approximately 70% in the furcations (Fig. 54-3). About 50% of the treated defects were completely filled with bone and had no remaining horizontal component to the furcation defect (Gantes et al., 1988). These results are favorable and may indicate that substantial regeneration is possible if adequate wound closure and clot stabilization can be achieved. With coronal positioning of the flap, the wound margin is moved to a position where it does not directly approximate the critical healing area. This margin is the area that seems the most susceptible to trauma, mechanical or otherwise, which would lead to breakdown of the initial root surface–coagulum interface, resulting in failure of the regenerative attempt. Moving this margin away enables the critical area to heal without complications. However, it is just as logical to relate the success of this study to the flap coverage

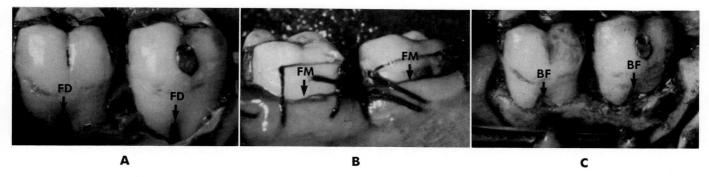

Fig. 54-3. A, Mandibular first and second molars with Class II furcation defects *(FD).* **B,** Same molar teeth after treatment and coronal positioning of flap margins *(FM).* Flap is secured by sutures attached to crown with composite resin. **C,** Reentry 1 year after regenerative surgery. Note bone fill *(BF)* in furcations. (From Gantes B et al: J Clin Periodontol 15:232, 1988. © 1988 Munksgaard International Publishers, Ltd., Copenhagen, Denmark.)

of the wound and/or to the flap support provided by the crown-attached sutures. In addition, the wound protection provided by the flap coverage may have affected wound healing positively in some way other than clot adhesion. These comments are made to demonstrate how little we know about the reasons for the initial success with this procedure and to emphasize that the concept of stability of the root surface–coagulum interface is a hypothesis only at this time.

Another method of wound stabilization that may be applicable in both flat-surface and interproximal defects, as well as furcations, is the technique of placing barrier membranes between the flap and the healing wound. The root surface–healing wound interface is then separated from the flap by the membrane and left to heal with less influence from the adjacent flap. The barrier membrane becomes an artificial flap, so to speak, which protects the healing wound until the membrane is removed or, in the case of biodegradable membranes, resorbed. This technique is discussed in detail in the section of this chapter dealing with guided tissue regeneration. In addition to its applications in guided tissue regeneration, it may be an effective mechanism of wound protection.

GUIDED CELL REPOPULATION

In 1976, reviewing the repair potential of periodontal tissues, Melcher suggested that the cells that repopulate the root surface after periodontal surgery may determine the type of attachment that will form on that root surface (Melcher, 1976). If this is true, there are apparently four sources of cells that can populate the root surface following regenerative periodontal surgery. These are (1) epithelial cells, (2) gingival connective tissue cells from the surgical flap, (3) bone cells from the alveolar bone and/or periosteum, and (4) connective tissue cells from the periodontal ligament (for review see Gottlow, 1986).

Research has demonstrated the healing events that result

from a root surface repopulated by cells of various origins. *Conventional periodontal regenerative attempts,* without any attempts at root surface augmentation other than root planing, seem to *routinely heal with a long junctional epithelium to the base of the original pocket* (Caton et al., 1980). There is evidence that even with substantial bone regeneration, epithelium may be found between the bone and the root surface (Listgarten and Rosenberg, 1979; Caton et al., 1980). Migration of the epithelium along the root surface is completed early in healing sites (Polson and Proye, 1983) and, of course, forms a barrier that prevents any new connective tissue attachment to the root surface. It is often assumed that this form of healing, with an epithelial layer between the root and the bone in an angular or vertical defect, represents an inadequate form of healing and may lead to recurrence. However, Pontoriero et al. (1988a) found that angular bone defects treated conventionally were no more susceptible to recurrent destructive periodontal disease than treated control sites that showed horizontal patterns of alveolar bone loss.

If the granulation tissue that populates the root surface originates from the gingival connective tissue, there will be a connective tissue–root surface interface. However, studies of the healing between this connective tissue and the root surface show a pattern that is generally dominated by ankylosis and resorption of the root surface. This resorption has been repeatedly demonstrated in animal studies (see Gottlow, 1986).

A bone–root surface interface is defined as *ankylosis.* Ankylosis has been studied in animals by extraction of teeth, removing the periodontal ligament or destroying its vitality, followed by the replantation of the teeth. The ankylosis seems to be followed by root resorption. In regenerative attempts, should the root surface be populated with bone cells, ankylosis and eventual resorption seem to occur (Egelberg, 1987).

If the root surface is repopulated with cells from the

periodontal ligament, this should favor the formation of a new periodontal ligament. This premise seems to be substantiated by animal studies using fenestration or window-type surgical defects. These defects are created by reflecting a full-thickness flap. Alveolar bone, periodontal ligament, and cementum are then removed in a specified area of the root, apical to the crest of the alveolar bone. The created surgical defect is circumscribed by intact periodontal ligament. Healing of smaller defects of this type is uneventful, with reestablishment of a new periodontal ligament and normal attachment apparatus. Cells from the surrounding periodontal ligament seem to be able to migrate across this root surface and produce the desired regeneration (Register, 1973; Andreasen and Kristersson, 1981; Nyman et al., 1982b).

In summary, there is research to support the hypothesis that the cell types that repopulate the root surface will determine the subsequent healing events and whether or not regeneration is achieved.

Guided tissue regeneration

The question arises, what can we do clinically to promote population of the root surface by cells and granulation tissue from the periodontal ligament? One such technique involves the placement of Teflon membranes that bridge the space between the alveolar crest and the cervical portion of the tooth. The membrane functions as a barrier that prevents access of cells from the surgical flap to the root surface. This reduces the possibility of the root surface being populated by cells from epithelium or the gingival connective tissue and may facilitate repopulation of the root surface by cells from the periodontal ligament. Membranes have been used in the treatment of dehiscence-type defects in animal models. Results from these studies have shown increased regeneration of cementum, alveolar bone, and periodontal ligament as compared with non–membrane treated controls. In addition, the healing aberrations associated with gingival connective tissue and bone cell repopulation of the root surface (i.e., resorption and ankylosis) were significantly reduced as compared with non–membrane treated controls (Nyman et al., 1982b; Aukhil et al., 1983, 1986; Gottlow et al., 1984; Magnusson et al., 1985).

This technique has been applied in preliminary human studies with successful results both clinically and histologically (Nyman et al., 1982a; Gottlow et al., 1986). In the material presented by Gottlow et al. (1986), 12 teeth in 10 human subjects were treated with polytetrafluoroethylene membranes. Five of the 12 teeth were examined histologically, and 7 were examined clinically. Clinical results showed a range of probing attachment gain of 4 to 7 mm at 3 months. Bone fill ranged from 3 to 8 mm at a reentry procedure 3 months after initial surgery. All five specimens examined histologically showed evidence of new connective tissue attachment. Five of the 12 teeth had furcation involvements, which showed successful bone fill. These limited human results are promising. Most likely, the membrane helped to produce a wound-healing environment that favored the formation of new connective tissue attachment and bone fill. This may be due to the membrane's enhancing the opportunity for repopulation of the root surface by periodontal ligament cells. It could also be a result of stabilization of the root surface–clot interface, as previously noted, or of some yet-undetermined effect of the membrane.

Presently, these results are being substantiated by controlled human studies with and without membranes. For example, Pontoriero et al. (1988b) tested the regenerative potential of guided tissue regeneration using Teflon membranes in a controlled study on humans with Class II mandibular molar defects. Each patient received a series of full-mouth scalings and root planings, and 2 to 3 months later, their furcation defects were treated by flap reflection and placement of a Teflon membrane covering the entrance to the furcation, as well as the bone apical to the crest. A second surgical procedure was performed after 1 to 2 months to remove the Teflon membranes. The controls were treated identically except that no Teflon membranes were placed. Early healing results in 3 to 6 months showed that in the control subjects, 20% of the sites showed complete clinical resolution of the defect, whereas in the experimental group, 90% of the sites showed disappearance of the anatomic defect. These early healing results are encouraging; however, long-term studies are needed to evaluate the stability of the healing and possible adverse effects such as root resorption and ankylosis.

A clinical sequence of a vertical defect and Class II furcation defect treated by the guided tissue regeneration technique using a biodegradable barrier membrane is shown in Fig. 54-4. At reentry 9 months after the initial surgery, both the furcation defect and the vertical defect showed substantial bone fill.

Another approach to guided tissue regeneration may eventually result from in vitro studies in which it now appears possible to influence migration and adhesion of cells that repopulate root surfaces by the use of biologically active extracellular matrix proteins or growth factors (for review, see Terranova and Wikesjö, 1987). For example, fibronectin, a large glycoprotein that is found in blood and connective tissues, enhances the migration and proliferation of fibroblasts on dentin surfaces, particularly dentin surfaces that have undergone surface demineralization prior to fibronectin application. Proliferation and movement of periodontal ligament fibroblasts can be further enhanced by treating the demineralized dentin surfaces with a combination of fibronectin and endothelial cell growth factor (Terranova and Wikesjö, 1987).

Whether or not there will be similar results from in vivo

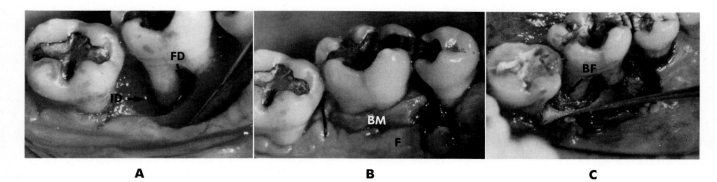

Fig. 54-4. A, Lingual surface of mandibular first molar demonstrating an intraosseous defect *(ID)* and furcation defect *(FD).* **B,** Surgical wound closed with a biodegradable barrier membrane *(BM)* interposed between surgical flap *(F)* and periodontal defects. **C,** Reentry 9 months following regenerative surgery showing bone fill *(BF)* in intraosseous defect and furcation.

experimentation remains to be seen. The complicated series of multiple events associated with in vivo wound healing may simply reflect the advantages seen with the application of these elements in the controlled in vitro environment. Animal studies wherein fibronectin was applied to demineralized root surfaces and the results compared with demineralized surfaces without fibronectin have been inconclusive. One study showed increases in connective tissue attachment on the fibronectin-treated surfaces (Caffesse et al., 1985). A second study also showed an advantage with fibronectin treatment (Wikesjö, 1987), and in this study the effectiveness of a tetracycline solution in addition to fibronectin in preparation of the root surface for regeneration was established. The possibility of directing specific cell populations to the root surface by conditioning the root surfaces with substances from the extracellular matrix and/or growth factors is an interesting approach for future research. It may be that agents such as fibronectin that are chemotactic for fibroblasts could best be used along with barrier membranes that would exclude fibroblasts from the gingival connective tissue.

SUMMARY

Predictable regeneration has been a goal of periodontal therapy for decades. Over the years researchers have investigated many promising avenues that on more complete study have demonstrated equivocal success. Stabilization of the root surface–blood clot interface and guided cell repopulation show promise for regenerative therapy. Further in the future is perhaps a biochemical approach using matrix components and growth factors to enhance the regenerative potential of the tissues.

REFERENCES

Andreasen JG and Kristersson L: Interrelation between alveolar bone and periodontal ligament repair after replantation of mature permanent incisors in monkeys, J Periodont Res 16:228, 1981.

Aukhil I, Simpson DM, and Schaberg TV: An experimental study of new attachment procedure in beagle dogs, J Periodont Res 18:643, 1983.

Aukhil I, Pettersson E, and Suggs C: Guided tissue regeneration: an experimental procedure in beagle dogs, J Periodont Res 57:727, 1986.

Bogle G et al: New connective tissue attachment in beagles with advanced natural periodontitis, J Periodont Res 18:220, 1983.

Bowers GM et al: Histologic evaluation of new attachment in humans: a preliminary report, J Periodontol 56:381, 1985.

Caffesse RG et al: The effect of citric acid and fibronectin application on healing following surgical treatment of naturally occurring periodontal disease in beagle dogs, J Clin Periodontol 12:578, 1985.

Caton J, Nyman S, and Zander H: Histometric evaluation of periodontal surgery. II. Connective tissue attachment levels after four regenerative procedures, J Clin Periodontol 7:224, 1980.

Cole RT et al: Connective tissue regeneration to periodontally diseased teeth: a histological study, J Periodont Res 15:1, 1980.

Cole RT et al: Pilot clinical studies on the effect of topical citric acid application on healing after replaced periodontal flap surgery, J Periodont Res 16:117, 1981.

Crigger M et al: The effect of topical citric acid application on healing after replaced flap surgery, J Periodont Res 13:538, 1978.

Egelberg J: Regeneration and repair of periodontal tissues, J Periodont Res 22:233, 1987.

Gantes B et al: Treatment of periodontal furcation defects. II. Bone regeneration in mandibular Class II defects, J Clin Periodontol 15:232, 1988.

Gottlow J: New attachment formation by guided tissue regeneration, thesis, Goteberg, Sweden, 1986, University of Goteberg.

Gottlow J et al: New attachment formation as the result of controlled tissue regeneration, J Clin Periodontol 11:494, 1984.

Gottlow J et al: New attachment formation in the human periodontium by guided tissue regeneration: case reports, J Clin Periodontol 13:604, 1986.

Klinge B, Nilveus R, and Egelberg J: Effect of crown-attached sutures on healing of experimental furcation defects in dogs, J Clin Periodontol 12:369, 1985.

Klinge B et al: Effect of flap placement and defect size on healing of experimental furcation defects, J Periodont Res 16:236, 1981.

Listgarten MA and Rosenberg MM: Histological study of repair following new attachment procedures in human periodontal lesions, J Periodontol 50:333, 1979.

Magnusson I et al: Root resorption following periodontal flap procedures in monkeys, J Periodont Res 20:79, 1985.

Martin M et al: Treatment of periodontal furcation defects. I. Review of the literature and description of a regenerative surgical procedure, J Clin Periodontol 15:227, 1988.

Melcher AH: On the repair potential of periodontal tissues, J Periodontol 47:256, 1976.

Nyman S et al: New attachment following surgical treatment of human periodontal disease, J Clin Periodontol 9:290, 1982a.

Nyman S et al: The regenerative potential of the periodontal ligament: an experimental study in the monkey, J Clin Periodontol 9:257, 1982b.

Polson AM and Proye MP: Effect of root alterations on periodontal healing. II. Citric acid treatment of the denuded root, J Clin Periodontol 9:441, 1982.

Polson AM and Proye MP: Fibrin linkage: a precursor for new attachment, J Periodontol 54:141, 1983.

Pontoriero R, Nyman S, and Lindhe J: The angular bony defect in the maintenance of the periodontal ligament, J Clin Periodontol 15:200, 1988a.

Pontoriero R et al: Guided tissue regeneration in degree II furcation–involved mandibular molars: a clinical study, J Clin Periodontol 15:247, 1988b.

Register AA: Bone and cementum induction by dentin, demineralized in situ, J Periodontol 44:49, 1973.

Register AA and Burdick FA: Accelerated reattachment with cementogenesis to dentin, demineralized in situ. I. Optimum range, J Periodontol 46:646, 1975.

Renvert S and Egelberg J: Healing after treatment of periodontal intraosseous defects. II. Effect of citric acid conditioning of the root surface, J Clin Periodontol 8:459, 1981.

Ririe CM, Crigger M, and Selvig KA: Healing of periodontal connective tissues following surgical wounding and application of citric acid in dogs, J Periodont Res 15:314, 1980.

Stahl SS and Froum SJ: Human clinical and histologic repair responses following the use of citric acid in periodontal therapy, J Periodontol 48: 261, 1977.

Terranova VP and Wikesjö UME: Extracellular matrices and polypeptide growth factors as mediators of functions of cells of the periodontium: a review, J Periodontol 58:371, 1987.

Wikesjö UME: Personal communcation, 1987.

Wikesjö UME et al: Repair of periodontal furcation defects in beagle dogs following reconstructive surgery including root surface demineralization with tetracycline hydrochloride and topical fibronectin application, J Clin Periodontol 15:73, 1988.

Chapter 55

FUTURE DIRECTIONS IN ANTIINFLAMMATORY THERAPY

Ray C. Williams

It is well established that periodontal disease is the result of bacterial buildup on the teeth and subgingivally. It is also apparent that although bacteria are essential agents, their presence alone on the tooth is not sufficient to explain the periodontal disease process. Rather, the reaction of the host to these inciting agents must be involved if disease is to develop and progress. Recent research already presented in this textbook has made considerable progress in determining how the immunoinflammatory system mediates periodontal destruction. With new awareness of which host mechanisms are involved in periodontal destruction, there is increasing interest in how these host responses, particularly pathways of destruction, may be modulated or blocked to alter the progression of periodontal disease. The ability to modulate specific cellular and humoral factors involved in the periodontal disease process should lead in the future to new and more effective prevention and treatment methods for periodontal disease.

This chapter focuses on one host response implicated in periodontal tissue destruction, the local production of prostaglandins and other arachidonic acid metabolites in the periodontal tissues. These pathways are diagrammed in

Fig. 55-1. In brief, following local tissue damage such as might occur in the gingival tissues, phospholipids in the plasma membranes of cells become available for action by phospholipase, leading to free arachidonic acid released into the area. The arachidonic acid can then be metabolized via either the cyclo-oxygenase pathway to the prostaglandins, prostacyclin, and thromboxane, or the lipoxygenase pathway to the leukotrienes. The prostaglandins, prostacyclins, thromboxane, and the leukotrienes have been implicated in a wide range of events that are associated with disease such as platelet aggregation, vasodilation and vasoconstriction, chemotaxis of neutrophils, increased vascular permeability, and bone resorption. In periodontal disease these metabolites are believed to be closely associated with gingivitis and alveolar bone resorption. This

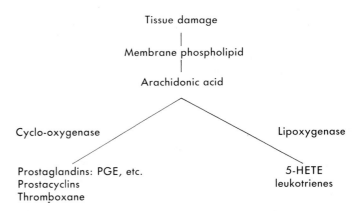

Fig. 55-1. Simplified schematic representation of metabolism of arachidonic acid locally within tissues via either cyclo-oxygenase pathway to prostaglandins or lipoxygenase pathway to leukotrienes.

chapter also examines the future role that blockage of this pathway with nonsteroidal antiinflammatory drugs (NSAIDs), as inhibitors of the enzyme cyclo-oxygenase, may have in controlling the periodontal disease process. Although the use of NSAIDs in the treatment of periodontal disease is in the early stages of evaluation, the research in this area is promising, and the prospects for using NSAIDs in the prevention and treatment of periodontal disease have great promise.

Evidence that local production of arachidonic acid metabolites is important in periodontal tissue destruction is reviewed first. Second, evidence suggesting that NSAIDs, as inhibitors of arachidonic acid metabolism, may also inhibit or decrease periodontal disease progression is reviewed. The final part of this chapter suggests research needs for the future.

EVIDENCE LINKING ARACHIDONIC ACID METABOLITES AND PERIODONTAL DISEASE

Two main lines of research have supported the hypothesis that prostaglandins and other arachidonic acid metabolites are important in the pathogenesis of periodontal disease. First, data clearly indicate that production of arachidonic acid metabolites within the periodontal tissues has the potential to be a major mediator of the pathologic events of periodontal disease: gingival inflammation and alveolar bone resorption. Second, analysis of periodontal tissue samples from humans and animals has demonstrated that in the diseased periodontal tissues, arachidonic acid metabolites are present and their levels are significantly elevated as compared with those in healthy tissue, suggesting a role for these metabolites in the periodontal disease process.

Local arachidonic acid metabolite production

Reports in the early 1970s that local production of prostaglandins within tissue may mediate the inflammatory response first linked prostaglandins and other arachidonic acid metabolites with gingival inflammation. Of particular interest to periodontal investigators was research into local regulation of bone resorption and the possibility that mediators of bone resorption in other osteolytic diseases might be similar to mediators of the alveolar bone resorption of periodontitis.

In this era periodontal researchers were studying the ability of various substances to stimulate bone resorption in tissue culture, including human gingival tissue, blood cells, media from cultures of gingival tissue, and bacterial endotoxin. One finding from these investigators linked local prostaglandin production with the periodontal disease process. Since then, a growing body of data has substantiated that concept considerably.

It was first found that tissues from several diseased conditions could stimulate bone resorption in vitro. Of particular interest was the finding that fragments of human gingival tissues, as well as the media from cultured fragments, markedly enhanced bone resorption of mouse calvaria in tissue culture (Goldhaber, 1971). Simultaneously it was reported that prostaglandins could stimulate bone resorption in tissue culture. This prompted investigators in bone physiology to examine the possibility that bone resorption–stimulating factors from a variety of tissues might be influenced by prostaglandin production, either in the particular tissue itself or in the bone organ culture system.

Goldhaber et al. (1973) reported that indomethacin inhibited bone resorption in tissue culture stimulatd by media from gingival fragments. From this research two concepts emerged. First, since human gingival tissues could produce a factor that was a potent stimulator of bone resorption in tissue culture, gingival tissues might be linked with the underlying bone resorption of periodontitis in vivo. Second, since the gingival bone resorption–stimulating factor was inhibited by indomethacin, it must be related to the production of arachidonic acid metabolites such as prostaglandin E_2 (PGE_2). These findings suggested that PGE_2 was a mediator of bone resorption in several osteolytic diseases.

Human dental cysts were found to produce prostaglandins that might be responsible for the bone resorption occurring around such cysts (Harris and Goldhaber, 1973). In addition, the bone resorption in tissue culture stimulated by a factor elaborated from mouse fibrosarcoma was found to be due to the production of PGE_2, and it was inhibited by indomethacin (Tashjian et al., 1972). Other investigators found that the ability of complement to enhance bone resorption in tissue culture could be explained by the enhanced synthesis of prostaglandins by bone (Raisz et al., 1974). PGE_2 also inhibited bone collagen synthesis in organ culture. Thus within a brief time period a relationship was established between prostaglandin production and bone resorption in several osteolytic diseases.

Goodson et al. (1974b) reported that solutions containing prostaglandin E_1 (PGE_1) injected under the skin overlying the calvarium of adult rats stimulated rapid resorption of bone, indicating that prostaglandins also have the capacity to induce bone resorption in vivo. Robinson et al. (1975) reported that synovial tissue from patients with rheumatoid arthritis produced a potent bone resorption–stimulating factor in tissue culture that was identified as PGE_2. They proposed that the bone resorption seen in the course of rheumatoid arthritis may be mediated by the production of prostaglandins.

Gomes et al. (1976) extended the concept that gingival tissues were able to stimulate bone resorption in experiments that used healthy and diseased gingiva from *Macaca speciosa* monkeys. Culture medium from gingival fragments of the monkey stimulated bone resorption. When cultured, the fragments released prostaglandins into the medium that could be blocked by up to 90% with the addition of indomethacin to the media. Unlike human gingival tissue, the bone resorption-stimulating ability of monkey gingival fragment media could be almost completely explained by the production of prostaglandins.

Prostacyclins and their metabolites have also been found to stimulate bone resorption in tissue culture. Since vessel walls produce prostacyclin and since increased vascularity is associated with inflammation and bone resorption, prostacyclin release could be responsible for the frequent association between increased vascularity and resorption of bone seen in many pathologic forms of osteolysis.

In summary, the research findings since 1970 have provided convincing evidence that several metabolites of arachidonic acid and their precursors can stimulate bone resorption in bone organ culture systems. Table 55-1 summarizes these research findings. If this is true in vivo, such as in the periodontal tissues, arachidonic acid metabolites may prove to be powerful local mediators of the alveolar bone resorption of periodontitis.

Arachidonic acid metabolite levels in periodontal tissues

A second line of evidence linking local arachidonic acid metabolite production and the pathogenesis of periodontal disease is derived from an examination of human and ani-

Table 55-1. Evidence that prostaglandins and other arachidonic acid metabolites may be mediators of bone resorption

Research findings	References
PGE_1 and PGE_2 stimulate resorption of fetal rat bone in tissue culture	Klein and Raisz (1970)
In tissue culture human gingival fragments and culture medium stimulate resorption of fetal rat bone that is inhibited by indomethacin	Goldhaber (1971)
	Goldhaber et al. (1973)
Dental cysts produce prostaglandins in tissue culture that in turn stimulate resorption of fetal rat bone	Harris and Goldhaber (1973)
Mouse fibrosarcoma produces a potent bone resorption stimulating factor in tissue culture that is inhibited by indomethacin	Tashjian et al. (1972)
Complement-mediated bone resorption in tissue culture is dependent on prostaglandin production	Raisz et al. (1974)
Arachidonic acid and phospholipase A_2 stimulate bone resorption in tissue culture	Goldhaber and Rabadjija (1982)
Injection of PGE_1 solutions over the calvarium in rats leads to bone resorption	Goodson et al. (1974b)
Prostaglandins E, F, A, and B stimulate resorption of fetal rat bone	Dietrich et al. (1975)
Rheumatoid synovial tissue and cells in culture produce PGE_2, which stimulates bone resorption of mouse calvaria	Robinson et al. (1975)
Monkey gingival fragments produce prostaglandins that stimulate bone resorption in tissue culture	Gomes et al. (1976)
Prostacyclin and metabolites of prostacyclin stimulate bone resorption in tissue culture	Ali et al. (1979)
	Dewhirst (1984)
	Neuman and Raisz (1984)

Table 55-2. Evidence that prostaglandins and other arachidonic acid metabolites are present in the periodontal tissues

Research findings	References
PGE_2 is elevated 10-fold in diseased human gingival tissues as compared with healthy gingiva	Goodson et al. (1974a)
PGE_2 is elevated as much as 20-fold in diseased human gingival tissues as compared with healthy gingiva	ElAttar (1976)
Prostacyclins are present in human gingiva	Wong et al. (1980)
PGE levels are markedly increased in established gingival lesions	Loning et al. (1980)
PGE and PGF levels are both elevated in human gingiva	ElAttar and Lin (1981)
PGE_2 crevicular fluid levels are elevated in patients with periodontitis, and PGE_2 levels are 3-fold higher in patients with juvenile periodontitis than in patients with adult periodontitis	Offenbacher et al. (1981, 1984, 1986)
Thromboxane B_2 levels are 2-fold higher in gingivitis versus normal tissues; levels are 3.5-fold higher in periodontitis as compared with gingivitis in beagles	Rifkin and Tai (1981)
Human gingival tissue converts exogenous arachidonic acid to metabolites via the lipoxygenase pathway	Sidhagen et al. (1982)
	ElAttar and Lin (1983)
Tissue samples from deep periodontal pockets contain prostaglandin E_2, thromboxane B_2, and 6-keto-PGFl∂	Dewhirst et al. (1983)
Eight different prostaglandin levels increase during advancing periodontal destruction; thomboxane B_2 and 6-keto-PGFl∂ are the most elevated	Ohm et al. (1984)

mal periodontal tissues, both healthy and diseased. These data indicate that metabolites of arachidonic acid are present in gingival biopsy specimens and are significantly elevated in diseased tissue as compared with healthy gingival tissue. At present, it seems clear that when proper experimental conditions are used, a number of arachidonic acid metabolites, via both the cyclo-oxygenase pathway and the lipoxygenase pathway, may be found in gingival tissue and crevicular fluid. These findings are summarized in Table 55-2. It seems likely that the presence of these metabolites within the gingival tissues contributes to the periodontal disease process. However, the overall contribution of these individual metabolites in the pathogenesis of periodontal tissue destruction is not known.

Goodson et al. (1974a), examining human gingival tissue samples excised during surgery, measured PGE_2 levels and found a tenfold elevation of PGE_2 in diseased tissue as compared with healthy tissue. Subsequently PGE_2 levels were found as much as 20 times higher in inflamed gingivae than in healthy gingivae (ElAttar, 1976). Offenbacher et al. (1981) have begun to provide some clues as to how levels of PGE_2 may relate to periodontal destruction. These investigators measured crevicular fluid prostaglandin E (PGE) concentrations in patients with periodontal disease. Patients with periodontitis had significantly higher crevicular fluid PGE concentrations than patients with gingivitis. In addition, PGE levels in periodontitis sites varied considerably. Some sites of periodontal destruction had low crevicular fluid PGE levels, whereas other sites of destruction had crevicular fluid PGE concentrations that were elevated tenfold. The reason for this difference was not known, but one explanation could be that elevated PGE levels are associated with ongoing active destruction at the time of sampling. Low PGE levels could reflect a site in remission. Subsequently these findings were extended to a study of individuals with adult periodontitis or juvenile periodontitis. The mean crevicular fluid PGE level in patients with juvenile periodontitis was almost threefold higher than that present in patients with adult periodontitis. Since alveolar bone resorption is likely to be actively progressing in patients with juvenile periodontitis at the time of study, these findings may be consistent with the association of elevated PGE levels with active periodontal bone loss (Offenbacher et al., 1984).

Recently patients with adult periodontitis were studied over a period of 18 to 36 months. The mean crevicular fluid level of PGE_2 was significantly elevated in those patients who had attachment loss over the time period studied as compared with the level in patients who did not lose attachment. Thus elevated levels of crevicular fluid PGE_2 have been linked with "active" periodontal tissue destruction (Offenbacher et al., 1986).

EFFECT OF NONSTEROIDAL ANTIINFLAMMATORY DRUGS ON PERIODONTAL DISEASE

The next question to be answered in a study of the relationship between arachidonic acid metabolite production and the pathogenesis of periodontal disease is whether inhibitors of arachidonic acid metabolism, such as NSAIDs, will slow the periodontal disease process. Investigators have begun to examine the effect of NSAIDs on blocking

Table 55-3. Evidence that nonsteroidal antiinflammatory drugs alter or diminish the periodontal disease process

Research findings	References
Indomethacin reduces alveolar bone uptake of technetium 99m in ligature-induced periodontal disease in rats	Nichols et al. (1979)
Indomethacin reduces inflammation and the onset of alveolar bone resorption in ligature-induced periodontal disease in dogs	Nyman et al. (1979)
Indomethacin is associated with less bone loss in diet-induced periodontal disease in hamsters	Lasfarques and Saffer (1983)
Indomethacin reduces loss of alveolar bone, loss of bone height, and increases osteoclast density in ligature-induced periodontal disease in monkeys	Weaks-Dybvig et al. (1982)
Flurbiprofen reduces the rate of alveolar bone loss in naturally occurring periodontal disease in beagles and rhesus monkeys	Williams et al. (1985) Jeffcoat et al. (1986) Offenbacher et al. (1987)
Indomethacin reduces the rate of alveolar bone loss in naturally occurring periodontal disease in beagles	Williams et al. (1987)
A substituted oxazolopyridine derivative topically applied inhibits gingivitis and loss of attachment in squirrel monkeys	Vogel et al. (1986)
Topical flurbiprofen reduces the rate of alveolar bone loss in beagles	Williams et al. (1988c)
Ibuprofen reduces the rate of alveolar bone loss in naturally occurring periodontal disease in beagles	Williams et al. (1988a)
Patients taking NSAIDs have a lower gingival index and shallower periodontal pockets	Waite et al. (1981)
Patients taking aspirin or aspirin plus indomethacin for at least 5 years have fewer sites with 10% or greater proximal bone loss	Feldman et al. (1983)
Patients taking flurbiprofen have a lower rate of alveolar bone loss than placebo-treated patients	Williams et al. (1988b, 1989)

or slowing the progression of periodontal disease, and although limited data are available, the reports are quite encouraging (Table 55-3).

The evidence available so far that NSAIDs can inhibit the periodontal disease process has come from animal model studies using both ligature-induced and naturally occurring periodontal disease. There have also been limited studies in humans indicating that NSAIDs may reduce the periodontal disease process.

Periodontal disease induced with ligatures in rats was reduced with injections of indomethacin, 1 mg/kg subcutaneously. The data from this early study suggested that in the rat, indomethacin administered subcutaneously could suppress alveolar bone loss (Nichols et al., 1979). Nyman et al. (1979) induced periodontal disease in beagles with ligatures. During a 28-day treatment period each dog was given 1 mg/kg indomethacin twice daily. With daily administration of indomethacin, the course of periodontal disease progression was altered as compared with the course of the disease without indomethacin administration. The initial inflammatory response was diminished, the onset of osteoclastic bone resorption delayed, and the total degree of alveolar bone resorption reduced. Periodontal disease induced in golden hamsters with a dietary regimen that promoted microbial buildup was treated with indomethacin, 2 mg/kg daily by gastric intubation. Bone loss was reduced by 28%, and the number of osteoclasts was reduced by 55% with indomethacin treatment (Lasfarques and Saffar, 1983).

Weaks-Dybvig et al. (1982) induced periodontitis in adult squirrel monkeys with ligatures over a 2-week period. Administration of indomethacin (5 mg/kg) to three animals reduced the loss of alveolar bone mass, the loss of bone height, and the increase in osteoclast density as compared with findings in the untreated controls.

Our laboratory is studying the effect of several NSAIDs, administered systemically daily, on the progression of naturally occurring periodontal disease in the adult beagle. In an initial 2-year study of the effect of the NSAID flurbiprofen, a potent cyclo-oxygenase inhibitor, we found that daily administration of flurbiprofen dramatically reduced the rate of alveolar bone loss in a 12-month treatment period by up to 66% as compared with a pretreatment baseline rate of bone loss (Williams et al., 1984, 1985; Jeffcoat et al., 1986).

In a second longitudinal study in beagles, we confirmed flurbiprofen's potent effect on inhibiting alveolar bone loss in beagles and found that indomethacin also inhibited bone loss in the beagle (Williams et al., 1987). Flurbiprofen has also been found to be a potent inhibitor of both ligature-induced and naturally occurring bone loss in the rhesus monkey, *Macaca mulatta* (Offenbacher et al., 1988). Recently we have examined the effect of ibuprofen on the course of bone loss in beagles and have found that ibuprofen is also a significant inhibitor of naturally occurring

bone loss in beagles (Williams et al., 1988a). Collectively, the data from animal studies conducted in several laboratories clearly indicate that several NSAIDs can significantly slow down the periodontal disease process.

Periodontal investigators must now determine the efficacy of NSAIDs in the treatment of human periodontal disease. There are limited data from human studies that indicate that NSAID administration is associated with less periodontal disease. Waite et al. (1981) investigated the prevalence of periodontal disease in a group of 22 patients taking several NSAIDs for arthritis or ankylosing spondylitis and compared the periodontal status with that of 22 age-matched individuals not taking NSAIDs. Patients taking NSAIDs had a lower gingival index (less gingivitis) and shallower periodontal pocket depths than individuals not taking NSAIDs. In another retrospective study 75 patients who had taken aspirin or aspirin plus indomethacin for at least 5 years for the treatment of arthritis had significantly fewer sites of 10% or greater proximal bone loss on radiographs as compared with 75 healthy control subjects (Feldman et al., 1983).

Our laboratory is concluding the first prospective longitudinal trial in humans to examine the effect of an NSAID on alveolar bone loss (Williams et al., 1988b, 1989). Fifty-six patients were studied for a 3-year period. The rate of alveolar bone loss in a 6-month baseline pretreatment period was measured radiographically for each patient. Patients were then separated into two groups with a similar mean rate of bone loss. Thereafter, one group was treated with a placebo for 2 years while the other group of patients was given flurbiprofen (Ansaid), 50 mg twice daily for 2 years. The rate of bone loss at 6, 12, 18, and 24 months of treatment was compared with the baseline rate of bone loss in the two patient groups (Fig. 55-2). The rate of bone loss in the patients treated with a placebo was less than the baseline rate at 6 and 12 months of treatment, most likely indicating that these patients responded to the increased care and were more attentive to their oral hy-

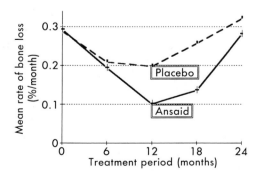

Fig. 55-2. Rate of alveolar bone loss in placebo- versus flurbiprofen-treated patients over a 2-year treatment period compared with rate of bone loss over a 6-month baseline pretreatment period.

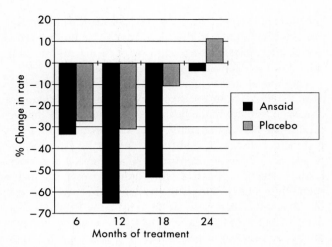

Fig. 55-3. Comparison of percentage change in rate of bone loss from baseline in placebo- versus flurbiprofen-treated patients at 6, 12, 18, and 24 months of treatment.

giene. Patients treated with flurbiprofen had a reduction in the rate of bone loss that was significantly better than the reduction in the placebo group at 12 and 18 months of treatment. At 24 months of treatment, the effect was lost, which we believe is a reflection of the fact that patients were no longer regularly taking the medication. The 66% reduction in the rate of bone loss from baseline at 12 months of treatment in the flurbiprofen-treated patients was the same reduction in the rate of bone loss that we have reported in our animal studies (Fig. 55-3). These findings from the human trial indicate that at least one NSAID, flurbiprofen, can significantly slow the progression of periodontitis in humans by preserving alveolar bone.

FUTURE DIRECTIONS

Well-controlled longitudinal studies in humans on the effect of NSAIDs on periodontal disease progression and the usefulness of these drugs in both treating and preventing the periodontal disease process are needed. This avenue of investigation is well underway, with both flurbiprofen and naproxen being studied in multicenter trials for their effect on human periodontal disease. It will be important to determine the adjunctive effects of NSAIDs on antiinfective therapy and on regenerative therapy in carefully controlled double-blind studies. It will also be interesting to see if other routes of administration of NSAIDs such as topical application will be effective in altering the course of periodontal disease progression. Recent reports have indicated that topical application of a substituted oxazolopyridine derivative significantly inhibits bone resorption in the squirrel monkey (Vogel et al., 1986). Also flurbiprofen applied topically significantly inhibits the rate of bone loss in beagles (Williams et al., 1988c).

In addition, research needs to look at possible mechanisms whereby NSAIDs alter the course of periodontal disease progression. Presently it is presumed that NSAIDs inhibit cyclo-oxygenase, thus inhibiting the metabolism of arachidonic acid to a number of possible metabolites. Also, it is presumed that inhibition of prostaglandin, as well as other metabolite production, will lead to a reduction in periodontal disease. This may not be the entire story. For example, are NSAIDs exerting an effect on cell populations per se, such as osteoclasts? NSAIDs could lead to an increase of certain arachidonic acid metabolites in the periodontal tissues, and this increase could affect the periodontal disease process. Hopefully, the research emanating from a study of NSAIDs and periodontal disease in the next several years will provide new ways to prevent and treat periodontal disease.

REFERENCES

ElAttar TMA: Prostaglandin E_2 in human gingival health and disease and its stimulation by female sex hormones, Prostaglandins 11:331, 1976.

Feldman R et al: Non-steroidal anti-inflammatory drugs in the reduction of human alveolar bone loss, J Clin Periodontol 10:131, 1983.

Goldhaber P: Tissue culture of bone as a model system for periodontal research, J Dent Res 50:278, 1971.

Goldhaber P et al: Bone resorption in tissue culture and its relevance to periodontal disease, J Am Dent Assoc 87(special issue):1027, 1973.

Gomes BC et al: Prostaglandins: bone resorption stimulating factors released from monkey gingiva, Calcif Tissue Res 19:285, 1976.

Goodson JM et al: Prostaglandin E_2 levels and human periodontal disease, Prostaglandins 6:81, 1974a.

Goodson JM et al: Prostaglandin-induced resorption of the adult rat calvarium, J Dent Res 53:670, 1974b.

Harris M and Goldhaber P: The production of bone resorbing factor by dental cysts in vitro, Br J Oral Surg 10:334, 1973.

Jeffcoat MK et al: Flurbiprofen treatment of periodontal disease in beagles, J Periodont Res 21:624, 1986.

Lasfarques JL and Saffar JL: Effect of indomethacin on bone destruction during experimental periodontal disease in the hamster, J Periodont Res 18:110, 1983.

Nichols FC et al: Bone imaging of experimentally induced periodontal disease: effects of indomethacin, J Dent Res 58:1298, 1979 (abstract).

Nyman S et al: Suppression of inflammation and bone resorption by indomethacin during experimental periodontitis in dogs, J Periodontol 50:450, 1979.

Offenbacher S et al: Measurement of prostaglandin E in crevicular fluid, J Clin Periodontol 8:359, 1981.

Offenbacher S et al: Crevicular fluid prostaglandin E levels as a measure of the periodontal disease status of adult and juvenile periodontitis patients, J Periodont Res 19:1, 1984.

Offenbacher S et al: The crevicular fluid prostaglandin E_2 levels as a predictor of periodontal attachment loss, J Periodont Res 21:101, 1986.

Offenbacher S et al: Effects of flurbiprofen on the progression of periodontitis in *Macaca mulatta,* J Periodont Res 22:473, 1987.

Raisz LG et al: Complement-dependent stimulation of prostaglandin synthesis and bone resorption, Science 185:789, 1974.

Robinson DR et al: Prostaglandin-stimulated bone resorption by rheumatoid synovia, J Clin Invest 56:1181, 1975.

Tashjian AH et al: Evidence that the bone resorption stimulating factor produced by mouse fibrosarcoma cells is prostaglandin E_2, J Exp Med 136:1329, 1972.

Vogel RI et al: The effects of a topically active non-steroidal anti-inflammatory drug on ligature-induced periodontal disease in the squirrel monkey, J Clin Periodontol 13:139, 1986.

Waite IM et al: The periodontal status of subjects receiving non-steroidal anti-inflammatory drugs, J Periodont Res 16:100, 1981.

Weaks-Dybvig M et al: The effect of indomethacin on alveolar bone loss in experimental periodontitis, J Periodont Res 17:90, 1982.

Williams RC et al: Non-steroidal anti-inflammatory drug treatment of periodontitis in beagles, J Periodont Res 19:633, 1984.

Williams RC et al: Flurbiprofen: a potent inhibitor of alveolar bone resorption in beagles, Science 227:640, 1985.

Williams RC et al: Indomethacin or flurbiprofen treatment of periodontitis in beagles: comparison of effect on bone loss, J Periodont Res 22:403, 1987.

Williams RC et al: Ibuprofen inhibits alveolar bone resorption in beagles, J Periodont Res 23:225, 1988a.

Williams RC et al: Three-year clinical trial of flurbiprofen treatment of human periodontitis: preliminary analysis, J Dent Res 67, 1988b (abstract).

Williams RC et al: Topical flurbiprofen treatment of periodontitis in beagles, J Periodont Res 23:166, 1988c.

Williams RC et al: Altering the course of human periodontal disease with the non-steroidal anti-inflammatory drug flurbiprofen: a three-year clinical trial, J Periodontol 60:485, 1989.

SUGGESTED READINGS

Ali NN et al: Effect of prostacyclin and its breakdown product 6-oxo-PGF$_1$ on bone resorption in vitro. In Vane JR, editor: Prostacyclin, New York, 1979, Raven Press.

Dietrich JW et al: Stimulation of bone resorption by various prostaglandins in organ culture, Prostaglandins 10:231, 1975.

Dewhirst FE: 6-Keto-prostaglandin E$_1$–stimulated bone resorption in organ culture, Calcif Tissue Int 36:380, 1984.

Dewhirst FE et al: Levels of prostaglandin E$_2$, thromboxane, and prostacyclin in periodontal tissues, J Periodont Res 18:156, 1983.

ElAttar TMA and Lin HS: Prostaglandins in gingiva of patients with periodontal disease, J Periodontol 52:16, 1981.

ElAttar TMA and Lin HS: Relative conversion of arachidonic acid through lipoxygenase and cyclooxygenase pathways by homogenates of diseased periodontal tissues, J Oral Pathol 12:7, 1983.

Goldhaber P and Rabadjija L: Influence of pharmacological agents on bone resorption. In Genco RJ and Mergerhagen SE, editors: Host-parasite interactions in periodontal diseases, Washington, DC, 1982, American Society of Microbiology.

Klein DC and Raisz LG: Prostaglandins: stimulation of bone resorption in tissue culture, Endocrinology 86:1436, 1970.

Loning TH et al: Prostaglandin E and the local immune response in chronic periodontal disease, J Periodont Res 15:525, 1980.

Neuman SD and Raisz LG: Effects of the prostacyclin products 6-keto prostaglandin E$_1$ and 6-keto prostaglandin F$_1$ on bone resorption in vitro, Prostaglandins Leukotrienes Med 15:103, 1984.

Ohm K et al: Measurement of eight prostaglandins in human gingival and periodontal disease using high pressure liquid chromatography and radioimmunoassay, J Periodont Res 19:501, 1984.

Rifkin BR and Tai HH: Elevated thromboxane B$_2$ levels in periodontal disease, J Periodont Res 16:194, 1981.

Sidhagen B et al: Formation of 12-L-hydroxyeicosatetraenoic acid (12-HETE) by gingival tissue, J Dent Res 61:761, 1982.

Wong PYK et al: Metabolism of arachidonic acid in inflamed human gingivae. I. Formation of 6-keto-prostaglandin F$_1\alpha$, J Dent Res 59:670, 1980.

Chapter 56

FUTURE DIRECTIONS IN MEASUREMENT OF PERIODONTAL DISEASES

Marjorie Jeffcoat

Periodontitis is characterized by loss of hard and soft tissue attachment to the tooth. Recent research has indicated that once the disease process has begun, attachment loss or "disease activity" may not occur at a steady rate, but rather in spurts of disease activity followed by remission (Socransky et al., 1984).

Conventional tests for periodontal disease are based on the clinical examination, periodontal probing, and radiographs. While providing information about the current degree of inflammation and bone and soft tissue attachment loss, these tests do not determine whether a tooth is actively losing bone. The aim of current research into diagnostic systems is to produce tests that are capable of detecting smaller amounts of destruction, earlier than previously thought possible.

Tests for the measurement of periodontal diseases may be classified into three categories as follows:

Etiologic factors. These tests provide the earliest information concerning the bacterial initiation of periodontal disease.

Metabolic changes. These tests measure early physiologic and biochemical responses to the disease. Theoretically, evidence of active disease may be present in a single examination prior to the time it may be detected clinically or radiographically.

Anatomic consequences. These tests measure the anatomic changes that occur as a result of disease activity. Anatomic changes are later manifestations of disease activity, and more than one examination is needed to make a diagnosis of active disease progression.

ETIOLOGIC FACTORS
Pathogen detection

Techniques have been developed that detect the presence of putative periodontopathic organisms, either by direct culture, the use of antibody-based detection systems, the use of DNA probes, the use of bacterial enzymes released into the gingival fluid, or the presence of antibodies to these bacteria in the blood or crevicular fluids (Haffajee et al., 1984; Listgarten et al., 1984; Zambon et al., 1985; Suido et al., 1988). These pathogens and tests to detect their presence are described elsewhere in this book. Although all of the pathogenic organism(s) for each type of periodontal disease have not been definitely identified, these tests offer promise for detecting the major known pathogens before structural damage to the periodontium has occurred. Under these circumstances intervention by the clinician may be most effective.

Host predisposition to disease

It has been well established that alterations in the host response are well correlated with specific periodontal diseases (Cianciola et al., 1977; Page and Schroeder, 1981; Tew et al., 1985). For example, alterations in neutrophil chemotaxis are commonly found in patients with juvenile periodontitis. These tests (Genco et al., 1985; Iacono et al., 1985), which are described elsewhere in this text, may in the not-too-distant future be used to identify individuals at risk for developing periodontal disease and allow early treatment.

METABOLIC CHANGES

The advantage of methods that measure metabolic or physiologic changes lies in the fact that active disease may be detected in a single examination during a spurt of disease activity. This is in contrast to tests that detect anatomic changes, such as radiographs, which require comparison of two or more examinations to determine that active disease has already occurred between the examinations. Thus tests that measure metabolic or physiologic changes can allow the investigator or clinician to quickly detect sites or teeth with active periodontal disease and intervene with treatment before additional anatomic destruction occurs.

Nuclear medicine

Nuclear medicine is the branch of radiology that uses very small doses of a short-lived radioactive element to detect sites of disease. In the case of bone, the radioactive element technetium 99m, with a 6-hour physical half-life, is coupled to a bone-seeking compound such as a diphosphonate. The resultant bone-seeking radiopharmaceutical has a 3-hour biologic half-life and detects areas of altered bone metabolism because it is taken up by areas of bone formation. Since bone resorption is generally coupled to formation behind the resorbing front, bone scans are used to detect both diseases characterized by resorption and those characterized by formation prior to the time the disease is visible radiographically. Nuclear medicine is used to detect a wide range of osseous defects, including stress fractures, infections, and tumors. Altered bone metabolism, as indicated by increased radiopharmaceutical uptake, has been shown to be associated with active progression of periodontal disease, as measured radiographically, in both untreated and treated beagles. In a preliminary study in human patients (Jeffcoat et al., 1986a), a single nuclear medicine examination was able to detect which tooth sites were actively losing bone with a high degree of accuracy. Active sites presented as "hot spots," or areas of increased bone-seeking radiopharmaceutical uptake. These hot spots may be represented pictorially with the use of a

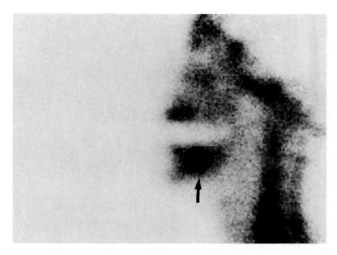

LT lateral

Fig. 56-1. Nuclear medicine bone scan. "Hot spot" in posterior mandible *(arrow)* was localized to second molar with use of a miniaturized probe radiation detector. Second molar was undergoing active bone loss.

gamma camera or localized to specific tooth sites with the use of a miniaturized semiconductor probe radiation detector (Fig. 56-1), which is similar in principle to a geiger counter on a contra-angle handpiece. Clinical studies are presently using nuclear medicine technology to rapidly assess the effect of drugs on the progression of periodontal disease.

Magnetic resonance imaging

Magnetic resonance imaging (MRI) is founded on the principles of nuclear magnetic resonance (Luiten, 1984). In this context the term *nuclear* applies to the nucleus of the atoms of the body, not to the use of ionizing radiation. In the presence of an external magnetic field, the spinning atomic nuclei tend to line up in the direction of the field. After excitation by an external resonance frequency (RF) radiation pulse, RF radiation is emitted by these vibrating nuclei. It is possible to reconstruct an MRI image based on this emitted radiation. In MRI the image contrast depends on the proton density and on the state of excitation determined by the spin lattice (T_1) or spin-spin (T_2) relaxation times. In biologic tissues, hydrogen nuclei protons are the only nuclei present in concentrations high enough to allow mathematical reconstruction of images with a reasonable degree of spacial resolution. Thus protons in water molecules are the primary contributors to the detected MRI signal. In contrast to conventional radiographs that detect osseous structures with a high degree of contrast, with MRI, bone and teeth are observed as black areas with minimal contrast (Fig. 56-2). By varying the parameters used to create the image, differences in contrast can readily be observed between various soft tissues and between normal

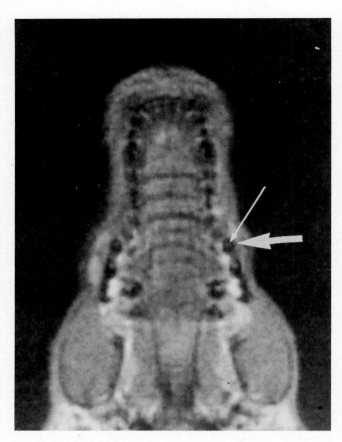

Fig. 56-2. Magnetic resonance image. This image is an occlusal view through a beagle's maxilla. Note that teeth and bone show little contrast *(large arrows)*. Soft tissue, including pulp tissue *(small arrow)* and palatal rugae, shows greater contrast.

and tumor or edematous tissue. To date, MRI appears to offer greatest promise for detection of salivary activity and for imaging the meniscus within the temporomandibular joint; however, at present the level of resolution is not adequate for detection of periodontal destruction.

Monitoring crevicular fluid and its components

The amount of gingival crevicular fluid present has been shown to be associated with gingival inflammation. More recently, however, investigators have assessed components of gingival fluid that are known or hypothesized to be related to periodontal breakdown. These include prostaglandins, collagenase, arylsulfatases, glucuronidases, and others (Cimasoni et al., 1983; Offenbacher et al., 1984; Golub et al., 1985; Lamster et al., 1985). The advantage of this approach is that a small amount of crevicular fluid can be obtained noninvasively, frozen, and stored for subsequent analysis. Ongoing studies at several laboratories will determine which of these tests will have sufficient specificity and sensitivity to provide evidence of active disease prior to physical evidence of disease progression. Detection of enzymes derived from periodontal pathogens in gingival fluid also holds promise for diagno-

sis and monitoring of periodontal destruction (Suido et al., 1988).

ANATOMIC CONSEQUENCES

The hallmark of tests that detect anatomic changes is that two or more examinations must be compared in order to determine if active destruction is occurring. This is the case because anatomy is the net result of both past disease activity and healing. Thus bone loss, visible radiographically, could represent a previously treated site now in remission or a site actively losing bone. Only two or more examinations separated in time can distinguish between these two alternatives. One goal of current research is to develop more sensitive tests capable of detecting smaller increments of disease progression. Such tests will be of value to the clinician who seeks to detect and treat sites of active disease before significant destruction has occurred.

Radiographic methods

Subtraction radiography. Conventional radiographic methods provide a two-dimensional picture of the structure of the periodontium. Overlap of structures not affected by periodontal disease, such as the teeth, make detection of small amounts of alveolar bone loss especially difficult. Subtraction radiography addresses just this problem. The process may be most easily understood in terms of photographic subtraction. In this case the original radiograph is photographically made into a positive print. After a period of time, a second radiographic film is taken using identical projection geometry. The second film, a negative, is overlaid on the first. The positive and negative prints cancel each other out to achieve a uniformly gray color wherever there has been no architectural change between the time of the two radiographs. Areas of bone loss or gain will stand out as darkened or lightened areas, respectively, on a uniform gray background. Such techniques have been used in medicine for decades to subtract overlying structures from angiograms.

The development of the image-processing computer has made the application of subtraction radiography to dental problems more convenient. With an image-processing computer, a video camera is used to input the radiographs into the computer. The computer then electronically manipulates the two images as described above to display only the area of change (Webber et al., 1982; Gröndahl et al., 1983). The computer can then be used to locate and highlight areas of change as shown in Fig. 56-3. Such technology has been applied to the study of periodontal disease (Hausmann et al., 1985, 1986). It has been used successfully to monitor the progress of untreated periodontitis (Hausmann et al., 1985) and to monitor the effects of therapy (Rosling et al., 1983). It has been shown that subtraction radiography is a highly sensitive and specific indicator of areas of bony change. In fact, defects may be detected when only 1% to 5% of the mineral is lost (Haus-

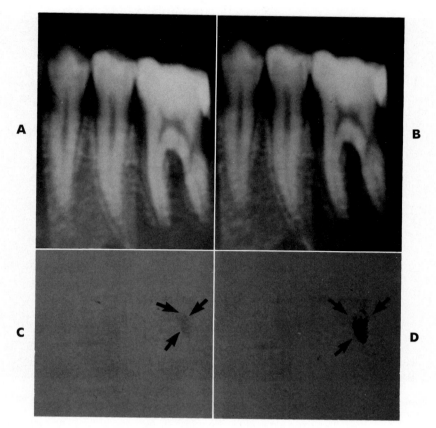

Fig. 56-3. Subtraction radiography. **A,** Original radiograph. **B,** Radiograph taken after a small amount of bone was lost. **C,** Subtraction radiograph. Note that area of bone loss appears as a dark region *(arrows)*; areas that have not changed appear as a uniformly gray background. **D,** Computer localization and enhancement of bone loss shown in **C.**

mann et al., 1986), when there is less than 0.5 mm of bone loss along the tooth root, or when there is less than 1 mm^3 of bone loss.

Although the procedure is used successfully in clinical research centers, application to dental office practice will require the development of technology for taking dental radiographs with reproducible geometry in a practice setting (Jeffcoat et al., 1987). Also, further refinement of the computer-assisted analysis will be necessary for routine use in a dental practice. These developments are likely to occur within the next few years, since the major elements in the technique have been developed.

Three-dimensional imaging. Extraction of three-dimensional information from radiographs requires taking multiple exposures from different angles. These different radiographic views of a region of interest may be used to provide information to a computer in order to reconstruct two-dimensional images of any desired slice of tissue lying within the region. The ability to reconstruct a particular "slice" after the fact is especially important, because the slice could be designed to be thin enough to eliminate anatomic surfaces that would overlie the region of interest in

a conventional radiograph, thereby obscuring an anatomic abnormality. Fig. 56-4 demonstrates the use of this technique to visualize an aberrant third root on a molar. A second advantage of this technique is the ability to reconstruct images from any angle to allow standardization of image geometry for subtraction radiography.

Probing methods

Physical detection of the soft tissue attachment, or periodontal probing, lies at the heart of the detection of periodontal disease. For purposes of detection of disease progression, simple comparison of pocket depth is inadequate because the location of the gingival margin reference may change. To circumvent this problem in research, the probing attachment level is defined as the distance from the cementoenamel junction (CEJ) to the pocket base. Because conventional probing measurements are affected by probing force, probe size and shape, and the degree of gingival inflammation, researchers have found that a conventional probe can be used to reliably determine attachment loss only if a change of 2 mm or more has occurred between examinations.

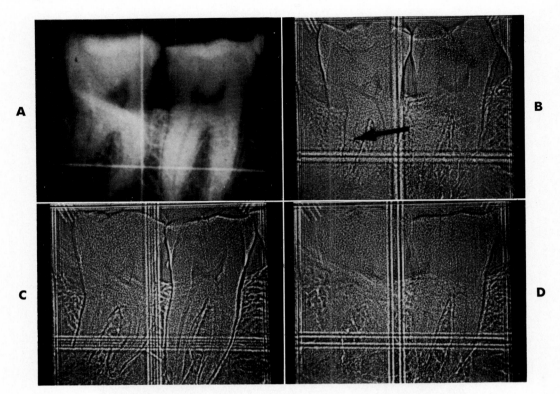

Fig. 56-4. Three-dimensional radiography. **A,** Conventional radiograph. **B,** Reconstructed "slice" through lingual aspect of mandible. Note that aberrant third root on third molar *(arrow)* is easily seen. **C,** "Slice" through midmandible. Note that aberrant third root is no longer visible, but mesial and distal roots are clearly visualized. **D,** "Slice" through buccal aspect of mandible. Note that second molar is no longer in focus. (Courtesy Dr. Richard Webber, National Institutes of Dental Research.)

One experimental instrument combines miniature sensors and signal processing to improve the sensitivity of the use of attachment level measurement for the detection of disease progression. Essentially, the CEJ is detected by automatically running a controlled force probe over the tooth surface into the pocket. When the CEJ is crossed, the probe tip motion momentarily slows. This is equivalent to the catch a clinician feels when an explorer is run over the CEJ. Appropriate sensors, electronics, and software (Baumgarten, 1988) can then detect the CEJ and automatically determine the attachment level, or distance from the CEJ to the pocket base. An automated periodontal probe with automatic CEJ detection is in use in clinical trials. Preliminary evidence indicates that these instruments are capable of determining attachment with a repeatability of 0.2 mm (Jeffcoat et al., 1986b). Several automated probes are likely to be available for use in dental practice in the future.

SUMMARY

Several new tests offer promise for clinical use in the future. These new capabilities will also bring to the clinician new responsibilities in identifying those patients who will benefit from each of the new tests. The clinician will not simply perform each available test on every new patient but will, after a careful history and clinical examination, perform specific tests. In this respect, the diagnosis of periodontal disease will be more like the diagnosis of many other skeletal abnormalities. For example, immunologic tests may be useful in detecting "at risk" adolescents with a family history of juvenile periodontitis. Physiologic tests such as nuclear medicine or enzyme analysis may be used to assess quickly which teeth are actively losing attachment in a patient with clinical evidence of periodontitis. Finally, the tests that detect changes in anatomy will be able to detect disease progression after only a very small amount of attachment has been lost. These tests may be most useful in the continuing evaluation of patients.

REFERENCES

Baumgarten H: A voice input computerized dental examination system using high resolution graphics, Compend Contin Educ Dent 9:446, 1988.

Cianciola LJ et al: Defective polymorphonuclear leukocyte function in a human periodontal disease, Nature 265(5593):445, 1977.

Cimasoni G: Crevicular fluid updated, Monogr Oral Sci 12, 1983.

Genco RJ et al: Serum and gingival fluid antibodies as adjuncts in the diagnosis of *Actinobacillus actinomycetemcomitans*–associated periodontal disease, J Periodontol 56:41, 1985.

Golub LM et al: Further evidence that tetracyclines inhibit collagenase activity in human crevicular fluid and from other mamalian sources, J Periodont Res 20:12, 1985.

Gröndahl HG et al: A digital subtraction technique for dental radiography, Oral Surg 55:96, 1983.

Haffajee AD et al: Clinical microbiological and immunologic features associated with the treatment of active periodontosis lesions, J Clin Periodontol 11:600, 1984.

Hausmann E et al: Usefulness of subtraction radiography in the evaluation of periodontal therapy, J Periodontol 56:4, 1985.

Hausmann E et al: Progression of untreated periodontitis as assessed by subtraction radiography, J Periodont Res 6:716, 1986.

Iacono VJ et al: In vivo assay of crevicular leukocyte migration: its development and potential applications, J Periodontol 56:56, 1985.

Jeffcoat MK et al: Detection of active alveolar bone destruction by analysis of radiopharmaceutical uptake after a single injection of 99m-Tc-methylene diphosphonate, J Periodont Res 6:677, 1986a.

Jeffcoat MK et al: A new periodontal probe with automated cemento-enamel junction detection, J Clin Periodontol 13:276, 1986b.

Jeffcoat MK et al: Extraoral control of geometry for digital subtraction radiography, J Periodont Res 22:396, 1987.

Lamster IB et al: Development of a biochemical profile for gingival crevicular fluid: methodological considerations and evaluation of collagen-degrading and ground substance–degrading enzyme activity during experimental gingivitis, J Periodontol 56:13, 1985.

Listgarten MA et al: Comparative differential dark field microscopy of subgingival bacteria from tooth surfaces with recent evidence of recurring periodontitis and from nonaffected surfaces, J Periodontol 55:398, 1984.

Luiten AL: Fundamentals of NMR imaging, Diagn Imag Clin Med 53:4, 1984.

Offenbacher S et al: Crevicular fluid prostaglandin E levels as a measure of the periodontal disease status of adult and juvenile periodontitis patients, J Periodont Res 19:1, 1984.

Page RC and Schroeder HE: Current status of the host response in chronic marginal periodontitis, J Periodontol 52:477, 1981.

Rosling BG et al: Microbiological and clinical effects of topical subgingival antimicrobial treatment on human periodontal disease, J Clin Periodontol 10(5):487, 1983.

Socransky SS et al: New concepts of destructive periodontal disease, J Clin Periodontol 11:21, 1984.

Suido H et al: Correlations between gingival crevicular fluid enzymes and the subgingival microflora, J Dent Res 67:1070, 1988.

Tew JG et al: Relationship between gingival crevicular fluid and serum antibody titers in young adults with generalized and localized periodontitis, Infect Immun 49:487, 1985.

Webber RL et al: X-ray image subtraction as a basis for assessment of periodontal changes, J Periodont Res 17:509, 1982.

Zambon JJ et al: Rapid identification of periodontal pathogens in subgingival dental plaque: comparison of direct immunofluorescence microscopy with bacterial culture for detection of *Bacteroides gingivalis*, J Periodontol 56:32, 1985.

Chapter 57

FUTURE PATTERNS IN PERIODONTAL DISEASE

Brian A. Burt

Future age structure of society
Tooth retention
Oral hygiene
Use of dental services
Future trends
Conclusions

Since the dawn of recorded history, humans have attempted to control disease by methods ranging from religious ritual to sophisticated modern technology. Success has been infrequent, at least until quite recently, because of a lack of understanding of the diseases concerned. That the human species has survived the ravages of various epidemic onslaughts can mostly be attributed to ecologic adaptation, both of humans to the organisms causing disease and of the organisms to their human hosts (Dubos, 1959; Dingle, 1973). Because successful adaptation is often manifested as chronic bacterial disease, predictions of future patterns of bacterial diseases are subject to the vagaries of ecologic adaptation of both host and agent, with the increasing degree of medical manipulation of the environment adding further uncertainty.

The periodontal diseases are infections; their manifestations represent the reactions of the human hosts to these infections, mediated by the environments in which they have occurred (Newman, 1985; Page, 1986). Fig. 57-1 displays an ecologic model of periodontal diseases, emphasizing their multifactorial nature.

This chapter seeks to identify some future epidemiologic patterns of the periodontal diseases by looking at trends in risk factors, which are those inherent, environmental, social, or behavioral characteristics known to be associated with the risk of developing the condition under study. Risk factors to be examined in this chapter include age structure of the population, trends in tooth retention, oral hygiene status, and use of dental services. (There are no doubt other determinants of periodontal diseases, such as genetic factors and the immune response, but because they cannot yet be quantified, they cannot be factored into future trends.) "The future," for purposes of this chapter, is from approximately the turn of the century to the year 2020.

Discussion in this chapter is concerned with gingivitis and adult periodontitis, the most common forms of periodontal disease, and does not deal with specific infections such as acute necrotizing ulcerative gingivitis (ANUG) and localized juvenile periodontitis (LJP). It also assumes no major technologic breakthroughs in the near future, such as a vaccine for the most common periodontal infections, which could fundamentally alter likely trends. The outlook is global. There is no evidence that the periodontal diseases are etiologically different from one country to another, though distribution and severity of gingivitis and periodontitis vary with national levels of general education, economic development, and living standards.

The starting point for a look at the future should be the present situation, which is presented elsewhere in this book as the epidemiology of periodontal diseases. In brief, these diseases are infections that affect a majority of all populations to some extent. Some degree of gingivitis is widespread globally, and adult periodontitis is common. Most cases of periodontitis are limited to certain sites in

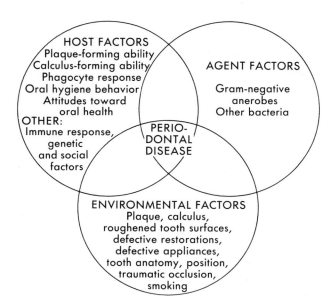

Fig. 57-1. Ecologic model of periodontal disease.

the mouth, can be inactive for long periods, and do not lead to massive loss of bony support for the teeth. A minority of individuals, however, ranging from 10% to 20% of the population, suffer from severe and extensive periodontitis, which can lead to tooth loss in spite of treatment. It is against this current epidemiologic background that the various risk factors are considered.

FUTURE AGE STRUCTURE OF SOCIETY

Trends in age distribution within developed countries are exemplified by data from the United States, where the "graying of America" has received considerable publicity in recent years. American society is growing older; the median age by 1980 was over 30 for the first time and continues to increase. The proportion of persons aged 65 or more, 11.3% in 1980, is estimated to reach 17.3% by the year 2020 (U.S. Department of Commerce, 1984).

The changes in age distribution in the population of the United States are shown graphically in Fig. 57-2. The expression "population pyramid" is used for this type of graphic because historically this representation of population has taken on a pyramidal shape, meaning larger numbers of younger persons than older ones. Population pyramids for developing countries today are of classical pyramidal structure, reflecting high birth rates and limited life expectancy. Fig. 57-2 shows the population structure in the United States in 1982, with predictions for the years 2000, 2030, and 2080. The main feature of the 1982 pyramid is the outgrowth in the 20- to 34-year age range, representing the "baby boomers" and the post–World War II increase in birth rates and family size, which tailed off around 1962. The shorter bars in the 1982 pyramid below the 20- to 34-year age range come from the sharply re-

duced birth rates of more recent years. By the year 2000, the baby boomers will be well into what is now considered middle age. In the long term, the pyramid becomes more and more like a rectangle, with substantial increases in the proportion of people above age 65.

Other populations effects can be seen from the pyramids in Fig. 57-2. The predominance of females in the older age groups will continue, but there will be a continuing increase in life expectancy, with considerable growth in the numbers and proportions of what are now considered very old people. In 1982 0.7% of the U.S. population was aged 90 or more. This proportion will have doubled by the year 2020, when the over-90 population will number nearly 3.5 million (U.S. Department of Commerce, 1984).

While population growth rates have slowed to less than 1% per year in the United States, that is still a net increase of over 2 million persons per year. In other developed countries, population growth is more static, though their populations are also aging. Indeed, the population pyramid is closer to a rectangle in several western European countries than it is in the United States.

To summarize age-distribution trends, the numbers and proportions of older persons in developed countries will continue to increase. Life expectancy will also continue to extend, and those now thought of as the very old will constitute a significant proportion of society by the turn of the century. These trends are not yet evident in developing countries, where population continues to grow at a more rapid rate and life expectancy is lower.

TOOTH RETENTION

Along with an aging of populations in developed countries, more teeth are being retained into the later years of life. A generation ago old age was virtually synonomous with total tooth loss in developed countries, reflecting the standards of dental practice at the time and the influence of the "focal infection" theory on medical and dental practice (Burt, 1978). The focal infection theory, which dominated dental practice during the 1910 to 1950 period, held that "oral sepsis" was a source of numerous bodily ailments and that, accordingly, a first line of treatment was to remove diseased teeth or teeth suspected of being diseased. Almost certainly, a large number of nondiseased teeth were extracted as well during this period, since total tooth loss came to be considered normal by middle age. The end result was a high proportion of older people in many developed countries who were edentulous (U.S. Public Health Service, 1960; Burgess and Beck, 1969; Gray et al., 1970; von der Fehr, 1982).

With the decline of the focal infection theory in the 1950s, however, standards of dental practice began to change. In particular, teeth were not extracted nearly as liberally as they formerly were. As a result, the four decades since the 1950s have seen the emergence of a new

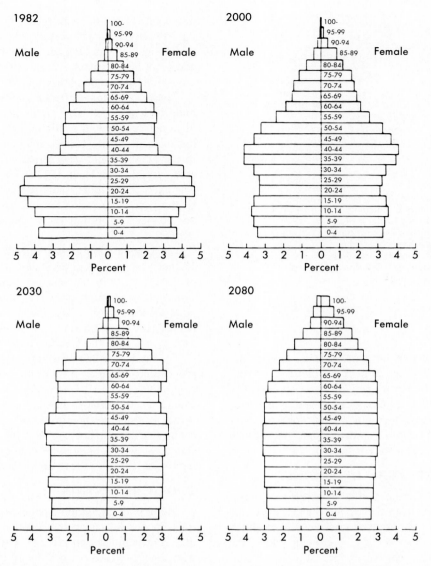

Fig. 57-2. Distribution of population by age and sex in United States in 1982, with predictions for 2000, 2030, and 2080. (From US Department of Commerce, Bureau of the Census: Projections of the population of the United States, by age, sex, and race: 1985 to 2080, series P-25, No 952, Washington, DC, 1984, US Government Printing Office.)

generation of older persons who have retained many of their teeth. In countries where total tooth loss in older persons was common, data are now showing reduced prevalence of this condition (Todd and Walker, 1980; Cutress et al., 1983; Baerum et al., 1985). In the United States, the change has been striking: total tooth loss was found in 13% of the population in 1957 to 1958, in 11.2% in 1971, and in only 8.7% by 1983 (Ismail et al., 1987).

It is perhaps ironic that evidence now exists to suggest that the focal infection theory may not have been all wrong and that several of the bacteria associated with destructive periodontal disease might be associated with serious systemic illness (Thoden Van Velzen et al., 1984). Even if

this is so, however, it is unlikely to lead to the wholesale extraction of teeth that characterized the first focal infection period, because more specific treatments for severe periodontal disease will be employed.

It has been estimated that total tooth loss in the United States by the year 2020 will decline to the extent that only some 10% of the 65- to 74-year age group will be affected (Weintraub and Burt, 1985), a substantial decline from the 34.1% of this age group that was edentulous in 1983 (Ismail et al., 1987). The predicted distribution of total tooth loss at that time, contrasted with the same data for 1971 to 1974, is shown in Fig. 57-3. As discussed in the previous section, the population aged 75 or more will be consider-

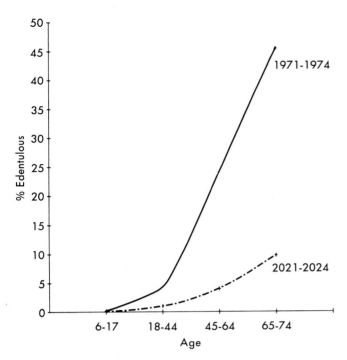

Fig. 57-3. Distribution of edentulous persons by age in United States, 1971 to 1974, with estimates for 2021 to 2024. (From Weintraub JA and Burt BA: Oral health status in the United States: tooth loss and edentulism, J Dent Educ 49:368, 1985; data for 1971 to 1974 from US Public Health Service, National Center for Health Statistics: Basic data on dental examination findings of persons 1-74 years, DHEW Pub No 79-1662, series 11, No 214, Washington, DC, US Government Printing Office.)

ably greater in 2020 than it is today, and it is not easy to predict what the trends in total tooth loss will be among those who today are looked on as the very old. Even so, it can be stated with confidence that the proportion of older people who still have a functioning dentition will continue to increase.

To summarize, not only is the number of older people increasing in developed countries, but they are retaining more teeth than ever before. This means that the number of teeth potentially at risk for developing periodontal infection is increasing substantially.

ORAL HYGIENE

It is quite likely that oral hygiene has been the subject of more dental health educational efforts worldwide than any other one aspect related to oral health, but data on trends in oral hygiene in populations are not easy to find. There are several reasons for this. Noncomparable measuring systems and examiner variability are two major problems, but a deeper problem might be that education for oral hygiene may take a long time to show a permanent change in habits. Oral hygiene is closely associated with personal hygiene practices and general living standards, so

improvements might be more influenced by improving economies than by any other single factor.

There is limited evidence, however, that oral hygiene in developed countries is continuing to improve. Douglass et al. (1983a) compared national survey data from 1960 to 1962 with data from 1971 to 1974 in the United States and concluded that an improvement had been demonstrated. The improvement was concentrated in scores for debris (plaque), with little change in calculus scores, suggesting that personal toothbrushing habits may have improved between the two studies but that the frequency of dental office visits, necessary for calculus removal, did not. This picture, however, has not been borne out by a comparison of two statewide studies in North Carolina (1960 to 1963 and 1976 to 1977), which suggested that oral hygiene standards had deteriorated over that time. The North Carolina studies found that plaque scores had increased and calculus scores had remained essentially the same (Hughes et al., 1982), just the opposite of what Douglass et al. concluded from the national surveys. The North Carolina studies might represent a local aberration, for earlier national studies in the United States had suggested that some improvements in oral hygiene were taking place among young people (U.S. Public Health Service, 1975).

It might be helpful to look at sales figures for oral hygiene aids in the United States and compare them with sales for soap, shampoo, and deodorant used in personal cleanliness and grooming. Fig. 57-4 shows these sales comparisons, adjusted for cost-of-living and population increases. With minor fluctuations in the late 1970s, which could be attributed to price changes relative to overall shifts in the Consumer Price Index, the essential picture is of a series of more-or-less parallel lines. This suggests that oral hygiene is perceived as an essential part of personal hygiene in the United States and can therefore be expected to improve further as standards of personal hygiene and grooming continue to creep upward. Continued improvement in oral hygiene standards will be assisted by the more efficient dentifrices and improved plaque-inhibitory mouth rinses being developed and marketed.

Common sense suggests that influences such as the barrage of advertising for fluoride-containing and "antiplaque" toothpastes and "antigingivitis" mouth rinses, plus the public education campaigns sponsored by various national dental associations, must be having some effect. However, "hard" evidence to demonstrate these effects remains elusive. If these efforts do have some impact over a period of time, however, they provide another reason why levels of personal oral hygiene status generally can be expected to continue to improve in developed countries.

In summary, it is thought by many that standards of oral hygiene in developed countries are continuing to improve. This improvement could be ascribed to rising health consciousness in these countries (seen in such activities as fitness movements and antismoking legislation), to rising

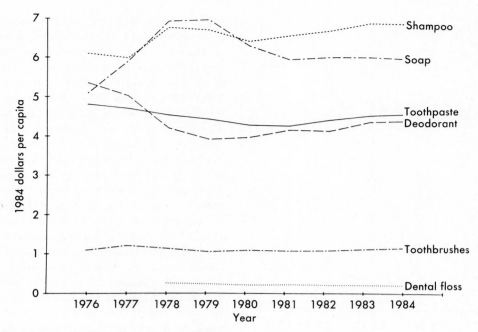

Fig. 57-4. Per capita expenditures for personal hygiene and grooming materials in constant 1984 dollars: United States, 1976 to 1984. (Data from various issues of *Drug Topics* for sales; U.S. Bureau of the Census reports for population data; and *Monthly Labor Review* for Consumer Price Index used to standardize expenditures.)

standards of personal hygiene and grooming, to technologically improved products for oral hygiene, and perhaps to the broader adoption of middle-class values.

USE OF DENTAL SERVICES

Tooth retention, higher levels of oral hygiene, and higher levels of gingival health are all associated with higher socioeconomic status, regardless of whether that status is measured by education, income, or occupation (Gray et al., 1970; Todd and Walker, 1980; Arnljot et al., 1985; Burt et al., 1985). Use of dental services is also strongly associated with socioeconomic status (U.S. Public Health Service, 1982; Arnljot et al., 1985). Gingival health is therefore associated with a greater frequency of dental visits, though a cause-effect relationship cannot necessarily be accepted; perhaps people with cleaner mouths visit the dentist more often. Whether the frequency of dental visits per se is associated with retention of bone and attachment levels is more difficult to demonstrate. The study of Suomi et al. (1971) concluded that frequent prophylaxes led to better maintenance of attachment levels, but the improvement over 3 years was small. Results could also have been influenced by a selection bias resulting from conditions of corporate participation; special treatment and control groups, selected from the same work site to get around the bias problem, showed no difference in attachment loss. All treatment groups showed some loss of attachment, so frequent professional care did not prevent it

entirely. At the other extreme, the studies of Löe et al. (1986) on the natural history of periodontal disease in an untreated group of Sri Lankan tea workers showed that in this group, where oral hygiene was uniformly poor, there was a small group (11%) that showed no progression of disease at all.

The relationship between frequency of dental office visits and retention of bony support and attachment levels is almost certainly multidimensional; factors such as the availability and accessibility of dental care, the nature and quality of that care, and the attitudes of dentist and patient affect the outcome.

While numerous clinical studies have shown that frequent dental visits, assuming good-quality periodontal care, slow down the rate of attachment loss in diagnosed patients, it cannot be stated for sure that frequent visits make any difference to nonsusceptible or uninfected individuals. The most that can be stated is that frequent dental office visits are associated with greater tooth retention and better gingival health. If the ultimate outcome of efforts to prevent and control periodontal disease is tooth retention, rather than bone height and attachment levels, then it can be accepted that frequent dental office visits are associated with better periodontal health.

One clear fact on the use of dental services is that edentulous people do not visit the dentist nearly as often as do dentate persons (Gray et al., 1970; Hunt et al., 1985; Palmqvist, 1986; Ismail et al., 1987). The frequency of

Table 57-1. Dental visits reported within the last year and average number of visits per year in the United States: various years from 1957 to 1983

	Proportion visiting within last year			Average visits per year		
	45-64 years	**65+ years**	**All ages**	**45-64 years**	**65+ years**	**All ages**
1983	51.9*	37.8	53.7	2.0*	1.5	1.9
1981	49.6	34.6	50.1	1.8	1.5	1.7
1979	49.0	32.8	50.1	1.9	1.4	1.7
1977	48.7	31.4	49.8	1.8	1.3	1.6
1975	48.2	30.3	50.3	1.8	1.2	1.6
1973	46.9	27.3	48.9	1.7	1.1	1.6
1969	42.3	23.2	44.9	1.6	1.0	1.5
1963-1964	38.4	20.8	42.0	1.7	0.8	1.6
1957-1958	32.3	16.2	36.6	1.7	0.8	1.6

Compiled from reports from the National Center for Health Statistics (NCHS), series B, No. 14; series 10, Nos. 23, 29, 76, 95, 115, 126, 136, 141; advance data No. 122.

*Estimation because of different age groups presented in NCHS report.

dental visits is usually considered to decline with increasing age, but data showing this decline (U.S. Public Health Service, 1982) usually make no adjustment for the greater proportion of edentulous individuals in the current generation of older persons. When that adjustment is made, data from the 1983 National Health Interview Survey in the United States show that older dentate persons continue to visit the dentist almost as often as younger ones do, with only a slight decline after age 74 (Ismail et al., 1987).

Data on the use of dental services, taken from the National Health Interview Surveys, are displayed for the period 1957 to 1983 in Table 57-1. The trend for increasing numbers of older persons to visit the dentist at least once each year seems consistent. These data are for all older persons, regardless of whether they have lost all their teeth or not, so the increasing use of services that the data suggest may be primarily a reflection of diminishing total tooth loss among older persons. (Again, other factors such as increasing insurance coverage are certain to be involved in a complex relationship, so the suggested link here should not be oversimplified.)

The trend toward a relative increase in the use of dental services among older persons seems likely to continue, and as the numbers of such persons in the population grow, there will be an absolute increase as well. Use of dental services by the 45- to 64-year age group now approximates the national average and may even rise above it as caries needs among younger persons decline further. Use of dental services by the 65 and older age group still lags behind the national average, but it can be expected that this, too, will approximate the national average as the proportion of dentate persons in this age group increases.

Use of dental services in developing countries is a totally different matter from that just described. Most of these countries are grossly deficient in dental manpower, and many of their economies cannot support more than very small private or public dental sectors. In such cases the use of dental services as a factor in the future disposition of periodontal diseases does not apply.

In summary, the use of dental services at present is likely to be associated with a higher level of periodontal health, at least as measured by tooth retention and gingival health, though this conclusion was certainly not correct during the time when mass extractions were normal treatment for periodontal disease.

FUTURE TRENDS

The risk factors discussed suggest trends in opposite directions for periodontal disease, and there are a number of imponderables, such as public awareness of periodontal conditions and how dentists may treat them, which are difficult to factor in. Predictions are always hazardous.

Looking at the demographics, it is clear that the numbers and proportions of older persons in developed countries are increasing, and their degree of tooth retention is improving. Douglass et al. (1983b), basing their conclusions on demographics and periodontal disease data from national surveys in the United States in 1960 to 1962 and 1971 to 1974, argued that the amount of periodontal disease to be treated in the future is thereby increased. Similar arguments have been advanced in other countries (Craft, 1984). While the demographics are clear, the way that indices have been used to measure periodontal disease in previous national surveys, especially with regard to the absence of probing to determine the presence of pockets, produces data that must be of doubtful validity to some extent. This problem raises a question as to the precision of these assessments of the extent of periodontal disease in the future.

The effect of age on susceptibility to periodontal disease requires further study, for it will clearly have a major impact on future trends. Current evidence is that destructive periodontal disease is not a disease of aging, at least up to age 74 (Page, 1984; Burt et al., 1985; Abdellatif and Burt, 1987). Indeed, periodontitis has been shown to begin early rather than late (Clerehugh and Lennon, 1986), and age has been shown not to be a factor in healing following periodontal surgery (Lindhe et al., 1985). Several epidemiologic studies, prior to the 1985 to 1986 adult survey in the United States, have demonstrated that older age groups show no greater degree of bone loss and deep pockets than younger age groups (Hugoson and Jorgan, 1982; Beck et al., 1984). The poorer levels of periodontal health historically reported in older age groups stem from the use of composite indices and are probably most related to increased gingivitis from long-term plaque and calculus accumulations. If the oral hygiene status of populations continues to improve, this improvement could partly counteract the threat posed by the increasing number of teeth at risk.

However, many people do accumulate plaque over a long period of time, and many will no doubt continue to do so even if general levels of oral hygiene improve. The considerable future increase in the numbers of older persons, and in teeth at risk, will probably mean an increased amount of periodontal disease to be treated in the future. In addition, it is possible that the periodontal response to the challenge of infection is more severe in elderly people (aged 75 or above), in whom the immune response is diminished and whose ability to practice good oral hygiene may have faded. If that happens, then a large number of previously nonsusceptible people might become susceptible in the later years of life, though the extent to which persons of this age would demand treatment for periodontal diseases is conjectural.

The nature of "susceptibility" requires further definition, which current research could well provide by the turn of the century. Traditionally, susceptibility has been virtually synonomous with poor oral hygiene and lack of professional care, but studies of diagnosed patients who declined care have suggested that not all suffer functional declines in periodontal health (Becker et al., 1979, 1984b). In addition, recent epidemiologic studies, including some in developing countries where oral hygiene is poor and there is virtually no clinical care available, have shown that the presence or absence of periodontitis (though not gingivitis) is not always related to oral hygiene status (Cutress et al., 1982; Beck et al., 1984; Buckley and Crowley, 1984; Powell, 1984; Baelum et al., 1986; Cutress, 1986; Hoover and Tynan, 1986; Ismail et al., 1986; Löe et al., 1986). These epidemiologic studies, which used indices differentiating between gingivitis and periodontitis, have suggested a less dominant etiologic role for oral hygiene in destructive periodontal disease. These and other epidemiologic studies (Cushing and Sheiham, 1985) have also suggested a concentration of destructive disease in a minority of those examined, enhancing the concept that

susceptibility is related to other factors in addition to oral hygiene status.

The view that the most serious disease is concentrated in a relatively small number of people is strengthened by recent clinical research in periodontal therapy (Haffajee et al., 1986). Long-term studies of periodontal patients have shown that while the majority respond well to modern forms of treatment, substantial tooth loss still occurs among a minority who do not respond (Hirschfield and Wasserman, 1978; McFall, 1982; Becker et al., 1984a; Goldman et al., 1986). This response/nonresponse cannot all be attributed to patients' failure to maintain stringent oral hygiene during their maintenance care, for while good oral hygiene is necessary to help prevent reinfection (Nyman et al., 1975; Rosling et al., 1976; Westfelt et al., 1983; Lindhe et al., 1984; Devore et al., 1986), exactly how meticulous this oral hygiene level must be is still a subject for debate (Pihlstrom et al., 1981; Morrison et al., 1982; Ramfjord et al., 1982). Reinfection seems to be related to factors other than the oral hygiene levels of the patient (Greenwell and Bissada, 1984).

In interpreting the findings of these clinical and epidemiologic studies, it must be remembered that *clinical* studies are conducted on diagnosed patients, in other words on "susceptibles," whereas *epidemiologic* studies include susceptibles and nonsusceptibles. Results of both kinds of study are consistent in suggesting that the nature of the plaque infection and the individual's response to it (i.e., susceptibility) are the main determinants of disease and will continue to be so in the future.

Oral hygiene in the United States appears to be improving, and it is thought to be improving also in other developed countries. That trend is to be encouraged, for it will continue to help reduce the rate of periodontal destruction. The clinical studies described, however, have suggested that the nature of the plaque infection and the host response to that infection are more precise determinants of periodontitis susceptibility among the patients studied than is the quantity of plaque.

The host response to periodontal infection has been extensively studied, and it is clear that, in general, lymphocytes, macrophages, and their end products mediate much of the tissue destruction seen in periodontitis (Genco and Slots, 1984). On the other hand, neutrophils and their accessory factors, antibodies and complement, are key factors in protection against periodontal infections (Genco and Slots, 1984). Reduction in neutrophil function is clearly a risk factor increasing the susceptibility to periodontal disease, and this is manifested most clearly by the severe periodontitis seen in juveniles who also suffer from neutrophil disorders such as agranulocytosis and cyclic neutropenia, or from diseases with secondary neutrophil abnormalities such as diabetes mellitus and Down syndrome (Genco et al., 1986).

Haffajee et al. (1985) found elevated humoral antibody

responses to three or more gram-negative bacterial species among patients who responded poorly to periodontal therapy, and they speculated as to whether difficult-to-treat patients might be identified in this manner. If a reliable method of identifying susceptible persons could be developed by these or other means (Listgarten, 1986; Johnson et al., 1988), then future treatment of periodontal diseases could become vastly more rational than it is today.

The future distribution of periodontal disease will depend on a number of factors that are not fully understood just yet. For example, it has been argued that periodontal diseases should be viewed more as social/behavioral conditions than as classical infections (Sheiham, 1977; Cushing et al., 1986); this argument is strengthened by data supporting oral hygiene's association with living standards and economic levels. At the same time, recent epidemiologic data have rendered uncertain the causal relationship between oral hygiene status and destructive periodontal disease. General levels of oral hygiene and the frequency of dental office visits among older persons can be expected to continue their upward trends, but future research must clarify the role of oral hygiene and its etiologic contribution to destructive periodontal disease relative to that of other host, agent, and environmental factors. A major issue in future disease distribution might be whether susceptibility is increased in persons aged 75 or more; if it is, then periodontal disease will clearly be a larger problem in the future as the numbers and proportions of such persons increase.

CONCLUSIONS

1. The numbers and proportions of older persons in developed countries will increase substantially in the future. To the extent that age is a factor in susceptibility to periodontal disease, the periodontal disease load will be increased as a result.
2. Tooth retention is steadily improving, so that the growing number of older people will have more teeth per person that are potentially at risk of developing periodontal disease.
3. General levels of oral hygiene are improving. To the extent that oral hygiene is a determinant of destructive periodontal disease, rather than of gingivitis only, this trend could help counteract, to some extent, the growing number of teeth at risk.
4. The frequency of dental office visits among older persons should continue to increase as the proportion of edentulous persons among them drops. To the extent that more frequent dental office visits help prevent destructive periodontal disease, this trend could also help counteract the growing number of teeth at risk.
5. The nature of susceptibility to periodontal disease requires further research. The respective roles of specific infections, immune response (especially phagocytic competence), personal oral hygiene, and frequency of

dental office visits cannot yet be specified. At present, it cannot be estimated whether the proportion of susceptible persons will increase in the future. The question is important because a relatively small number of susceptible persons require a major share of treatment resources.
6. A major factor in future periodontal disease trends will be the extent to which advanced age, 75 years or more, increases susceptibility to destructive periodontal disease. Further research on this issue is required.

REFERENCES

Abdellatif HM and Burt BA: An epidemiological investigation into the relative importance of age and oral hygiene status as determinants of periodontitis, J Dent Res 56:13, 1987.

Arnljot HA et al: Oral health care systems: an international collaborative study, Chicago, 1985, Quintessence Publishing Co, Inc.

Baelum V, Fejerskov O, and Karring T: Oral hygiene, gingivitis, and periodontal breakdown in adult Tanzanians, J Periodont Res 21:221, 1986.

Baerum P, Holst D, and Rise J: Dental health in Trondelag: changes from 1973-1983, Oslo, Norway, 1983, Directorate of Health.

Beck JD et al: Risk factors for various levels of periodontal disease and treatment needs of Iowa, Community Dent Oral Epidemiol 12:17, 1984.

Becker W, Berg L, and Becker BE: Untreated periodontal disease: a longitudinal study, J Periodontol 50:234, 1979.

Becker W, Berg L, and Becker BE: The long term evaluation of periodontal treatment and maintenance in 95 patients, Int J Periodontics Restorative Dent 4:54, 1984a.

Becker W et al: Periodontal treatment without maintenance: a retrospective study in 44 patients, J Periodontol 55:505, 1984b.

Buckley LA and Crowley MJ: A longitudinal study of untreated periodontal disease, J Clin Periodontol 11:523, 1984.

Burgess WC and Beck DJ: Survey of denture wearers in New Zealand, 1968, NZ Dent J 65:223, 1969.

Burt BA: Influences for change in the dental health status of populations: an historical perspective, J Public Health Dent 38:272, 1978.

Burt BA et al: Periodontal disease, tooth loss, and oral hygiene among older Americans, Community Dent Oral Epidemiol 13:93, 1985.

Clerehugh V and Lennon MA: A two-year longitudinal study of early periodontitis in 14- to 16-year-old school children, Community Dent Health 3:135, 1986.

Craft M: Dental health education and periodontal disease: health policies, disease trends, target groups and strategies. In Frandsen A, editor: Public health aspects of periodontal disease, Chicago, 1984, Quintessence Publishing Co, Inc.

Cushing AM and Sheiham A: Assessing periodontal treatment needs and periodontal status in a study of adults in north-west England, Community Dent Health 2:187, 1985.

Cushing AM, Sheiham A, and Maizels J: Developing sociodental indicators—the social impact of dental disease, Community Dent Health 3:3, 1986.

Cutress TW: Periodontal health and periodontal disease in young people: global epidemiology, Int Dent J 36:146, 1986.

Cutress TW, Hunter PBV, and Hoskins DIH: Adult oral health in New Zealand, 1976-1982, Wellington, NZ, 1983, Medical Research Council of New Zealand.

Cutress TW, Powell RN, and Ball ME: Differing profiles of periodontal disease in two similar South Pacific island populations, Community Dent Oral Epidemiol 10:193, 1982.

Devore CH et al: Bone loss following periodontal therapy in subjects without frequent periodontal maintenance, J Periodontol 57:354, 1986.

Dingle JH: The ills of man, Sci Am 229:77, 1973.

Douglass CW et al: National trends in the prevalence and severity of the periodontal diseases, J Am Dent Assoc 107:403, 1983a.

Douglass CW et al: The potential for increase in the periodontal diseases of the aged population, J Periodontol 54:721, 1983b.

Dubos R: The mirage of health, New York, 1959, Doubleday.

Genco RJ, Christersson LA, and Zambon JJ: Juvenile periodontitis, Int Dent J 36:168, 1986.

Genco RJ and Slots J: Host responses in periodontal diseases, J Dent Res 63:441, 1984.

Goldman MJ, Ross IF, and Goteiner D: Effect of periodontal therapy on patients maintained for 15 years or longer, J Periodontol 57:347, 1986.

Gray PG et al: Adult dental health in England and Wales in 1968, London, 1970, Her Majesty's Stationery Office.

Greenwell H and Bissada NF: Variations in subgingival microflora from healthy and intervention sites using probing depth and bacteriologic identification criteria, J Periodontol 55:391, 1984.

Haffajee AD and Socransky SS: Frequency distributions of periodontal attachment loss: critical and microbiological features, J Clin Periodontol 13:625, 1986.

Haffajee AD, Socransky SS, and Ebersole JL: Survival analysis of periodontal sites before and after periodontal therapy, J Clin Periodontol 12:553, 1985.

Hirschfield L and Wasserman B: A long-term survey of tooth loss in 600 treated periodontal patients, J Periodontol 49:225, 1978.

Hoover JN and Tynan JJ: Periodontal status of a group of Canadian adults, J Can Dent Assoc 52:761, 1986.

Hughes JT, Rozier RG, and Ramsey DL: Natural history of dental diseases in North Carolina, 1976-1977, Durham, NC, 1982, Carolina Academic Press.

Hugoson A and Jordan T: Frequency distribution of individuals aged 20-70 years according to severity of periodontal disease, Community Dent Oral Epidemiol 10:187, 1982.

Hunt RJ et al: Edentulism and oral health problems among elderly rural Iowans: the Iowa 65+ rural health study, Am J Public Health 75:1177, 1985.

Ismail AI et al: Prevalence of deep periodontal pockets in New Mexico adults aged 27 to 74 years, J Public Health Dent 46:199, 1986.

Ismail AI et al: Findings from the dental care supplement of the National Health Interview Survey, 1983, J Am Dent Assoc 114:617, 1987.

Johnson NW et al: Detection of high-risk groups and individuals for periodontal diseases: evidence for the resistance of high risk groups and individuals and approaches to their detection, J Clin Periodontol 15:276, 1988.

Lindhe J et al: Long-term effect of surgical/non-surgical treatment of periodontal disease, J Clin Periodontol 11:448, 1984.

Lindhe J et al: Effect of age on healing following periodontal therapy, J Clin Periodontol 12:774, 1985.

Listgarten MA: A perspective on periodontal diagnosis, J Clin Periodontol 13:175, 1986.

Löe H et al: Natural history of periodontal disease in man: rapid, moderate, and no loss of attachment in Sri Lankan laborers 14 to 46 years of age, J Clin Periodontol 13:431, 1986.

McFall WT Jr: Tooth loss in 100 treated patients with periodontal disease, J Periodontol 53:539, 1982.

Morrison EC et al: The significance of gingivitis during the maintenance phase of periodontal treatment, J Periodontol 53:31, 1982.

Newman MG: Current concepts of the pathogenesis of periodontal disease: microbiology emphasis, J Periodontol 56:734, 1985.

Nyman S, Rosling B, and Lindhe J: Effect of professional tooth cleaning on healing after periodontal surgery, J Clin Periodontol 2:80, 1975.

Page RC: Periodontal diseases in the elderly: a critical evaluation of current information, Gerontology 3:63, 1984.

Page RC: Current understanding of the aetiology and progression of periodontal disease, Int Dent J 36:153, 1986.

Palmqvist S: Oral health patterns in a Swedish county population aged 65 and above, Swed Dent J Suppl 32, 1986.

Pihlstrom BL, Ortiz-Campos C, and McHugh RB: A randomized four-year study of periodontal therapy, J Periodontol 52:227, 1981.

Powell RN: The natural history of periodontal diseases, Ann R Aust Coll Dent Surg 8:26, 1984.

Ramfjord SP et al: Oral hygiene and maintenance of periodontal support, J Periodontol 53:26, 1982.

Rosling B, Nyman S, and Lindhe J: The effect of systematic plaque control on bone regeneration in infrabony pockets, J Clin Periodontol 3:38, 1976.

Sheiham A: Prevention and control of periodontal disease. In Klavan B et al, editors: International conference on research in the biology of periodontal disease, Chicago, 1977, University of Illinois.

Suomi JD et al: The effect of controlled oral hygiene procedures on the progression of periodontal disease in adults: results after third and final year, J Periodontol 42:152, 1971.

Thoden Van Velzen SK, Abramhan-Inpijn L, and Moorer WR: Plaque and systemic disease: a reappraisal of the focal infection concept, J Clin Periodontol 11:209, 1984.

Todd JE and Walker AM: Adult dental health, vol 1, England and Wales, 1968-1978, London, 1980, Her Majesty's Stationery Office.

US Department of Commerce, Bureau of the Census: Projections of the population of the United States, by age, sex, and race: 1983 to 2080, series P-25, No 952, Washington, DC, 1984, US Government Printing Office.

US Public Health Service, National Center for Health Statistics: Loss of teeth, United States, June 1957–June 1958, PHS Pub No 584-822, Washington, DC, 1960, US Government Printing Office.

US Public Health Service, National Center for Health Statistics: Oral hygiene among youths 12-17 years, United States, DHEW Pub No (HRA) 76-1633, series 11, No 151, Washington, DC, 1975, US Government Printing Office.

US Public Health Service, National Center for Health Statistics: Dental visits: volume and interval since last visit; United States, 1978 and 1979, DHHS Pub No (PHS) 82-1566, series 10, No 138, Washington, DC, 1982, US Government Printing Office.

von der Fehr F: Dental disease in Scandinavia. In Frandsen A, editor: Dental health care in Scandinavia: achievements and future strategies, Chicago, 1982, Quintessence Publishing Co, Inc.

Weintraub JA and Burt BA: Oral health status in the United States: tooth loss and edentulism, J Dent Educ 49:368, 1985.

Westfelt E et al: Significance of frequency of professional tooth cleaning for healing following periodontal surgery, J Clin Periodontol 10:148, 1983.

Chapter 58

CONTROVERSIES IN PERIODONTICS

Aubrey Sheiham

The growth of knowledge is usually associated with controversy. Statements and scientific theories are constantly challenged and defended. Ideally, when a scientific theory is refuted by new evidence, the theory should be discarded. In practice, the refutation is seldom conclusive or the proponents of the theory cling to their beliefs despite conclusive evidence to the contrary.

Periodontics, like any other scientific endeavor, has had its fair share of controversy. The writings of Pierre Fouchard, the "Father of Dentistry," provoked much controversy in the eighteenth century, as did those of Gottlieb in this century. The role of systemic factors in the etiology of periodontal disease was hotly debated, as was the importance of occlusal trauma. The contribution of occlusal factors to the initiation and progression of periodontal disease was one of the most controversial issues in periodontics until 1966. In 1966 the committee report on etiology at the World Workshop in Periodontics (Ramfjord et al., 1966) concluded that occlusal forces did not initiate gingivitis but may aggravate the destruction of the periodontium. The issue was hotly debated at the workshop. Since then, the general view on the response of the periodontium to occlusal factors has been that there is a physiologic adaptation that can result in increased mobility. Apical progression of the epithelial attachment is not related to the occlusal factors (Ranney, 1977).

Three controversial subjects are discussed in this chapter. They are as follows:

1. The scientific basis for regular 6-month dental examinations
2. The high-risk versus population strategy for controlling periodontal disease
3. The role of iatrogenesis in periodontal disease

SCIENTIFIC BASIS FOR REGULAR 6-MONTH PERIODONTAL EXAMINATIONS

The 6-month dental examination has been recommended by dental professionals for over 100 years. It is therefore surprising that there has not been adequate scientific appraisal of the necessity for regular examinations or of the optimal interval between periodontal examinations for the general public. The scientific basis for the 6-month examination was questioned, and it was concluded that there was no scientific basis for the recommended interval (Sheiham, 1977). Longer intervals between examinations were recommended. The questioning of such a well-accepted recommendation led to a widescale debate—a debate that continues despite the absence of any new evidence to support the 6-month interval. On the other hand, there is more reason to question the need for regular 6-month examinations for all people in light of new evidence on the natural history of periodontal disease.

Objectives of regular periodontal examinations

There are three main objectives for recalling a person regularly for a periodontal examination. The first is to detect periodontal disease or a predisposition to it in order to institute treatment that will have a favorable effect on the disease. The second is to reinforce oral hygiene behaviors. The third is to evaluate the response to therapy. It is clear that frequent professional oral hygiene is important in the maintenance of periodontal health in a patient who has had periodontal treatment and that lack of such maintenance can lead to recurrence of periodontitis (see Chapter 41). The following discussion deals with regular examination of the general dental clinic population who have not had periodontal treatment.

Criterion for deciding on the interval between examinations

The main criterion for deciding on the interval between periodontal examinations is the patient's risk of developing periodontitis, which will not regress without therapy and for which an effective therapeutic treatment exists.

Assessment of those at risk

There is no reliable method of predicting who will develop periodontitis. Neither is it known which sites will progress from gingival inflammation to periodontitis. Indeed, one may question whether gingival inflammation is a disease. Considerable controversy surrounds the definition of normal, healthy periodontal tissue. There does not appear to be a clearly defined density of leukocytes in the gingiva that is consistent with health. In addition, the clinical criteria for diagnosing gingivitis are not available, and there is a wide variation in diagnostic abilities between examiners. In addition to the problems of defining gingivitis, the new concepts of periodontal disease indicate that gingival inflammation does not inevitably lead to destructive progressive periodontitis. The term *contained gingivitis* can be used in cases where gingival inflammation is limited to the gingiva and does not progress to periodontitis.

Further modification of the traditional continuous disease model of periodontal disease has important implications for periodontal therapy in general and for deciding on the optimal interval between periodontal examinations. The new concepts of periodontal disease outlined by Goodson et al. (1982), Haffajee et al. (1983), and Socransky et al. (1984) suggest that certain gingival sites could be free of destructive periodontal disease for a lifetime. These sites experience one or more bursts of destructive disease followed by a period of repair or remission. The length of time a burst lasts has not been adequately established. Neither are there methods available for predicting when a burst will occur. The remission following a burst may be permanent or intermittent. One of the main findings in the studies related to the new burst models concerns the large number of sites that showed no change in status for long periods. Another finding is that even severe, rapidly destructive periodontal disease stops suddenly for unknown reasons without therapy. Socransky et al. (1984) have called their models the "random burst" and the "asynchronous burst" models. Acceptance of either of their two models or of the continuous progressive disease model will require a radical change in the concepts of periodontal treatment. If the traditional continuous progressive disease model is correct, then the basis for treating periodontal disease by conventional methods is open to question because the rate of loss of attachment is very slow in the majority of people. The average loss per year is approximately 0.05 to 0.1 mm a year (Selikowitz et al., 1981).

The slow rates of progression cast doubts on the necessity for 6-month recall examinations. The amounts of destruction per year are so small that they will not be accurately detected at intervals shorter than 2 to 3 years. In addition, scaling and root planing will frequently deepen periodontal pockets of 4 mm or less (Lindhe et al., 1982a, 1982b).

If either of the burst models is correct, then the indications for routine periodontal examinations are not justified until more evidence is available on the range of patterns of bursts and the periodicity of the bursts.

According to the burst theory, a burst can occur at any moment and last for a short period. Therefore very frequent screenings at intervals of less than a month would be required to detect a burst. But most of the bursts stop spontaneously, and some repair themselves. In addition, the dogma that all gingival inflammation must be eliminated and that any periodontal pocket deeper than 3 mm must be treated should be seriously questioned. Treating patients with periodontal pockets that are not in an active destructive phase of the disease is analogous to treating a person for pneumonia who had the disease some years earlier but still has the consequences of the disease.

In summary, the traditional continuous destructive periodontal disease model is being questioned particularly because it assumes that all gingival inflammation progresses to periodontitis and ultimately to severe bone loss. Even if the disease process is progressive, the rates of progression are generally very slow.

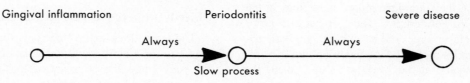

CONTINUOUS DISEASE MODEL

Gingival inflammation   Periodontitis   Severe disease

Always   Always

Slow process

BURST MODEL

Gingival inflammation   Periodontitis   Severe disease

Sometimes   Sometimes

Variable rates

The burst models suggest that gingival inflammation leads to periodontitis and that at some sites the periodontitis progresses rapidly to deep pocketing.

Prevalence and severity of periodontal disease

Evidence from epidemiologic research has lead to a reappraisal of the periodontal disease problem. In my opinion, it is becoming increasingly clear that periodontal disease is not an important public health problem and that although many people have some gingival inflammation, the probability of the inflammation progressing to severe loss of periodontal support and to tooth loss is not great.

Periodontal disease is not the major cause of tooth loss in adults, as has been previously assumed (Schaub, 1984). In addition, the prevalence and severity of periodontal disease is decreasing in the United States, England, and Sweden (Hugoson et al., 1980; Douglass et al., 1983; Sheiham et al., 1986). In the United States 57% of women and 45% of men were periodontally healthy in 1971 to 1974. In 1960 to 1962 the comparable percentages were 31% and 21%, respectively (Douglass et al., 1983).

A false impression of the extent of periodontal disease is given by scoring as positive any individual with one or more inflamed gingival sites. The number of inflamed gingival sites is seldom presented. If the same criterion for disease, namely the presence of inflammation in a square millimeter of skin or mucosa, were adopted, then almost all of the population would be categorized as diseased.

In the United States gingival inflammation has been reported in 95% of children aged 5 to 17 years. However, 65% had inflammation affecting less than half their teeth, only 2.5% had severe gingivitis, and only 0.5% had true periodontal pocketing. These data are not sufficiently precise. More precise data are provided on the periodontal status of New Zealanders (Cutress et al., 1983). Less than 4% of the surveyed population aged 15 to 19, 25 to 29, and 35 to 44 years had noninflamed gums. At age 15 to 19 years 19% had gingivitis, 29% were periodontally healthy, and 1% had periodontitis. When the data were presented by the number and percentage of teeth affected, 65% of teeth had noninflamed gingivae and 0.4% of teeth per person had periodontitis. Presenting data in this manner gives a more favorable and more accurate picture of periodontal health.

Low levels of periodontal disease as found in the United States, Sweden, and New Zealand are relatively in-

significant health problems and cannot justify a high priority for financial resources. Neither do they justify frequent periodontal examinations. Few gingival sites are inflamed per person. Those that are inflamed do not always progress to periodontitis in many sites or individuals. A few gingival sites and individuals are at greater risk of developing severe periodontal disease, but until a reliable prognostic indicator of who will develop severe periodontal disease is developed, routine periodontal examinations for all people at intervals of 6 months should not be recommended.

Altering the natural history of periodontal disease for the better

While there is no doubt that the frequent removal of dental plaque by professionals will prevent and control the development of periodontal disease (Nyman et al., 1975; Axelsson et al., 1976; Rosling et al., 1976), there is no evidence that removal of plaque at intervals of more than 4 weeks is of significant therapeutic benefit. Yet the public are told to see their dentist every 6 months for an examination and to have their teeth scaled and polished. Two studies have been carried out to test how frequently scaling and polishing is required. Lightner et al. (1968, 1971) found no difference in clinical significance in gingival health in persons having two or four preventive periodontal treatments a year—a finding confirmed by Suomi et al. (1973), who found that there was no difference in periodontal status in groups treated once or three times a year.

Further confirmation that there is a need to reevaluate treatment or preventive maintenance schemes that have been introduced without adequate data to support their claims of safety and efficacy has been provided by Listgarten et al. (1985; 1986a). In a 3-year longitudinal study of adults with gingivitis, they found that 25 of the 30 subjects in the treatment group required recall intervals of 12 to 24 months. Eleven subjects reached the end of the study without receiving a single prophylaxis during the entire 3-year period. Yet their periodontal status was no worse than the status of those receiving an examination or prophylaxis every 6 months. The study also demonstrated how few gingival sites progress to pocketing over a 3-year period. Of the 38,228 sites probed, only 21 exhibited an increase in probing depth from a baseline of 3 mm or more; an increase in probing depth could be expected to occur by chance in 19 sites (Listgarten et al., 1985).

The uncritical acceptance of the recommendation for

routine 6-month examinations for periodontal disease and to do a prophylaxis and give oral hygiene instruction is no longer acceptable by rational clinicians. Persistence with such an outdated regimen is tantamount to overtreatment. The unnecessary efforts expended on individuals who do not need attention can be directed more beneficially to those who are undertreated. Furthermore, repetition and reinforcement of oral hygiene instruction and prophylaxis may have a dampening effect on motivation for both patients and educators and so reduce the motivation for self-care (Hamp and Johansson, 1982). Patients become dependent on the dentist for maintenance of their periodontal health and take on the role of perpetual patients—an unhealthy behavior (Sheiham, 1983).

HIGH-RISK VERSUS POPULATION STRATEGY FOR CONTROLLING PERIODONTAL DISEASE

There are two principal strategies that can control periodontal disease. One strategy is to increase the amount of periodontal treatment and oral hygiene instruction given to individuals at high risk of developing periodontal disease. The other strategy is to concentrate on health education of communities, with dentists reinforcing the community health education and acting as advisors on the scientific basis for dental health education. The practice of periodontics is strongly biased toward the high-risk, dentist-centered strategy. On the other hand, health educators and public health dentists subscribe to the population strategy. With the decline in the incidence of dental caries in industrialized countries, dentists are concentrating more on periodontal disease. This shift coincides with the reappraisal of the traditional continuous destructive disease model of periodontal disease and the acceptance of the burst models, which stress that severe periodontal disease occurs in a few sites in a small number of people. The question is, which of these two strategies is the most appropriate for improving the periodontal health of the whole population (Sheiham, 1984)?

The current practice of periodontics is based on the theory of specific etiology and a manipulative engineering approach to the maintenance of periodontal health. Such an approach suggests that an individual's periodontal health can be influenced mainly by dental intervention. Some of the salient notions derived from this dental model are as follows:

Periodontal diseases are discrete entities constituting specific problems and needing specific solutions.

Periodontal diseases are primarily biologic problems to be dealt with by the existing types of dental procedures.

Biologic problems are essentially those of an individual, with activities based on interaction with the individual and on risk factors, instead of on comprehensive behavior patterns.

Dental health education focuses on dentally defined problems and is essentially a dental activity. The consequence of this concept is that the appropriate way and place to impart dental health education is via the dentist or hygienist in the dental practice setting (Sheiham, 1985).

This dental model of periodontal disease differs from a social model. The social model does not define health as the absence of disease but as a state of social and psychologic well-being. Thus factors influencing health are to be found not only in pathologic conditions that may or may not result from personal behavior patterns, but also in social and environmental conditions frequently outside the individual's control, and in culturally determined forces that affect the development of interpersonal relationships and the acquisition of life-style.

The social model questions the implicit goal of the dental model, namely that all clinically and subclinically detected periodontal disease should be eliminated and the idea that periodontal health is the absence of gingivitis, no loss of attachment, and anatomically perfect gingival contours. The adoption of the social model, with its orientation toward lay competence, the interrelatedness of health and dental health behaviors, and primary and secondary socialization, involves three conceptual reorientations (Kickbusch, 1981):

From dental orientation to lay competence

From authoritarian instruction to supportive health education

From individualistic behavior modification to a systematic population strategy using public health approaches

The social model of periodontal health concentrates on the causes of the causes. Instead of focusing solely on microorganisms in dental plaque, more emphasis is given to the reasons why individuals have high or low plaque scores. In addition, attention is focused on the sociopsychologic factors that influence the immune response. How do adverse life events such as bereavement, unemployment, or divorce affect the immune response on the one hand and oral cleanliness on the other? The social model recognizes that oral cleanliness is related to general body cleanliness, which is influenced by primary and secondary socialization. Socialization stimulates copying behavior in young children, and in older children, grooming behavior is an important motivating force for oral hygiene (Rayner and Cohen, 1971; Hodge et al., 1982; Sheiham, 1983).

In practical terms, according to the social model of periodontal health, the evidence that individuals with more plaque have more severe periodontal disease than those with less plaque suggests the appropriateness of a population strategy aimed at lowering the level of plaque in all people to a level compatible with retaining a natural, functional, socially acceptable dentition for the lifetime of most people. The objective does not imply that all 32 teeth will have physiologically and anatomically perfect periodontal support. A level of structural change can be tolerated if it is acceptable to the patient and does not affect such social and biologic functions as self-esteem, appearance, speech, chewing, taste, and comfort (Pilot, 1980).

A detailed outline of the population strategy has been published (Sheiham, 1980, 1984; Frandsen, 1984). The population and high-risk strategies should not be seen as alternative strategies. There is a small percentage of persons (10% to 20% of adults) with severe progressive periodontal disease. In these cases appropriate antimicrobial therapy could be used to change the bacterial flora. The other groups of individuals who require a high-risk strategy are those with medical or sociopsychologic conditions that would be affected by periodontal disease. Both the periodontal and medical high-risk groups should be assessed by sociopsychologic, as well as clinical and bacteriologic, methods because there is evidence that psychologic states can affect the immune response and alter the bacterial flora of the mouth.

The high-risk strategy has a number of unwanted side effects, including clinical and social iatrogenesis.

CLINICAL AND SOCIAL IATROGENESIS

Physicians and dentists, in their efforts to improve health, sometimes inadvertently cause damage. This damage can be clinical and social and is called iatrogenesis— physican- or dentist-made disease. Clinical iatrogenesis comprises all clinical conditions for which therapies, physicians, dentists, and hygienists are to blame. The most common forms of dental clinical iatrogenesis are caused by operative procedures and dental materials. Periodontists have recognized for some time that the most important factor determining whether a dental restoration adversely affects periodontal health is the physical relationship between the two. Subgingivally placed cervical margins, especially those not able to be kept plaque free, are deleterious to gingival health. In particular, overhanging restorations function as plaque retention areas and commonly initiate and enhance periodontal disease (Ramfjord et al., 1966), and there is growing evidence that overhanging restorations, poorly contoured restorations, and partial dentures are important dental public health problems. The situation is summed up by a quote attributed to Professor Jens Waerhaug that dentists "extend the cavity for the prevention of caries but inadvertently promote periodontal disease."

A less well known form of clinical iatrogenesis is the damage caused by subgingival scaling, root planing, and surgical periodontal procedures. In a recent overview of the current status of nonsurgical and surgical periodontal treatment, Lang (1984) concluded that with all the procedures employed, some clinical attachment is lost in sulci with an initial probing depth of 1 to 3 mm. This conclusion is based on the longitudinal studies conducted by Ramfjord et al. (1968), Morrison et al. (1980), and Lindhe et al. (1982a, 1982b). Since sulci 1 to 3 mm deep are the most commonly found, care should be taken not to deepen them iatrogenically by unnecessary scaling, root planing, and surgical procedures. In particular, regular instrumentation and polishing should not be directed at disease-free areas except where esthetically important (Committee Report on Prevention and Control of Periodontal Disease, 1977).

Unnecessary and clinically damaging dental procedures have an additional drawback. They lead to social iatrogenesis. People become dependent on dental care and chemotherapeutic agents. They become dependent on the dentist because they are led to believe that only by regular periodontal care will they achieve periodontal health. This attitude decreases self-care because people believe that they are incapable of achieving the unrealistic levels of plaque control demanded by dental health professionals. Patients become passive.

SUMMARY

In this chapter an outline is given of subjects that are considered by some to be of a controversial nature. In any discipline there is a dominant set of values and beliefs. These beliefs are frequently challenged, and through critical analysis the discipline improves. As health professionals, we should always insist that treatment and preventive programs be based on a sound scientific rationale. The optimal interval between recall visits, the high-risk versus population strategy for controlling periodontal disease, and iatrogenesis, with its implications of overtreatment and the establishment of dependence on dental care, are subjects with a central theme, namely that unnecessary procedures are clinically and socially harmful. Most periodontal disease can be prevented or controlled by the individual without much professional intervention. Emphasis should therefore be given to the population strategy complemented by a high-risk strategy to deal with the small percentage of individuals and teeth affected by rapidly progressing periodontal disease.

REFERENCES

Axelsson P et al: The effect of various plaque control measures on gingivitis and caries in school children, Community Dent Oral Epidemiol 4:232, 1976.

Committee Report on Prevention and Control of Periodontal Disease. In International Conference on Research in the Biology of Periodontal Disease, Chicago, 1977, College of Dentistry, University of Illinois.

Cutress TW et al: Adult dental health in New Zealand 1976-1982, Wellington, 1983, Medical Research Council of New Zealand.

Douglass CW et al: National trends in the prevalence and severity of periodontal disease, J Am Dent Assoc 107:403, 1983.

Frandsen A, editor: Public health aspects of periodontal disease, Chicago, 1984, Quintessence Publishing Co, pp 241-250.

Goodson JM et al: Patterns of progression and regression of advanced destructive periodontal disease, J Clin Periodontol 9:472, 1982.

Haffajee AD et al: Comparison of different data analyses for detecting changes in attachment level, J Clin Periodontol 10:298, 1983.

Hamp SE and Johansson LA: Dental prophylaxis for youths in their late teens, J Clin Periodontol 9:2, 1982.

Hodge HC et al: Factors associated with toothbrushing behavior in adolescents, Br Dent J 152:48, 1982.

Hugoson A et al: Dental health 1973 and 1978 in individuals aged 3-20 years in the community of Jonkoping, Sweden, Swed Dent J 4:217, 1980.

Kickbusch L: Involvement in health: a social concept of health education, Int J Health Educ (suppl 14), p 3, 1981.

Lang NP: Current status of nonsurgical and surgical periodontal treatment. In Frandsen A, editor: Public health aspects of periodontal disease, Chicago, 1984, Quintessence Publishing Co, Inc.

Lightner LM et al: Preventive periodontic treatment procedures: results after one year, J Am Dent Assoc 78:1043, 1968.

Lightner LM et al: Preventive periodontic treatment procedures: results after 46 months, J Periodontol 42:555, 1971.

Lindhe J et al: Healing following surgical-nonsurgical treatment of periodontal disease, J Clin Periodontol 9:115, 1982a.

Lindhe J et al: Scaling and root planing in shallow pockets, J Clin Periodontol 9:415, 1982b.

Listgarten MA et al: 3-year longitudinal study of the periodontal status of an adult population with gingivitis, J Clin Periodontol 12:225, 1985.

Listgarten MA et al: Comparative longitudinal study of 2 methods of scheduling maintenance visits: 2 year data, J Clin Periodontol 13:692, 1986a.

Listgarten MA et al: Failure of a microbial assay to reliably predict disease recurrence in a treated periodontitis population receiving regularly scheduled prophylaxes, J Clin Periodontol 13:768, 1986b.

Morrison EC et al: Short term effects of initial nonsurgical periodontal treatment, J Clin Periodontol 7:199, 1980.

Nyman S et al: Effect of professional tooth cleaning on healing after periodontal surgery, J Clin Periodontol 2:80, 1975.

Pilot T: Analysis of the overall effectiveness of treatment of periodontal disease. In Shanley DB, editor: Efficacy of treatment procedures in periodontics, Chicago, 1980, Quintessence Publishing Co, Inc.

Ramfjord SP et al, editors: World workshop in periodontics, Ann Arbor, 1966, University of Michigan.

Ramfjord SP et al: Subgingival curettage versus surgical elimination of periodontal pockets, J Periodontol 39:167, 1968.

Ranney RR: Pathogenesis of periodontal disease. In International conference on research in the biology of periodontal disease, Chicago, 1977, College of Dentistry, University of Illinois.

Rayner JF and Cohen LK: School dental health education. In Richards ND and Cohen LK, editors: Social sciences and dentistry, London, 1971, Federation Dentaire Internationale.

Rosling B et al: The healing potential of the periodontal tissues following different techniques of periodontal surgery in plaque-free dentitions: a 2 year clinical study, J Clin Periodontol 3:233, 1976.

Schaub RMH: Barriers to effective periodontal care, Groningen, 1984, Ryksuniversiteit te Groningen.

Selikowitz HS et al: Retrospective longitudinal study of the rate of alveolar bone loss in humans using bite-wing radiographs, J Clin Periodontol 8:431, 1981.

Sheiham A: Is there a scientific basis for six-monthly dental examinations? Lancet 2:442, 1977.

Sheiham A: Prevention and control of periodontal disease. In International conference on research in the biology of periodontal disease, Chicago, 1977, College of Dentistry, University of Illinois.

Sheiham A: Current concepts in health education. In Shanley D, editor: Efficacy of treatment procedures in periodontics, Chicago, 1980, Quintessence Publishing Co, Inc.

Sheiham A: Promoting periodontal health-effective programmes of education and promotion, Int Dent J 33:182, 1983.

Sheiham A: An analysis of existing dental services in relation to periodontal care. In Frandsen A, editor: Public health aspects of periodontal disease, Chicago, 1984, Quintessence Publishing Co, Inc.

Sheiham A: The future of periodontology. In Derrick DD, editor: The dental annual, Bristol, UK, 1985, John Wright.

Sheiham A et al: Changes in periodontal health in a cohort of British workers over a 14 year period, Br Dent J 160:125, 1986.

Socransky SS et al: Changing concepts of destructive periodontal disease, J Clin Periodontol 11:21, 1984.

Suomi JD et al: Study of the effect of different prophylaxis frequencies on the periodontium of young adults, J Periodontol 44:406, 1973.

INDEX

Page numbers in *italics* indicate illustrations; page numbers followed by t indicate tables.

Cultures, bacterial, scope of, and procedure for, 454-455
Curettage
    chemical, 559, 562
    gingival, 557-559, *558, 559*
    in regenerative therapy
        closed, with root planing, *586,* 586-587, *587*
        open-flap, with root planing, 587, *588,* 589
Curettes, 402-404, *403*
    effects of sterilization on, 538
    for scaling and root planing, 527, *527, 528,* 528-529, *529*
    sharpening, 534, *535, 536,* 538
Cuticle, dental, 23
Cyclosporine
    gingival effects of, 273
    side effects of, 273
Cystatins, salivary, 120
Cysts, 287-288
    gingival, 288
    lateral periodontal, 288
    odontogenic, 287
    periodontal, 479, *479*
    radicular, 288
    radiologic features of, 287
Cytokines in bone resorption, 189
Cytometry, flow, scope of, and technique for, 457

D

Dalmane; *see* Flurazepam
Dapsone, side effects of, 232
Dead spaces, avoidance of, during surgery, 546
Dental calculus; *see* Calculus
Dental cuticle, 23
    formation of, in periodontal disease, *93,* 93-94
Dental floss, *364*
Dental history, 331-332
Dental implants, 653-667
    future directions in, 666-667
    patient selection for, 658-659
    postsurgical problems, procedures, and maintenance in, 664-666
    presurgical evaluation in, 659, 663
    Screw-Vent, *658,* 659
    surgical techniques for, 663-664
    systems of, 654, 657-658
Dental pellicles, 121-124
    colonization of, 189-190
    defined, 121
    distinguished from plaque, 126
    early, 121-122
        compared with saliva, 122t
    formation of, 121
    function of, 117
    later, 122
    protective functions of, 121-122
Dental plaque; *see* Plaque
Dental services
    future patterns in use of, 700-701
    use of, 700-701
Dentifrices, 432

Dentin
    demineralization of, 53
    hypersensitivity of, agents for, 379
Dentinal tubules, 607-608
Dentinocemental junction, 36, *37,* 38
Dentistry, reconstructive, preparation margins in, 170-173
Dentogingival fibers of supraalveolar connective tissue, 16
Dentogingival junction
    apical shift of, 29-30
    histogenesis of, *21,* 21-23, *22, 23*
Dentoperiosteal fibers of supraalveolar connective tissue, 16, *18*
Deoxycycline, bacterial resistance to, 166
Dermatoses, histopathology and immunopathology in, 229t; *see also* Skin disorders
Desciclovir for hairy leukoplakia, 304
Desmosomes, gingival, 10, *11, 13*
Diabetes mellitus
    complications of, 213
    as contraindication to periodontal surgery, 557
    gestational, 212
    insulin-dependent (type I)
        clinical symptoms of, 212
        periodontal disease in, 213, *214,* 214t
    neutrophil defects in, 203, 212-217
    non-insulin-dependent (type II), clinical symptoms of, 212
    periodontal disease in, 213, *214,* 215-217, *216*
    secondary, 212
    treatment of, 212-213
Diazepam
    dose and administration of, 378t
    during pregnancy, 224
Dihydropyridines, gingival effects of, 273-274
Disinfectants, 374
Distolingual grooves, periodontal disease and, 180
DNA probes, procedure for, 457
Down's syndrome
    characteristics of, 217
Dressings after scaling and root planing, 415
Drugs; *see also* Analgesics; Antiinfective therapy; Medications; specific drugs
    antianxiety; *see* Antianxiety drugs
    choice of, 672-673, 673t
    gingival changes from, 69
    periodontal tissue and, 269-276
    during pregnancy, 224
Dysplasia
    epithelial, histopathology of, 280, *281*
    periapical cemental, 289

E

Edentulous ridge
    deformed
        with fixed prostheses, *638,* 638-640, *639, 640, 641*
        reconstruction of, 643-652
        with removable prostheses, 640, *641,* 642
        surgical correction of, 629, 632
    in fixed and removable prosthetic treatment, 637-643
    normal, 637-638
Edlan-Mejchar procedure, 575-576